SAUNDERS
INTERNATIONAL
MEDICAL
WORD BOOK

1991 W.B. SAUNDERS COMPANY
Harcourt Brace Jovanovich, Inc.
Philadelphia   London   Toronto   Montreal   Sydney   Tokyo

W.B. Saunders Company
Harcourt Brace Jovanovich, Inc.

The Curtis Center
Independence Square West
Philadelphia, PA 19106

Saunders International Medical Word Book   ISBN 0-7216-3620-9

Copyright 1991 Radcliffe Medical Press

Saunders international medical word book.
   p.   cm.
   ISBN 0-7216-3620-9
   1. Medicine—Dictionaries—Polyglot.   2. Dictionaries, Polyglot.
   I. W.B. Saunders Company.
   [DNLM: 1. Medicine—abbreviations—multilingual.   2. Nomenclature—multilingual. W 15 S257]
   R121.S325 1991
   610'.3—sx20
   DNLM/DLC   91-18589

Typeset by Advance Typesetting Ltd., Oxford
Printed in Great Britain by Billing & Sons Ltd., Worcester

CONTENTS

Introduction

INTRODUCTION

The growth in information exchange throughout the world has increased the need for a reference of this kind. It has been compiled with the help of an extensive team of medically qualified personnel from a wide range of disciplines who are native speakers of the languages included in the work.

The International Medical Word Book covers the principal key words in medicine — over 3,500 terms in all. Each of the five sections begins with these key words appearing in alphabetical order in English, French, German, Italian and Spanish — and immediate translation into any of the other four is achieved by referring to the appropriate column across the page. This single volume therefore enables the reader to translate from English to French just as easily as from Spanish to German.

As a further aid to international understanding, the standard anatomical drawings are reproduced with the main features translated into all five languages. Similarly, the standard medical abbreviations in each language are also listed.

In compiling the word book we intended primarily to meet the needs of those in clinical and laboratory medicine and in medical research and education. However, it has become apparent that it could be a fundamental source of reference in nursing, pharmacy and all the other professions allied to medicine. We also believe that it contains valuable information for those providing pharmaceutical and other health care services wherever a European language is spoken.

The Saunders International Medical Word Book is intended to evolve with the developments in the professions it serves, and with the needs of its users. We therefore welcome suggestions on material that could be added or omitted in future editions.

Publisher's note

For the sake of simplicity it was decided not to include grammatical information in the first edition of the Word Book. Where a word might occur, for example, as both noun and adjective, the most commonly used form in the context of medicine has been translated. However, certain words have been identified which might be used as both noun and adjective, or both noun and verb; in these cases translations for the two alternatives have been provided, and identified by *(n)*—noun, *(a)*—adjective and *(v)*—verb following the word in question.

ENGLISH
French
German
Italian
Spanish
ENGLISH

A

ENGLISH	FRENCH	GERMAN
abdomen	abdomen	Abdomen
abdominal	abdominal	abdominal
abdomino-perineal	abdomino-périnéal	abdominoperineal
abduct	produire l'abduction	abduzieren
abduction	abduction	Abduktion
abductor	abducteur	Abduktor
aberrant	aberrant	aberrans, abartig
aberration	aberration	Aberration, Abweichung
ability	capacité, aptitude, compétence	Fähigkeit
ablation	ablation	Ablatio, Absetzung
abnormal	anormal	abnormal
abort	avorter	fehlgebären
abortion	avortement	Abort, Fehlgeburt
abrasion	abrasion	Abschabung, Ausschabung
abreaction	abréaction	Abreaktion
abscess	abcès	Abszeß
absorption	absorption	Absorption
abuse	abus	Abusus, Mißbrauch
accommodation	accommodation	Akkommodation
acetabulum	acétabule	Azetabulum, Hüftgelenkspfanne
achalasia	achalasie	Achalasie
Achilles tendon	tendon d'Achille	Achillessehne
achondroplasia	achondroplasie	Achondroplasie
acid (n)	acide (n)	Säure (n)
acid (a)	acide (a)	sauer (a)
acid-alcohol-fast	résistant à l'alcool et à l'acide	säurealkoholbeständig
acid-fast	acido-résistant	säurebeständig
acidity	acidité	Säuregehalt
acidosis	acidose	Azidose
acne	acné	Akne
acoustic	acoustique	akustisch, Gehör-
acquired immune deficiency syndrome (AIDS)	syndrome d'immuno-déficience acquise (SIDA)	erworbenes Immundefektsyndrom (AIDS)
acromegaly	acromégalie	Akromegalie
acromioclavicular	acromio-claviculaire	akromioklavikular
acromion	acromion	Akromion
actinomycosis	actinomycose	Aktinomykose
action	action	Tätigkeit
active	actif	aktiv, wirksam
acuity	acuité	Schärfe
acupuncture	acupuncture	Akupunktur
acute	aigu(ë)	spitz, scharf
acute febrile respiratory disease/illness (AFRD/I)	affection/maladie respiratoire fébrile aiguë	Atemwegsinfekt (akut fieberhaft)
Adam's apple	pomme d'Adam	Adamsapfel
addiction	accoutumance	Sucht, Gewöhnung

2

ITALIAN	SPANISH	ENGLISH
addome	abdomen	**abdomen**
addominale	abdominal	**abdominal**
addomino-perineale	abdominoperineal	**abdomino-perineal**
abdurre	abducir	**abduct**
abduzione	abducción	**abduction**
abduttore	abductor	**abductor**
aberrante	aberrante, desviado	**aberrant**
aberrazione	aberración	**aberration**
abilità, capacità	habilidad, capacidad	**ability**
ablazione	ablación, excisión	**ablation**
anormale	anormal	**abnormal**
abortire	abortar	**abort**
aborto	aborto	**abortion**
abrasione	abrasión	**abrasion**
abreazione, catarsi	abreacción, catarsis	**abreaction**
ascesso	absceso	**abscess**
assorbimento	absorción	**absorption**
abuso	abuso	**abuse**
accomodazione	acomodación	**accommodation**
acetabolo	acetábulo	**acetabulum**
acalasia	acalasia	**achalasia**
tendine di Achille	tendón de Aquiles	**Achilles tendon**
acondroplasia	acondroplasia	**achondroplasia**
acido (n)	ácido (n)	**acid** (n)
acido (a)	ácido (a)	**acid** (a)
alcool-acido-resistente	ácido-alcohol-resistente	**acid-alcohol-fast**
acido resistente	ácido-resistente	**acid-fast**
acidità	acidez	**acidity**
acidosi	acidosis	**acidosis**
acne	acné	**acne**
acustico	acústico	**acoustic**
sindrome da immunodeficienza acquisita (AIDS)	síndrome de inmunodeficiencia adquirida (SIDA)	**acquired immune deficiency syndrome (AIDS)**
acromegalia	acromegalia	**acromegaly**
acromioclavicolare	acromioclavicular	**acromioclavicular**
acromion	acromion	**acromion**
actinomicosi	actinomicosis	**actinomycosis**
azione	acción	**action**
attivo	activo	**active**
acuità	agudeza	**acuity**
agopuntura	acupuntura	**acupuncture**
acuto	agudo	**acute**
malattia respiratoria acuta febbrile	enfermedad respiratoria febril aguda	**acute febrile respiratory disease/illness (AFRD/I)**
pomo di Adamo	huez de Adán	**Adam's apple**
tossicomania	adicción, toxicomanía	**addiction**

ENGLISH	FRENCH	GERMAN
Addison's disease	maladie d'Addison	Addison Krankheit
adduct	produire l'adduction	adduzieren, zusammenziehen
adduction	adduction	Adduktion
adductor	adducteur	Adduktor
adenocarcinoma	adénocarcinome	Adenokarzinom
adenoidectomy	adénoïdectomie	Adenoidektomie, Polypenentfernung
adenoids	végétations adénoïdes	Adenoide, Nasenpolypen
adenoma	adénome	Adenom
adenomyoma	adénomyome	Adenomyom
adenotonsillectomy	adéno-amygdalectomie	Adenotonsillektomie
adenovirus	adénovirus	Adenovirus
adhesion	adhésion	Adhäsion, Anhaften
adipose	adipeux	adipös, fettleibig
adjuvant	adjuvant	Adjuvans
adnexa	annexes	Adnexe
adolescence	adolescence	Adoleszenz, Jugendalter
adoption	adoption	Adoption
adrenal	surrénale	Nebennieren-
adrenal cortical hormone (ACH)	hormone cortico-surrénale	Nebennierenrindenhormon (ACH)
adrenaline	adrénaline	Adrenalin
adrenergic	adrénergique	adrenerg
adrenocorticotrophic hormone (ACTH)	hormone adrénocorticotrope (ACTH)	adrenokortikotropes Hormon (ACTH)
adsorption	adsorption	Adsorption
adverse drug reaction (ADR)	réaction médicamenteuse indésirable	unerwünschte Arzneimittelreaktion
aerobe	aérobie	Aerobier
aerophagia	aérophagie	Aerophagie, Luftschlucken
aerosol	aérosol	Aerosol
aetiology	étiologie	Ätiologie
afebrile	afébrile	fieberfrei
affect (n)	affect (n)	Affekt (n), Erregung (n)
affect (v)	affecter (v)	befallen (v)
affective	affectif	affektiv
afferent	afférent	afferent, zuführend
afterbirth	arrière-faix	Plazenta, Nachgeburt
aftercare	postcure	Nachbehandlung, Nachsorge
afterpains	tranchées utérines	Nachwehen
ageing	vieillissement	Altern
agenesis	agénésie	Agenesie
agglutination	agglutination	Agglutination
agglutinin	agglutinine	Agglutinin
aggression	agression	Aggression
agitated depression	dépression anxieuse	agitierte Depression
agnathia	agnathie	Agnathie
agnosia	agnosie	Agnosie
agonist	agoniste	Agonist

morbo di Addison	enfermedad de Addison	Addison's disease
addurre	aducir	adduct
adduzione	aducción	adduction
adduttore	aductor	adductor
adenocarcinoma	adenocarcinoma	adenocarcinoma
adenoidectomia	adenoidectomía	adenoidectomy
adenoidi	adenoides	adenoids
adenoma	adenoma	adenoma
adenomioma	adenomioma	adenomyoma
adenotonsillectomia	amigdaloadenoidectomía	adenotonsillectomy
adenovirus	adenovirus	adenovirus
adesione	adherencia	adhesion
adiposo	adiposo, graso	adipose
adiuvante	coadyuvante	adjuvant
annessi	anejos, anexos	adnexa
adolescenza	adolescencia	adolescence
adozione	adopción	adoption
surrenale	adrenal	adrenal
ormone corticosurrenale	hormona corticosuprarrenal (HCS)	adrenal cortical hormone (ACH)
adrenalina	adrenalina	adrenaline
adrenergico	adrenérgico	adrenergic
ormone corticotropo (ACTH)	hormona adrenocorticotropa (ACTH)	adrenocorticotrophic hormone (ACTH)
adsorbimento	adsorción	adsorption
reazione dannosa (indesiderata) da farmaci	reacción adversa a un medicamento	adverse drug reaction (ADR)
aerobio	aerobio, aeróbico	aerobe
aerofagia	aerofagia	aerophagia
aerosol	aerosol	aerosol
eziologia	etiología	aetiology
afebbrile	apirético, afebril	afebrile
emozione (n)	afecto (n)	affect (n)
attaccare (v), influenzare (v)	afectar (v)	affect (v)
affettivo	afectivo	affective
afferente	aferente	afferent
secondine, membrane fetali e placenta	secundinas, expulsión de la placenta y membranas	afterbirth
assistenza post-operatoria	cuidados postoperatorios	aftercare
contrazioni uterine post partum	entuertos	afterpains
senescenza, invecchiamento	envejecimiento	ageing
agenesia	agenesia	agenesis
agglutinazione	aglutinación	agglutination
agglutinine	aglutinina	agglutinin
aggressività	agresión	aggression
depressione agitata	depresión agitada	agitated depression
agnazia	agnatia	agnathia
agnosia	agnosia	agnosia
agonista	agonista	agonist

ENGLISH	FRENCH	GERMAN
agoraphobia	agoraphobie	Agoraphobie, Platzangst
agranulocytosis	agranulocytose	Agranulozytose
AIDS-related complex	para-SIDA	AIDS-related complex
airway breathing and circulation (ABC)	intubation, ventilation et circulation	Luftwege Atmung und Kreislauf (ABC-Regel)
akinetic	acinétique	akinetisch
albumin	albumine	Albumin
albuminuria	albuminurie	Albuminurie
alcohol	alcool	Alkohol
alcohol-fast	résistant à l'alcool	alkoholresistent
alcoholism	alcoolisme	Alkoholismus, Alkoholvergiftung
alcohol syndrome	syndrome d'alcoolisme	Alkoholsyndrom
alimentation	alimentation	Ernährung
alkali	alcali	Alkali, Lauge, Base
alkaline	alcalin	alkalisch, basisch
alkalosis	alcalose	Alkalose
allergen	allergène	Allergen
allergy	allergie	Allergie
allopurinol	allopurinol	Allopurinol
alopecia	alopécie	Alopezie, Haarausfall
alpha-fetoprotein (AFP)	alpha-foetoprotéine	Alpha-Fetoprotein
alternative medicine	médecine complémentaire	Alternativmedizin
altitude sickness	mal d'altitude, mal des montagnes	Höhenkrankheit
alveolitis	alvéolite	Alveolitis
alveolus	alvéole	Alveole
Alzheimer's disease	maladie d'Alzheimer	Alzheimer Krankheit
amaurosis	amaurose	Amaurose
amblyopia	amblyopie	Amblyopie, Sehschwäche
ambulant	ambulant	ambulant
ambulatory	ambulatoire	ambulant
ameba (Am)	amibe	Amöbe
amebiasis (Am)	amibiase	Amöbenkrankheit, Amöbiasis
ameboma (Am)	amibome	Amöbengranulom
amelioration	amélioration	Besserung
amenorrhea (Am)	aménorrhée	Amenorrhoe
amenorrhoea (Eng)	aménorrhée	Amenorrhoe
amino acid	acide aminé	Aminosäure
amnesia	amnésie	Amnesie
amniocentesis	amniocentèse	Amniozentese
amnion	amnion	Amnion
amnioscopy	amnioscopie	Amnioskopie
amniotic cavity	cavité amniotique	Amnionhöhle
amniotic fluid	liquide amniotique	Amnionflüssigkeit, Fruchtwasser
amniotomy	amniotomie	Amnionpunktur
amoeba (Eng)	amibe	Amöbe
amoebiasis (Eng)	amibiase	Amöbenkrankheit, Amöbiasis
amoeboma (Eng)	amibome	Amöbengranulom

ITALIAN	SPANISH	ENGLISH
agorafobia	agorafobia	agoraphobia
agranulocitosi	agranulocitosis	agranulocytosis
complesso AIDS-correlato	complejo relacionado con SIDA	AIDS-related complex
ventilazione e respirazione nelle vie respiratorie	vías respiratorias y circulación	airway breathing and circulation (ABC)
acinetico	acinético	akinetic
albumina	albúmina	albumin
albuminuria	albuminuria	albuminuria
alcool	alcohol	alcohol
alcool-resistente	resistente al alcohol	alcohol-fast
alcolismo	alcoholismo	alcoholism
sindrome da alcool	síndrome alcohólico	alcohol syndrome
alimentazione	alimentación	alimentation
alcali	álcali	alkali
alcalino	alcalino	alkaline
alcalosi	alcalosis	alkalosis
allergene	alérgeno	allergen
allergia	alergia	allergy
allopurinolo	alopurinol	allopurinol
alopecia	alopecia, calvicie	alopecia
alfafetoproteina	alfafetoproteína (AFP)	alpha-fetoprotein (AFP)
medicina alternativa	medicina alternativa	alternative medicine
mal di montagna	mal de altura	altitude sickness
alveolite	alveolitis	alveolitis
alveolo	alvéolo	alveolus
morbo di Alzheimer	enfermedad de Alzheimer	Alzheimer's disease
amaurosi	amaurosis, ceguera	amaurosis
ambliopia	ambliopía	amblyopia
ambulatorio	ambulante	ambulant
ambulatoriale	ambulatorio	ambulatory
ameba	ameba	ameba (Am)
amebiasi	amebiasis	amebiasis (Am)
ameboma	ameboma	ameboma (Am)
miglioramento	mejoría	amelioration
amenorrea	amenorrea	amenorrhea (Am)
amenorrea	amenorrea	amenorrhoea (Eng)
aminoacido	aminoácido	amino acid
amnesia	amnesia	amnesia
amniocentesi	amniocentesis	amniocentesis
amnios	amnios	amnion
amnioscopia	amnioscopia	amnioscopy
cavità amniotica	cavidad amniótica	amniotic cavity
fluido amniotico	líquido amniótico	amniotic fluid
amniotomia	amniotomía	amniotomy
ameba	ameba	amoeba (Eng)
amebiasi	amebiasis	amoebiasis (Eng)
ameboma	ameboma	amoeboma (Eng)

ENGLISH	FRENCH	GERMAN
amorphous	amorphe	amorph
ampoule (Eng)	ampoule	Ampulle
ampule (Am)	ampoule	Ampulle
ampulla	ampoule	Ampulle
amputation	amputation	Amputation
amputee	amputé	Amputierter
amyloid (n)	amyloïde (n)	Amyloid (n)
amyloid (a)	amyloïde (a)	amyloid (a), stärkehaltig (a)
amyloidosis	amylose	Amyloidose
anabolism	anabolisme	Anabolismus, Aufbaustoffwechsel
anaemia (Eng)	anémie	Anämie
anaerobe (Eng)	anaérobie	Anaerobier
anaerobic respiration (Eng)	respiration anaérobie	anaerobe Respiration
anaesthesia (Eng)	anesthésie	Anästhesie, Betäubung, Narkose
anaesthetic (Eng) (n)	anesthésique (n)	Anästhetikum (n), Betäubungsmittel (n), Narkosemittel (n)
anaesthetic (Eng) (a)	anesthésique (a)	anästhetisch (a), betäubend (a), gefühllos (a)
analeptic (n)	analeptique (n)	Analeptikum (n)
analeptic (a)	analeptique (a)	analeptisch (a)
analgesia	analgésie	Analgesie, Schmerzlosigkeit
analgesic (n)	analgésique (n)	Analgetikum (n), Schmerzmittel (n)
analgesic (a)	analgésique (a)	analgetisch (a), schmerzlindernd (a), schmerzunempfindlich (a)
analysis	analyse	Analyse
anaphylactic reaction	réaction anaphylactique	anaphylaktische Reaktion
anaphylaxis	anaphylaxie	Anaphylaxie
anaplasia	anaplasie	Anaplasie
anarthria	anarthrie	Anarthrie
anastomosis	anastomose	Anastomose
anatomy	anatomie	Anatomie
androgens	androgènes	Androgene
anemia (Am)	anémie	Anämie
anencephaly	anencéphalie	Anenzephalie
anerobe (Am)	anaérobie	Anaerobier
anerobic respiration (Am)	respiration anaérobie	anaerobe Respiration
anesthesia (Am)	anesthésie	Anästhesie, Betäubung, Narkose
anesthetic (Am) (n)	anesthésique (n)	Anästhetikum (n), Betäubungsmittel (n), Narkosemittel (n)
anesthetic (Am) (a)	anesthésique (a)	anästhetisch (a), betäubend (a), gefühllos (a)
aneurysm	anévrisme	Aneurysma
angina	angor	Angina
angioneurotic edema (solidus) (Am)	oedème angioneurotique	Quincke-Ödem
angioneurotic oedema (solidus) (Eng)	oedème angioneurotique	Quincke-Ödem
angioplasty	angioplastie	Angioplastie
angiotensin	angiotensine	Angiotensin
anisocytosis	anisocytose	Anisozytose
ankle	cheville	Knöchel, Talus

ITALIAN	SPANISH	ENGLISH
amorfo	amorfo	amorphous
ampolla, fiala	ampolla, vial	ampoule (Eng)
ampolla, fiala	ampolla, vial	ampule (Am)
ampolla, fiala	ampolla	ampulla
amputazione	amputación	amputation
amputato	amputado	amputee
amiloide (n)	amiloide (n)	amyloid (n)
amiloide (a)	amiloideo (a)	amyloid (a)
amiloidosi	amiloidosis	amyloidosis
anabolismo	anabolismo	anabolism
anemia	anemia	anaemia (Eng)
anaerobio	anaerobio	anaerobe (Eng)
respirazione anaerobica	respiración anaerobia	anaerobic respiration (Eng)
anestesia	anestesia	anaesthesia (Eng)
anestetico (n)	anestésico (n)	anaesthetic (Eng) (n)
anestetico (a)	anestésico (a)	anaesthetic (Eng) (a)
analettico (n)	analéptico, estimulante (n)	analeptic (n)
analettico (a)	analéptico, estimulante (a)	analeptic (a)
analgesia	analgesia	analgesia
analgesico (n)	analgésico (n)	analgesic (n)
analgesico (a)	analgésico (a)	analgesic (a)
analisi	análisis	analysis
reazione anafilattica	reacción anafiláctica	anaphylactic reaction
anafilassi	anafilaxis	anaphylaxis
anaplasia	anaplasia	anaplasia
anartria	anartria	anarthria
anastomosi	anastómosis	anastomosis
anatomia	anatomía	anatomy
androgeni	andrógenos	androgens
anemia	anemia	anemia (Am)
anencefalia	anencefalia	anencephaly
anaerobio	anaerobio	anerobe (Am)
respirazione anaerobica	respiración anaerobia	anerobic respiration (Am)
anestesia	anestesia	anesthesia (Am)
anestetico (n)	anestésico (n)	anesthetic (Am) (n)
anestetico (a)	anestésico (a)	anesthetic (Am) (a)
aneurisma	aneurisma	aneurysm
angina	angina	angina
edema angioneurotico	edema angioneurótico (sólido)	angioneurotic edema (solidus) (Am)
edema angioneurotico	edema angioneurico (sólido)	angioneurotic oedema (solidus) (Eng)
angioplastica	angioplastia	angioplasty
angiotensina	angiotensina	angiotensin
anisocitosi	anisocitosis	anisocytosis
caviglia	tobillo	ankle

ENGLISH	FRENCH	GERMAN
ankylosis	ankylose	Ankylose, Versteifung
annular	annulaire	ringförmig
anogenital	anogénital	anogenital
anomaly	anomalie	Anomalie, Fehlbildung
anorectal	anorectal	anorektal
anorectic (n)	anorexique (n)	Anorektiker(in) (n), Magersüchtige(r) (n), Apettitzügler (n)
anorectic (a)	anorexique (a)	anorektisch (a), magersüchtig (a)
anorexia	anorexie	Anorexie, Magersucht
anosmia	anosmie	Anosmie
anovular	anovulaire	anovulatorisch
anoxia	anoxie	Anoxie, Sauerstoffmangel
antacid	antiacide	Antazidum
antagonism	antagonisme	Antagonismus
antagonist	antagoniste	Antagonist
antenatal	anténatal	pränatal
ante-partum	ante partum	ante partum, vor der Entbindung
anterior	antérieur	anterior, Vorder-
anterograde	antérograde	anterograd
anteversion	antéversion	Anteversion
anthrax	anthrax	Anthrax, Milzbrand
anthropoid	anthropoïde	anthropoid
anthropology	anthropologie	Anthropologie
anti-arrhythmic	antiarythmique	antiarrhythmisch
antibacterial	antibactérien	antibakteriell
antibiotics	antibiotiques	Antibiotika
antibodies (Ab)	anticorps	Antikörper
anticholinergic	anticholinergique	anticholinerg
anticoagulant	anticoagulant	Antikoagulans, Gerinnungshemmer
anticonvulsant (n)	anticonvulsant (n)	Antiepileptikum (n), Antikonvulsivum (n)
anticonvulsant (a)	anticonvulsant (a)	antiepileptisch (a), antikonvulsiv (a)
anti-D	anti-D	Anti-D-Immununglobulin
antidepressant	antidépresseur	Antidepressivum
antidote	antidote	Antidot
antiemetic (n)	antiémétique (n)	Antiemetikum (n)
antiemetic (a)	antiémétique (a)	antiemetisch (a)
anti-epileptic (n)	antiépileptique (n)	Antiepileptikum (n), Antikonvulsivum (n)
anti-epileptic (a)	antiépileptique (a)	antiepileptisch (a), antikonvulsiv (a)
antigen	antigène	Antigen
antigen binding capacity (ABC)	capacité de liaison d'un antigène, capacité de fixation d'un antigène	Antigen-Bindungskapazität
antihistamine	antihistamine	Antihistamine
antihypertensive (n)	antihypertenseur (n)	Antihypertonikum (n), Antihypertensivum (n)
antihypertensive (a)	antihypertensif (a)	blutdrucksenkend (a), antihypertensiv (a)
anti-inflammatory	anti-inflammatoire	entzündungshemmend

10

anchilosi	anquilosis	**ankylosis**
anulare	anular	**annular**
anogenitale	anogenital	**anogenital**
anomalia	anomalía	**anomaly**
anorettale	anorrectal	**anorectal**
anoressico (n)	anoréxico (n)	**anorectic** (n)
anoressico (a)	anoréxico (a)	**anorectic** (a)
anoressia	anorexia	**anorexia**
anosmia	anosmia	**anosmia**
anovulare	anovular	**anovular**
anossia	anoxia	**anoxia**
antiacido	antiácido	**antacid**
antagonismo	antagonismo	**antagonism**
antagonista	antagonista	**antagonist**
prenatale	antenatal	**antenatal**
preparto	ante partum, preparto	**ante-partum**
anteriore	anterior	**anterior**
anterogrado	anterógrado	**anterograde**
antiversione	anteversión	**anteversion**
antrace, carbonchio	carbunco	**anthrax**
antropoide	antropoide	**anthropoid**
antropologia	antropología	**anthropology**
anti aritmico	antiarrítmico	**anti-arrhythmic**
antibatterico	antibacteriano	**antibacterial**
antibiotici	antibióticos	**antibiotics**
anticorpi (Ac)	anticuerpos	**antibodies (Ab)**
anticolinergico	anticolinérgico	**anticholinergic**
anticoagulante	anticoagulante	**anticoagulant**
anticonvulsivante (n)	anticonvulsivo (n)	**anticonvulsant** (n)
anticonvulsivante (a)	anticonvulsivo (a)	**anticonvulsant** (a)
anti-D	anti-D	**anti-D**
antidepressivo	antidepresivo	**antidepressant**
antidoto	antídoto	**antidote**
anti-emetico (n)	antiemético (n)	**antiemetic** (n)
anti-emetico (a)	antiemético (a)	**antiemetic** (a)
anticomiziale (n)	antiepiléptico (n)	**anti-epileptic** (n)
anticomiziale (a)	antiepiléptico (a)	**anti-epileptic** (a)
antigene	antígeno	**antigen**
capacità di legame dell'antigene	capacidad de unión con antígenos	**antigen binding capacity (ABC)**
anti-istaminico	antihistamínico	**antihistamine**
anti-ipertensivo (n)	hipotensor (n)	**antihypertensive** (n)
anti-ipertensivo (a)	hipotensor (a)	**antihypertensive** (a)
anti infiammatorio	antiinflamatorio	**anti-inflammatory**

ENGLISH	FRENCH	GERMAN
antimalarial *(n)*	antipaludique *(n)*	Antimalariamittel *(n)*, Malariamittel *(n)*
antimalarial *(a)*	antipaludique *(a)*	Antimalaria- *(a)*
antimetabolite	antimétabolite	Antimetabolit
antimicrobial	antimicrobien	antimikrobiell
antimycotic *(n)*	antimycotique *(n)*	Antimykotikum *(n)*
antimycotic *(a)*	antimycotique *(a)*	antimykotisch *(a)*
antiparkinson(ism) drugs	médicaments contre la maladie de Parkinson	Antiparkinsonmittel
antipruritic *(n)*	antiprurigineux *(n)*	Antipruriginosum *(n)*
antipruritic *(a)*	antiprurigineux *(a)*	antipruriginös *(a)*, juckreizlindernd *(a)*
antipsychotic *(n)*	antipsychotique *(n)*	Antipsychotikum *(n)*, Neuroleptikum *(n)*
antipsychotic *(a)*	antipsychotique *(a)*	antipsychotisch *(a)*, neuroleptisch *(a)*
antipyretic *(n)*	antipyrétique *(n)*	Antipyretikum *(n)*, Fiebermittel *(n)*
antipyretic *(a)*	antipyrétique *(a)*	antipyretisch *(a)*, fiebersenkend *(a)*
antisepsis	antisepsie	Antisepsis
antiseptic *(n)*	antiseptique *(n)*	Antiseptikum *(n)*
antiseptic *(a)*	antiseptique *(a)*	antiseptisch *(a)*
antiserum	anti-serum	Antiserum, Immunserum
antisocial	antisocial	dissozial
antisocial personality	personnalité psychopathique	asoziale Persönlichkeit
antispasmodic *(n)*	antispasmodique *(n)*	Spasmolytikum *(n)*
antispasmodic *(a)*	antispasmodique *(a)*	spasmolytisch *(a)*, krampflösend *(a)*
antitoxin	antitoxine	Antitoxin, Gegengift
antitussive *(n)*	antitussif *(n)*	Antitussivum *(n)*, Hustenmittel *(n)*
antitussive *(a)*	antitussif *(a)*	antitussiv *(a)*
antivenin	sérum antivenimeux	Schlangenserum
antrostomy	antrostomie	Antrumeröffnung
antrum	antre	Antrum
anuria	anurie	Anurie, Harnverhaltung
anus	anus	Anus, After
anxiety	anxiété	Angst
anxiolytic *(n)*	anxiolytique *(n)*	Anxiolytikum *(n)*
anxiolytic *(a)*	anxiolytique *(a)*	anxiolytisch *(a)*
aorta	aorte	Aorta, Hauptschlagader
apathy	apathie	Apathie
aperient *(n)*	laxatif *(n)*	Abführmittel *(n)*, Laxans *(n)*
aperient *(a)*	laxatif *(a)*	abführend *(a)*, laxierend *(a)*
apex	apex	Apex, Spitze
Apgar score	indice d'Apgar	Apgar-Index
aphasia	aphasie	Aphasie
aphthae	aphtes	Aphthe
apnea (Am)	apnée	Apnoe, Atemstillstand
apnoea (Eng)	apnée	Apnoe, Atemstillstand
apocrine gland	glande apocrine	apokrine Drüse
appendectomy	appendicectomie	Appendektomie, Blinddarmoperation
appendicectomy	appendicectomie	Appendektomie, Blinddarmoperation

ITALIAN	SPANISH	ENGLISH
antimalarico *(n)*	antipalúdico *(n)*	antimalarial *(n)*
antimalarico *(a)*	antipalúdico *(a)*	antimalarial *(a)*
antimetabolita	antimetabolito	antimetabolite
antimicrobico	antimicrobiano	antimicrobial
antimicotico *(n)*	antimicótico *(n)*	antimycotic *(n)*
antimicotico *(a)*	antimicótico *(a)*	antimycotic *(a)*
farmaci antiparkinsoniani	farmacos antiparkinsonianos	antiparkinson(ism) drugs
antipruriginoso *(n)*	antipruriginoso *(n)*	antipruritic *(n)*
antipruriginoso *(a)*	antipruriginoso *(a)*	antipruritic *(a)*
antipsicotico *(n)*	antipsicótico *(n)*	antipsychotic *(n)*
antipsicotico *(a)*	antipsicótico *(a)*	antipsychotic *(a)*
anti-piretico *(n)*	antipirético *(n)*	antipyretic *(n)*
anti-piretico *(a)*	antipirético *(a)*	antipyretic *(a)*
antisepsi	antisepsia	antisepsis
antisettico *(n)*	antiséptico *(n)*	antiseptic *(n)*
antisettico *(a)*	antiséptico *(a)*	antiseptic *(a)*
anti-siero	antisuero	antiserum
antisociale	antisocial	antisocial
personalità antisociale	personalidad antisocial	antisocial personality
antispastico *(n)*	antiespasmódico *(n)*	antispasmodic *(n)*
antispastico *(a)*	antiespasmódico *(a)*	antispasmodic *(a)*
antitossina	antitoxina	antitoxin
antibechico *(n)*	antitusígeno *(n)*	antitussive *(n)*
antibechico *(a)*	antitusígeno *(a)*	antitussive *(a)*
antiveleno, contravveleno	antídoto	antivenin
antrostomia	antrostomía	antrostomy
antro	antro	antrum
anuria	anuria	anuria
ano	ano	anus
ansietà	ansiedad	anxiety
ansiolitico *(n)*	ansiolítico *(n)*	anxiolytic *(n)*
ansiolitico *(a)*	ansiolítico *(a)*	anxiolytic *(a)*
aorta	aorta	aorta
apatia	apatía	apathy
lassativo *(n)*	laxante *(n)*	aperient *(n)*
lassativo *(a)*	laxante *(a)*	aperient *(a)*
apice	ápex	apex
indice di Apgar	índice de Apgar	Apgar score
afasia	afasia	aphasia
afte	aftas	aphthae
apnea	apnea	apnea *(Am)*
apnea	apnea	apnoea *(Eng)*
ghiandola apocrina	glándula apocrina	apocrine gland
appendicectomia	apendicectomía	appendectomy
appendicectomia	apendicectomía	appendicectomy

appendicitis	appendicite	Appendizitis, Blinddarmentzündung
appendix	appendice	Appendix, Blinddarm
applicator	applicateur	Applikator
apposition	apposition	Apposition
apraxia	apraxie	Apraxie
apyrexia	apyrexie	Apyrexie
aqueduct	aqueduc	Aquädukt
aqueous	aqueux	wässrig, wasserhaltig
arachnoid	arachnoïde	arachnoid
arbovirus	arbovirus	ARBO-Virus
areola	aréole	Areola, Brustwarzenhof
arm	bras	Arm
Arnold-Chiari malformation	malformation d'Arnold Chiari	Arnold-Chiari-Mißbildung
arrhythmia	arythmie	Arrhythmie, Rhythmusstörung
artefact (Eng)	artefact	Artefakt
arteriole	artériole	Arteriole
arteriopathy	artériopathie	Arteriopathie, Arterienerkrankung
arteriosclerosis	artériosclérose	Arteriosklerose, Arterienverkalkung
arteriovenous	artérioveineux	arteriovenös
arteritis	artérite	Arteriitis
artery	artère	Arterie, Schlagader
arthralgia	arthralgie	Arthralgie, Gelenkschmerz
arthritis	arthrite	Arthritis, Gelenkentzündung
arthrodesis	arthrodèse	Arthrodese
arthrography	arthrographie	Arthrographie
arthropathy	arthropathie	Arthropathie, Gelenkleiden
arthroplasty	arthroplastie	Arthroplastik, Gelenkplastik
arthroscopy	arthroscopie	Arthroskopie, Gelenkendoskopie
articular	articulaire	Gelenk-
articulation	articulation	Artikulation
artifact (Am)	artefact	Artefakt
artificial insemination (AI)	insémination artificielle (IA)	künstliche Befruchtung
artificial insemination by donor (AID)	insémination hétérologue	heterologe Insemination
asbestos	asbeste	Asbest
asbestosis	asbestose	Asbestose
ascaris	ascaris	Spulwurm
ascending colon	côlon ascendant	Colon ascendens
ascites	ascite	Aszites
asepsis	asepsie	Asepsis
aseptic technique	technique aseptique	aseptische Technik
aspergillosis	aspergillose	Aspergillose
asphyxia	asphyxie	Asphyxie
aspiration	aspiration	Aspiration
assimilation	assimilation	Assimilation
association	association	Assoziation
astereognosis	astéréognosie	Astereognosie

ITALIAN	SPANISH	ENGLISH
appendicite	apendicitis	appendicitis
appendice	apéndice	appendix
applicatore	aplicador	applicator
apposizione	aposición	apposition
aprassia	apraxia	apraxia
apiressia	apirexia	apyrexia
acquedotto	acueducto	aqueduct
acquoso	acuoso	aqueous
aracnoidea	aracnoideo	arachnoid
arbovirus	arbovirus	arbovirus
areola	areola	areola
braccio	brazo	arm
sindrome di Arnold Chiari	malformación de Arnold-Chiari	Arnold-Chiari malformation
aritmia	arritmia	arrhythmia
artefatto	artefacto	artefact (Eng)
arteriola	arteriola	arteriole
arteriopatia	arteriopatía	arteriopathy
arteriosclerosi	arteriosclerosis	arteriosclerosis
arterovenosa	arteriovenoso	arteriovenous
arterite	arteritis	arteritis
arteria	arteria	artery
artralgia	artralgia	arthralgia
artrite	artritis	arthritis
artrodesi	artrodesis	arthrodesis
artrografia	artrografía	arthrography
artropatia	artropatía	arthropathy
artroplastica	artroplastia	arthroplasty
artroscopia	artroscopia	arthroscopy
articolare	articular	articular
articolazione	articulación	articulation
artefatto	artefacto	artifact (Am)
inseminazione artificiale	inseminación artificial	artificial insemination (AI)
fecondazione artificiale tramite donatore	inseminación artificial por donante (AID)	artificial insemination by donor (AID)
asbesto	asbesto	asbestos
asbestosi	asbestosis	asbestosis
ascaride	áscaris	ascaris
colon ascendente	colon ascendente	ascending colon
ascite	ascitis	ascites
asepsi	asepsia	asepsis
tecnica asettica	técnica aséptica	aseptic technique
aspergillosi	aspergilosis	aspergillosis
asfissia	asfixia	asphyxia
aspirazione	aspiración	aspiration
assimilazione	asimilación	assimilation
associazione	asociación	association
astereognosia	astereognosia	astereognosis

ENGLISH	FRENCH	GERMAN
asthma	asthme	Asthma
astigmatism	astigmatisme	Astigmatismus
astringent	astringent	adstringierend
asymmetry	asymétrie	Asymmetrie
asymptomatic	asymptomatique	asymptomatisch
ataxia	ataxie	Ataxie, Koordinationsstörung
atelectasis	atélectasie	Atelektase
atherogenic	athérogène	atherogen
atheroma	athérome	Atherom, Grützbeutel
atherosclerosis	athérosclérose	Atherosklerose
athetosis	athétose	Athetose
athlete's foot	pied d'athlète	Fußpilz
atom	atome	Atom
atomic weight (at wt)	poids atomique	Atomgewicht
atonic	atonique	atonisch
atresia	atrésie	Atresie
atrial fibrillation	fibrillation auriculaire	Vorhofflimmern
atrial flutter	flutter auriculaire	Vorhofflattern
atrial septal defect (ASD)	communication auriculaire	Vorhofseptumdefekt
atrioventricular (AV)	atrio-ventriculaire	atrioventrikulär
atrium	oreillette	Atrium, Vorhof
atrophy	atrophie	Atrophie
atropine	atropine	Atropin
attack	attaque	Anfall, Attacke
attenuation	atténuation	Verdünnung, Abschwächung
atypical	atypique	atypisch, heterolog
audiogram	audiogramme	Audiogramm, Hörkurve
audiology	audiologie	Audiologie
auditory	auditif	Gehör-, Hör-
aura	aura	Aura
aural	aural	Gehör-, Ohr-, Aura-
auriscope	auriscope	Ohrenspiegel
auscultation	auscultation	Auskultation, Abhören
Australian antigen	antigène australien	Australia-Antigen (HBsAG)
autism	autisme	Autismus
autistic	autiste	autistisch
autoantibody	auto-anticorps	Autoantikörper
autoantigen	auto-antigène	Autoantigen
autoclave	autoclave	Autoklav, Sterilisationsapparat
autograft	autogreffe	Autoplastik
autoimmune disease	maladie auto-immune	Autoimmunerkrankung
autoimmunity	auto-immunisation	Autoimmunität
autologous	autologue	autolog
autolysis	autolyse	Autolyse
autonomic	autonome	autonom
autopsy	autopsie	Autopsie, Sektion

ITALIAN	SPANISH	ENGLISH
asma	asma	**asthma**
astigmatismo	astigmatismo	**astigmatism**
astringente	astringente	**astringent**
asimmetria	asimetría	**asymmetry**
asintomatico	asintomático	**asymptomatic**
atassia	ataxia	**ataxia**
atelettasia	atelectasia	**atelectasis**
aterogenico	aterogénico	**atherogenic**
ateroma	ateroma	**atheroma**
aterosclerosi	aterosclerosis	**atherosclerosis**
atetosi	atetosis	**athetosis**
piede di atleta	pie de atleta	**athlete's foot**
atomo	átomo	**atom**
peso atomico	peso atómico	**atomic weight (at wt)**
atonico	atono	**atonic**
atresia	atresia	**atresia**
fibrillazione atriale	fibrilación auricular	**atrial fibrillation**
flutter atriale	aleteo auricular	**atrial flutter**
difetto atriosettale	defecto del septum auricular	**atrial septal defect (ASD)**
atrioventricolare	atrioventricular, aurículo-ventricular (AV)	**atrioventricular (AV)**
atrio	aurícula	**atrium**
atrofia	atrofia	**atrophy**
atropina	atropina	**atropine**
attacco	ataque	**attack**
attenuazione	atenuación	**attenuation**
atipico	atípico	**atypical**
audiogramma	audiograma	**audiogram**
audiologia	audiología	**audiology**
acustico, auditivo	auditorio	**auditory**
aura	aura	**aura**
auricolare	aural	**aural**
otoscopio	auriscopio	**auriscope**
auscultazione	auscultación	**auscultation**
antigene Australia	antígeno Australia	**Australian antigen**
autismo	autismo	**autism**
autistico	persona autística	**autistic**
autoanticorpo	autoanticuerpo	**autoantibody**
autoantigene	autoantígeno	**autoantigen**
autoclave	autoclave	**autoclave**
autoinnesto	autoinjerto	**autograft**
malattia autoimmune	enfermedad autoinmune	**autoimmune disease**
autoimmunizzazione	autoinmunización	**autoimmunity**
autologo	autólogo	**autologous**
autolisi	autólisis	**autolysis**
autonomo	autónomo	**autonomic**
autopsia	autopsia	**autopsy**

ENGLISH	FRENCH	GERMAN
avascular	avasculaire	gefäßlos
aversion therapy	cure de dégoût	Aversionstherapie
avulsion	avulsion	Abriß, Ausreißen
axilla	aisselle	Axilla, Achsel(höhle)
axis	axe	Achse
axon	axone	Axon
axonotmesis	axonotmésis	Axonotmesis
azygous	azygos	azygos

ITALIAN	SPANISH	ENGLISH
avascolare	avascular	**avascular**
decondizionamento	tratamiento por aversión	**aversion therapy**
avulsione	avulsión	**avulsion**
ascella	axila	**axilla**
asse, colonna vertebrale	eje	**axis**
cilindrasse, assone	axón	**axon**
degenerazione del cilindrasse, con possibile rigenerazione	axonotmesis	**axonotmesis**
azygos	ácigos	**azygous**

B

English	French	German
Babinski's reflex	réflexe de Babinski	Babinski-Reflex
bacille Calmette-Guérin (BCG)	bacille de Calmette-Guérin (BCG)	Bacillus Calmette-Guérin (BCG)
bacillus	bacille	Bazillus
bacteraemia (Eng)	bactériémie	Bakteriämie
bacteremia (Am)	bactériémie	Bakteriämie
bacteria	bactérie	Bakterien
bactericide	bactéricide	Bakterizid
bacteriology	bactériologie	Bakteriologie
bacteriostasis	bactériostase	Bakteriostase
bacteriuria	bactériurie	Bakteriurie
balanitis	balanite	Balanitis
balanoposthitis	balanoposthite	Balanoposthitis
ballottement	ballottement	Ballottement
bandage	bandage	Verband
barium enema	lavement au baryte	Bariumeinlauf
barrier nursing	nursage de protection	Isolierung (auf Isolierstation)
Bartholin's glands	glandes de Bartholin	Bartholini-Drüsen
basal ganglia	noyau lenticulaire, noyau caudé, avant-mur et noyau amygdalien	Basalganglien
basal metabolic rate (BMR)	taux du métabolisme basal	Grundumsatz
basic life support	équipement de survie	Vitalfunktionserhaltung
basilar-vertebral insufficiency	insuffisance basilaire vertébrale	Basilarvertebralinsuffizienz
bath	bain	Bad
battered baby syndrome	syndrome des enfants maltraités	Kindesmißhandlung (Folgen)
bearing down	efforts expulsifs	Pressen
bedsore	escarre de décubitus	Dekubitus, Durchliegen
bedwetting	incontinence nocturne	Bettnässen
behavior (Am)	comportement	Verhalten
behaviour (Eng)	comportement	Verhalten
Behçet syndrome	syndrome de Behçet	Behçet-Syndrom
belching	éructation	Aufstoßen
'belle indifference'	indifférence	belle indifference
Bell's palsy	paralysie de Bell	Bell-Fazialisparese
belly	ventre	Bauch
Bence-Jones protein (BJ)	protéine de Bence Jones (BJ)	Bence-Jones-Proteine
benign	bénin (bénigne)	benigne, gutartig
beri-beri	béribéri	Beriberi
beta blocker	bêtabloquant	Betablocker
biceps	biceps	Bizeps
bicornuate	bicorne	bicornis
bicuspid	bicuspide	bicuspidal
bifid	bifide	bifidus
bifurcation	bifurcation	Bifurkation
bilateral	bilatéral	zweiseitig
bile	bile	Galle

riflesso di Babinski	reflejo de Babinski	**Babinski's reflex**
bacillo di Calmette e Guérin	bacilo de Calmette-Guérin (BCG)	**bacille Calmette-Guérin (BCG)**
bacillo	bacilo	**bacillus**
batteriemia	bacteriemia	**bacteraemia** (Eng)
batteriemia	bacteriemia	**bacteremia** (Am)
batteri	bacteria	**bacteria**
battericida	bactericida	**bactericide**
batteriologia	bacteriología	**bacteriology**
batteriostasi	bacteriostasis	**bacteriostasis**
batteriuria	bacteriuria	**bacteriuria**
balanite	balanitis	**balanitis**
balanopostite	balanopostitis	**balanoposthitis**
ballottamento	peloteo	**ballottement**
benda	vendaje	**bandage**
clisma opaco	enema de bario	**barium enema**
isolamento	enfermería por aislamiento	**barrier nursing**
ghiandole di Bartolini	glándulas de Bartolino	**Bartholin's glands**
gangli basali	ganglios basales	**basal ganglia**
indice del metabolismo basale (MB)	tasa de metabolismo basal (MB)	**basal metabolic rate (BMR)**
mantenimento delle funzioni vitali	soporte de vida básico	**basic life support**
insufficienza vertebrobasilare	insuficiencia vertebrobasilar	**basilar-vertebral insufficiency**
bagno	baño	**bath**
sindrome del bambino maltrattato	síndrome del niño apaleado	**battered baby syndrome**
fase espulsiva del parto	postración	**bearing down**
piaga da decubito	úlcera por decúbito	**bedsore**
enuresi notturna	enuresis nocturna	**bedwetting**
comportamento	comportamiento	**behavior** (Am)
comportamento	comportamiento	**behaviour** (Eng)
sindrome di Behçet	síndrome de Behçet	**Behçet syndrome**
eruttazione	eructo	**belching**
'belle indifference'	la belle indifférence	**'belle indifference'**
paralisi di Bell	parálisis de Bell	**Bell's palsy**
addome, ventre	vientre	**belly**
proteina di Bence-Jones	proteína de Bence-Jones	**Bence-Jones protein (BJ)**
benigno	benigno	**benign**
beri-beri	beri-beri	**beri-beri**
beta-bloccante	beta-bloqueador	**beta blocker**
bicipite	bíceps	**biceps**
bicorne	bicornio	**bicornuate**
bicuspide	bicúspide	**bicuspid**
bifido	bífido	**bifid**
biforcazione	bifurcación	**bifurcation**
bilaterale	bilateral	**bilateral**
bile	bilis	**bile**

ENGLISH	FRENCH	GERMAN
biliary	biliaire	biliär
bilious	bilieux	biliös
bilirubin	bilirubine	Bilirubin
biliuria	biliurie	Bilirubinurie
Billroth's operation	opération de Billroth	Billroth-Magenresektion
bimanual	bimanuel	bimanuell, beidhändig
binocular vision	vision binoculaire	binokulares Sehen, beidäugiges Sehen
biological	biologique	biologisch
biopsy	biopsie	Biopsie
biorhythm	biorythme	Biorhythmus
bipolar	bipolaire	bipolar
birth	naissance	Geburt
birthmark	naevus, envie	Muttermal, Storchenbiß
bisexual	bisexuel	bisexuell
bivalve	bivalve	zweiklappig
blackwater fever	hématurie	Schwarzwasserfieber
bladder	vessie	Blase, Harnblase
bleb	phlyctène	Bläschen
bleed	saigner	bluten
'bleeding time'	temps de saignement	Blutungszeit
blepharitis	blépharite	Blepharitis, Lidentzündung
blepharospasm	blépharospasme	Blepharospasmus, Lidkrampf
blind loop syndrome	syndrome de l'anse borgne	Syndrom der blinden Schlinge
blindness	cécité	Blindheit
blind spot	tache aveugle	blinder Fleck, Papille
blister	ampoule	Blase, Hautblase, Brandblase
blood	sang	Blut
blood bank	banque de sang	Blutbank
blood-brain barrier (BBB)	barrière hémato-encéphalique	Blut-Hirn-Schranke
blood clotting	coagulation du sang	Blutgerinnung
blood coagulation	coagulation sanguine	Blutgerinnung
blood count	dénombrement des hématies	Blutbild
blood culture	hémoculture	Blutkultur
blood group	groupe sanguin	Blutgruppe
blood pressure (BP)	tension artérielle (TA)	Blutdruck
blood sedimentation rate (BSR)	vitesse de sédimentation sanguine	Blutkörperchen-Senkungsgeschwindigkeit (BSG, BKS)
blood sugar	glycémie	Blutzucker
blood urea	urée du sang	Blutharnstoff
blood volume (BV)	masse sanguine	Blutvolumen
blue baby	enfant bleu, enfant atteint de la maladie bleue	zyanotisches Neugeborenes
body mass index (BMI)	indice de masse corporelle (IMC)	Körpermassenindex
boil	furoncle	Furunkel, Eiterbeule
bolus	bol	Bolus
bonding	attachement	Bindung

ITALIAN	SPANISH	ENGLISH
biliare	biliar	**biliary**
biliare	bilioso	**bilious**
bilirubina	bilirrubina	**bilirubin**
biliuria	biliuria	**biliuria**
operazione di Billroth	operación de Billroth	**Billroth's operation**
bimanuale	bimanual	**bimanual**
visione binoculare	visión binocular	**binocular vision**
biologico	biológico	**biological**
biopsia	biopsia	**biopsy**
bioritmo	biorritmo	**biorhythm**
bipolare	bipolar	**bipolar**
nascita	nacimiento, parto	**birth**
nevo congenito	mancha de nacimiento	**birthmark**
bisessuale	bisexual	**bisexual**
bivalve	bivalvo	**bivalve**
febbre emoglobinurica da Plasmodium falciparum	fiebre hemoglobinúrica	**blackwater fever**
vescica	vejiga	**bladder**
vescichetta, flittena	vesícula, bulla, ampolla	**bleb**
sanguinare	sangrar	**bleed**
tempo di sanguinamento	tiempo de sangría	**'bleeding time'**
blefarite	blefaritis	**blepharitis**
blefarospasmo	blefarospasmo	**blepharospasm**
sindrome dell'ansa cieca	síndrome del asa ciega	**blind loop syndrome**
cecità	ceguera	**blindness**
punto cieco	mancha ciega	**blind spot**
vescicola, bolla	vesícula, ampolla, flictena	**blister**
sangue	sangre	**blood**
banca del sangue	banco de sangre	**blood bank**
barriera ematoencefalica	barrera hematoencefálica (BHE)	**blood-brain barrier (BBB)**
coagulazione ematica	coagulación de la sangre	**blood clotting**
coagulazione del sangue	coagulación de la sangre	**blood coagulation**
emocitometria	recuento sanguíneo	**blood count**
emocoltura	hemocultivo	**blood culture**
gruppo sanguigno	grupo sanguíneo	**blood group**
pressione arteriosa	presión arterial (PA)	**blood pressure (BP)**
velocità di eritrosedimentazione (VES)	velocidad de sedimentación globular (VSG)	**blood sedimentation rate (BSR)**
glicemia	glucemia	**blood sugar**
azotemia	urea sérica	**blood urea**
volume sanguigno	volumen hemático	**blood volume (BV)**
'blue baby' (cianosi da cardiopatia congenita)	niño azul	**blue baby**
indice di massa corporea (IMC)	índice de masa corporal (IMC)	**body mass index (BMI)**
foruncolo	forúnculo	**boil**
bolo	bolo	**bolus**
legame	vinculación	**bonding**

ENGLISH	FRENCH	GERMAN
bone	os	Knochen, Gräte
bone graft	greffe osseuse	Osteoplastik, Knochentransplantation
bone marrow	moelle osseuse	Knochenmark
Bornholm disease	maladie de Bornholm	Bornholm-Krankheit
borreliosis	borréliose	Borreliose
botulism	botulisme	Botulismus
bovine spongiform encephalitis (BSE)	encéphalite spongiforme bovine	Rinderwahnsinn, Bovine Spongiforme Enzephalitis (BSE)
bowel	intestin	Darm
brachial	brachial	Arm-
bradycardia	bradycardie	Bradykardie
brain	cerveau	Gehirn, Verstand
bran	son	Kleie
branchial	branchial	branchial-
breast	sein	Brust
breast self-examination (BSE)	auto-examen des seins	Selbstuntersuchung der Brust
breath	haleine, souffle	Atem, Atemzug
breech	siège	Steiß, Gesäß
breech-birth presentation	présentation, naissance par le siège	Steißlage
broad ligament	ligaments larges	ligamentum latum uteri
Broca's area	centre moteur de Broca	Broca-Sprachzentrum
Brompton's mixture	liquide de Brompton	Brompton-Lösung (Alkohol, Morphin, Kokain)
bronchi	bronches	Bronchien
bronchial asthma	asthme bronchique	Asthma bronchiale
bronchiectasis	bronchectasie	Bronchiektase
bronchiole	bronchiole	Bronchiolus, Bronchiole
bronchiolitis	bronchiolite	Bronchiolitis
bronchitis	bronchite	Bronchitis
bronchoconstrictor	bronchoconstricteur	Bronchokonstriktor
bronchodilator	bronchodilatateur	Bronchodilatator
bronchopneumonia	bronchopneumonie	Bronchopneumonie
bronchopulmonary	bronchopulmonaire	bronchopulmonal
bronchoscope	bronchoscope	Bronchoskop
bronchospasm	bronchospasme	Bronchospasmus
bronchus	bronche	Bronchus
brow	front, sourcil	Augenbraue
brucellosis	brucellose	Brucellose
bruise (n)	contusion (n)	Quetschung (n), Prellung (n)
bruise (v)	contusionner (v)	stoßen (v), quetschen (v)
buccal	buccal	bukkal
bulbar	bulbaire	bulbär
bulimia	boulimie	Bulimie
bulla	bulle	Bulla, Blase
bunion	hallux valgus	entzündeter Fußballen
burn (n)	brûlure (n)	Verbrennung (n), Brandwunde (n)
burn (v)	brûler (v)	brennen (v), verbrennen (v)

ITALIAN	SPANISH	ENGLISH
osso	hueso	**bone**
trapianto osseo	injerto óseo, osteoplastia	**bone graft**
midollo osseo	médula ósea	**bone marrow**
malattia di Bornholm, mialgia epidemica	enfermedad de Bornholm	**Bornholm disease**
borreliosi	borreliosis	**borreliosis**
botulismo	botulismo	**botulism**
encefalite spongiforme bovina	encefalitis espongiforme bovina	**bovine spongiform encephalitis (BSE)**
intestino	intestino	**bowel**
brachiale	braquial	**brachial**
bradicardia	bradicardia	**bradycardia**
cervello	cerebro	**brain**
crusca	salvado	**bran**
branchiale	branquial	**branchial**
mammella	mama, pecho	**breast**
autopalpazione mammaria	autoexamen de la mama	**breast self-examination (BSE)**
respiro	aliento	**breath**
natica	nalgas	**breech**
presentazione podalica	presentación de nalgas	**breech-birth presentation**
legamento largo	ligamento ancho	**broad ligament**
area di Broca	área de Broca	**Broca's area**
soluzione di Brompton	mezcla de Brompton	**Brompton's mixture**
bronchi	bronquios	**bronchi**
asma bronchiale	asma bronquial	**bronchial asthma**
bronchiettasia	bronquiectasia	**bronchiectasis**
bronchiolo	bronquiolo	**bronchiole**
bronchiolite	bronquiolitis	**bronchiolitis**
bronchite	bronquitis	**bronchitis**
broncocostrittore	broncoconstrictor	**bronchoconstrictor**
broncodilatatore	broncodilatador	**bronchodilator**
broncopolmonite	bronconeumonia	**bronchopneumonia**
broncopolmonare	broncopulmonar	**bronchopulmonary**
broncoscopio	broncoscopio	**bronchoscope**
broncospasmo	broncospasmo	**bronchospasm**
bronco	bronquio	**bronchus**
arcata soppracciliare, sopracciglio	ceja	**brow**
brucellosi	brucelosis	**brucellosis**
contusione (n)	contusión (n), equimosis (n)	**bruise** (n)
ammaccare (v)	magullar (v), contundir (v)	**bruise** (v)
buccale	bucal	**buccal**
bulbare	bulbar	**bulbar**
bulimia	bulimia	**bulimia**
bolla	bulla	**bulla**
borsite dell'alluce	juanete	**bunion**
ustione (n), scottatura (n)	quemadura (n)	**burn** (n)
bruciare (v)	quemar (v)	**burn** (v)

burnout syndrome	syndrome de 'surmenage'	Helfer-Syndrom
bursa	bourse	Bursa
bursitis	bursite	Bursitis, Schleimbeutelentzündung
buttock	fesse	Gesäßbacke

ITALIAN	SPANISH	ENGLISH
incapacità ad agire, sindrome di esaurimento professionale	surmenage, neurastenia	**burnout syndrome**
borsa	bolsa	**bursa**
borsite	bursitis	**bursitis**
natica	nalga	**buttock**

C

English	French	German
cachexia	cachexie	Kachexie
cadaver	cadavre	Kadaver, Leiche
caecostomy (Eng)	caecostomie	Zökostomie
caecum (Eng)	caecum	Zökum
caesarean section (Eng)	césarienne	Kaiserschnitt, Sectio
caffeine	caféine	Koffein
calcification	calcification	Kalzifikation, Verkalkung
calcium	calcium	Kalzium
calculus	calcul	Stein
Caldwell-Luc operation	opération de Caldwell-Luc	Caldwell-Luc-Operation
calf	mollet	Wade
caliper	armature orthopédique	Schiene
callosity	callosité	Schwiele, Hornhaut
callus	cal	Kallus
calor	chaleur	Fieber, Hitze
caloric test	essai calorique	kalorische Prüfung
calorie	calorie	Kalorie
canal	canal	Kanal, Gang
cancellous	spongieux	spongiös, schwammartig
cancer	cancer	Karzinom, Krebs
candidiasis	candidose	Candidiasis
canine	canin	Hunde-
cannula	canule	Kanüle
capillary	capillaire	Kapillare
capsule	capsule	Kapsel
capsulitis	capsulite	Kapselentzündung
caput succedaneum	caput succedaneum	Geburtsgeschwulst
carbohydrate (CHO)	glucide	Kohlenhydrat, Kohlenwasserstoff
carboxyhaemoglobin (Eng)	carboxyhémoglobine	Carboxyhämoglobin
carboxyhemoglobin (Am)	carboxyhémoglobine	Carboxyhämoglobin
carbuncle	charbon	Karbunkel
carcinogen	carcinogène	Karzinogen
carcinogenesis	carcinogenèse	Karzinogenese
carcinoid syndrome	syndrome carcinoïde	Karzinoid-Syndrom
carcinoma	carcinome	Karzinom, Krebs
carcinomatosis	carcinomatose	Karzinose, Karzinomatose
cardia	cardia	Kardia, Mageneingang
cardiac	cardiaque	Herz-
cardiogenic	cardiogène	kardiogen
cardiology	cardiologie	Kardiologie
cardiomegaly	cardiomégalie	Kardiomegalie
cardiomyopathy	cardiomyopathie	Kardiomyopathie
cardiopulmonary	cardiopulmonaire	kardiopulmonal, Herz-Lungen-
cardiopulmonary resuscitation (CPR)	réanimation cardiorespiratoire	Herz-Lungen-Wiederbelebung, Reanimation

ITALIAN	SPANISH	ENGLISH
cachessia	caquexia	**cachexia**
cadavere	cadáver	**cadaver**
ciecostomia	cecostomía	**caecostomy** (Eng)
intestino cieco	ciego	**caecum** (Eng)
taglio cesareo	cesárea	**caesarean section** (Eng)
caffeina	cafeína	**caffeine**
calcificazione	calcificación	**calcification**
calcio	calcio	**calcium**
calcolo	cálculo	**calculus**
operazione di Caldwell-Luc	operación de Caldwell-Luc	**Caldwell-Luc operation**
polpaccio	pantorrilla	**calf**
compasso per pelvi-craniometria	compás, calibrador	**caliper**
callosità	callosidad	**callosity**
callo	callo	**callus**
calore	calor	**calor**
test calorico	prueba calórica	**caloric test**
caloria	caloría	**calorie**
canale	canal	**canal**
spugnoso, trabecolare	esponjoso, reticulado	**cancellous**
cancro	cáncer	**cancer**
candidiasi	candidiasis	**candidiasis**
canino	canino	**canine**
cannula	cánula	**cannula**
capillare	capilar	**capillary**
capsula	cápsula	**capsule**
capsulite	capsulitis	**capsulitis**
tumore da parto	caput succedaneum	**caput succedaneum**
carboidrato	hidrato de carbono	**carbohydrate (CHO)**
carbossiemoglobina	carboxihemoglobina	**carboxyhaemoglobin** (Eng)
carbossiemoglobina	carboxihemoglobina	**carboxyhemoglobin** (Am)
carbonchio, antrace, favo	ántrax	**carbuncle**
carcinogeno	carcinogénico	**carcinogen**
carcinogenesi	carcinogénesis	**carcinogenesis**
sindrome da carcinoide	síndrome carcinoide	**carcinoid syndrome**
carcinoma	carcinoma	**carcinoma**
carcinomatosi	carcinomatosis	**carcinomatosis**
cardias	cardias	**cardia**
cardiaco	cardíaco	**cardiac**
cardiogeno	cardiógenico	**cardiogenic**
cardiologia	cardiología	**cardiology**
cardiomegalia	cardiomegalia	**cardiomegaly**
cardiomiopatia	cardiomiopatía, miocardiopatía	**cardiomyopathy**
cardiopolmonàre	cardiopulmonar	**cardiopulmonary**
rianimazione cardiorespiratoria	resucitación cardiopulmonar	**cardiopulmonary resuscitation (CPR)**

ENGLISH	FRENCH	GERMAN
cardiorespiratory	cardiorespiratoire	kardiorespiratorisch
cardiospasm	cardiospasme	Kardiospasmus
cardiothoracic	cardiothoracique	kardiothorakal
cardiotocograph	cardiotocographe	Kardiotokograph
cardiotoxic	cardiotoxique	kardiotoxisch, herzschädigend
cardiovascular	cardiovasculaire	kardiovaskulär, Kreislauf-
cardioversion	cardioversion	Kardioversion
caries	carie	Karies
carina	carène	Carina
carminative (n)	carminatif (n)	Karminativum (n)
carminative (a)	carminatif (a)	karminativ (a), entblähend (a)
carotene	carotène	Karotin
carotid	carotide	Karotis-
carpal tunnel syndrome	syndrome du canal carpien	Karpaltunnelsyndrom
carpometacarpal	carpo-métarcarpien	karpometakarpal
carpopedal	carpo-pédal	karpopedal
carrier	porteur	Ausscheider, Trägerstoff
cartilage	cartilage	Knorpel
caruncle	caroncule	Karunkel
cast	plâtre	Abdruck, Gipsverband
castration	castration	Kastration
catabolism	catabolisme	Katabolismus, Abbaustoffwechsel
catalyst	catalyseur	Katalysator
cataract	cataracte	Katarakt, grauer Star
catarrh	catarrhe	Katarrh
catatonic	catatonique	kataton
catgut	catgut	Catgut
catheter	cathéter	Katheter
catheterization	cathétérisme	Katheterisierung
causalgia	causalgie	Kausalgie, brennender Schmerz
cause of death (COD)	cause du décès	Todesursache
caustic (n)	caustique (n)	Ätzmittel (n), Kaustikum (n)
caustic (a)	caustique (a)	ätzend (a), brennend (a)
cauterize	cautériser	kauterisieren, ätzen, brennen
cavernous	caverneux	kavernös
cavity	cavité	Höhle
cecostomy (Am)	caecostomie	Zökostomie
cecum (Am)	caecum	Zökum
celiac (Am)	coeliaque	abdominal
cell	cellule	Zelle
cell membrane	membrane cellulaire	Zellmembran
cellulitis	cellulite	Zellulitis
centigrade	centigrade	Celsiusgrad
central nervous system (CNS)	système nerveux central (CNS)	Zentralnervensystem (ZNS)
central venous pressure (CVP)	tension veineuse centrale	zentraler Venendruck (ZVD)
centrifugal	centrifuge	zentrifugal
centrifuge (n)	centrifugeur (n)	Zentrifuge (n)

ITALIAN	SPANISH	ENGLISH
cardiorespiratorio	cardiorespiratorio	**cardiorespiratory**
spasmo cardiale, acalasia esofagea	cardiospasmo	**cardiospasm**
cardiotoracico	cardiotorácico	**cardiothoracic**
cardiotocografia	tococardiógrafo	**cardiotocograph**
cardiotossico	cardiotóxico	**cardiotoxic**
cardiovascolare	cardiovascular	**cardiovascular**
cardioversione	cardioversión	**cardioversion**
carie	caries	**caries**
carena tracheale	carina	**carina**
carminativo *(n)*	carminativo *(n)*	**carminative** *(n)*
carminativo *(a)*	carminativo *(a)*	**carminative** *(a)*
carotene	carotenos	**carotene**
carotide	carótida	**carotid**
sindrome del tunnel carpale	síndrome del túnel carpiano	**carpal tunnel syndrome**
carpometacarpale	carpometacarpiano	**carpometacarpal**
carpopedalico	carpopedal	**carpopedal**
portatore	portador	**carrier**
cartilagine	cartílago	**cartilage**
caruncola	carúncula	**caruncle**
ingessatura, steccatura	enyesado, vendaje de yeso	**cast**
castrazione	castración	**castration**
catabolismo	catabolismo	**catabolism**
catalizzatore	catalizador	**catalyst**
cataratta	catarata	**cataract**
catarro	catarro	**catarrh**
catatonico	catatónico	**catatonic**
catgut	catgut	**catgut**
catetere	catéter	**catheter**
cateterizzazione	cateterismo	**catheterization**
causalgia	causalgia	**causalgia**
causa di morte	causa de la muerte	**cause of death (COD)**
caustico *(n)*	cáustico *(n)*	**caustic** *(n)*
caustico *(a)*	cáustico *(a)*	**caustic** *(a)*
cauterizzare	cauterizar	**cauterize**
cavernoso	cavernoso	**cavernous**
cavità	cavidad	**cavity**
ciecostomia	cecostomía	**cecostomy** (Am)
intestino cieco	ciego	**cecum** (Am)
celiaco	celiaco	**celiac** (Am)
cellula	célula	**cell**
membrana cellulare	membrana celular	**cell membrane**
cellulite	celulitis	**cellulitis**
centigrado	centígrado	**centigrade**
sistema nervoso centrale	sistema nervioso central (SNC)	**central nervous system (CNS)**
pressione venosa centrale	presión venosa central (PVC)	**central venous pressure (CVP)**
centrifugo	centrífugo	**centrifugal**
centrifuga *(n)*	centrífugo *(n)*	**centrifuge** *(n)*

ENGLISH	FRENCH	GERMAN
centrifuge *(v)*	centrifuger *(v)*	zentrifugieren *(v)*
centripetal	centripète	zentripetal
cephalhaematoma (Eng)	céphalhématome	Kephalhämatom
cephalhematoma (Am)	céphalhématome	Kephalhämatom
cephalic	céphalique	Kopf-, Schädel-
cephalometry	céphalométrie	Kephalometrie, Schädelmessung
cerebellum	cervelet	Cerebellum, Kleinhirn
cerebral	cérébral	zerebral, Gehirn-
cerebral palsy	infirmité motrice cérébrale	Zerebralparese
cerebrospinal	cérébrospinal	zerebrospinal
cerebrospinal fluid (CSF)	liquide céphalo-rachidien	Liquor
cerebrovascular	cérébrovasculaire	zerebrovaskulär
cerebrovascular accident (CVA)	accident cérébrovasculaire	Schlaganfall, Apoplex
cerebrum	cerveau	Gehirn, Großhirn
cervical	cervical	zervikal
cervical intraepithelial neoplasia (CIN)	néoplasie intra-épithéliale cervicale	zervikale intraepitheliale Neoplasie (CIN)
cervix	cou	Zervix, Gebärmutterhals
cesarean section (Am)	césarienne	Kaiserschnitt, Sectio
chalazion	chalazion	Chalazion, Hagelkorn
chancre	chancre	Schanker
character	caractère	Charakter, Merkmal
charcoal	charbon	Holzkohle
Charcot's joint	arthropathie neurogène	Charcot-Gelenk
cheek	joue	Wange, Backe
cheilosis	chéilose	Mundeckenschrunden
chelating agent	agent chélateur	Chelatbildner
chemoprophylaxis	chimioprophylaxie	Chemoprophylaxe
chemoreceptor	chimiorécepteur	Chemorezeptor
chemosis	chémosis	Chemosis
chemotaxis	chimiotaxie	Chemotaxis
chemotherapy	chimiothérapie	Chemotherapie
Cheyne-Stokes respiration	dyspnée de Cheyne-Stokes	Cheyne-Stokes-Atmung
chiasma	chiasma	Chiasma
chickenpox	varicelle	Varizellen, Windpocken
chilblain	engelure	Frostbeule, Pernio
child abuse	sévices infligés aux enfants, martyre d'enfants	Kindesmißhandlung
chin	menton	Kinn
chiropodist	pédicure	Fußpfleger
chiropody	chiropodie	Pediküre, Fußpflege
chiropractic	chiropractique	Chiropraktik
chiropractor	chiropracteur	Chiropraktiker
chloasma	chloasma	Chloasma, Hyperpigmentierung
chocolate cyst	kyste chocolat	Schokoladenzyste, Teerzyste
cholangiography	cholangiographie	Cholangiographie

ITALIAN	SPANISH	ENGLISH
centrifugare *(v)*	centrifugar *(v)*	**centrifuge** *(v)*
centripeto	centrípeto	**centripetal**
cefaloematoma	hematoma cefálico	**cephalhaematoma** (Eng)
cefaloematoma	hematoma cefálico	**cephalhematoma** (Am)
cefalico	cefálico	**cephalic**
cefalometria	cefalometría	**cephalometry**
cervelletto	cerebelo	**cerebellum**
cerebrale	cerebral	**cerebral**
paralisi cerebrale	parálisis cerebral	**cerebral palsy**
cerebrospinale	cerebroespinal	**cerebrospinal**
liquido cerebrospinale (LCS)	liquido cefalorraquídeo (LCR)	**cerebrospinal fluid (CSF)**
cerebrovascolare	cerebrovascular	**cerebrovascular**
ictus, accidente cerebrovascolare (ACV)	accidente vascular cerebral (ACV)	**cerebrovascular accident (CVA)**
cervello	cerebro	**cerebrum**
cervicale	cervical	**cervical**
neoplasia intraepiteliale della cervice uterina (CIN)	neoplasia intraepitelial cervical	**cervical intracpithelial neoplasia (CIN)**
cervice	cuello uterino	**cervix**
taglio cesareo	cesárea	**cesarean section** (Am)
calazion	chalacio, orzuelo	**chalazion**
cancroide, ulcera venerea	chancro	**chancre**
carattere	carácter	**character**
carbone vegetale	carbón vegetal	**charcoal**
artropatia di Charcot	articulación de Charcot	**Charcot's joint**
guancia	mejilla	**cheek**
cheilosi	queilosis	**cheilosis**
agente chelante	quelantes	**chelating agent**
chemioprofilassi	quimioprofilaxis	**chemoprophylaxis**
chemorecettore	quimiorreceptor	**chemoreceptor**
chemosi	quemosis	**chemosis**
chemiotassi	quimiotaxis	**chemotaxis**
chemioterapia	quimioterapia	**chemotherapy**
respiro di Cheyne-Stokes	respiración de Cheyne-Stokes	**Cheyne-Stokes respiration**
chiasma	quiasma	**chiasma**
varicella	varicela	**chickenpox**
gelone	sabañón	**chilblain**
maltrattamento a bambini	abuso de menores	**child abuse**
mento	barbilla	**chin**
callista	callista, podólogo	**chiropodist**
chiropodia	podología	**chiropody**
chiropratica	quiropráctica	**chiropractic**
chiropratico	quiropractor	**chiropractor**
cloasma	cloasma	**chloasma**
cisti cioccolato (c. emosiderinica dell'endometriosi)	quiste de chocolate	**chocolate cyst**
colangiografia	colangiografía	**cholangiography**

ENGLISH	FRENCH	GERMAN
cholangitis	cholangite	Cholangitis
cholecystectomy	cholécystectomie	Cholezystektomie
cholecystitis	cholécystite	Cholezystitis
cholecystography	cholécystographie	Cholezystographie
choledochography	cholédochographie	Choledochographie
choledocholithiasis	cholédocholithiase	Choledocholithiasis
cholelithiasis	cholélithiase	Cholelithiasis, Gallensteinleiden
cholera	choléra	Cholera
cholestasis	cholestase	Cholestase, Gallenstauung
cholesteatoma	cholestéatome	Cholesteatom
cholesterol (chol)	cholestérol	Cholesterin
cholinergic	cholinergique	cholinergisch
chondritis	chondrite	Chondritis
chondroma	chondrome	Chondrom
chondromalacia	chondromalacie	Chondromalazie
chorea	chorée	Chorea, Veitstanz
chorion	chorion	Chorion
chorionic villi	villosités du chorion	Chorionzotten
chorionic villus biopsy	biopsie du villus chorionique	Chorionzottenbiopsie
choroid	choroïde	Choroidea, Aderhaut
choroiditis	choroïdite	Choroiditis
chromatography	chromatographie	Chromatographie
chromosome	chromosome	Chromosom
chronic	chronique	chronisch
chronic brain syndrome (CBS)	syndrome chronique du cerveau	chronisches Gehirnsyndrom
chronic coronary insufficiency (CCI)	insuffisance coronarienne chronique	chronische Koronarinsuffizienz
chronic obstructive airway disease (COAD)	bronchopneumopathie chronique obstructive, syndrome respiratoire	chronische obstruktive Lungenerkrankung
Chvostek's sign	signe de Chvostek	Chvostek-Zeichen
chyle	chyle	Chylus
cilia	cils	Zilien, Wimpern
ciliary	ciliaire	ziliar, Wimpern-
circinate	circinal	kreisförmig
circulation	circulation	Kreislauf, Zirkulation, Durchblutung
circumcision	circoncision	Zirkumzision, Beschneidung
circumoral	péribuccal	zirkumoral
cirrhosis	cirrhose	Zirrhose
claudication	claudication	Hinken, Claudicatio
claustrophobia	claustrophobie	Klaustrophobie
clavicle	clavicule	Schlüsselbein
cleft palate	fente palatine	Gaumenspalte
climacteric	climatérique	Klimakterium, Wechseljahre
clinical	clinique	klinisch
clitoris	clitoris	Klitoris
clone	clone	Klonus
clonus	clonus	Klonus
clot (n)	caillot (n)	Blutgerinnsel (n), Koagel (n)

ITALIAN	SPANISH	ENGLISH
colangite	colangitis	**cholangitis**
colecistectomia	colecistectomía	**cholecystectomy**
colecistite	colecistitis	**cholecystitis**
colecistografia	colecistografía	**cholecystography**
coledocografia	coledocografía	**choledochography**
coledocolitiasi	coledocolitiasis	**choledocholithiasis**
colelitiasi	colelitiasis	**cholelithiasis**
colera	cólera	**cholera**
colestasi	colestasis	**cholestasis**
colesteatoma	colesteatoma	**cholesteatoma**
colesterolo	colesterol	**cholesterol (chol)**
colinergico	colinérgico	**cholinergic**
condrite	condritis	**chondritis**
condroma	condroma	**chondroma**
condromalacia	condromalacia	**chondromalacia**
corea	corea	**chorea**
corion	corion	**chorion**
villi coriali	vellosidades coriónicas	**chorionic villi**
biopsia dei villi coriali	biopsia de las vellosidades coriónicas	**chorionic villus biopsy**
coroide	coroides	**choroid**
coroidite	coroiditis	**choroiditis**
cromatografia	cromatografía	**chromatography**
cromosoma	cromosoma	**chromosome**
cronico	crónico	**chronic**
sindrome cerebrale cronica	síndrome cerebral crónico	**chronic brain syndrome (CBS)**
insufficienza coronarica cronica	insuficiencia coronaria crónico	**chronic coronary insufficiency (CCI)**
malattia ostruttiva cronica delle vie respiratorie	enfermedad obstructiva crónica de las vias respiratorias	**chronic obstructive airway disease (COAD)**
segno di Chvostek	signo de Chvostek	**Chvostek's sign**
chilo	quilo	**chyle**
ciglia	cilios	**cilia**
ciliare	ciliar	**ciliary**
circinato	circinado	**circinate**
circolazione	circulación	**circulation**
circoncisione	circuncisión	**circumcision**
circumorale	circumoral, peroral	**circumoral**
cirrosi	cirrosis	**cirrhosis**
claudicazione	claudicación	**claudication**
claustrofobia	claustrofobia	**claustrophobia**
clavicola	clavícula	**clavicle**
palatoschisi	paladar hendido	**cleft palate**
climaterio	climatérico	**climacteric**
clinico	clínico	**clinical**
clitoride	clítoris	**clitoris**
clone	clono	**clone**
clono	clono, clonus	**clonus**
coagulo *(n)*	coágulo *(n)*	**clot** *(n)*

ENGLISH	FRENCH	GERMAN
clot (v)	coaguler (v)	gerinnen (v), koagulieren (v)
clubbing	hippocratisme digital	Trommelschlegelfinger
club-foot	pied bot	Klumpfuß
coalesce	se combiner	zusammenwachsen
coal tar	coaltar	Steinkohlenteer
coarctation	coarctation	Coarctatio
coccyx	coccyx	Steißbein
cochlea	limaçon osseux	Cochlea, Schnecke
coeliac (Eng)	coeliaque	abdominal
cognition	cognition	Erkennungsvermögen, Wahrnehmung
coitus	coït	Koitus, Geschlechtsverkehr
cold (n)	rhume (n)	Kälte (n), Erkältung (n)
cold (a)	froid (a)	kalt (a)
cold abscess	abcès froid	kalter Abszeß
cold sore	herpès	Herpes
colectomy	colectomie	Kolektomie, Kolonresektion
colic	colique	Kolik
coliform	coliforme	coliform
colitis	colite	Kolitis
collagen	collagène	Kollagen
collapse (n)	affaissement (n)	Kollaps (n)
collapse (v)	s'affaisser (v)	kollabieren (v)
collateral circulation	circulation collatérale	Kollateralkreislauf
Colles' fracture	fracture de Pouteau-Colles	distale Radiusfraktur
colloid	colloïde	Kolloid
coloboma	colobome, coloboma	Kolobom
colon	côlon	Kolon
colonize	coloniser	kolonisieren
colonoscopy	coloscopie	Koloskopie
color blindness (Am)	daltonisme	Farbenblindheit
colorectal	colorectal	kolorektal
colostomy	colostomie	Kolostomie
colostrum	colostrum	Kolostrum, Vormilch
colour blindness (Eng)	daltonisme	Farbenblindheit
colporrhaphy	colporraphie	Kolporrhaphie
colposcope	colposcope	Kolposkop
coma	coma	Koma
comatose	comateux	komatös
combined oral contraceptive	contraceptif oral combiné	orales Kontrazeptivum (Kombinationspräparat)
comminuted fracture	fracture esquilleuse	Splitterbruch
commissure	commissure	Kommissur
compatibility	compatibilité	Kompatibilität, Verträglichkeit
compensation	compensation	Kompensation, Entschädigung
complement	complément	Komplement
complementary medicine	traitement complémentaire	komplementäre Medizin
complete blood count (CBC)	numération globulaire	großes Blutbild

ITALIAN	SPANISH	ENGLISH
coagulare (v)	coagular (v)	clot (v)
dita a clava, ippocratismo	dedos en palillo de tambor, dedos hipocráticos	clubbing
piede torto	pie zambo	club-foot
aggregarsi	coalescer	coalesce
catrame	alquitrán, brea	coal tar
coartazione	coartación	coarctation
coccige	cóccix	coccyx
coclea	cóclea	cochlea
celiaco	celíaco	coeliac (Eng)
cognizione	cognición	cognition
coito	coito	coitus
raffreddore (n)	resfriado (n)	cold (n)
freddo (a)	frío (a)	cold (a)
ascesso freddo	absceso frío	cold abscess
herpes, labialis	herpes labial	cold sore
colectomia	colectomía	colectomy
colica	cólico	colic
coliforme	coliforme	coliform
colite	colitis	colitis
collageno	colágeno	collagen
collasso (n)	colapso (n)	collapse (n)
collassarsi (v), crollare (v)	colapsar (v)	collapse (v)
circolazione collaterale	circulación colateral	collateral circulation
frattura di Colles	fractura de Colles	Colles' fracture
colloide	coloide	colloid
coloboma	coloboma	coloboma
colon	colon	colon
colonizzare	colonizar	colonize
colonscopia	colonoscopia	colonoscopy
cecità ai colori, acromatopsia	daltonismo, ceguera de colores	color blindness (Am)
colorettale	colorrectal	colorectal
colostomia	colostomía	colostomy
colostro	calostro	colostrum
cecità ai colori, acromatopsia	daltonismo, ceguera de colores	colour blindness (Eng)
colporrafia	colporrafia	colporrhaphy
colposcopio	colposcopio	colposcope
coma	coma	coma
comatoso	comatoso	comatose
contraccettivo orale estro-progestinico	anticonceptivo oral combinado	combined oral contraceptive
frattura comminuta	fractura conminuta	comminuted fracture
commessura	comisura	commissure
compatibilità	compatibilidad	compatibility
compenso	compensación	compensation
complemento	complemento	complement
medicina complementare	medicina complementaria	complementary medicine
esame emocromocitometrico	hemograma completo	complete blood count (CBC)

ENGLISH	FRENCH	GERMAN
compos mentis	compos mentis	zurechnungsfähig
compound	composé	Verbindung, Zusammensetzung
compression	compression	Kompression
compulsion	compulsion	Zwang
computerized axial tomography (CAT)	tacographie	axiale Computertomographie
computerized tomography	tomographie avec ordinateur, scanographie	Computertomographie (CT)
conception	conception	Empfängnis
concussion	commotion	Erschütterung, Commotio
conditioned reflex	réflexe conditionné	bedingter Reflex, konditionierter Reflex
condom	préservatif	Kondom, Präservativ
confusion	confusion	Verwirrung
congenital	congénital	angeboren
congestion	congestion	Stauung
congestive cardiac failure (CCF)	insuffisance cardiaque globale	Stauungsherz, Herzinsuffizienz mit Stauungszeichen
congestive heart failure (CHF)	insuffisance cardiaque globale	Stauungsherz, Herzinsuffizienz mit Stauungszeichen
conjugate (n)	diamètre conjugué (n)	Beckendurchmesser (n)
conjugate (a)	conjugué (a)	konjugiert (a)
conjunctiva	conjonctive	Konjunktiva, Bindehaut
conjunctivitis	conjonctivite	Konjunktivitis, Bindehautentzündung
conscious	conscient	bewußt, bei Bewußtsein
consolidation	consolidation	Konsolidierung, Festigung
constipation	constipation	Verstopfung
constriction	constriction	Konstriktion, Einengung
consumption	consommation	Konsum, Verbrauch
contact	contact	Kontakt, Berührung
contact lens	verre de contact	Kontaktlinse
contagious	contagieux	kontagiös, ansteckend
continuous positive airway pressure (CPAP)	ventilation spontanée en pression positive continue	kontinuierlich positiver Atemwegsdruck
contraceptive (n)	contraceptif (n)	Kontrazeptivum (n), Verhütungsmittel (n)
contraceptive (a)	contraceptif (a)	kontrazeptiv (a), Verhütungs- (a)
contraction	contraction	Kontraktion
contracture	contracture	Kontraktur
contraindication	contre-indication	Kontraindikation, Gegenanzeige
contralateral	controlatéral	kontralateral
contrecoup	contrecoup	contre coup
controlled drug	médicament contrôlé	Betäubungsmittel (gemäß BTM)
convulsion	convulsion	Krampf, Zuckung, Konvulsion
cord	cordon	Strang, Schnur, Ligament
cordotomy	cordotomie	Stimmbandresektion
corn	cor	Klavus, Hühnerauge
cornea	cornée	Kornea, Hornhaut (des Auges)
corneal graft	greffe de la cornée	Korneaplastik

ITALIAN	SPANISH	ENGLISH
mentalmente sano	compos mentis, de espíritu sano	compos mentis
composto	compuesto	compound
compressione	compresión	compression
compulsione	compulsión, apremio	compulsion
tomografia assiale computerizzata (TAC)	tomografía axial computerizada (TAC)	computerized axial tomography (CAT)
tomografia computerizzata	tomografía computerizada	computerized tomography
concepimento	concepción	conception
commozione	concusión, contusión violenta	concussion
riflesso condizionato	reflejo condicionado	conditioned reflex
profilattico maschile	condón	condom
confusione	confusión	confusion
congenito	congénito	congenital
congestione	congestión	congestion
insufficienza cardiaca congestizia	insuficiencia cardíaca congestiva (ICC)	congestive cardiac failure (CCF)
scompenso cardiaco congestizio	insuficiencia cardíaca congestiva (ICC)	congestive heart failure (CHF)
coniugata (n)	conjugado (n)	conjugate (n)
coniugato (a)	conjugado (a)	conjugate (a)
congiuntiva	conjuntiva	conjunctiva
congiuntivite	conjuntivitis	conjunctivitis
conscio	consciente	conscious
solidificazione, addensamento	consolidación	consolidation
stipsi	estreñimiento	constipation
costrizione	constricción	constriction
consunzione	consunción, tisis	consumption
contatto	contacto	contact
lente a contatto	lente de contacto	contact lens
contagioso	contagioso, trasmisible	contagious
pressione continua positiva delle vie aeree	presión continua positiva de las vías respiratorias	continuous positive airway pressure (CPAP)
anticoncezionale (n)	anticonceptivo (n)	contraceptive (n)
anticoncezionale (a)	anticonceptivo (a)	contraceptive (a)
contrazione	contracción	contraction
contrattura	contractura	contracture
controindicazione	contraindicación	contraindication
controlaterale	contralateral	contralateral
contraccolpo	contragolpe	contrecoup
farmaco sottoposto a controllo	fármaco controlado	controlled drug
convulsione	convulsión	convulsion
corda, cordone, notocorda	cordón, cuerda, médula espinal	cord
cordotomia	cordotomía	cordotomy
callo	callo, papiloma	corn
cornea	córnea	cornea
trapianto corneale	injerto corneal	corneal graft

ENGLISH	FRENCH	GERMAN
coronary (n)	coronaire (n)	Koronararterie (n)
coronary (a)	coronaire (a), coronarien (a)	koronar (a)
coronary artery disease (CAD)	coronaropathie, cardiopathie ischémique, insuffisance coronarienne globale	Koronaropathie
coronary care unit (CCU)	unité de soins intensifs coronaires	Infarktpflegestation
coronary heart disease (CHD)	insuffisance coronarienne cardiaque	koronare Herzkrankheit (KHK)
coronary heart failure (CHF)	insuffisance coronarienne cardiaque	Herzinfarkt
coroner	médecin légiste	Leichenbeschauer
corpse	cadavre	Leiche, Toter
cor pulmonale	coeur pulmonaire	Cor pulmonale
corpus	corps	Corpus
corpuscle	corpuscule	Corpusculum
cortex	cortex	Cortex, Rinde
corticosteroid	corticostéroïde	Kortikosteroide
coryza	coryza	Koryza, Schnupfen
costal	costal	kostal, Rippen-
costochondral	costochondral	Rippenknorpel-
costochondritis	costochondrite	Tietze Syndrom
cot death	mort subite de nourrisson	plötzlicher Säuglingstod
cough (n)	toux (n)	Husten (n)
cough (v)	tousser (v)	husten (v)
counselling	consultation	Beratung
Coxsackie virus	virus Coxsackie	Coxsackie-Virus
cradle cap	casque séborrhéique	Milchschorf
cramp	crampe	Krampf
cranial nerve	nerf crânien	Hirnnerv
cranio-synostosis	craniosynostose	Kraniosynostose
cranium	boîte crânienne	Schädel, Kranium
C-reactive protein (CRP)	test de protéine C-réactive	C-reaktives Protein (CRP)
creatine	créatine	Kreatin
creatinine	créatinine	Kreatinin
crepitation	crépitation	Krepitation, Rasseln
cretinism	crétinisme	Kretinismus
cricoid	cricoïde	krikoid
crisis	crise	Krise
Crohn's disease	mal de Crohn	Morbus Crohn
croup	croup	Krupp
cryosurgery	cryochirurgie	Kryochirurgie
cryotherapy	cryothérapie	Kryotherapie
crypt	crypte	Krypte
cryptogenic	cryptogène	kryptogenetisch, unbekannten Ursprungs
cryptomenorrhea (Am)	cryptoménorrhée	Kryptomenorrhoe
cryptomenorrhoea (Eng)	cryptoménorrhée	Kryptomenorrhoe

ITALIAN	SPANISH	ENGLISH
coronaria (n)	coronario (n)	coronary (n)
coronarico (a)	coronario (a)	coronary (a)
malattia delle arterie coronarica (MAC)	enfermadad arterial coronaria, cardiopatía isquémica	coronary artery disease (CAD)
reparto coronarico	unidad de cuidados coronarios (UCC)	coronary care unit (CCU)
malattia cardiaca coronarica (MCC)	enfermedad coronaria, cardiopatía isquémica	coronary heart disease (CHD)
insufficienza cardiaca coronarica	insuficiencia coronaria	coronary heart failure (CHF)
medico legale	médico forense	coroner
cadavere	cadáver	corpse
cuore polmonare	cor pulmonale	cor pulmonale
corpo	cuerpo	corpus
corpuscolo	corpúsculo	corpuscle
corteccia	corteza	cortex
corticosteroide	corticosteroide	corticosteroid
coriza	coriza	coryza
costale	costal	costal
costocondrale	costocondral	costochondral
costocondrite	costocondritis	costochondritis
sindrome da morte improvvisa del lattante	muerte en la cuna, muerte súbita infantil	cot death
tosse (n)	tos (n)	cough (n)
tossire (v)	toser (v)	cough (v)
consulenza eugenetica	ascsoramiento, consejo, consulta psicológica	counselling
virus Coxsackie	virus Coxsackie	Coxsackie virus
stecca, rima di frattura	costra láctea, dermatitis del cuero cabelludo	cradle cap
crampo	calambre, espasmo	cramp
nervo craniale	nervio craneal	cranial nerve
craniosinostosi	craneosinostosis	cranio-synostosis
cranio	cráneo	cranium
proteina C reattiva	proteína C-reactiva	C-reactive protein (CRP)
creatina	creatina	creatine
creatinina	creatinina	creatinine
crepitazione	crepitación	crepitation
cretinismo	cretinismo	cretinism
cricoide	cricoideo	cricoid
crisi	crisis	crisis
malattia di Crohn	enfermedad de Crohn	Crohn's disease
ostruzione laringea	garrotillo, crup, difteria laríngea	croup
criochirurgia	criocirugía	cryosurgery
crioterapia	crioterapia	cryotherapy
cripta	cripta	crypt
criptogenico	criptogénico	cryptogenic
criptomenorrea	criptomenorrea	cryptomenorrhea (Am)
criptomenorrea	criptomenorrea	cryptomenorrhoea (Eng)

cubital vein	veine de l'avant-bras	Unterarmvene
culture	culture	Bakterienkultur, Kultur
curet (Am) *(n)*	curette *(n)*	Kürette *(n)*
curet (Am) *(v)*	cureter *(v)*	kürettieren *(v)*
curettage	curetage	Kürettage, Ausschabung
curette (Eng) *(n)*	curette *(n)*	Kürette *(n)*
curette (Eng) *(v)*	cureter *(v)*	kürettieren *(v)*
curetting	curetages	Kürettage, Ausschabung
Cushing's syndrome	syndrome de Cushing	Cushing-Syndrom
cutaneous	cutané	kutan, Haut-
cuticle	cuticule	Cuticula, Häutchen
cyanosis	cyanose	Zyanose
cycle	cycle	Zyklus
cyclical vomiting	vomissement cyclique	zyklisches Erbrechen
cyesis	grossesse	Schwangerschaft
cyst	kyste	Zyste
cystectomy	cystectomie	Zystektomie, Zystenentfernung
cystic fibrosis (CF)	fibrose cystique	Mukoviszidose
cystitis	cystite	Zystitis, Blasenentzündung
cystocele	cystocèle	Zystozele
cystometry	cystométrie	Zystometrie, Blasendruckmessung
cystopexy	cystopexie	Zystopexie
cystoscope	cystoscope	Zystoskop, Blasenspiegel
cystoscopy	cystoscopie	Zystoskopie, Blasenspiegelung
cytology	cytologie	Zytologie
cytomegalovirus (CMV)	cytomégalovirus	Zytomegalie-Virus (CMV)
cytotoxic	cytotoxique	zytotoxisch, zellschädigend

vena cubitale	vena cubital	**cubital vein**
coltura	cultivo	**culture**
curette *(n)*, cucchiaio chirurgico *(n)*	cureta, cucharilla de legrado *(n)*	**curet** (Am) *(n)*
raschiare *(v)*, scarificare *(v)*	legrar *(v)*	**curet** (Am) *(v)*
curettage, raschiamento	raspado, legrado, curetaje	**curettage**
curette *(n)*, cucchiaio chirurgico *(n)*	cureta, cucharilla de legrado *(n)*	**curette** (Eng) *(n)*
raschiare *(v)*, scarificare *(v)*	legrar *(v)*	**curette** (Eng) *(v)*
curettage, raschiamento	raspados, material de legrado	**curetting**
sindrome di Cushing	síndrome de Cushing	**Cushing's syndrome**
cutaneo	cutáneo	**cutaneous**
cuticola	cutícula	**cuticle**
cianosi	cianosis	**cyanosis**
ciclo	ciclo	**cycle**
vomito ciclico	vómito cíclico	**cyclical vomiting**
gravidanza	ciesis, embarazo	**cyesis**
cisti	quiste	**cyst**
cistectomia	quistectomía	**cystectomy**
mucoviscidosi, malattia fibrocistica del pancreas	fibrosis quística	**cystic fibrosis (CF)**
cistite	cistitis	**cystitis**
cistocele	cistocele	**cystocele**
cistometria	cistometría	**cystometry**
cistopessia	cistopexia	**cystopexy**
cistoscopio	citoscopio	**cystoscope**
cistoscopia	citoscopía	**cystoscopy**
citologia	citología	**cytology**
citomegalovirus	citomegalovirus	**cytomegalovirus (CMV)**
citotossico	citotóxico	**cytotoxic**

43

D

ENGLISH	FRENCH	GERMAN
dacryocystitis	dacryocystite	Dakryozystitis
dandruff	pellicules	Schuppen
date of birth (DOB)	date de naissance	Geburtsdatum
date of conception (DOC)	date du rapport fécondant	Empfängnisdatum
day hospital	hôpital de jour	Tagesklinik
dead	mort	tot
dead on arrival (DOA)	mort à l'arrivée	tot bei Einlieferung
deaf	sourd	taub, schwerhörig
deafness	surdité	Taubheit, Schwerhörigkeit
death	mort	Tod, Todesfall
debility	débilité	Schwäche
debridement	débridement	Debridement, Wundtoilette
decerebrate	décérébré	dezerebriert
decidua	caduque	Dezidua
decompensation	décompensation	Dekompensation, Insuffizienz
decompression	décompression	Dekompression, Drucksenkung
decongestant	décongestionnant	Dekongestionsmittel
deep vein thrombosis (DVT)	thrombose veineuse profonde (TVP)	tiefe Venenthrombose
defaecation (Eng)	défécation	Defäkation, Darmentleerung
defecation (Am)	défécation	Defäkation, Darmentleerung
defect	anomalie, défaut	Defekt, Mangel, Störung
defibrillation	défibrillation	Defibrillierung
defibrillator	défibrillateur	Defibrillator
degeneration	dégénération	Degeneration, Verfall
dehiscence	déhiscence	Dehiszenz, Schlitz
dehydration	déshydratation	Dehydration, Flüssigkeitsmangel
delirium	délire	Delirium, Fieberwahn
delivery	livraison, accouchement	Entbindung, Geburt
deltoid	deltoïde	Deltoides, Deltamuskel
delusion	hallucination	Wahn, Wahnvorstellung
demarcation	démarcation	Demarkation
dementia	démence	Demenz
demography	démographie	Demographie
demyelination	démyélinisation	Demyelinisierung, Entmarkung
dendritic ulcer	ulcère dendritique	verzweigtes Geschwür
denervation	énervation	Denervierung
dengue	dengue	Denguefieber
dentist	dentiste	Zahnarzt
dentistry	médecine dentaire, dentisterie	Zahnheilkunde, Zahntechnik
dentition	dentition	Dentition, Zahnung
denture	dentier	Gebiß
deodorant (n)	déodorant (n)	Deodorant (n)
deodorant (a)	déodorant (a)	desodorierend (a)
deoxygenation	désoxygénation	Desoxydation, Sauerstoffentzug

ITALIAN	SPANISH	ENGLISH
dacriocistite	dacriocistitis	dacryocystitis
forfora	caspa	dandruff
data di nascita	fecha de nacimiento	date of birth (DOB)
data del concepimento	fecha de concepción	date of conception (DOC)
ospedale diurno	hospital de día	day hospital
morto	muerto	dead
deceduto all'arrivo in ospedale	muerto al llegar	dead on arrival (DOA)
sordo	sordo	deaf
sordità	sordera	deafness
morte	muerte	death
debilità	debilidad	debility
sbrigliamento	desbridamiento	debridement
decerebrato	descerebrado	decerebrate
decidua	decidua	decidua
decompensazione	descompensación	decompensation
decompressione	descompresión	decompression
decongestionante	descongestivo	decongestant
trombosi venosa profonda (TVP)	trombosis venosa profunda	deep vein thrombosis (DVT)
defecazione	defecación	defaecation (Eng)
defecazione	defecación	defecation (Am)
difetto	defecto	defect
defibrillazione	desfibrilación	defibrillation
defibrillatore	desfibrilador	defibrillator
degenerazione	degeneración	degeneration
deiscenza	dehiscencia	dehiscence
deidratazione	deshidratación	dehydration
delirio	delirio	delirium
parto	parto	delivery
deltoide	deltoides	deltoid
allucinazione, fissazione	idea delusiva, delirio	delusion
demarcazione	demarcación	demarcation
demenza	demencia	dementia
demografia	demografia	demography
demielinizzazione	desmielinización	demyelination
ulcera dendritica	úlcera dendrítica	dendritic ulcer
denervazione	denervación	denervation
dengue, infezione da Flavivirus ('febbre rompiossa')	dengue	dengue
dentista	dentista	dentist
odontolatria	odontologia	dentistry
dentizione	dentición	dentition
dentiera	dentadura	denture
deodorante (n)	desodorante (n)	deodorant (n)
deodorante (a)	desodorante (a)	deodorant (a)
deossigenazione	desoxigenación	deoxygenation

deoxyribonucleic acid (DNA)	acide désoxyribonucléique (ADN)	Desoxyribonukleinsäure (DNS)
depressed fracture	enfoncement localisé	Impressionsfraktur
depression	dépression	Depression
derealization	déréalisation	Derealisation
dermatitis	dermatite	Dermatitis
dermatologist	dermatologue	Dermatologe
dermatology	dermatologie	Dermatologie
dermatome	dermatome	Dermatom, Hautmesser
dermatomyositis	dermatomyosite	Dermatomyositis
dermatosis	dermatose	Dermatose, Hauterkrankung
dermis	derme	Haut
dermoid	dermoïde	Dermoid, Dermoidzyste
descending colon	côlon descendant	Colon descendens
desensitization	désensibilisation	Desensibilisierung
desloughing	curetage	Schorfabtragung
desquamation	desquamation	Desquamation, Schuppung
detached retina	rétine décollée	abgelöste Netzhaut
detergent	détergent	Reinigungsmittel
deterioration	détérioration	Verschlechterung
dextrocardia	dextrocardie	Dextrokardie
diabetes	diabète	Diabetes
diabetes insipidus	diabète insipide	Diabetes insipidus
diabetes mellitus (DM)	diabète sucré	Diabetes mellitus, Zuckerkrankheit
diagnosis	diagnostic	Diagnose
diagnostic	diagnostique	diagnostisch
dialysate	dialysat	Dialysat
dialyser (Eng)	dialyseur	Dialysator
dialysis	dialyse	Dialyse
dialyzer (Am)	dialyseur	Dialysator
diaper rash (Am)	érythème fessier du nourrisson, érythème papulo-érosif	Windeldermatitis
diaphoresis	diaphorèse	Diaphorese, Schweißabsonderung
diaphragm	diaphragme	Diaphragma, Zwerchfell
diaphysis	diaphyse	Diaphyse, Knochenschaft
diarrhea (Am)	diarrhée	Diarrhoe, Durchfall
diarrhea and vomiting (D & V) (Am)	diarrhées et vomissements	Brechdurchfall
diarrhoea (Eng)	diarrhée	Diarrhoe, Durchfall
diarrhoea and vomiting (D & V) (Eng)	diarrhées et vomissements	Brechdurchfall
diastasis	diastasis	Diastase
diastole	diastole	Diastole
diathermy	diathermie	Diathermie
diet	régime	Ernährung, Diät
dietary fiber (Am)	fibre alimentaire	Ballaststoff
dietary fibre (Eng)	fibre alimentaire	Ballaststoff
dietetics	diététique	Diätlehre, Ernährungskunde
dietitian	diététicien	Diätspezialist

ITALIAN	SPANISH	ENGLISH
acido deossiribonucleico	ácido desoxirribonucléico (ADN)	deoxyribonucleic acid (DNA)
frattura con infossamento dei frammenti	fractura con hundimiento	depressed fracture
depressione	depresión	depression
derealizzazione	desrealización	derealization
dermatite	dermatitis	dermatitis
dermatologo	dermatólogo	dermatologist
dermatologia	dermatología	dermatology
dermatomo	dermátomo	dermatome
dermatomiosite	dermatomiositis	dermatomyositis
dermatosi	dermatosis	dermatosis
derma	dermis	dermis
dermoide	dermoide	dermoid
colon discendente	colon descendente	descending colon
desensibilizzazione	desensibilización	desensitization
rimozione di escara da una ferita	desesfacelación	desloughing
desquamazione	desescamación	desquamation
distacco di retina	desprendimiento de retina	detached retina
detergente	detergente	detergent
deterioramento	deterioro	deterioration
destrocardia	dextrocardia	dextrocardia
diabete	diabetes	diabetes
diabete insipido	diabetes insípida	diabetes insipidus
diabete mellito	diabetes mellitus	diabetes mellitus (DM)
diagnosi	diagnóstico	diagnosis
diagnostico	diagnóstico	diagnostic
dialisato	dializado	dialysate
dializzatore	dializador	dialyser (Eng)
dialisi	diálisis	dialysis
dializzatore	dializador	dialyzer (Am)
eruzione cutanea da pannolino	exantema del pañal	diaper rash (Am)
diaforesi	diaforesis	diaphoresis
diaframma	diafragma	diaphragm
diafisi	diáfisis	diaphysis
diarrea	diarrea	diarrhea (Am)
diarrea e vomito	diarrea y vómitos	diarrhea and vomiting (D & V) (Am)
diarrea	diarrea	diarrhoea (Eng)
diarrea e vomito	diarrea y vómitos	diarrhoea and vomiting (D & V) (Eng)
diastasi, amilasi	diastasis	diastasis
diastole	diástole	diastole
diatermia	diatermia	diathermy
regime, dieta	régimen	diet
fibra dietetica	fibra dietética	dietary fiber (Am)
fibra dietetica	fibra dietética	dietary fibre (Eng)
dietetica	dietética	dietetics
dietista, dietologo	dietista	dietitian

ENGLISH	FRENCH	GERMAN
differential blood count	formule leucocytaire	Differentialblutbild
differential diagnosis	diagnostic différentiel	Differentialdiagnose
digestion	digestion	Verdauung
digestive system	système digestif	Verdauungsapparat
digital compression	compression digitale	Fingerdruck
digitalis	digitale	Digitalis, Fingerhut
digitalization	digitalisation	Digitalisierung
dilatation (Eng)	dilatation	Dilatation, Erweiterung
dilatation and curettage (D & C) (Eng)	dilatation et curetage	Dilatation und Kürettage
dilation (Am)	dilatation	Dilatation, Erweiterung
dilation and curettage (D & C) (Am)	dilatation et curetage	Dilatation und Kürettage
diphtheria	diphtérie	Diphtherie
diplegia	diplégie	Diplegie, doppelseitige Lähmung
diplopia	diplopie	Diplopie, Doppelsehen
disarticulation	désarticulation	Exartikulation
discectomy (Eng)	discectomie	Diskektomie
discrete	discret	diskret
disease	maladie	Krankheit, Leiden
disimpaction	désimpaction	Fragmentlösung
disinfect	désinfecter	desinfizieren
disinfectant	désinfectant	Desinfektionsmittel
disinfection	désinfection	Desinfektion
disinfestation	désinfestation	Entwesung, Entlausung
diskectomy (Am)	discectomie	Diskektomie
dislocation	dislocation	Dislokation, Verrenkung
disorientation	désorientation	Desorientiertheit
dissection	dissection	Sektion, Obduktion
disseminated	disséminé	disseminiert, verstreut
disseminated intravascular coagulation (DIC)	coagulation intravasculaire disséminée (CID)	disseminierte intravasale Gerinnung (DIC)
dissociation	dissociation	Dissoziation, Trennung
distal	distal	distal
diuresis	diurèse	Diurese
diuretic (n)	diurétique (n)	Diuretikum (n)
diuretic (a)	diurétique (a)	diuretisch (a)
diverticulitis	diverticulite	Divertikulitis
diverticulosis	diverticulose	Divertikulose
diverticulum	diverticulum	Divertikel
dizziness	étourdissement	Schwindel
doctor	médecin	Arzt
dolor	douleur	Schmerz
dominant	dominant	dominant, vorherrschend
donor	donneur	Spender
dopamine	dopamine	Dopamin
Doppler ultrasound technique	échographie de Doppler	Doppler-Sonographie

ITALIAN	SPANISH	ENGLISH
formula leucocitaria	fórmula leucocitaria	differential blood count
diagnosi differenziale	diagnóstico diferencial	differential diagnosis
digestione	digestión	digestion
sistema digestivo	aparato digestivo	digestive system
compressione digitale	compresión digital	digital compression
digitale	digital	digitalis
digitalizzazione	digitalización	digitalization
dilatazione	dilatación	dilatation (Eng)
dilatazione e raschiamento	dilatación y raspado/legrado	dilatation and curettage (D & C) (Eng)
dilatazione	dilatación	dilation (Am)
dilatazione e raschiamento	dilatación y raspado/legrado	dilation and curettage (D & C) (Am)
difterite	difteria	diphtheria
diplegia	diplejía, parálisis bilateral	diplegia
diplopia	diplopia	diplopia
disarticolazione	desarticulación	disarticulation
discectomia, asportazione di disco intervertebrale	disquectomía	discectomy (Eng)
discreto	discreto	discrete
malattia, affezione, infermità	enfermedad	disease
riduzione	desimpactación	disimpaction
disinfettare	desinfectar	disinfect
disinfettante	desinfectante	disinfectant
disinfezione	desinfección	disinfection
disinfestazione	desinfestación	disinfestation
discectomia, asportazione di disco intervertebrale	disquectomía	diskectomy (Am)
dislocazione	dislocación	dislocation
disorientamento	desorientación	disorientation
dissezione	disección	dissection
disseminato	diseminado	disseminated
coagulazione intravascolare disseminata (CID)	coagulación intravascular diseminada (CID)	disseminated intravascular coagulation (DIC)
dissociazione	disociación	dissociation
distale	distal	distal
diuresi	diuresis	diuresis
diuretico (n)	diurético (n)	diuretic (n)
diuretico (a)	diurético (a)	diuretic (a)
diverticolite	diverticulitis	diverticulitis
diverticolosi	diverticulosis	diverticulosis
diverticolo	divertículo	diverticulum
stordimento, capogiro, vertigini	desvanecimiento, mareo	dizziness
dottore, medico	médico	doctor
dolore	dolor	dolor
dominante	dominante	dominant
donatore	donante	donor
dopammina	dopamina	dopamine
tecnica ultrasonografica Doppler	técnica de ultrasonidos Doppler	Doppler ultrasound technique

ENGLISH	FRENCH	GERMAN
dorsal	dorsal	dorsal, Rücken-
dorsiflexion	dorsiflexion	Dorsalflexion
double vision	double vision	Doppelsehen, Diplopie
douche	douche	Dusche, Spülung
Down's syndrome	trisomie 21	Down-Syndrom, Mongolismus
drain (n)	drain (n)	Drain (n)
drain (v)	drainer (v)	drainieren (v)
drawsheet	alèse	Unterziehtuch
dressing	pansement	Verband, Umschlag
drip (n)	perfusion (n)	Tropfinfusion (n)
drip (v)	perfuser (v)	tröpfeln (v), tropfen (v)
drop attack	chute brusque par dérobement des jambes	Drop attack
drug	médicament	Arzneimittel, Rauschgift
drug abuse	toxicomanie	Arzneimittelmißbrauch, Drogenmißbrauch
duct	conduit	Ductus, Gang
ductus arteriosus	canal artériel	Ductus arteriosus
dumping syndrome	syndrome de chasse	Dumping-Syndrom
duodenal ulcer	ulcère duodénal	Duodenalulkus, Zwölffingerdarmgeschwür
duodenitis	duodénite	Duodenitis, Zwölffingerdarmentzündung
duodenum	duodénum	Duodenum, Zwölffingerdarm
dwarfism	nanisme	Zwergwuchs
dysarthria	dysarthrie	Dysarthrie
dyscrasia	dyscrasie	Dyskrasie
dysentery	dysenterie	Dysenterie, Ruhr
dysfunction	dysfonctionnement	Dysfunktion, Funktionsstörung
dysfunctional uterine bleeding (DUB)	ménométrorragies fonctionnelles	dysfunktionale Uterusblutung
dyskaryosis	dyskaryose	Kernanomalie, Dysplasie
dyskinesia	dyskinésie	Dyskinesie
dyslexia	dyslexie	Dyslexie
dysmenorrhea (Am)	dysménorrhée	Dysmenorrhoe
dysmenorrhoea (Eng)	dysménorrhée	Dysmenorrhoe
dyspareunia	dyspareunie	Dyspareunie
dyspepsia	dyspepsie	Dyspepsie, Verdauungsstörung
dysphagia	dysphagie	Dysphagie, Schluckbeschwerden
dysphasia	dysphasie	Dysphasie
dysplasia	dysplasie	Dysplasie, Fehlbildung
dyspnea (Am)	dyspnée	Dyspnoe, Atemnot
dyspnoea (Eng)	dyspnée	Dyspnoe, Atemnot
dyspraxia	dyspraxie	Dyspraxie
dysrhythmia	dysrythmie	Dysrhythmie, Rhythmusstörung
dystrophy	dystrophie	Dystrophie
dysuria	dysurie	Dysurie

ITALIAN	SPANISH	ENGLISH
dorsale	dorsal	**dorsal**
dorsiflessione	dorsiflexión	**dorsiflexion**
diplopia	visión doble	**double vision**
lavanda vaginale	ducha	**douche**
mongoloidismo, sindrome di Down	síndrome de Down	**Down's syndrome**
drenaggio *(n)*	drenaje *(n)*	**drain** *(n)*
drenare *(v)*	drenar *(v)*	**drain** *(v)*
traversa	alezo, faja	**drawsheet**
medicazione	cura, vendaje	**dressing**
fleboclisi *(n)*	gota a gota intravenoso *(n)*	**drip** *(n)*
gocciolare *(v)*, far gocciolare *(v)*	infundir *(v)*	**drip** *(v)*
improvvisa perdita della postura ad insorgenza periodica	ataque isquémico transitorio (AIT), caida	**drop attack**
farmaco, medicinale, droga	fármaco	**drug**
abuso di droga, abuso di farmaci	abuso de drogas	**drug abuse**
dotto	conducto	**duct**
dotto arterioso	ductus arteriosus	**ductus arteriosus**
sindrome del gastroresecato	síndrome de dumping, síndrome del vaciamiento en gastrectomizados	**dumping syndrome**
ulcera duodenale	úlcera duodenal	**duodenal ulcer**
duodenite	duodenitis	**duodenitis**
duodeno	duodeno	**duodenum**
nanismo	enanismo	**dwarfism**
disartria	disartria	**dysarthria**
discrasia	discrasia	**dyscrasia**
dissenteria	disentería	**dysentery**
disfunzione	disfunción	**dysfunction**
sanguinamento uterino funzionale	hemorragia uterina funcional	**dysfunctional uterine bleeding (DUB)**
discariosi	discariosis	**dyskaryosis**
discinesia	discinesia	**dyskinesia**
dislessia	dislexia	**dyslexia**
dismenorrea	dismenorrea	**dysmenorrhea** (Am)
dismenorrea	dismenorrea	**dysmenorrhoea** (Eng)
dispareunia	dispareunia	**dyspareunia**
dispepsia	dispepsia	**dyspepsia**
disfagia	disfagia	**dysphagia**
disfasia	disfasia	**dysphasia**
displasia	displasia	**dysplasia**
dispnea	disnea	**dyspnea** (Am)
dispnea	disnea	**dyspnoea** (Eng)
disprassia	dispraxia	**dyspraxia**
disritmia	disritmia	**dysrhythmia**
distrofia	distrofia	**dystrophy**
disuria	disuria	**dysuria**

E

English	French	German
ear	oreille	Ohr
eardrum	tympan	Trommelfell
ear nose and throat (ENT)	oto-rhino-laryngologie (ORL)	Hals- Nasen- Ohren-
ear wax	cérumen	Zerumen, Ohrenschmalz
ecchymosis	ecchymose	Ekchymose
echocardiography	échocardiographie	Echokardiographie
echoencephalography	écho-encéphalographie	Echoenzephalographie
echolalia	écholalie	Echolalie
echovirus	échovirus	ECHO-Virus
eclampsia	éclampsie	Eklampsie
ectoderm	ectoderme	Ektoderm
ectoparasite	ectoparasite	Ektoparasit
ectopic	ectopique	ektop
ectopic pregnancy	grossesse ectopique	ektope Schwangerschaft
ectropion	ectropion	Ektropion
eczema	eczéma	Ekzem
edema (Am)	oedème	Ödem, Flüssigkeitsansammlung
edentulous	édenté	zahnlos
efferent	efférent	efferent
effusion	effusion	Erguß
egg	oeuf	Ei, Ovum
ejaculation	éjaculation	Ejakulation, Samenerguß
elastin	élastine	Elastin
electrocardiogram (ECG)	électrocardiogramme (ECG)	Elektrokardiogramm (EKG)
electroconvulsive therapy (ECT)	électrochoc	Elektroschocktherapie
electrode	électrode	Elektrode
electroencephalogram (EEG)	électroencéphalogramme (EEG)	Elektroenzephalogramm (EEG)
electrolysis	électrolyse	Elektrolyse
electrolyte	électrolyte	Elektrolyt
electromyography	électromyographie	Elektromyographie
elephantiasis	éléphantiasis	Elephantiasis
elimination	élimination	Elimination, Ausscheidung
elixir	élixir	Elixier
elliptocytosis	elliptocytose	Elliptozytose
emaciation	émaciation	Auszehrung
embolic	embolique	embolisch
embolism	embolisme	Embolie
embolus	embole	Embolus
embryo	embryon	Embryo
embryology	embryologie	Embryologie
embryopathy	embryopathie	Embryopathie
emergency treatment/trauma unit (ETU)	service des urgences/des traumatismes	Notfallstation
emesis	vomissement	Erbrechen
emetic (n)	émétique (n)	Emetikum (n), Brechmittel (n)

ITALIAN	SPANISH	ENGLISH
orecchio	oído	ear
timpano	tímpano	eardrum
orecchio naso e gola, otorinolaringoiatria	otorrinolaringología (ORL)	ear nose and throat (ENT)
cerume	cerumen	ear wax
ecchimosi	equímosis	ecchymosis
ecocardiografia	ecocardiografía	echocardiography
ecoencefalografia	ecoencefalografía	echoencephalography
ecolalia	ecolalia	echolalia
echovirus	virus ECHO	echovirus
eclampsia	eclampsia	eclampsia
ectoderma	ectodermo	ectoderm
ectoparassita	ectoparásito	ectoparasite
ectopico	ectópico	ectopic
gravidanza ectopica	embarazo ectópico	ectopic pregnancy
ectropion	ectropión	ectropion
eczema	eccema	eczema
edema	edema	edema (Am)
edentulo	dcsdentado	edentulous
efferente	eferente	efferent
effusione	derrame	effusion
uovo	huevo	egg
eiaculazione	eyaculación	ejaculation
elastina	elastina	elastin
elettrocardiogramma (ECG)	electrocardiograma (ECG)	electrocardiogram (ECG)
terapia elettroconvulsiva, elettroshock	electrochoqueterapia (ECT)	electroconvulsive therapy (ECT)
elettrodo	electrodo	electrode
elettroencefalogramma (EEG)	electroencefalograma (EEG)	electroencephalogram (EEG)
elettrolisi	electrólisis	electrolysis
elettrolito	electrólito	electrolyte
elettromiografia	electromiografía	electromyography
elefantiasi	elefantiasis	elephantiasis
eliminazione	eliminación	elimination
elisir	elixir	elixir
ellissocitosi	eliptocitosis	elliptocytosis
emaciazione	emaciación	emaciation
embolico	embólico	embolic
embolia	embolia	embolism
embolo	émbolo	embolus
embrione	embrión	embryo
embriologia	embriología	embryology
embriopatia	embriopatía	embryopathy
pronto soccorso	servicio de urgencias/traumatologia	emergency treatment/trauma unit (ETU)
vomito, emesi	emesis	emesis
emetico (n)	emético (n)	emetic (n)

ENGLISH	FRENCH	GERMAN
emetic (a)	émétique (a)	emetisch (a)
emollient (n)	émollient (n)	Emollientium (n)
emollient (a)	émollient (a)	erweichend (a)
emotion	émotion	Emotion, Gefühl
emotional	émotionnel	emotional
empathy	empathie	Empathie, Einfühlungsvermögen
emphysema	emphysème	Emphysem
empirical	empirique	empirisch
empyema	empyème	Empyem
emulsion	émulsion	Emulsion
enamel	émail	Emaille
encapsulation	capsulage	Verkapselung
encephalin (Eng)	encéphaline	Enzephalin
encephalitis	encéphalite	Enzephalitis
encephalomyelitis	encéphalomyélite	Enzephalomyelitis
encephalopathy	encéphalopathie	Enzephalopathie
encopresis	encoprésie	Enkopresis, Einkoten
endarterectomy	endartériectomie	Endarteriektomie
endarteritis	endartérite	Endarteriitis
endemic (n)	endémie (n)	Endemie (n)
endemic (a)	endémique (a)	endemisch (a)
endocarditis	endocardite	Endokarditis
endocervical	endocervical	endozervikal
endocrine	endocrine	endokrin
endocrinology	endocrinologie	Endokrinologie
endogenous	endogène	endogen
endometriosis	endométriose	Endometriose
endometritis	endométrite	Endometritis
endometrium	endomètre	Endometrium
endoneurium	endonèvre	Endoneurium
endoparasite	endoparasite	Endoparasit
endorphin	endorphine	Endorphin
endoscope	endoscope	Endoskop
endoscopic retrograde cholangiopancreatography (ERCP)	cholangio-pancréatographie rétrograde endoscopique (CPRE)	endoskopische retrograde Cholangiopankreatographie (ERCP)
endoscopy	endoscopie	Endoskopie
endothelium	endothélium	Endothel
endotoxin	endotoxine	Endotoxin
endotracheal	endotrachéique	endotracheal
enema	lavement	Klistier, Einlauf
engorgement	engorgement	Stauung, Anschoppung
enkephalin (Am)	encéphaline	Enzephalin
enophthalmos	énophtalmie	Enophtalmus
enteral	entéral	enteral
enteric	entérique	enterisch
enteric-coated tablet (ECT)	dragée entérosoluble, comprimé à délitement entérique	magensaftresistente Tablette

ITALIAN	SPANISH	ENGLISH
emetico *(a)*	emético *(a)*	**emetic** *(a)*
emoliente *(n)*	emoliente *(n)*	**emollient** *(n)*
emoliente *(a)*	emoliente *(a)*	**emollient** *(a)*
emozione	emoción	**emotion**
emotivo	emocional	**emotional**
immedesimazione, identificazione	empatía	**empathy**
enfisema	enfisema	**emphysema**
empirico	empírico	**empirical**
empiema	empiema	**empyema**
emulsione	emulsión	**emulsion**
smalto	esmalte	**enamel**
incapsulamento	encapsulación	**encapsulation**
encefalina	encefalina	**encephalin** (Eng)
encefalite	encefalitis	**encephalitis**
encefalomielite	encefalomielitis	**encephalomyelitis**
encefalopatia	encefalopatía	**encephalopathy**
encopresi	encopresis	**encopresis**
endoarterectomia	endarterectomía	**endarterectomy**
endoarterite	endarteritis	**endarteritis**
endemia *(n)*	endémico *(n)*	**endemic** *(n)*
endemico *(a)*	endémico *(a)*	**endemic** *(a)*
endocardite	endocarditis	**endocarditis**
endocervicale	endocervical	**endocervical**
endocrino	endocrino	**endocrine**
endocrinologia	endocrinología	**endocrinology**
endogeno	endógeno	**endogenous**
endometriosi	endometriosis	**endometriosis**
endometrite	endometritis	**endometritis**
endometrio	endometrio	**endometrium**
endonevrio	endoneuro	**endoneurium**
endoparassita	endoparásito	**endoparasite**
endorfina	endorfina	**endorphin**
endoscopio	endoscopio	**endoscope**
colangio-pancreatografia retrograda endoscopica (ERCP)	colangiopancreatografía endoscópica retrógrada	**endoscopic retrograde cholangiopancreatography (ERCP)**
endoscopia	endoscopia	**endoscopy**
endotelio	endotelio	**endothelium**
endotossina	endotoxina	**endotoxin**
endotracheale	endotraqueal	**endotracheal**
clistere	enema	**enema**
congestione	estancamiento	**engorgement**
encefalina	encefalina	**enkephalin** (Am)
enoftalmo	enoftalmos	**enophthalmos**
enterale, intestinale	enteral	**enteral**
enterico	entérico	**enteric**
compressa enterica rivestita (passano lo stomaco senza sciogliersi)	comprimido entérico	**enteric-coated tablet (ECT)**

ENGLISH	FRENCH	GERMAN
enteritis	entérite	Enteritis
enteroanastomosis	entéro-anastomose	Enteroanastomose
enterocele	entérocèle, hernie intestinale	Enterozele
enterocolitis	entérocolite	Enterokolitis
enterostomy	entérostomie	Enterostomie
enterovirus	entérovirus	Enterovirus
entropion	entropion	Entropion
enucleation	énucléation	Enukleation, Ausschälung
enuresis	énurèse	Enuresis, Bettnässen
environment	milieu	Umgebung, Umwelt
enzyme	enzyme	Enzym
enzyme-linked immunosorbent assay (ELISA)	dosage par la méthode (ELISA)	enzyme-linked immunosorbent assay (ELISA)
enzymology	enzymologie	Enzymologie
eosinophil (n)	éosinophile (n)	Eosinophiler (n)
eosinophil (a)	éosinophile (a)	eosinophil (a)
eosinophilia	éosinophilie	Eosinophilie
ependymoma	épendymome	Ependymom
ephedrine	éphédrine	Ephedrin
epicanthus	épicanthus	Epikanthus
epicardium	épicarde	Epikard
epidemic (n)	épidémie (n)	Epidemie (n)
epidemic (a)	épidémique (a)	epidemisch (a)
epidemiology	épidémiologie	Epidemiologie
epidermis	épiderme	Epidermis
epididymis	épididyme	Epididymis, Nebenhoden
epididymitis	épididymite	Epididymitis, Nebenhodenentzündung
epididymo-orchitis	orchi-épididymite	Epididymoorchitis
epidural	épidural	epidural
epigastrium	épigastre	Epigastrium, Oberbauch
epiglottis	épiglotte	Epiglottis
epiglottitis	épiglottite	Epiglottitis
epilepsy	épilepsie	Epilepsie
epileptic	épileptique	epileptisch
epileptiform	épileptiforme	epileptiform
epileptogenic	épileptogène	epileptogen
epinephrine	adrénaline, épinéphrine	Adrenalin
epiphysis	épiphyse	Epiphyse, Zirbeldrüse
episclera	épisclérotique	Episklera
episcleritis	épisclérite	Episkleritis
episiotomy	épisiotomie	Episiotomie, Dammschnitt
epistaxis	épistaxis	Epistaxis, Nasenbluten
epithelioma	épithélioma	Epitheliom
epithelium	épithélium	Epithel
Epstein-Barr virus (EBV)	virus d'Epstein-Barr	Epstein-Barr-Virus (EBV)
erectile	érectile	erektil
erection	érection	Erektion

ITALIAN	SPANISH	ENGLISH
enterite	enteritis	enteritis
enteroanastomosi	enteroanastómosis	enteroanastomosis
enterocele	enterocele	enterocele
enterocolite	enterocolitis	enterocolitis
enterostomia	enterostomía	enterostomy
enterovirus	enterovirus	enterovirus
entropion	entropión	entropion
enucleazione	enucleación	enucleation
enuresi	enuresis	enuresis
ambiente	ambiente	environment
enzima	enzima	enzyme
test di immunoassorbimento enzimatico	análisis enzimático por inmunoabsorción	enzyme-linked immunosorbent assay (ELISA)
enzimologia	enzimología	enzymology
eosinofilo (n)	eosinófilo (n)	eosinophil (n)
eosinofilo (a)	eosinófilo (a)	eosinophil (a)
eosinofilia	eosinofilia	eosinophilia
ependimoma	ependimoma	ependymoma
efedrina	efedrina	ephedrine
epicanto	epicanto	epicanthus
epicardio	epicardio	epicardium
epidemia (n)	epidemia (n)	epidemic (n)
epidemico (a)	epidémico (a)	epidemic (a)
epidemiologia	epidemiología	epidemiology
epidermide	epidermis	epidermis
epididimo	epidídimo	epididymis
epididimite	epididimitis	epididymitis
epididimo-orchite	epididimoorquitis	epididymo-orchitis
epidurale	epidural	epidural
epigastrio	epigastrio	epigastrium
epiglottide	epiglotis	epiglottis
epiglottite	epiglotitis	epiglottitis
epilessia	epilepsia	epilepsy
epilettico	epiléptico	epileptic
epilettiforme	epileptiforme	epileptiform
epilettogeno	epileptógeno	epileptogenic
adrenalina	epinefrina	epinephrine
epifisi	epífisis	epiphysis
episclera	episclera	episclera
episclerite	escleritis	episcleritis
episiotomia	episiotomía	episiotomy
epistassi	epistaxis	epistaxis
epitelioma	epitelioma	epithelioma
epitelio	epitelio	epithelium
virus di Epstein Barr	virus de Epstein-Barr	Epstein-Barr virus (EBV)
erettile	eréctil	erectile
erezione	erección	erection

eruption	éruption	Ausbruch, Ausschlag
erysipelas	érysipèle	Erysipel, Wundrose
erythema	érythème	Erythem
erythroblast	érythroblaste	Erythroblast
erythrocyte	érythrocyte	Erythrozyt, rotes Blutkörperchen
erythrocyte sedimentation rate (ESR)	vitesse de sédimentation globulaire	Blutkörperchen-Senkungsgeschwindigkeit (BSG, BKS)
erythroderma	érythroderme	Erythrodermie
erythropoiesis	érythropoïèse	Erythropoese
erythropoietin	érythropoïétine	Erythropoetin, erythropoetischer Faktor
eschar	escarre	Brandschorf
esophageal (Am)	oesophagien	ösophageal
esophagitis (Am)	oesophagite	Ösophagitis
esophagus (Am)	oesophage	Ösophagus, Speiseröhre
essence	essence	Essenz
essential amino acid	acide aminé essentiel	essentielle Aminosäure
essential fatty acid	acide gras essentiel	essentielle Fettsäure
estradiol (Am)	oestradiol	Östradiol
estriol (Am)	oestriol	Östriol
estrogen (Am)	oestrogène	Östrogen
ethmoid	ethmoïde	Ethmoid, Siebbein
ethnic	ethnique	ethnisch, rassisch
euphoria	euphorie	Euphorie
Eustachian tube	trompe d'Eustache	Eustachische Röhre
euthanasia	euthanasie	Euthanasie, Sterbehilfe
evacuation	évacuation	Ausleerung, Stuhlgang
evaporate	évaporer	verdampfen, verdunsten
eversion	éversion	Auswärtskehrung, Umstülpung
Ewing's tumour	tumeur d'Ewing	Ewing-Sarkom
exacerbation	exacerbation	Verschlimmerung
excision	excision	Exzision
excitability	excitabilité	Reizbarkeit, Erregbarkeit
excitation	excitation	Reizung, Erregung
excoriation	excoriation	Exkoriation, Abschürfung
excretion	excrétion	Exkretion, Ausscheidung
exfoliation	exfoliation	Exfoliation
exhibitionism	exhibitionnisme	Exhibitionismus
exocrine	exocrine	exokrin
exogenous	exogène	exogen
exomphalos	exomphale	Exomphalos, Nabelbruch
exophthalmos	exophthalmie	Exophthalmus
exostosis	exostose	Exostose
exotoxin	exotoxine	Exotoxin
expected date of confinement (EDC)	date présumée de l'accouchement	errechneter Geburtstermin
expected date of delivery (EDD)	date présumée de l'accouchement	errechneter Geburtstermin

ITALIAN	SPANISH	ENGLISH
eruzione	erupción	eruption
erisipela	erisipela	erysipelas
eritema	eritema	erythema
eritroblasto	eritroblasto	erythroblast
eritrocito	eritrocito	erythrocyte
velocità di eritrosedimentazione (VES)	velocidad de sedimentación globular (VSG)	erythrocyte sedimentation rate (ESR)
eritrodermia	eritrodermia	erythroderma
eritropoiesi	eritropoyesis	erythropoiesis
eritropoietina	eritropoyetina	erythropoietin
escara	escara, costra	eschar
esofageo	esofágico	esophageal (Am)
esofagite	esofagitis	esophagitis (Am)
esofago	esófago	esophagus (Am)
essenza	esencia	essence
aminoacido essenziale	aminoácido esencial	essential amino acid
acido grasso essenziale	ácido graso esencial	essential fatty acid
estradiolo	estradiol	estradiol (Am)
estriolo	estriol	estriol (Am)
estrogeno	estrógeno	estrogen (Am)
etmoide	etmoides	ethmoid
etnico	étnico	ethnic
euforia	euforia	euphoria
tuba d'Eustachio	trompa de Eustaquio	eustachian tube
eutanasia	eutanasia	euthanasia
evacuazione	evacuación	evacuation
evaporare	evaporar	evaporate
eversione, estrofia	eversión	eversion
tumore di Ewing	sarcoma de Ewing	Ewing's tumour
esacerbazione	exacerbación	exacerbation
escissione	excisión	excision
eccitabilità	excitabilidad	excitability
eccitazione	excitación	excitation
escoriazione	excoriación	excoriation
escrezione	excreción	excretion
esfoliazione	exfoliación	exfoliation
esibizionismo	exhibicionismo	exhibitionism
esocrino	exocrino	exocrine
esogeno	exógeno	exogenous
ernia ombelicale, protrusione dell'ombelico	exónfalo, hernia umbilical	exomphalos
esoftalmo	exoftalmía	exophthalmos
esostosi	exostosis	exostosis
esotossina	exotoxina	exotoxin
data presunta delle doglie	fecha esperada del parto	expected date of confinement (EDC)
data prevista per il parto	fecha probable del parto (FPP)	expected date of delivery (EDD)

ENGLISH	FRENCH	GERMAN
expectorant *(n)*	expectorant *(n)*	Expektorans *(n)*, Sekretolytikum *(n)*
expectorant *(a)*	expectorant *(a)*	schleimlösend *(a)*
extension	extension	Extension, Streck-
extensor	extenseur	Extensor, Streckmuskel
external cephalic version (ECV)	version céphalique externe	äußere Wendung auf den Kopf
extra-articular	extra-articulaire	extraartikulär
extracellular	extracellulaire	extrazellulär
extraction	extraction	Extraktion
extradural	extradural	extradural
extramural	extramural	extramural
extrapyramidal side effects	effets latéraux extrapyramidaux	extrapyramidale Nebenwirkungen
extrasystole	extrasystole	Extrasystole
extrauterine	extra-utérin	extrauterin
extravasation	extravasation	Extravasat
extrinsic	extrinsèque	exogen
exudate	exsudat	Exsudat
eye	oeil	Auge

ITALIAN	SPANISH	ENGLISH
espettorante *(n)*	expectorante *(n)*	**expectorant** *(n)*
espettorante *(a)*	expectorante *(a)*	**expectorant** *(a)*
estensione	extensión	**extension**
estensore	extensor	**extensor**
versione cefalica esterna	versión cefálica externa	**external cephalic version (ECV)**
extraarticolare	extraarticular	**extra-articular**
extracellulare	extracelular	**extracellular**
estrazione	extracción	**extraction**
extradurale	extradural	**extradural**
extramurale	extramural	**extramural**
reazioni collaterali extrapiramidali da farmaci	efectos secundarios extrapiramidales	**extrapyramidal side effects**
extrasistole	extrasístole	**extrasystole**
extrauterino	extrauterino	**extrauterine**
stravaso	extravasación	**extravasation**
estrinseco	extrínseco	**extrinsic**
essudato	exudado	**exudate**
occhio	ojo	**eye**

F

ENGLISH	FRENCH	GERMAN
facet	facette	Facette
facial	facial	Gesichts-
facies	faciès	Facies, Gesicht
facultative	facultatif	fakultativ
faecal (Eng)	fécal	fäkal, kotig
faecalith (Eng)	concrétion fécale	Kotstein
faecal occult blood (FOB) (Eng)	sang occulte fécal	okkultes Blut (im Stuhl)
faeces (Eng)	fèces	Fäzes, Kot
failure to thrive (FTT)	absence de développement pondéro-statural normal	Gedeihstörung
faint (n)	syncope (n)	Ohnmacht (n)
faint (v)	s'évanouir (v)	ohmächtig werden (v)
falciform	falciforme	falciformis
Fallopian tube	trompe de Fallope	Tube, Eileiter
Fallot's tetralogy	trilogie de Fallot	Fallot-Tetralogie
familial	familial	familiär
family planning	contrôle des naissances	Familienplanung
fascia	fascia	Faszie
fasciculation	fasciculation	Faszikulation
fasting blood sugar (FBS)	glycémie à jeun	Nüchternblutzucker (NBZ)
fat (n)	graisse (n)	Fett (n)
fat (a)	gras (a), obèse (a)	fett (a), fetthaltig (a)
fatigue	fatigue	Ermüdung
fatty acid	acide gras	Fettsäure
fatty degeneration	dégénérescence graisseuse	fettige Degeneration, Verfettung
fauces	fosse gutturale	Rachen, Schlund
febrile	fébrile	Fieber-, fieberhaft
fecal (Am)	fécal	fäkal, kotig
fecalith (Am)	concrétion fécale	Kotstein
fecal occult blood (FOB) (Am)	sang occulte fécal	okkultes Blut (im Stuhl)
feces (Am)	fèces	Fäzes, Kot
female	femelle	weiblich
femoral artery	artère fémorale	Arteria femoralis
femoral vein	veine fémorale	Vena femoralis
femur	fémur	Femur
fenestration	fenestration	Fensterung
ferrous (Eng)	ferreux	Eisen-
ferrus (Am)	ferreux	Eisen-
fertilization	fertilisation	Befruchtung
fetal alcohol syndrome	syndrome d'alcoolisme foetal	fetales Alkoholsyndrom
fetal circulation	circulation foetale	fetaler Kreislauf
fetal heart rate (FHR)	fréquence cardiaque foetale	fetale Herzfrequenz
fetoscopy	fétoscopie	Fetoskopie
fetus	foetus	Fetus
fever	fièvre	Fieber

ITALIAN	SPANISH	ENGLISH
faccetta	faceta	facet
facciale	facial	facial
facies	facies	facies
facoltativo	facultativo	facultative
fecale	fecal	faecal (Eng)
fecalito	fecalito	faecalith (Eng)
sangue occulto fecale	sangre oculta fecal	faecal occult blood (FOB) (Eng)
feci	heces	faeces (Eng)
marasma infantile	desmedro, marasmo	failure to thrive (FTT)
svenimento (n)	vahído (n), síncope (n)	faint (n)
sverire (v)	desmayar (v)	faint (v)
falciforme	falciforme	falciform
tuba di Falloppio	trompa de Falopio	Fallopian tube
tetralogia di Fallot	tetralogía de Fallot	Fallot's tetralogy
familiare	familiar	familial
controllo delle nascite	planificación familiar	family planning
fascia	fascia, aponeurosis	fascia
fascicolazione	fasciculación	fasciculation
glicemia a digiuno	glucemia en ayunas	fasting blood sugar (FBS)
adipe (n)	grasa (n)	fat (n)
grasso (a)	graso (a)	fat (a)
stanchezza, astenia	fatiga, cansancio	fatigue
acido grasso	ácido graso	fatty acid
degenerazione grassa	degeneración grasa	fatty degeneration
fauci	fauces	fauces
febbrile	febril	febrile
fecale	fecal	fecal (Am)
fecalito	fecalito	fecalith (Am)
sangue occulto fecale	sangre oculta fecal	fecal occult blood (FOB) (Am)
feci	heces	feces (Am)
femmina	hembra	female
arteria femorale	arteria femoral	femoral artery
vena femorale	vena femoral	femoral vein
femore	fémur	femur
fenestrazione	fenestración	fenestration
ferroso	ferroso	ferrous (Eng)
ferroso	ferroso	ferrus (Am)
fertilizzazione	fertilización	fertilization
sindrome da alcolismo materno	síndrome alcohólico fetal	fetal alcohol syndrome
circolazione fetale	circulación fetal	fetal circulation
battito cardiaco fetale	frecuencia cardíaca fetal (FCF)	fetal heart rate (FHR)
fetoscopia	fetoscopia	fetoscopy
feto	feto	fetus
febbre	fiebre	fever

fiber (Am)	fibre	Faser
fibre (Eng)	fibre	Faser
fibril	fibrille	Fibrille, Fäserchen
fibrillation	fibrillation	Fibrillieren
fibrin	fibrine	Fibrin
fibrinogen	fibrinogène	Fibrinogen
fibroadenoma	fibroadénome	Fibroadenom
fibroblast	fibroblaste	Fibroblast
fibrocystic	fibrokystique	fibrozystisch
fibroma	fibrome	Fibrom
fibromyoma	fibromyome	Fibromyom
fibrosarcoma	fibrosarcome	Fibrosarkom
fibrosis	fibrose	Fibrose
fibrositis	fibrosite	Fibrositis, Bindegewebsentzündung
fibula	fibula	Fibula, Wadenbein
field of vision	champ de vision	Gesichtsfeld
filariasis	filariose	Filariasis, Fadenwurmbefall
filtrate	filtrat	Filtrat
filtration	filtration	Filtrieren, Filtration
fimbria	fimbria	Fimbrie
fine tremor	tremblement fin	feinschlägiger Tremor
finger	doigt	Finger
first aid	secourisme, premiers soins	Erste Hilfe
fission	fission	Spaltung
fistula	fistule	Fistel
fit	attaque	Anfall
fixation	fixation	Fixation, Fixierung
flaccid	mou	schlaff
flail chest	volet thoracique	Flatterbrust
flap	lambeau	Lappen, Hautlappen
flat-foot	pied plat	Plattfuß
flatulence	flatulence	Flatulenz, Blähung
flatus	flatuosité	Flatus, Wind
flea	puce	Floh
flex	fléchir	beugen, flektieren
flexion	flexion	Flexion, Beugung
flexor	fléchisseur	Flexor, Beugemuskel
flexure	angle	Flexur
flight of ideas	fuite des idées	Ideenflucht
floaters	flottants	Mouches volantes
flora	flore	Flora
florid	coloré	floride
fluctuation	variation	Fluktuation
fluke	douve	Trematode
fluorescein	fluorescéine	Fluorescin

| --- | --- | --- |
fibra	fibra	**fiber** (Am)
fibra	fibra	**fibre** (Eng)
fibrilla	fibrilla	**fibril**
fibrillazione	fibrilación	**fibrillation**
fibrina	fibrina	**fibrin**
fibrinogeno	fibrinógeno	**fibrinogen**
fibroadenoma	fibroadenoma	**fibroadenoma**
fibroblasto	fibroblasto	**fibroblast**
fibrocistico	fibrocístico	**fibrocystic**
fibroma	fibroma	**fibroma**
fibromioma	fibromioma	**fibromyoma**
fibrosarcoma	fibrosarcoma	**fibrosarcoma**
fibrosi	fibrosis	**fibrosis**
fibrosite	fibrositis	**fibrositis**
fibula	peroné	**fibula**
campo visivo	campo de visión	**field of vision**
filariasi	filariasis	**filariasis**
filtrato	filtrado	**filtrate**
filtrazione	filtración	**filtration**
fimbria	fimbria, franja	**fimbria**
tremore fino	temblor fino	**fine tremor**
dito	dedo de la mano	**finger**
pronto soccorso	primeros auxilios	**first aid**
fissione	fisión	**fission**
fistola	fístula	**fistula**
convulsione	ataque, acceso	**fit**
fissazione	fijación	**fixation**
flaccido	fláccido	**flaccid**
anomala motilità respiratoria della cassa toracica in conseguenza di fratture	volet torácico	**flail chest**
lembo, innesto	colgajo, injerto	**flap**
piede piatto	pie plano	**flat-foot**
flatulenza	flatulencia	**flatulence**
flatulenza, gas intestinale	flato	**flatus**
pulce	pulga	**flea**
flettere	flexionar	**flex**
flessione	flexión	**flexion**
flessore	flexor	**flexor**
flessura	flexura	**flexure**
fuga delle idee	fuga de ideas	**flight of ideas**
corpuscoli vitreali sospesi visibili	flotadores	**floaters**
flora	flora	**flora**
florido	florido, bien desarrollado	**florid**
fluttuazione	fluctuación	**fluctuation**
trematode, Digeneum	trematodo	**fluke**
fluoresceina	fluoresceína	**fluorescein**

fluorescent treponemal antibody (FTA)	test d'immunofluorescence absorbée pour le diagnostic	Fluoreszenz-Treponemen-Antikörper
fluoride	fluorure	Fluorid
flush	rougeur	Flush
folic acid	acide folique	Folsäure
follicle	follicule	Follikel
follicle stimulating hormone (FSH)	hormone folliculo-stimulante, gonadotrophine A	follikelstimulierendes Hormon (FSH)
folliculitis	folliculite	Follikulitis
fontanelle	fontanelle	Fontanelle
food allergy	allergie alimentaire	Nahrungsmittelallergie
food poisoning	intoxication alimentaire	Nahrungsmittelvergiftung
foot	pied	Fuß
foramen	orifice	Foramen
forced expiratory volume (FEV)	volume expiratoire maximum (VEM)	forciertes Exspirationsvolumen, Atemstoßwert
forceps	forceps	Zange, Pinzette, Klemme
forearm	avant-bras	Unterarm
forehead	front	Stirn
forensic medicine	médecine légale	Gerichtsmedizin, Rechtsmedizin
foreskin	prépuce	Präputium, Vorhaut
formula	formule	Formel, Milchzusammensetzung
formulary	formulaire	Formelnbuch
fornix	fornix	Fornix
fostering	prise en nourrice	Pflege
fourchette	fourchette	hintere Schamlippenkommissur
fovea	fovea	Fovea
fracture (n)	fracture (n)	Fraktur (n), Knochenbruch (n)
fracture (v)	fracturer (v)	frakturieren (v), brechen (v)
free thyroxine (FT)	thyroxine libre (TL)	freies Thyroxin (FT)
free thyroxine index (FTI)	index de thyroxine libre	freier Thyroxinindex (FTi)
frenotomy	frénotomie	Frenotomie, Zungenbändchendurchtrennung
frenum	frein	Frenulum
friable	friable	bröckelig, brüchig
friction	friction	Friktion, Reibung
Friedreich's ataxia	maladie de Friedreich	Friedreich Ataxie
frigidity	frigidité	Frigidität, Kälte
frontal	frontal	Stirn-, frontal
frostbite	gelure	Erfrierung
frozen shoulder	épaule ankylosée	Frozen shoulder, Periarthritis humeroscapularis
fugue	fugue	Fugue
fulguration	fulguration	Fulguration
full-term	à terme	ausgetragen
fulminant	fulminant	fulminant
function (n)	fonction (n)	Funktion (n)
function (v)	fonctionner (v)	funktionieren (v)
functional disorder	fonctionnel	funktionelle Störung

ITALIAN	SPANISH	ENGLISH
anticorpo immino-fluorescente anti-treponema	anticuerpo anti-treponema fluorescente	fluorescent treponemal antibody (FTA)
fluoruro	flúor	fluoride
eritema vasomotorio	rubor	flush
acido folico	ácido fólico	folic acid
follicolo	folículo	follicle
ormone follicolostimolante (FSH)	hormona estimulante del folículo (FSH)	follicle stimulating hormone (FSH)
follicolite	foliculitis	folliculitis
fontanella	fontanela	fontanelle
allergia alimentare	alergia alimentaria	food allergy
avvelenamento alimentare	intoxicación alimentaria	food poisoning
piede	pie	foot
foramen	foramen	foramen
volume espiratorio forzato	volumen espiratorio forzado (VEF)	forced expiratory volume (FEV)
forcipe	fórceps	forceps
avambraccio	antebrazo	forearm
fronte	frente	forehead
medicina forense	medicina forense	forensic medicine
prepuzio	prepucio	foreskin
formula	fórmula, receta	formula
formulario	formulario	formulary
fornice	fórnix, bóveda	fornix
affido	adopción	fostering
forchetta	horquilla, frenillo pudendo	fourchette
fovea	fóvea	fovea
frattura (n)	fractura (n)	fracture (n)
fratturare (v)	fracturar (v)	fracture (v)
tiroxina libera (FT)	tiroxina libre	free thyroxine (FT)
indice di tiroxina libera	indice de tiroxina libre	free thyroxine index (FTI)
frenulotomia	frenotomía	frenotomy
freno	frenillo	frenum
friabile	friable	friable
attrito, frizione	fricción	friction
malattia di Friedreich	ataxia de Friedreich	Friedreich's ataxia
frigidità	frigidez	frigidity
frontale	frontal	frontal
congelamento	congelación, sabañón	frostbite
'spalla congelata', periartrite scapoloomerale	hombro conqelando/rígido	frozen shoulder
fuga	fuga	fugue
folgorazione	fulguración	fulguration
gravidanza a termine	embarazo a término	full-term
fulminante	fulminante	fulminant
funzione (n)	función (n)	function (n)
funzionare (v)	funcionar (v)	function (v)
disturbo funzionale	trastorno funcional	functional disorder

ENGLISH	FRENCH	GERMAN
fundoplication	fundoplication	Fundoplikatio(n)
fundus	fond	Fundus, Augenhintergrund
fungus	mycète	Pilz
furuncle	furoncle	Furunkel

ITALIAN	SPANISH	ENGLISH
fundoplicazione	fundoplicatura	**fundoplication**
fondo	fundus	**fundus**
fungo	hongo	**fungus**
foruncolo	forúnculo	**furuncle**

G

ENGLISH	FRENCH	GERMAN
gait	démarche	Gang
galactagogue	galactagogue	Galaktagogum
galactorrhea (Am)	galactorrhée	Galaktorrhoe
galactorrhoea (Eng)	galactorrhée	Galaktorrhoe
galactosaemia (Eng)	galactosémie	Galaktosämie
galactose	galactose	Galaktose
galactosemia (Am)	galactosémie	Galaktosämie
gall bladder	vésicule biliaire	Gallenblase
gallipot	petit pot	Salbentopf
gallstones	calculs biliaires	Gallensteine
gamete	gamète	Gamete
gammaglobulin	gamma-globuline	Gammaglobulin
gamma glutamyl transferase (GGT)	gamma-glutamyl-transférase (GGT)	Gammaglutamyltransferase (gGT)
ganglion	ganglion	Ganglion, Überbein
gangrene	gangrène	Gangrän
gargle (n)	gargarisme (n)	Gurgelmittel (n)
gargle (v)	se gargariser (v)	gurgeln (v)
gas	gaz	Gas, Wind
gastrectomy	gastrectomie	Magenresektion
gastric	gastrique	gastrisch, Magen-
gastrin	gastrine	Gastrin
gastritis	gastrite	Gastritis, Magenschleimhautentzündung
gastrocnemius	gastrocnémien	gastrocnemius
gastrocolic	gastrocolique	gastrokolisch
gastrodynia	gastrodynie	Magenschmerz
gastroenteritis	gastro-entérite	Gastroenteritis
gastroenterology	gastro-entérologie	Gastroenterologie
gastroenteropathy	gastro-entéropathie	Gastroenteropathie
gastroenterostomy	gastro-entérostomie	Gastroenterostomie
gastroesophageal (Am)	gastro-oesophagien	gastroösophageal
gastrointestinal	gastro-intestinal	gastrointestinal, Magendarm-
gastrojejunostomy	gastrojéjunostomie	Gastrojejunostomie
gastro-oesophageal (Eng)	gastro-oesophagien	gastroösophageal
gastroschisis	gastroschisis	Gastroschisis
gastroscope	gastroscope	Gastroskop, Magenspiegel
gastrostomy	gastrostomie	Gastrostomie
gauze	gaze	Gaze, Mull
gelatin (Am)	gélatine	Gelatine, Gallerte
gelatine (Eng)	gélatine	Gelatine, Gallerte
gene	gène	Gen
general paralysis of the insane	paralysie générale des aliénés	progressive Paralyse
generative	génératif	fertil, Fortpflanzungs-
generic (n)	dénomination commune d'un médicament (n)	Substanznahme (n), Generic (n)
generic (a)	générique (a)	generisch (a)

andatura	marcha	**gait**
galattagogo	galactogogo	**galactagogue**
galattorrea	galactorrea	**galactorrhea** (Am)
galattorrea	galactorrea	**galactorrhoea** (Eng)
galattosemia	galactosemia	**galactosaemia** (Eng)
galattosio	galactosa	**galactose**
galattosemia	galactosemia	**galactosemia** (Am)
cistifellea	vesícula biliar	**gall bladder**
ampolla o vasetto unguentario	bote	**gallipot**
calcoli biliari	cálculos biliares	**gallstones**
gamete	gameto	**gamete**
gammaglobulina	gammaglobulina	**gammaglobulin**
transaminasi, transferasi glutammica	gamma glutamil transferasa (GGT)	**gamma glutamyl transferase (GGT)**
ganglio	ganglio	**ganglion**
gangrena	gangrena	**gangrene**
gargarismi (n)	gárgara (n), colutorio (n)	**gargle** (n)
gargarizzare (v)	gargajear (v)	**gargle** (v)
gas	gas	**gas**
gastrectomia	gastrectomía	**gastrectomy**
gastrico	gástrico	**gastric**
gastrina	gastrina	**gastrin**
gastrite	gastritis	**gastritis**
gastrocnemio	gastrocnemio, gemelos	**gastrocnemius**
gastrocolico	gastrocólico	**gastrocolic**
gastrodinia	gastrodinia	**gastrodynia**
gastroenterite	gastroenteritis	**gastroenteritis**
gastroenterologia	gastroenterología	**gastroenterology**
gastroenteropatia	gastroenteropatía	**gastroenteropathy**
gastroenterostomia	gastroenterostomía	**gastroenterostomy**
gastroesofageo	gastroesofágico	**gastroesophageal** (Am)
gastrointestinale	gastrointestinal	**gastrointestinal**
gastrodigiunostomia	gastroyeyunostomía	**gastrojejunostomy**
gastroesofageo	gastroesofágico	**gastro-oesophageal** (Eng)
gastroschisi	gastrosquisis	**gastroschisis**
gastroscopio	gastroscopio	**gastroscope**
gastrostomia	gastrotomía	**gastrostomy**
garza	gasa	**gauze**
gelatina	gelatina	**gelatin** (Am)
gelatina	gelatina	**gelatine** (Eng)
gene	gen	**gene**
paralisi progressiva luetica	parálisis cerebral	**general paralysis of the insane**
riproduttivo	generador	**generative**
medico generico (n)	genérico (n)	**generic** (n)
generico (a)	genérico (a)	**generic** (a)

ENGLISH	FRENCH	GERMAN
genetic	génétique	genetisch
genetics	génétique	Genetik
genital	génital	genital, Geschlechts-
genitalia	organes génitaux	Genitalien
genitourinary (GU)	génito-urinaire (GT)	urogenital
genome	génome	Genom
genotype	génotype	Genotyp
genus	genre	Genus, Gattung
genu valgum	genu valgum	Genu valgum, X-Bein
genu varum	genu varum	Genu varum, O-Bein
geriatric	gériatrique	geriatrisch
geriatrician	gériatre	Geriater
geriatrics	gériatrie	Geriatrie
germ	germe	Erreger, Keim, Bazillus
German measles	rubéole	Rubella, Röteln
gestation	gestation	Gestation, Schwangerschaft
giant cell arteritis	artérite temporale	Riesenzellarteriitis
giardiasis	giardiase	Lambliasis
giddy	pris de vertige	schwindlig
gingiva	gencive	Gingiva, Zahnfleisch
gingivitis	gingivite	Gingivitis, Zahnfleischentzündung
girdle	ceinture	Gürtel
gland	glande	Glandula, Drüse
glandular fever	fièvre glandulaire	Mononukleose, Pfeiffersches Drüsenfieber
glaucoma	glaucome	Glaukom, grüner Star
glenohumeral	gléno-huméral	glenohumeral
glenoid	glénoïde	Schultergelenk-
glioma	gliome	Gliom
globus hystericus	boule hystérique	Globus hystericus, Globusgefühl
glomerular filtration rate (GFR)	taux de filtration glomérulaire	glomeruläre Filtrationsrate (GFR)
glomerulitis	glomérulite	Glomerulitis
glomerulonephritis	glomérulonéphrite	Glomerulonephritis
glomerulosclerosis	glomérulosclérose	Glomerulosklerose
glomerulus	glomérule	Glomerulus
glossa	langue	Zunge
glossitis	glossite	Glossitis
glossodynia	glossodynie	Glossodynie, Zungenschmerz
glossopharyngeal	glossopharyngien	glossopharyngeal
glottis	glotte	Glottis, Stimmritze
glucagon	glucagon	Glukagon
glucocorticoid	glucocorticoïde	Glukokortikoid
glucogenesis	glucogenèse	Glukogenese
gluconeogenesis	gluconéogenèse	Glukoneogenese
glucose	glucose	Glukose, Traubenzucker

ITALIAN	SPANISH	ENGLISH
genetico	genético	genetic
genetica	genética	genetics
genitale	genital	genital
organi genitali	genitales	genitalia
genito-urinario	genitourinario	genitourinary (GU)
genoma	genoma	genome
genotipo	genotipo	genotype
genere	género	genus
ginocchio valgo	genu valgum	genu valgum
ginocchio varo	genu varum	genu varum
geriatrico	geriátrico	geriatric
geriatra	geriatra	geriatrician
geriatria	geriatría	geriatrics
germe	gérmen	germ
rosolia	rubéola	German measles
gestazione	gestación	gestation
arterite a cellule giganti	arteritis de células gigantes	giant cell arteritis
giardiasi	giardiasis	giardiasis
stordito, affetto da vertigini o cupogiro	mareado	giddy
gengiva	encía	gingiva
gengivite	gingivitis	gingivitis
cintura	cintura	girdle
ghiandola	glándula	gland
mononucleosi infettiva	fiebre glandular	glandular fever
glaucoma	glaucoma	glaucoma
gleno-omerale	glenohumeral	glenohumeral
glenoide	glenoide	glenoid
glioma	glioma	glioma
bolo isterico	globo histérico	globus hystericus
volume di filtrazione glomerulare (VFG)	tasa de filtración glomerular (FG)	glomerular filtration rate (GFR)
glomerulite	glomerulitis	glomerulitis
glomerulonefrite	glomerulonefritis	glomerulonephritis
glomerulosclerosi	glomerulosclerosis	glomerulosclerosis
glomerulo	glomérulo	glomerulus
lingua	lengua	glossa
glossite	glositis	glossitis
glossodinia	glosodinia	glossodynia
glossofaringeo	glosofaríngeo	glossopharyngeal
glottide	glotis	glottis
glucagone	glucagón	glucagon
glicocorticoide	glucocorticoide	glucocorticoid
glucogenesi	glucogénesis	glucogenesis
gluconeogenesi	gluconeogénesis	gluconeogenesis
glucosio	glucosa	glucose

ENGLISH	FRENCH	GERMAN
glucose insulin tolerance test (GITT)	épreuve de tolérance au glucose et à l'insuline	Glukose-Insulin-Toleranztest
glucose tolerance test (GTT)	épreuve d'hyperglycémie provoquée	Glukose-Toleranztest
glue ear	otite moyenne adhésive	glue ear
glue sniffing	intoxication par inhalation de solvant	Schnüffeln, Leimschnüffeln
gluteal	fessier	gluteal
gluten	gluten	Gluten
gluten-induced enteropathy	maladie coeliaque	Zöliakie
gluteus muscles	muscles fessiers	Glutealmuskulatur, Gesäßmuskulatur
glycogenesis	glycogenèse	Glykogenese
glycolysis	glycolyse	Glykolyse, Glukoseabbau
glycosuria	glycosurie	Glykosurie, Glukoseausscheidung im Urin
goiter (Am)	goitre	Struma, Kropf
goitre (Eng)	goitre	Struma, Kropf
gonad	gonade	Gonade
gonadotrophin (Eng)	gonadotrophine	Gonadotropin
gonadotropin (Am)	gonadotrophine	Gonadotropin
gonorrhea (Am)	gonorrhée	Gonorrhoe, Tripper
gonorrhoea (Eng)	gonorrhée	Gonorrhoe, Tripper
gout	goutte	Gicht
Graafian follicle	follicule de De Graaf	Graaf-Follikel
graft (n)	greffe (n)	Transplantat (n), Transplantation (n), Plastik (n)
graft (v)	greffer (v)	transplantieren (v), übertragen (v)
Gram stain	coloration de Gram	Gramfärbung
grand mal	grand mal	Grand mal
granulation	granulation	Granulation
granulocyte	granulocyte	Granulozyt
granuloma	granulome	Granulom, Granulationsgeschwulst
Graves' disease	goitre exophtalmique	Basedow-Krankheit
gravitational	gravitationnel	Gravitations-
gravity	gravité	Schwere (der Erkrankung)
greenstick fracture	fracture incomplète	Grünholzfraktur
gripe	colique	Kolik, Bauchschmerzen
groin	aine	Leiste
grommet	grommet	Öse
growth	croissance	Wachstum, Zunahme, Geschwulst, Tumor
growth hormone (GH)	hormone de croissance (HGH), somatotrophine (STH)	Wachstumshormon
gullet	oesophage	Speiseröhre
gumma	gomme	Gumma
gut	intestin	Darm
Guthrie test	test de Guthrie	Guthrie-Test
gynaecology (Eng)	gynécologie	Gynäkologie, Frauenheilkunde
gynaecomastia (Eng)	gynécomastie	Gynäkomastie

ITALIAN	SPANISH	ENGLISH
test insulinico di tolleranza al glucosio	prueba de resistencia a la insulina	**glucose insulin tolerance test (GITT)**
test di tolleranza al glucosio (TTG)	prueba de tolerancia a la glucosa	**glucose tolerance test (GTT)**
cerume nell orecchio	otitis media exudativa crónica, tapon de oído	**glue ear**
inalazione di toluene o collanti	inhalación de pegamento	**glue sniffing**
gluteo	glúteo	**gluteal**
glutine	gluten	**gluten**
enteropatia da glutine	enteropatía provocada por glúten	**gluten-induced enteropathy**
muscoli glutei	músculos glúteos	**gluteus muscles**
glicogenesi	glucogénesis	**glycogenesis**
glicolisi	glucolisis	**glycolysis**
glicosuria	glucosuria	**glycosuria**
gozzo	bocio	**goiter** (Am)
gozzo	bocio	**goitre** (Eng)
gonade	gónada	**gonad**
gonadotropina	gonadotropina	**gonadotrophin** (Eng)
gonadotropina	gonadotropina	**gonadotropin** (Am)
gonorrea	gonorrea	**gonorrhea** (Am)
gonorrea	gonorrea	**gonorrhoea** (Eng)
gotta	gota	**gout**
follicolo di Graaf	folículo de De Graaf	**Graafian follicle**
trapianto (n), innesto (n)	injerto (n)	**graft** (n)
trapiantare (v)	injertar (v)	**graft** (v)
colorazione di Gram	tinción de Gram	**Gram stain**
grande male	gran mal	**grand mal**
granulazione	granulación	**granulation**
granulocita	granulocito	**granulocyte**
granuloma	granuloma	**granuloma**
morbo di Graves	enfermedad de Graves	**Graves' disease**
gravitazionale	gestacional	**gravitational**
gravità	gravedad	**gravity**
frattura a legno verde	fractura en tallo verde	**greenstick fracture**
colica addominale	cólico intestinal	**gripe**
inguine	ingle	**groin**
catetere per drenaggio auricolare	cánula ótica	**grommet**
crescita	crecimiento	**growth**
ormone della crescita (GH)	hormona del crecimiento (HC)	**growth hormone (GH)**
esofago (gola)	gaznate	**gullet**
gomma	goma	**gumma**
intestino	intestino	**gut**
test di Guthrie per la fenilchetonuria	prueba de Guthrie	**Guthrie test**
ginecologia	ginecología	**gynaecology** (Eng)
ginecomastia	ginecomastia	**gynaecomastia** (Eng)

ENGLISH	FRENCH	GERMAN
gynecology (Am)	gynécologie	Gynäkologie, Frauenheilkunde
gynecomastia (Am)	gynécomastie	Gynäkomastie
gypsum	gypse	Gips

ITALIAN	SPANISH	ENGLISH
ginecologia	ginecología	**gynecology** (Am)
ginecomastia	ginecomastia	**gynecomastia** (Am)
gesso, solfato di calcio	yeso	**gypsum**

H

ENGLISH	FRENCH	GERMAN
H2 antagonist	antagoniste H2	H2-Antagonist
habit	habitude	Gewohnheit
habituation	accoutumance	Habituation, Gewöhnung
haemangioma (Eng)	hémangiome	Hämangiom
haemarthrosis (Eng)	hémarthrose	Hämarthros
haematemesis (Eng)	hématémèse	Hämatemesis, Bluterbrechen
haematocolpos (Eng)	hématocolpos	Hämatokolpos
haematocrit (Eng)	hématocrite	Hämatokrit (HKT)
haematology (Eng)	hématologie	Hämatologie
haematoma (Eng)	hématome	Hämatom, Bluterguß
haematuria (Eng)	hématurie	Hämaturie, Blut im Urin
haemochromatosis (Eng)	hémochromatose	Hämochromatose, Bronzediabetes
haemodialysis (Eng)	hémodialyse	Hämodialyse
haemoglobin (Hb) (Hg) (Eng)	hémoglobine (Hb) (Hg)	Hämoglobin
haemoglobinopathy (Eng)	hémoglobinopathie	Hämoglobinopathie
haemoglobinuria (Eng)	hémoglobinurie	Hämoglobinurie
haemolysis (Eng)	hémolyse	Hämolyse
haemolytic disease of the newborn (HDN) (Eng)	hémolyse des nouveau-nés	Morbus haemolyticus neonatorum
haemolytic uraemic syndrome (HUS) (Eng)	hémolyse urémique des nouveau-nés	hämolytisch-urämisches Syndrom
haemopericardium (Eng)	hémopéricarde	Hämatoperikard
haemoperitoneum (Eng)	hémopéritoine	Hämatoperitoneum
haemophilia (Eng)	hémophilie	Hämophilie, Bluterkrankheit
haemopneumothorax (Eng)	hémopneumothorax	Hämatopneumothorax
haemopoiesis (Eng)	hémopoïèse	Hämatopoese
haemoptysis (Eng)	hémoptysie	Hämoptoe, Bluthusten
haemorrhage (Eng)	hémorragie	Hämorrhagie, Blutung
haemorrhagic disease of the newborn (Eng)	hémorragies des nouveau-nés	Morbus haemorrhagicus neonatorum
haemorrhoid (Eng)	hémorroïde	Hämorrhoide
haemorrhoidectomy (Eng)	hémorroïdectomie	Hämorrhoidektomie, Hämorrhoidenoperation
haemostasis (Eng)	hémostase	Hämostase, Blutgerinnung
haemothorax (Eng)	hémothorax	Hämatothorax
hair	poil	Haar
halitosis	halitose	Foetor ex ore, Mundgeruch
hallucination	hallucination	Halluzination
hallux	hallux	Hallux, Großzeh
hamstring	tendon du jarret	Kniesehne
hand	main	Hand
handicap	handicapé	Behinderung
harelip	bec-de-lièvre	Hasenscharte
Harrington rod	tige de Harrington	Harrington Stab
Hartmann's solution	liquide de Hartmann	Hartmann-Lösung
Hashimoto's disease	maladie d'Hashimoto	Hashimoto-Struma

ITALIAN	SPANISH	ENGLISH
antagonista H2	antagonista H2	**H2 antagonist**
abitudine	hábito	**habit**
assuefazione	habituación	**habituation**
emangioma	hemangioma	**haemangioma** (Eng)
emartrosi	hemartrosis	**haemarthrosis** (Eng)
ematemesi	hematemesis	**haematemesis** (Eng)
ematocolpo	hematocolpos	**haematocolpos** (Eng)
ematrocrito	hematócrito	**haematocrit** (Eng)
ematologia	hematología	**haematology** (Eng)
ematoma	hematoma	**haematoma** (Eng)
ematuria	hematuria	**haematuria** (Eng)
emocromatosi	hemocromatosis	**haemochromatosis** (Eng)
emodialisi	hemodiálisis	**haemodialysis** (Eng)
emoglobina (E)	hemoglobina (Hb)	**haemoglobin (Hb) (Hg)** (Eng)
emoglobinopatia	hemoglobinopatía	**haemoglobinopathy** (Eng)
emoglobinuria	hemoglobinuria	**haemoglobinuria** (Eng)
emolisi	hemólisis	**haemolysis** (Eng)
ittero dei neonati, eritroblastosi fetale (da incompatibilità Rh)	enfermedad hemolítica del recién nacido	**haemolytic disease of the newborn (HDN)** (Eng)
sindrome emolitico-uremica	síndrome hemolítico urémico	**haemolytic uraemic syndrome (HUS)** (Eng)
emopericardio	hemopericardio	**haemopericardium** (Eng)
emoperitoneo	hemoperitoneo	**haemoperitoneum** (Eng)
emofilia	hemofilia	**haemophilia** (Eng)
emopneumotorace	hemoneumotórax	**haemopneumothorax** (Eng)
ematopoiesi	hemopoyesis	**haemopoiesis** (Eng)
cartilagine costale	hemoptisis	**haemoptysis** (Eng)
emorragia	hemorragia	**haemorrhage** (Eng)
malattia emorragica del neonato	enfermedad hemorrágica neonatal	**haemorrhagic disease of the newborn** (Eng)
emorroide	hemorroide	**haemorrhoid** (Eng)
emorroidectomia	hemorroidectomía	**haemorrhoidectomy** (Eng)
emostasi	hemostasis	**haemostasis** (Eng)
emotorace	hemotórax	**haemothorax** (Eng)
pelo, capello	pelo	**hair**
alitosi	halitosis	**halitosis**
allucinazione	alucinación	**hallucination**
alluce	dedo gordo del pie	**hallux**
tendine del ginocchio	tendón del hueso poplíteo	**hamstring**
mano	mano	**hand**
handicappato, minorato	disminución, minusvalía	**handicap**
labbro leporino	labio leporino	**harelip**
bastoncello retiníco (per anestetizzare la dentina)	varilla de Harrington	**Harrington rod**
soluzione di Hartmann	solución de Hartmann	**Hartmann's solution**
tiroidite di Hashimoto	enfermedad de Hashimoto	**Hashimoto's disease**

ENGLISH	FRENCH	GERMAN
hay fever	rhume des foins	Heuschnupfen
head	tête	Kopf
headache	mal de tête, céphalée	Kopfschmerzen
Heaf test	cuti-réaction de Heaf	Heaf-Test
healing	curatif	Heilung
health	santé	Gesundheit
hearing	audition	Gehör, Hören
hearing test	test auditif	Hörtest
heart	coeur	Herz
heartbeat	pulsation (de coeur)	Herzschlag
heartburn	aigreurs	Sodbrennen
heart disease	insuffisance cardiaque	Herzerkrankung, Herzleiden
heart failure	cardiopathie, maladie du coeur	Herzinsuffizienz, Herzversagen
heart-lung machine	poumon d'acier	Herzlungenmaschine
heat exhaustion	échauffement	Hitzschlag
heatstroke	coup de chaleur	Hitzschlag
hebephrenia	hébéphrénie	Hebephrenie
heel	talon	Ferse
hemangioma (Am)	hémangiome	Hämangiom
hemarthrosis (Am)	hémarthrose	Hämarthros
hematemesis (Am)	hématémèse	Hämatemesis, Bluterbrechen
hematocolpos (Am)	hématocolpos	Hämatokolpos
hematocrit (Am)	hématocrite	Hämatokrit (HKT)
hematology (Am)	hématologie	Hämatologie
hematoma (Am)	hématome	Hämatom, Bluterguß
hematuria (Am)	hématurie	Hämaturie, Blut im Urin
hemicolectomy	hémicolectomie	Hemikolektomie
hemiparesis	hémiparésie	Hemiparese, unvollständige Halbseitenlähmung
hemiplegia	hémiplégie	Hemiplegie, Halbseitenlähmung
hemochromatosis (Am)	hémochromatose	Hämochromatose, Bronzediabetes
hemodialysis (Am)	hémodialyse	Hämodialyse
hemoglobin (Hb) (Hg) (Am)	hémoglobine (Hb) (Hg)	Hämoglobin
hemoglobinopathy (Am)	hémoglobinopathie	Hämoglobinopathie
hemoglobinuria (Am)	hémoglobinurie	Hämoglobinurie
hemolysis (Am)	hémolyse	Hämolyse
hemolytic disease of the newborn (HDN) (Am)	hémolyse des nouveau-nés	Morbus haemolyticus neonatorum
hemolytic uremic syndrome (HUS) (Am)	hémolyse urémique des nouveau-nés	hämolytisch-urämisches Syndrom
hemopericardium (Am)	hémopéricarde	Hämatoperikard
hemoperitoneum (Am)	hémopéritoine	Hämatoperitoneum
hemophilia (Am)	hémophilie	Hämophilie, Bluterkrankheit
hemopneumothorax (Am)	hémopneumothorax	Hämatopneumothorax
hemopoiesis (Am)	hémopoïèse	Hämatopoese
hemoptysis (Am)	hémoptysie	Hämoptoe, Bluthusten
hemorrhage (Am)	hémorragie	Hämorrhagie, Blutung

ITALIAN	SPANISH	ENGLISH
febbre da fieno, raffreddore da fieno	fiebre del heno	**hay fever**
testa	cabeza	**head**
mal di testa	cefalea	**headache**
test alla tubercolina	prueba de Heaf	**Heaf test**
cicatrizzazione, guarigione	curación	**healing**
salute	salud	**health**
udito	oído	**hearing**
test audiometrici	prueba auditiva	**hearing test**
cuore	corazón	**heart**
battito cardiaco	patido cardíaco	**heartbeat**
pirosi	ardor de estómago, pirosis	**heartburn**
malattia cardiaca	cardiopatía	**heart disease**
scompenso cardiaco	insuficiencia cardíaca	**heart failure**
macchina cuore-polmone	máquina de circulación extracorpórea	**heart-lung machine**
collasso da colpo di calore	agotamiento por calor	**heat exhaustion**
colpo di calore	insolación	**heatstroke**
ebefrenia	hebefrenia	**hebephrenia**
tallone	talón	**heel**
emangioma	hemangioma	**hemangioma** (Am)
emartrosi	hemartrosis	**hemarthrosis** (Am)
ematemesi	hematemesis	**hematemesis** (Am)
ematocolpo	hematocolpos	**hematocolpos** (Am)
ematrocrito	hematócrito	**hematocrit** (Am)
ematologia	hematología	**hematology** (Am)
ematoma	hematoma	**hematoma** (Am)
ematuria	hematuria	**hematuria** (Am)
emicolectomia	hemocolectomía	**hemicolectomy**
emiparesi	hemiparesia	**hemiparesis**
emiplegia	hemiplejía	**hemiplegia**
emocromatosi	hemocromatosis	**hemochromatosis** (Am)
emodialisi	hemodiálisis	**hemodialysis** (Am)
emoglobina (E)	hemoglobina (Hb)	**hemoglobin (Hb) (Hg)** (Am)
emoglobinopatia	hemoglobinopatía	**hemoglobinopathy** (Am)
emoglobinuria	hemoglobinuria	**hemoglobinuria** (Am)
emolisi	hemólisis	**hemolysis** (Am)
ittero dei neonati, eritroblastosi fetale (da incompatibilità Rh)	enfermedad hemolítica del recién nacido	**hemolytic disease of the newborn (HDN)** (Am)
sindrome emolitico-uremica	síndrome hemolítico urémico	**hemolytic uremic syndrome (HUS)** (Am)
emopericardio	hemopericardio	**hemopericardium** (Am)
emoperitoneo	hemoperitoneo	**hemoperitoneum** (Am)
emofilia	hemofilia	**hemophilia** (Am)
emopneumotorace	hemoneumotórax	**hemopneumothorax** (Am)
ematopoiesi	hemopoyesis	**hemopoiesis** (Am)
cartilagine costale	hemoptisis	**hemoptysis** (Am)
emorragia	hemorragia	**hemorrhage** (Am)

ENGLISH	FRENCH	GERMAN
hemorrhagic disease of the newborn (Am)	hémorragies des nouveau-nés	Morbus haemorrhagicus neonatorum
hemorrhoid (Am)	hémorroïde	Hämorrhoide
hemorrhoidectomy (Am)	hémorroïdectomie	Hämorrhoidektomie, Hämorrhoidenoperation
hemostasis (Am)	hémostase	Hämostase, Blutgerinnung
hemothorax (Am)	hémothorax	Hämatothorax
Henoch-Schönlein purpura	purpura rhumatoïde	Purpura Schönlein-Henoch
hepatic	hépatique	hepatisch, Leber-
hepatitis	hépatite	Hepatitis
hepatocellular	hépatocellulaire	hepatozellulär
hepatoma	hépatome	Hepatom
hepatomegaly	hépatomégalie	Hepatomegalie
hepatosplenomegaly	hépatosplénomégalie	Hepatosplenomegalie
hepatotoxic	hépatotoxique	leberschädigend
hereditary	héréditaire	hereditär, erblich
heredity	hérédité	Erblichkeit, Vererbung
hermaphrodite	hermaphrodite	Hermaphrodit, Zwitter
hernia	hernie	Hernie, Bruch
herniorraphy	herniorrhaphie	Bruchoperation
herniotomy	herniotomie	Herniotomie
herpes	herpès	Herpes, Bläschenausschlag
herpes-like virus (HLV)	virus de type herpétique (HLV)	Herpes-ähnlicher Virus
herpes simplex virus (HSV)	virus de l'herpès simplex (HSV)	Herpes simplex-Virus (HSV)
heterogenous	hétérogène	heterogen
heterosexual	hétérosexuel	heterosexuell
hiccup	hoquet	Schluckauf
hidrosis	transpiration	Hidrosis, Schweißabsonderung
high density lipoprotein (HDL)	lipoprotéine de haute densité (LHD)	high density lipoprotein (HDL)
high density lipoprotein cholesterol (HDLC)	cholestérol composé de lipoprotéines de haute densité	high density lipoprotein-cholesterol (HDL-Cholesterol)
hilum	hile	Hilus
hip	hanche	Hüfte
hip bone	os coxal	Hüftknochen
Hirschsprung's disease	maladie de Hirschsprung	Hirschsprung-Krankheit
hirsuties	hirsutisme	Hirsutismus
hirsutism	hirsutisme	Hirsutismus
histiocyte	histiocyte	Histiozyt
histiocytoma	histiocytome	Histiozytom
histocompatibility antigen	antigène d'histocompatibilité	Histokompatibilitäts-Antigen
histology	histologie	Histologie
histolysis	histolyse	Histolyse
hives	éruption	Ausschlag, Nesselfieber
Hodgkin's disease	maladie de Hodgkin	Morbus Hodgkin
homeopathy (Am)	homéopathie	Homöopathie
homeostasis	homéostasie	Homöostase
homicide	homicide	Totschlag, Mord
homoeopathy (Eng)	homéopathie	Homöopathie

malattia emorragica del neonato	enfermedad hemorrágica neonatal	hemorrhagic disease of the newborn (Am)
emorroide	hemorroide	hemorrhoid (Am)
emorroidectomia	hemorroidectomía	hemorrhoidectomy (Am)
emostasi	hemostasis	hemostasis (Am)
emotorace	hemotórax	hemothorax (Am)
porpora di Schönlein-Henoch	púrpura de Schönlein-Henoch	Henoch-Schönlein purpura
epatico	hepático	hepatic
epatite	hepatitis	hepatitis
epatocellulare	hepatocelular	hepatocellular
epatoma	hepatoma	hepatoma
epatomegalia	hepatomegalia	hepatomegaly
epatosplenomegalia	hepatosplenomegalia	hepatosplenomegaly
epatotossico	hepatotóxico	hepatotoxic
ereditario	hereditario	hereditary
eredità	herencia	heredity
ermafrodito	hermafrodita	hermaphrodite
ernia	hernia	hernia
erniorrafia	herniorrafia	herniorraphy
erniotomia	herniotomía	herniotomy
herpes	herpes	herpes
virus della famiglia dell'herpes	virus semejante al del herpes (HLV)	herpes-like virus (HLV)
virus herpes simplex	virus del herpes simple (VHS)	herpes simplex virus (HSV)
eterogenico	heterogéneo	heterogenous
eterosessuale	heterosexual	heterosexual
singhiozzo	hipo	hiccup
idrosi, sudorazione	hidrosis	hidrosis
lipoproteina ad alta densità (LAD)	lipoproteína de alta densidad (HDL)	high density lipoprotein (HDL)
colesterolo legato a lipoproteina ad alta densità	colesterol unido a las lipoproteínas de alta densidad (HDLC)	high density lipoprotein cholesterol (HDLC)
ilo	hilio	hilum
anca	cadera	hip
osso iliaco	hueso coxal o ilíaco	hip bone
malattia di Hirschsprung	enfermedad de Hirschsprung	Hirschsprung's disease
irsutismo	hirsutismo	hirsuties
irsutismo	hirsutismo	hirsutism
istiocito	histiocito	histiocyte
istiocitoma	histiocitoma	histiocytoma
antigene di istocompatibilità	antígeno de histocompatibilidad	histocompatibility antigen
istologia	histología	histology
istolisi	histólisis	histolysis
orticaria	urticaria	hives
malattia di Hodgkin	enfermedad de Hodgkin	Hodgkin's disease
omeopatia	homeopatía	homeopathy (Am)
omeostasi	homeostasis	homeostasis
omicidio	homicidio	homicide
omeopatia	homeopatía	homoeopathy (Eng)

ENGLISH	FRENCH	GERMAN
homogeneous (Eng)	homogène	homogen
homogenous (Am)	homogène	homogen
homologous	homologue	homolog
homonymous	homonyme	homonym
homosexual (n)	homosexuel (n)	Homosexueller (n)
homosexual (a)	homosexuel (a)	homosexuell (a)
homovanillic acid (HVA)	acide homovanillique	Homovanillinsäure
homozygous	homozygote	homozygot
hookworm	ankylostome	Hakenwurm
hormone	hormone	Hormon
hormone replacement therapy (HRT)	traitement hormonal substitutif, hormonothérapie supplétive	Hormonsubstitutionstherapie
Horner's syndrome	syndrome de Bernard-Horner, syndrome oculaire sympathique	Horner-Syndrom
hospice	hospice, asile	Hospiz
hospital	hôpital	Krankenhaus, Hospital
host	hôte	Wirt
human chorionic gonadotrophin (HCG) (Eng)	gonadotrophine chorionique humaine (GCH)	Choriongonadotropin (HCG)
human chorionic gonadotropin (HCG) (Am)	gonadotrophine chorionique humaine (GCH)	Choriongonadotropin (HCG)
human chorionic somatomammotrophin (HCS) (Eng)	somatomammotropine chorionique humaine (HCS), somatoprolactine	human chorionic somatomammotropin (HCS)
human chorionic somatomammotropin (HCS, HPL) (Am)	somatomammotropine chorionique humaine (HCS), somatoprolactine	human chorionic somatomammotropin (HCS)
human erythrocyte antigen (HEA)	antigène humain des erythrocytes	menschliches Erythrozyten-Antigen
human gamma globulin (HGG)	gamma-globuline humaine (GGH), globuline humaine	Human-Gammaglobulin
human immunodeficiency virus (HIV)	virus de l'immunodéficience humaine	human immunodeficiency virus (HIV), AIDS-Virus
human lymphocytic antigen (HLA)	antigène lymphocytaire humain	human lymphocytic antigen (HLA)
human T-cell leukaemia virus (HTLV) (Eng)	leucémie humaine à lymphocytes T	human T-cell leukemia virus (HTLV)
human T-cell leukemia virus (HTLV) (Am)	leucémie humaine à lymphocytes T	human T-cell leukemia virus (HTLV)
humerus	humérus	Humerus, Oberarmknochen
hunger	faim	Hunger
Huntington's chorea	chorée de Huntington	Chorea Huntington
hyaline membrane disease	maladie des membranes hyalines	Hyalinmembrankrankheit
hyalitis	hyalite	Hyalitis
hyaloid	hyaloïde	Glaskörper-
hydatid	kyste hydatique	Hydatide
hydatidiform mole	hydatidiforme	Blasenmole
hydramnios	hydramnios	Hydramnion
hydrate (n)	hydrate (n)	Hydrat (n)
hydrate (v)	hydrater (v)	hydrieren (v), hydratisieren (v)
hydrocele	hydrocèle	Hydrozele, Wasserbruch
hydrocephalus	hydrocéphale	Hydrozephalus
hydrolysis	hydrolyse	Hydrolyse

ITALIAN	SPANISH	ENGLISH
omogeneo	homogéneo	homogeneous (Eng)
omogeneo	homogéneo	homogenous (Am)
omologo	homólogo	homologous
omonimo	homónimo	homonymous
omosessuale (n)	homosexual (n)	homosexual (n)
omosessuale (a)	homosexual (a)	homosexual (a)
acido omovanillico	ácido homovaníllico	homovanillic acid (HVA)
omozigote	homocigoto	homozygous
strongiloide	anquilostoma duodenal	hookworm
ormone	hormona	hormone
terapia sostitutiva ormonale	terapéutica de reposición de hormonas	hormone replacement therapy (HRT)
sindrome di Horner	síndrome de Horner	Horner's syndrome
ricovero	hospicio	hospice
ospedale	hospital	hospital
ospite	huésped	host
gonadotropina corionica umana (GCU)	gonadotropina coriónica humana (GCH)	human chorionic gonadotrophin (HCG) (Eng)
gonadotropina corionica umana (GCU)	gonadotropina coriónica humana (GCH)	human chorionic gonadotropin (HCG) (Am)
somatomammotropina corionica umana	somatomamotropina corionica humana	human chorionic somatomammotrophin (HCS) (Eng)
somatomammotropina corionica umana	somatomamotropina corionica humana	human chorionic somatomammotropin (HCS, HPL) (Am)
antigene eritrocitico umano	antígeno eritrocitario humano	human erythrocyte antigen (HEA)
gammaglobulina umana	gammaglobulina humana	human gamma globulin (HGG)
virus dell'immunodeficienza umana (HIV)	virus de la inmunodeficiencia humana (VIH)	human immunodeficiency virus (HIV)
antigene linfocitario umano	antígeno linfocitario humano (HLA)	human lymphocytic antigen (HLA)
virus della leucemia a cellule T	leucemia por virus humano de las células T	human T-cell leukaemia virus (HTLV) (Eng)
virus della leucemia a cellule T	leucemia por virus humano de las células T	human T-cell leukemia virus (HTLV) (Am)
omero	húmero	humerus
fame	hambre	hunger
corea di Huntington	corea de Huntington	Huntington's chorea
malattia delle membrane ialine	enfermedad de la membrana hialina	hyaline membrane disease
ialinite	hialitis	hyalitis
ialoideo	hialoide	hyaloid
cisti idatidea	quiste hidatídico	hydatid
idatiforme	mola hidatidiforme	hydatidiform mole
idramnios	hidramnios	hydramnios
idrato (n)	hidrato (n)	hydrate (n)
idratare (v)	hidratar (v)	hydrate (v)
idrocele	hidrocele	hydrocele
idrocefalo	hidrocéfalo	hydrocephalus
idrolisi	hidrólisis	hydrolysis

ENGLISH	FRENCH	GERMAN
hydronephrosis	hydronéphrose	Hydronephrose
hydrops fetalis	anasarque foeto-placentaire	Hydrops fetalis
hydrosalpinx	hydrosalpinx	Hydrosalpinx
hygiene	hygiène	Hygiene
hygroma	hygroma	Hygrom
hymen	hymen	Hymen
hymenectomy	hymenectomie	Hymenektomie
hyoid	hyoïde	(os) hyeoideum
hyperacidity	hyperacidité	Hyperazidität
hyperactivity	hyperactivité	Überaktivität
hyperaemia (Eng)	hyperémie	Hyperämie
hyperaesthesia (Eng)	hyperesthésie	Hyperästhesie
hyperalgesia	hyperalgie, hyperalgésie	Hyperalgesie
hyperbaric oxygen treatment	oxygénothérapie hyperbase	hyperbare Sauerstoffbehandlung
hyperbilirubinaemia (Eng)	hyperbilirubinémie	Hyperbilirubinämie
hyperbilirubinemia (Am)	hyperbilirubinémie	Hyperbilirubinämie
hypercalcaemia (Eng)	hypercalcémie	Hyperkalzämie
hypercalcemia (Am)	hypercalcémie	Hyperkalzämie
hypercalciuria	hypercalciurie	Hyperkalziurie
hypercapnia	hypercapnie	Hyperkapnie
hypercholesterolaemia (Eng)	hypercholestérolémie	Hypercholesterinämie
hypercholesterolemia (Am)	hypercholestérolémie	Hypercholesterinämie
hyperemesis	hyperémèse	Hyperemesis
hyperemia (Am)	hyperémie	Hyperämie
hyperesthesia (Am)	hyperesthésie	Hyperästhesie
hyperextension	hyperextension	Überdehnung, Überstreckung
hyperflexion	hyperflexion	Hyperflexion
hyperglycaemia (Eng)	hyperglycémie	Hyperglykämie
hyperglycemia (Am)	hyperglycémie	Hyperglykämie
hyperidrosis	hyperhidrose	Hyperhidrosis
hyperkalaemia (Eng)	hyperkaliémie	Hyperkaliämie
hyperkalemia (Am)	hyperkaliémie	Hyperkaliämie
hyperkinetic syndrome	syndrome hyperkinétique	hyperkinetisches Syndrom
hyperlipaemia (Eng)	hyperlipémie	Hyperlipämie
hyperlipemia (Am)	hyperlipémie	Hyperlipämie
hyperlipoproteinaemia (Eng)	hyperlipoprotéinémie	Hyperlipoproteinämie
hyperlipoproteinemia (Am)	hyperlipoprotéinémie	Hyperlipoproteinämie
hypermetropia	hypermétropie	Hypermetropie, Weitsichtigkeit
hypernephroma	hypernéphrome	Hypernephrom
hyperparathyroidism	hyperparathyroïdisme	Hyperparathyreoidismus
hyperplasia	hyperplasie	Hyperplasie
hyperpnea (Am)	hyperpnoïa	Hyperpnoe
hyperpnoea (Eng)	hyperpnoïa	Hyperpnoe
hyperpyrexia	hyperpyrexie	Hyperpyrexie
hypersensitive	hypersensibilité	Hypersensibilität, Überempfindlichkeit
hypertelorism	hypertélorisme	Hypertelorismus

ITALIAN	SPANISH	ENGLISH
idronefrosi	hidronefrosis	hydronephrosis
idrope fetale	hydrops fetal	hydrops fetalis
idrosalpinge	hidrosálpinx	hydrosalpinx
igiene	higiene	hygiene
igroma	higroma	hygroma
imene	himen	hymen
imenectomia	himenectomía	hymenectomy
ioide	hioides	hyoid
iperacidità	hiperacidez	hyperacidity
iperattività	hiperactividad	hyperactivity
iperemia	hiperemia	hyperaemia (Eng)
iperestesia	hiperestesia	hyperaesthesia (Eng)
iperalgesia	hiperalgesia	hyperalgesia
ossigenoterapia iperbarica	tratamiento con oxígeno hiperbárico	hyperbaric oxygen treatment
iperbilirubinemia	hiperbilirrubinemia	hyperbilirubinaemia (Eng)
iperbilirubinemia	hiperbilirrubinemia	hyperbilirubinemia (Am)
ipercalcemia	hipercalcemia	hypercalcaemia (Eng)
ipercalcemia	hipercalcemia	hypercalcemia (Am)
ipercalciuria	hipercalciuria	hypercalciuria
ipercapnia	hipercapnia	hypercapnia
ipercolesterolemia	hipercolesterolemia	hypercholesterolaemia (Eng)
ipercolesterolemia	hipercolesterolemia	hypercholesterolemia (Am)
iperemesi	hiperemesis	hyperemesis
iperemia	hiperemia	hyperemia (Am)
iperestesia	hiperestesia	hyperesthesia (Am)
iperestensione	hiperextensión	hyperextension
iperflessione	hiperflexión	hyperflexion
iperglicemia	hiperglucemia	hyperglycaemia (Eng)
iperglicemia	hiperglucemia	hyperglycemia (Am)
iperidrosi	hiperhidrosis	hyperidrosis
iperkaliemia, iperpotassiemia	hipercaliemia	hyperkalaemia (Eng)
iperkaliemia, iperpotassiemia	hipercaliemia	hyperkalemia (Am)
sindrome ipercinetica	síndrome hipercinético	hyperkinetic syndrome
iperlipemia	hiperlipemia	hyperlipaemia (Eng)
iperlipemia	hiperlipemia	hyperlipemia (Am)
iperlipoproteinemia	hiperlipoproteinemia	hyperlipoproteinaemia (Eng)
iperlipoproteinemia	hiperlipoproteinemia	hyperlipoproteinemia (Am)
ipermetropia	hipermetropía	hypermetropia
ipernefroma	hipernefroma	hypernephroma
iperparatiroidismo	hiperparatiroidismo	hyperparathyroidism
iperplasia	hiperplasia	hyperplasia
iperpnea	hiperpnea	hyperpnea (Am)
iperpnea	hiperpnea	hyperpnoea (Eng)
iperpiressia	hiperpirexia	hyperpyrexia
ipersensitività, ipersensibilità	hipersensibilidad	hypersensitive
ipertelorismo	hipertelorismo	hypertelorism

ENGLISH	FRENCH	GERMAN
hypertension	hypertension	Hypertonie
hyperthermia	hyperthermie	Hyperthermie
hyperthyroidism	hyperthyroïdisme	Hyperthyreoidismus,. Schilddrüsenüberfunktion
hypertonia	hypertonie	Hypertension, Hypertonus
hypertonic	hypertonique	hyperton
hypertrophy	hypertrophie	Hypertrophie
hyperventilation	hyperventilation	Hyperventilation
hypervolaemia (Eng)	hypervolémie	Hypervolämie
hypervolemia (Am)	hypervolémie	Hypervolämie
hyphaema (Eng)	hyphéma	Hyphaema
hyphema (Am)	hyphéma	Hyphaema
hypnosis	hypnose	Hypnose
hypnotherapy	hypnothérapie	Hypnotherapie
hypnotic (n)	hypnotique (n)	Schlafmittel (n), Hypnotikum (n)
hypnotic (a)	hypnotique (a)	hypnotisch (a)
hypoaesthesia (Eng)	hypoesthésie, hypesthésie	Hypästhesie
hypocalcaemia (Eng)	hypocalcémie	Hypokalzämie
hypocalcemia (Am)	hypocalcémie	Hypokalzämie
hypocapnia	hypocapnie	Hypokapnie
hypochondria	hypocondrie	Hypochondrie
hypochondrium	hypocondre	Hypochondrium
hypochromic	hypochromique	hypochrom, farbarm
hypodermic	hypodermique	subkutan
hypoesthesia (Am)	hypoesthésie, hypesthésie	Hypästhesie
hypofunction	hypofonction	Unterfunktion
hypogastrium	hypogastre	Hypogastrium
hypoglossal nerve	hypoglosse	Nervus hypoglossus
hypoglycaemia (Eng)	hypoglycémie	Hypoglykämie
hypoglycemia (Am)	hypoglycémie	Hypoglykämie
hypoidrosis	hypohidrose	Hypohidrosis, Schweißmangel
hypokalaemia (Eng)	hypokalémie	Hypokaliämie
hypokalemia (Am)	hypokalémie	Hypokaliämie
hypomania	hypomanie	Hypomanie
hypoparathyroidism	hypoparathyroïdisme	Hypoparathyreoidismus
hypopharynx	hypopharynx	Hypopharynx
hypopituitarism	hypopituitarisme	Hypopituitarismus
hypoplasia	hypoplasie	Hypoplasie
hypopnea (Am)	hypopnée	flache Atmung
hypopnoea (Eng)	hypopnée	flache Atmung
hypoproteinaemia (Eng)	hypoprotéinémie	Hypoproteinämie
hypoproteinemia (Am)	hypoprotéinémie	Hypoproteinämie
hypopyon	hypopyon	Hypopyon
hyposecretion	hyposécrétion	Sekretionsmangel, Sekretionsschwäche
hyposensitive	hyposensibilité	hyposensibel, unterempfindlich
hypospadias	hypospadias	Hypospadie
hypostasis	hypostase	Hypostase

ITALIAN	SPANISH	ENGLISH
ipertensione	hipertensión	**hypertension**
ipertermia	hipertermia	**hyperthermia**
ipertiroidismo	hipertiroidismo	**hyperthyroidism**
ipertonia	hipertonía	**hypertonia**
ipertonico	hipertónico	**hypertonic**
ipertrofia	hipertrofia	**hypertrophy**
iperventilazione	hiperventilación	**hyperventilation**
ipervolemia	hipervolemia	**hypervolaemia** (Eng)
ipervolemia	hipervolemia	**hypervolemia** (Am)
ifema	hipema	**hyphaema** (Eng)
ifema	hipema	**hyphema** (Am)
ipnosi	hipnosis	**hypnosis**
ipnoterapia	hipnoterapia	**hypnotherapy**
ipnotico (n)	hipnótico (n)	**hypnotic** (n)
ipnotico (a)	hipnótico (a)	**hypnotic** (a)
ipoestesia	hipoestesia	**hypoaesthesia** (Eng)
ipocalcemia	hipocalcemia	**hypocalcaemia** (Eng)
ipocalcemia	hipocalcemia	**hypocalcemia** (Am)
ipocapnia	hipocapnia	**hypocapnia**
ipocondria	hipocondría	**hypochondria**
ipocondrio	hipocondrio	**hypochondrium**
ipocromico	hipocrómico	**hypochromic**
ipodermico	hipodérmico	**hypodermic**
ipoestesia	hipoestesia	**hypoesthesia** (Am)
ipofunzione	hipofunción	**hypofunction**
ipogastrio	hipogastrio	**hypogastrium**
ipoglosso	hipogloso	**hypoglossal nerve**
ipoglicemia	hipoglucemia	**hypoglycaemia** (Eng)
ipoglicemia	hipoglucemia	**hypoglycemia** (Am)
ipoidrosi	hipohidrosis	**hypoidrosis**
ipokalemia	hipocaliemia	**hypokalaemia** (Eng)
ipokalemia	hipocaliemia	**hypokalemia** (Am)
ipomania	hipomanía	**hypomania**
ipoparatiroidismo	hipoparatiroidismo	**hypoparathyroidism**
ipofaringe	hipofaringe	**hypopharynx**
ipopituitarismo	hipopituitarismo	**hypopituitarism**
ipoplasia	hipoplasia	**hypoplasia**
ipopnea	hipopnea	**hypopnea** (Am)
ipopnea	hipopnea	**hypopnoea** (Eng)
ipoproteinemia	hipoproteinemia	**hypoproteinaemia** (Eng)
ipoproteinemia	hipoproteinemia	**hypoproteinemia** (Am)
ipopion	hipopión	**hypopyon**
iposecrezione	hiposecreción	**hyposecretion**
iposensitività, iposensibilità	hiposensibilidad	**hyposensitive**
ipospadia	hipospadias	**hypospadias**
ipostasi	hipostasis	**hypostasis**

ENGLISH	FRENCH	GERMAN
hypotension	hypotension	Hypotonie
hypothalamus	hypothalamus	Hypothalamus
hypothenar eminence	éminence hypothénar	Antithenar
hypothermia	hypothermie	Hypothermie
hypothyroidism	hypothyroïdisme	Hypothyreose
hypotonia	hypotonie	Hypotonie
hypotonic	hypotonique	hypoton
hypoventilation	hypoventilation	Hypoventilation
hypovolaemia (Eng)	hypovolémie	Hypovolämie
hypovolemia (Am)	hypovolémie	Hypovolämie
hypoxaemia (Eng)	hypoxémie	Hypoxämie
hypoxemia (Am)	hypoxémie	Hypoxämie
hypoxia	hypoxie	Hypoxie
hysterectomy	hystérectomie	Hysterektomie
hysteria	hystérie	Hysterie
hysterosalpingectomy	hystérosalpingectomie	Hysterosalpingektomie
hysterosalpingography	hystérosalpingographie	Hysterosalpingographie
hysterotomy	hystérotomie	Hysterotomie

ipotensione	hipotensión	**hypotension**
ipotalamo	hipotálamo	**hypothalamus**
eminenza ipotenar	eminencia hipotenar	**hypothenar eminence**
ipotermia	hipotermia	**hypothermia**
ipotiroidismo	hipotiroidismo	**hypothyroidism**
ipotonia	hipotonía	**hypotonia**
ipotonico	hipotónico	**hypotonic**
ipoventilazione	hipoventilación	**hypoventilation**
ipovolemia	hipovolemia	**hypovolaemia** (Eng)
ipovolemia	hipovolemia	**hypovolemia** (Am)
ipossiemia	hipoxemia	**hypoxaemia** (Eng)
ipossiemia	hipoxemia	**hypoxemia** (Am)
ipossia	hipoxia	**hypoxia**
isterectomia	histerectomía	**hysterectomy**
isteria	histeria	**hysteria**
isterosalpingectomia	histerosalpingectomía	**hysterosalpingectomy**
isterosalpingografia	histerosalpingografía	**hysterosalpingography**
isterotomia	histerotomía	**hysterotomy**

I

English	French	German
iatrogenic	iatrogène	iatrogen
ichthyosis	ichthyose	Ichthyosis
icterus	ictère	Ikterus, Gelbsucht
id	ça	Es
idea	idée	Gedanke, Vorstellung
identical twins	jumeaux univitellins	eineiige Zwillinge
identification	identification	Identifizierung
idiopathic	idiopathique	idiopathisch, essentiell
idiosyncrasy	idiosyncrasie	Idiosynkrasie
ileal conduit	conduit iléal	Ileumconduit
ileectomy	iléoctomie	Ileumresektion
ileitis	iléite	Ileitis
ileocaecal (Eng)	iléocaecal	ileozäkal
ileocecal (Am)	iléocaecal	ileozäkal
ileostomy	iléostomie	Ileostomie
ileum	iléon	Ileum
ileus	iléus	Ileus, Darmverschluß
iliac	iliaque	ileo-
ilium	ilion	Os ilium
illness	maladie	Krankheit
illusion	illusion	Illusion
imbalance	déséquilibre	Gleichgewichtsstörung
immediately after onset (IAO)	immédiatement après le début	unmittelbar nach Krankheitsausbruch
immune	immun	immun
immune reaction	réaction immunitaire	Immunreaktion
immunity	immunité	Immunität
immunization	immunisation	Immunisierung, Schutzimpfung
immunoassay	dosage immunologique, immunodosage	Immunoassay
immunocompromised patient	malade à déficit immunitaire	immungestörter Patient
immunodeficiency	immunodéficience	Immundefekt
immunofluorescence	immunofluorescence	Immunfluoreszenz
immunoglobulin (Ig)	immunoglobuline (lg)	Immunglobulin
immunology	immunologie	Immunologie
immunosuppressed patient	malade à suppression immunitaire	immunsupprimierter Patient
immunosuppression	immunosuppression	Immunsuppression
impacted	enclavé	impaktiert
imperforate	imperforé	nicht perforiert
impetigo	impétigo	Impetigo
implant (n)	implant (n)	Implantat (n)
implant (v)	implanter (v)	implantieren (v)
implantation	implantation	Implantation
impotence	impotence	Impotenz

iatrogeno	yatrógeno	**iatrogenic**
ittiosi	ictiosis	**ichthyosis**
ittero	ictericia	**icterus**
incoscio	id	**id**
idea	idea	**idea**
gemelli omozigoti	gemelos idénticos	**identical twins**
indentificazione	identificación	**identification**
idiopatico	idiopático	**idiopathic**
idiosincrasia	idiosincrasia	**idiosyncrasy**
vescica ileale (protesi mediante segmento ileale)	conducto ileal	**ileal conduit**
ileectomia	ileoctomía	**ileectomy**
ileite	ileítis	**ileitis**
ileocecale	ileocecal	**ileocaecal** (Eng)
ileocecale	ileocecal	**ileocecal** (Am)
ileostomia	ileostomía	**ileostomy**
ileo	ileón	**ileum**
ileo, occlusione intestinale acuta	íleo	**ileus**
iliaco	iliaco	**iliac**
ilio, osso dell'anca	ilion	**ilium**
malattia	enfermedad	**illness**
illusione	ilusión	**illusion**
squilibrio	desequilibrio	**imbalance**
immediatamente dopo l'attacco	inmediatamente después del comienzo	**immediately after onset (IAO)**
immune	inmune	**immune**
immunoreazione, reazione immune	reacción inmunológica	**immune reaction**
immunità	inmunidad	**immunity**
immunizzazione	inmunización	**immunization**
dosaggio immunologico	inmunoensayo	**immunoassay**
paziente immunocompromesso	paciente inmunocomprometido	**immunocompromised patient**
immunodeficienza	inmunodeficiencia	**immunodeficiency**
immunofluorescenza	inmunofluorescencia	**immunofluorescence**
immunoglobulina (Ig)	inmunoglobulina (Ig)	**immunoglobulin (Ig)**
immunologia	inmunología	**immunology**
paziente immunosoppresso	paciente inmunosuprimido	**immunosuppressed patient**
immunosoppressione	inmunosupresión	**immunosuppression**
impatto, compresso, incuneato	impactado	**impacted**
imperforato	imperforado	**imperforate**
impetigine	impétigo	**impetigo**
impianto chirurgico sottocutaneo di farmaci (n)	implante (n)	**implant** (n)
impiantare (v)	implantar (v)	**implant** (v)
impianto	implantación	**implantation**
impotenza	impotencia	**impotence**

ENGLISH	FRENCH	GERMAN
impulse	impulsion	Impuls, Reiz
incarcerated	incarcéré	inkarzeriert, eingeklemmt
incest	inceste	Inzest
incidence	fréquence	Inzidenz
incipient	débutant	beginnend
incision	incision	Inzision, Einschnitt
incisor	incisive	Schneidezahn
incompatibility	incompatibilité	Inkompatibilität, Unverträglichkeit
incompetence	incompétence	Insuffizienz
incontinence	incontinence	Inkontinenz
incoordination	incoordination	Inkoordination
incubation	incubation	Inkubation
incubator	incubateur	Inkubator, Brutkasten
incus	enclume	Incus, Amboß
indicator	indicateur	Indikator
indigenous	indigène	eingeboren, einheimisch
indigestion	indigestion	Verdauungsstörung, Magenverstimmung
induced abortion	avortement provoqué	Abtreibung, künstlicher Abort
induction	induction	Induktion, Einleitung
induration	induration	Induration, Verhärtung
industrial disease	maladie professionnelle	Berufskrankheit
inertia	inertie	Trägheitsmoment, Untätigkeit
infant	enfant, nourrisson	Kleinkind, Säugling
infantile	infantile	infantil, kindlich
infarction	infarcissement	Infarzierung
infection	infection	Infektion
infectious disease	maladie infectieuse	Infektionskrankheit
infectious mononucleosis	mononucléose infectieuse	Pfeiffersches Drüsenfieber, infektiöse Mononukleose
infective	infectieux	infektiös, ansteckend
inferior	inférieur	tiefer gelegen, minderwertig
infertility	infertilité	Infertilität
infestation	infestation	Befall
infiltration	infiltration	Infiltration
inflammation	inflammation	Entzündung
influenza	grippe	Influenza, Grippe
infusion	infusion	Infusion
ingestion	ingestion	Einnahme, Aufnahme
inguinal	inguinal	inguinal, Leisten-
inhalation	inhalation	Inhalation, Einatmen
inhale	inhaler	inhalieren, einatmen
inherent	inhérent	eigen, angeboren
inhibition	inhibition	Inhibierung, Hemmung
inject	injecter	injizieren, spritzen
injection	injection	Injektion, Spritze
injury	blessure	Verletzung
innate	endogène	kongenital, angeboren

ITALIAN	SPANISH	ENGLISH
impulso	impulso	**impulse**
incarcerato	incarcerado	**incarcerated**
incesto	incesto	**incest**
incidenza	incidencia	**incidence**
incipiente	incipiente	**incipient**
incisione	incisión	**incision**
incisore	incisivo	**incisor**
incompatibilità	incompatibilidad	**incompatibility**
incompetenza	incompetencia	**incompetence**
incontinenza	incontinencia	**incontinence**
incoordinazione	incoordinación	**incoordination**
incubazione	incubación	**incubation**
incubatore	incubadora	**incubator**
incudine	incus, yunque	**incus**
indicatore	indicador	**indicator**
indigeno	indígena	**indigenous**
indigestione	indigestión	**indigestion**
aborto procurato	aborto inducido	**induced abortion**
induzione	inducción	**induction**
indurimento	Induración	**induration**
malattia industriale	enfermedad industrial	**industrial disease**
inerzia	inercia	**inertia**
infante	lactante	**infant**
infantile	infantil	**infantile**
infarto	infarto	**infarction**
infezione	infección	**infection**
malattia infettiva	enfermedad infecciosa	**infectious disease**
mononucleosi infettiva	mononucleosis infecciosa	**infectious mononucleosis**
infettivo	infeccioso	**infective**
inferiore	inferior	**inferior**
infertilità	infertilidad	**infertility**
infestazione	infestación	**infestation**
infiltrazione	infiltración	**infiltration**
infiammazione	inflamación	**inflammation**
influenza	influenza	**influenza**
infusione	infusión	**infusion**
ingestione	ingestión	**ingestion**
inguinale	inguinal	**inguinal**
inalazione	inhalación	**inhalation**
inalare	inhalar	**inhale**
inerente	inherente	**inherent**
inibizione	inhibición	**inhibition**
iniettare	inyectar	**inject**
iniezione	inyección	**injection**
lesione	lesión	**injury**
innato	innato	**innate**

ENGLISH	FRENCH	GERMAN
innervation	innervation	Innervation
innocent	innocent	unschuldig, unschädlich
innocuous	inoffensif	unschädlich, harmlos
inoculation	inoculation	Impfung
inorganic	inorganique	anorganisch
inotropic	inotrope	inotrop
insanity	aliénation	Geisteskrankheit
insemination	insémination	Befruchtung
insensible	insensible	bewußtlos, unempfindlich
insertion	insertion	Insertion
insidious	insidieux	heimtückisch, schleichend
in situ	in situ	in situ
insomnia	insomnie	Schlaflosigkeit
inspiration	inspiration	Inspiration, Einatmung
inspissated	épaissir	kondensiert, eingedickt
instep	tarse	Fußrücken, Spann
instillation	instillation	Einträufelung, Einflößung
instinct	instinct	Instinkt
institutionalization	institutionalisation	Institutionalisierung
insufflation	insufflation	Insufflation
insulin	insuline	Insulin
insulin dependent diabetes mellitus (IDDM)	diabète sucré insulinodépendant	insulinabhängiger Diabetes mellitus
insulin tolerance test (ITT)	épreuve de tolérance à l'insuline	Insulintoleranztest
intellect	intellect	Intellekt
intelligence	intelligence	Intelligenz
intensive care unit (ICU)	unité de soins intensifs	Intensivstation
intensive therapy unit (ITU)	service de réanimation	Intensivstation
interaction	interaction	Wechselwirkung
interarticular	interarticulaire	interartikulär
intercostal	intercostal	interkostal
intercourse	rapports	Koitus, Geschlechtsverkehr
intercurrent	intercurrent	interkurrent
interleukin	interleukine	Interleukin
intermenstrual	intermenstruel	intermenstruel
intermittent	intermittent	intermittierend
internal	interne	intern, innerlich
interosseous	interosseux	interossär
interspinous	interépineux	interspinal
interstitial	interstitiel	interstitiell
intertrigo	intertrigo	Intertrigo
intertrochanteric	intertrochantérien	intertrochantär
intervertebral	intervertébral	intervertebral, Zwischenwirbel-
intestine	intestin	Darm
intima	intima	Intima
intolerance	intolérance	Intoleranz, Unverträglichkeit
intra-abdominal	intra-abdominal	intraabdominal

ITALIAN	SPANISH	ENGLISH
innervazione	inervación	innervation
innocente	inocente	innocent
innocuo	inocuo	innocuous
inoculazione	inoculación	inoculation
inorganico	inorgánico	inorganic
inotropo	inotrópico	inotropic
pazzia	locura, demencia	insanity
inseminazione	inseminación	insemination
insensibile	insensible	insensible
inserzione	inserción	insertion
insidioso	insidioso	insidious
in situ	in situ	in situ
insonnia	insomnio	insomnia
inspirazione	inspiración	inspiration
inspessito	espesado	inspissated
dorso del piede	empeine	instep
istillazione	instilación	instillation
istinto	instinto	instinct
istituzionalizzazione	institucionalización	institutionalization
insufflazione	insuflación	insufflation
insulina	insulina	insulin
diabete mellito insulinodipendente	diabetes mellitus insulinodependiente	insulin dependent diabetes mellitus (IDDM)
test di tolleranza all' insulina	prueba de la tolerancia a la insulina	insulin tolerance test (ITT)
intelletto	intelecto	intellect
intelligenza	inteligencia	intelligence
unità di cura intensiva	unidad de cuidados intensivos (UCI)	intensive care unit (ICU)
unità di terapia intensiva	unidad de cuidados intensivos (UCI)	intensive therapy unit (ITU)
interazione	interacción	interaction
interarticolare	interarticular	interarticular
intercostale	intercostal	intercostal
coito	coito	intercourse
intercorrente	intercurrente	intercurrent
interleuchina	interleucina	interleukin
intermestruale	intermenstrual	intermenstrual
intermittente	intermitente	intermittent
interno	interno	internal
interosseo	interóseo	interosseous
interspinoso	interespinoso	interspinous
interstiziale	intersticial	interstitial
intertrigine	intertrigo	intertrigo
intertrocanterico	intertrocantéreo	intertrochanteric
intervertebrale	intervertebral	intervertebral
intestino	intestino	intestine
intima	íntima	intima
intolleranza	intolerancia	intolerance
intra-addominale	intraabdominal	intra-abdominal

ENGLISH	FRENCH	GERMAN
intra-arterial	intra-artériel	intraarteriell
intracapsular	intracapsulaire	intrakapsulär
intracellular	intracellulaire	intrazellulär
intracranial pressure (ICP)	pression intracrânienne	Hirndruck, intrakranieller Druck
intradermal	intradermique	intradermal, intrakutan
intramural	intramural	intramural
intramuscular (IM)	intramusculaire (IM)	intramuskulär
intranasal	intranasal	intranasal
intraocular	intra-oculaire	intraokulär
intraoral	intra-oral	intraoral
intrapartum	intrapartum	intra partum
intraperitoneal	intrapéritonéal	intraperitoneal
intrathecal	intrathécal	intrathekal
intrauterine	intra-utérin	intrauterin
intrauterine contraceptive device (IUD, IUCD)	dispositif intra-utérin (DIU), stérilet	Intrauterinpessar (IUP)
intravaginal	intravaginal	intravaginal
intravenous (IV)	intraveineux (IV)	intravenös, endovenös
intravenous pyelogram (IVP)	urographie intraveineuse (UIV)	i.v. - Pyelogramm
intrinsic	intrinsèque	intrinsisch, endogen
introitus	orifice	Introitus
introspection	introspection	Introspektion
introversion	introversion	Introversion
introvert	introverti	Introvertierter
intubation	intubation	Intubation
intussusception	intussusception	Intussuszeption
invagination	invagination	Invagination
invasion	invasion	Invasion
inversion	inversion	Inversion, Umkehrung
in vitro	in vitro	in vitro
in vitro fertilization (IVF)	fertilisation in vitro	In-vitro-Fertilisation
in vivo	in vivo	in vivo
involuntary	involontaire	unabsichtlich, unwillkürlich
involution	involution	Involution, Rückbildung
iodine	iode	Jod
ion	ion	Ion
ipsilateral	ipsilatéral	ipsilateral
iris	iris	Iris
iritis	iritis	Iritis
iron binding capacity (IBC)	pouvoir sidéropexique, capacité de fixation du fer	Eisenbindungskapazität
iron binding protein (IBP)	sidérophyline	eisenbindendes Protein
irradiation	irradiation	Bestrahlung
irreducible	irréductible	unreduzierbar
irrigation	irrigation	Spülung
irritable	irritable	reizbar, erregbar
irritable bowel syndrome	syndrome de l'intestin irritable	Reizdarm
irritant	irritant	reizend

ITALIAN	SPANISH	ENGLISH
intra-arterioso	intraarterial	intra-arterial
intracapsulare	intracapsular	intracapsular
intracellulare	intracelular	intracellular
pressione intracranica	presión intracraneal (PIC)	intracranial pressure (ICP)
intradermico	intradérmico	intradermal
intramurale	intramural	intramural
intramuscolare (IM)	intramuscular (im)	intramuscular (IM)
intranasale	intranasal	intranasal
intraoculare	intraocular	intraocular
intraorale	intraoral	intraoral
intraparto	intra partum	intrapartum
intraperitoneale	intraperitoneal	intraperitoneal
intratecale	intratecal	intrathecal
intrauterino	intrauterino	intrauterine
dispositivo anticoncezionale intrauterino (IUD)	dispositivo intrauterino anticonceptivo (DIU)	intrauterine contraceptive device (IUD, IUCD)
intravaginale	intravaginal	intravaginal
endovenoso (EV)	intravenoso (IV)	intravenous (IV)
pielografia endovenosa (PE)	pielograma intravenoso	intravenous pyelogram (IVP)
intrinseco	intrínseco	intrinsic
introito	introito	introitus
introspezione	introspección	introspection
introversione	introversión	introversion
introverso	introvertido	introvert
intubazione	intubación	intubation
intussuscezione	intususcepción	intussusception
invaginazione	invaginación	invagination
invasione	invasión	invasion
inversione	inversión	inversion
in vitro	in vitro	in vitro
fertilizzazione in vitro	fertilización in vitro (FIV)	in vitro fertilization (IVF)
in vivo	in vivo	in vivo
involontario	involuntario	involuntary
involuzione	involución	involution
iodio	yodo	iodine
ione	ión	ion
ipsilaterale, omolaterale	ipsilateral	ipsilateral
iride	iris	iris
irite	iritis	iritis
capacità di legame del ferro	capacidad de unión con el hierro	iron binding capacity (IBC)
proteina che lega il ferro	proteína de unión con el hierro	iron binding protein (IBP)
irradiazione	irradiación	irradiation
irriducibile	irreductible	irreducible
irrigazione	irrigación	irrigation
irritabile	irritable	irritable
sindrome dell'intestino irritabile	síndrome del intestino irritable	irritable bowel syndrome
irritante	irritante	irritant

ENGLISH	FRENCH	GERMAN
ischaemia (Eng)	ischémie	Ischämie
ischaemic heart disease (IHD) (Eng)	cardiopathie ischémique	ischämische Herzkrankheit (IHK)
ischemia (Am)	ischémie	Ischämie
ischemic heart disease (IHD) (Am)	cardiopathie ischémique	ischämische Herzkrankheit (IHK)
ischiorectal	ischio-rectal	ischiorektal
ischium	ischion	Ischium, Sitzbein
islets of Langerhans	îlots de Langerhans, îlots pancréatiques	Langerhans-Inseln
isoimmunization	iso-immunisation	Isoimmunisierung
isolation	isolement	Isolierung
isometric	isométrique	isometrisch
isotonic	isotonique	isotonisch
isthmus	isthme	Isthmus, Verengung
itch	démangeaison	Jucken

J

jaundice	jaunisse	Ikterus, Gelbsucht
jaw-bone	mâchoire	Kieferknochen
jejunal biopsy	biopsie jéjunale	Jejunumbiopsie
jejunum	jéjunum	Jejunum
joint	articulation	Gelenk
jugular vein	veine jugulaire	Vena jugularis
junk food	aliments non nutritifs	ungesunde Nahrung

ITALIAN	SPANISH	ENGLISH
ischemia	isquemia	**ischaemia** (Eng)
cardiopatia ischemica	cardiopatía isquémica	**ischaemic heart disease (IHD)** (Eng)
ischemia	isquemia	**ischemia** (Am)
cardiopatia ischemica	cardiopatía isquémica	**ischemic heart disease (IHD)** (Am)
ischiorettale	isquiorrectal	**ischiorectal**
ischio	isquión	**ischium**
isole di Langerhans	islotes de Langerhans	**islets of Langerhans**
isoimmunizzazione	isoinmunización	**isoimmunization**
isolamento	aislamiento	**isolation**
isometrico	isométrico	**isometric**
isotonico	isotónico	**isotonic**
istmo	istmo	**isthmus**
prurito	picor	**itch**
ittero	ictericia	**jaundice**
osso mandibolare	mandíbula	**jaw-bone**
biopsia digiunale	biopsia del yeyuno	**jejunal biopsy**
digiuno	yeyuno	**jejunum**
articolazione	articulación	**joint**
vena giugulare	vena yugular	**jugular vein**
cibo contenente additivi chimici	comidas preparadas poco nutritivas	**junk food**

K

kala-azar	kala-azar	Kala-Azar
Kaposi's sarcoma	sarcome de Kaposi	Kaposi-Sarkom
karyotype	karyotype	Karyotyp
keloid	chéloïde	Keloid
keratin	kératine	Keratin
keratinization	kératinisation	Keratinisation, Verhornung
keratitis	kératite	Keratitis, Hornhautentzündung
keratocele	kératocèle	Keratozele
keratoconjunctivitis	kératoconjonctivite	Keratokonjunktivitis
keratomalacia	kératomalacie	Keratomalazie
keratome	kératome	Keratotom
keratosis	kératose	Keratose
kernicterus	ictère cérébral	Kernikterus
Kernig's sign	signe de Kernig	Kernig Zeichen
ketoacidosis	céto-acidose	Ketoazidose
ketogenesis	cétogenèse	Ketogenese
ketogenic diet	régime cétogène	ketogene Ernährung
ketone	cétone	Keton, Ketonkörper
ketonuria	cétonurie	Ketonurie
ketosis	cétose	Ketose
kidney	rein	Niere
kinase	kinase	Kinase
kiss of life	bouche-à-bouche	Mund-zu-Mund-Wiederbelebung
Klinefelter's syndrome	syndrome de Klinefelter	Klinefelter-Syndrom
knee	genou	Knie
knock-knee	genou cagneux	Genu valgum, X-Bein
knuckle	jointure	Knöchel
koilonychia	koïlonychie	Koilonychie, Löffelnagel
Koplik's spots	points de Koplik	Koplik-Flecken
Korsakoff's psychosis	psychose de Korsakoff	Korsakow-Psychose
kraurosis vulvae	kraurosis de la vulve	Craurosis vulvae
Kveim test	test de Kveim	Kveim-Test
kwashiorkor	kwashiorkor	Kwashiorkor
kypholordosis	cypholordose	Kypholordose
kyphoscoliosis	cyphoscoliose	Kyphoskoliose
kyphosis	cyphose	Kyphose

ITALIAN	SPANISH	ENGLISH
kala-azar	kala-azar	**kala-azar**
sarcoma di Kaposi	sarcoma de Kaposi	**Kaposi's sarcoma**
cariotipo	cariotipo	**karyotype**
cheloide	queloide	**keloid**
cheratina	queratina	**keratin**
cheratinizzazione	queratinización	**keratinization**
cheratite	queratitis	**keratitis**
cheratocele	queratocele	**keratocele**
cheratocongiuntivite	queratoconjuntivitis	**keratoconjunctivitis**
cheratomalacia	queratomalacia	**keratomalacia**
cheratomo	queratoma	**keratome**
cheratosi	queratosis	**keratosis**
ittero nucleare	ictericia nuclear	**kernicterus**
segno di Kernig	signo de Kernig	**Kernig's sign**
chetoacidosi	cetoacidosis	**ketoacidosis**
chetogenesi	cetogénesis	**ketogenesis**
dieta chetogenica	dieta cetógena	**ketogenic diet**
chetoni	acetona	**ketone**
chetonuria	cetonuria	**ketonuria**
chetosi	cetosis	**ketosis**
rene	riñón	**kidney**
chinasi	cinasa	**kinase**
respirazione bocca a bocca	beso de vida	**kiss of life**
sindrome di Klinefelter	síndrome de Klinefelter	**Klinefelter's syndrome**
ginocchio	rodilla	**knee**
ginocchio valgo	genu valgum	**knock-knee**
articolazione interfalangea	nudillo	**knuckle**
coilonichia	coiloniquia	**koilonychia**
segni di Koplik	manchas de Koplik	**Koplik's spots**
psicosi di Korsakoff	psicosis de Korsakoff	**Korsakoff's psychosis**
craurosi vulvare	craurosis vulvar	**kraurosis vulvae**
test di Kveim	prueba de Kveim	**Kveim test**
kwashiorkor	kwashiorkor	**kwashiorkor**
cifolordosi	cifolordosis	**kypholordosis**
cifoscoliosi	cifoscoliosis	**kyphoscoliosis**
cifosi	cifosis	**kyphosis**

L

English	French	German
labia	lèvres	Labia
labile	labile	labil
lability	labilité	Labilität
labor (Am)	travail	Wehen
labour (Eng)	travail	Wehen
labyrinth	labyrinthe	Labyrinth
labyrinthitis	labyrinthite	Labyrinthitis
lacerated	lacéré	eingerissen, zerrissen
lacrimal	lacrymal	Tränen-, Tränengangs-
lactase	lactase	Laktase
lactate	lactate	Laktat
lactation	lactation	Laktation, Milchbildung, Stillen
lactic acid	acide lactique	Milchsäure
lactose	lactose	Laktose, Milchzucker
lactulose	lactulose	Laktulose
lamina	lame	Lamina
laminectomy	laminectomie	Laminektomie, Wirbelbogenresektion
Lancefield's groups	groupes de streptocoques suivant la classification de Lancefield	Lancefield-Gruppen
lanugo	lanugo	Lanugo
laparoscopy	coelioscopie	Laparoskopie, Bauchspiegelung
laparotomy	laparotomie	Laparotomie
laryngeal	laryngien	laryngeal, Kehlkopf-
laryngitis	laryngite	Laryngitis
laryngology	laryngologie	Laryngologie
laryngoscope	laryngoscope	Laryngoskop, Kehlkopfspiegel
laryngospasm	laryngospasme	Laryngospasmus
laryngotracheobronchitis	laryngotrachéobronchite	Laryngo-Tracheobronchitis
larynx	larynx	Larynx, Kehlkopf
laser	laser	Laser
lash	mèche, lanière	Wimper
Lassa fever	fièvre de Lassa	Lassafieber
last menstrual period (LMP)	dernières règles	letzte Menstruationsperiode
lateral	latéral	lateral, seitlich
lavage	lavage	Spülung
laxative (n)	laxatif (n)	Laxans (n), Abführmittel (n)
laxative (a)	laxatif (a)	laxierend (a), abführend (a)
lead	plomb	Ableitung
lecithin	lécithine	Lezithin
left-handed	gaucher	linkshändig
left occipito-anterior (LOA)	occipito-antérieur gauche	linke vordere Hinterhauptslage
leg	jambe	Bein
legionnaires' disease	maladie des légionnaires	Legionärskrankheit
Leishman-Donovan body	Leishmania donovani	Leishman-Donovan-Körper
leishmaniasis	leishmaniose	Leishmaniose

ITALIAN	SPANISH	ENGLISH
labbra	labios	**labia**
labile	lábil	**labile**
labilità	labilidad	**lability**
travaglio di parto	parto	**labor** (Am)
travaglio di parto	parto	**labour** (Eng)
labirinto	laberinto	**labyrinth**
labirintite	laberintitis	**labyrinthitis**
lacerato	lacerado	**lacerated**
lacrimale	lagrimal	**lacrimal**
lattasi	lactasa	**lactase**
lattato	lactato	**lactate**
lattazione	lactación	**lactation**
acido lattico	ácido láctico	**lactic acid**
lattosio	lactosa	**lactose**
lattulosio	lactulosa	**lactulose**
lamina	lámina	**lamina**
laminectomia	laminectomía	**laminectomy**
gruppi di Lancefield	grupos de Lancefield	**Lancefield's groups**
lanugine	lanugo	**lanugo**
laparoscopia	laparoscopia	**laparoscopy**
laparotomia	laparotomía	**laparotomy**
laringeo	laríngeo	**laryngeal**
laringite	laringitis	**laryngitis**
laringologia	laringología	**laryngology**
laringoscopio	laringoscopio	**laryngoscope**
laringospasmo	laringospasmo	**laryngospasm**
laringotracheobronchite	laringotraqueobronquitis	**laryngotracheobronchitis**
laringe	laringe	**larynx**
laser	láser	**laser**
ciglio	pestaña	**lash**
febbre di Lassa	fiebre de Lassa	**Lassa fever**
ultimo periodo mestruale	fecha última regla (FUR)	**last menstrual period (LMP)**
laterale	lateral	**lateral**
lavaggio	lavado	**lavage**
lassativo (n)	laxante (n)	**laxative** (n)
lassativo (a)	laxativo (a)	**laxative** (a)
piombo derivazione	plomo	**lead**
lecitina	lecitina	**lecithin**
mancino	zurdo	**left-handed**
occipitoanteriore sinistro (OAS)	occipito anterior izquierdo	**left occipito-anterior (LOA)**
arto, gamba, membro	pierna	**leg**
malattia dei legionari	enfermedad del legionario	**legionnaires' disease**
corpi di Leishman-Donovan	cuerpo de Leishman-Donovan	**Leishman-Donovan body**
leishmaniosi	leishmaniasis	**leishmaniasis**

ENGLISH	FRENCH	GERMAN
lens	lentille	Linse
lentigo	lentigo	Lentigo
leprosy	lèpre	Lepra, Aussatz
leptospirosis	leptospirose	Leptospirose
lesbian	lesbien	lesbisch
lesion	lésion	Läsion, Verletzung
lethal	létal, léthal	letal, tödlich
lethargy	léthargie	Lethargie
leucocyte (Eng)	leucocyte	Leukozyt
leucocytosis (Eng)	leucocytose	Leukozytose
leucopenia (Eng)	leucopénie	Leukopenie
leucoplakia (Eng)	leucoplasie	Leukoplakie
leucorrhea (Eng)	leucorrhée	Leukorrhoe
leucotomy (Eng)	leucotomie	Leukotomie
leukaemia (Eng)	leucémie	Leukämie
leukemia (Am)	leucémie	Leukämie
leukocyte (Am)	leucocyte	Leukozyt
leukocytosis (Am)	leucocytose	Leukozytose
leukopenia (Am)	leucopénie	Leukopenie
leukoplakia (Am)	leucoplasie	Leukoplakie
leukorrhea (Am)	leucorrhée	Leukorrhoe
leukotomy (Am)	leucotomie	Leukotomie
levator	releveur	Levator
LH-releasing factor (LHRF)	substance libératrice de l'hormone lutéotrope	LH-luteinizing hormone releasing factor (LHRF)
libido	libido	Libido
lichen	lichen	Lichen
lichenification	lichénification	Lichenifikation
ligament	ligament	Ligament, Band
ligate	ligaturer	abbinden
ligature	ligature	Ligatur, Gefäßunterbindung
limb	membre	Glied, Extremität
linctus	linctus	Linctus
linea	ligne	Linea, Linie
liniment	liniment	Liniment, Einreibemittel
lip	lèvre	Lippe
lipaemia (Eng)	lipémie	Lipämie
lipase	lipase	Lipase
lipemia (Am)	lipémie	Lipämie
lipid	lipide	Lipid
lipidosis	lipidose, dyslipoïdose	Lipidose
lipochondrodystrophy	maladie de Hurler, lipochondrodystrophie	Lipochondrodystrophie
lipodystrophy	lipodystrophie	Lipodystrophie
lipolysis	lipolyse	Lipolyse
lipoma	lipome	Lipom
lipoprotein	lipoprotéine	Lipoprotein
lipotrophic	hormone lipotrope hypophysaire	lipotroph

ITALIAN	SPANISH	ENGLISH
lente	cristalino	lens
lentiggine	lentigo	lentigo
lebbra	lepra	leprosy
leptospirosi	leptospirosis	leptospirosis
lesbismo	lesbiana	lesbian
lesione	lesión	lesion
letale	letal	lethal
letargia	letargo	lethargy
leucocito	leucocito	leucocyte (Eng)
leucocitosi	leucocitosis	leucocytosis (Eng)
leucopenia	leucopenia	leucopenia (Eng)
leucoplachia	leucoplasia	leucoplakia (Eng)
leucorrea	leucorrea	leucorrhea (Eng)
leucotomia	leucotomía	leucotomy (Eng)
leucemia	leucemia	leukaemia (Eng)
leucemia	leucemia	leukemia (Am)
leucocito	leucocito	leukocyte (Am)
leucocitosi	leucocitosis	leukocytosis (Am)
leucopenia	leucopenia	leukopenia (Am)
leucoplachia	leucoplasia	leukoplakia (Am)
leucorrea	leucorrea	leukorrhea (Am)
leucotomia	leucotomía	leukotomy (Am)
muscolo elevatore	elevador	levator
releasing factor dell'ormone LH	factor liberador de la hormona luteinizante	LH-releasing factor (LHRF)
desiderio sessuale	líbido	libido
lichene	líquen	lichen
lichenificazione	liquenificación	lichenification
ligamento	ligamento	ligament
legare	ligar	ligate
legatura	ligadura	ligature
braccio	extremidad	limb
sciroppo	linctus	linctus
linea	línea	linea
linimento	linimento	liniment
labbro	labio	lip
lipemia	lipemia	lipaemia (Eng)
lipasi	lipasa	lipase
lipemia	lipemia	lipemia (Am)
lipide	lípido	lipid
lipoidosi	lipidosis	lipidosis
lipocondrodistrofia	lipocondrodistrofia	lipochondrodystrophy
lipodistrofia	lipodistrofia	lipodystrophy
lipolisi	lipolisis	lipolysis
lipoma	lipoma	lipoma
lipoproteina	lipoproteína	lipoprotein
lipotrofico	lipotrófico	lipotrophic

liquor	liquide	Liquor, Flüssigkeit
lithonephrotomy	lithonéphrotomie	Nephrolithotomie
lithotomy	lithotomie	Lithotomie
lithotripsy	lithotripsie, lithotritie	Lithotripsie
lithotriptor	lithotriteur	Lithotriptor
lithotrite	lithotriteur	Lithotriptor
litmus	tournesol	Lackmus
liver	foie	Leber
liver function test (LFT)	test de la fonction hépatique (TFH)	Leberfunktionstest
liver spot	tache hépatique	Leberfleck
livid	livide	livide, bleich
lobe	lobe	Lappen (Organ-)
lobectomy	lobectomie	Lobektomie, Lungenlappenresektion
lobotomy	lobotomie	Lobotomie, Leukotomie
lobule	lobule	Lobulus, Läppchen
localize	localiser	lokalisieren
lochia	lochies	Lochien, Wochenfluß
lock jaw	tétanos	Kiefersperre
locomotor	locomoteur	fortbewegend, Bewegungs-
loculated	loculé	gekammert
loin	région lombaire	Lende
lordosis	lordose	Lordose
louse	pou	Laus
low back pain	douleurs lombaires basses	Kreuzschmerzen
low birth weight (LBW)	hypotrophie	niedriges Geburtsgewicht
low density lipoprotein (LDL)	lipoprotéine de basse densité (LBD)	low density lipoprotein (LDL)
lower respiratory tract infection (LRTI)	infection du poumon profond	Atemwegsinfekt (untere)
lozenge	pastille	Pastille
lucid	lucide	glänzend, bei Bewußtsein
lumbago	lumbago	Lumbago, Hexenschuß
lumbar	lombaire	Lumbal-, Lenden-
lumbar puncture (LP)	ponction lombaire	Lumbalpunktion
lumbosacral	lombo-sacré	lumbosakral
lumen	lumière	Lumen, Durchmesser
lumpectomy	exérèse locale d'une tumeur du sein	Lumpektomie
lung	poumon	Lunge
lupus	lupus	Lupus
lupus erythematosus	lupus érythémateux	Lupus erythematodes
luteinizing hormone (LH)	hormone lutéinisante (HL)	luteinisierendes Hormon
luteum	corps jaune	Luteom, Luteinom
Lyme disease	arthrite de Lyme, maladie de Lyme	Lyme-Arthritis, Lyme-Borreliose
lymph	lymphe	Lymphe
lymphadenectomy	lymphadénectomie	Lymphadenektomie
lymphadenitis	lymphadénite	Lymphadenitis
lymphadenopathy	lymphadénopathie	Lymphadenopathie
lymphangitis	lymphangite	Lymphangitis

ITALIAN	SPANISH	ENGLISH
liquido	licor	**liquor**
litonefrotomia	litonefrotomía	**lithonephrotomy**
litotomia	litotomía	**lithotomy**
litotripsia	litotripsia	**lithotripsy**
litotritore	litotriptor	**lithotriptor**
litotritore	litotritor	**lithotrite**
tornasole	tornasol	**litmus**
fegato	hígado	**liver**
test di funzionalità epatica (TFE)	prueba de función hepática	**liver function test (LFT)**
cloasma	cloasma	**liver spot**
livido	lívido	**livid**
lobo	lóbulo	**lobe**
lobectomia	lobectomía	**lobectomy**
lobotomia	lobotomía	**lobotomy**
lobulo	lóbulo	**lobule**
localizzare	localizar	**localize**
lochi puerperali	loquios	**lochia**
tetano, trisma	trismo	**lock jaw**
locomotore	locomotor	**locomotor**
loculato	loculado	**loculated**
regione lombare	lomo	**loin**
lordosi	lordosis	**lordosis**
pidocchio	piojo	**louse**
rachialgia lombosacrale	lumbalgia	**low back pain**
basso peso alla nascita	bajo peso al nacer	**low birth weight (LBW)**
lipoproteina a bassa densità (LBD)	lipoproteína de baja densidad (LDL)	**low density lipoprotein (LDL)**
infezione del tratto respiratorio inferiore (LRTI)	infección de las vías respiratorias bajas	**lower respiratory tract infection (LRTI)**
pastiglia	pastilla	**lozenge**
lucido	lúcido	**lucid**
lombaggine	lumbago	**lumbago**
lombare	lumbar	**lumbar**
puntura lombare, rachicentesi	punción lumbar (PL)	**lumbar puncture (LP)**
lombosacrale	lumbosacro	**lumbosacral**
lume	luz	**lumen**
mastectomia parziale	exéresis de tumores benignos de la mama	**lumpectomy**
polmoni	pulmón	**lung**
lupus	lupus	**lupus**
lupus eritematoso	lupus eritematoso	**lupus erythematosus**
ormone luteinizzante (LH)	hormona luteinizante (LH)	**luteinizing hormone (LH)**
luteo	lúteo	**luteum**
malattia di Lyme	enfermedad de Lyme	**Lyme disease**
linfa	linfa	**lymph**
linfoadenectomia	linfadenectomía	**lymphadenectomy**
linfadenite	linfadenitis	**lymphadenitis**
linfadenopatia	linfadenopatía	**lymphadenopathy**
linfangite	linfangitis	**lymphangitis**

ENGLISH	FRENCH	GERMAN
lymphatic	lymphatique	lymphatisch, Lymph-
lymphedema (Am)	lymphoedème	Lymphödem
lymph node	ganglion lymphatique	Lymphknoten
lymphoblast	lymphoblaste	Lymphoblast
lymphocyte	lymphocyte	Lymphozyt
lymphocytosis	lymphocytose	Lymphozytose
lymphoedema (Eng)	lymphoedème	Lymphödem
lymphogranuloma inguinale	lymphogranulome vénérien	Lymphogranuloma inguinale
lymphokine	lymphokine	Lymphokine
lymphoma	lymphome	Lymphom
lymphosarcoma	lymphosarcome	Lymphosarkom
lysis	lyse	Lysis
lysosome	lysosome	Lysosom
lysozyme	lysozyme	Lysozym

ITALIAN	SPANISH	ENGLISH
linfatico	linfático	**lymphatic**
linfedema	linfedema	**lymphedema** (Am)
linfonodo	ganglio linfático	**lymph node**
linfoblasto	linfoblasto	**lymphoblast**
linfocito	linfocito	**lymphocyte**
linfocitosi	linfocitosis	**lymphocytosis**
linfedema	linfedema	**lymphoedema** (Eng)
linfogranuloma inguinale	linfogranuloma inguinal	**lymphogranuloma inguinale**
linfochina	linfocinesis	**lymphokine**
linfoma	linfoma	**lymphoma**
linfosarcoma	linfosarcoma	**lymphosarcoma**
lisi	lisis	**lysis**
lisosoma	lisosoma	**lysosome**
lisozima	lisozima	**lysozyme**

M

ENGLISH	FRENCH	GERMAN
maceration	macération	Mazeration
macrocephaly	macrocéphalie	Makrozephalie
macrocyte	macrocyte	Makrozyt
macrophage	macrophage	Phagozyt
macroscopic	macroscopique	makroskopisch
macula	macule	Makula, Fleck
macule	macule	Makula, Fleck
maculopapular	maculopapuleux	makulopapulär
maggot	asticot	Larve, Made
magnetic resonance imaging (MRI)	imagerie par résonance magnétique	Kernspintomographie (NMR)
mal	mal	Übel, Leiden
malabsorption	malabsorption	Malabsorption
malacia	malacie	Malazie, Erweichung
maladjustment	inadaptation	Fehlanpassung
malaise	malaise	Unwohlsein
malar	malaire	Backe betr, Backen-
malaria	paludisme	Malaria
malathion	malathion	Malathion
malformation	malformation	Mißbildung
malignancy	malignité	Malignität, Bösartigkeit
malignant	malin	maligne, bösartig
malingering	simulation	scheinkrank
malleolus	malléole	Malleolus, Knöchel
malleus	marteau	Malleus, Hammer
malnutrition	malnutrition	Unterernährung, Fehlernährung
malocclusion	malocclusion	Malokklusion
malposition	malposition	Lageanomalie
malpractice	faute professionnelle	Kunstfehler
malpresentation	présentation vicieuse	anomale Kindslage
maltose	maltose	Maltose
malunion	cal vicieux	Fehlstellung (Frakturenden)
mammography	mammographie	Mammographie
mammoplasty	mammoplastie	Mammaplastik
mandible	mandibule	Mandibula, Unterkiefer
mania	manie	Manie
manic-depressive psychosis	psychose maniacodépressive	manisch-depressive Psychose
manipulation	manipulation	Manipulation, Handhabung
manubrium	manubrium	Manubrium
marasmus	athrepsie	Marasmus
marsupialization	marsupialisation	Marsupialisation
massage	massage.	Massage
mastalgia	mastalgie, mammalgie	Mastodynie
mastectomy	mastectomie	Mastektomie, Brustamputation
mastication	mastication	Kauen, Kauvermögen

ITALIAN	SPANISH	ENGLISH
macerazione	maceración	maceration
macrocefalia	macrocefalia	macrocephaly
macrocito	macrocito	macrocyte
macrofago	macrófago	macrophage
macroscopico	macroscópico	macroscopic
macula	mácula	macula
macula	mácula	macule
maculopapulare	maculopapular	maculopapular
larva	antojo	maggot
indagine morfologica con risonanza magnetica	formación de imágenes por resonancia magnética	magnetic resonance imaging (MRI)
male, malattia	mal	mal
malassorbimento	malabsorción	malabsorption
malacia	malacia	malacia
assestamento difettoso	inadaptación	maladjustment
indisposizione, malessere	destemplanza, malestar	malaise
malare	malar	malar
malaria	paludismo	malaria
malathion	malathion	malathion
malformazione	malformación	malformation
neoplasia maligna	malignidad	malignancy
maligno	maligno	malignant
simulazione di malattia	simulación de síntomas	malingering
malleolo	maléolo	malleolus
martello	martillo	malleus
malnutrizione	desnutrición	malnutrition
malocclusione	maloclusión	malocclusion
malposizione	malposición	malposition
pratica errata o disonesta	malpraxis	malpractice
presentazione fetale anomala	malpresentación	malpresentation
maltosio	maltosa	maltose
unione difettosa	unión defectuosa	malunion
mammografia	mamografía	mammography
mammoplastica	mamoplastia	mammoplasty
mandibola	mandíbula	mandible
mania	manía	mania
psicosi maniaco-depressiva	psicosis maniacodepresiva	manic-depressive psychosis
manipolazione	manipulación	manipulation
manubrio	manubrio	manubrium
marasma	marasmo	marasmus
marsupializzazione	marsupialización	marsupialization
massaggio	masaje	massage
mastalgia	mastalgia	mastalgia
mastectomia	mastectomía	mastectomy
masticazione	masticación	mastication

ENGLISH	FRENCH	GERMAN
mastitis	mastite	Mastitis, Brustdrüsenentzündung
mastoid	mastoïde	mastoideus
mastoidectomy	mastoïdectomie	Mastoidektomie
mastoiditis	mastoïdite	Mastoiditis
masturbation	masturbation	Masturbation, Selbstbefriedigung
matrix	matrice	Matrix
maxilla	maxillaire	Maxilla, Oberkieferknochen
maxillofacial	maxillofacial	maxillofazial
McBurney's point	point de McBurney	McBurney-Punkt
mean corpuscular volume (MCV)	volume globulaire moyen (VGM)	mittleres Erythrozytenvolumen (MCV)
measles	rougeole	Masern
measles mumps and rubella (MMR)	oreillons rougeole et rubéole	Masern Mumps und Röteln
Meckel's diverticulum	diverticule de Meckel	Meckel-Divertikel
meconium	méconium	Mekonium
medial	interne	medial
median	médian	Median-
mediastinitis	médiastinite	Mediastinitis
mediastinum	médiastin	Mediastinum
medicament	médicament	Medikament, Arzneimittel
medicated	médicamenté	medizinisch
medicine	médecine	Medizin, Arznei
medicolegal	médico-légal	rechtsmedizinisch
medicosocial	médico-social	sozialmedizinisch
medium	milieu	Medium
medulla	moelle	Medulla, Mark
medulloblastoma	médulloblastome	Medulloblastom
megacolon	mégacôlon	Megacoloncongenitum, Hirschsprung-Krankheit
megaloblast	mégaloblaste	Megaloblast
meiosis	méiose	Meiose
melaena (Eng)	méléna	Meläna, Blutstuhl
melancholia	mélancolie	Melancholie
melanin	mélanine	Melanin
melanoma	mélanome	Melanom
melena (Am)	méléna	Meläna, Blutstuhl
membrane	membrane	Membran
memory	mémoire	Gedächtnis, Erinnerungsvermögen
menarche	établissement de la menstruation	Menarche
Mendelson's syndrome	syndrome de Mendelson	Mendelson-Syndrom
Ménière's disease	syndrome de Ménière	Morbus Ménière
meninges	méninges	Meningen, Hirnhäute
meningioma	méningiome	Meningiom
meningism	méningisme	Meningismus
meningitis	méningite	Meningitis, Gehirnhautentzündung
meningocele	méningocèle	Meningozele
meningoencephalitis	méningo-encéphalite	Meningoenzephalitis

ITALIAN	SPANISH	ENGLISH
mastite	mastitis	**mastitis**
mastoide, mastoideo	mastoideo	**mastoid**
mastoidectomia	mastoidectomía	**mastoidectomy**
mastoidite	mastoiditis	**mastoiditis**
masturbazione	masturbación	**masturbation**
matrice	matriz	**matrix**
mascella superiore	maxilar	**maxilla**
maxillofacciale	maxilofacial	**maxillofacial**
punto di McBurney	punto de McBurney	**McBurney's point**
volume corpuscolare medio (VCM)	volumen corpuscular medio (VCM)	**mean corpuscular volume (MCV)**
morbillo	sarampión	**measles**
parotide epidemica morbillo e rosolia	sarampión parotiditis y rubéola	**measles mumps and rubella (MMR)**
diverticolo di Meckel	divertículo de Meckel	**Meckel's diverticulum**
meconio	meconio	**meconium**
mediale	medial	**medial**
mediano	mediana	**median**
mediastinite	mediastinitis	**mediastinitis**
mediastino	mediastino	**mediastinum**
medicamento	medicamento	**medicament**
medicato, medicamentoso	medicado	**medicated**
medicina	medicina	**medicine**
medicolegale	médicolegal	**medicolegal**
medicosociale	médicosocial	**medicosocial**
mezzo	medio	**medium**
midollo	médula	**medulla**
medulloblastoma	meduloblastoma	**medulloblastoma**
megacolon	megacolon	**megacolon**
megaloblasto	megaloblasto	**megaloblast**
meiosi	meiossis	**meiosis**
melena	melena	**melaena** (Eng)
melanconia	melancolía	**melancholia**
melanina	melanina	**melanin**
melanoma	melanoma	**melanoma**
melena	melena	**melena** (Am)
membrana	membrana	**membrane**
memoria	memoria	**memory**
menarca	menarquía	**menarche**
sindrome di Mendelson	síndrome de Mendelson	**Mendelson's syndrome**
sindrome di Ménière	enfermedad de Ménière	**Ménière's disease**
meningi	meninges	**meninges**
meningioma	meningioma	**meningioma**
meningismo	meningismo	**meningism**
meningite	meningitis	**meningitis**
meningocele	meningocele	**meningocele**
meningoencefalite	meningoencefalitis	**meningoencephalitis**

ENGLISH	FRENCH	GERMAN
meningomyelocele	méningomyélocèle	Meningomyelozele
meniscectomy	méniscectomie	Meniskusentfernung
meniscus	ménisque	Meniskus
menopause	ménopause	Menopause, Wechseljahre
menorrhagia	ménorrhagie	Menorrhagie
menorrhea (Am)	ménorrhée	Monatsblutung, Menstruation
menorrhoea (Eng)	ménorrhée	Monatsblutung, Menstruation
menstrual	menstruel	menstruell
menstruation	menstruation	Menstruation, Monatsblutung
mental	mental	geistig, seelisch
mentoanterior	posture antéromentonnière	mentoanterior
mentoposterior	posture postmentonnière	mentoposterior
mentum	menton	Kinn
mercury	mercure	Quecksilber
mesentery	mésentère	Mesenterium
mesothelioma	mésothéliome	Mesotheliom
metabolic	métabolique	metabolisch, Stoffwechsel-
metabolism	métabolisme	Metabolismus, Stoffwechsel
metabolite	métabolite	Metabolit, Stoffwechselprodukt
metacarpophalangeal	métacarpophalangien	metakarpophalangeal
metacarpus	métacarpe	Metakarpus, Mittelhand
metastasis	métastase	Metastase
metatarsalgia	métatarsalgie	Metatarsalgie
metatarsophalangeal	métatarsophalangien	metatarsophalangeal
metatarsus	métatarse	Metatarsus, Mittelfuß
methaemoglobin (Eng)	méthémoglobine	Methämoglobin
methaemoglobinaemia (Eng)	méthémoglobinémie	Methämoglobinämie
methemoglobin (Am)	méthémoglobine	Methämoglobin
methemoglobinemia (Am)	méthémoglobinémie	Methämoglobinämie
methylcellulose	méthylcellulose	Methylzellulose
metropathia haemorrhagica (Eng)	métropathie hémorragique	Metropathia haemorrhagica
metropathia hemorrhagica (Am)	métropathie hémorragique	Metropathia haemorrhagica
metrorrhagia	métrorragie	Metrorrhagie, Zwischenblutung
microbiology	microbiologie	Mikrobiologie
microcephaly	microcéphalie	Mikrozephalie
microcirculation	microcirculation	Mikrozirkulation
microcyte	microcyte	Mikrozyt
microfilaria	microfilaire	Mikrofilarie
microorganism	micro-organisme	Mikroorganismus
microscope	microscope	Mikroskop
microscopic	microscopique	mikroskopisch
microsurgery	microchirurgie	Mikrochirurgie
microvilli	micropoils	Mikrovilli
micturition	micturition	Wasserlassen, Blasenentleerung
midbrain	mésencéphale	Mittelhirn
midriff	diaphragme	Zwerchfell, Diaphragma

ITALIAN	SPANISH	ENGLISH
meningomielocele	mielomeningocele	**meningomyelocele**
meniscectomia	meniscectomía	**meniscectomy**
menisco	menisco	**meniscus**
menopausa	menopausia	**menopause**
menorragia	menorragia	**menorrhagia**
menorrea	menorrea	**menorrhea** (Am)
menorrea	menorrea	**menorrhoea** (Eng)
mestruale	menstrual	**menstrual**
mestruazione	menstruación	**menstruation**
mentale	mental	**mental**
mentoanteriore	mentoanterior	**mentoanterior**
mentoposteriore	mentoposterior	**mentoposterior**
mento	mentón	**mentum**
mercurio	mercurio	**mercury**
mesentere	mesenterio	**mesentery**
mesotelioma	mesotelioma	**mesothelioma**
metabolico	metabólico	**metabolic**
metabolismo	metabolismo	**metabolism**
metabolita	metabolito	**metabolite**
metacarpofalangeo	metacarpofalángico	**metacarpophalangeal**
metacarpo	metacarpo	**metacarpus**
metastasi	metástasis	**metastasis**
metatarsalgia	metatarsalgia	**metatarsalgia**
metatarsofalangeo	metatarsofalángico	**metatarsophalangeal**
metatarso	metatarso	**metatarsus**
metemoglobina	metahemoglobina	**methaemoglobin** (Eng)
metemoglobinemia	metahemoglobinemia	**methaemoglobinaemia** (Eng)
metemoglobina	metahemoglobina	**methemoglobin** (Am)
metemoglobinemia	metahemoglobinemia	**methemoglobinemia** (Am)
metilcellulosa	metilcelulosa	**methylcellulose**
metropatia emorragica	metropatía hemorrágica	**metropathia haemorrhagica** (Eng)
metropatia emorragica	metropatía hemorrágica	**metropathia hemorrhagica** (Am)
metrorragia	metrorragia	**metrorrhagia**
microbiologia	microbiología	**microbiology**
microcefalia	microcefalia	**microcephaly**
microcircolazione	microcirculación	**microcirculation**
microcita	microcito	**microcyte**
microfilaria	microfilaria	**microfilaria**
microoganismo	microorganismo	**microorganism**
microscopio	microscopio	**microscope**
microscopico	microscópico	**microscopic**
microchirurgia	microcirugía	**microsurgery**
microvilli	microvellosidad	**microvilli**
minzione	micción	**micturition**
mesencefelo	mesencéfalo	**midbrain**
parte bassa del torace, diaframma	diafragma	**midriff**

ENGLISH	FRENCH	GERMAN
midstream urine specimen (MUS)	urine du milieu du jet	Mittelstrahlurin
midwife	sage-femme	Hebamme
migraine	migraine	Migräne
miliaria	miliaire	Miliaria
miliary	miliaire	miliar
milk	lait	Milch
milliequivalent (mEq)	milliéquivalent (mEq)	Milli-Äquivalent
mineralocorticoid	minéralocorticoïde	Mineralokortikoid
miosis	myosis	Miosis, Pupillenverengung
miscarriage	fausse couche	Fehlgeburt
missed abortion	rétention foetale	verhaltener Abort, missed abortion
mitochondrion	mitochondrie	Mitochondrium
mitosis	mitose	Mitose
mitral	mitral	mitral
mittelschmerz	crise intermenstruelle	Mittelschmerz
molar	molaire	molar
mole	naevus	Mole, Muttermal
molecule	molécule	Molekül
molluscum	molluscum	Molluscum
monoamine oxidase inhibitor (MAOI)	inhibiteur de la monoamine-oxydase (IMAO)	Monoaminoxydase-Hemmer
monochromat	monochromat	Monochromat, monochrom Farbenblinder
monoclonal antibody	anticorps monoclonal	monoklonaler Antikörper
mononuclear	mononucléaire	mononukleär
mononucleosis	mononucléose	Mononukleose, Pfeiffersches Drüsenfieber
monoplegia	monoplégie	Monoplegie
morbidity	morbidité	Morbidität, Krankhaftigkeit
morbilliform	morbilliforme	morbilliform, masernähnlich
moribund	moribond	moribund, sterbend
morning sickness	nausées matinales	morgendliche Übelkeit der Schwangeren
Moro reflex	réflexe de Moro	Moro-Reflex
morphology	morphologie	Morphologie
mortality	mortalité	Mortalität, Sterblichkeit
motile	mobile	bewegungsfähig, beweglich
motion	mouvement	Bewegung, Stuhlgang
motor	moteur	motorisch
motor nerve	nerf moteur	motorischer Nerv
motor neurone	neurone moteur	Motoneuron
mouth	bouche	Mund
mouth to mouth resuscitation	réanimation au bouche-à-bouche	Mund-zu-Mund-Wiederbelebung
mucin	mucine	Muzin
mucocele (Am)	mucocèle	Mukozele
mucocoele (Eng)	mucocèle	Mukozele
mucocutaneous	mucocutané	mukokutan
mucoid	mucoïde	mukoid

ITALIAN	SPANISH	ENGLISH
campione urinario del mitto intermedio (CUM)	muestra de orina de la parte media de la micción	midstream urine specimen (MUS)
levatrice	comadrona	midwife
emicrania	migraña	migraine
miliaria, esantema miliare	miliaria	miliaria
miliare	miliar	miliary
latte	leche	milk
milliequivalente (mEq)	miliequivalente (mEq)	milliequivalent (mEq)
mineralcorticoide	mineralocorticoide	mineralocorticoid
miosi	miosis	miosis
aborto	aborto	miscarriage
aborto interno, aborto ritenuto	aborto diferido	missed abortion
mitocondrio	mitocondria	mitochondrion
mitosi	mitosis	mitosis
mitrale, mitralico	mitral	mitral
dolore intermestruale	mittelschmerz	mittelschmerz
molare	molar	molar
neo	nevo	mole
molecula	molécula	molecule
mollusco	molusco	molluscum
inibitore monoaminoossidasi (IMAO)	inhibidor de la monoaminooxidasa (IMAO)	monoamine oxidase inhibitor (MAOI)
monocromatico	monocromato	monochromat
anticorpo monoclonale	anticuerpo monoclonal	monoclonal antibody
mononucleare	mononuclear	mononuclear
mononucleosi	mononucleosis	mononucleosis
monoplegia	monoplegia	monoplegia
morbilità	morbilidad	morbidity
morbilliforme	morbiliforme	morbilliform
moribondo	moribundo	moribund
malessere mattutino	náuseas matinales	morning sickness
riflesso di Moro	reflejo de Moro	Moro reflex
morfologia	morfología	morphology
mortalità	mortalidad	mortality
mobile	móvil	motile
movimento	movimiento	motion
motore	motor	motor
nervo motore	nervio motor	motor nerve
neurone motore	neurona motora	motor neurone
bocca	boca	mouth
rianimazione bocca a bocca	respiración boca a boca	mouth to mouth resuscitation
mucina	mucina	mucin
mucocele	mucocele	mucocele (Am)
mucocele	mucocele	mucocoele (Eng)
mucocutaneo	mucocutáneo	mucocutaneous
mucoide	mucoide	mucoid

ENGLISH	FRENCH	GERMAN
mucolytic	mucolytique	schleimlösendes Mittel
mucopolysaccharidosis	mucopolysaccharidose	Mukopolysaccharidose
mucopurulent	mucopurulent	mukopurulent, schleimig-eitrig
mucosa	muqueuse	Mukosa, Schleimhaut
mucous (Eng)	muqueux	mukös, schleimig
mucus (Am)	muqueux	mukös, schleimig
multigravida	multigeste	Multigravida
multilocular	multiloculaire	multilokulär
multiple sclerosis (MS)	sclérose en plaques	multiple Sklerose (MS)
mumps	oreillons	Mumps, Ziegenpeter
Münchhausen's syndrome	syndrome de Münchhausen	Münchhausen-Syndrom
mural	pariétal	mural
murmur	murmure	Herzgeräusch, Geräusch
muscle	muscle	Muskel
muscular dystrophy	dystrophie musculaire	Muskeldystrophie
musculocutaneous	musculo-cutané	muskulokutan
musculoskeletal	musculo-squelettique	Skelettmuskulatur betr.
mutagen	mutagène	Mutagen
mutant	mutant	Mutante
mutation	mutation	Mutation
mutilation	mutilation	Verstümmelung
mutism	mutisme	Mutismus, Stummheit
myalgia	myalgie	Myalgie, Muskelschmerz
myalgic encephalomyelitis (ME)	encéphalomyélite myalgique	myalgische Enzephalomyelitis
myasthenia	myasthénie	Myasthenie, Muskelschwäche
myasthenic crisis	crise myasthénique	myasthenische Krise
mycosis	mycose	Mykose, Pilzinfektion
mydriasis	mydriase	Mydriasis, Pupillenerweiterung
mydriatic (n)	mydriatique (n)	Mydriatikum (n)
mydriatic (a)	mydriatique (a)	mydriatisch (a), pupillenerweiternd (a)
myelin	myéline	Myelin
myelitis	myélite	Myelitis
myelofibrosis	myélofibrose	Myelofibrose
myelography	myélographie	Myelographie
myeloid	myéloïde	myeloisch
myeloma	myélome	Myelom
myelomatosis	myélomatose	Myelomatose
myelopathy	myélopathie	Myelopathie
myocardial infarction (MI)	infarctus du myocarde	Myokardinfarkt, Herzinfarkt
myocarditis	myocardite	Myokarditis, Herzmuskelentzündung
myocardium	myocarde	Myokard, Herzmuskel
myofibrosis	myofibrose	Myofibrose
myoma	myome	Myom
myomectomy	myomectomie	Myomektomie
myometrium	myomètre	Myometrium
myopathy	myopathie	Myopathie, Muskelerkrankung
myope	myope	Myoper, Kurzsichtiger

ITALIAN	SPANISH	ENGLISH
mucolitico	mucolítico	mucolytic
mucopolisaccaridosi	mucopolisacaridosis	mucopolysaccharidosis
mucopurulento	mucopurulento	mucopurulent
mucosa	mucosa	mucosa
mucoso	moco	mucous (Eng)
mucoso	moco	mucus (Am)
plurigravida	multípara	multigravida
multiloculare	multilocular	multilocular
sclerosi multipla	esclerosis múltiple	multiple sclerosis (MS)
parotite epidemica	paperas	mumps
sindrome di Münchhausen	síndrome de Münchhausen	Münchhausen's syndrome
murale, parietale	mural	mural
soffio, rullio	soplo	murmur
muscolo	músculo	muscle
distrofia muscolare	distrofia muscular	muscular dystrophy
muscolocutaneo	musculocutáneo	musculocutaneous
muscoloscheletrico	musculoesquelético	musculoskeletal
mutageno	mutágeno	mutagen
mutante	mutante	mutant
mutazione	mutación	mutation
mutilazione	mutilación	mutilation
mutismo	mutismo	mutism
mialgia	mialgia	myalgia
encefalomielite mialgica	encefalomielitis miálgica	myalgic encephalomyelitis (ME)
miastenia	miastenia	myasthenia
crisi miastenica	crisis miasténica	myasthenic crisis
micosi	micosis	mycosis
midriasi	midriasis	mydriasis
midriatico (n)	midriático (n)	mydriatic (n)
midriatico (a)	midriático (a)	mydriatic (a)
mielina	mielina	myelin
mielite	mielitis	myelitis
mielofibrosi	mielofibrosis	myelofibrosis
mielografia	mielografía	myelography
mieloide	mieloide	myeloid
mieloma, plasmacitoma maligno	mieloma	myeloma
mielomatosi	mielomatosis	myelomatosis
mielopatia	mielopatía	myelopathy
infarto miocardico	infarto de miocardio (IM)	myocardial infarction (MI)
miocardite	miocarditis	myocarditis
miocardio	miocardio	myocardium
miosite	miofibrosis	myofibrosis
leiomioma dell'utero, mioma	mioma	myoma
miomectomia	miomectomía	myomectomy
miometrio	miometrio	myometrium
miopatia	miopatía	myopathy
miope	miope	myope

ENGLISH	FRENCH	GERMAN
myopia	myopie	Myopie, Kurzsichtigkeit
myositis	myosite	Myositis
myringotomy	myringotomie	Parazentese
myxedema (Am)	myxoedème	Myxödem
myxoedema (Eng)	myxoedème	Myxödem
myxoma	myxome	Myxom
myxovirus	myxovirus	Myxovirus

ITALIAN	SPANISH	ENGLISH
miopia	miopía	**myopia**
miosite	miositis	**myositis**
miringotomia	miringotomía	**myringotomy**
mixedema	mixedema	**myxedema** (Am)
mixedema	mixedema	**myxoedema** (Eng)
mixoma	mixoma	**myxoma**
myxovirus	mixovirus	**myxovirus**

N

English	French	German
nabothian follicles	oeufs de Naboth	Naboth-Eier
naevus (Eng)	naevus	Nävus, Muttermal
nail	ongle	Nagel
nape	nuque	Nacken
napkin rash (Eng)	érythème fessier du nourrisson, érythème papulo-érosif	Windeldermatitis
narcolepsy	narcolepsie	Narkolepsie
narcosis	narcose	Narkose, Anästhesie
narcotic (n)	narcotique (n)	Narkosemittel (n), Betäubungsmittel (n), Rauschgift (n)
narcotic (a)	narcotique (a)	narkotisch (a)
nasal	nasal	nasal
nasogastric	nasogastrique	nasogastrisch
nasolacrimal	nasolacrymal	nasolakrimal
nasopharynx	rhinopharynx	Nasopharynx, Nasenrachenraum
nausea	nausée	Nausea, Übelkeit, Brechreiz
navel	nombril	Nabel
nebulizer	nébuliseur	Zerstäuber, Vernebler
neck	cou	Nacken, Hals
necrosis	nécrose	Nekrose
necrotizing enterocolitis (NEC)	entérocolite nécrosante	nekrotisierende Enterokolitis
needle	aiguille	Nadel, Kanüle
negligence	négligence	Nachlässigkeit
nematode	nématode	Nematode, Fadenwurm
neonatal intensive care unit (NICU) (Am)	service de soins intensifs néonatals	Frühgeborenen-Intensivstation
neonatal period	période néonatale	Neonatalperiode, Neugeborenenperiode
neonate (n)	nouveau-né (n)	Neugeborenes (n)
neonate (a)	nouveau-né (a)	neugeboren (a)
neoplasia	néoplasie	Neoplasie
neoplasm	néoplasme	Neoplasma, Tumor
nephralgia	néphralgie	Nephralgie
nephrectomy	néphrectomie	Nephrektomie
nephritis	néphrite	Nephritis, Nierenentzündung
nephrogenic	d'origine rénale	nephrogen
nephrology	néphrologie	Nephrologie
nephron	néphron	Nephron
nephrosis	néphrose	Nephrose
nephrostomy	néphrostomie	Nephrostomie
nephrotic syndrome	syndrome néphrotique	nephrotisches Syndrom
nephrotoxic	néphrotoxique	nephrotoxisch, nierenschädigend
nerve	nerf	Nerv
nerve block	anesthésie par blocage nerveux	Leitungsanästhesie
nerve ending	terminaison nerveuse	Nervenendigung
nettle rash	urticaire	Nesselfieber

follicoli di Naboth	folículos de Naboth	**nabothian follicles**
nevo	nevo	**naevus** (Eng)
unghia	uña	**nail**
nuca	nuca	**nape**
eruzione cutanea da pannolino	exantema del pañal	**napkin rash** (Eng)
narcolessia	narcolepsia	**narcolepsy**
narcosi	narcosis	**narcosis**
narcotico (n)	narcótico (n)	**narcotic** (n)
narcotico (a)	narcótico (a)	**narcotic** (a)
nasale	nasal	**nasal**
nasogastrico	nasogástrico	**nasogastric**
nasolacrimale	nasolacrimal	**nasolacrimal**
nasofaringe	nasofaringe	**nasopharynx**
nausea	náusea	**nausea**
ombelico	ombligo	**navel**
nebulizzatore, atomizzatore	nebulizador	**nebulizer**
collo	cuello	**neck**
necrosi	necrosis	**necrosis**
enterocolite necrotizzante	enterocolitis necrotizante	**necrotizing enterocolitis (NEC)**
ago	aguja	**needle**
negligenza	negligencia	**negligence**
nematode	nematodo	**nematode**
reparto di terapia intensiva neonatale	unidad de cuidados intensivos para recién nacidos	**neonatal intensive care unit (NICU)** (Am)
periodo neonatale	período neonatal	**neonatal period**
neonato (n)	neonato (n)	**neonate** (n)
neonato (a)	neonato (a)	**neonate** (a)
neoplasia	neoplasia	**neoplasia**
neoplasma	neoplasma	**neoplasm**
nevralgia	nefralgia	**nephralgia**
nefrectomia	nefrectomía	**nephrectomy**
nefrite	nefritis	**nephritis**
nefrogenico	nefrógeno	**nephrogenic**
nefrologia	nefrologia	**nephrology**
nefrone	nefrona	**nephron**
nefrosi, nefropatia	nefrosis	**nephrosis**
nefrostomia	nefrostomía	**nephrostomy**
sindrome nefrosica	síndrome nefrótico	**nephrotic syndrome**
nefrotossico	nefrotóxico	**nephrotoxic**
nervo	nervio	**nerve**
blocco nervoso	bloqueo nervioso	**nerve block**
terminazione nervosa	terminación nerviosa	**nerve ending**
orticaria	urticaria	**nettle rash**

ENGLISH	FRENCH	GERMAN
neural	neural	neural
neuralgia	névralgie	Neuralgie
neurapraxia	neurapraxie	Neurapraxie
neurasthenia	neurasthénie	Neurasthenie
neuritis	névrite	Neuritis, Nervenentzündung
neuroblastoma	neuroblastome	Neuroblastom
neurofibromatosis	neurofibromatose	Neurofibromatose
neurogenic	neurogène	neurogen
neurolemma	neurilemme	Neurolemm
neuroleptic (n)	neuroleptique (n)	Neuroleptikum (n)
neuroleptic (a)	neuroleptique (a)	neuroleptisch (a)
neurology	neurologie	Neurologie
neuromuscular	neuromusculaire	neuromuskulär
neuron	neurone	Neuron
neuropathy	neuropathie	Neuropathie
neuropharmacology	neuropharmacologie	Neuropharmakologie
neuropsychiatry	neuropsychiatrie	Neuropsychiatrie
neurosis	névrose	Neurose
neurosurgery	neurochirurgie	Neurochirurgie
neurosyphilis	neurosyphilis	Neurosyphilis
neurotropic	neurotrope	neurotrop
neutropenia	neutropénie	Neutropenie
neutrophil (n)	polynucléaire neutrophile (n)	Neutrophiler (n)
neutrophil (a)	neutrophile (a)	neutrophil (a)
nevus (Am)	naevus	Nävus, Muttermal
newborn (n)	nouveau-né (n)	Neugeborenes (n)
newborn (a)	nouveau-né (a)	neugeboren (a)
nicotine	nicotine	Nikotin
nidus	foyer morbide	Nidus
night blindness	cécité nocturne	Nachtblindheit
night sweat	sueurs nocturnes	Nachtschweiß
nipple	mamelon	Brustwarze, Mamille
nit	lente	Nisse
nocturia	nycturie	Nykturie
nocturnal	nocturne	nächtlich, Nacht-
node	noeud	Knoten
nodule	nodule	Nodulus, Knötchen
non-accidental injury (NAI)	traumatisme non accidentel	nicht unfallbedingte Verletzung
noncompliance	non observance	Noncompliance
non-gonococcal urethritis (NGU)	urétrite non gonococcique	nicht durch Gonokokken bedingte Urethritis
non-insulin dependent diabetes mellitus (NIDDM)	diabète sucré non insulinodépendant	Diabetes mellitus Typ II, non-insulin dependent diabetes mellitus (NIDDM)
non-invasive	non invasif	nichtinvasiv
non-specific urethritis (NSU)	urétrite aspécifique	unspezifische Urethritis
non-steroidal anti-inflammatory drug (NSAID)	anti-inflammatoire non stéroïdien	nichtsteroidales Antiphlogistikum

ITALIAN	SPANISH	ENGLISH
neurale	nervioso	**neural**
nevralgia	neuralgia	**neuralgia**
neuroaprassia	neuropraxia	**neurapraxia**
neuroastenia	neurastenia	**neurasthenia**
neurite	neuritis	**neuritis**
neuroblastoma	neuroblastoma	**neuroblastoma**
neurofibromatosi	neurofibromatosis	**neurofibromatosis**
neurogenico	neurógeno	**neurogenic**
neurilemma	neurolema	**neurolemma**
neurolettico *(n)*	neuroléptico *(n)*	**neuroleptic** (n)
neurolettico *(a)*	neuroléptico *(a)*	**neuroleptic** (a)
neurologia	neurología	**neurology**
neuromuscolare	neuromuscular	**neuromuscular**
neurone	neurona	**neuron**
neuropatia	neuropatia	**neuropathy**
neurofarmacologia	neurofarmacología	**neuropharmacology**
neuropsichiatria	neuropsiquiatría	**neuropsychiatry**
nevrosi	neurosis	**neurosis**
neurochirurgia	neurocirugía	**neurosurgery**
neurosifilide	neurosífilis	**neurosyphilis**
neurotropo	neurotrópico	**neurotropic**
neutropenia	neutropenia	**neutropenia**
granulocito neutrofilo *(n)*	neutrófilo *(n)*	**neutrophil** (n)
neutrofilo *(a)*	neutrófilo *(a)*	**neutrophil** (a)
nevo	nevo	**nevus** (Am)
neonato *(n)*	neonato *(n)*	**newborn** (n)
neonato *(a)*	neonato *(a)*	**newborn** (a)
nicotina	nicotina	**nicotine**
nido	nido	**nidus**
emeralopia	ceguera nocturna	**night blindness**
sudorazione notturna	sudoración nocturna	**night sweat**
capezzolo	pezón	**nipple**
lendine	liendre	**nit**
nicturia	nicturia	**nocturia**
notturno	nocturno	**nocturnal**
nodo	nodo	**node**
nodulo	nódulo	**nodule**
lesione non accidentale	lesión no accidental	**non-accidental injury (NAI)**
inadempienza a prescrizioni	incumplimiento	**noncompliance**
uretrite non gonococcica	uretritis no gonocócica	**non-gonococcal urethritis (NGU)**
diabete mellito non insulinodipendente	diabetes mellitus no insulinodependiente	**non-insulin dpendent diabetes mellitus (NIDDM)**
non invasivo	no invasivo	**non-invasive**
uretrite aspecifica	uretritis inespecífica	**non-specific urethritis (NSU)**
farmaco antinfiammatorio non steroideo (FANS)	fármaco antiinflamatorio no esteroide (AINE)	**non-steroidal anti-inflammatory drug (NSAID)**

ENGLISH	FRENCH	GERMAN
noradrenaline	noradrénaline	Noradrenalin
norepinephrine	norépinéphrine, noradrénaline	Norepinephrin, Noradrenalin
normoblast	normoblaste	Normoblast
normocyte	normocyte	Normozyt
normoglycaemic (Eng)	normoglycémique	Normoglykämie
normoglycemic (Am)	normoglycémique	Normoglykämie
normotonic	normotonique	normoton
nose	nez	Nase
nosebleed	saignement de nez, épistaxis	Nasenbluten, Epistaxis
nostril	narine	Nasenloch
notifiable disease	maladie à déclaration obligatoire	meldepflichtige Erkrankung
not yet diagnosed (NYD)	non encore diagnostiqué	noch nicht diagnostiziert
nucleus	noyau	Nukleus, Kern
nullipara	nullipare	Nullipara
nurse (n)	infirmière (n)	Krankenschwester (n), Schwester (n), Pflegerin (n)
nurse (v)	soigner (v)	stillen (v), pflegen (v)
nutrient (n)	nutriment (n)	Nahrungsmittel (n)
nutrient (a)	nourricier (a)	nahrhaft (a)
nutrition	nutrition	Ernährung
nyctalgia	nyctalgie	Nyktalgie
nycturia	nycturie	Nykturie
nystagmus	nystagmus	Nystagmus

ITALIAN	SPANISH	ENGLISH
noradrenalina	noradrenalina	**noradrenaline**
norepinefrina	norepinefrina	**norepinephrine**
normoblasto	normoblasto	**normoblast**
normocito	normocito	**normocyte**
normoglicemico	normoglucémico	**normoglycaemic** (Eng)
normoglicemico	normoglucémico	**normoglycemic** (Am)
normotonico	normotónico	**normotonic**
naso	nariz	**nose**
epistassi	epistaxis	**nosebleed**
narice	fosa nasale	**nostril**
malattia da denunciare alle autorità sanitarie	enfermedad declarable	**notifiable disease**
non ancora diagnosticato	todavía no diagnosticado	**not yet diagnosed (NYD)**
nucleo	núcleo	**nucleus**
nullipara	nulípara	**nullipara**
infermiere (n)	enfermera (n)	**nurse** (n)
assistere (v)	cuidar (v)	**nurse** (v)
sostanza nutritiva (n)	nutriente (n)	**nutrient** (n)
nutriente (a)	nutriente (a)	**nutrient** (a)
nutrizione	nutrición	**nutrition**
nictalgia	nictalgia	**nyctalgia**
nicturia	nicturia	**nycturia**
nistagmo	nistagmo	**nystagmus**

O

ENGLISH	FRENCH	GERMAN
oat cell cancer	épithélioma à petites cellules	kleinzelliges Bronchialkarzinom
obesity	obésité	Adipositas, Obesitas
obsessional neurosis	névrose obsessionnelle	Zwangsneurose
obstetrics	obstétrique	Geburtshilfe
obstructive	obstructif	obstruktiv
obturator	obturateur	Obturator, Gaumenverschlußplatte
occipital	occipital	okzipital
occipitoanterior	occipito-antérieur	vordere Hinterhauptslage
occipitofrontal	occipito-frontal	okzipitofrontal
occipitoposterior	occipito-postérieur	hintere Hinterhauptslage
occiput	occiput	Okziput, Hinterkopf
occlusion	occlusion	Okklusion, Verschluß
occult	occulte	okkult
occult blood	sang occulte	okkultes Blut
occupational disease	maladie professionnelle	Berufskrankheit
occupational health	hygiène du travail	Gewerbehygiene
occupational therapy	ergothérapie	Beschäftigungstherapie
ocular	oculaire	okular
oculogyric	oculogyre	Bewegung der Augen betr.
oculomotor	oculomoteur	Oculomotorius-
odontic	dentaire	Odonto-, Zahn-
odontoid	odontoïde	odontoid
oedema (Eng)	oedème	Ödem, Flüssigkeitsansammlung
oesophageal (Eng)	oesophagien	ösophageal
oesophagitis (Eng)	oesophagite	Ösophagitis
oesophagus (Eng)	oesophage	Ösophagus, Speiseröhre
oestradiol (Eng)	oestradiol	Östradiol
oestriol (Eng)	oestriol	Östriol
oestrogen (Eng)	oestrogène	Östrogen
ointment	pommade	Salbe
old age pensioner (OAP)	retraité(e)	Rentner
olecranon (process)	olécrane	Olekranon, Ellenbozen
olfactory	olfactif	olfaktorisch
oligaemia (Eng)	hypovolémie	Oligämie, Blutmangel
oligemia (Am)	hypovolémie	Oligämie, Blutmangel
oligomenorrhea (Am)	spanioménorrhée	Oligomenorrhoe
oligomenorrhoea (Eng)	spanioménorrhée	Oligomenorrhoe
oliguria	oligurie	Oligurie
omentum	épiploon	Omentum, Netz
onchocerciasis	onchocercose	Onchozerkose
oncogene	oncogène	Onkogen
oncology	oncologie	Onkologie
onychogryphosis	onychogryphose	Onychogryposis
onycholysis	onycholyse	Onycholyse, Nagelablösung

ITALIAN	SPANISH	ENGLISH
microcitoma, carcinoma a piccole cellule	carcinoma de células de avena	oat cell cancer
obesità	obesidad	obesity
nevrosi ossessiva	neurosis obsesiva	obsessional neurosis
ostetricia	obstetricia	obstetrics
ostruttivo	obstructivo	obstructive
otturatorio	obturador	obturator
occipitale	occipital	occipital
occipitoanteriore	occipitoanterior	occipitoanterior
occipitofrontale	occipitofrontal	occipitofrontal
occipitoposteriore	occipitoposterior	occipitoposterior
occipite	occipucio	occiput
occlusione	oclusión	occlusion
occulto	oculta	occult
sangue occulto	sangre oculta	occult blood
malattia professionale	enfermedad profesional	occupational disease
medicina del lavoro	higiene profesional	occupational health
ergoterapia	terapéutica ocupacional	occupational therapy
oculare	ocular	ocular
oculogiro	oculógiro	oculogyric
oculomotore	oculomotor	oculomotor
dentario	dentario	odontic
odontoide	odontoides	odontoid
edema	edema	oedema (Eng)
esofageo	esofágico	oesophageal (Eng)
esofagite	esofagitis	oesophagitis (Eng)
esofago	esófago	oesophagus (Eng)
estradiolo	estradiol	oestradiol (Eng)
estriolo	estriol	oestriol (Eng)
estrogeno	estrógeno	oestrogen (Eng)
unguento	ungüento	ointment
anziano pensionato	jubilado	old age pensioner (OAP)
olecrano	olécranon	olecranon (process)
olfattorio	olfatorio	olfactory
oligoemia	oligohemia	oligaemia (Eng)
oligoemia	oligohemia	oligemia (Am)
oligomenorrea	oligomenorrea	oligomenorrhea (Am)
oligomenorrea	oligomenorrea	oligomenorrhoea (Eng)
oliguria	oliguria	oliguria
omento	epiplón	omentum
oncocerchiasi	oncocerciasis	onchocerciasis
oncogene	oncogén	oncogene
oncologia	oncología	oncology
onicogrifosi	onicogriposis	onychogryphosis
onicolisi	onicólisis	onycholysis

ENGLISH	FRENCH	GERMAN
oophorectomy	ovariectomie	Oophorektomie
opacity	opacité	Opazität
opaque	opaque	undurchsichtig, verschattet (radiolog)
operating microscope	microscope opératoire	Operationsmikroskop
operation	opération	Operation, Einwirkung, Eingriff
ophthalmia	ophtalmie	Ophthalmie
ophthalmic	ophtalmique	Augen-
ophthalmology	ophtalmologie	Ophthalmologie, Augenheilkunde
ophthalmoplegia	ophtalmoplégie	Ophthalmoplegie, Augenmuskellähmung
ophthalmoscope	ophtalmoscope	Ophthalmoskop, Augenspiegel
opportunistic infection	infection opportuniste	opportunistische Infektion
optic	optique	optisch, Seh-
optician	opticien	Optiker
optimum	optimum	optimal
oral	oral	oral
orbit	orbite	Orbita, Augenhöhle
orchidectomy	orchidectomie	Orchidektomie
orchidopexy	orchidopexie	Orchidopexie
orchidotomy	orchodotomie	Orchidotomie
orchiopexy	orchidopexie	Orchipexie
orchis	testicule	Hoden
orchitis	orchite	Orchitis
organic	organique	organisch
organism	organisme	Organismus, Keim
orgasm	orgasme	Orgasmus
orientation	orientation	Orientierung
orifice	orifice	Öffnung
origin	origine	Ursprung
oropharynx	oropharynx	Mundrachenhöhle
orthodontics	orthodontie	Kieferorthopädie
orthopaedic (Eng)	orthopédique	orthopädisch
orthopedic (Am)	orthopédique	orthopädisch
orthopnea (Am)	orthopnée	Orthopnoe
orthopnoea (Eng)	orthopnée	Orthopnoe
orthoptics	orthoptique	Orthoptik
orthosis	orthèse	Orthose
orthostatic	orthostatique	orthostatisch
oscillation	oscillation	Oszillation, Schwankung
Osgood-Schlatter disease	maladie d'Osgood-Schlatter	Osgood-Schlatter-Krankheit
Osler's nodes	nodules d'Osler	Osler-Knötchen
osmolality	osmolalité	Osmolalität
osmolarity	osmolarité	Osmolarität
osmosis	osmose	Osmose
osmotic pressure	pression osmotique	osmotischer Druck
osseous	osseux	knöchern, Knochen-
ossicle	osselet	Gehörknöchelchen, Ossikel

ovariectomia, ooforectomia	ooforectomía	oophorectomy
opacità	opacidad	opacity
opaco	opaco	opaque
microscopio chirurgico	microscopio quirúrgico	operating microscope
operazione	intervención quirúrgica	operation
oftalmia	oftalmía	ophthalmia
oftalmico	oftálmico	ophthalmic
oftalmologia	oftalmología	ophthalmology
oftalmoplegia	oftalmoplejía	ophthalmoplegia
oftalmoscopio	oftalmoscopio	ophthalmoscope
infezione opportunista	infección oportunista	opportunistic infection
ottico	óptico	optic
ottico	óptico	optician
optimum	óptimo	optimum
orale	oral	oral
orbita	órbita	orbit
orchidectomia	orquidectomía	orchidectomy
orchidopessia	orquidopexia	orchidopexy
orchidectomia	orquidotomía	orchidotomy
orchidopessia	orquiopexia	orchiopexy
testicolo	testículo	orchis
orchite	orquitis	orchitis
organico	orgánico	organic
organismo	organismo	organism
orgasmo	orgasmo	orgasm
orientamento	orientación	orientation
orifizio	orificio	orifice
origine	origen	origin
orofaringe	orofaringe	oropharynx
ortodonzia	ortodoncia	orthodontics
ortopedia	ortopedia	orthopaedic (Eng)
ortopedia	ortopedia	orthopedic (Am)
ortopnea	ortopnea	orthopnea (Am)
ortopnea	ortopnea	orthopnoea (Eng)
ortottica	ortóptica	orthoptics
raddrizzamento, correzione di una deformità	ortosis	orthosis
ortostatico	ortostático	orthostatic
oscillazione	oscilación	oscillation
malattia di Osgood-Schlatter	enfermedad de Osgood-Schlatter	Osgood-Schlatter disease
noduli di Osler	nódulos de Osler	Osler's nodes
osmolalità	osmolalidad	osmolality
osmolarità	osmolaridad	osmolarity
osmosi	osmosis	osmosis
pressione osmotica	presión osmótica	osmotic pressure
osseo	óseo	osseous
ossicino	huesecillos	ossicle

ENGLISH	FRENCH	GERMAN
osteitis	ostéite	Ostitis, Knochenentzündung
osteoarthritis (OA)	ostéo-arthrite	Osteoarthritis
osteoarthropathy	ostéo-arthropathie	Osteoarthrose
osteoblast	ostéoblaste	Osteoblast
osteochondritis	ostéochondrite	Osteochondritis
osteochondroma	ostéochondrome	Osteochondrom
osteochondrosis	ostéochondrose	Osteochondrose
osteoclast	ostéoclaste	Osteoklast
osteocyte	ostéocyte	Osteozyt
osteodystrophy	ostéodystrophie	Osteodystrophie
osteogenic	ostéogène	osteogen
osteolytic	ostéolytique	osteolytisch
osteoma	ostéome	Osteom
osteomalacia	ostéomalacie	Osteomalazie
osteomyelitis	ostéomyélite	Osteomyelitis, Knochenmarksentzündung
osteopathy	ostéopathie	Osteopathie
osteopetrosis	ostéopétrose	Osteopetrose
osteophyte	ostéophyte	Osteophyt
osteoporosis	ostéoporose	Osteoporose
osteosarcoma	ostéosarcome	Osteosarkom, Knochensarkom
osteosclerosis	ostéosclérose	Osteosklerose, Eburnifikation
osteotomy	ostéotomie	Osteotomie
ostomy	ostéotomie	Osteotomie
otalgia	otalgie	Otalgie, Ohrenschmerz
otitis	otite	Otitis, Mittelohrentzündung
otolaryngology	otolaryngologie	Otolaryngologie
otology	otologie	Otologie, Ohrenheilkunde
otorrhea (Am)	otorrhée	Otorrhoe, Ohrenfluß
otorrhoea (Eng)	otorrhée	Otorrhoe, Ohrenfluß
otosclerosis	otospongiose	Otosklerose
otoscope	otoscope	Otoskop, Ohrenspiegel
ototoxic	ototoxique	ototoxisch
ovarian	ovarien	ovarial, Eierstock-
ovary	ovaire	Ovarium, Eierstock
over the counter (OTC)	spécialités pharmaceutiques grand public	rezeptfrei
ovulation	ovulation	Ovulation, Eisprung
ovum	ovule, ovocyte de premier ordre, oeuf	Ovum, Ei
oxidation	oxydation	Oxydation
oxygenation	oxygénation	Sauerstoffsättigung, Oxygenierung
oxytocin	oxytocine	Oxytozin

ITALIAN	SPANISH	ENGLISH
osteite	osteítis	osteitis
osteoartrosi (OA)	osteoartritis	osteoarthritis (OA)
osteoartropatia	osteoartropatía	osteoarthropathy
osteoblasto	osteoblasto	osteoblast
osteocondrite	osteocondritis	osteochondritis
osteocondroma	osteocondroma	osteochondroma
osteocondrosi	osteocondrosis	osteochondrosis
osteoclasto	osteoclasto	osteoclast
osteocito	osteocito	osteocyte
osteodistrofia	osteodistrofia	osteodystrophy
osteogenico	osteogénico	osteogenic
osteolitico	osteolítico	osteolytic
osteoma	osteoma	osteoma
osteomalacia	osteomalacia	osteomalacia
osteomielite	osteomielitis	osteomyelitis
osteopatia	osteopatía	osteopathy
osteoporosi	osteopetrosis	osteopetrosis
osteofito	osteofito	osteophyte
osteoporosi	osteoporosis	osteoporosis
sarcoma osteogenico	osteosarcoma	osteosarcoma
osteosclerosi	osteosclerosis	osteosclerosis
osteotomia	osteotomía	osteotomy
otalgia	ostomía	ostomy
otite	otalgia	otalgia
otite	otitis	otitis
otolaringologia	otolaringología	otolaryngology
otologia	otología	otology
otorrea	otorrea	otorrhea (Am)
otorrea	otorrea	otorrhoea (Eng)
otosclerosi	otosclerosis	otosclerosis
otoscopio	otoscopio	otoscope
ototossico	ototóxico	ototoxic
ovarico	ovárico	ovarian
ovaio	ovario	ovary
(farmaco) ottenibile senza prescrizione medica	sin receta médica	over the counter (OTC)
ovulazione	ovulación	ovulation
uovo, gamete femminile	óvulo	ovum
ossidazione	oxidación	oxidation
ossigenazione	oxigenación	oxygenation
ossitocina	oxitocina	oxytocin

P

ENGLISH	FRENCH	GERMAN
pacemaker	stimulateur cardiaque	Schrittmacher
packed cell volume (PCV)	hématocrite	Hämatokrit (HKT)
paediatrics (Eng)	pédiatrie	Pädiatrie, Kinderheilkunde
Paget's disease	maladie de Paget	Morbus Paget
pain	douleur	Schmerz
palate	palais	Gaumen
palatine	palatin	palatal
palliative (n)	palliatif (n)	Palliativum (n)
palliative (a)	palliatif (a)	palliativ (a)
pallor	pâleur	Blässe
palm	paume	Handinnenfläche
palmar	palmaire	palmar
palpable	palpable	palpabel, tastbar
palpation	palpation	Palpation
palpebra	paupière	Palpebra, Lid
palpitation	palpitation	Palpitation, Herzklopfen
palsy	paralysie	Paralyse, Lähmung
pancreas	pancréas	Pankreas, Bauchspeicheldrüse
pancreatic islets	îlots pancréatiques, îlots de Langerhans	Langerhans-Inseln
pancreatitis	pancréatite	Pankreatitis, Bauchspeicheldrüsenentzündung
pancytopenia	pancytopénie	Panzytopenie
pandemic (n)	pandémie (n)	Pandemie (n)
pandemic (a)	pandémique (a)	pandemisch (a)
Papanicolaou's stain test (Pap test)	test de Papanicolaou	Papanicolaou-Färbung (Pap)
papillary	papillaire	papillär
papilledema (Am)	oedème papillaire	Papillenödem
papilloedema (Eng)	oedème papillaire	Papillenödem
papilloma	papillome	Papillom
papule	papule	Papel, Knötchen
paraesthesia (Eng)	paresthésie	Parästhesie
paralysis	paralysie	Paralyse, Lähmung
paralytic	paralytique	paralytisch, gelähmt
paramedical	paramédical	paramedizinisch
paranoia	paranoïa	Paranoia
paranoid schizophrenia	schizophrénie paranoïaque	paranoide Schizophrenie
paraphimosis	paraphimosis	Paraphimose
paraphrenia	paraphrénie	Paraphrenie
paraplegia	paraplégie	Paraplegie, Querschnittslähmung
parasite	parasite	Parasit, Schmarotzer
parasuicide	parasuicide	parasuizidale Handlung
parasympathetic	parasympathique	parasympathisch
parathormone	parathormone	Parathormon
parathyroidectomy	parathyroïdectomie	Parathyreoidektomie
parathyroid gland	glande parathyroïde	Nebenschilddrüse, Parathyreoidea

ITALIAN	SPANISH	ENGLISH
pacemaker	marcapasos	**pacemaker**
volume cellulare (VC)	volumen de células agregadas	**packed cell volume (PCV)**
pediatria	pediatría	**paediatrics** (Eng)
malattia di Paget	enfermedad de Paget	**Paget's disease**
dolore	dolor	**pain**
palato	paladar	**palate**
palatale, palatino	palatino	**palatine**
palliativo (n)	paliativo (n)	**palliative** (n)
palliativo (a)	paliativo (a)	**palliative** (a)
pallore	palidez	**pallor**
palmo	palma	**palm**
palmare	palmar	**palmar**
palpabile	palpable	**palpable**
palpazione	palpación	**palpation**
palpebra	párpado	**palpebra**
palpitazione	palpitación	**palpitation**
paralisi	parálisis	**palsy**
pancreas	páncreas	**pancreas**
isolotti pancreatici	islotes pancreáticos	**pancreatic islets**
pancreatite	pancreatitis	**pancreatitis**
pancitopenia	pancitopenia	**pancytopenia**
pandemia (n)	pandémico (n)	**pandemic** (n)
pandemico (a)	pandémico (a)	**pandemic** (a)
test di Papanicolaou (Pap test)	prueba de tinción de Papanicolaou	**Papanicolaou's stain test (Pap test)**
papillare	papilar	**papillary**
papilledema	papiledema	**papilledema** (Am)
papilledema	papiledema	**papilloedema** (Eng)
papilloma	papiloma	**papilloma**
papula	pápula	**papule**
parestesia	parestesia	**paraesthesia** (Eng)
paralisi	parálisis	**paralysis**
paralitico	paralítico	**paralytic**
paramedico	paramédico	**paramedical**
paranoia	paranoia	**paranoia**
schizofrenia paranoide	esquizofrenia paranoica	**paranoid schizophrenia**
parafimosi	parafimosis	**paraphimosis**
parafrenia	parafrenia	**paraphrenia**
paraplegia	paraplejía	**paraplegia**
parassita	parásito	**parasite**
suicidio figurato	parasuicidio	**parasuicide**
parasimpatico	parasimpático	**parasympathetic**
paratormone	parathormona	**parathormone**
paratiroidectomia	paratiroidectomía	**parathyroidectomy**
ghiandola paratiroide	glándula paratiroidea	**parathyroid gland**

| --- | --- | --- |
paratyphoid fever	fièvre paratyphoïde	Paratyphus
paravertebral	paravertébral	paravertebral
parenchyma	parenchyme	Parenchym
parenteral	parentéral	parenteral
paresis	parésie	Parese, Lähmung
paresthesia (Am)	paresthésie	Parästhesie
pareunia	coït	Koitus, Geschlechtsverkehr
parietal	pariétal	parietal, wandständig
parity	parité	Gebärfähigkeit, Ähnlichkeit
parkinsonism	parkinsonisme	Parkinsonismus
paronychia	panaris superficiel	Paronychie
parotid gland	glande parotide	Parotis, Ohrspeicheldrüse
parotitis	parotite	Parotitis
parous	poreux	geboren habend
paroxysmal	paroxysmal	paroxysmal, krampfartig
partial pressure	pression partielle	Partialdruck
partly soluble (p.sol)	partiellement soluble	teilweise löslich
parts per million (ppm)	parties par million (ppm)	ppm, mg/l
parturient	parturient	gebärend
parturition	parturition	Gebären, Geburt
passive	passif	passiv, teilnahmslos
paste	pâte	Paste, Salbe
pasteurization	pasteurisation	Pasteurisierung
patch test	tache, plaque, pièce	Läppchenprobe, Einreibeprobe
patella	rotule	Patella, Kniescheibe
patent	libre	offen, durchgängig
pathogen	pathogène	Krankheitserreger, Erreger
pathogenesis	pathogenèse	Pathogenese
pathogenicity	pouvoir pathogène	Pathogenität
pathognomonic	pathognomonique	pathognomonisch
pathological fracture	fracture spontanée	pathologische Fraktur
pathology	pathologie	Pathologie
patient compliance	observance du patient	Compliance
Paul-Bunnell test	réaction de Paul et Bunnell	Paul-Bunnell-Reaktion
peak expiratory flow meter (PEFM)	appareil de mesure du débit expiratoire de pointe	Peak-Flowmeter
peak expiratory flow rate (PEFR)	débit expiratoire de pointe	maximale exspiratorische Atemstromstärke
peak expiratory velocity (PEV)	volume expiratoire maximum (VEM)	maximale exspiratorische Atemgeschwindigkeit
peau d'orange	peau d'orange	Orangenhaut
pectoral	pectoral	pektoral, Brust-
pedal	pédieux	Fuß-
pediatrics (Am)	pédiatrie	Pädiatrie, Kinderheilkunde
pediculosis	pédiculose	Pedikulose, Läusebefall
peduncle	pédoncule	Stiel
peeling	desquamation	Schälen (Haut), Schuppung

febbre paratifoide	fiebre paratifoidea	paratyphoid fever
paravertebrale	paravertebral	paravertebral
parenchima	parénquima	parenchyma
parenterale	parenteral	parenteral
paresi	paresia	paresis
parestesia	parestesia	paresthesia (Am)
coito	pareunia	pareunia
parietale	parietal	parietal
parità, numero di gravidanze pregresse	paridad	parity
parkinsonismo	parkinsonismo	parkinsonism
paronichia	paroniquia	paronychia
ghiandola parotide	glándula parótida	parotid gland
parotite	parotiditis	parotitis
che ha avuto figli	parir	parous
parossistico	paroxístico	paroxysmal
pressione parziale	presión parcial	partial pressure
parzialmente solubile	semisoluble	partly soluble (p.sol)
parti per milione (ppm)	partes por millón (ppm)	parts per million (ppm)
partoriente	parturienta	parturient
parto	parturición, parto	parturition
passivo	pasivo	passive
pasta, pasta gelificante	pasta	paste
pastorizzazione	pasteurización	pasteurization
test epicutaneo	prueba del parche	patch test
patella, rotula	rótula	patella
aperto, esposto	permeable	patent
patogeno	patógeno	pathogen
patogenesi	patogenia	pathogenesis
patogeneticità	patogenicidad	pathogenicity
patognomonico	patognomónico	pathognomonic
frattura patologica	fractura patológica	pathological fracture
patologia	patología	pathology
acquiescenza alle prescrizioni	cumplimiento del paciente	patient compliance
test di Paul-Bunnell	prueba de Paul-Bunnell	Paul-Bunnell test
misuratore del flusso espiratorio massimo	medida de la velocidad máxima del flujo espiratorio	peak expiratory flow meter (PEFM)
tasso di picco del flusso espiratorio	velocidad máxima del flujo espiratorio (VMFE)	peak expiratory flow rate (PEFR)
velocità espiratoria massima (VEM)	velocidad espiratoria máxima (VEM)	peak expiratory velocity (PEV)
buccia d'arancia	piel de naranja	peau d'orange
pettorale	pectoral	pectoral
del piede	pedal	pedal
pediatria	pediatria	pediatrics (Am)
pediculosi	pediculosis	pediculosis
peduncolo	pedúnculo	peduncle
desquamazione	exfoliación	peeling

ENGLISH	FRENCH	GERMAN
pellagra	pellagre	Pellagra
pelvic floor	plancher pelvien	Beckenboden
pelvic girdle	ceinture pelvienne	Beckengürtel
pelvic inflammatory disease (PID)	pelvipéritonite	Salpingitis
pelvimetry	pelvimétrie	Pelvimetrie
pelvis	pelvis	Pelvis, Becken
pemphigoid	pemphigoïde	pemphigoid
pemphigus	pemphigus	Pemphigus
pendulous	pendant	hängend, gestielt
penetrating wound	plaie par pénétration	penetrierende Verletzung
penis	pénis	Penis
pepsin	pepsine	Pepsin
peptic	peptique	peptisch
peptide	peptide	Peptide
perception	perception	Perzeption, Wahrnehmung
percussion	percussion	Perkussion
percutaneous	percutané	perkutan
perforation	perforation	Perforation
perfusion	perfusion	Durchblutung
perianal	périanal	perianal
pericarditis	péricardite	Perikarditis
pericardium	péricarde	Perikard, Herzbeutel
perichondrium	périchondre	Perichondrium, Knorpelhaut
perinatal	périnatal	perinatal
perineum	périnée	Perineum, Damm
periodontal disease	paradontolyse	Periodontitis, Wurzelhautentzündung
perioperative	périopératoire	perioperativ
perioral	périoral	perioral
periosteum	périoste	Periost, Knochenhaut
peripheral	périphérique	peripher
peristalsis	péristaltisme	Peristaltik
peritoneal dialysis	dialyse péritonéale	Peritonealdialyse
peritoneum	péritoine	Peritoneum, Bauchfell
peritonitis	péritonite	Peritonitis
peritonsillar abscess	abcès périamygdalien	Peritonsillarabszeß
periumbilical	périombilical	periumbilikal
permeable	perméable	permeabel, durchlässig
pernicious anaemia (Eng)	anémie pernicieuse	perniziöse Anämie
pernicious anemia (Am)	anémie pernicieuse	perniziöse Anämie
peroneal nerve	nerf péronier	Nervus peroneus
peroneus muscles	muscles péroniers	Musculi peronei
peroral	peroral	peroral
perseveration	persévération	Perseveration
personality	personnalité	Persönlichkeit
perspiration	perspiration	Schweiß
Perthes' disease	coxa plana	Perthes-Krankheit

| --- | --- | --- |
pellagra	pelagra	**pellagra**
pavimento pelvico	suelo de la pelvis	**pelvic floor**
cingolo pelvico	cintura pélvica	**pelvic girdle**
malattia infiammatoria della pelvi (PID)	enfermedad inflamatoria de la pelvis	**pelvic inflammatory disease (PID)**
pelvimetria	pelvimetría	**pelvimetry**
pelvi	pelvis	**pelvis**
pemfigoide	penfigoide	**pemphigoid**
pemfigo	pénfigo	**pemphigus**
pendulo	péndulo	**pendulous**
ferita penetrante	herida penetrante	**penetrating wound**
pene	pene	**penis**
pepsina	pepsina	**pepsin**
peptico	péptico	**peptic**
peptide	péptido	**peptide**
percezione	percepción	**perception**
percussione	percusión	**percussion**
percutaneo	percutáneo	**percutaneous**
perforazione	perforación	**perforation**
perfusione	perfusión	**perfusion**
perianale	perianal	**perianal**
pericardite	pericarditis	**pericarditis**
pericardio	pericardio	**pericardium**
pericondrio	pericondrio	**perichondrium**
perinatale	perinatal	**perinatal**
perineo	perineo	**perineum**
periodontopatia	enfermedad periodontal	**periodontal disease**
perioperatorio	perioperatorio	**perioperative**
periorale	perioral	**perioral**
periostio	periostio	**periosteum**
periferico	periférico	**peripheral**
peristalsi	peristalsis	**peristalsis**
dialisi peritoneale	diálisis peritoneal	**peritoneal dialysis**
peritoneo	peritoneo	**peritoneum**
peritonite	peritonitis	**peritonitis**
ascesso peritonsillare	absceso periamigdalino	**peritonsillar abscess**
periombelicale	periumbilical	**periumbilical**
permeabile	permeable	**permeable**
anemia perniciosa	anemia perniciosa	**pernicious anaemia** (Eng)
anemia perniciosa	anemia perniciosa	**pernicious anemia** (Am)
nervo peroneo	nervio peroneo	**peroneal nerve**
muscoli peronei	músculos peroneos	**peroneus muscles**
perorale	peroral	**peroral**
perseverazione	perseverancia	**perseveration**
personalità	personalidad	**personality**
perspirazione	sudor	**perspiration**
malattia di Perthes	enfermedad de Perthes	**Perthes' disease**

ENGLISH	FRENCH	GERMAN
pertussis	pertussis	Pertussis, Keuchhusten
pessary	pessaire	Pessar
petechia	pétéchie	Petechie
petit mal	petit mal	Petit mal
Petri dish	boîte de Pétri	Petrischale
Peyer's patches	plaques de Peyer	Peyer Plaques
Peyronie's disease	maladie de La Peyronie	Induratio penis plastica
phaeochromocytoma (Eng)	phéochromocytome	Phäochromozytom
phagocyte	phagocyte	Phagozyt
phagocytosis	phagocytose	Phagozytose
phalanges	phalanges	Fingerglieder, Zehenglieder
phallus	phallus	Phallus, Penis
phantom pregnancy	fausse grossesse	Scheinschwangerschaft, hysterische Schwangerschaft
pharmaceutical	pharmaceutique	pharmazeutisch, Apotheker-
pharmacist	pharmacien	Apotheker, Pharmazeut
pharmacogenetics	pharmacogénétique	Pharmakogenetik
pharmacokinetics	pharmacocinétique	Pharmakokinetik
pharmacology	pharmacologie	Pharmakologie
pharyngeal pouch	poche ectobranchiale et entobranchiale	Schlundtasche
pharyngitis	pharyngite	Pharyngitis
pharyngotomy	pharyngotomie	Pharyngotomie
pharynx	pharynx	Pharynx, Rachen
phenotype	phénotype	Phänotyp
phenylketonuria (PKU)	phénylcétonurie	Phenylketonurie (PKU)
pheochromocytoma (Am)	phéochromocytome	Phäochromozytom
phimosis	phimosis	Phimose
phlebectomy	phlébectomie	Phlebektomie
phlebitis	phlébite	Phlebitis, Venenentzündung
phlebolith	phlébolithe	Phlebolith
phlebotomy	phlébotomie	Venae sectio
phlegm	phlegme	Phlegma
phobia	phobie	Phobie
phocomelia	phocomélie	Phokomelie
photophobia	photophobie	Photophobie, Lichtscheue
photosensitive	photosensible	lichtempfindlich
phototherapy	photothérapie	Phototherapie
phrenic	psychique	diaphragmatisch, Zwerchfell-
physician	médecin	Arzt
physiological	physiologique	physiologisch
pica	pica	Pica
pigeon chest	thorax en carène	Hühnerbrust
pigment	pigment	Pigment, Farbstoff
pigmentation	pigmentation	Pigmentierung, Färbung
piles	hémorroïdes	Hämorrhoiden
pill	pilule	Pille
pilonidal	pilonidal	pilonidal

ITALIAN	SPANISH	ENGLISH
pertosse	tos ferina	**pertussis**
pessario	pesario	**pessary**
petecchia	petequia	**petechia**
piccolo male	petit mal	**petit mal**
capsula di Petri	disco de Petri	**Petri dish**
placche di Peyer	placas de Peyer	**Peyer's patches**
malattia di Peyronie	enfermedad de Peyronie	**Peyronie's disease**
feocromocitoma	feocromocitoma	**phaeochromocytoma** (Eng)
fagocito	fagocito	**phagocyte**
fagocitosi	fagocitosis	**phagocytosis**
falangi	falanges	**phalanges**
fallo	falo	**phallus**
pseudociesi	embarazo fantasma	**phantom pregnancy**
farmaceutico	farmacéutico	**pharmaceutical**
farmacista	farmacéutico	**pharmacist**
farmacogenetica	farmacogenético	**pharmacogenetics**
farmacocinetica	farmacocinética	**pharmacokinetics**
farmacologia	farmacología	**pharmacology**
tasca faringea	bolsa faringea	**pharyngeal pouch**
faringite	faringitis	**pharyngitis**
faringotomia	faringotomía	**pharyngotomy**
faringe	faringe	**pharynx**
fenotipo	fenotipo	**phenotype**
fenilchetonuria	fenilcetonuria	**phenylketonuria (PKU)**
feocromocitoma	feocromocitoma	**pheochromocytoma** (Am)
fimosi	fimosis	**phimosis**
flebectomia	flebectomía	**phlebectomy**
flebite	flebitis	**phlebitis**
flebolito	flebolito	**phlebolith**
flebotomia	flebotomía	**phlebotomy**
flemma	flema	**phlegm**
fobia	fobia	**phobia**
focomelia	focomelia	**phocomelia**
fotofobia	fotofobia	**photophobia**
fotosensibile	fotosensible	**photosensitive**
fototerapia	fototerapia	**phototherapy**
frenico (diaframmatico mentale)	frénico	**phrenic**
medico	facultativo, médico	**physician**
fisiologico	fisiológico	**physiological**
picacismo	pica	**pica**
torace carenato	tórax de pichón	**pigeon chest**
pigmento	pigmento	**pigment**
pigmentazione	pigmentación	**pigmentation**
emorroidi	hemorroides	**piles** .
pillola	píldora	**pill**
pilonidale	pilonidal	**pilonidal**

ENGLISH	FRENCH	GERMAN
pimple	bouton	Pickel, Mitesser
pineal body	glande pinéale	Epiphyse
pinguecula	pinguécula	Pinguekula
pinkeye	conjonctivite aiguë contagieuse	epidemische Konjunktivitis
pinna	pavillon de l'oreille	Ohrmuschel
pinta	pinta	Pinta
pitting	formation de godet	Dellenbildung
pituitary gland	hypophyse	Hypophyse
pityriasis	pityriasis	Pityriasis
placebo	placebo	Plazebo
placenta	placenta	Plazenta, Nachgeburt
placental abruption	rupture placentaire	Plazentaablösung
placental insufficiency	insuffisance placentaire	Plazentainsuffizienz
plague	peste	Pest, Seuche
plantar	plantaire	plantar
plaque	plaque	Plaque, Zahnbelag
plasma	plasma	Plasma
plasmapheresis	plasmaphérèse	Plasmapherese
plaster	plâtre	Gips, Pflaster
plaster of Paris	sulfate de calcium hydraté, plâtre	Gips
platelet	plaquette	Thrombozyt, Blutplättchen
platelet aggregation test (PAT)	test d'agrégation plaquettaire (PAT)	Plättchen-Aggregations-Test (PAT)
plethora	pléthore	Plethora
pleura	plèvre	Pleura
pleurisy (pleuritis)	pleurésie	Pleuritis, Rippenfellentzündung
pleurodesis	pleurodèse	Pleurodese
pleurodynia	pleurodynie	Pleuralgie
plexus	plexus	Plexus
plication	plicature	Faltenbildung
plumbism	saturnisme	Bleivergiftung
pneumaturia	pneumaturie	Pneumaturie
pneumocephalus	pneumo-encéphale, pneumocéphale	Pneumozephalus
pneumoconiosis	pneumoconiose	Pneumokoniose, Staublunge
pneumocyte	cellule alvéolaire	Pneumozyt
pneumonectomy	pneumonectomie	Pneumonektomie, Lungenresektion
pneumonia	pneumonie	Pneumonie, Lungenentzündung
pneumonitis	pneumonite	Pneumonitis
pneumoperitoneum	pneumopéritoine	Pneumoperitoneum
pneumothorax	pneumothorax	Pneumothorax
poison (n)	poison (n)	Gift (n)
poison (v)	empoisonner (v)	vergiften (v)
poliomyelitis	poliomyélite	Poliomyelitis, Kinderlähmung
poliovirus	poliovirus	Poliovirus
polyarteritis	polyartérite	Polyarteritis
polyarthralgia	polyarthralgie	Polyarthralgie

ITALIAN	SPANISH	ENGLISH
pustola, piccolo foruncolo	grano	**pimple**
ghiandola pineale	cuerpo pineal	**pineal body**
pinguecula	pinguécula	**pinguecula**
congiuntivite batterica acuta contagiosa, congiuntivite catarrale	conjuntivitis	**pinkeye**
padiglione auricolare	pabellón de la oreja	**pinna**
pinta, spirochetosi discromica	mal de pinto	**pinta**
depressioni puntiformi, fovea	cavitación	**pitting**
ghiandola pituitaria, ipofisi	hipófisis	**pituitary gland**
pitiriasi	pitiriasis	**pityriasis**
placebo	placebo	**placebo**
placenta	placenta	**placenta**
distacco prematuro della placenta	desprendimiento prematuro de la placenta	**placental abruption**
insufficienza placentare	insuficiencia placentaria	**placental insufficiency**
peste	peste, plaga	**plague**
plantare	plantar	**plantar**
placca	placa	**plaque**
plasma	plasma	**plasma**
plasmaferesi	plasmaféresis	**plasmapheresis**
gesso	yeso	**plaster**
gesso di Parigi (calcio solfato diidrato)	escayola	**plaster of Paris**
piastrina	plaqueta	**platelet**
test di aggregazione piastrinico	prueba de la agregación plaquetaria	**platelet aggregation test (PAT)**
pletora	plétora	**plethora**
pleura	pleura	**pleura**
pleurite	pleuresia, pleuritis	**pleurisy (pleuritis)**
pleurodesi	pleurodesis	**pleurodesis**
pleurodinia	pleurodinia	**pleurodynia**
plesso	plexo	**plexus**
plicazione, piegatura	plicatura	**plication**
intossicazione da piombo	plumbismo, saturnismo	**plumbism**
pneumaturia	neumaturia	**pneumaturia**
pneumocefalo	neumocéfalo	**pneumocephalus**
pneumoconiosi	neumoconiosis	**pneumoconiosis**
pneumocito	neumocito	**pneumocyte**
pneumonectomia	neumonectomía	**pneumonectomy**
polmonite	neumonía	**pneumonia**
polmonite	neumonitis	**pneumonitis**
pneumoperitoneo	neumoperitoneo	**pneumoperitoneum**
pneumotorace	neumotórax	**pneumothorax**
veleno *(n)*	veneno *(n)*	**poison** *(n)*
avvelenare *(v)*	envenenar *(v)*	**poison** *(v)*
poliomielite	poliomielitis	**poliomyelitis**
virus della poliomielite	poliovirus	**poliovirus**
poliarterite	poliarteritis	**polyarteritis**
poliartralgia	poliartralgia	**polyarthralgia**

ENGLISH	FRENCH	GERMAN
polyarthritis	polyarthrite	Polyarthritis
polycystic	polykystique	polyzystisch
polycythaemia (Eng)	polycythémie	Polyzythämie
polycythemia (Am)	polycythémie	Polyzythämie
polydipsia	polydipsie	Polydipsie
polymyalgia rheumatica	polymyalgie rhumatismale	Polymyalgia rheumatica
polymyositis	polymyosite	Polymyositis
polyneuritis	polynévrite	Polyneuritis
polyp	polype	Polyp
polypectomy	polypectomie	Polypektomie
polypharmacy	polypharmacie	Polypragmasie
polyposis	polypose	Polyposis
polysaccharide	polysaccharide	Polysaccharid
polyuria	polyurie	Polyurie
pompholyx	pompholyx	Pompholyx
popliteal	poplité	popliteal
popliteus	poplité	popliteus
pore	pore	Pore
porphyria	porphyrie	Porphyrie
porphyrin	porphyrine	Porphyrin
porta	porte	Eingang
portacaval	porto-cave	portokaval
portahepatitis	porto-hépatite	Porta hepatis, Leberpforte
portal circulation	hypertension porte	Portalkreislauf, Pfortaderkreislauf
portal hypertension	circulation porte	Pfortaderhochdruck
portal vein	veine porte	Pfortader
positive pressure ventilation	ventilation à pression positive	Überdruckbeatmung
posseting	régurgitation	Regurgitation bei Säuglingen
postcoital	après rapport	Postkoital-
postencephalitic	postencéphalitique	postenzephalitisch
posterior	postérieur	posteriore, hintere, Gesäß-
posthepatic	posthépatique	posthepatisch
postherpetic	postherpétique	postherpetisch
postmaturity	postmature	Überreife
postmenopausal	postménopausique	postmenopausal
post-mortem	post mortem	postmortal
postnasal	rétronasal	postnasal
postnatal	postnatal	postnatal
postoperative	postopératoire	postoperativ
postpartum	postpartum	post partum
postprandial	postprandial	postprandial
postural	postural	Lage-
Pott's disease	mal de Pott	Malum Potti
Pott's fracture	fracture de Pott	Pott-Fraktur
pouch	poche	Beutel, Tasche
pounds per square inch (psi)	livres par pouce carré (psi)	pounds per square inch (psi)

poliartrite	poliartritis	**polyarthritis**
policistico	poliquístico	**polycystic**
policitemia	policitemia	**polycythaemia** (Eng)
policitemia	policitemia	**polycythemia** (Am)
polidipsia	polidipsia	**polydipsia**
polimialgia reumatica	polimialgia reumática	**polymyalgia rheumatica**
polimiosite	polimiositis	**polymyositis**
polineurite	polineuritis	**polyneuritis**
polipo	pólipo	**polyp**
polipectomia	polipectomía	**polypectomy**
prescrizione multipla di farmaci, abuso di farmaci	polifarmacia	**polypharmacy**
poliposi	poliposis	**polyposis**
polisaccaride	polisacárido	**polysaccharide**
poliuria	poliuria	**polyuria**
ponfolice (disidrosi vescicolare)	ponfólix	**pompholyx**
popliteo	poplíteo	**popliteal**
popliteo	poplíteo	**popliteus**
poro	poro	**pore**
porfiria	porfiria	**porphyria**
porfirina	porfirinas	**porphyrin**
porta	porta	**porta**
portocavale	portocava	**portacaval**
portaepatite	portohepatitis	**portanepatitis**
circolazione portale	circulación portal	**portal circulation**
ipertensione portale	hipertensión portal	**portal hypertension**
vena porta	vena porta	**portal vein**
ventilazione a pressione positiva	ventilación con presión positiva	**positive pressure ventilation**
rigurgito	regurgitación láctea del neonato	**posseting**
postcoitale	postcoital	**postcoital**
postencefalitico	postencefalítico	**postencephalitic**
posteriore	posterior	**posterior**
postepatico	posthepático	**posthepatic**
posterpetico	postherpético	**postherpetic**
postmaturo, ipermaturo	postmaduro	**postmaturity**
postmenopausale	postmenopáusico	**postmenopausal**
post mortem	postmortem	**post-mortem**
retronasale	postnasal	**postnasal**
postnatale	postnatal	**postnatal**
postoperatorio	postoperatorio	**postoperative**
post partum	postpartum	**postpartum**
postprandiale	postprandial	**postprandial**
posturale	postural	**postural**
malattia di Pott	enfermedad de Pott	**Pott's disease**
frattura di Pott	fractura de Pott	**Pott's fracture**
tasca	bolsa	**pouch**
libbre per pollici quadrati	libras por pulgada cuadrada (psi)	**pounds per square inch (psi)**

ENGLISH	FRENCH	GERMAN
precancerous	précancéreux	präkanzerös
preconceptual	préconceptuel	vor Empfängnis
precordial	précordial	präkordial
precursor	précurseur	Vorzeichen, Vorstufe, Präkursor
predisposition	prédisposition	Prädisposition, Anfälligkeit
pre-eclampsia	éclampsisme	Präeklampsie, Eklampsiebereitschaft
pregnancy	grossesse	Schwangerschaft, Gravidität
premature	prématuré	frühreif, vorzeitig
premedication	prémédication	Prämedikation
premenstrual	prémenstruel	prämenstruell
premenstrual tension (PMT)	syndrome de tension prémenstruelle	prämenstruelles Syndrom
prenatal	prénatal	pränatal, vorgeburtlich
preoperative	préopératoire	präoperativ
prepubertal	prépubertaire	Präpubertäts-
prepuce	prépuce	Präputium, Vorhaut
prerenal	prérénal	prärenal
prescription	ordonnance	Rezept, Verschreibung
presenile dementia	démence présénile	präsenile Demenz
presentation	présentation	Lage, Kindslage
pressor	pressif	blutdruckerhöhend, vasopressorisch
pressure area	zone particulièrement sensible	Druckfläche
pressure point	point particulièrement sensible	Druckpunkt, Dekubitus
pressure sore	plaie de décubitus	Druckgeschwür, Dekubitus
primary care	soins de santé primaires	Primärversorgung
primary complex	complexe primaire	Primärkomplex
primigravida	primigeste	Primigravida
primipara	primipare	Primipara, Erstgebärende
procidentia	procidence	Prolaps, Vorfall
proctalgia	proctalgie	Proktalgie
proctitis	rectite	Proktitis
proctocolectomy	proctocolectomie	Proktokolektomie
proctocolitis	rectocolite	Proktokolitis
proctoscope	rectoscope	Rektoskop
prodromal	prodromique	prodromal
pro-drug	précurseur de médicament	pro-drug (Pharmakon-Vorform)
prognosis	pronostic	Prognose
prolapse	prolapsus	Prolaps, Vorfall
proliferate	proliférer	proliferieren
pronate	mettre en pronation	pronieren
pronator	pronateur	Pronator
prone	en pronation	veranlagt, empfänglich
prophylaxis	prophylaxie	Prophylaxe, Vorbeugung
proprietary name	nom de marque	Markenname
proptosis	proptose	Vorfall, Exophthalmus
prostaglandin	prostaglandine	Prostaglandine
prostate	prostate	Prostata

ITALIAN	SPANISH	ENGLISH
precanceroso	precanceroso	precancerous
precedente il concepimento	preconceptual	preconceptual
precordiale, epigastrico	precordial	precordial
precursore	precursor	precursor
predisposizione	predisposición	predisposition
preeclampsia	preeclampsia	pre-eclampsia
gravidanza	embarazo	pregnancy
preamaturo	prematuro	premature
premedicazione, preanestesia	premedicación	premedication
premestruale	premenstrual	premenstrual
tensione premenstruale	tensión premenstrual	premenstrual tension (PMT)
prenatale	prenatal	prenatal
preoperatorio	preoperatorio	preoperative
prepubertale	prepubertal	prepubertal
prepuzio	prepucio	prepuce
prerenale	prerrenal	prerenal
prescrizione, ricetta	receta	prescription
demenza presenile	demencia presenil	presenile dementia
presentazione	presentación	presentation
pressorio	presor	pressor
area di pressione	zona de decúbito	pressure area
punto cutaneo sensibile alla pressione	punto de presión	pressure point
ulcera da decubito	úlcera de decúbito	pressure sore
primaria, neoplasia primitiva	asistencia primaria	primary care
complesso primario, complesso di Ghon	complejo primario	primary complex
primigravida	primigrávida	primigravida
primipara	primípara	primipara
procidenza	procidencia	procidentia
proctalgia	proctalgia	proctalgia
proctite	proctitis	proctitis
proctocolectomia, rettocolectomia	proctocolectomia	proctocolectomy
proctocolite	proctocolitis	proctocolitis
proctoscopio	proctoscopio	proctoscope
prodromico	prodrómico	prodromal
profarmaco (precursore inattivo)	profármaco	pro-drug
prognosi	pronóstico	prognosis
prolasso	prolapso	prolapse
proliferare	proliferar	proliferate
pronare	pronar	pronate
pronatore	pronador	pronator
prono	prono, inclinado	prone
profilassi	profilaxis	prophylaxis
marchio depositato	nombre de patente	proprietary name
proptosi	proptosis	proptosis
prostaglandina	prostaglandina	prostaglandin
prostata	próstata	prostate

ENGLISH	FRENCH	GERMAN
prostatectomy	prostatectomie	Prostatektomie
prostatism	prostatisme	chronisches Prostataleiden
prosthesis	prothèse	Prothese
protein	protéine	Protein
proteinuria	protéinurie	Proteinurie
proteolytic enzyme	enzyme protéolytique	proteolytisches Enzym
protozoa	protozoaires	Protozoe
proximal	proximal	proximal
pruritus	prurit	Pruritus, Jucken
pseudopolyposis	pseudopolypose	Pseudopolypse
psittacosis	psittacose	Psittakose, Ornithose
psoas	psoas	Psoas
psoralen	psoralène	Psoralen
psoriasis	psoriasis	Psoriasis, Schuppenflechte
psoriatic arthritis	rhumatisme psoriasique	Arthritis psoriatica
psychiatric	psychiatrique	psychiatrisch
psychiatry	psychiatrie	Psychiatrie
psychic	psychique	psychisch, seelisch
psychoanalysis	psychanalyse	Psychoanalyse
psychodynamics	psychodynamique	Psychodynamik
psychogenic	psychogène	psychogen
psychogeriatric	psychogériatrique	gerontopsychiatrisch
psychology	psychologie	Psychologie
psychomotor	psychomoteur	psychomotorisch
psychopath	psychopathe	Psychopath
psychopathic personality	personnalité psychopathique	psychopathische Persönlichkeit
psychopathology	psychopathologie	Psychopathologie
psychopathy	psychopathie	Psychopathie
psychosis	psychose	Psychose
psychosomatic	psychosomatique	psychosomatisch, Leib-Seele-
psychotherapy	psychothérapie	Psychotherapie
psychotropic	psychotrope	psychotrop
pterygium	ptérygion	Pterygium
ptosis	ptose	Ptose
puberty	puberté	Pubertät
pubis	pubis	Os pubis, Schambein
pudendal block	vulve	Pudendusblock
puerperal	puerpéral	puerperal, Kindbett-
puerperium	puerpérium	Wochenbett, Puerperium
pulmonary	pulmonaire	Lungen-
pulmonary capillary pressure (PCP)	pression capillaire pulmonaire (PCP), pression artérielle bloquée moyenne	Lungenkapillardruck
pulmonary embolism (PE)	embolie pulmonaire (EP)	Lungenembolie
pulmonary vascular disease (PVD)	pneumopathie vasculaire	Lungengefäßerkrankung
pulsatile	pulsatile	pulsierend
pulsation	pulsation	Pulsieren, Pulsschlag

ITALIAN	SPANISH	ENGLISH
prostatectomia	prostatectomía	prostatectomy
prostatismo	prostatismo	prostatism
protesi	prótesis	prosthesis
proteina	proteína	protein
proteinuria	proteinuria	proteinuria
enzima proteolitico, proteasi	enzima proteolítico	proteolytic enzyme
protozoi	protozoos	protozoa
prossimale	proximal	proximal
prurito	prurito	pruritus
pseudopoliposi	pseudopoliposis	pseudopolyposis
psittacosi	psitacosis	psittacosis
psoas	psoas	psoas
psoralene	psoralen	psoralen
psoriasi	psoriasis	psoriasis
artropatia psoriasica, psoriasi artropatica	artritis psoriásica	psoriatic arthritis
psichiatrico	psiquiátrico	psychiatric
psichiatria	psiquiatría	psychiatry
psichico	psíquico	psychic
psicoanalisi	psicoanálisis	psychoanalysis
psicodinamica	psicodinámica	psychodynamics
psicogenico	psicógeno	psychogenic
psicogeriatrico	psicogeriátrico	psychogeriatric
psicologia	psicología	psychology
psicomotorio	psicomotor	psychomotor
psicopatico	psicópata	psychopath
personalità psicopatica	personalidad psicopática	psychopathic personality
psicopatologia	psicopatología	psychopathology
psicopatia	psicopatía	psychopathy
psicosi	psicosis	psychosis
psicosomatico	psicosomático	psychosomatic
psicoterapia	psicoterapia	psychotherapy
psicotropo	psicotrópico	psychotropic
pterigio, eponichio	pterigión	pterygium
ptosi	ptosis	ptosis
pubertà	pubertad	puberty
pube	pubis	pubis
anestesia della regione pubica	bloqueo del pudendo	pudendal block
puerperale	puerperal	puerperal
puerperio	puerperio	puerperium
polmonare	pulmonar	pulmonary
pressione polmonare di incuneamento	presión capilar pulmonar (PCP)	pulmonary capillary pressure (PCP)
embolia polmonare (EP)	embolismo pulmonar	pulmonary embolism (PE)
vasculopatia polmonare	vasculopatia pulmonar	pulmonary vascular disease (PVD)
pulsatile	pulsátil	pulsatile
pulsazione	pulsación	pulsation

ENGLISH	FRENCH	GERMAN
pulse	pouls	Puls
pulseless disease	syndrome de Takayashu	Pulsloskrankheit
pulsus alternans	pouls alternant	Pulsus alternans
pulsus paradoxus	pouls paradoxal	Pulsus paradoxus
puncture *(n)*	ponction *(n)*	Stich *(n)*, Injektion *(n)*
puncture *(v)*	ponctionner *(v)*	stechen *(v)*, injizieren *(v)*
pupil	pupille	Pupille
pupillary	pupillaire	pupillar, Pupillen-
purgative *(n)*	purgatif *(n)*	Purgativum *(n)*, Abführmittel *(n)*
purgative *(a)*	purgatif *(a)*	purgierend *(a)*, abführend *(a)*
purpura	purpura	Purpura
purulent	purulent	purulent, eitrig
pus	pus	Eiter
pustule	pustule	Pustel, Pickel
putrefaction	putréfaction	Verwesung, Fäulnis
pyaemia (Eng)	septicopyohémie	Pyämie
pyarthrosis	pyarthrose	Pyarthrose, eitrige Gelenkentzündung
pyelitis	pyélite	Pyelitis, Nierenbeckenentzündung
pyelography	pyélographie	Pyelographie
pyelonephritis	pyélonéphrite	Pyelonephritis
pyemia (Am)	septicopyohémie	Pyämie
pyloromyotomy	pylorotomie	Pyloromyotomie
pyloroplasty	pyloroplastie	Pyloroplastik
pylorospasm	pylorospasme	Pylorospasmus
pylorus	pylore	Pylorus
pyoderma	pyodermie	Pyodermie
pyogenic	pyogène	pyogen
pyometra	pyométrie	Pyometra
pyonephrosis	pyonéphrose	Pyonephrose
pyosalpinx	pyosalpinx	Pyosalpinx
pyramidal	pyramidal	pyramidal
pyrexia	pyrexie	Fieber
pyrexia of unknown origin (PUO, FUO)	fièvre d'origine inconnue	Fieber unklarer Genese
pyrosis	pyrosis	Sodbrennen
pyuria	pyurie	Pyurie

ITALIAN	SPANISH	ENGLISH
polso	pulso	**pulse**
sindrome dell'arco aortico	enfermedad sin pulso	**pulseless disease**
polso alternante	pulso alternante	**pulsus alternans**
polso paradosso	pulso paradójico	**pulsus paradoxus**
puntura (n)	punción (n)	**puncture** (n)
pungere (v)	pinchar (v)	**puncture** (v)
pupilla	pupila	**pupil**
pupillare	pupilar	**pupillary**
lassativo (n)	purga (n)	**purgative** (n)
purgante (a)	purgante (a)	**purgative** (a)
porpora	púrpura	**purpura**
purulento	purulento	**purulent**
pus	pus	**pus**
pustola	pústula	**pustule**
putrefazione	putrefacción	**putrefaction**
piemia	piemia	**pyaemia** (Eng)
pioartrosi, piartro	piartrosis	**pyarthrosis**
pielite	pielitis	**pyelitis**
pielografia	pielografía	**pyelography**
pielonefrite	pielonefritis	**pyelonephritis**
piemia	piemia	**pyemia** (Am)
piloromiotomia, intervento di Ramstedt	piloromiotomía	**pyloromyotomy**
piloroplastica	piloroplastia	**pyloroplasty**
pilorospasmo	pilorospasmo	**pylorospasm**
piloro	píloro	**pylorus**
piodermite, pioderma	pioderma	**pyoderma**
piogenico	piógeno	**pyogenic**
piometra	piómetra	**pyometra**
pionefrosi	pionefrosis	**pyonephrosis**
piosalpinge	piosalpinx	**pyosalpinx**
piramidale	piramidal	**pyramidal**
piressia	pirexia, fiebre	**pyrexia**
piressia di origine sconosciuta (POS)	fiebre de origen desconocido	**pyrexia of unknown origin (PUO, FUO)**
pirosi	pirosis	**pyrosis**
piuria	piuria	**pyuria**

Q

ENGLISH	FRENCH	GERMAN
Q fever	fièvre Q	Q-Fieber
quadriceps	quadriceps	Quadrizeps
quadriplegia	quadriplégie	Tetraplegie
qualitative	qualitatif	qualitativ
quantitative	quantitatif	quantitativ
quarantine	quarantaine	Quarantäne
quartan	quarte	quartana (Malaria)
queasy	indigeste, délicat	unwohl, übel
quinsy	phlegmon amygdalien ou périamygdalien	Peritonsillarabszeß

ITALIAN	SPANISH	ENGLISH
febbre Q	fiebre Q	**Q fever**
quadricipite	cuádriceps	**quadriceps**
tetraplegia	cuadriplejía	**quadriplegia**
qualitativo	cualitativo	**qualitative**
quantitativo	cuantitativo	**quantitative**
quarantena	cuarentena	**quarantine**
quartana	cuartana	**quartan**
nauseabondo, nauseato, a disagio	nauseabundo	**queasy**
ascesso peritonsillare	absceso periamigdalino, angina	**quinsy**

R

ENGLISH	FRENCH	GERMAN
rabies	rage	Tollwut
radial artery	artère radiale	Arteria radialis
radial vein	veine radiale	Vena radialis
radical	radical	radikal, Wurzel-
radioactive	radioactif	radioaktiv
radioallergosorbent test (RAST)	technique du RAST	Radio-Allergo-Sorbent-Test (RAST)
radiograph	radiographe	Röntgenaufnahme
radiography	radiographie	Röntgen
radioisotope	radio-isotope	Radioisotop
radiology	radiologie	Radiologie, Röntgenologie
radio-opaque	radio-opaque	röntgendicht
radiosensitive	radiosensible	strahlenempfindlich
radiotherapy	radiothérapie	Strahlentherapie, Radiotherapie
radius	radius	Radius, Halbmesser
Ramsay Hunt syndrome	maladie de Ramsay Hunt	Ramsay-Hunt-Syndrom
Ramstedt's operation	opération de Ramstedt	Weber-Ramstedt-Operation, Ramstedt-(Weber)-Operation
rapid eye movement (REM)	période des mouvements oculaires	rapid eye movement (REM)
rash	rash	Ausschlag, Hautausschlag
Raynaud's disease	maladie de Raynaud	Raynaud-Krankheit
reaction	réaction	Reaktion
reagent	réactif	Reagens
rebore	désobstruction	Desobliteration
recall (n)	évocation (n)	Errinerung (n), Errinerungsvermögen (n)
recall (v)	évoquer (v)	(sich) erinnern (v)
receptor	récepteur	Rezeptor
recessive	récessif	rezessiv
recipient	receveur	Empfänger
recommended daily allowance (RDA)	taux quotidien recommandé	empfohlene Tagesdosis
rectocele	rectocèle	Rektozele
rectum	rectum	Rektum
recumbent	couché	liegend, ruhend
recurrence	répétition, réapparition	Rezidiv
red blood cell (RBC)	globule rouge	Erythrozyt
red blood cell count (RBC)	numération érythrocytaire	rotes Blutbild
referred pain	douleur irradiée	ausstrahlender Schmerz, fortgeleiteter Schmerz
reflex	réflexe	Reflex
reflux	reflux	Reflux
refraction	réfraction	Refraktion, Brechung
refractory	réfractaire	refraktär
regeneration	régénération	Regeneration
regimen	régime	Diät

ITALIAN	SPANISH	ENGLISH
rabbia	rabia	rabies
arteria radiale	arteria radial	radial artery
vena radiale	vena radial	radial vein
radicale	radical	radical
radioattivo	radiactivo	radioactive
test di radioallergoassorbimento (RAST)	prueba radioalergosorbente (RAST)	radioallergosorbent test (RAST)
immagine radiologica	radiografía	radiograph
radiografia	radiografía	radiography
radioisotopo	radioisótopo	radioisotope
radiologia	radiología	radiology
radioopaco	radiopaco	radio-opaque
radiosensibile	radiosensible	radiosensitive
radioterapia	radioterapia	radiotherapy
radio	radio	radius
sindrome di Ramsay Hunt	síndrome de Ramsay-Hunt	Ramsay Hunt syndrome
intervento di Ramstedt, piloromiotomia	operación de Ramstedt	Ramstedt's operation
fase REM del sonno, movimento oculare rapido	movimiento rápido de los ojos (REM)	rapid eye movement (REM)
eruzione cutanea	exantema	rash
malattia di Raynaud	enfermedad de Raynaud	Raynaud's disease
reazione	reacción	reaction
reagente	reactivo	reagent
disobliterazione	desobliteración, repermeabilización	rebore
memoria (n)	recuerdo (n)	recall (n)
ricordare (v)	recordar (v)	recall (v)
recettore	receptor	receptor
recessivo	recesivo	recessive
ricevente	recipiente	recipient
dose giornaliera raccomandata	dosis diaria recomendada	recommended daily allowance (RDA)
rettocele	rectocele	rectocele
retto	recto	rectum
supino, sdraiato	recumbente, de pie	recumbent
recidiva	periódico	recurrence
eritrocito, globulo rosso (RBC)	eritrocito, glóbulo rojo	red blood cell (RBC)
conteggio dei globuli rossi (CGR)	recuento de glóbulos rojos	red blood cell count (RBC)
dolore riferito	dolor referido	referred pain
riflesso	reflejo	reflex
reflusso	reflujo	reflux
rifrazione	refracción	refraction
refrattario	refractario	refractory
rigenerazione	regeneración	regeneration
prescrizione dietetica, dieta	régimen	regimen

ENGLISH	FRENCH	GERMAN
regional ileitis	iléite régionale	Ileitis regionalis
regression	régression	Regression, Rückbildung
regurgitation	régurgitation	Regurgitieren
rehabilitation	réadaptation	Rehabilitation
Reiter's syndrome	syndrome de Fiessinger-Leroy-Reiter	Reiter-Syndrom
rejection	rejet	Abstoßung
relapse (n)	rechute (n)	Rückfall (n), Rezidiv (n)
relapse (v)	rechuter (v)	rezidivieren (v), Rückfall erleiden (v)
relaxant (n)	relaxant (n)	Relaxans (n)
relaxant (a)	relaxant (a)	entspannend (a), relaxierend (a)
remission	rémission	Remission
remittent	rémittent	remittierend, abfallend
REM sleep	sommeil paradoxal	REM-Schlaf
renal	rénal	renal, Nieren-
renal blood flow (RBF)	débit sanguin rénal	Nierendurchblutung, renaler Blutfluß (RBF)
renin	rénine	Renin
repression	répression	Unterdrückung, Verdrängung
reproductive system	système reproducteur	Fortpflanzungsapparat
resection	résection	Resektion
resectoscope	résectoscope	Resektoskop, Resektionszystoskop
residual	résiduel	Residual-
resolution	résolution	Auflösung, Rückgang
resonance	résonance	Resonanz, Schall
resorption	résorption	Resorption
respiration	respiration	Respiration, Atmung
respirator	respirateur	Respirator, Beatmungsgerät
respiratory distress syndrome (RDS)	syndrome de membrane hyaline et de souffrance respiratoire	Respiratory-distress-Syndrom, Atemnotsyndrom
respiratory failure	insuffisance respiratoire	respiratorische Insuffizienz
respiratory function test	test de la fonction respiratoire	Atemfunktionstest
respiratory syncytial virus (RSV)	virus respiratoire syncytial	RS-Virus
respiratory system	système respiratoire	Atmungsapparat, Atmungsorgane
restless legs syndrome	syndrome d'impatience musculaire	Wittmaack-Ekbom-Syndrom
resuscitation	ressuscitation	Reanimation, Wiederbelebung
retardation	retard	Verzögerung, Hemmung
retching	haut-le-coeur	Würgen, Brechreiz
retention	rétention	Retention
reticular	réticulaire	retikulär
reticulocyte	réticulocyte	Retikulozyt
reticulocytosis	réticulocytose	Retikulozytose
reticuloendothelial system (RES)	système réticulo-endothélial	retikuloendotheliales System
retina	rétine	Retina, Netzhaut
retinitis	rétinite	Retinitis, Netzhautentzündung
retinoblastoma	rétinoblastome	Retinoblastom
retinopathy	rétinopathie	Retinopathie

ITALIAN	SPANISH	ENGLISH
ileite regionale	ileítis regional	**regional ileitis**
regressione	regresión	**regression**
regurgito	regurgitación	**regurgitation**
riabilitazione	rehabilitación	**rehabilitation**
sindrome di Reiter	síndrome de Reiter	**Reiter's syndrome**
rigetto	rechazo	**rejection**
ricaduta *(n)*, recidiva *(n)*	recidiva *(n)*	**relapse** *(n)*
recidivare *(v)*	recaer *(v)*	**relapse** *(v)*
rilassante *(n)*	relajante *(n)*	**relaxant** *(n)*
rilassante *(a)*	relajante *(a)*	**relaxant** *(a)*
remissione	remisión	**remission**
remittente	remitente	**remittent**
sonno REM, fase dei movimenti oculari rapidi	sueño REM	**REM sleep**
renale	renal	**renal**
perfusione renale	flujo sanguíneo renal (FSR)	**renal blood flow (RBF)**
renina	renina	**renin**
repressione	represión	**repression**
sistema riproduttivo	aparato reproductor	**reproductive system**
resezione	resección	**resection**
resettore endoscopico	resectoscopio	**resectoscope**
residuo	residual	**residual**
risoluzione	resolución	**resolution**
risonanza	resonancia	**resonance**
riassorbimento	resorción	**resorption**
respirazione	respiración	**respiration**
respiratore	respirador	**respirator**
sindrome di sofferenza respiratoria	síndrome de distress respiratorio	**respiratory distress syndrome (RDS)**
insufficienza respiratoria	insuficiencia respiratoria	**respiratory failure**
test di funzionalità respiratoria	prueba de función respiratoria	**respiratory function test**
virus respiratorio sinciziale (RSV)	virus sincitial respiratorio (VSR)	**respiratory syncytial virus (RSV)**
sistema respiratorio	aparato respiratorio	**respiratory system**
sindrome delle gambe irrequiete, sindrome di Ekbom	síndrome de piernas inquietas	**restless legs syndrome**
rianimazione	resucitación	**resuscitation**
ritardo mentale, psicomotorio	retraso	**retardation**
conati di vomito	arcadas	**retching**
ritenzione	retención	**retention**
reticolare	reticular	**reticular**
reticolocito	reticulocito	**reticulocyte**
reticolocitosi	reticulocitosis	**reticulocytosis**
sistema reticoloendoteliale (RES)	sistema reticuloendotelial (SRE)	**reticuloendothelial system (RES)**
retina	retina	**retina**
retinite	retinitis	**retinitis**
retinoblastoma	retinoblastoma	**retinoblastoma**
retinopatia	retinopatía	**retinopathy**

ENGLISH	FRENCH	GERMAN
retractile	rétractile	retraktionsfähig
retractor	rétracteur	Wundhaken, Spreizer, Retraktor
retrobulbar	rétrobulbaire	retrobulbär
retrocaecal (Eng)	rétrocaecal	retrozökal
retrocecal (Am)	rétrocaecal	retrozökal
retrograde	rétrograde	retrograd, rückläufig
retrolental fibroplasia	fibroplasie rétrolentale	retrolentale Fibroplasie
retroperitoneal	rétropéritonéal	retroperitoneal
retropharyngeal	rétropharyngien	retropharyngeal
retroplacental	rétroplacentaire	retroplazentar
retrosternal	rétrosternal	retrosternal
retroversion	rétroversion	Retroversion
revascularization	revascularisation	Revaskularisation
Reye's syndrome	syndrome de Reye	Reye-Syndrom
Rhesus factor	facteur Rhésus	Rhesusfaktor
Rhesus incompatibility	incompatibilité Rhésus	Rh-Unverträglichkeit
rhesus negative (Rh−)	rhésus négatif (Rh−)	Rh-negativ
rhesus positive (Rh+)	rhésus positif (Rh+)	Rh-positiv
rheumatic fever	rhumatisme articulaire aigu	rheumatisches Fieber
rheumatism	rhumatisme	Rheumatismus
rheumatoid	rhumatoïde	rheumatisch
rheumatoid arthritis (RA)	polyarthrite rhumatoïde (PR), polyarthrite chronique évolutive (PCE)	Polyarthritis rheumatica (PCP), Rheumatoide Arthritis
rheumatology	rhumatologie	Rheumatologie
rhinitis	rhinite	Rhinitis
rhinophyma	rhinophyma	Rhinophym
rhinoplasty	rhinoplastie	Rhinoplastik
rhinorrhea (Am)	rhinorrhée	Rhinorrhoe
rhinorrhoea (Eng)	rhinorrhée	Rhinorrhoe
rhinovirus	rhinovirus	Rhinovirus
rhonchus	ronchus	Rhonchus, Rasselgeräusch
rib	côte	Rippe
ribonucleic acid (RNA)	acide ribonucléique (RNA)	Ribonukleinsäure (RNA)
rickets	rachitisme	Rachitis
rickety rosary	chapelet costal	rachitischer Rosenkranz
rigor	rigor	Rigor, Starre
ringworm	dermatophytose	Tinea, Fadenpilzerkrankung, Onchozerkose
river blindness	cécité des rivières	Flußblindheit
road traffic accident (RTA)	accident de la route	Verkehrsunfall
Rocky Mountain spotted fever	fièvre pourprée des montagnes Rocheuses	Rocky Mountain spotted fever
rodent ulcer	ulcus rodens	Ulcus rodens
rosacea	acné rosacée	Rosacea
roseola	roséole	Roseole
rotator	rotateur	Rotator
rotavirus	rotavirus	Rotavirus

ITALIAN	SPANISH	ENGLISH
retrattile	retráctil	retractile
divaricatore	retractor	retractor
retrobulbare	retrobulbar	retrobulbar
retrociecale	retrocecal	retrocaecal (Eng)
retrociecale	retrocecal	retrocecal (Am)
retrogrado	retrógrado	retrograde
fibroplasia retrolenticolare	fibroplasia retrolental	retrolental fibroplasia
retroperitoneale	retroperitoneal	retroperitoneal
retrofaringeo	retrofaríngeo	retropharyngeal
retroplacentare	retroplacentario	retroplacental
retrosternale	retrosternal	retrosternal
retroversione	retroversión	retroversion
rivascolarizzazione	revascularización	revascularization
sindrome di Reye	síndrome de Reye	Reye's syndrome
fattore Rh	factor Rhesus	Rhesus factor
incompatibilità Rh	incompatibilidad Rhesus	Rhesus incompatibility
Rh negativo (Rh−)	rhesus negativo (Rh−)	rhesus negative (Rh−)
Rh positivo (Rh+)	rhesus positivo (Rh+)	rhesus positive (Rh+)
febbre reumatica	fiebre reumática	rheumatic fever
reumatismo	reumatismo	rheumatism
reumatoide	reumatoide	rheumatoid
artrite reumatoide (AR)	artritis reumatoide (AR)	rheumatoid arthritis (RA)
reumatologia	reumatología	rheumatology
rinite	rinitis	rhinitis
rinofima	rinofima	rhinophyma
rinoplastica	rinoplastia	rhinoplasty
rinorrea	rinorrea	rhinorrhea (Am)
rinorrea	rinorrea	rhinorrhoea (Eng)
rhinovirus	rinovirus	rhinovirus
ronco	roncus	rhonchus
costa	costilla	rib
acido ribonucleico (RNA)	ácido ribonucléico (ARN)	ribonucleic acid (RNA)
rachitismo	raquitismo	rickets
rosario rachitico	rosario raquítico	rickety rosary
rigor, ipertonia extrapiramidale	rigor	rigor
tricofizia, tinea	tiña	ringworm
oncocerchiasi, cecità fluviale	oncocerciasis ocular	river blindness
incidente stradale	accidente de circulacion	road traffic accident (RTA)
febbre purpurica delle Montagne Rocciose	fiebre manchada de las Montañas Rocosas	Rocky Mountain spotted fever
ulcus rodens, basalioma	úlcera corrosiva	rodent ulcer
rosacea, acne rosacea	rosácea	rosacea
roseola	roséola	roseola
muscolo rotatore	rotatorio	rotator
rotavirus	rotavirus	rotavirus

ENGLISH	FRENCH	GERMAN
roughage	ballant intestinal	Ballaststoff
rouleaux	rouleaux	Geldrollenagglutination
roundworm	ascaris	Rundwurm, Spulwurm
rubella	rubéole	Rubella, Röteln
rubor	rougeur	Rubor, Rötung
rupture	hernie	Riß, Bruch

ITALIAN	SPANISH	ENGLISH
alimento ricco di fibre	fibra alimentaria	**roughage**
colonne di eritrociti	rollos	**rouleaux**
ascaride, nematelminto	áscaris	**roundworm**
rosolia	rubéola	**rubella**
arrossamento infiammatorio	rubor	**rubor**
rottura	ruptura	**rupture**

S

ENGLISH	FRENCH	GERMAN
sac	sac	Sack, Beutel
sacral	sacré	sakral, Kreuzbein-
sacrococcygeal	sacrococcygien	sakrokokkygeal
sacroiliac	sacro-iliaque	Iliosakral-
sacroiliitis	sacro-ilite	Sakroiliitis
sacrum	sacrum	Sakrum, Kreuzbein
sagittal	sagittal	sagittal
saline (n)	solution physiologique (n)	Kochsalzlösung (n)
saline (a)	salin (a)	salinisch (a)
saliva	salive	Speichel
salivary gland	glande salivaire	Speicheldrüse
salpingectomy	salpingectomie	Salpingektomie
salpingitis	salpingite	Salpingitis, Eileiterentzündung
salve	pommade	Salbe
sanity	santé mentale	geistige Gesundheit
saphenous	saphène	saphenus
sarcoid	sarcoïde	fleischähnlich
sarcoidosis	sarcoïdose	Sarkoidose, Morbus Boeck
sarcoma	sarcome	Sarkom
scab (n)	croûte (n)	Schorf (n), Kruste (n)
scab (v)	former une croûte (v)	verkrusten (v)
scabies	gale	Skabies, Krätze
scald	échaudure	Verbrühung, Brandwunde
scalp	épicrâne	Kopfhaut
scalpel	scalpel	Skalpell
scan	échogramme	Scan
scaphoid	scaphoïde	Scaphoid
scapula	omoplate	Skapula, Schulterblatt
scar	cicatrice	Narbe
scarlet fever	scarlatine	Scharlach
Schick test	réaction de Schick	Schick-Test
schistosomiasis	schistosomiase	Schistosomiasis, Bilharziose
schizoid personality	personnalité schizoïde	schizoide Persönlichkeit
schizophrenia	schizophrénie	Schizophrenie
Schlatter's disease	maladie d'Osgood-Schlatter	Schlatter-Krankheit
sciatic	sciatique	ischiadicus
sciatica	sciatique	Ischias
sciatic nerve	nerf grand sciatique	Ischiasnerv, Nervus ischiadicus
sclera	sclérotique	Sklera
scleredema (Am)	scléroderme	Sklerödem
scleredoema (Eng)	scléroderme	Sklerödem
scleritis	sclérite	Skleritis
scleroderma	scléroderme	Sklerodermie
sclerosis	sclérose	Sklerose
sclerotherapy	sclérothérapie	Sklerotherapie

ITALIAN	SPANISH	ENGLISH
sacco, sacca	saco	sac
sacrale	sacral	sacral
sacrococcigeo	sacrococcígeo	sacrococcygeal
sacroiliaco	sacroíliaco	sacroiliac
sacroiliite	sacroileítis	sacroiliitis
sacro	sacro	sacrum
sagittale	sagital	sagittal
soluzione fisiologica (n)	solución salina (n)	saline (n)
salino (a)	salino (a)	saline (a)
saliva	saliva	saliva
ghiandola salivare	glándula salivar	salivary gland
salpingectomia	salpingectomía	salpingectomy
salpingite	salpingitis	salpingitis
unguento	ungüento	salve
sanità	cordura	sanity
safeno	safeno	saphenous
sarcoideo	sarcoideo	sarcoid
sarcoidosi	sarcoidosis	sarcoidosis
sarcoma	sarcoma	sarcoma
crosta (n), escara (n)	costra (n)	scab (n)
ricoprirsi di croste (v)	formar una costra (v)	scab (v)
scabbia	sarna	scabies
scottatura	escaldadura	scald
cuoio capelluto	cuero cabelludo	scalp
bisturi	escalpelo	scalpel
ecografia, scintigrafia	exploración, barrido	scan
scafoide	escafoides	scaphoid
scapola	omoplato	scapula
cicatrice	cicatriz	scar
scarlattina	escarlatina	scarlet fever
test di Schick	prueba de Schick	Schick test
schistosomiasi	esquistosomiasis	schistosomiasis
personalità schizoide	personalidad esquizoide	schizoid personality
schizofrenia	esquizofrenia	schizophrenia
malattia di Schlatter	enfermedad de Schlatter	Schlatter's disease
sciatico	ciático	sciatic
sciatica	ciática	sciatica
nervo sciatico	nervio ciático	sciatic nerve
sclera, sclerotica	esclerótica	sclera
scleredema	escleredema	scleredema (Am)
scleredema	escleredema	scleredoema (Eng)
sclerite	escleritis	scleritis
sclerodermia	escleroderma	scleroderma
sclerosi	esclerosis	sclerosis
scleroterapia	escleroterapia	sclerotherapy

ENGLISH	FRENCH	GERMAN
sclerotic	sclérotique	sklerotisch, Sklera-
scoliosis	scoliose	Skoliose
scotoma	scotome	Skotom, Gesichtsfeldausfall
screening	dépistage	Screening, Reihenuntersuchung
scrofula	scrofule	Skrofula, Lymphknotentuberkulose
scrotum	scrotum	Skrotum, Hodensack
scurvy	scorbut	Skorbut
sebaceous	sébacé	Talg-, talgig
seborrhea (Am)	séborrhée	Seborrhoe
seborrheic dermatitis (Am)	eczéma	seborrhoisches Ekzem
seborrhoea (Eng)	séborrhée	Seborrhoe
seborrhoeic dermatitis (Eng)	eczéma	seborrhoisches Ekzem
sebum	sébum	Talg
secretion	sécrétion	Sekretion
secretory	secréteur	sekretorisch
sedation	sédation	Sedierung
sedative (n)	sédatif (n)	Sedativum (n), Beruhigungsmittel (n)
sedative (a)	sédatif (a)	sedierend (a), beruhigend (a)
sedentary	sédentaire	sitzend, seßhaft
sedimentation rate (SR)	vitesse de sédimentation (VS)	Blutkörperchen-Senkungsgeschwindigkeit (BSG, BKS)
segment	segment	Segment
seizure	accès	Anfall
self-harm	automutilation	Selbstschädigung
self-poisoning	intoxication volontaire	Selbstvergiftung
semeiotic	sémiologique	semiotisch
semen	sperme	Samen
semicircular canal	canal semi-circulaire	Bogengang
semilunar	semi-lunaire	semilunar, halbmondförmig
seminal	séminal, spermatique	Samen-, Spermien-
seminoma	séminome	Seminom
semipermeable	semi-perméable	semipermeabel
senescence	sénescence	Seneszenz, Altern
senile	sénile	senil, Alters-
sensation	sensation	Sinneswahrnehmung, Gefühl
sense	sens	Sinn
sensitive	sensible	sensitiv, empfindlich
sensitivity	sensibilité	Empfindlichkeit, Feingefühl
sensitization	sensibilisation	Sensitivierung, Allergisierung
sensorineural	de perception	Sinne u. Nerven betr.
sensory	sensitif	sensorisch, Sinnes-
sepsis	septicémie	Sepsis
septicaemia (Eng)	septicémie	Septikämie
septicemia (Am)	septicémie	Septikämie
septum	septum	Septum, Scheidewand
sequela	séquelle	Folgeerscheinung, Folgezustand
sequestrum	séquestre	Sequester

ITALIAN	SPANISH	ENGLISH
sclerotico	esclerótico	sclerotic
scoliosi	escoliosis	scoliosis
scotoma	escotoma	scotoma
selezione	criba, despistaje	screening
scrofola, linfadenite tubercolare	escrófula	scrofula
scroto	escroto	scrotum
scorbuto	escorbuto	scurvy
sebaceo	sebáceo	sebaceous
seborrea	seborrea	seborrhea (Am)
dermatite seborroica	dermatitis seborréica	seborrheic dermatitis (Am)
seborrea	seborrea	seborrhoea (Eng)
dermatite seborroica	dermatitis seborréica	seborrhoeic dermatitis (Eng)
sebo	sebo	sebum
secrezione	secreción	secretion
secretorio	secretorio	secretory
sedazione	sedación	sedation
sedativo (n)	sedante (n)	sedative (n)
sedativo (a)	sedante (a)	sedative (a)
sedentario	sedentario	sedentary
velocità di eritrosedimentazione (VES)	velocidad de sedimentación globular (VSG)	sedimentation rate (SR)
segmento	segmento	segment
attacco, convulsione	acceso, ataque	seizure
autolesionismo	autolesión	self-harm
autoavvelenamento	autointoxicación	self-poisoning
semiotico	semiótica	semeiotic
seme	semen	semen
canale semicircolare	conducto semicircular	semicircular canal
semilunare	semilunar	semilunar
seminale	seminal	seminal
seminoma	seminoma	seminoma
semipermeabile	semipermeable	semipermeable
senescenza	senescencia	senescence
senile	senil	senile
sensazione, sensibilità	sensación	sensation
sensi	sentido	sense
sensibile	sensible	sensitive
sensibilità	sensibilidad	sensitivity
sensibilizzazione	sensibilización	sensitization
neurosensoriale	sensorineural	sensorineural
sensoriale	sensorio	sensory
sepsi	sepsis	sepsis
setticemia	septicemia	septicaemia (Eng)
setticemia	septicemia	septicemia (Am)
setto	septo, tabique	septum
sequela	secuela	sequela
sequestro	secuestro	sequestrum

ENGLISH	FRENCH	GERMAN
serology	sérologie	Serologie
seropositive	séropositif	seropositiv
serosa	séreuse	Serosa
serous	séreux	serös, Serum-
serum	sérum	Serum, Blutserum
sex-linked	lié au sexe	geschlechtsgebunden
sexual abuse	sévices sexuels	sexueller Mißbrauch
sexual intercourse	rapports sexuels	Geschlechtsverkehr, Koitus
sexually transmitted disease (STD)	maladie sexuellement transmissible (MST)	Geschlechtskrankheit
shin bone	tibia	Schienbein
shingles	zona	Herpes zoster, Gürtelrose
Shirodkar's operation	opération de Shirodkar	Shirodkar-Operation
shock	choc	Schock
shortness of breath	essoufflement	Kurzatmigkeit
shoulder	épaule	Schulter
shoulder girdle	ceinture scapulaire	Schultergürtel
'show'	eaux de l'amnios	Geburtsbeginn (Anzeichen)
shunt	dérivation	Shunt
sibling	frère ou soeur	Geschwister
sickle-cell anaemia (Eng)	drépanocytose	Sichelzellanämie
sickle-cell anemia (Am)	drépanocytose	Sichelzellanämie
side effect	effet latéral	Nebenwirkung
sigmoid	sigmoïde	sigmoid
sigmoidoscope	sigmoïdoscope	Sigmoidoskop
sigmoidostomy	sigmoïdostomie	Sigmoidostomie
sign	signe	Zeichen, Symptom
silicosis	silicose	Silikose
Sims' position	position de Sim	Sims-Lage
Sims' speculum	spéculum de Sim	Sims-Spekulum
sinoatrial node	noeud sinusal de Keith et Flack	Sinusknoten
sinus	sinus	Sinus, Nebenhöhle
sinusitis	sinusite	Sinusitis
Sjögren-Larsson syndrome	syndrome de Sjögren	Sjögren-Syndrom
skeleton	squelette	Skelett
skin	peau	Haut
skull	crâne	Schädel
sleep	sommeil	Schlaf
slipped disc	hernie discale	Bandscheibenvorfall
slipped epiphysis	épiphysiolyse	Epiphyseolyse
slough	escarre	Schorf
slow release drug	médicament retard	Retardmittel
small-for-dates (SFD)	présentant un retard de croissance	termingemäß klein
smallpox	variole	Variola, Pocken
smear	frottis	Belag, Abstrich

ITALIAN	SPANISH	ENGLISH
sierologia	serología	serology
siero-positivo	seropositivo	seropositive
sierosa, membrana sierosa	serosa	serosa
sieroso	seroso	serous
siero	suero	serum
legato al sesso	vinculado al sexo	sex-linked
violenza sessuale, violenza carnale	abuso sexual	sexual abuse
coito	coito	sexual intercourse
malattia a trasmissione sessuale (STD)	enfermedad de transmisión sexual (ETS)	sexually transmitted disease (STD)
tibia	tibia	shin bone
herpes zoster	herpes zóster	shingles
intervento di Shirodkar	operación de Shirodkar	Shirodkar's operation
shock	shock	shock
respiro affannoso	disnea	shortness of breath
spalla	hombro	shoulder
cingolo scapolare	cintura escapular	shoulder girdle
perdita ematica che precede il parto o la mestruazione	'señal sanguinolenta menstrual'	'show'
derivazione	derivación	shunt
fratello germano	hermano no gemelo	sibling
anemia drepanocitica	anemia drepanocítica	sickle-cell anaemia (Eng)
anemia drepanocitica	anemia drepanocítica	sickle-cell anemia (Am)
effetto collaterale	efecto secundario	side effect
sigmoide	sigmoideo	sigmoid
sigmoidoscopio	sigmoidoscopio	sigmoidoscope
sigmoidostomia	sigmoidostomía	sigmoidostomy
segno	signo	sign
silicosi	silicosis	silicosis
posizione di Sim	posición de Sim	Sims's position
speculum di Sim	espéculo de Sim	Sim's speculum
nodo sinoatriale	nodo sinoauricular	sinoatrial node
seno, fistula suppurante	seno	sinus
sinusite	sinusitis	sinusitis
sindrome di Sjögren-Larsson (eritrodermia ittiosiforme con oligofrenia spastica)	síndrome de Sjögren	Sjögren-Larsson syndrome
scheletro	esqueleto	skeleton
pelle	piel	skin
cranio	cráneo	skull
sonno	sueño	sleep
ernia discale	hernia de disco	slipped disc
distacco epifisario	epífisis desplazada	slipped epiphysis
crosta, escara	esfacelo	slough
farmaco a lenta dismissione	medicamento de liberación lenta	slow release drug
basso peso alla nascita	útero pequeño para la edad gestacional	small-for-dates (SFD)
vaiolo	viruela	smallpox
striscio	frotis	smear

ENGLISH	FRENCH	GERMAN
sneeze (n)	éternuement (n)	Niesen (n)
sneeze (v)	éternuer (v)	niesen (v)
snore (n)	ronflement (n)	Schnarchen (n)
snore (v)	ronfler (v)	schnarchen (v)
sociomedical	sociomédical	sozialmedizinisch
soft palate	voile du palais	weicher Gaumen
solar plexus	plexus solaire	Solarplexus
solution	solution	Lösung, Auflösung
solvent	solvant	Lösungsmittel
somatic	somatique	somatisch, körperlich
somnambulism	somnambulisme	Somnambulismus, Schlafwandeln
soporific (n)	soporifique (n)	Schlafmittel (n)
soporific (a)	soporifique (a)	einschläfernd (a)
sore	douloureux	wund, schmerzhaft
sound	son	Ton, Klang
spasm	spasme	Spasmus, Krampf
spasmodic dysmenorrhoea	dysménorrhée spasmodique	spastische Dysmenorrhoe
spastic	spastique	spastisch, krampfhaft
spatula	spatule	Spatel
special care baby unit (SCBU)	pavillon de soins spéciaux aux nouveau-nés	Säuglings-Intensivstation
special care unit (SCU)	unité de soins spéciaux	Intensivstation
species	espèce	Spezies, Art
specific	spécifique	spezifisch, speziell
speculum	spéculum	Spekulum, Spiegel
speech therapy	orthophonie	Sprachtherapie
sperm	sperme	Sperma, Samen
spermatic	spermatique	Sperma-, Samen-
spermatocele	spermatocèle	Spermatozele
spermicide	spermicide	Spermizid
sphenoid	sphénoïde	Sphenoid, Keilbein
spherocytosis	sphérocytose	Sphärozytose, Kugelzellanämie
sphincter	sphincter	Sphinkter, Schließmuskel
sphygmomanometer	sphygmomanomètre	Blutdruckmeßgerät
spica	spica	Kornährenverband, Sporn
spicule	spicule	Spikulum
spider naevus (Eng)	naevi	Spider naevus, Naevus arachnoideus
spider nevus (Am)	naevi	Spider naevus, Naevus arachnoideus
spina bifida	spina bifida	Spina bifida
spinal	spinal	spinal, Rückenmarks-, Wirbelsäulen-
spine	colonne vertébrale	Wirbelsäule, Rückgrat
spinhaler	turbo-inhalateur	Drehinhaliergerät
spirochaete (Eng)	spirochète	Spirochäte
spirochete (Am)	spirochète	Spirochäte
spirograph	spirographe	Spirograph
spirometer	spiromètre	Spirometer
spittle	crachat	Speichel

ITALIAN	SPANISH	ENGLISH
starnuto (n)	estornudo (n)	sneeze (n)
starnutire (v)	estornudar (v)	sneeze (v)
russo (n)	ronquido (n)	snore (n)
russare (v)	roncar (v)	snore (v)
sociosanitario	médico-social	sociomedical
palato molle	paladar blando	soft palate
plesso solare, plesso celiaco	plexo solar	solar plexus
soluzione	solución	solution
solvente	disolvente	solvent
somatico	somático	somatic
sonnambulismo	sonambulismo	somnambulism
ipnotico (n)	soporífero (n)	soporific (n)
ipnotico (a)	soporífero (a)	soporific (a)
dolente	doloroso	sore
suono	sonido	sound
spasmo	espasmo	spasm
dismenorrea spastica	dismenorrea espasmódica	spasmodic dysmenorrhoea
spastico	espástico	spastic
spatola	espátula	spatula
unità di cure speciali pediatriche	unidad para cuidados especiales neonatales	special care baby unit (SCBU)
unità pediatrica di cure speciali	unidad de cuidados especiales	special care unit (SCU)
specie	especie	species
specifico	específico	specific
speculum	espéculo	speculum
terapia del linguaggio	logopedia	speech therapy
sperma	esperma	sperm
spermatico	espermático	spermatic
spermatocele	espermatocele	spermatocele
spermicida	espermicida	spermicide
sfenoide	esfenoides	sphenoid
sferocitosi	esferocitosis	spherocytosis
sfintere	esfínter	sphincter
sfigmomanometro	esfigmomanómetro	sphygmomanometer
spiga	espica	spica
spicola, picco	espícula	spicule
angioma stellare	araña vascular	spider naevus (Eng)
angioma stellare	araña vascular	spider nevus (Am)
spina bifida	espina bífida	spina bifida
spinale	espinal	spinal
spina	raquis	spine
nebulizzatore per farmaci	inhalador spinhaler	spinhaler
spirocheta	espiroqueta	spirochaete (Eng)
spirocheta	espiroqueta	spirochete (Am)
spirografo	espirografía	spirograph
spirometro	espirómetro	spirometer
saliva	salivazo	spittle

ENGLISH	FRENCH	GERMAN
splanchnic	splanchnique	viszeral, Eingeweide-
spleen	rate	Milz
splenectomy	splénectomie	Splenektomie
splenomegaly	splénomégalie	Splenomegalie
splint	attelle	Schiene
spondylitis	spondylite	Spondylitis
spondylolisthesis	spondylolisthésis	Spondylolisthesis
sporadic	sporadique	sporadisch
spot	bouton	Flecken, Pickel
sprain (n)	foulure (n)	Verstauchung (n)
sprain (v)	se fouler (v)	verstauchen (v)
sprue	sprue	Sprue
sputum	salive	Sputum, Auswurf
squamous	squameux	squamös, schuppig
squint	strabisme	Schielen
stammer	bégaiement	Stottern
stapedectomy	stapédectomie	Stapedektomie
stapes	étrier	Stapes, Steigbügel
stasis	stase	Stase
status	statut	Status, Zustand
steatorrhea (Am)	stéatorrhée	Steatorrhoe, Fettstuhl
steatorrhoea (Eng)	stéatorrhée	Steatorrhoe, Fettstuhl
Stein-Leventhal syndrome	syndrome de Stein-Leventhal	Stein-Leventhal-Syndrom
Steinmann's pin	broche de Steinmann	Steinmann Knochennagel
stenosis	sténose	Stenose
sterile	stérile	steril, keimfrei, unfruchtbar
sterilization	stérilisation	Sterilisation, Sterilisierung
sternal puncture	ponction sternale	Sternalpunktion
sternocleidomastoid muscle	muscle sternocléidomastoïdien	Musculus sternocleidomastoideus
sternocostal	sternocostal	sternokostal
sternum	sternum	Sternum, Brustbein
steroid	stéroïde	Steroid
stethoscope	stéthoscope	Stethoskop
Stevens-Johnson syndrome	syndrome de Stevens-Johnson	Stevens-Johnson-Syndrom
stigmata	stigmate	Stigmata, Kennzeichen
stilbestrol (Am)	stilboestrol	Diäthylstilboestrol
stilboestrol (Eng)	stilboestrol	Diäthylstilboestrol
stillborn	mort-né	totgeboren
Still's disease	maladie de Still	Still-Krankheit
stimulant (n)	stimulant (n)	Stimulans (n)
stimulant (a)	stimulant (a)	stimulierend (a)
sting	piqûre	Stachel, Stich
stitch	point de suture	Stechen
Stokes-Adams syndrome	syndrome de Stokes-Adams	Morgagni-Stokes-Adams-Syndrom
stoma	stoma	Stoma, Mund
stomach	estomac	Magen
stomatitis	stomatite	Stomatitis, Mundhöhlenentzündung

ITALIAN	SPANISH	ENGLISH
splancnico	esplácnico	splanchnic
milza	bazo	spleen
splenectomia	esplenectomía	splenectomy
splenomegalia	esplenomegalia	splenomegaly
stecca ortopedica	astilla	splint
spondilite	espondilitis	spondylitis
spondilolistesi	espondilolistesis	spondylolisthesis
sporadico	esporádico	sporadic
foruncolo	mancha	spot
distorsione (n)	esguince (n)	sprain (n)
distorcere (v)	torcer (v)	sprain (v)
sprue	esprue	sprue
sputo, escreato	esputo	sputum
squamoso	escamoso	squamous
strabismo	estrabismo	squint
balbuzie	tartamudeo	stammer
stapedectomia	estapedectomía	stapedectomy
staffa	estribo	stapes
stasi, ristagno	estasis	stasis
stato	status	status
steatorrea, seborrea	esteatorrea	steatorrhea (Am)
steatorrea, seborrea	esteatorrea	steatorrhoea (Eng)
sindrome di Stein-Leventhal	síndrome de Stein-Leventhal	Stein-Leventhal syndrome
chiodo per estensione di Steinmann	clavo de Steinmann	Steinmann's pin
stenosi	estenosis	stenosis
sterile	estéril	sterile
sterilizzazione	esterilización	sterilization
puntura sternale	punción esternal	sternal puncture
muscolo sternocleidomastoideo	músculo esternocleidomastoideo	sternocleidomastoid muscle
sternocostale	esternocostal	sternocostal
sterno	esternón	sternum
steroide	esteroide	steroid
stetoscopio	estetoscopio	stethoscope
sindrome di Stevens-Johnson	síndrome de Stevens-Johnson	Stevens-Johnson syndrome
stigmate	estigmas	stigmata
stilbestrolo	estilbestrol	stilbestrol (Am)
stilbestrolo	estilbestrol	stilboestrol (Eng)
nato morto	mortinato, nacido muerto	stillborn
malattia di Still	enfermedad de Still	Still's disease
stimolante (n)	estimulante (n)	stimulant (n)
stimolante (a)	estimulante (a)	stimulant (a)
dolore acuto, puntura	picadura	sting
punto	punto de sutura	stitch
sindrome di Stokes-Adams	síndrome de Stokes-Adams	Stokes-Adams syndrome
stoma, orifizio	estoma	stoma
stomaco	estómago	stomach
stomatite	estomatitis	stomatitis

ENGLISH	FRENCH	GERMAN
stone	caillou	Stein
stool	selle	Stuhl, Stuhlgang, Kot
strabismus	strabisme	Strabismus, Schielen
strain	entorse	Anstrengung, Belastung
strangulated hernia	hernie étranglée	inkarzerierte Hernie
strangulation	strangulation	Strangulation, Einklemmung
strangury	strangurie	Harnzwang
stratum	couche	Stratum, Schicht
stress	stress	Belastung, Streß
striae	stries	Striae, Streifen
stricture	rétrécissement	Striktur
stridor	stridor	Stridor
stroke	apoplexie	Schlag, Schlaganfall
stupor	stupeur	Stupor, Benommenheit
stye	orgelet	Hordeolum, Gerstenkorn
styloid	styloïde	Styloid-
subacute	subaigu	subakut
subacute bacterial endocarditis (SBE)	endocardite lente	Endocarditis lenta
subarachnoid haemorrhage (Eng)	hémorragie sous-arachnoïdienne	Subarachnoidalblutung
subarachnoid hemorrhage (Am)	hémorragie sous-arachnoïdienne	Subarachnoidalblutung
subarachnoid space	espace sous-arachnoïdien	Subarachnoidalraum
subclavian	sous-clavier	Subklavia-
subclinical	sous-clinique	subklinisch
subconjunctival	sous-conjonctival	subkonjunktival
subconscious	subconscient	unterbewußt
subcostal	sous-costal	subkostal
subcutaneous (SC, SQ)	sous-cutané (SC)	subkutan
subdural	sous-dural	subdural
subfertility	sous-fertilité	Subfertilität
subjective	subjectif	subjektiv
sublimate	sublimé	Sublimat, Quicksilberchlorid
subliminal	subliminal	unterschwellig
sublingual	sublingual	sublingual
subluxation	subluxation	Subluxation
submandibular	submandibulaire	submandibulär
submucosa	tissu sous-muqueux	Submukosa
subnormality	subnormalité	Subnormalität
suboccipital	sous-occipital	subokzipital
subphrenic	sous-phrénique	subdiaphragmatisch
succussion	succussion	Erschütterung, Schütteln
sudden infant death syndrome (SIDS)	syndrome de mort subite de nourrisson	plötzlicher Säuglingstod, Sudden-infant-death-Syndrom (SIDS)
suffocation	suffocation	Ersticken, Erstickung
suggestion	suggestion	Vorschlag, Suggestion
suicide	suicide	Suizid, Selbstmord
sulcus	sillon, gouttière, scissure	Sulcus, Furche

calcolo	cálculo	**stone**
feci	deposición	**stool**
strabismo	estrabismo	**strabismus**
tensione	cepa	**strain**
ernia strozzata	hernia estrangulada	**strangulated hernia**
strangolamento	estrangulación	**strangulation**
stranguria	estranguria	**strangury**
strato	estrato	**stratum**
stress	stress, estrés	**stress**
stria	estrias	**striae**
stenosi, restringimento	estrictura	**stricture**
stridore	estridor	**stridor**
ictus, colpo apoplettico, accidente cerebrovascolare	ictus	**stroke**
stupore	estupor	**stupor**
orzaiolo	orzuelo	**stye**
stiloide, stiloideo	estiloides	**styloid**
subacuto	subagudo	**subacute**
endocardite batterica subacuta	endocarditis bacteriana subaguda	**subacute bacterial endocarditis (SBE)**
emorragia subaracnoidea	hemorragia subaracnoidea	**subarachnoid haemorrhage** (Eng)
emorragia subaracnoidea	hemorragia subaracnoidea	**subarachnoid hemorrhage** (Am)
spazio subaracnoideo	espacio subaracnoideo	**subarachnoid space**
succlavio, sottoclavicolare	subclavia	**subclavian**
subclinico	subclínico	**subclinical**
sottocongiuntivale	subconjuntival	**subconjunctival**
subconscio	subconsciente	**subconscious**
sottocostale	subcostal	**subcostal**
sottocutaneo	subcutáneo (SC)	**subcutaneous (SC, SQ)**
subdurale, sottodurale	subdural	**subdural**
subfertilità	subfertilidad	**subfertility**
soggettivo	subjetivo	**subjective**
sublimato	sublimado	**sublimate**
subliminale	subliminal	**subliminal**
sublinguale	sublingual	**sublingual**
sublussazione	subluxación	**subluxation**
sottomandibolare	submandibular	**submandibular**
sottomucosa	submucosa	**submucosa**
subnormalità	subnormalidad	**subnormality**
suboccipitale	suboccipital	**suboccipital**
subfrenico, sottodiaframmatico	subfrénico	**subphrenic**
succussione, scuotimento	sucusión	**succussion**
sindrome della morte neonatale improvvisa (SIDS)	síndrome de muerte súbita infantil	**sudden infant death syndrome (SIDS)**
soffocamento	asfixia	**suffocation**
suggestione	sugestión	**suggestion**
suicidio	suicidio	**suicide**
solco	surco	**sulcus**

ENGLISH	FRENCH	GERMAN
sulfonamide (Am)	sulfamide	Sulfonamid
sulfonylurea (Am)	sulfonylurée	Sulfonylharnstoff
sulphonamide (Eng)	sulfamide	Sulfonamid
sulphonylurea (Eng)	sulfonylurée	Sulfonylharnstoff
sunstroke	insolation	Sonnenstich
superior	supérieur	oben, überlegen
supination	supination	Supination
supinator	supinateur	Supinator
supine	en supination	supiniert
suppository	suppositoire	Suppositorium, Zäpfchen
suppression	suppression	Unterdrückung, Verdrängung
suppuration	suppuration	Suppuration, Eiterung
supraclavicular	supraclaviculaire	supraklavikulär
supracondylar	supracondylaire	suprakondylär
suprapubic	suprapubien	suprapubisch
suprasternal	suprasternal	suprasternal
surfactant	surfactant	Surfactant-Faktor
surgeon	chirurgien	Chirurg
surgery	chirurgie	Chirurgie
susceptibility	susceptibilité	Anfälligkeit, Empfindlichkeit
suture (n)	suture (n)	Naht (n)
suture (v)	suturer (v)	nähen (v)
swab	tampon	Tupfer, Abstrichtupfer
swallow	avaler	schlucken
sweat (n)	sueur (n)	Schweiß (n)
sweat (v)	suer (v)	schwitzen (v)
sweat test	test de sueur	Schweißtest
swollen	enflé	geschwollen, vergrößert
symbiosis	symbiose	Symbiose
sympathectomy	sympathector:ie	Sympathektomie
sympathetic nervous system	système nerveux sympathique	sympathisches Nervensystem
sympathomimetic (n)	sympathomimétique (n)	Sympathomimetikum (n)
sympathomimetic (a)	sympathomimétique (a)	sympathomimetisch (a)
symphysis	symphyse	Symphyse
symptom	symptôme	Symptom
synapse	synapse	Synapse
syncope	syncope	Synkope
syndrome	syndrome	Syndrom
synechia	synéchie	Synechie, Verwachsung
synergy	synergie	Synergie
synovial fluid	fluide synovial	Synovialflüssigkeit
synovial membrane	membrane synoviale	Synovia
syphilis	syphilis	Syphilis, Lues
syringe	seringue	Spritze
syringomyelia	syringomyélie	Syringomyelie
systemic circulation	circulation systémique	Großer Kreislauf

ITALIAN	SPANISH	ENGLISH
sulfonammide	sulfonamida	**sulfonamide** (Am)
sulfonilurea	sulfonilurea	**sulfonylurea** (Am)
sulfonammide	sulfonamida	**sulphonamide** (Eng)
sulfonilurea	sulfonilurea	**sulphonylurea** (Eng)
colpo di sole	insolación	**sunstroke**
superiore	superior	**superior**
supinazione	supinar	**supination**
supinatore	supinador	**supinator**
supino	supino	**supine**
supposta	supositorio	**suppository**
soppressione	supresión	**suppression**
suppurazione	supuración	**suppuration**
sopraclavicolare	supraclavicular	**supraclavicular**
sopracondiloideo, epicondiloideo	supracondilar	**supracondylar**
soprapubico	suprapúbico	**suprapubic**
soprasternale	supraesternal	**suprasternal**
tensioattivo, surfattante	tensoactivo	**surfactant**
chirurgo	cirujano	**surgeon**
chirurgia	cirugía	**surgery**
suscettibilità	susceptibilidad	**susceptibility**
sutura (n)	sutura (n)	**suture** (n)
suturare (v), cucire (v)	suturar (v)	**suture** (v)
tampone	torunda	**swab**
inghiottire	tragar	**swallow**
sudore (n)	sudor (n)	**sweat** (n)
sudare (v)	sudar (v)	**sweat** (v)
test del sudore, prova del sudore	prueba del sudor	**sweat test**
gonfio, tumefatto	hinchado	**swollen**
simbiosi	simbiosis	**symbiosis**
simpatectomia, simpaticectomia	simpatectomía	**sympathectomy**
sistema nervoso simpatico	sistema nervioso simpático	**sympathetic nervous system**
simpaticomimetico (n)	simpaticomimético (n)	**sympathomimetic** (n)
simpaticomimetico (a)	simpaticomimético (a)	**sympathomimetic** (a)
sinfisi	sínfisis	**symphysis**
sintomo	síntoma	**symptom**
sinapsi, giunzione	sinapsis	**synapse**
sincope	síncope	**syncope**
sindrome	síndrome	**syndrome**
sinechia, aderenza	sinequia	**synechia**
sinergia	sinergia	**synergy**
liquido sinoviale	líquido sinovial	**synovial fluid**
membrana sinoviale	membrana sinovial	**synovial membrane**
sifilide	sífilis	**syphilis**
siringa	jeringuilla	**syringe**
siringomielia	siringomielia	**syringomyelia**
circolazione sistemica	circulación sistémica	**systemic circulation**

ENGLISH	FRENCH	GERMAN
systemic lupus erythematosus (SLE)	lupus érythémateux systémique	systemischer Lupus erythematodes, Lupus erythematodes visceralis (SLE)
systole	systole	Systole
systolic murmur	murmure systolique	systolisches Geräusch, Systolikum

ITALIAN	SPANISH	ENGLISH
lupus eritematoso sistemico (LES)	lupus eritematoso sistémico (LES)	**systemic lupus erythematosus (SLE)**
sistole	sístole	**systole**
soffio sistolico	soplo sistólico	**systolic murmur**

T

ENGLISH	FRENCH	GERMAN
tabes	tabès	Auszehrung, Schwindsucht
tablet	comprimé	Tablette
tachycardia	tachycardie	Tachykardie
tachypnea (Am)	tachypnée	Tachypnoe
tachypnoea (Eng)	tachypnée	Tachypnoe
tactile	tactile	taktil, tastbar
Taenia	ténia	Bandwurm, Tänia
talc	talc	Talkum
talipes	pied bot	Klumpfuß, pes equinovarus
talus	astragale	Talus
tamponade	tamponnement	Tamponade
tapeworm	ténia	Bandwurm, Tänia
tapping	ponction	Abzapfen, Punktieren, Perkutieren
tarsalgia	tarsalgie	Tarsalgie
tarsorrhaphy	tarsorraphie	Tarsorrhaphie
tarsus	tarse	Fußwurzel, Lidknorpel
Tay-Sachs disease	maladie de Tay-Sachs	Tay-Sachs-Krankheit
tears	larmes	Tränen
tease	défilocher	zupfen
teeth	dents	Zähne, Gebiß
telangiectasis	télangiectasie	Teleangiektasie
temperament	tempérament	Temperament, Gemütsart
temple	tempe	Schläfe
temporal	temporal	temporal, Schläfen-
temporomandibular joint syndrome	syndrome de Costen	Costen-Syndrom
tendinitis (Am)	tendinite	Tendinitis, Sehnenentzündung
tendon	tendon	Sehne
tendonitis (Eng)	tendinite	Tendinitis, Sehnenentzündung
tenesmus	ténesme	Tenesmus
tennis elbow	'tennis elbow'	Tennisellenbogen
tenosynovitis	ténosynovite	Tendovaginitis, Tendosynovitis, Sehnenscheidenentzündung
tenotomy	ténotomie	Tenotomie
tension headache	céphalée due à la tension	Spannungskopfschmerz
teratogen	tératogène	Teratogen
teratoma	tératome	Teratom
terminal care	soins pour malades en phase terminale	Pflege Sterbender
termination of pregnancy (TOP)	interruption de grossesse (IG)	Schwangerschaftsabbruch
tertiary	tertiaire	tertiär, dritten Grades
test (n)	test (n)	Test (n), Untersuchung (n)
test (v)	tester (v)	testen (v), untersuchen (v)
testis	testicule	Hoden
test tube	tube à essai, éprouvette	Reagenzglas

ITALIAN	SPANISH	ENGLISH
tabe dorsale	tabes	**tabes**
pasticca, compressa	comprimido	**tablet**
tachicardia	taquicardia	**tachycardia**
tachipnea	taquipnea	**tachypnea** (Am)
tachipnea	taquipnea	**tachypnoea** (Eng)
tattile	táctil	**tactile**
Tenia	tenia	**Taenia**
talco	talco	**talc**
piede talo	talipes	**talipes**
astragalo, talo	astrágalo	**talus**
tamponamento	taponamiento	**tamponade**
cestode	tenia solitaria	**tapeworm**
aspirazione di fluido	paracentesis	**tapping**
tarsalgia	tarsalgia	**tarsalgia**
tarsorrafia	tarsorrafia	**tarsorrhaphy**
tarso	tarso	**tarsus**
malattia di Tay-Sachs	enfermedad de Tay-Sachs	**Tay-Sachs disease**
lacrime	lágrimas	**tears**
dissociare i tessuti	separar con aguja	**tease**
denti	dientes	**teeth**
telangectasia	telangiectasia	**telangiectasis**
temperamento	temperamento	**temperament**
tempia	sien	**temple**
temporale	temporal	**temporal**
sindrome dell'articolazione temporomandibolare	síndrome de la articulación temporomandibular	**temporomandibular joint syndrome**
tendinite	tendinitis	**tendinitis** (Am)
tendine	tendón	**tendon**
tendinite	tendinitis	**tendonitis** (Eng)
tenesmo	tenesmo	**tenesmus**
epicondilite radio-omerale, gomito del tennista	codo del tenista	**tennis elbow**
tenosinovite	tenosinovitis	**tenosynovitis**
tenotomia	tenotomía	**tenotomy**
cefalea muscolotensiva	cefalea por tensión	**tension headache**
teratogeno	teratógeno	**teratogen**
teratoma	teratoma	**teratoma**
cura terminale	cuidados terminales	**terminal care**
interruzione di gravidanza (IG)	interrupción del embarazo	**termination of pregnancy (TOP)**
terziario	terciario	**tertiary**
test (n), prova (n)	prueba (n)	**test** (n)
valutare (v)	probar (v)	**test** (v)
testicolo	testículo	**testis**
provetta	tubo de ensayo	**test tube**

ENGLISH	FRENCH	GERMAN
tetanus	tétanos	Tetanus, Wundstarrkrampf
tetany	tétanie	Tetanie
tetralogy of Fallot	tétralogie de Fallot	Fallot-Tetralogie
tetraplegia	tétraplégie	Tetraplegie
thalamus	thalamus	Thalamus
thalassaemia (Eng)	thalassémie	Thalassämie, Mittelmeeranämie
thalassemia (Am)	thalassémie	Thalassämie, Mittelmeeranämie
thenar	thénar	Thenar-
therapeutic abortion	avortement thérapeutique	indizierter Abort
therapeutics	thérapeutique	Therapeutik, -therapie
therapy	thérapie	Therapie, Behandlung
thermal	thermique	thermal, Wärme-
thermometer	thermomètre	Thermometer
thirst	soif	Durst
thoracic	thoracique	thorakal, Brust-
thoracoplasty	thoracoplastie	Thorakoplastik
thoracotomy	thoracotomie	Thorakotomie
thorax	thorax	Thorax, Brustkorb
threadworm	ascaride	Fadenwurm
threatened abortion	risque d'avortement	drohender Abort
thrill	murmure respiratoire	Vibrieren, Schwirren
thrombectomy	thrombectomie	Thrombektomie
thrombocyte	thrombocyte	Thrombozyt, Blutplättchen
thrombocythaemia (Eng)	thrombocytémie	Thrombozythämie
thrombocythemia (Am)	thrombocytémie	Thrombozythämie
thrombocytopenia	thrombopénie	Thrombopenie
thrombocytosis	thrombocytose	Thrombozytose
thromboembolic	thrombo-embolique	thromboembolisch
thrombolytic	thrombolytique	thrombolytisch
thrombophlebitis	thrombophlébite	Thrombophlebitis
thrombosis	thrombose	Thrombose
thrombus	thrombus	Thrombus
thrush	aphte	Soor, Sprue
thumb	pouce	Daumen
thymus	thymus	Thymus
thyroglossal	thyroglossien	thyreoglossus
thyroid	thyroïde	Thyreoidea, Schilddrüse
thyroidectomy	thyroïdectomie	Thyreoidektomie
thyroiditis	thyroïdite	Thyreoiditis
thyroid stimulating hormone (TSH)	thyrotrophine, thyréostimuline	Thyreotropin
thyrotoxic crisis	crise thyrotoxique	thyreotoxische Krise
thyrotoxicosis	thyrotoxicose	Thyreotoxikose
tibia	tibia	Tibia, Schienbein
tibiofibular	tibiofibulaire	tibiofibular
tic	tic	Tic
tic douloureux	tic douloureux	Tic douloureux

ITALIAN	SPANISH	ENGLISH
tetano	tétanos	tetanus
tetania	tetania	tetany
tetralogia di Fallot	tetralogía de Fallot	tetralogy of Fallot
tetraplegia	tetraplejía	tetraplegia
talamo	tálamo	thalamus
talassemia	talasemia	thalassaemia (Eng)
talassemia	talasemia	thalassemia (Am)
pertinente al palmo della mano	tenar	thenar
aborto terapeutico	aborto terapéutico	therapeutic abortion
terapia	terapéutica	therapeutics
terapia	terapéutica	therapy
termale	termal	thermal
termometro	termómetro	thermometer
sete	sed	thirst
toracico	torácico	thoracic
toracoplastica	toracoplastia	thoracoplasty
toracotomia	toracotomía	thoracotomy
torace	tórax	thorax
ossiuro	enterobius vermincularis, oxiuros	threadworm
minaccia d'aborto	amenaza de aborto	threatened abortion
fremito	frémito	thrill
trombectomia	trombectomía	thrombectomy
trombocito	trombocito	thrombocyte
trombocitemia	trombocitemia	thrombocythaemia (Eng)
trombocitemia	trombocitemia	thrombocythemia (Am)
trombocitopenia	trombocitopenia	thrombocytopenia
trombocitosi	trombocitosis	thrombocytosis
tromboembolico	tromboembólico	thromboembolic
trombolitico	trombolítico	thrombolytic
tromboflebite	tromboflebitis	thrombophlebitis
trombosi	trombosis	thrombosis
trombo	trombo	thrombus
stomatite de Candida albicans, mughetto	muguet	thrush
pollice	pulgar	thumb
timo	timo	thymus
tireoglosso	tirogloso	thyroglossal
tiroide	tiroides	thyroid
tiroidectomia	tiroidectomía	thyroidectomy
tiroidite	tiroiditis	thyroiditis
ormone tireotropo (TSH)	hormona estimulante del tiroides (TSH)	thyroid stimulating hormone (TSH)
crisi tireotossica	crisis tirotóxica	thyrotoxic crisis
tireotossicosi, ipertiroidismo	tirotoxicosis	thyrotoxicosis
tibia	tibia	tibia
tibiofibulare	tibioperoneo	tibiofibular
tic	tic	tic
tic doloroso, nevralgia del trigemino	tic doloroso	tic douloureux

ENGLISH	FRENCH	GERMAN
tick	tique	Zecke
tinea	teigne	Tinea
tinnitus	tintement	Tinnitus
tissue	tissu	Gewebe
titer (Am)	titre	Titer
titration	titrage	Titration
titre (Eng)	titre	Titer
toe	orteil	Zehe
tolerance	tolérance	Toleranz
tone	tonus	Ton, Laut
tongue	langue	Zunge
tonic	tonique	Tonikum, Stärkungsmittel
tonometer	tonomètre	Tonometer
tonsils	amygdales	Tonsillen, Mandeln
tonsillectomy	amygdalectomie	Tonsillektomie, Mandelentfernung
tonsillitis	angine	Tonsillitis, Mandelentzündung
tooth	dent	Zahn
tophus	tophus	Tophus, Gichtknoten
topical	topique	topisch, örtlich
torsion	torsion	Torsion
total body weight (TBW)	poids corporel total	Körpergewicht
total iron binding capacity (TIBC)	capacité totale de fixation du fer	totale Eisenbindungskapazität (TEBK)
total lung capacity (TLC)	capacité pulmonaire totale	Totalkapazität (TK)
total parenteral nutrition (TPN)	alimentation parentérale totale	parenterale Ernährung
tourniquet	tourniquet	Tourniquet
toxaemia (Eng)	toxémie	Toxämie, Toxikämie, Blutvergiftung
toxemia (Am)	toxémie	Toxämie, Toxikämie, Blutvergiftung
toxic	toxique	toxisch, giftig
toxicity	toxicité	Toxizität
toxic shock syndrome	syndrome de choc toxique staphylococcique	toxisches Schocksyndrom (TSS)
toxin	toxine	Toxin
toxoid	toxoïde	Toxoid
toxoplasmosis	toxoplasmose	Toxoplasmose
tracer	traceur	Tracer
trachea	trachée	Trachea, Luftröhre
tracheitis	trachéite	Tracheitis
tracheoesophageal (Am)	trachéo-oesophagien	Tracheoösophageal-
tracheo-oesophageal (Eng)	trachéo-oesophagien	Tracheoösophageal-
tracheostomy	trachéostomie	Tracheostomie
tracheotomy	trachéotomie	Tracheotomie, Luftröhrenschnitt
trachoma	trachome	Trachom, ägyptische Augenkrankheit
trachoma inclusion conjunctivitis (TRIC)	conjonctivite à inclusions trachomateuses	Trachom, Einschluß(körperchen)-konjunktivitis
traction	traction	Traktion, Zug
trait	trait	Zug, Charakterzug, Eigenschaft
tranquilizer	tranquillisant	Tranquilizer, Beruhigungsmittel

ITALIAN	SPANISH	ENGLISH
zecca	garrapata	tick
tigna	tiña	tinea
tinnito	tinnitus	tinnitus
tessuto	tejido	tissue
titolo	titulo	titer (Am)
titolazione	titulación	titration
titolo	titulo	titre (Eng)
dito del piede	dedo del pie	toe
tolleranza	tolerancia	tolerance
tono	tono	tone
lingua	lengua	tongue
tonico	tónico	tonic
tonometro	tonómetro	tonometer
tonsille	amígdalas	tonsils
tonsillectomia	tonsilectomía	tonsillectomy
tonsillite	amigdalitis	tonsillitis
dente	diente	tooth
tofo, concrezione tofacea	tofo	tophus
topico, locale	tópico	topical
torsione	torsión	torsion
peso corporeo totale	peso corporal total	total body weight (TBW)
capacità totale di legame del ferro (TIBC)	capacidad total de unión con el hierro	total iron binding capacity (TIBC)
capacità polmonare totale	capacidad pulmonar total (CPT)	total lung capacity (TLC)
nutrizione parenterale totale	nutrición parenteral total	total parenteral nutrition (TPN)
laccio emostatico	torniquete	tourniquet
tossiemia	toxemia	toxaemia (Eng)
tossiemia	toxemia	toxemia (Am)
tossico	tóxico	toxic
tossicità	toxicidad	toxicity
sindrome da shock tossico	síndrome de shock tóxico	toxic shock syndrome
tossina	toxina	toxin
tossoide	toxoide	toxoid
toxoplasmosi	toxoplasmosis	toxoplasmosis
tracciante	trazador	tracer
trachea	tráquea	trachea
tracheite	traqueitis	tracheitis
tracheoesofageo	traqueoesofágico	tracheoesophageal (Am)
tracheoesofageo	traqueoesofágico	tracheo-oesophageal (Eng)
tracheostomia	traqueostomía	tracheostomy
tracheotomia	traqueotomía	tracheotomy
tracoma	tracoma	trachoma
congiuntivite tracomatosa	conjuntivitis de inclusión por tracomas	trachoma inclusion conjunctivitis (TRIC)
trazione, attrazione	tracción	traction
tratto, carattere ereditario	rasgo	trait
tranquillante	tranquilizante	tranquilizer

ENGLISH	FRENCH	GERMAN
transabdominal	transabdominal	transabdominal
transamniotic	transamniotique	transamniotisch
transcutaneous	transcutané	transkutan
transection	transsection	Querschnitt
transfusion	transfusion	Transfusion, Bluttransfusion
transient ischaemic attack (TIA) (Eng)	accès ischémique transitoire cérébral	transitorische ischämische Attacke (TIA)
transient ishemic attack (TIA) (Am)	accès ischémique transitoire cérébral	transitorische ischämische Attacke (TIA)
translocation	translocation	Translokation
translucent	translucide	durchscheinend, durchsichtig
transmural	transmural	transmural
transplant (n)	transplantation (n)	Transplantat (n), Transplantation (n)
transplant (v)	transplanter (v)	transplantieren (v)
transthoracic	transthoracique	transthorakal
transudate	transsudat	Transsudat
transurethral	transurétral	transurethral
transverse colon	côlon transversal	Colon transversum
trapezius muscles	muscles trapèzes	Musculi trapezii
trauma	traumatisme	Trauma
tremor	tremblement	Tremor
trench foot	pied gelé	Schützengrabenfuß
Trendelenburg sign	signe de Trendelenburg	Trendelenburg-Zeichen
trephine (n)	tréphine (n)	Trepan (n)
trephine (v)	trépaner (v)	trepanieren (v)
triage	triage	Triage
triceps	triceps	Trizeps
trichotillomania	trichotillomanie	Trichotillomanie
tricuspid	tricuspide	Trikuspidal
trigeminal	trigéminal	Trigeminus-
trigger finger	index	schnellender Finger
trimester	trimestre	Trimester
triple antigen	triple antigène	Dreifachantigen
triple vaccine	triple vaccin	Dreifachimpfstoff
trisomy	trisomie	Trisomie
trochanter	trochanter	Trochanter
trophic ulcer	ulcère trophique	trophisches Ulkus
tropical disease	maladie tropicale	Tropenkrankheit
trypanosomiasis	trypanosomiase	Trypanosomiasis
tsetse	mouche tsé-tsé	Tsetsefliege
tubal	tubaire	Tuben-, Eileiter-
tubercle	tubercule	Tuberkel
tuberculoid	tuberculoïde	tuberkuloid
tuberculosis (TB)	tuberculose (TB)	Tuberkulose
tuberosity	tubérosité	Tuberositas
tuberous sclerosis	sclérose tubéreuse du cerveau	tuberöse Sklerose
tubular necrosis	nécrose tubulaire	Tubulusnekrose
tubule	tube	Tubulus, Röhrchen

ITALIAN	SPANISH	ENGLISH
transaddominale	transabdominal	transabdominal
transamniotico	transamniótico	transamniotic
percutaneo	transcutáneo	transcutaneous
sezione trasversale	transección	transection
trasfusione	transfusión	transfusion
attacco ischemico transitorio	ataque isquémico transitorio (AIT)	transient ischaemic attack (TIA) (Eng)
attacco ischemico transitorio	ataque isquémico transitorio (AIT)	transient ishemic attack (TIA) (Am)
traslocazione	translocación	translocation
translucido	translúcido	translucent
transmurale	transmural	transmural
trapianto (n)	trasplante (n)	transplant (n)
trapiantare (v)	trasplantar (v)	transplant (v)
transtoracico	transtorácico	transthoracic
trasudato	trasudado	transudate
transuretrale	transuretral	transurethral
colon trasverso	colon transverso	transverse colon
muscoli trapezi	músculos trapecios	trapezius muscles
trauma	trauma	trauma
tremore	temblor	tremor
piede da trincea	pie de trinchera	trench foot
segno di Trendelenburg	signo de Trendelenburg	Trendelenburg sign
trapano (n)	trépano (n)	trephine (n)
trapanare (v)	trepanar (v)	trephine (v)
selezione e distribuzione dei malati	triage	triage
tricipite	tríceps	triceps
tricotíllomania	tricotilomanía	trichotillomania
tricuspide	tricúspide	tricuspid
trigemino	trigémino	trigeminal
dito a scatto	dedo en gatillo	trigger finger
trimestre	trimestre	trimester
antigene triplo	antígeno triple	triple antigen
triplo vaccino	vacuna triple	triple vaccine
trisomia	trisomía	trisomy
trocantere	trocánter	trochanter
ulcera trofica	úlcera trófica	trophic ulcer
malattia tropicale	enfermedad tropical	tropical disease
tripanosomiasi	tripanosomiasis	trypanosomiasis
tse-tse	mosca tsetsé	tsetse
tubarico	tubárico	tubal
tubercolo	tubérculo	tubercle
tubercoloide	tuberculoide	tuberculoid
tubercolosi (TBC)	tuberculosis (TB)	tuberculosis (TB)
tuberosità	tuberosidad	tuberosity
sclerosi tuberosa	esclerosis tuberosa	tuberous sclerosis
necrosi tubulare	necrosis tubular	tubular necrosis
tubulo	túbulo	tubule

ENGLISH	FRENCH	GERMAN
tumescence	tumescence	Tumeszenz, diffuse Anschwellung
tumor (Am)	tumeur	Tumor
tumour (Eng)	tumeur	Tumor
turbinate	cornet	Nasenmuschel
turgid	enflé	geschwollen
Turner's syndrome	syndrome de Turner	Turner-Syndrom
twin	jumeau	Zwilling
tympanic	tympanique	Trommelfell-
tympanoplasty	tympanoplastie	Tympanoplastik
tympanum	tympan	Tympanon, Trommelfell
type	type	Typ, Art
typhoid fever	fièvre typhoïde	Typhus
typhus	typhus	Typhus, Fleckfieber

ITALIAN	SPANISH	ENGLISH
tumefazione	tumescencia	tumescence
tumore, tumefazione	tumor	tumor (Am)
tumore, tumefazione	tumor	tumour (Eng)
turbinato	turbinado	turbinate
turgido	túrgido	turgid
sindrome di Turner, disgenesia gonadica	síndrome de Turner	Turner's syndrome
gemello	mellizo	twin
timpanico, risonante	timpánico	tympanic
timpanoplastica	timpanoplastia	tympanoplasty
timpano	tímpano	tympanum
tipo	tipo	type
febbre tifoide, tifo addominale, ileotifo	fiebre tifoidea	typhoid fever
tifo	tifus	typhus

U

English	French	German
ulcer	ulcère	Ulkus, Geschwür
ulcerative	ulcératif	ulzerierend, geschwürig
ulna	cubitus	Ulna, Elle
ultrasonography	échographie	Sonographie, Ultraschallmethode
ultraviolet (UV)	ultraviolet (UV)	ultraviolett
umbilical cord	cordon ombilical	Nabelschnur
umbilical hernia	hernie ombilicale	Nabelbruch
umbilicus	nombril	Nabel
unconscious	sans connaissance	bewußtlos
undescended testes	ectopie testiculaire	Kryptorchismus
unilateral	unilatéral	einseitig
uniocular	unioculé	einäugig
upper respiratory tract infection (URTI)	infection des voies respiratoires supérieures	Atemwegsinfekt
uraemia (Eng)	urémie	Urämie, Harnvergiftung
urate	urate	Urat
urea	urée	Urea, Harnstoff
uremia (Am)	urémie	Urämie
ureter	uretère	Ureter, Harnleiter
ureterocolic	urétérocolique	Ureterkolik
urethra	urètre	Urethra, Harnröhre
urethral syndrome	syndrome urétral	Urethralsyndrom
urethritis	urétrite	Urethritis
urethrocele	urétrocèle	Urethrozele
uric acid	acide urique	Harnsäure
uricaemia (Eng)	uricémie	Urikämie
uricemia (Am)	uricémie	Urikämie
uricosuria	uricosurique	Urikosurie
urinalysis	analyse d'urine	Urinanalyse, Urinuntersuchung
urinary tract infection (UTI)	infection des voies urinaires	Harnwegsinfekt
urine	urine	Urin, Harn
urography	urographie	Urographie
urology	urologie	Urologie
urticaria	urticaire	Urtikaria, Nesselsucht
uterosacral	utéro-sacré	uterosakral
uterovesical	utéro-vésical	uterovesikal
uterus	utérus	Uterus, Gebärmutter
uveitis	uréite	Uveitis
uvula	uvule	Uvula, Zäpfchen
uvulitis	uvulite	Uvulitis

ITALIAN	SPANISH	ENGLISH
ulcera	úlcera	ulcer
ulcerativo, ulceroso	ulcerativo	ulcerative
ulna	cúbito	ulna
ultrasonografia, ecografia	ultrasonografía, ecografía	ultrasonography
ultravioletto (UV)	ultravioleta (UV)	ultraviolet (UV)
cordone ombelicale	cordón umbilical	umbilical cord
ernia ombelicale	hernia umbilical	umbilical hernia
ombelico	ombligo	umbilicus
inconscio	inconsciente, sin sentido	unconscious
testicoli ritenuti	testículos no descendidos	undescended testes
unilaterale	unilateral	unilateral
monoculare	uniocular	uniocular
infezione del tratto respiratorio superiore (URTI)	infección de las vías respiratorias altas	upper respiratory tract infection (URTI)
uremia	uremia	uraemia (Eng)
urato	urato	urate
urea, carbammide	urea	urea
uremia	uremia	uremia (Am)
uretere	uréter	ureter
ureterocolico	ureterocólico	ureterocolic
uretra	uretra	urethra
sindrome uretrale	síndrome uretral	urethral syndrome
uretrite	uretritis	urethritis
uretrocele	uretrocele	urethrocele
acido urico	ácido úrico	uric acid
uricemia	uricemia	uricaemia (Eng)
uricemia	uricemia	uricemia (Am)
uricuria	uricosúrico	uricosuria
esame dell'urina	urinálisis	urinalysis
infezione delle vie urinarie (IVU)	infección de las vías urinarias (IVU)	urinary tract infection (UTI)
urina	orina	urine
urografia	urografía	urography
urologia	urología	urology
orticaria	urticaria	urticaria
uterosacrale	uterosacro	uterosacral
uterovescicale	uterovesical	uterovesical
utero	útero	uterus
uveite	uveitis	uveitis
ugola	úvula	uvula
stafilite	uvulitis	uvulitis

V

vaccination	vaccination	Impfung, Vakzination
vaccine	vaccin	Vakzine, Impfstoff
vacuum extractor	ventouse obstétricale	Vakuumextraktor, Saugglocke
vagal	vague	vagal, Vagus-
vagina	vagin	Vagina, Scheide
vaginismus	vaginisme	Vaginismus
vaginitis	vaginite	Vaginitis
vagotomy	vagotomie	Vagotomie
valgus	valgus	valgus
valve	valve	Klappe, Ventil
valvotomy	valvulotomie	Valvotomie
vanyl mandelic acid (VMA)	acide vanillyl-mandélique	Vanillylmandelsäure
varicella	varicelle	Varizellen, Windpocken
varicose veins	varices	Varizen, Krampfadern
varus	varus	varus
vascular	vasculaire	vaskulär, Gefäß-
vasculitis	vasculite	Vaskulitis
vasectomy	vasectomie	Vasektomie, Vasoresektion
vasoconstrictor (n)	vasoconstricteur (n)	Vasokonstriktor (n)
vasoconstrictor (a)	vasoconstricteur (a)	vasokonstriktorisch (a)
vasodilator (n)	vasodilatateur (n)	Vasodilatator (n)
vasodilator (a)	vasodilatateur (a)	vasodilatatorisch (a)
vasomotor nerves	nerfs vasomoteurs	vasomotorische Nerven
vasopressor (n)	vasopresseur (n)	Vasopressor (n)
vasopressor (a)	vasopresseur (a)	vasopressorisch (a)
vasospasm	spasme d'un vaisseau	Vasospasmus
vasovagal attack	malaise vasovagal	vasovagale Synkope
vector	vecteur	Überträger, Vektor
vein	veine	Vene
vena cava	veine cave	Vena cava
venepuncture	ponction d'une veine	Venenpunktion
venereal	vénérien	venerisch
venereal disease (VD)	maladie vénérienne (MV)	Geschlechtskrankheit
venereology	vénéréologie	Venerologie
venesection	phlébotomie	Venae sectio
venipuncture	ponction d'une veine	Venenpunktion
venography	phlébographie	Phlebographie
ventilator	appareil de ventilation artificielle	Ventilator
ventouse extraction	extraction par ventouse	Schröpfkopf
ventral	ventral	ventral, Bauch-
ventricle	ventricule	Ventrikel, Kammer
ventrofixation	hystéropexie abdominale	Hysteropexie
ventrosuspension	ventro-suspension	Ventrofixation, Ligamentopexie
venule	veinule	Venula
verruca	verrue	Warze, Verruca

ITALIAN	SPANISH	ENGLISH
vaccinazione	vacunación	vaccination
vaccino	vacuna	vaccine
ventosa ostetrica, ventosa cefalica	extractor al vacío	vacuum extractor
vagale	vagal	vagal
vagina	vagina	vagina
vaginismo	vaginismo	vaginismus
vaginite	vaginitis	vaginitis
vagotomia	vagotomía	vagotomy
valgo	valgus	valgus
valvola	válvula	valve
valvulotomia	valvotomía	valvotomy
acido vanilmandelico	ácido vanilmandélico (AVM)	vanyl mandelic acid (VMA)
varicella	varicela	varicella
vene varicose	varices	varicose veins
varo	varus	varus
vascolare	vascular	vascular
vasculite	vasculitis	vasculitis
vasectomia	vasectomía	vasectomy
vasocostrittore (n)	vasoconstrictor (n)	vasoconstrictor (n)
vasocostrittore (a)	vasoconstrictor (a)	vasoconstrictor (a)
vasodilatatore (n)	vasodilatador (n)	vasodilator (n)
vasodilatatore (a)	vasodilatador (a)	vasodilator (a)
nervi vasomotori	nervios vasomotores	vasomotor nerves
vasopressore (n)	vasopresor (n)	vasopressor (n)
vasopressore (a)	vasopresor (a)	vasopressor (a)
vasospasmo, angiospasmo	vasospasmo	vasospasm
crisi vagale	ataque vasovagal	vasovagal attack
vettore	vector	vector
vena	vena	vein
vena cava	vena cava	vena cava
puntura di vena	venopuntura	venepuncture
venereo	venéreo	venereal
malattia venerea (MV)	enfermedad venérea	venereal disease (VD)
venereologia	venereología	venereology
flebotomia	venisección	venesection
puntura di vena	venipuntura	venipuncture
flebografia	venografía	venography
ventilatore	ventilador	ventilator
estrazione con ventosa ostetrica	extracción con ventosa	ventouse extraction
ventrale	ventral	ventral
ventricolo	ventrículo	ventricle
ventro-fissazione	ventrofijación	ventrofixation
ventrosospensione, ventrofissazione	ventrosuspensión	ventrosuspension
venula	vénula	venule
verruca	verruga	verruca

ENGLISH	FRENCH	GERMAN
version	version	Versio, Wendung
vertebra	vertèbre	Wirbel
vertebral column	colonne vertébrale	Wirbelsäule, Rückgrat
vertebrobasilar insufficiency (VBI)	insuffisance vertébro-basilaire	vertebrobasiläre Insuffizienz
vertex	vertex	Vertex, Scheitel
vertigo	vertige	Schwindel, Vertigo
very low density lipoprotein (VLDL)	lipoprotéine de très faible densité	Lipoprotein sehr geringer Dichte
vesicle	vésicule	Vesikula, Bläschen
vesicoureteric	vésico-urétérique	vesikoureteral
vesicovaginal	vésico-vaginal	vesikovaginal
vessel	vaisseau	Gefäß, Ader
vestibule	vestibule	Vestibulum, Vorhof
viable	viable	lebensfähig
vibration syndrome	syndrome de vibrations	Vibrationssyndrom
villus	villosité	Zotte
viraemia (Eng)	virémie	Virämie
viral hepatitis	hépatite virale	Virushepatitis
viremia (Am)	virémie	Virämie
virilism	virilisme	Virilismus
virology	virologie	Virologie
virulence	virulence	Virulenz
virus	virus	Virus
viscera	viscères	Eingeweide, Viszera
viscid	visqueux	zäh, klebrig
visual	visuel	visuell, Seh-
visual acuity	acuité visuelle	Sehschärfe
vital capacity	capacité vitale	Vitalkapazität
vitamin	vitamine	Vitamin
vitiligo	vitiligo	Vitiligo
vitreous body	vitré	Glaskörper
vocal cord	corde vocale	Stimmband
Volkmann's ischaemic contracture (Eng)	contracture ischémique de Volkmann	Volkmann-Kontraktur
Volkmann's ischemic contracture (Am)	contracture ischémique de Volkmann	Volkmann-Kontraktur
volvulus	volvulus	Volvulus
vomit	vomir	sich übergeben, erbrechen
von Recklinghausen's disease	maladie de von Recklinghausen	Morbus von Recklinghausen
von Willebrand's disease	maladie de von Willebrand	Willebrand-Krankheit
vulva	vulve	Vulva
vulvitis	vulvite	Vulvitis
vulvovaginal	vulvo-vaginal	vulvovaginal

|---------|---------|---------|
versione	versión	version
vertebra	vértebra	vertebra
colonna vertebrale	columna vertebral	vertebral column
insufficienza vertebrobasilare	insuficiencia vertebrobasilar	vertebrobasilar insufficiency (VBI)
vertice	vértice	vertex
vertigine	vértigo	vertigo
lipoproteina a bassissima densità	lipoproteína de muy baja densidad (VLDL)	very low density lipoprotein (VLDL)
vescicola	vesícula	vesicle
vescicoureterale	vesicoureteral	vesicoureteric
vescicovaginale	vesicovaginal	vesicovaginal
vaso	vaso	vessel
vestibolo	vestíbulo	vestibule
vitale, in grado di vivere	viable	viable
sindrome vibratoria	síndrome de vibración	vibration syndrome
villo	vellosidad	villus
viremia	viremia	viraemia (Eng)
epatite virale	hepatitis vírica	viral hepatitis
viremia	viremia	viremia (Am)
virilismo	virilismo	virilism
virologia	virología	virology
virulenza	virulencia	virulence
virus	virus	virus
visceri	visceras	viscera
viscido	viscoso	viscid
visivo	visual	visual
acutezza visiva	agudeza visual	visual acuity
capacità vitale	capacidad vital	vital capacity
vitamina	vitamina	vitamin
vitiligine	vitíligo	vitiligo
corpo vitreo	vítreo	vitreous body
corda vocale	cuerda vocal	vocal cord
paralisi ischemica di Volkmann	contractura isquémica de Volkmann	Volkmann's ischaemic contracture (Eng)
paralisi ischemica di Volkmann	contractura isquémica de Volkmann	Volkmann's ischemic contracture (Am)
volvolo	vólvulo	volvulus
vomitare	vomitar	vomit
malattia di von Recklinghausen, neurofibromatosi	enfermedad de von Recklinghausen	von Recklinghausen's disease
malattia di von Willebrand	enfermedad de von Willebrand	von Willebrand's disease
vulva	vulva	vulva
vulvite	vulvitis	vulvitis
vulvovaginale	vulvovaginal	vulvovaginal

W

English	French	German
waiting list	liste d'attente	Warteliste
wart	verrue	Warze
Wassermann reaction	réaction de Wassermann	Wassermann-Reaktion
wasting away	dépérissement	Schwinden
weakness	faiblesse	Schwäche
weal	marque	Schwiele, Striemen
weight loss	perte de poids	Gewichtsverlust
Weil's disease	maladie de Weil	Weil Krankheit
wheeze	wheezing	Giemen
whiplash	coup de fouet	Peitschenhiebsyndrom, Mediansyndrom
whipworm	flagellé	Oxyuris, Peitschenwurm
white blood cell count (WBC)	nombre de globules blancs (NGB)	weißes Blutbild
whitlow	panaris	Panaritium
whooping cough	coqueluche	Keuchhusten
Widal reaction	réaction de Widal	Widal-Reaktion
Wilms' tumor (Am)	tumeur de Wilms	Wilms-Tumor
Wilms' tumour (Eng)	tumeur de Wilms	Wilms-Tumor
Wilson's disease	maladie de Wilson	Wilson-Krankheit
wind	gaz	Blähung, Wind
windpipe	trachée	Luftröhre, Trachea
wisdom tooth	dent de sagesse	Weisheitszahn
withdrawal	retrait, sevrage, suppression	Entzug
womb	utérus	Uterus, Gebärmutter
worm	ver	Wurm
wound	plaie	Wunde, Verletzung
wound dressing	pansements	Verbandmaterial
wrist	poignet	Handgelenk, Karpus
wry-neck	torticolis	Tortikollis, (angeborener) Schiefhals

ITALIAN	SPANISH	ENGLISH
lista d'attesa	lista de espera	waiting list
verruca volgare	verruga	wart
reazione di Wassermann	reacción de Wassermann	Wassermann reaction
cachessia	consunción	wasting away
debolezza	debilidad	weakness
pomfo	verdugón	weal
perdita di peso	pérdida de peso	weight loss
malattia di Weil	enfermedad de Weil	Weil's disease
sibilo	jadeo	wheeze
colpo di frusta	latigazo	whiplash
verme a frusta, tricocefalo	trichuris trichiura	whipworm
conteggio dei globuli bianchi (CGB, WBC)	recuento de leucocitos	white blood cell count (WBC)
patereccio	panadizo	whitlow
pertosse	tos ferina	whooping cough
reazione di Widal	reacción de Widal	Widal reaction
tumore di Wilms	tumor de Wilms	Wilms' tumor (Am)
tumore di Wilms	tumor de Wilms	Wilms' tumour (Eng)
malattia di Wilson	enfermedad de Wilson	Wilson's disease
flatulenza, ventosità	flatulencia, ventosidad	wind
trachea	tráquea	windpipe
dente del giudizio	muela del juicio	wisdom tooth
ritiro, astinenza, sospensione	supresión, abstinencia	withdrawal
utero	matriz	womb
verme	lombriz	worm
ferita	herida	wound
medicazione di ferita	curas para heridas	wound dressing
polso	muñeca	wrist
torcicollo	tortícolis	wry-neck

X

xanthaemia (Eng)	xanthémie, caroténémie	Xanthämie
xanthelasma	xanthélasma	Xanthelasma
xanthemia (Am)	xanthémie, caroténémie	Xanthämie
xanthoma	xanthome	Xanthom
xeroderma	xérodermie	Xerodermie
xerophthalmia	xérophtalmie	Xerophthalmie
X-rays	rayons X	Röntgenstrahlen, Röntgenaufnahmen

Y

yawn	bâillement	Gähnen
yaws	pian	Frambösie
yeast	levure	Hefe, Hefepilz
yellow fever	fièvre jaune	Gelbfieber

Z

zoonosis	zoonose	Zoonose, Tierkrankheit
zoster	zona	Herpes zoster, Gürtelrose
zygoma	zygoma	Zygoma, Jochbein
zygote	zygote	Zygote

xantemia	xantemia	**xanthaemia** (Eng)
xantelasma	xantelasma	**xanthelasma**
xantemia	xantemia	**xanthemia** (Am)
xantoma, malattia di Rayer	xantoma	**xanthoma**
xerodermia	xeroderma	**xeroderma**
xeroftalmia	xeroftalmia	**xerophthalmia**
raggi X	rayos X	**X-rays**

sbadiglio	bostezo	**yawn**
framboesia, pian	yaws, pian	**yaws**
lievito	levadura	**yeast**
febbre gialla	fiebre amarilla	**yellow fever**

zoonosi	zoonosis	**zoonosis**
herpes zoster	zóster	**zoster**
zigomo, osso zigomatico	cigoma	**zygoma**
zigote	cigoto	**zygote**

ABRÉVIATIONS ANGLAISES
ENGLISCHE ABKÜRZUNGEN
ABBREVIAZIONE INGLESI
ABREVIATURAS INGLESAS

Ab	antibodies
ABC	airway, breathing and circulation
ABC	antigen binding capacity
ACH	adrenal cortical hormone
ACTH	adrenocorticotrophic hormone
ADR	adverse drug reaction
AFP	alpha-fetoprotein
AFRD/I	acute febrile respiratory disease/illness
AI	artificial insemination
AID	artificial insemination by donor
AIDS	acquired immune deficiency syndrome
ASD	atrial septal defect
at wt	atomic weight
AV	atrioventricular
BBB	blood-brain barrier
BCG	bacille Calmette-Guérin
BJ	Bence Jones (protein)
BMI	body mass index
BMR	basal metabolic rate
BP	blood pressure
BSE	bovine spongiform encephalitis
BSE	breast self-examination
BSR	blood sedimentation rate
BV	blood volume
CAD	coronary artery disease
CAT	computerized axial tomography
CBC	complete blood count
CBS	chronic brain syndrome
CCF	congestive cardiac failure
CCI	chronic coronary insufficiency
CCU	coronary care unit
CF	cystic fibrosis
CHD	coronary heart disease
CHF	congestive heart failure
CHF	coronary heart failure
CHO	carbohydrate
chol	cholesterol
CIN	cervical intraepithelial neoplasia
CMV	cytomegalovirus
CNS	central nervous system
COAD	chronic obstructive airway disease
COD	cause of death
CPAP	continuous positive airway pressure
CPR	cardiopulmonary resuscitation
CRP	C-reactive protein
CSF	cerebrospinal fluid
CVA	cerebrovascular accident
CVP	central venous pressure
D & C	dilatation/dilation and curettage

D & V	diarrhoea/diarrhea and vomiting
DIC	disseminated intravascular coagulation
DM	diabetes mellitus
DNA	deoxyribonucleic acid
DOA	dead on arrival
DOB	date of birth
DOC	date of conception
DUB	dysfunctional uterine bleeding
DVT	deep vein thrombosis
EBV	Epstein-Barr virus
ECG	electrocardiogram
ECT	electroconvulsive therapy
ECT	enteric-coated tablet
ECV	external cephalic version
EDC	expected date of confinement
EDD	expected date of delivery
EEG	electroencephalogram
ELISA	enzyme-linked immunosorbent assay
ENT	ear, nose and throat
ERCP	endoscopic retrograde cholangiopancreatography
ESR	erythrocyte sedimentation rate
ETU	emergency treatment/trauma unit
FBS	fasting blood sugar
FEV	forced expiratory volume
FHR	fetal heart rate
FOB	faecal/fecal occult blood
FSH	follicle stimulating hormone
FT	free thyroxine
FTA	fluorescent treponemal antibody
FTI	free thyroxine index
FTT	failure to thrive
FUO	fever of unknown origin
GFR	glomerular filtration rate
GGT	gamma glutamyl transferase
GH	growth hormone
GITT	glucose insulin tolerance test
GTT	glucose tolerance test
GU	genitourinary
Hb	haemoglobin/hemoglobin
HCG	human chorionic gonadotrophin/gonadotropin
HCS	human chorionic somatomammotrophin/ somatomammotropin
HDL	high density lipoprotein
HDLC	high density lipoprotein cholesterol
HDN	haemolytic/hemolytic disease of the newborn
HEA	human erythroctye antigen
Hg	haemoglobin/hemoglobin
HGG	human gamma globulin
HIV	human immunodeficiency virus
HLA	human lymphocytic antigen
HLV	herpes-like virus
HPL	human placental lactogen
HRT	hormone replacement therapy
HSV	herpes simplex virus
HUS	haemolytic uraemic/hemolytic uremic syndrome
HVA	homovanillic acid
IAO	immediately after onset

IBC	iron binding capacity
IBP	iron binding protein
ICP	intracranial pressure
ICU	intensive care unit
IDDM	insulin dependent diabetes mellitus
Ig	immunoglobulin
IHD	ischaemic/ischemic heart disease
IM	intramuscular
ITT	insulin tolerance test
ITU	intensive therapy unit
IUCD	intrauterine contraceptive device
IUD	intrauterine device
IV	intravenous
IVF	in vitro fertilization
IVP	intravenous pyelogram
LBW	low birth weight
LDL	low density lipoprotein
LFT	liver function test
LH	luteinizing hormone
LHRF	LH-releasing factor
LMP	last menstrual period
LOA	left occipito-anterior
LP	lumbar puncture
LRTI	lower respiratory tract infection
MAOI	monoamine oxidase inhibitor
MCV	mean corpuscular volume
ME	myalgic encephalomyelitis
mEq	milliequivalent
MI	myocardial infarction
MMR	measles, mumps and rubella
MRI	magnetic resonance imaging
MS	multiple sclerosis
MUS	midstream urine specimen
NAI	non-accidental injury
NEC	necrotizing enterocolitis
NGU	non-gonococcal urethritis
NICU	neonatal intensive care unit
NIDDM	non-insulin dependent diabetes mellitus
NSAID	non-steroidal anti-inflammatory drug
NSU	nonspecific urethritis
NYD	not yet diagnosed
OA	osteoarthritis
OAP	old age pensioner
OTC	over the counter
PAT	platelet aggregation test
PCP	pulmonary capillary pressure
PCV	packed cell volume
PE	pulmonary embolism
PEFM	peak expiratory flow meter
PEFR	peak expiratory flow rate
PEV	peak expiratory velocity
PID	pelvic inflammatory disease
PKU	phenylketonuria
PMT	premenstrual tension
ppm	parts per million
psi	pounds per square inch
p.sol	partly soluble

PUO	pyrexia of unknown origin
PVD	pulmonary vascular disease
RA	rheumatoid arthritis
RAST	radioallergosorbent test
RBC	red blood cell/count
RBF	renal blood flow
RDA	recommended daily allowance
RDS	respiratory distress syndrome
REM	rapid eye movement
RES	reticuloendothelial system
Rh−	rhesus negative
Rh+	rhesus positive
RNA	ribonucleic acid
RSV	respiratory syncytial virus
RTA	road traffic accident
SBE	subacute bacterial endocarditis
SC	subcutaneous
SCBU	special care baby unit
SCU	special care unit
SFD	small for dates
SIDS	sudden infant death syndrome
SLE	systemic lupus erythematosus
SQ	subcutaneous
SR	sedimentation rate
STD	sexually transmitted disease
TB	tuberculosis
TBW	total body weight
TIA	transient ischaemic/ischemic attack
TIBC	total iron binding capacity
TLC	total lung capacity
TOP	termination of pregnancy
TPN	total parenteral nutrition
TRIC	trachoma inclusion conjunctivitis
TSH	thyroid stimulating hormone
URTI	upper respiratory tract infection
UTI	urinary tract infection
UV	ultraviolet
VBI	vertebrobasilar insufficiency
VD	venereal disease
VLDL	very low density lipoprotein
VMA	vanyl mandelic acid
WBC	white blood cell count

FRENCH
English
Spanish
Italian
German
FRENCH

A

FRENCH	ENGLISH	SPANISH
abcès	abscess	absceso
abcès froid	cold abscess	absceso frío
abcès périamygdalien	peritonsillar abscess	absceso periamigdalino
abdomen	abdomen	abdomen
abdominal	abdominal	abdominal
abdomino-périnéal	abdomino-perineal	abdominoperineal
abducteur	abductor	abductor
abduction	abduction	abducción
aberrant	aberrant	aberrante, desviado
aberration	aberration	aberración
ablation	ablation	ablación, excisión
abrasion	abrasion	abrasión
abréaction	abreaction	abreacción, catarsis
absence de développement pondéro-statural normal	failure to thrive (FTT)	desmedro, marasmo
absorption	absorption	absorción
abus	abuse	abuso
accès	seizure	acceso, ataque
accès ischémique transitoire cérébral	transient ischaemic attack (TIA) (Eng), transient ishemic attack (TIA) (Am)	ataque isquémico transitorio (AIT)
accident cérébrovasculaire	cerebrovascular accident (CVA)	accidente vascular cerebral (ACV)
accident de la route	road traffic accident (RTA)	accidente de circulacion
accommodation	accommodation	acomodación
accouchement	delivery	parto
accoutumance	addiction, habituation	adicción, toxicomanía, habituación
acétabule	acetabulum	acetábulo
achalasie	achalasia	acalasia
achondroplasie	achondroplasia	acondroplasia
acide (n)	acid (n)	ácido (n)
acide (a)	acid (a)	ácido (a)
acide aminé	amino acid	aminoácido
acide aminé essentiel	essential amino acid	aminoácido esenciale
acide désoxyribonucléique (ADN)	deoxyribonucleic acid (DNA)	ácido desoxirribonucléico (ADN)
acide folique	folic acid	ácido fólico
acide gras	fatty acid	ácido graso
acide gras essentiel	essential fatty acid	ácido graso esenciale
acide homovanillique	homovanillic acid (HVA)	ácido homovaníllico
acide lactique	lactic acid	ácido láctico
acide ribonucléique (RNA)	ribonucleic acid (RNA)	ácido ribonucléico (ARN)
acide urique	uric acid	ácido úrico
acide vanillyl-mandélique	vanyl mandelic acid (VMA)	ácido vanilmandélico (AVM)
acidité	acidity	acidez
acido-résistant	acid-fast	ácido-resistente
acidose	acidosis	acidosis
acinétique	akinetic	acinético

ascesso	Abszeß	abcès
ascesso freddo	kalter Abszeß	abcès froid
ascesso peritonsillare	Peritonsillarabszeß	abcès périamygdalien
addome	Abdomen	abdomen
addominale	abdominal	abdominal
addomino-perineale	abdominoperineal	abdomino-périnéal
abduttore	Abduktor	abducteur
abduzione	Abduktion	abduction
aberrante	aberrans, abartig	aberrant
aberrazione	Aberration, Abweichung	aberration
ablazione	Ablatio, Absetzung	ablation
abrasione	Abschabung, Ausschabung	abrasion
abreazione, catarsi	Abreaktion	abréaction
marasma infantile	Gedeihstörung	absence de développement pondéro-statural normal
assorbimento	Absorption	absorption
abuso	Abusus, Mißbrauch	abus
attacco, convulsione	Anfall	accès
attacco ischemico transitorio	transitorische ischämische Attacke (TIA)	accès ischémique transitoire cérébral
ictus, accidente cerebrovascolare (ACV)	Schlaganfall, Apoplex	accident cérébrovasculaire
incidente stradale	Verkehrsunfall	accident de la route
accomodazione	Akkommodation	accommodation
parto	Entbindung, Geburt	accouchement
tossicomania, assuefazione	Sucht, Gewöhnung, Habituation	accoutumance
acetabolo	Azetabulum, Hüftgelenkspfanne	acétabule
acalasia	Achalasie	achalasie
acondroplasia	Achondroplasie	achondroplasie
acido (n)	Säure (n)	acide (n)
acido (a)	sauer (a)	acide (a)
aminoacido	Aminosäure	acide aminé
aminoacido essenziale	essentielle Aminosäure	acide aminé essentiel
acido deossiribonucleico	Desoxyribonukleinsäure (DNS)	acide désoxyribonucléique (ADN)
acido folico	Folsäure	acide folique
acido grasso	Fettsäure	acide gras
acido grasso essenziale	essentielle Fettsäure	acide gras essentiel
acido omovanillico	Homovanillinsäure	acide homovanillique
acido lattico	Milchsäure	acide lactique
acido ribonucleico (RNA)	Ribonukleinsäure (RNA)	acide ribonucléique (RNA)
acido urico	Harnsäure	acide urique
acido vanilmandelico	Vanillylmandelsäure	acide vanillyl-mandélique
acidità	Säuregehalt	acidité
acido resistente	säurebeständig	acido-résistant
acidosi	Azidose	acidose
acinetico	akinetisch	acinétique

FRENCH	ENGLISH	SPANISH
acné	acne	acné
acné rosacée	rosacea	rosácea
acoustique	acoustic	acústico
acromégalie	acromegaly	acromegalia
acromio-claviculaire	acromioclavicular	acromioclavicular
acromion	acromion	acromion
actif	active	activo
actinomycose	actinomycosis	actinomicosis
action	action	acción
acuité	acuity	agudeza
acuité visuelle	visual acuity	agudeza visual
acupuncture	acupuncture	acupuntura
adducteur	adductor	aductor
adduction	adduction	aducción
adéno-amygdalectomie	adenotonsillectomy	amigdaloadenoidectomía
adénocarcinome	adenocarcinoma	adenocarcinoma
adénoïdectomie	adenoidectomy	adenoidectomía
adénome	adenoma	adenoma
adénomyome	adenomyoma	adenomioma
adénovirus	adenovirus	adenovirus
adhésion	adhesion	adherencia
adipeux	adipose	adiposo, graso
adjuvant	adjuvant	coadyuvante
adolescence	adolescence	adolescencia
adoption	adoption	adopción
adrénaline	adrenaline, epinephrine	adrenalina, epinefrina
adrénergique	adrenergic	adrenérgico
adsorption	adsorption	adsorción
aérobie	aerobe	aerobio, aeróbico
aérophagie	aerophagia	aerofagia
aérosol	aerosol	aerosol
afébrile	afebrile	apirético, afebril
affaissement	collapse	colapso
affect	affect	afecto
affecter	affect	afectar
affectif	affective	afectivo
affection/maladie respiratoire fébrile aiguë	acute febrile respiratory disease/illness (AFRD/I)	enfermedad respiratoria febril aguda
afférent	afferent	aferente
agénésie	agenesis	agenesia
agent chélateur	chelating agent	quelantes
agglutination	agglutination	aglutinación
agglutinine	agglutinin	aglutinina
agnathie	agnathia	agnatia
agnosie	agnosia	agnosia
agoniste	agonist	agonista
agoraphobie	agoraphobia	agorafobia

ITALIAN	GERMAN	FRENCH
acne	Akne	acné
rosacea, acne rosacea	Rosacea	acné rosacée
acustico	akustisch, Gehör-	acoustique
acromegalia	Akromegalie	acromégalie
acromioclavicolare	akromioklavikular	acromio-claviculaire
acromion	Akromion	acromion
attivo	aktiv, wirksam	actif
actinomicosi	Aktinomykose	actinomycose
azione	Tätigkeit	action
acuità	Schärfe	acuité
acutezza visiva	Sehschärfe	acuité visuelle
agopuntura	Akupunktur	acupuncture
adduttore	Adduktor	adducteur
adduzione	Adduktion	adduction
adenotonsillectomia	Adenotonsillektomie	adéno-amygdalectomie
adenocarcinoma	Adenokarzinom	adénocarcinome
adenoidectomia	Adenoidektomie, Polypenentfernung	adénoïdectomie
adenoma	Adenom	adénome
adenomioma	Adenomyom	adénomyome
adenovirus	Adenovirus	adénovirus
adesione	Adhäsion, Anhaften	adhésion
adiposo	adipös, fettleibig	adipeux
adiuvante	Adjuvans	adjuvant
adolescenza	Adoleszenz, Jugendalter	adolescence
adozione	Adoption	adoption
adrenalina	Adrenalin	adrénaline
adrenergico	adrenerg	adrénergique
adsorbimento	Adsorption	adsorption
aerobio	Aerobier	aérobie
aerofagia	Aerophagie, Luftschlucken	aérophagie
aerosol	Aerosol	aérosol
afebbrile	fieberfrei	afébrile
collasso	Kollaps	affaissement
emozione	Affekt, Erregung	affect
attaccare, influenzare	befallen	affecter
affettivo	affektiv	affectif
malattia respiratoria acuta febbrile	Atemwegsinfekt (akut fieberhaft)	affection/maladie respiratoire fébrile aiguë
afferente	afferent, zuführend	afférent
agenesia	Agenesie	agénésie
agente chelante	Chelatbildner	agent chélateur
agglutinazione	Agglutination	agglutination
agglutinine	Agglutinin	agglutinine
agnazia	Agnathie	agnathie
agnosia	Agnosie	agnosie
agonista	Agonist	agoniste
agorafobia	Agoraphobie, Platzangst	agoraphobie

FRENCH	ENGLISH	SPANISH
agranulocytose	agranulocytosis	agranulocitosis
agression	aggression	agresión
aigreurs	heartburn	ardor de estómago, pirosis
aigu(ë)	acute	agudo
aiguille	needle	aguja
aine	groin	ingle
aisselle	axilla	axila
albumine	albumin	albúmina
albuminurie	albuminuria	albuminuria
alcali	alkali	álcali
alcalin	alkaline	alcalino
alcalose	alkalosis	alcalosis
alcool	alcohol	alcohol
alcoolisme	alcoholism	alcoholismo
alèse	drawsheet	alezo, faja
aliénation	insanity	locura, demencia
alimentation	alimentation	alimentación
alimentation parentérale totale	total parenteral nutrition (TPN)	nutrición parenteral total
aliments non nutritifs	junk food	comidas preparadas poco nutritivas
allergène	allergen	alérgeno
allergie	allergy	alergia
allergie alimentaire	food allergy	alergia alimentaria
allopurinol	allopurinol	alopurinol
alopécie	alopecia	alopecia, calvicie
alpha-foetoprotéine	alpha-fetoprotein (AFP)	alfafetoproteína (AFP)
alvéole	alveolus	alvéolo
alvéolite	alveolitis	alveolitis
amaurose	amaurosis	amaurosis, ceguera
amblyopie	amblyopia	ambliopía
ambulant	ambulant	ambulante
ambulatoire	ambulatory	ambulatorio
amélioration	amelioration	mejoría
aménorrhée	amenorrhea (Am), amenorrhoea (Eng)	amenorrea
amibe	ameba (Am), amoeba (Eng)	ameba
amibiase	amebiasis (Am), amoebiasis (Eng)	amebiasis
amibome	ameboma (Am), amoeboma (Eng)	ameboma
amnésie	amnesia	amnesia
amniocentèse	amniocentesis	amniocentesis
amnion	amnion	amnios
amnioscopie	amnioscopy	amnioscopia
amniotomie	amniotomy	amniotomía
amorphe	amorphous	amorfo
ampoule	ampoule (Eng), ampule (Am), ampulla, blister	ampolla, víal, vesícula, flictena
amputation	amputation	amputación
amputé	amputee	amputado
amygdalectomie	tonsillectomy	tonsilectomía

ITALIAN	GERMAN	FRENCH
agranulocitosi	Agranulozytose	agranulocytose
aggressività	Aggression	agression
pirosi	Sodbrennen	aigreurs
acuto	spitz, scharf	aigu(ë)
ago	Nadel, Kanüle	aiguille
inguine	Leiste	aine
ascella	Axilla, Achsel(höhle)	aisselle
albumina	Albumin	albumine
albuminuria	Albuminurie	albuminurie
alcali	Alkali, Lauge, Base	alcali
alcalino	alkalisch, basisch	alcalin
alcalosi	Alkalose	alcalose
alcool	Alkohol	alcool
alcolismo	Alkoholismus, Alkoholvergiftung	alcoolisme
traversa	Unterziehtuch	alèse
pazzia	Geisteskrankheit	aliénation
alimentazione	Ernährung	alimentation
nutrizione parenterale totale	parenterale Ernährung	alimentation parentérale totale
cibo contenente additivi chimici	ungesunde Nahrung	aliments non nutritifs
allergene	Allergen	allergène
allergia	Allergie	allergie
allergia alimentare	Nahrungsmittelallergie	allergie alimentaire
allopurinolo	Allopurinol	allopurinol
alopecia	Alopezie, Haarausfall	alopécie
alfafetoproteina	Alpha-Fetoprotein	alpha-foetoprotéine
alveolo	Alveole	alvéole
alveolite	Alveolitis	alvéolite
amaurosi	Amaurose	amaurose
ambliopia	Amblyopie, Sehschwäche	amblyopie
ambulatorio	ambulant	ambulant
ambulatoriale	ambulant	ambulatoire
miglioramento	Besserung	amélioration
amenorrea	Amenorrhoe	aménorrhée
ameba	Amöbe	amibe
amebiasi	Amöbenkrankheit, Amöbiasis	amibiase
ameboma	Amöbengranulom	amibome
amnesia	Amnesie	amnésie
amniocentesi	Amniozentese	amniocentèse
amnios	Amnion	amnion
amnioscopia	Amnioskopie	amnioscopie
amniotomia	Amnionpunktur	amniotomie
amorfo	amorph	amorphe
ampolla, fiala, vescicola, bolla	Ampulle, Blase, Hautblase, Brandblase	ampoule
amputazione	Amputation	amputation
amputato	Amputierter	amputé
tonsillectomia	Tonsillektomie, Mandelentfernung	amygdalectomie

FRENCH	ENGLISH	SPANISH
amygdales	tonsils	amígdalas
amyloïde (n)	amyloid (n)	amiloide (n)
amyloïde (a)	amyloid (a)	amiloideo (a)
amylose	amyloidosis	amiloidosis
anabolisme	anabolism	anabolismo
anaérobie	anaerobe (Eng), anerobe (Am)	anaerobio
analeptique (n)	analeptic (n)	analéptico, estimulante (n)
analeptique (a)	analeptic (a)	analéptico, estimulante (a)
analgésie	analgesia	analgesia
analgésique (n)	analgesic (n)	analgésico (n)
analgésique (a)	analgesic (a)	analgésico (a)
analyse	analysis	análisis
analyse d'urine	urinalysis	urinálisis
anaphylaxie	anaphylaxis	anafilaxis
anaplasie	anaplasia	anaplasia
anarthrie	anarthria	anartria
anasarque foeto-placentaire	hydrops fetalis	hydrops fetal
anastomose	anastomosis	anastómosis
anatomie	anatomy	anatomía
androgènes	androgens	andrógenos
anémie	anaemia (Eng), anemia (Am)	anemia
anémie pernicieuse	pernicious anaemia (Eng), pernicious anemia (Am)	anemia perniciosa
anencéphalie	anencephaly	anencefalia
anesthésie	anaesthesia (Eng), anesthesia (Am)	anestesia
anesthésie par blocage nerveux	nerve block	bloqueo nervioso
anesthésique (n)	anaesthetic (Eng) (n), anesthetic (Am) (n)	anestésico (n)
anesthésique (a)	anaesthetic (Eng) (a), anesthetic (Am) (a)	anestésico (a)
anévrisme	aneurysm	aneurisma
angine	tonsillitis	amigdalitis
angioplastie	angioplasty	angioplastia
angiotensine	angiotensin	angiotensina
angle	flexure	flexura
angor	angina	angina
anisocytose	anisocytosis	anisocitosis
ankylose	ankylosis	anquilosis
ankylostome	hookworm	anquilostoma duodenal
annexes	adnexa	anejos, anexos
annulaire	annular	anular
anogénital	anogenital	anogenital
anomalie	anomaly, defect	anomalía, defecto
anorectal	anorectal	anorrectal
anorexie	anorexia	anorexia

ITALIAN	GERMAN	FRENCH
tonsille	Tonsillen, Mandeln	amygdales
amiloide (n)	Amyloid (n)	amyloïde (n)
amiloide (a)	amyloid (a), stärkehaltig (a)	amyloïde (a)
amiloidosi	Amyloidose	amylose
anabolismo	Anabolismus, Aufbaustoffwechsel	anabolisme
anaerobio	Anaerobier	anaérobie
analettico (n)	Analeptikum (n)	analeptique (n)
analettico (a)	analeptisch (a)	analeptique (a)
analgesia	Analgesie, Schmerzlosigkeit	analgésie
analgesico (n)	Analgetikum (n), Schmerzmittel (n)	analgésique (n)
analgesico (a)	analgetisch (a), schmerzlindernd (a), schmerzunempfindlich (a)	analgésique (a)
analisi	Analyse	analyse
esame dell'urina	Urinanalyse, Urinuntersuchung	analyse d'urine
anafilassi	Anaphylaxie	anaphylaxie
anaplasia	Anaplasie	anaplasie
anartria	Anarthrie	anarthrie
idrope fetale	Hydrops fetalis	anasarque foeto-placentaire
anastomosi	Anastomose	anastomose
anatomia	Anatomie	anatomie
androgeni	Androgene	androgènes
anemia	Anämie	anémie
anemia perniciosa	perniziöse Anämie	anémie pernicieuse
anencefalia	Anenzephalie	anencéphalie
anestesia	Anästhesie, Betäubung, Narkose	anesthésie
blocco nervoso	Leitungsanästhesie	anesthésie par blocage nerveux
anestetico (n)	Anästhetikum (n), Betäubungsmittel (n), Narkosemittel (n)	anesthésique (n)
anestetico (a)	anästhetisch (a), betäubend (a), gefühllos (a)	anesthésique (a)
aneurisma	Aneurysma	anévrisme
tonsillite	Tonsillitis, Mandelentzündung	angine
angioplastica	Angioplastie	angioplastie
angiotensina	Angiotensin	angiotensine
flessura	Flexur	angle
angina	Angina	angor
anisocitosi	Anisozytose	anisocytose
anchilosi	Ankylose, Versteifung	ankylose
strongiloide	Hakenwurm	ankylostome
annessi	Adnexe	annexes
anulare	ringförmig	annulaire
anogenitale	anogenital	anogénital
anomalia, difetto	Anomalie, Fehlbildung, Defekt, Mangel, Störung	anomalie
anorettale	anorektal	anorectal
anoressia	Anorexie, Magersucht	anorexie

anorexique *(n)*	anorectic *(n)*	anoréxico *(n)*
anorexique *(a)*	anorectic *(a)*	anoréxico *(a)*
anormal	abnormal	anormal
anosmie	anosmia	anosmia
anovulaire	anovular	anovular
anoxie	anoxia	anoxia
antagonisme	antagonism	antagonismo
antagoniste	antagonist	antagonista
antagoniste H2	H2 antagonist	antagonista H2
anténatal	antenatal	antenatal
ante partum	ante-partum	ante partum, preparto
antérieur	anterior	anterior
antérograde	anterograde	anterógrado
antéversion	anteversion	anteversión
anthrax	anthrax	carbunco
anthropoïde	anthropoid	antropoide
anthropologie	anthropology	antropología
antiacide	antacid	antiácido
antiarythmique	anti-arrhythmic	antiarrítmico
antibactérien	antibacterial	antibacteriano
antibiotiques	antibiotics	antibióticos
anticholinergique	anticholinergic	anticolinérgico
anticoagulant	anticoagulant	anticoagulante
anticonvulsant *(n)*	anticonvulsant *(n)*	anticonvulsivo *(n)*
anticonvulsant *(a)*	anticonvulsant *(a)*	anticonvulsivo *(a)*
anticorps	antibodies (Ab)	anticuerpos
anticorps monoclonal	monoclonal antibody	anticuerpo monoclonal
anti-D	anti-D	anti-D
antidépresseur	antidepressant	antidepresivo
antidote	antidote	antídoto
antiémétique *(n)*	antiemetic *(n)*	antiemético *(n)*
antiémétique *(a)*	antiemetic *(a)*	antiemético *(a)*
antiépileptique *(n)*	anti-epileptic *(n)*	antiepiléptico *(n)*
antiépileptique *(a)*	anti-epileptic *(a)*	antiepiléptico *(a)*
antigène	antigen	antígeno
antigène australien	Australian antigen	antígeno Australia
antigène d'histocompatibilité	histocompatibility antigen	antígeno de histocompatibilidad
antigène humain des erythrocytes	human erythrocyte antigen (HEA)	antígeno eritrocitario humano
antigène lymphocytaire humain	human lymphocytic antigen (HLA)	antígeno linfocitario humano (HLA)
antihistamine	antihistamine	antihistamínico
antihypertenseur	antihypertensive	hipotensor
antihypertensif	antihypertensive	hipotensor
anti-inflammatoire	anti-inflammatory	antiinflamatorio

ITALIAN	GERMAN	FRENCH
anoressico (n)	Anorektiker(in) (n), Magersüchtige(r) (n), Apettitzügler (n)	anorexique (n)
anoressico (a)	anorektisch (a), magersüchtig (a)	anorexique (a)
anormale	abnormal	anormal
anosmia	Anosmie	anosmie
anovulare	anovulatorisch	anovulaire
anossia	Anoxie, Sauerstoffmangel	anoxie
antagonismo	Antagonismus	antagonisme
antagonista	Antagonist	antagoniste
antagonista H2	H2-Antagonist	antagoniste H2
prenatale	pränatal	anténatal
preparto	ante partum, vor der Entbindung	ante partum
anteriore	anterior, Vorder-	antérieur
anterogrado	anterograd	antérograde
antiversione	Anteversion	antéversion
antrace, carbonchio	Anthrax, Milzbrand	anthrax
antropoide	anthropoid	anthropoïde
antropologia	Anthropologie	anthropologie
antiacido	Antazidum	antiacide
anti-aritmico	antiarrhythmisch	antiarythmique
antibatterico	antibakteriell	antibactérien
antibiotici	Antibiotika	antibiotiques
anticolinergico	anticholinerg	anticholinergique
anticoagulante	Antikoagulans, Gerinnungshemmer	anticoagulant
anticonvulsivante (n)	Antiepileptikum (n), Antikonvulsivum (n)	anticonvulsant (n)
anticonvulsivante (a)	antiepileptisch (a), antikonvulsiv (a)	anticonvulsant (a)
anticorpi (Ac)	Antikörper	anticorps
anticorpo monoclonale	monoklonaler Antikörper	anticorps monoclonal
anti-D	Anti-D-Immununglobulin	anti-D
antidepressivo	Antidepressivum	antidépresseur
antidoto	Antidot	antidote
anti-emetico (n)	Antiemetikum (n)	antiémétique (n)
anti-emetico (a)	antiemetisch (a)	antiémétique (a)
anticomiziale (n)	Antiepileptikum (n), Antikonvulsivum (n)	antiépileptique (n)
anticomiziale (a)	antiepileptisch (a), antikonvulsiv (a)	antiépileptique (a)
antigene	Antigen	antigène
antigene Australia	Australia-Antigen (HBsAG)	antigène australien
antigene di istocompatibilità	Histokompatibilitäts-Antigen	antigène d'histocompatibilité
antigene eritrocitico umano	menschliches Erythrozyten-Antigen	antigène humain des erythrocytes
antigene linfocitario umano	human lymphocytic antigen (HLA)	antigène lymphocytaire humain
anti-istaminico	Antihistamine	antihistamine
anti-ipertensivo	Antihypertonikum, Antihypertensivum	antihypertenseur
anti-ipertensivo	blutdrucksenkend, antihypertensiv	antihypertensif
anti-infiammatorio	entzündungshemmend	anti-inflammatoire

FRENCH	ENGLISH	SPANISH
anti-inflammatoire non stéroïdien	non-steroidal anti-inflammatory drug (NSAID)	fármaco antiinflamatorio no esteroide (AINE)
antimétabolite	antimetabolite	antimetabolito
antimicrobien	antimicrobial	antimicrobiano
antimycotique (n)	antimycotic (n)	antimicótico (n)
antimycotique (a)	antimycotic (a)	antimicótico (a)
antipaludique (n)	antimalarial (n)	antipalúdico (n)
antipaludique (a)	antimalarial (a)	antipalúdico (a)
antiprurigineux (n)	antipruritic (n)	antipruriginoso (n)
antiprurigineux (a)	antipruritic (a)	antipruriginoso (a)
antipsychotique (n)	antipsychotic (n)	antipsicótico (n)
antipsychotique (a)	antipsychotic (a)	antipsicótico (a)
antipyrétique (n)	antipyretic (n)	antipirético (n)
antipyrétique (a)	antipyretic (a)	antipirético (a)
antisepsie	antisepsis	antisepsia
antiseptique (n)	antiseptic (n)	antiséptico (n)
antiseptique (a)	antiseptic (a)	antiséptico (a)
anti-serum	antiserum	antisuero
antisocial	antisocial	antisocial
antispasmodique (n)	antispasmodic (n)	antiespasmódico (n)
antispasmodique (a)	antispasmodic (a)	antiespasmódico (a)
antitoxine	antitoxin	antitoxina
antitussif (n)	antitussive (n)	antitusígeno (n)
antitussif (a)	antitussive (a)	antitusígeno (a)
antre	antrum	antro
antrostomie	antrostomy	antrostomía
anurie	anuria	anuria
anus	anus	ano
anxiété	anxiety	ansiedad
anxiolytique (n)	anxiolytic (n)	ansiolítico (n)
anxiolytique (a)	anxiolytic (a)	ansiolítico (a)
aorte	aorta	aorta
apathie	apathy	apatía
apex	apex	ápex
aphasie	aphasia	afasia
aphte	thrush	muguet
aphtes	aphthae	aftas
apnée	apnea (Am), apnoea (Eng)	apnea
apoplexie	stroke	ictus
appareil de mesure du débit expiratoire de pointe	peak expiratory flow meter (PEFM)	medida de la velocidad máxima del flujo espiratorio
appareil de ventilation artificielle	ventilator	ventilador
appendice	appendix	apéndice
appendicectomie	appendectomy, appendicectomy	apendicectomía
appendicite	appendicitis	apendicitis

ITALIAN	GERMAN	FRENCH
farmaco antinfiammatorio non steroideo (FANS)	nichtsteroidales Antiphlogistikum	anti-inflammatoire non stéroïdien
antimetabolita	Antimetabolit	antimétabolite
antimicrobico	antimikrobiell	antimicrobien
antimicotico (n)	Antimykotikum (n)	antimycotique (n)
antimicotico (a)	antimykotisch (a)	antimycotique (a)
antimalarico (n)	Antimalariamittel (n), Malariamittel (n)	antipaludique (n)
antimalarico (a)	Antimalaria- (a)	antipaludique (a)
antipruriginoso (n)	Antipruriginosum (n)	antiprurigineux (n)
antipruriginoso (a)	antipruriginös (a), juckreizlindernd (a)	antiprurigineux (a)
antipsicotico (n)	Antipsychotikum (n), Neuroleptikum (n)	antipsychotique (n)
antipsicotico (a)	antipsychotisch (a), neuroleptisch (a)	antipsychotique (a)
anti-piretico (n)	Antipyretikum (n), Fiebermittel (n)	antipyrétique (n)
anti-piretico (a)	antipyretisch (a), fiebersenkend (a)	antipyrétique (a)
antisepsi	Antisepsis	antisepsie
antisettico (n)	Antiseptikum (n)	antiseptique (n)
antisettico (a)	antiseptisch (a)	antiseptique (a)
anti-siero	Antiserum, Immunserum	anti-serum
antisociale	dissozial	antisocial
antispastico (n)	Spasmolytikum (n)	antispasmodique (n)
antispastico (a)	spasmolytisch (a), krampflösend (a)	antispasmodique (a)
antitossina	Antitoxin, Gegengift	antitoxine
antibechico (n)	Antitussivum (n), Hustenmittel (n)	antitussif (n)
antibechico (a)	antitussiv (a)	antitussif (a)
antro	Antrum	antre
antrostomia	Antrumeröffnung	antrostomie
anuria	Anurie, Harnverhaltung	anurie
ano	Anus, After	anus
ansietà	Angst	anxiété
ansiolitico (n)	Anxiolytikum (n)	anxiolytique (n)
ansiolitico (a)	anxiolytisch (a)	anxiolytique (a)
aorta	Aorta, Hauptschlagader	aorte
apatia	Apathie	apathie
apice	Apex, Spitze	apex
afasia	Aphasie	aphasie
stomatite de Candida albicans, mughetto	Soor, Sprue	aphte
afte	Aphthe	aphtes
apnea	Apnoe, Atemstillstand	apnée
ictus, colpo apoplettico, accidente cerebrovascolare	Schlag, Schlaganfall	apoplexie
misuratore del flusso espiratorio massimo	Peak-Flowmeter	appareil de mesure du débit expiratoire de pointe
ventilatore	Ventilator	appareil de ventilation artificielle
appendice	Appendix, Blinddarm	appendice
appendicectomia	Appendektomie, Blinddarmoperation	appendicectomie
appendicite	Appendizitis, Blinddarmentzündung	appendicite

FRENCH	ENGLISH	SPANISH
applicateur	applicator	aplicador
apposition	apposition	aposición
apraxie	apraxia	apraxia
après rapport	postcoital	postcoital
aptitude	ability	habilidad, capacidad
apyrexie	apyrexia	apirexia
aqueduc	aqueduct	acueducto
aqueux	aqueous	acuoso
arachnoïde	arachnoid	aracnoideo
arbovirus	arbovirus	arbovirus
aréole	areola	areola
armature orthopédique	caliper	compás, calibrador
arrière-faix	afterbirth	secundinas, expulsión de la placenta y membranas
artefact	artefact (Eng), artifact (Am)	artefacto
artère	artery	arteria
artère fémorale	femoral artery	arteria femoral
artère radiale	radial artery	arteria radial
artériole	arteriole	arteriola
artériopathie	arteriopathy	arteriopatía
artériosclérose	arteriosclerosis	arteriosclerosis
artérioveineux	arteriovenous	arteriovenoso
artérite	arteritis	arteritis
artérite temporale	giant cell arteritis	arteritis de células gigantes
arthralgie	arthralgia	artralgia
arthrite	arthritis	artritis
arthrite de Lyme	Lyme disease	enfermedad de Lyme
arthrodèse	arthrodesis	artrodesis
arthrographie	arthrography	artrografía
arthropathie	arthropathy	artropatía
arthropathie neurogène	Charcot's joint	articulación de Charcot
arthroplastie	arthroplasty	artroplastia
arthroscopie	arthroscopy	artroscopia
articulaire	articular	articular
articulation	articulation, joint	articulación
arythmie	arrhythmia	arritmia
asbeste	asbestos	asbesto
asbestose	asbestosis	asbestosis
ascaride	threadworm	enterobius vermincularis, oxiuros
ascaris	ascaris, roundworm	áscaris
ascite	ascites	ascitis
asepsie	asepsis	asepsia
asile	hospice	hospicio
aspergillose	aspergillosis	aspergilosis
asphyxie	asphyxia	asfixia
aspiration	aspiration	aspiración
assimilation	assimilation	asimilación

ITALIAN	GERMAN	FRENCH
applicatore	Applikator	applicateur
apposizione	Apposition	apposition
aprassia	Apraxie	apraxie
postcoitale	Postkoital-	après rapport
abilità, capacità	Fähigkeit	aptitude
apiressia	Apyrexie	apyrexie
acquedotto	Aquädukt	aqueduc
acquoso	wässrig, wasserhaltig	aqueux
aracnoidea	arachnoid	arachnoïde
arbovirus	ARBO-Virus	arbovirus
areola	Areola, Brustwarzenhof	aréole
compasso per pelvi-craniometria	Schiene	armature orthopédique
secondine, membrane fetali e placenta	Plazenta, Nachgeburt	arrière-faix
artefatto	Artefakt	artefact
arteria	Arterie, Schlagader	artère
arteria femorale	Arteria femoralis	artère fémorale
arteria radiale	Arteria radialis	artère radiale
arteriola	Arteriole	artériole
arteriopatia	Arteriopathie, Arterienerkrankung	artériopathie
arteriosclerosi	Arteriosklerose, Arterienverkalkung	artériosclérose
arterovenosa	arteriovenös	artérioveineux
arterite	Arteriitis	artérite
arterite a cellule giganti	Riesenzellarteriitis	artérite temporale
artralgia	Arthralgie, Gelenkschmerz	arthralgie
artrite	Arthritis, Gelenkentzündung	arthrite
malattia di Lyme	Lyme-Arthritis, Lyme-Borreliose	arthrite de Lyme
artrodesi	Arthrodese	arthrodèse
artrografia	Arthrographie	arthrographie
artropatia	Arthropathie, Gelenkleiden	arthropathie
artropatia di Charcot	Charcot-Gelenk	arthropathie neurogène
artroplastica	Arthroplastik, Gelenkplastik	arthroplastie
artroscopia	Arthroskopie, Gelenkendoskopie	arthroscopie
articolare	Gelenk-	articulaire
articolazione	Artikulation, Gelenk	articulation
aritmia	Arrhythmie, Rhythmusstörung	arythmie
asbesto	Asbest	asbeste
asbestosi	Asbestose	asbestose
ossiuro	Fadenwurm	ascaride
ascaride, nematelminto	Rundwurm, Spulwurm	ascaris
ascite	Aszites	ascite
asepsi	Asepsis	asepsie
ricovero	Hospiz	asile
aspergillosi	Aspergillose	aspergillose
asfissia	Asphyxie	asphyxie
aspirazione	Aspiration	aspiration
assimilazione	Assimilation	assimilation

FRENCH	ENGLISH	SPANISH
association	association	asociación
astéréognosie	astereognosis	astereognosia
asthme	asthma	asma
asthme bronchique	bronchial asthma	asma bronquial
asticot	maggot	antojo
astigmatisme	astigmatism	astigmatismo
astragale	talus	astrágalo
astringent	astringent	astringente
asymétrie	asymmetry	asimetría
asymptomatique	asymptomatic	asintomático
ataxie	ataxia	ataxia
atélectasie	atelectasis	atelectasia
à terme	full-term	embarazo a término
athérogène	atherogenic	aterogénico
athérome	atheroma	ateroma
athérosclérose	atherosclerosis	aterosclerosis
athétose	athetosis	atetosis
athrepsie	marasmus	marasmo
atome	atom	átomo
atonique	atonic	atono
atrésie	atresia	atresia
atrio-ventriculaire	atrioventricular (AV)	atrioventricular, aurículo-ventricular (AV)
atrophie	atrophy	atrofia
atropine	atropine	atropina
attachement	bonding	vinculación
attaque	attack, fit	ataque, acceso
attelle	splint	astilla
atténuation	attenuation	atenuación
atypique	atypical	atípico
audiogramme	audiogram	audiograma
audiologie	audiology	audiología
auditif	auditory	auditorio
audition	hearing	oído
aura	aura	aura
aural	aural	aural
auriscope	auriscope	auriscopio
auscultation	auscultation	auscultación
autisme	autism	autismo
autiste	autistic	persona autística
auto-anticorps	autoantibody	autoanticuerpo
auto-antigène	autoantigen	autoantígeno
autoclave	autoclave	autoclave
auto-examen des seins	breast self-examination (BSE)	autoexamen de la mama
autogreffe	autograft	autoinjerto
auto-immunisation	autoimmunity	autoinmunización
autologue	autologous	autólogo

ITALIAN	GERMAN	FRENCH
associazione	Assoziation	association
astereognosia	Astereognosie	astéréognosie
asma	Asthma	asthme
asma bronchiale	Asthma bronchiale	asthme bronchique
larva	Larve, Made	asticot
astigmatismo	Astigmatismus	astigmatisme
astragalo, talo	Talus	astragale
astringente	adstringierend	astringent
asimmetria	Asymmetrie	asymétrie
asintomatico	asymptomatisch	asymptomatique
atassia	Ataxie, Koordinationsstörung	ataxie
atelettasia	Atelektase	atélectasie
gravidanza a termine	ausgetragen	à terme
aterogenico	atherogen	athérogène
ateroma	Atherom, Grützbeutel	athérome
aterosclerosi	Atherosklerose	athérosclérose
atetosi	Athetose	athétose
marasma	Marasmus	athrepsie
atomo	Atom	atome
atonico	atonisch	atonique
atresia	Atresie	atrésie
atrioventricolare	atrioventrikulär	atrio-ventriculaire
atrofia	Atrophie	atrophie
atropina	Atropin	atropine
legame	Bindung	attachement
attacco, convulsione	Anfall, Attacke	attaque
stecca ortopedica	Schiene	attelle
attenuazione	Verdünnung, Abschwächung	atténuation
atipico	atypisch, heterolog	atypique
audiogramma	Audiogramm, Hörkurve	audiogramme
audiologia	Audiologie	audiologie
acustico, auditivo	Gehör-, Hör-	auditif
udito	Gehör, Hören	audition
aura	Aura	aura
auricolare	Gehör-, Ohr-, Aura-	aural
otoscopio	Ohrenspiegel	auriscope
auscultazione	Auskultation, Abhören	auscultation
autismo	Autismus	autisme
autistico	autistisch	autiste
autoanticorpo	Autoantikörper	auto-anticorps
autoantigene	Autoantigen	auto-antigène
autoclave	Autoklav, Sterilisationsapparat	autoclave
autopalpazione mammaria	Selbstuntersuchung der Brust	auto-examen des seins
autoinnesto	Autoplastik	autogreffe
autoimmunizzazione	Autoimmunität	auto-immunisation
autologo	autolog	autologue

FRENCH	ENGLISH	SPANISH
autolyse	autolysis	autólisis
automutilation	self-harm	autolesión
autonome	autonomic	autónomo
autopsie	autopsy	autopsia
avaler	swallow	tragar
avant-bras	forearm	antebrazo
avasculaire	avascular	avascular
avortement	abortion	aborto
avortement provoqué	induced abortion	aborto inducido
avortement thérapeutique	therapeutic abortion	aborto terapéutico
avorter	abort	abortar
avulsion	avulsion	avulsión
axe	axis	eje
axone	axon	axón
axonotmésis	axonotmesis	axonotmesis
azygos	azygous	ácigos

ITALIAN	GERMAN	FRENCH
autolisi	Autolyse	autolyse
autolesionismo	Selbstschädigung	automutilation
autonomo	autonom	autonome
autopsia	Autopsie, Sektion	autopsie
inghiottire	schlucken	avaler
avambraccio	Unterarm	avant-bras
avascolare	gefäßlos	avasculaire
aborto	Abort, Fehlgeburt	avortement
aborto procurato	Abtreibung, künstlicher Abort	avortement provoqué
aborto terapeutico	indizierter Abort	avortement thérapeutique
abortire	fehlgebären	avorter
avulsione	Abriß, Ausreißen	avulsion
asse, colonna vertebrale	Achse	axe
cilindrasse, assone	Axon	axone
degenerazione del cilindrasse, con possibile rigenerazione	Axonotmesis	axonotmésis
azygos	azygos	azygos

B

FRENCH	ENGLISH	SPANISH
bacille	bacillus	bacilo
bacille de Calmette-Guérin (BCG)	bacille Calmette-Guérin (BCG)	bacilo de Calmette-Guérin (BCG)
bactéricide	bactericide	bactericida
bactérie	bacteria	bacteria
bactériémie	bacteraemia (Eng), bacteremia (Am)	bacteriemia
bactériologie	bacteriology	bacteriología
bactériostase	bacteriostasis	bacteriostasis
bactériurie	bacteriuria	bacteriuria
bâillement	yawn	bostezo
bain	bath	baño
balanite	balanitis	balanitis
balanoposthite	balanoposthitis	balanopostitis
ballant intestinal	roughage	fibra alimentaria
ballottement	ballottement	peloteo
bandage	bandage	vendaje
banque de sang	blood bank	banco de sangre
barrière hémato-encéphalique	blood-brain barrier (BBB)	barrera hematoencefálica (BHE)
bec-de-lièvre	harelip	labio leporino
bégaiement	stammer	tartamudeo
bénin (bénigne)	benign	benigno
béribéri	beri-beri	beri-beri
bêtabloquant	beta blocker	beta-bloqueador
biceps	biceps	bíceps
bicorne	bicornuate	bicornio
bicuspide	bicuspid	bicúspide
bifide	bifid	bífido
bifurcation	bifurcation	bifurcación
bilatéral	bilateral	bilateral
bile	bile	bilis
biliaire	biliary	biliar
bilieux	bilious	bilioso
bilirubine	bilirubin	bilirrubina
biliurie	biliuria	biliuria
bimanuel	bimanual	bimanual
biologique	biological	biológico
biopsie	biopsy	biopsia
biopsie du villus chorionique	chorionic villus biopsy	biopsia de las vellosidades coriónicas
biopsie jéjunale	jejunal biopsy	biopsia del yeyuno
biorythme	biorhythm	biorritmo
bipolaire	bipolar	bipolar
bisexuel	bisexual	bisexual
bivalve	bivalve	bivalvo
blépharite	blepharitis	blefaritis
blépharospasme	blepharospasm	blefarospasmo
blessure	injury	lesión

ITALIAN	GERMAN	FRENCH
bacillo	Bazillus	bacille
bacillo di Calmette e Guérin	Bacillus Calmette-Guérin (BCG)	bacille de Calmette-Guérin (BCG)
battericida	Bakterizid	bactéricide
batteri	Bakterien	bactérie
batteriemia	Bakteriämie	bactériémie
batteriologia	Bakteriologie	bactériologie
batteriostasi	Bakteriostase	bactériostase
batteriuria	Bakteriurie	bactériurie
sbadiglio	Gähnen	bâillement
bagno	Bad	bain
balanite	Balanitis	balanite
balanopostite	Balanoposthitis	balanoposthite
alimento ricco di fibre	Ballaststoff	ballant intestinal
ballottamento	Ballottement	ballottement
benda	Verband	bandage
banca del sangue	Blutbank	banque de sang
barriera ematoencefalica	Blut-Hirn-Schranke	barrière hémato-encéphalique
labbro leporino	Hasenscharte	bec-de-lièvre
balbuzie	Stottern	bégaiement
benigno	benigne, gutartig	bénin (bénigne)
beri-beri	Beriberi	béribéri
beta-bloccante	Betablocker	bêtabloquant
bicipite	Bizeps	biceps
bicorne	bicornis	bicorne
bicuspide	bicuspidal	bicuspide
bifido	bifidus	bifide
biforcazione	Bifurkation	bifurcation
bilaterale	zweiseitig	bilatéral
bile	Galle	bile
biliare	biliär	biliaire
biliare	biliös	bilieux
bilirubina	Bilirubin	bilirubine
biliuria	Bilirubinurie	biliurie
bimanuale	bimanuell, beidhändig	bimanuel
biologico	biologisch	biologique
biopsia	Biopsie	biopsie
biopsia dei villi coriali	Chorionzottenbiopsie	biopsie du villus chorionique
biopsia digiunale	Jejunumbiopsie	biopsie jéjunale
bioritmo	Biorhythmus	biorythme
bipolare	bipolar	bipolaire
bisessuale	bisexuell	bisexuel
bivalve	zweiklappig	bivalve
blefarite	Blepharitis, Lidentzündung	blépharite
blefarospasmo	Blepharospasmus, Lidkrampf	blépharospasme
lesione	Verletzung	blessure

FRENCH	ENGLISH	SPANISH
boîte crânienne	cranium	cráneo
boîte de Pétri	Petri dish	disco de Petri
bol	bolus	bolo
borréliose	borreliosis	borreliosis
botulisme	botulism	botulismo
bouche	mouth	boca
bouche-à-bouche	kiss of life	beso de vida
boule hystérique	globus hystericus	globo histérico
boulimie	bulimia	bulimia
bourse	bursa	bolsa
bouton	pimple, spot	grano, mancha
brachial	brachial	braquial
bradycardie	bradycardia	bradicardia
branchial	branchial	branquial
bras	arm	brazo
broche de Steinmann	Steinmann's pin	clavo de Steinmann
bronche	bronchus	bronquio
bronchectasie	bronchiectasis	bronquiectasia
bronches	bronchi	bronquios
bronchiole	bronchiole	bronquiolo
bronchiolite	bronchiolitis	bronquiolitis
bronchite	bronchitis	bronquitis
bronchoconstricteur	bronchoconstrictor	broncoconstrictor
bronchodilatateur	bronchodilator	broncodilatador
bronchopneumonie	bronchopneumonia	bronconeumonia
bronchopneumopathie chronique obstructive	chronic obstructive airway disease (COAD)	enfermedad obstructiva crónica de las vias respiratorias
bronchopulmonaire	bronchopulmonary	broncopulmonar
bronchoscope	bronchoscope	broncoscopio
bronchospasme	bronchospasm	broncospasmo
brucellose	brucellosis	brucelosis
brûler	burn	quemar
brûlure	burn	quemadura
buccal	buccal	bucal
bulbaire	bulbar	bulbar
bulle	bulla	bulla
bursite	bursitis	bursitis

ITALIAN	GERMAN	FRENCH
cranio	Schädel, Kranium	**boîte crânienne**
capsula di Petri	Petrischale	**boîte de Pétri**
bolo	Bolus	**bol**
borreliosi	Borreliose	**borréliose**
botulismo	Botulismus	**botulisme**
bocca	Mund	**bouche**
respirazione bocca a bocca	Mund-zu-Mund-Wiederbelebung	**bouche-à-bouche**
bolo isterico	Globus hystericus, Globusgefühl	**boule hystérique**
bulimia	Bulimie	**boulimie**
borsa	Bursa	**bourse**
pustola, piccolo foruncolo, foruncolo	Pickel, Mitesser, Flecken	**bouton**
brachiale	Arm-	**brachial**
bradicardia	Bradykardie	**bradycardie**
branchiale	branchial-	**branchial**
braccio	Arm	**bras**
chiodo per estensione di Steinmann	Steinmann Knochennagel	**broche de Steinmann**
bronco	Bronchus	**bronche**
bronchiettasia	Bronchiektase	**bronchectasie**
bronchi	Bronchien	**bronches**
bronchiolo	Bronchiolus, Bronchiole	**bronchiole**
bronchiolite	Bronchiolitis	**bronchiolite**
bronchite	Bronchitis	**bronchite**
broncocostrittore	Bronchokonstriktor	**bronchoconstricteur**
broncodilatatore	Bronchodilatator	**bronchodilatateur**
broncopolmonite	Bronchopneumonie	**bronchopneumonie**
malattia ostruttiva cronica delle vie respiratorie	chronische obstruktive Lungenerkrankung	**bronchopneumopathie chronique obstructive**
broncopolmonare	bronchopulmonal	**bronchopulmonaire**
broncoscopio	Bronchoskop	**bronchoscope**
broncospasmo	Bronchospasmus	**bronchospasme**
brucellosi	Brucellose	**brucellose**
bruciare	brennen, verbrennen	**brûler**
ustione, scottatura	Verbrennung, Brandwunde	**brûlure**
buccale	bukkal	**buccal**
bulbare	bulbär	**bulbaire**
bolla	Bulla, Blase	**bulle**
borsite	Bursitis, Schleimbeutelentzündung	**bursite**

C

ça	id	id
cachexie	cachexia	caquexia
cadavre	cadaver, corpse	cadáver
caduque	decidua	decidua
caecostomie	caecostomy (Eng), cecostomy (Am)	cecostomía
caecum	caecum (Eng), cecum (Am)	ciego
caféine	caffeine	cafeína
caillot	clot	coágulo
caillou	stone	cálculo
cal	callus	callo
calcification	calcification	calcificación
calcium	calcium	calcio
calcul	calculus	cálculo
calculs biliaires	gallstones	cálculos biliares
callosité	callosity	callosidad
calorie	calorie	caloría
cal vicieux	malunion	unión defectuosa
canal	canal	canal
canal artériel	ductus arteriosus	ductus arteriosus
canal semi-circulaire	semicircular canal	conducto semicircular
cancer	cancer	cáncer
candidose	candidiasis	candidiasis
canin	canine	canino
canule	cannula	cánula
capacité	ability	habilidad, capacidad
capacité de fixation du fer	iron binding capacity (IBC)	capacidad de unión con el hierro
capacité de fixation d'un antigène	antigen binding capacity (ABC)	capacidad de unión con antígenos
capacité de liaison d'un antigène	antigen binding capacity (ABC)	capacidad de unión con antígenos
capacité pulmonaire totale	total lung capacity (TLC)	capacidad pulmonar total (CPT)
capacité totale de fixation du fer	total iron binding capacity (TIBC)	capacidad total de unión con el hierro
capacité vitale	vital capacity	capacidad vital
capillaire	capillary	capilar
capsulage	encapsulation	encapsulación
capsule	capsule	cápsula
capsulite	capsulitis	capsulitis
caput succedaneum	caput succedaneum	caput succedaneum
caractère	character	carácter
carboxyhémoglobine	carboxyhaemoglobin (Eng), carboxyhemoglobin (Am)	carboxihemoglobina
carcinogène	carcinogen	carcinogénico
carcinogenèse	carcinogenesis	carcinogénesis
carcinomatose	carcinomatosis	carcinomatosis
carcinome	carcinoma	carcinoma
cardia	cardia	cardias
cardiaque	cardiac	cardíaco

ITALIAN	GERMAN	FRENCH
incoscio	Es	ça
cachessia	Kachexie	cachexie
cadavere	Kadaver, Leiche, Toter	cadavre
decidua	Dezidua	caduque
ciecostomia	Zökostomie	caecostomie
intestino cieco	Zökum	caecum
caffeina	Koffein	caféine
coagulo	Blutgerinnse, Koagel	caillot
calcolo	Stein	caillou
callo	Kallus	cal
calcificazione	Kalzifikation, Verkalkung	calcification
calcio	Kalzium	calcium
calcolo	Stein	calcul
calcoli biliari	Gallensteine	calculs biliaires
callosità	Schwiele, Hornhaut	callosité
caloria	Kalorie	calorie
unione difettosa	Fehlstellung (Frakturenden)	cal vicieux
canale	Kanal, Gang	canal
dotto arterioso	Ductus arteriosus	canal artériel
canale semicircolare	Bogengang	canal semi-circulaire
cancro	Karzinom, Krebs	cancer
candidiasi	Candidiasis	candidose
canino	Hunde-	canin
cannula	Kanüle	canule
abilità, capacità	Fähigkeit	capacité
capacità di legame del ferro	Eisenbindungskapazität	capacité de fixation du fer
capacità di legame dell'antigene	Antigen-Bindungskapazität	capacité de fixation d'un antigène
capacità di legame dell'antigene	Antigen-Bindungskapazität	capacité de liaison d'un antigène
capacità polmonare totale	Totalkapazität (TK)	capacité pulmonaire totale
capacità totale di legame del ferro (TIBC)	totale Eisenbindungskapazität (TEBK)	capacité totale de fixation du fer
capacità vitale	Vitalkapazität	capacité vitale
capillare	Kapillare	capillaire
incapsulamento	Verkapselung	capsulage
capsula	Kapsel	capsule
capsulite	Kapselentzündung	capsulite
tumore da parto	Geburtsgeschwulst	caput succedaneum
carattere	Charakter, Merkmal	caractère
carbossiemoglobina	Carboxyhämoglobin	carboxyhémoglobine
carcinogeno	Karzinogen	carcinogène
carcinogenesi	Karzinogenese	carcinogenèse
carcinomatosi	Karzinose, Karzinomatose	carcinomatose
carcinoma	Karzinom, Krebs	carcinome
cardias	Kardia, Mageneingang	cardia
cardiaco	Herz	cardiaque

FRENCH	ENGLISH	SPANISH
cardiogène	cardiogenic	cardiógenico
cardiologie	cardiology	cardiología
cardiomégalie	cardiomegaly	cardiomegalia
cardiomyopathie	cardiomyopathy	cardiomiopatía, miocardiopatía
cardiopathie	heart failure	insuficiencia cardíaca
cardiopathie ischémique	coronary artery disease (CAD), ischaemic heart disease (IHD) (Eng) ischemic heart disease (IHD) (Am)	enfermadad arterial coronaria, cardiopatía isquémica
cardiopulmonaire	cardiopulmonary	cardiopulmonar
cardiorespiratoire	cardiorespiratory	cardiorespiratorio
cardiospasme	cardiospasm	cardiospasmo
cardiothoracique	cardiothoracic	cardiotorácico
cardiotocographe	cardiotocograph	tococardiógrafo
cardiotoxique	cardiotoxic	cardiotóxico
cardiovasculaire	cardiovascular	cardiovascular
cardioversion	cardioversion	cardioversión
carène	carina	carina
carie	caries	caries
carminatif (n)	carminative (n)	carminativo (n)
carminatif (a)	carminative (a)	carminativo (a)
caroncule	caruncle	carúncula
carotène	carotene	carotenos
caroténémie	xanthaemia (Eng), xanthemia (Am)	xantemia
carotide	carotid	carótida
carpo-métacarpien	carpometacarpal	carpometacarpiano
carpo-pédal	carpopedal	carpopedal
cartilage	cartilage	cartílago
casque séborrhéique	cradle cap	costra láctea, dermatitis del cuero cabelludo
castration	castration	castración
catabolisme	catabolism	catabolismo
catalyseur	catalyst	catalizador
cataracte	cataract	catarata
catarrhe	catarrh	catarro
catatonique	catatonic	catatónico
catgut	catgut	catgut
cathéter	catheter	catéter
cathétérisme	catheterization	cateterismo
causalgie	causalgia	causalgia
cause du décès	cause of death (COD)	causa de la muerte
caustique (n)	caustic (n)	cáustico (n)
caustique (a)	caustic (a)	cáustico (a)
cautériser	cauterize	cauterizar
caverneux	cavernous	cavernoso
cavité	cavity	cavidad
cavité amniotique	amniotic cavity	cavidad amniótica
cécité	blindness	ceguera
cécité des rivières	river blindness	oncocerciasis ocular

ITALIAN	GERMAN	FRENCH
cardiogeno	kardiogen	**cardiogène**
cardiologia	Kardiologie	**cardiologie**
cardiomegalia	Kardiomegalie	**cardiomégalie**
cardiomiopatia	Kardiomyopathie	**cardiomyopathie**
scompenso cardiaco	Herzinsuffizienz, Herzversagen	**cardiopathie**
malattia delle arterie coronarica (MAC), cardiopatia ischemica	Koronaropathie, ischämische Herzkrankheit (IHK)	**cardiopathie ischémique**
cardiopolmonare	kardiopulmonal, Herz-Lungen-	**cardiopulmonaire**
cardiorespiratorio	kardiorespiratorisch	**cardiorespiratoire**
spasmo cardiale, acalasia esofagea	Kardiospasmus	**cardiospasme**
cardiotoracico	kardiothorakal	**cardiothoracique**
cardiotocografia	Kardiotokograph	**cardiotocographe**
cardiotossico	kardiotoxisch, herzschädigend	**cardiotoxique**
cardiovascolare	kardiovaskulär, Kreislauf-	**cardiovasculaire**
cardioversione	Kardioversion	**cardioversion**
carena tracheale	Carina	**carène**
carie	Karies	**carie**
carminativo (n)	Karminativum (n)	**carminatif** (n)
carminativo (a)	karminativ (a), entblähend (a)	**carminatif** (a)
caruncola	Karunkel	**caroncule**
carotene	Karotin	**carotène**
xantemia	Xanthämie	**caroténémie**
carotide	Karotis-	**carotide**
carpometacarpale	karpometakarpal	**carpo-métarcarpien**
carpopedalico	karpopedal	**carpo-pédal**
cartilagine	Knorpel	**cartilage**
stecca, rima di frattura	Milchschorf	**casque séborrhéique**
castrazione	Kastration	**castration**
catabolismo	Katabolismus, Abbaustoffwechsel	**catabolisme**
catalizzatore	Katalysator	**catalyseur**
cataratta	Katarakt, grauer Star	**cataracte**
catarro	Katarrh	**catarrhe**
catatonico	kataton	**catatonique**
catgut	Catgut	**catgut**
catetere	Katheter	**cathéter**
cateterizzazione	Katheterisierung	**cathétérisme**
causalgia	Kausalgie, brennender Schmerz	**causalgie**
causa di morte	Todesursache	**cause du décès**
caustico (n)	Ätzmittel (n), Kaustikum (n)	**caustique** (n)
caustico (a)	ätzend (a), brennend (a)	**caustique** (a)
cauterizzare	kauterisieren, ätzen, brennen	**cautériser**
cavernoso	kavernös	**caverneux**
cavità	Höhle	**cavité**
cavità amniotica	Amnionhöhle	**cavité amniotique**
cecità	Blindheit	**cécité**
oncocerchiasi, cecità fluviale	Flußblindheit	**cécité des rivières**

FRENCH	ENGLISH	SPANISH
cécité nocturne	night blindness	ceguera nocturna
ceinture	girdle	cintura
ceinture pelvienne	pelvic girdle	cintura pélvica
ceinture scapulaire	shoulder girdle	cintura escapular
cellule	cell	célula
cellule alvéolaire	pneumocyte	neumocito
cellulite	cellulitis	celulitis
centigrade	centigrade	centígrado
centre moteur de Broca	Broca's area	área de Broca
centrifuge	centrifugal	centrífugo
centrifuger	centrifuge	centrifugar
centrifugeur	centrifuge	centrífugo
centripète	centripetal	centrípeto
céphalée	headache	cefalea
céphalée due à la tension	tension headache	cefalea por tensión
céphalhématome	cephalhaematoma (Eng), cephalhematoma (Am)	hematoma cefálico
céphalique	cephalic	cefálico
céphalométrie	cephalometry	cefalometría
cérébral	cerebral	cerebral
cérébrospinal	cerebrospinal	cerebroespinal
cérébrovasculaire	cerebrovascular	cerebrovascular
cérumen	ear wax	cerumen
cerveau	brain, cerebrum	cerebro
cervelet	cerebellum	cerebelo
cervical	cervical	cervical
césarienne	caesarean section (Eng), cesarean section (Am)	cesárea
céto-acidose	ketoacidosis	cetoacidosis
cétogenèse	ketogenesis	cetogénesis
cétone	ketone	acetona
cétonurie	ketonuria	cetonuria
cétose	ketosis	cetosis
chalazion	chalazion	chalacio, orzuelo
chaleur	calor	calor
champ de vision	field of vision	campo de visión
chancre	chancre	chancro
chapelet costal	rickety rosary	rosario raquítico
charbon	carbuncle, charcoal	ántrax, carbón vegetal
chéilose	cheilosis	queilosis
chéloïde	keloid	queloide
chémosis	chemosis	quemosis
cheville	ankle	tobillo
chiasma	chiasma	quiasma
chimioprophylaxie	chemoprophylaxis	quimioprofilaxis
chimiorécepteur	chemoreceptor	quimiorreceptor
chimiotaxie	chemotaxis	quimiotaxis

ITALIAN	GERMAN	FRENCH
emeralopia	Nachtblindheit	**cécité nocturne**
cintura	Gürtel	**ceinture**
cingolo pelvico	Beckengürtel	**ceinture pelvienne**
cingolo scapolare	Schultergürtel	**ceinture scapulaire**
cellula	Zelle	**cellule**
pneumocito	Pneumozyt	**cellule alvéolaire**
cellulite	Zellulitis	**cellulite**
centigrado	Celsiusgrad	**centigrade**
area di Broca	Broca-Sprachzentrum	**centre moteur de Broca**
centrifugo	zentrifugal	**centrifuge**
centrifugare	zentrifugieren	**centrifuger**
centrifuga	Zentrifuge	**centrifugeur**
centripeto	zentripetal	**centripète**
mal di testa	Kopfschmerzen	**céphalée**
cefalea muscolotensiva	Spannungskopfschmerz	**céphalée due à la tension**
cefaloematoma	Kephalhämatom	**céphalhématome**
cefalico	Kopf-, Schädel-	**céphalique**
cefalometria	Kephalometrie, Schädelmessung	**céphalométrie**
cerebrale	zerebral, Gehirn-	**cérébral**
cerebrospinale	zerebrospinal	**cérébrospinal**
cerebrovascolare	zerebrovaskulär	**cérébrovasculaire**
cerume	Zerumen, Ohrenschmalz	**cérumen**
cervello	Gehirn, Verstand, Großhirn	**cerveau**
cervelletto	Cerebellum, Kleinhirn	**cervelet**
cervicale	zervikal	**cervical**
taglio cesareo	Kaiserschnitt, Sectio	**césarienne**
chetoacidosi	Ketoazidose	**céto-acidose**
chetogenesi	Ketogenese	**cétogenèse**
chetoni	Keton, Ketonkörper	**cétone**
chetonuria	Ketonurie	**cétonurie**
chetosi	Ketose	**cétose**
calazion	Chalazion, Hagelkorn	**chalazion**
calore	Fieber, Hitze	**chaleur**
campo visivo	Gesichtsfeld	**champ de vision**
cancroide, ulcera venerea	Schanker	**chancre**
rosario rachitico	rachitischer Rosenkranz	**chapelet costal**
carbonchio, antrace, favo, carbone vegetale	Karbunkel, Holzkohle	**charbon**
cheilosi	Mundeckenschrunden	**chéilose**
cheloide	Keloid	**chéloïde**
chemosi	Chemosis	**chémosis**
caviglia	Knöchel, Talus	**cheville**
chiasma	Chiasma	**chiasma**
chemioprofilassi	Chemoprophylaxe	**chimioprophylaxie**
chemorecettore	Chemorezeptor	**chimiorécepteur**
chemiotassi	Chemotaxis	**chimiotaxie**

FRENCH	ENGLISH	SPANISH
chimiothérapie	chemotherapy	quimioterapia
chiropodie	chiropody	podología
chiropracteur	chiropractor	quiropractor
chiropractique	chiropractic	quiropráctica
chirurgie	surgery	cirugía
chirurgien	surgeon	cirujano
chloasma	chloasma	cloasma
choc	shock	shock
cholangiographie	cholangiography	colangiografía
cholangio-pancréatographie rétrograde endoscopique (CPRE)	endoscopic retrograde cholangiopancreatography (ERCP)	colangiopancreatografía endoscópica retrógrada
cholangite	cholangitis	colangitis
cholécystectomie	cholecystectomy	colecistectomía
cholécystite	cholecystitis	colecistitis
cholécystographie	cholecystography	colecistografía
cholédochographie	choledochography	coledocografía
cholédocholithiase	choledocholithiasis	coledocolitiasis
cholélithiase	cholelithiasis	colelitiasis
choléra	cholera	cólera
cholestase	cholestasis	colestasis
cholestéatome	cholesteatoma	colesteatoma
cholestérol	cholesterol (chol)	colesterol
cholestérol composé de lipoprotéines de haute densité	high density lipoprotein cholesterol (HDLC)	colesterol unido a las lipoproteínas de alta densidad (HDLC)
cholinergique	cholinergic	colinérgico
chondrite	chondritis	condritis
chondromalacie	chondromalacia	condromalacia
chondrome	chondroma	condroma
chorée	chorea	corea
chorée de Huntington	Huntington's chorea	corea de Huntington
chorion	chorion	corion
choroïde	choroid	coroides
choroïdite	choroiditis	coroiditis
chromatographie	chromatography	cromatografía
chromosome	chromosome	cromosoma
chronique	chronic	crónico
chute brusque par dérobement des jambes	drop attack	ataque isquémico transitorio (AIT), caida
chyle	chyle	quilo
cicatrice	scar	cicatriz
ciliaire	ciliary	ciliar
cils	cilia	cilios
circinal	circinate	circinado
circoncision	circumcision	circuncisión
circulation	circulation	circulación
circulation collatérale	collateral circulation	circulación colateral
circulation foetale	fetal circulation	circulación fetal
circulation porte	portal hypertension	hipertensión portal

ITALIAN	GERMAN	FRENCH
chemioterapia	Chemotherapie	**chimiothérapie**
chiropodia	Pediküre, Fußpflege	**chiropodie**
chiropratico	Chiropraktiker	**chiropracteur**
chiropratica	Chiropraktik	**chiropractique**
chirurgia	Chirurgie	**chirurgie**
chirurgo	Chirurg	**chirurgien**
cloasma	Chloasma, Hyperpigmentierung	**chloasma**
shock	Schock	**choc**
colangiografia	Cholangiographie	**cholangiographie**
colangio-pancreatografia retrograda endoscopica (ERCP)	endoskopische retrograde Cholangiopankreatographie	**cholangio-pancréatographie rétrograde endoscopique (CPRE)**
colangite	Cholangitis	**cholangite**
colecistectomia	Cholezystektomie	**cholécystectomie**
colecistite	Cholezystitis	**cholécystite**
colecistografia	Cholezystographie	**cholécystographie**
coledocografia	Choledochographie	**cholédochographie**
coledocolitiasi	Choledocholithiasis	**cholédocholithiase**
colelitiasi	Cholelithiasis, Gallensteinleiden	**cholélithiase**
colera	Cholera	**choléra**
colestasi	Cholestase, Gallenstauung	**cholestase**
colesteatoma	Cholesteatom	**cholestéatome**
colesterolo	Cholesterin	**cholestérol**
colesterolo legato a lipoproteina ad alta densità	high density lipoprotein-cholesterol (HDL-Cholesterol)	**cholestérol composé de lipoprotéines de haute densité**
colinergico	cholinergisch	**cholinergique**
condrite	Chondritis	**chondrite**
condromalacia	Chondromalazie	**chondromalacie**
condroma	Chondrom	**chondrome**
corea	Chorea, Veitstanz	**chorée**
corea di Huntington	Chorea Huntington	**chorée de Huntington**
corion	Chorion	**chorion**
coroide	Choroidea, Aderhaut	**choroïde**
coroidite	Choroiditis	**choroïdite**
cromatografia	Chromatographie	**chromatographie**
cromosoma	Chromosom	**chromosome**
cronico	chronisch	**chronique**
improvvisa perdita della postura ad insorgenza periodica	Drop attack	**chute brusque par dérobement des jambes**
chilo	Chylus	**chyle**
cicatrice	Narbe	**cicatrice**
ciliare	ziliar, Wimpern-	**ciliaire**
ciglia	Zilien, Wimpern	**cils**
circinato	kreisförmig	**circinal**
circoncisione	Zirkumzision, Beschneidung	**circoncision**
circolazione	Kreislauf, Zirkulation, Durchblutung	**circulation**
circolazione collaterale	Kollateralkreislauf	**circulation collatérale**
circolazione fetale	fetaler Kreislauf	**circulation foetale**
ipertensione portale	Pfortaderhochdruck	**circulation porte**

FRENCH	ENGLISH	SPANISH
circulation systémique	systemic circulation	circulación sistémica
cirrhose	cirrhosis	cirrosis
claudication	claudication	claudicación
claustrophobie	claustrophobia	claustrofobia
clavicule	clavicle	clavícula
climatérique	climacteric	climatérico
clinique	clinical	clínico
clitoris	clitoris	clítoris
clone	clone	clono
clonus	clonus	clono, clonus
coagulation du sang	blood clotting	coagulación de la sangre
coagulation intravasculaire disséminée (CID)	disseminated intravascular coagulation (DIC)	coagulación intravascular diseminada (CID)
coagulation sanguine	blood coagulation	coagulación de la sangre
coaguler	clot	coagular
coaltar	coal tar	alquitrán, brea
coarctation	coarctation	coartación
coccyx	coccyx	cóccix
coeliaque	celiac (Am), coeliac (Eng)	celíaco
coelioscopie	laparoscopy	laparoscopia
coeur	heart	corazón
coeur pulmonaire	cor pulmonale	cor pulmonale
cognition	cognition	cognición
coït	coitus, pareunia	coito, pareunia
colectomie	colectomy	colectomía
coliforme	coliform	coliforme
colique	colic, gripe	cólico, cólico intestinal
colite	colitis	colitis
collagène	collagen	colágeno
colloïde	colloid	coloide
coloboma	coloboma	coloboma
colobome	coloboma	coloboma
côlon	colon	colon
côlon ascendant	ascending colon	colon ascendente
côlon descendant	descending colon	colon descendente
coloniser	colonize	colonizar
colonne vertébrale	spine, vertebral column	raquis, columna vertebral
côlon transversal	transverse colon	colon transverso
coloration de Gram	Gram stain	tinción de Gram
coloré	florid	florido, bien desarrollado
colorectal	colorectal	colorrectal
coloscopie	colonoscopy	colonoscopia
colostomie	colostomy	colostomía
colostrum	colostrum	calostro
colporraphie	colporrhaphy	colporrafia
colposcope	colposcope	colposcopio
coma	coma	coma

ITALIAN	GERMAN	FRENCH
circolazione sistemica	Großer Kreislauf	circulation systémique
cirrosi	Zirrhose	cirrhose
claudicazione	Hinken, Claudicatio	claudication
claustrofobia	Klaustrophobie	claustrophobie
clavicola	Schlüsselbein	clavicule
climaterio	Klimakterium, Wechseljahre	climatérique
clinico	klinisch	clinique
clitoride	Klitoris	clitoris
clone	Klonus	clone
clono	Klonus	clonus
coagulazione ematica	Blutgerinnung	coagulation du sang
coagulazione intravascolare disseminata (CID)	disseminierte intravasale Gerinnung (DIC)	coagulation intravasculaire disséminée (CID)
coagulazione del sangue	Blutgerinnung	coagulation sanguine
coagulare	gerinnen, koagulieren	coaguler
catrame	Steinkohlenteer	coaltar
coartazione	Coarctatio	coarctation
coccige	Steißbein	coccyx
celiaco	abdominal	coeliaque
laparoscopia	Laparoskopie, Bauchspiegelung	coelioscopie
cuore	Herz	coeur
cuore polmonare	Cor pulmonale	coeur pulmonaire
cognizione	Erkennungsvermögen, Wahrnehmung	cognition
coito	Koitus, Geschlechtsverkehr	coït
colectomia	Kolektomie, Kolonresektion	colectomie
coliforme	coliform	coliforme
colica, colica addominale	Kolik, Bauchschmerzen	colique
colite	Kolitis	colite
collageno	Kollagen	collagène
colloide	Kolloid	colloïde
coloboma	Kolobom	coloboma
coloboma	Kolobom	colobome
colon	Kolon	côlon
colon ascendente	Colon ascendens	côlon ascendant
colon discendente	Colon descendens	côlon descendant
colonizzare	kolonisieren	coloniser
spina, colonna vertebrale	Wirbelsäule, Rückgrat	colonne vertébrale
colon trasverso	Colon transversum	côlon transversal
colorazione di Gram	Gramfärbung	coloration de Gram
florido	floride	coloré
colorettale	kolorektal	colorectal
colonscopia	Koloskopie	coloscopie
colostomia	Kolostomie	colostomie
colostro	Kolostrum, Vormilch	colostrum
colporrafia	Kolporrhaphie	colporraphie
colposcopio	Kolposkop	colposcope
coma	Koma	coma

FRENCH	ENGLISH	SPANISH
comateux	comatose	comatoso
commissure	commissure	comisura
commotion	concussion	concusión, contusión violenta
communication auriculaire	atrial septal defect (ASD)	defecto del septum auricular
compatibilité	compatibility	compatibilidad
compensation	compensation	compensación
compétence	ability	habilidad, capacidad
complément	complement	complemento
complexe primaire	primary complex	complejo primario
comportement	behavior (Am), behaviour (Eng)	comportamiento
composé	compound	compuesto
compos mentis	compos mentis	compos mentis, de espíritu sano
compression	compression	compresión
compression digitale	digital compression	compresión digital
comprimé	tablet	comprimido
comprimé à délitement entérique	enteric-coated tablet (ECT)	comprimido entérico
compulsion	compulsion	compulsión, apremio
conception	conception	concepción
concrétion fécale	faecalith (Eng), fecalith (Am)	fecalito
conduit	duct	conducto
conduit iléal	ileal conduit	conducto ileal
confusion	confusion	confusión
congénital	congenital	congénito
congestion	congestion	congestión
conjonctive	conjunctiva	conjuntiva
conjonctivite	conjunctivitis	conjuntivitis
conjonctivite aiguë contagieuse	pinkeye	conjuntivitis
conjonctivite à inclusions trachomateuses	trachoma inclusion conjunctivitis (TRIC)	conjuntivitis de inclusion por tracomas
conjugué	conjugate	conjugado
conscient	conscious	consciente
consolidation	consolidation	consolidación
consommation	consumption	consunción, tisis
constipation	constipation	estreñimiento
constriction	constriction	constricción
consultation	counselling	asesoramiento, consejo, consulta psicológica
contact	contact	contacto
contagieux	contagious	contagioso, trasmisible
contraceptif (n)	contraceptive (n)	anticonceptivo (n)
contraceptif (a)	contraceptive (a)	anticonceptivo (a)
contraceptif oral combiné	combined oral contraceptive	anticonceptivo oral combinado
contraction	contraction	contracción
contracture	contracture	contractura

ITALIAN	GERMAN	FRENCH
comatoso	komatös	comateux
commessura	Kommissur	commissure
commozione	Erschütterung, Commotio	commotion
difetto atriosettale	Vorhofseptumdefekt	communication auriculaire
compatibilità	Kompatibilität, Verträglichkeit	compatibilité
compenso	Kompensation, Entschädigung	compensation
abilità, capacità	Fähigkeit	compétence
complemento	Komplement	complément
complesso primario, complesso di Ghon	Primärkomplex	complexe primaire
comportamento	Verhalten	comportement
composto	Verbindung, Zusammensetzung	composé
mentalmente sano	zurechnungsfähig	compos mentis
compressione	Kompression	compression
compressione digitale	Fingerdruck	compression digitale
pasticca, compressa	Tablette	comprimé
compressa enterica rivestita (passano lo stomaco senza sciogliersi)	magensaftresistente Tablette	comprimé à délitement entérique
compulsione	Zwang	compulsion
concepimento	Empfängnis	conception
fecalito	Kotstein	concrétion fécale
dotto	Ductus, Gang	conduit
vescica ileale (protesi mediante segmento ileale)	Ileumconduit	conduit iléal
confusione	Verwirrung	confusion
congenito	angeboren	congénital
congestione	Stauung	congestion
congiuntiva	Konjunktiva, Bindehaut	conjonctive
congiuntivite	Konjunktivitis, Bindehautentzündung	conjonctivite
congiuntivite batterica acuta contagiosa, congiuntivite catarrale	epidemische Konjunktivitis	conjonctivite aiguë contagieuse
congiuntivite tracomatosa	Trachom, Einschluß(körperchen)-konjunktivitis	conjonctivite à inclusions trachomateuses
coniugato	konjugiert	conjugué
conscio	bewußt, bei Bewußtsein	conscient
solidificazione, addensamento	Konsolidierung, Festigung	consolidation
consunzione	Konsum, Verbrauch	consommation
stipsi	Verstopfung	constipation
costrizione	Konstriktion, Einengung	constriction
consulenza eugenetica	Beratung	consultation
contatto	Kontakt, Berührung	contact
contagioso	kontagiös, ansteckend	contagieux
anticoncezionale (n)	Kontrazeptivum (n), Verhütungsmittel (n)	contraceptif (n)
anticoncezionale (a)	kontrazeptiv (a), Verhütungs- (a)	contraceptif (a)
contraccettivo orale estro-progestinico	orales Kontrazeptivum (Kombinationspräparat)	contraceptif oral combiné
contrazione	Kontraktion	contraction
contrattura	Kontraktur	contracture

239

FRENCH	ENGLISH	SPANISH
contracture ischémique de Volkmann	Volkmann's ischaemic contracture (Eng), Volkmann's ischemic contracture (Am)	contractura isquémica de Volkmann
contrecoup	contrecoup	contragolpe
contre-indication	contraindication	contraindicación
controlatéral	contralateral	contralateral
contrôle des naissances	family planning	planificación familiar
contusion	bruise	contusión, equímosis
contusionner	bruise	magullar, contundir
convulsion	convulsion	convulsión
coqueluche	whooping cough	tos ferina
cor	corn	callo, papiloma
cordes vocales	vocal cord	cuerda vocal
cordon	cord	cordón, cuerda, médula espinal
cordon ombilical	umbilical cord	cordón umbilical
cordotomie	cordotomy	cordotomía
cornée	cornea	córnea
cornet	turbinate	turbinado
coronaire (n)	coronary (n)	coronario (n)
coronaire (a)	coronary (a)	coronario (a)
coronarien	coronary	coronario
coronaropathie	coronary artery disease (CAD)	enfermadad arterial coronaria, cardiopatía isquémica
corps	corpus	cuerpo
corps jaune	luteum	lúteo
corpuscule	corpuscle	corpúsculo
cortex	cortex	corteza
corticostéroïde	corticosteroid	corticosteroide
coryza	coryza	coriza
costal	costal	costal
costochondral	costochondral	costocondral
costochondrite	costochondritis	costocondritis
côte	rib	costilla
cou	cervix, neck	cuello uterino, cuello
couche	stratum	estrato
couché	recumbent	recumbente, de pie
coup de chaleur	heatstroke	insolación
coup de fouet	whiplash	latigazo
coxa plana	Perthes' disease	enfermedad de Perthes
crachat	spittle	salivazo
crampe	cramp	calambre, espasmo
crâne	skull	cráneo
craniosynostose	cranio-synostosis	craneosinostosis
créatine	creatine	creatina
créatinine	creatinine	creatinina
crépitation	crepitation	crepitación

paralisi ischemica di Volkmann	Volkmann-Kontraktur	contracture ischémique de Volkmann
contraccolpo	contre coup	contrecoup
controindicazione	Kontraindikation, Gegenanzeige	contre-indication
controlaterale	kontralateral	controlatéral
controllo delle nascite	Familienplanung	contrôle des naissances
contusione	Quetschung, Prellung	contusion
ammaccare	stoßen, quetschen	contusionner
convulsione	Krampf, Zuckung, Konvulsion	convulsion
pertosse	Keuchhusten	coqueluche
callo	Klavus, Hühnerauge	cor
corda vocale	Stimmband	cordes vocales
corda, cordone, notocorda	Strang, Schnur, Ligament	cordon
cordone ombelicale	Nabelschnur	cordon ombilical
cordotomia	Stimmbandresektion	cordotomie
cornea	Kornea, Hornhaut (des Auges)	cornée
turbinato	Nasenmuschel	cornet
coronaria (n)	Koronararterie (n)	coronaire (n)
coronarico (a)	koronar (a)	coronaire (a)
coronarico	koronar	coronarien
malattia delle arterie coronarica (MAC)	Koronaropathie	coronaropathie
corpo	Corpus	corps
luteo	Luteom, Luteinom	corps jaune
corpuscolo	Corpusculum	corpuscule
corteccia	Cortex, Rinde	cortex
corticosteroide	Kortikosteroide	corticostéroïde
coriza	Koryza, Schnupfen	coryza
costale	kostal, Rippen-	costal
costocondrale	Rippenknorpel-	costochondral
costocondrite	Tietze Syndrom	costochondrite
costa	Rippe	côte
cervice, collo	Zervix, Gebärmutterhals, Nacken, Hals	cou
strato	Stratum, Schicht	couche
supino, sdraiato	liegend, ruhend	couché
colpo di calore	Hitzschlag	coup de chaleur
colpo di frusta	Peitschenhiebsyndrom, Mediansyndrom	coup de fouet
malattia di Perthes	Perthes-Krankheit	coxa plana
saliva	Speichel	crachat
crampo	Krampf	crampe
cranio	Schädel	crâne
craniosinostosi	Kraniosynostose	craniosynostose
creatina	Kreatin	créatine
creatinina	Kreatinin	créatinine
crepitazione	Krepitation, Rasseln	crépitation

FRENCH	ENGLISH	SPANISH
crétinisme	cretinism	cretinismo
cricoïde	cricoid	cricoideo
crise	crisis	crisis
crise intermenstruelle	mittelschmerz	mittelschmerz
crise myasthénique	myasthenic crisis	crisis miasténica
crise thyrotoxique	thyrotoxic crisis	crisis tirotóxica
croissance	growth	crecimiento
croup	croup	garrotillo, crup, difteria laríngea
croûte	scab	costra
cryochirurgie	cryosurgery	criocirugía
cryothérapie	cryotherapy	crioterapia
crypte	crypt	cripta
cryptogène	cryptogenic	criptogénico
cryptoménorrhée	cryptomenorrhea (Am), cryptomenorrhoea (Eng)	criptomenorrea
cubitus	ulna	cúbito
culture	culture	cultivo
curatif	healing	curación
cure de dégoût	aversion therapy	tratamiento por aversión
curetage	curettage, desloughing	raspado, legrado, curetaje, desesfacelación
curetages	curetting	raspados, material de legrado
cureter	curette (Eng), curet (Am)	legrar
curette	curette (Eng), curet (Am)	cureta, cucharilla de legrado
cutané	cutaneous	cutáneo
cuticule	cuticle	cutícula
cuti-réaction de Heaf	Heaf test	prueba de Heaf
cyanose	cyanosis	cianosis
cycle	cycle	ciclo
cypholordose	kypholordosis	cifolordosis
cyphoscoliose	kyphoscoliosis	cifoscoliosis
cyphose	kyphosis	cifosis
cystectomie	cystectomy	quistectomía
cystite	cystitis	cistitis
cystocèle	cystocele	cistocele
cystométrie	cystometry	cistometría
cystopexie	cystopexy	cistopexia
cystoscope	cystoscope	citoscopio
cystoscopie	cystoscopy	citoscopía
cytologie	cytology	citología
cytomégalovirus	cytomegalovirus (CMV)	citomegalovirus
cytotoxique	cytotoxic	citotóxico

ITALIAN	GERMAN	FRENCH
cretinismo	Kretinismus	**crétinisme**
cricoide	krikoid	**cricoïde**
crisi	Krise	**crise**
dolore intermestruale	Mittelschmerz	**crise intermenstruelle**
crisi miastenica	myasthenische Krise	**crise myasthénique**
crisi tireotossica	thyreotoxische Krise	**crise thyrotoxique**
crescita	Wachstum, Zunahme, Geschwulst, Tumor	**croissance**
ostruzione laringea	Krupp	**croup**
crosta, escara	Schorf, Kruste	**croûte**
criochirurgia	Kryochirurgie	**cryochirurgie**
crioterapia	Kryotherapie	**cryothérapie**
cripta	Krypte	**crypte**
criptogenico	kryptogenetisch, unbekannten Ursprungs	**cryptogène**
criptomenorrea	Kryptomenorrhoe	**cryptoménorrhée**
ulna	Ulna, Elle	**cubitus**
coltura	Bakterienkultur, Kultur	**culture**
cicatrizzazione, guarigione	Heilung	**curatif**
decondizionamento	Aversionstherapie	**cure de dégoût**
curettage, raschiamento, rimozione di escara da una ferita	Kürettage, Ausschabung, Schorfabtragung	**curetage**
curettage, raschiamento	Kürettage, Ausschabung	**curetages**
raschiare, scarificare	kürettieren	**cureter**
curette, cucchiaio chirurgico	Kürette	**curette**
cutaneo	kutan, Haut-	**cutané**
cuticola	Cuticula, Häutchen	**cuticule**
test alla tubercolina	Heaf-Test	**cuti-réaction de Heaf**
cianosi	Zyanose	**cyanose**
ciclo	Zyklus	**cycle**
cifolordosi	Kypholordose	**cypholordose**
cifoscoliosi	Kyphoskoliose	**cyphoscoliose**
cifosi	Kyphose	**cyphose**
cistectomia	Zystektomie, Zystenentfernung	**cystectomie**
cistite	Zystitis, Blasenentzündung	**cystite**
cistocele	Zystozele	**cystocèle**
cistometria	Zystometrie, Blasendruckmessung	**cystométrie**
cistopessia	Zystopexie	**cystopexie**
cistoscopio	Zystoskop, Blasenspiegel	**cystoscope**
cistoscopia	Zystoskopie, Blasenspiegelung	**cystoscopie**
citologia	Zytologie	**cytologie**
citomegalovirus	Zytomegalie-Virus (CMV)	**cytomégalovirus**
citotossico	zytotoxisch, zellschädigend	**cytotoxique**

D

FRENCH	ENGLISH	SPANISH
dacryocystite	dacryocystitis	dacriocistitis
daltonisme	color blindness (Am), colour blindness (Eng)	daltonismo, ceguera de colores
date de naissance	date of birth (DOB)	fecha de nacimiento
date du rapport fécondant	date of conception (DOC)	fecha de concepción
date présumée de l'accouchement	expected date of confinement (EDC), expected date of delivery (EDD)	fecha esperada del parto, fecha probable del parto (FPP)
débilité	debility	debilidad
débit expiratoire de pointe	peak expiratory flow rate (PEFR)	velocidad máxima del flujo espiratorio (VMFE)
débit sanguin rénal	renal blood flow (RBF)	flujo sanguíneo renal (FSR)
débridement	debridement	desbridamiento
débutant	incipient	incipiente
décérébré	decerebrate	descerebrado
décompensation	decompensation	descompensación
décompression	decompression	descompresión
décongestionnant	decongestant	descongestivo
défaut	defect	defecto
défécation	defaecation (Eng), defecation (Am)	defecación
défibrillateur	defibrillator	desfibrilador
défibrillation	defibrillation	desfibrilación
défilocher	tease	separar con aguja
dégénération	degeneration	degeneración
dégénérescence graisseuse	fatty degeneration	degeneración grasa
déhiscence	dehiscence	dehiscencia
délicat	queasy	nauseabundo
délire	delirium	delirio
deltoïde	deltoid	deltoides
démangeaison	itch	picor
démarcation	demarcation	demarcación
démarche	gait	marcha
démence	dementia	demencia
démence présénile	presenile dementia	demencia presenil
démographie	demography	demografia
démyélinisation	demyelination	desmielinización
dengue	dengue	dengue
dénombrement des hématies	blood count	recuento sanguíneo
dénomination commune d'un médicament	generic	genérico
dent	tooth	diente
dentaire	odontic	dentario
dent de sagesse	wisdom tooth	muela del juicio
dentier	denture	dentadura
dentiste	dentist	dentista
dentisterie	dentistry	odontologia

dacriocistite	Dakryozystitis	**dacryocystite**
cecità ai colori, acromatopsia	Farbenblindheit	**daltonisme**
data di nascita	Geburtsdatum	**date de naissance**
data del concepimento	Empfängnisdatum	**date du rapport fécondant**
data presunta delle doglie, data prevista per il parto	errechneter Geburtstermin	**date présumée de l'accouchement**
debilità	Schwäche	**débilité**
tasso di picco del flusso espiratorio	maximale exspiratorische Atemstromstärke	**débit expiratoire de pointe**
perfusione renale	Nierendurchblutung, renaler Blutfluß (RBF)	**débit sanguin rénal**
sbrigliamento	Debridement, Wundtoilette	**débridement**
incipiente	beginnend	**débutant**
decerebrato	dezerebriert	**décérébré**
decompensazione	Dekompensation, Insuffizienz	**décompensation**
decompressione	Dekompression, Drucksenkung	**décompression**
decongestionante	Dekongestionsmittel	**décongestionnant**
difetto	Defekt, Mangel, Störung	**défaut**
defecazione	Defäkation, Darmentleerung	**défécation**
defibrillatore	Defibrillator	**défibrillateur**
defibrillazione	Defibrillierung	**défibrillation**
dissociare i tessuti	zupfen	**défilocher**
degenerazione	Degeneration, Verfall	**dégénération**
degenerazione grassa	fettige Degeneration, Verfettung	**dégénérescence graisseuse**
deiscenza	Dehiszenz, Schlitz	**déhiscence**
nauseabondo, nauseato, a disagio	unwohl, übel	**délicat**
delirio	Delirium, Fieberwahn	**délire**
deltoide	Deltoides, Deltamuskel	**deltoïde**
prurito	Jucken	**démangeaison**
demarcazione	Demarkation	**démarcation**
andatura	Gang	**démarche**
demenza	Demenz	**démence**
demenza presenile	präsenile Demenz	**démence présénile**
demografia	Demographie	**démographie**
demielinizzazione	Demyelinisierung, Entmarkung	**démyélinisation**
dengue, infezione da Flavivirus ('febbre romplossa')	Denguefieber	**dengue**
emocitometria	Blutbild	**dénombrement des hématies**
medico generico	Substanznahme, Generic	**dénomination commune d'un médicament**
dente	Zahn	**dent**
dentario	Odonto-, Zahn-	**dentaire**
dente del giudizio	Weisheitszahn	**dent de sagesse**
dentiera	Gebiß	**dentier**
dentista	Zahnarzt	**dentiste**
odontoiatria	Zahnheilkunde, Zahntechnik	**dentisterie**

FRENCH	ENGLISH	SPANISH
dentition	dentition	dentición
dents	teeth	dientes
déodorant (n)	deodorant (n)	desodorante (n)
déodorant (a)	deodorant (a)	desodorante (a)
de perception	sensorineural	sensorineural
dépérissement	wasting away	consunción
dépistage	screening	criba, despistaje
dépression	depression	depresión
dépression anxieuse	agitated depression	depresión agitada
déréalisation	derealization	desrealización
dérivation	shunt	derivación
dermatite	dermatitis	dermatitis
dermatologie	dermatology	dermatología
dermatologue	dermatologist	dermatólogo
dermatome	dermatome	dermátomo
dermatomyosite	dermatomyositis	dermatomiositis
dermatophytose	ringworm	tiña
dermatose	dermatosis	dermatosis
derme	dermis	dermis
dermoïde	dermoid	dermoide
dernières règles	last menstrual period (LMP)	fecha última regla (FUR)
désarticulation	disarticulation	desarticulación
désensibilisation	desensitization	desensibilización
déséquilibre	imbalance	desequilibrio
déshydratation	dehydration	deshidratación
désimpaction	disimpaction	desimpactación
désinfectant	disinfectant	desinfectante
désinfecter	disinfect	desinfectar
désinfection	disinfection	desinfección
désinfestation	disinfestation	desinfestación
désobstruction	rebore	desobliteración, repermeabilización
désorientation	disorientation	desorientación
désoxygénation	deoxygenation	desoxigenación
desquamation	desquamation, peeling	desescamación, exfoliación
détergent	detergent	detergente
détérioration	deterioration	deterioro
dextrocardie	dextrocardia	dextrocardia
diabète	diabetes	diabetes
diabète insipide	diabetes insipidus	diabetes insípida
diabète sucré	diabetes mellitus (DM)	diabetes mellitus
diabète sucré insulinodépendant	insulin dependent diabetes mellitus (IDDM)	diabetes mellitus insulinodependiente
diabète sucré noninsulinodépendant	non-insulin dependent diabetes mellitus (NIDDM)	diabetes mellitus no insulinodependiente
diagnostic	diagnosis	diagnóstico
diagnostic différentiel	differential diagnosis	diagnóstico diferencial

246

ITALIAN	GERMAN	FRENCH
dentizione	Dentition, Zahnung	dentition
denti	Zähne, Gebiß	dents
deodorante (n)	Deodorant (n)	déodorant (n)
deodorante (a)	desodorierend (a)	déodorant (a)
neurosensoriale	Sinne u Nerven betr	de perception
cachessia	Schwinden	dépérissement
selezione	Screening, Reihenuntersuchung	dépistage
depressione	Depression	dépression
depressione agitata	agitierte Depression	dépression anxieuse
derealizzazione	Derealisation	déréalisation
derivazione	Shunt	dérivation
dermatite	Dermatitis	dermatite
dermatologia	Dermatologie	dermatologie
dermatologo	Dermatologe	dermatologue
dermatomo	Dermatom, Hautmesser	dermatome
dermatomiosite	Dermatomyositis	dermatomyosite
tricofizia, tinea	Tinea, Fadenpilzerkrankung, Onchozerkose	dermatophytose
dermatosi	Dermatose, Hauterkrankung	dermatose
derma	Haut	derme
dermoide	Dermoid, Dermoidzyste	dermoïde
ultimo periodo mestruale	letzte Menstruationsperiode	dernières règles
disarticolazione	Exartikulation	désarticulation
desensibilizzazione	Desensibilisierung	désensibilisation
squilibrio	Gleichgewichtsstörung	déséquilibre
deidratazione	Dehydration, Flüssigkeitsmangel	déshydratation
riduzione	Fragmentlösung	désimpaction
disinfettante	Desinfektionsmittel	désinfectant
disinfettare	desinfizieren	désinfecter
disinfezione	Desinfektion	désinfection
disinfestazione	Entwesung, Entlausung	désinfestation
disobliterazione	Desobliteration	désobstruction
disorientamento	Desorientiertheit	désorientation
deossigenazione	Desoxydation, Sauerstoffentzug	désoxygénation
desquamazione	Desquamation, Schuppung, Schälen (Haut)	desquamation
detergente	Reinigungsmittel	détergent
deterioramento	Verschlechterung	détérioration
destrocardia	Dextrokardie	dextrocardie
diabete	Diabetes	diabète
diabete insipido	Diabetes insipidus	diabète insipide
diabete mellito	Diabetes mellitus, Zuckerkrankheit	diabète sucré
diabete mellito insulinodipendente	insulinabhängiger Diabetes mellitus	diabète sucré insulinodépendant
diabete mellito non insulinodipendente	Diabetes mellitus Typ II, non-insulin dependent diabetes mellitus (NIDDM)	diabète sucré noninsulinodépendant
diagnosi	Diagnose	diagnostic
diagnosi differenziale	Differentialdiagnose	diagnostic différentiel

FRENCH	ENGLISH	SPANISH
diagnostique	diagnostic	diagnóstico
dialysat	dialysate	dializado
dialyse	dialysis	diálisis
dialyse péritonéale	peritoneal dialysis	diálisis peritoneal
dialyseur	dialyser (Eng), dialyzer (Am)	dializador
diamètre conjugué	conjugate	conjugado
diaphorèse	diaphoresis	diaforesis
diaphragme	diaphragm, midriff	diafragma
diaphyse	diaphysis	diáfisis
diarrhée	diarrhea (Am), diarrhoea (Eng)	diarrea
diarrhées et vomissements	diarrhea and vomiting (D & V) (Am), diarrhoea and vomiting (D & V) (Eng)	diarrea y vómitos
diastasis	diastasis	diastasis
diastole	diastole	diástole
diathermie	diathermy	diatermia
diététicien	dietitian	dietista
diététique	dietetics	dietética
digestion	digestion	digestión
digitale	digitalis	digital
digitalisation	digitalization	digitalización
dilatation	dilatation (Eng), dilation (Am)	dilatación
dilatation et curetage	dilatation and curettage (D & C) (Eng), dilation and curettage (D & C) (Am)	dilatación y raspado/legrado
diphtérie	diphtheria	difteria
diplégie	diplegia	diplejía, parálisis bilateral
diplopie	diplopia	diplopia
discectomie	discectomy (Eng), diskectomy (Am)	disquectomía
discret	discrete	discreto
dislocation	dislocation	dislocación
dispositif intra-utérin (DIU)	intrauterine contraceptive device (IUD, IUCD)	dispositivo intrauterino anticonceptivo (DIU)
dissection	dissection	disección
disséminé	disseminated	diseminado
dissociation	dissociation	disociación
distal	distal	distal
diurèse	diuresis	diuresis
diurétique (n)	diuretic (n)	diurético (n)
diurétique (a)	diuretic (a)	diurético (a)
diverticule de Meckel	Meckel's diverticulum	divertículo de Meckel
diverticulite	diverticulitis	diverticulitis
diverticulose	diverticulosis	diverticulosis
diverticulum	diverticulum	divertículo
doigt	finger	dedo de la mano
dominant	dominant	dominante
donneur	donor	donante
dopamine	dopamine	dopamina

ITALIAN	GERMAN	FRENCH
diagnostico	diagnostisch	**diagnostique**
dialisato	Dialysat	**dialysat**
dialisi	Dialyse	**dialyse**
dialisi peritoneale	Peritonealdialyse	**dialyse péritonéale**
dializzatore	Dialysator	**dialyseur**
coniugata	Beckendurchmesser	**diamètre conjugué**
diaforesi	Diaphorese, Schweißabsonderung	**diaphorèse**
diaframma, parte bassa del torace	Diaphragma, Zwerchfell	**diaphragme**
diafisi	Diaphyse, Knochenschaft	**diaphyse**
diarrea	Diarrhoe, Durchfall	**diarrhée**
diarrea e vomito	Brechdurchfall	**diarrhées et vomissements**
diastasi, amilasi	Diastase	**diastasis**
diastole	Diastole	**diastole**
diatermia	Diathermie	**diathermie**
dietista, dietologo	Diätspezialist	**diététicien**
dietetica	Diätlehre, Ernährungskunde	**diététique**
digestione	Verdauung	**digestion**
digitale	Digitalis, Fingerhut	**digitale**
digitalizzazione	Digitalisierung	**digitalisation**
dilatazione	Dilatation, Erweiterung	**dilatation**
dilatazione e raschiamento	Dilatation und Kürettage	**dilatation et curetage**
difterite	Diphtherie	**diphtérie**
diplegia	Diplegie, doppelseitige Lähmung	**diplégie**
diplopia	Diplopie, Doppelsehen	**diplopie**
discectomia, asportazione di disco intervertebrale	Diskektomie	**discectomie**
discreto	diskret	**discret**
dislocazione	Dislokation, Verrenkung	**dislocation**
dispositivo anticoncezionale intrauterino (IUD)	Intrauterinpessar (IUP)	**dispositif intra-utérin (DIU)**
dissezione	Sektion, Obduktion	**dissection**
disseminato	disseminiert, verstreut	**disséminé**
dissociazione	Dissoziation, Trennung	**dissociation**
distale	distal	**distal**
diuresi	Diurese	**diurèse**
diuretico (n)	Diuretikum (n)	**diurétique (n)**
diuretico (a)	diuretisch (a)	**diurétique (a)**
diverticolo di Meckel	Meckel-Divertikel	**diverticule de Meckel**
diverticolite	Divertikulitis	**diverticulite**
diverticolosi	Divertikulose	**diverticulose**
diverticolo	Divertikel	**diverticulum**
dito	Finger	**doigt**
dominante	dominant, vorherrschend	**dominant**
donatore	Spender	**donneur**
dopammina	Dopamin	**dopamine**

FRENCH	ENGLISH	SPANISH
d'origine rénale	nephrogenic	nefrógeno
dorsal	dorsal	dorsal
dorsiflexion	dorsiflexion	dorsiflexión
dosage immunologique	immunoassay	inmunoensayo
dosage par la méthode (ELISA)	enzyme-linked immunosorbent assay (ELISA)	análisis enzimático por inmunoabsorción
double vision	double vision	visión doble
douche	douche	ducha
douleur	pain, dolor	dolor
douleur irradiée	referred pain	dolor referido
douleurs lombaires basses	low back pain	lumbalgia
douloureux	sore	doloroso
douve	fluke	trematodo
dragée entérosoluble	enteric-coated tablet (ECT)	comprimido entérico
drain	drain	drenaje
drainer	drain	drenar
drépanocytose	sickle-cell anaemia (Eng), sickle-cell anemia (Am)	anemia drepanocítica
duodénite	duodenitis	duodenitis
duodénum	duodenum	duodeno
dysarthrie	dysarthria	disartria
dyscrasie	dyscrasia	discrasia
dysenterie	dysentery	disentería
dysfonctionnement	dysfunction	disfunción
dyskaryose	dyskaryosis	discariosis
dyskinésie	dyskinesia	discinesia
dyslexie	dyslexia	dislexia
dyslipoïdose	lipidosis	lipidosis
dysménorrhée	dysmenorrhea (Am), dysmenorrhoea (Eng)	dismenorrea
dysménorrhée spasmodique	spasmodic dysmenorrhoea	dismenorrea espasmódica
dyspareunie	dyspareunia	dispareunia
dyspepsie	dyspepsia	dispepsia
dysphagie	dysphagia	disfagia
dysphasie	dysphasia	disfasia
dysplasie	dysplasia	displasia
dyspnée	dyspnea (Am), dyspnoea (Eng)	disnea
dyspnée de Cheyne-Stokes	Cheyne-Stokes respiration	respiración de Cheyne-Stokes
dyspraxie	dyspraxia	dispraxia
dysrythmie	dysrhythmia	disritmia
dystrophie	dystrophy	distrofia
dystrophie musculaire	muscular dystrophy	distrofia muscular
dysurie	dysuria	disuria

ITALIAN	GERMAN	FRENCH
nefrogenico	nephrogen	d'origine rénale
dorsale	dorsal, Rücken-	dorsal
dorsiflessione	Dorsalflexion	dorsiflexion
dosaggio immunologico	Immunoassay	dosage immunologique
test di immunoassorbimento enzimatico	enzyme-linked immunosorbent assay (ELISA)	dosage par la méthode (ELISA)
diplopia	Doppelsehen, Diplopie	double vision
lavanda vaginale	Dusche, Spülung	douche
dolore	Schmerz	douleur
dolore riferito	ausstrahlender Schmerz, fortgeleiteter Schmerz	douleur irradiée
rachialgia lombosacrale	Kreuzschmerzen	douleurs lombaires basses
dolente	wund, schmerzhaft	douloureux
trematode, Digeneum	Trematode	douve
compressa enterica rivestita (passano lo stomaco senza sciogliersi)	magensaftresistente Tablette	dragée entérosoluble
drenaggio	Drain	drain
drenare	drainieren	drainer
anemia drepanocitica	Sichelzellanämie	drépanocytose
duodenite	Duodenitis, Zwölffingerdarmentzündung	duodénite
duodeno	Duodenum, Zwölffingerdarm	duodénum
disartria	Dysarthrie	dysarthrie
discrasia	Dyskrasie	dyscrasie
dissenteria	Dysenterie, Ruhr	dysenterie
disfunzione	Dysfunktion, Funktionsstörung	dysfonctionnement
discariosi	Kernanomalie, Dysplasie	dyskaryose
discinesia	Dyskinesie	dyskinésie
dislessia	Dyslexie	dyslexie
lipoidosi	Lipidose	dyslipoïdose
dismenorrea	Dysmenorrhoe	dysménorrhée
dismenorrea spastica	spastische Dysmenorrhoe	dysménorrhée spasmodique
dispareunia	Dyspareunie	dyspareunie
dispepsia	Dyspepsie, Verdauungsstörung	dyspepsie
disfagia	Dysphagie, Schluckbeschwerden	dysphagie
disfasia	Dysphasie	dysphasie
displasia	Dysplasie, Fehlbildung	dysplasie
dispnea	Dyspnoe, Atemnot	dyspnée
respiro di Cheyne-Stokes	Cheyne-Stokes-Atmung	dyspnée de Cheyne-Stokes
disprassia	Dyspraxie	dyspraxie
disritmia	Dysrhythmie, Rhythmusstörung	dysrythmie
distrofia	Dystrophie	dystrophie
distrofia muscolare	Muskeldystrophie	dystrophie musculaire
disuria	Dysurie	dysurie

E

eaux de l'amnios	'show'	'señal sanguinolenta menstrual'
ecchymose	ecchymosis	equímosis
échaudure	scald	escaldadura
échauffement	heat exhaustion	agotamiento por calor
échocardiographie	echocardiography	ecocardiografía
écho-encéphalographie	echoencephalography	ecoencefalografía
échographie de Doppler	Doppler ultrasound technique	técnica de ultrasonidos Doppler
échogramme	scan	exploración, barrido
échographie	ultrasonography	ultrasonografía, ecografía
écholalie	echolalia	ecolalia
échovirus	echovirus	virus ECHO
éclampsie	eclampsia	eclampsia
éclampsisme	pre-eclampsia	preeclampsia
ectoderme	ectoderm	ectodermo
ectoparasite	ectoparasite	ectoparásito
ectopie testiculaire	undescended testes	testículos no descendidos
ectopique	ectopic	ectópico
ectropion	ectropion	ectropión
eczéma	eczema, seborrheic dermatitis (Am) seborrhoeic dermatitis (Eng)	eccema, dermatitis seborréica
édenté	edentulous	desdentado
efférent	efferent	eferente
effet latéral	side effect	efecto secundario
effets latéraux extrapyramidaux	extrapyramidal side effects	efectos secundarios extrapiramidales
efforts expulsifs	bearing down	postración
effusion	effusion	derrame
éjaculation	ejaculation	eyaculación
élastine	elastin	elastina
électrocardiogramme (ECG)	electrocardiogram (ECG)	electrocardiograma (ECG)
électrochoc	electroconvulsive therapy (ECT)	electrochoqueterapia (ECT)
électrode	electrode	electrodo
électroencéphalogramme (EEG)	electroencephalogram (EEG)	electroencefalograma (EEG)
électrolyse	electrolysis	electrólisis
électrolyte	electrolyte	electrólito
électromyographie	electromyography	electromiografía
éléphantiasis	elephantiasis	elefantiasis
élimination	elimination	eliminación
élixir	elixir	elixir
elliptocytose	elliptocytosis	eliptocitosis
émaciation	emaciation	emaciación
émail	enamel	esmalte
embole	embolus	émbolo
embolie pulmonaire (EP)	pulmonary embolism (PE)	embolismo pulmonar
embolique	embolic	embólico

ITALIAN	GERMAN	FRENCH
perdita ematica che precede il parto o la mestruazione	Geburtsbeginn (Anzeichen)	eaux de l'amnios
ecchimosi	Ekchymose	ecchymose
scottatura	Verbrühung, Brandwunde	échaudure
collasso da colpo di calore	Hitzschlag	échauffement
ecocardiografia	Echokardiographie	échocardiographie
ecoencefalografia	Echoenzephalographie	écho-encéphalographie
tecnica ultrasonografica Doppler	Doppler-Sonographie	échographie de Doppler
ecografia, scintigrafia	Scan	échogramme
ultrasonografia, ecografia	Sonographie, Ultraschallmethode	échographie
ecolalia	Echolalie	écholalie
echovirus	ECHO-Virus	échovirus
eclampsia	Eklampsie	éclampsie
preeclampsia	Präeklampsie, Eklampsiebereitschaft	éclampsisme
ectoderma	Ektoderm	ectoderme
ectoparassita	Ektoparasit	ectoparasite
testicoli ritenuti	Kryptorchismus	ectopie testiculaire
ectopico	ektop	ectopique
ectropion	Ektropion	ectropion
eczema, dermatite seborroica	Ekzem, seborrhoisches Ekzem	eczéma
edentulo	zahnlos	édenté
efferente	efferent	efférent
effetto collaterale	Nebenwirkung	effet latéral
reazioni collaterali extrapiramidali da farmaci	extrapyramidale Nebenwirkungen	effets latéraux extrapyramidaux
fase espulsiva del parto	Pressen	efforts expulsifs
effusione	Erguß	effusion
eiaculazione	Ejakulation, Samenerguß	éjaculation
elastina	Elastin	élastine
elettrocardiogramma (ECG)	Elektrokardiogramm (EKG)	électrocardiogramme (ECG)
terapia elettroconvulsiva, elettroshock	Elektroschocktherapie	électrochoc
elettrodo	Elektrode	électrode
elettroencefalogramma (EEG)	Elektroenzephalogramm (EEG)	électroencéphalogramme (EEG)
elettrolisi	Elektrolyse	électrolyse
elettrolito	Elektrolyt	électrolyte
elettromiografia	Elektromyographie	électromyographie
elefantiasi	Elephantiasis	éléphantiasis
eliminazione	Elimination, Ausscheidung	élimination
elisir	Elixier	élixir
ellissocitosi	Elliptozytose	elliptocytose
emaciazione	Auszehrung	émaciation
smalto	Emaille	émail
embolo	Embolus	embole
embolia polmonare (EP)	Lungenembolie	embolie pulmonaire (EP)
embolico	embolisch	embolique

FRENCH	ENGLISH	SPANISH
embolisme	embolism	embolia
embryologie	embryology	embriología
embryon	embryo	embrión
embryopathie	embryopathy	embriopatía
émétique (n)	emetic (n)	emético (n)
émétique (a)	emetic (a)	emético (a)
éminence hypothénar	hypothenar eminence	eminencia hipotenar
émollient (n)	emollient (n)	emoliente (n)
émollient (a)	emollient (a)	emoliente (a)
émotion	emotion	emoción
émotionnel	emotional	emocional
empathie	empathy	empatía
emphysème	emphysema	enfisema
empirique	empirical	empírico
empoisonner	poison	envenenar
empyème	empyema	empiema
émulsion	emulsion	emulsión
encéphaline	encephalin (Eng), enkephalin (Am)	encefalina
encéphalite	encephalitis	encefalitis
encéphalite spongiforme bovine	bovine spongiform encephalitis (BSE)	encefalitis espongiforme bovina
encéphalomyélite	encephalomyelitis	encefalomielitis
encéphalomyélite myalgique	myalgic encephalomyelitis (ME)	encefalomielitis miálgica
encéphalopathie	encephalopathy	encefalopatía
enclavé	impacted	impactado
enclume	incus	incus, yunque
encoprésie	encopresis	encopresis
endartériectomie	endarterectomy	endarterectomía
endartérite	endarteritis	endarteritis
endémie	endemic	endémico
endémique	endemic	endémico
endocardite	endocarditis	endocarditis
endocardite lente	subacute bacterial endocarditis (SBE)	endocarditis bacteriana subaguda
endocervical	endocervical	endocervical
endocrine	endocrine	endocrino
endocrinologie	endocrinology	endocrinología
endogène	endogenous, innate	endógeno, innato
endomètre	endometrium	endometrio
endométriose	endometriosis	endometriosis
endométrite	endometritis	endometritis
endonèvre	endoneurium	endoneuro
endoparasite	endoparasite	endoparásito
endorphine	endorphin	endorfina
endoscope	endoscope	endoscopio
endoscopie	endoscopy	endoscopia
endothélium	endothelium	endotelio
endotoxine	endotoxin	endotoxina

ITALIAN	GERMAN	FRENCH
embolia	Embolie	embolisme
embriologia	Embryologie	embryologie
embrione	Embryo	embryon
embriopatia	Embryopathie	embryopathie
emetico (n)	Emetikum (n), Brechmittel (n)	émétique (n)
emetico (a)	emetisch (a)	émétique (a)
eminenza ipotenar	Antithenar	éminence hypothénar
emoliente (n)	Emollientium (n)	émollient (n)
emoliente (a)	erweichend (a)	émollient (a)
emozione	Emotion, Gefühl	émotion
emotivo	emotional	émotionnel
immedesimazione, identificazione	Empathie, Einfühlungsvermögen	empathie
enfisema	Emphysem	emphysème
empirico	empirisch	empirique
avvelenare	vergiften	empoisonner
empiema	Empyem	empyème
emulsione	Emulsion	émulsion
encefalina	Enzephalin	encéphaline
encefalite	Enzephalitis	encéphalite
encefalite spongiforme bovina	Rinderwahnsinn, Bovine Spongiforme Enzephalitis (BSE)	encéphalite spongiforme bovine
encefalomielite	Enzephalomyelitis	encéphalomyélite
encefalomielite mialgica	myalgische Enzephalomyelitis	encéphalomyélite myalgique
encefalopatia	Enzephalopathie	encéphalopathie
impatto, compresso, incuneato	impaktiert	enclavé
incudine	Incus, Amboß	enclume
encopresi	Enkopresis, Einkoten	encoprésie
endoarterectomia	Endarteriektomie	endartériectomie
endoarterite	Endarteriitis	endartérite
endemia	Endemie	endémie
endemico	endemisch	endémique
endocardite	Endokarditis	endocardite
endocardite batterica subacuta	Endocarditis lenta	endocardite lente
endocervicale	endozervikal	endocervical
endocrino	endokrin	endocrine
endocrinologia	Endokrinologie	endocrinologie
endogeno, innato	endogen, kongenital, angeboren	endogène
endometrio	Endometrium	endomètre
endometriosi	Endometriose	endométriose
endometrite	Endometritis	endométrite
endonevrio	Endoneurium	endonèvre
endoparassita	Endoparasit	endoparasite
endorfina	Endorphin	endorphine
endoscopio	Endoskop	endoscope
endoscopia	Endoskopie	endoscopie
endotelio	Endothel	endothélium
endotossina	Endotoxin	endotoxine

endotrachéique	endotracheal	endotraqueal
énervation	denervation	denervación
enfant	infant	lactante
enfant atteint de la maladie bleue	blue baby	niño azul
enfant bleu	blue baby	niño azul
enflé	swollen, turgid	hinchado, túrgido
enfoncement localisé	depressed fracture	fractura con hundimiento
engelure	chilblain	sabañón
engorgement	engorgement	estancamiento
énophtalmie	enophthalmos	enoftalmos
en pronation	prone	prono, inclinado
en supination	supine	supino
entéral	enteral	enteral
entérique	enteric	entérico
entérite	enteritis	enteritis
entéro-anastomose	enteroanastomosis	enteroanastómosis
entérocèle	enterocele	enterocele
entérocolite	enterocolitis	enterocolitis
entérocolite nécrosante	necrotizing enterocolitis (NEC)	enterocolitis necrotizante
entérostomie	enterostomy	enterostomía
entérovirus	enterovirus	enterovirus
entorse	strain	cepa
entropion	entropion	entropión
énucléation	enucleation	enucleación
énurèse	enuresis	enuresis
envie	birthmark	mancha de nacimiento
enzyme	enzyme	enzima
enzyme protéolytique	proteolytic enzyme	enzima proteolítico
enzymologie	enzymology	enzimología
éosinophile (n)	eosinophil (n)	eosinófilo (n)
éosinophile (a)	eosinophil (a)	eosinófilo (a)
éosinophilie	eosinophilia	eosinofilia
épaissir	inspissated	espesado
épaule	shoulder	hombro
épaule ankylosée	frozen shoulder	hombro congelado/rígido
épendymome	ependymoma	ependimoma
éphédrine	ephedrine	efedrina
épicanthus	epicanthus	epicanto
épicarde	epicardium	epicardio
épicrâne	scalp	cuero cabelludo
épidémie	epidemic	epidemia
épidémiologie	epidemiology	epidemiología
épidémique	epidemic	epidémico
épiderme	epidermis	epidermis

endotracheale	endotracheal	endotrachéique
denervazione	Denervierung	énervation
infante	Kleinkind, Säugling	enfant
'blue baby' (cianosi da cardiopatia congenita)	zyanotisches Neugeborenes	enfant atteint de la maladie bleue
'blue baby' (cianosi da cardiopatia congenita)	zyanotisches Neugeborenes	enfant bleu
gonfio, tumefatto, turgido	geschwollen, vergrößert	enflé
frattura con infossamento dei frammenti	Impressionsfraktur	enfoncement localisé
gelone	Frostbeule, Pernio	engelure
congestione	Stauung, Anschoppung	engorgement
enoftalmo	Enophtalmus	énophtalmie
prono	veranlagt, empfänglich	en pronation
supino	supiniert	en supination
enterale, intestinale	enteral	entéral
enterico	enterisch	entérique
enterite	Enteritis	entérite
enteroanastomosi	Enteroanastomose	entéro-anastomose
enterocele	Enterozele	entérocèle
enterocolite	Enterokolitis	entérocolite
enterocolite necrotizzante	nekrotisierende Enterokolitis	entérocolite nécrosante
enterostomia	Enterostomie	entérostomie
enterovirus	Enterovirus	entérovirus
tensione	Anstrengung, Belastung	entorse
entropion	Entropion	entropion
enucleazione	Enukleation, Ausschälung	énucléation
enuresi	Enuresis, Bettnässen	énurèse
nevo congenito	Muttermal, Storchenbiß	envie
enzima	Enzym	enzyme
enzima proteolitico, proteasi	proteolytisches Enzym	enzyme protéolytique
enzimologia	Enzymologie	enzymologie
eosinofilo (n)	Eosinophiler (n)	éosinophile (n)
eosinofilo (a)	eosinophil (a)	éosinophile (a)
eosinofilia	Eosinophilie	éosinophilie
inspessito	kondensiert, eingedickt	épaissir
spalla	Schulter	épaule
'spalla congelata', periartrite scapoloomerale	Frozen shoulder, Periarthritis humeroscapularis	épaule ankylosée
ependimoma	Ependymom	épendymome
efedrina	Ephedrin	éphédrine
epicanto	Epikanthus	épicanthus
epicardio	Epikard	épicarde
cuoio capelluto	Kopfhaut	épicrâne
epidemia	Epidemie	épidémie
epidemiologia	Epidemiologie	épidémiologie
epidemico	epidemisch	épidémique
epidermide	Epidermis	épiderme

FRENCH	ENGLISH	SPANISH
épididyme	epididymis	epidídimo
épididymite	epididymitis	epididimitis
épidural	epidural	epidural
épigastre	epigastrium	epigastrio
épiglotte	epiglottis	epiglotis
épiglottite	epiglottitis	epiglotitis
épilepsie	epilepsy	epilepsia
épileptiforme	epileptiform	epileptiforme
épileptique	epileptic	epiléptico
épileptogène	epileptogenic	epileptógeno
épinéphrine	epinephrine	epinefrina
épiphyse	epiphysis	epífisis
épiphysiolyse	slipped epiphysis	epífisis desplazada
épiploon	omentum	epiplón
épisclérite	episcleritis	episcleritis
épisclérotique	episclera	episclera
épisiotomie	episiotomy	episiotomía
épistaxis	epistaxis, nosebleed	epistaxis
épithélioma	epithelioma	epitelioma
épithélioma à petites cellules	oat cell cancer	carcinoma de células de avena
épithélium	epithelium	epitelio
épreuve de tolérance à l'insuline	insulin tolerance test (ITT)	prueba de la tolerancia a la insulina
épreuve de tolérance au glucose et à l'insuline	glucose insulin tolerance test (GITT)	prueba de resistencia a la insulina
épreuve d'hyperglycémie provoquée	glucose tolerance test (GTT)	prueba de tolerancia a la glucosa
éprouvette	test tube	tubo de ensayo
équipement de survie	basic life support	soporte de vida básico
érectile	erectile	eréctil
érection	erection	erección
ergothérapie	occupational therapy	terapéutica ocupacional
éructation	belching	eructo
éruption	eruption, hives	erupción, urticaria
érysipèle	erysipelas	erisipela
érythème	erythema	eritema
érythème fessier du nourrisson	napkin rash (Eng), diaper rash (Am)	exantema del pañal
érythème papulo-érosif	napkin rash (Eng), diaper rash (Am)	exantema del pañal
érythroblaste	erythroblast	eritroblasto
érythrocyte	erythrocyte	eritrocito
érythroderme	erythroderma	eritrodermia
érythropoïèse	erythropoiesis	eritropoyesis
érythropoïétine	erythropoietin	eritropoyetina
escarre	eschar, slough	escara, costra, esfacelo
escarre de décubitus	bedsore	úlcera por decúbito
espace sous-arachnoïdien	subarachnoid space	espacio subaracnoideo
espèce	species	especie
essai calorique	caloric test	prueba calórica

ITALIAN	GERMAN	FRENCH
epididimo	Epididymis, Nebenhoden	épididyme
epididimite	Epididymitis, Nebenhodenentzündung	épididymite
epidurale	epidural	épidural
epigastrio	Epigastrium, Oberbauch	épigastre
epiglottide	Epiglottis	épiglotte
epiglottite	Epiglottitis	épiglottite
epilessia	Epilepsie	épilepsie
epilettiforme	epileptiform	épileptiforme
epilettico	epileptisch	épileptique
epilettogeno	epileptogen	épileptogène
adrenalina	Adrenalin	épinéphrine
epifisi	Epiphyse, Zirbeldrüse	épiphyse
distacco epifisario	Epiphyseolyse	épiphysiolyse
omento	Omentum, Netz	épiploon
episclerite	Episkleritis	épisclérite
episclera	Episklera	épisclérotique
episiotomia	Episiotomie, Dammschnitt	épisiotomie
epistassi	Epistaxis, Nasenbluten	épistaxis
epitelioma	Epitheliom	épithélioma
microcitoma, carcinoma a piccole cellule	kleinzelliges Bronchialkarzinom	épithélioma à petites cellules
epitelio	Epithel	épithélium
test di tolleranza all' insulina	Insulintoleranztest	épreuve de tolérance à l'insuline
test insulinico di tolleranza al glucosio	Glukose-Insulin-Toleranztest	épreuve de tolérance au glucose et à l'insuline
test di tolleranza al glucosio (TTG)	Glukose-Toleranztest	épreuve d'hyperglycémie provoquée
provetta	Reagenzglas	éprouvette
mantenimento delle funzioni vitali	Vitalfunktionserhaltung	équipement de survie
erettile	erektil	érectile
erezione	Erektion	érection
ergoterapia	Beschäftigungstherapie	ergothérapie
eruttazione	Aufstoßen	éructation
eruzione, orticaria	Ausbruch, Ausschlag, Nesselfieber	éruption
erisipela	Erysipel, Wundrose	érysipèle
eritema	Erythem	érythème
eruzione cutanea da pannolino	Windeldermatitis	érythème fessier du nourrisson
eruzione cutanea da pannolino	Windeldermatitis	érythème papulo-érosif
eritroblasto	Erythroblast	érythroblaste
eritrocito	Erythrozyt, rotes Blutkörperchen	érythrocyte
eritrodermia	Erythrodermie	érythroderme
eritropoiesi	Erythropoese	érythropoïèse
eritropoietina	Erythropoetin, erythropoetischer Faktor	érythropoïétine
escara, crosta	Brandschorf, Schorf	escarre
piaga da decubito	Dekubitus, Durchliegen	escarre de décubitus
spazio subaracnoideo	Subarachnoidalraum	espace sous-arachnoïdien
specie	Spezies, Art	espèce
test calorico	kalorische Prüfung	essai calorique

FRENCH	ENGLISH	SPANISH
essence	essence	esencia
essoufflement	shortness of breath	disnea
estomac	stomach	estómago
établissement de la menstruation	menarche	menarquía
éternuement	sneeze	estornudo
éternuer	sneeze	estornudar
ethmoïde	ethmoid	etmoides
ethnique	ethnic	étnico
étiologie	aetiology	etiología
étourdissement	dizziness	desvanecimiento, mareo
étrier	stapes	estribo
euphorie	euphoria	euforia
euthanasie	euthanasia	eutanasia
évacuation	evacuation	evacuación
évaporer	evaporate	evaporar
éversion	eversion	eversión
évocation	recall	recuerdo
évoquer	recall	recordar
exacerbation	exacerbation	exacerbación
excision	excision	excisión
excitabilité	excitability	excitabilidad
excitation	excitation	excitación
excoriation	excoriation	excoriación
excrétion	excretion	excreción
exérèse locale d'une tumeur du sein	lumpectomy	exéresis de tumores benignos de la mama
exfoliation	exfoliation	exfoliación
exhibitionnisme	exhibitionism	exhibicionismo
exocrine	exocrine	exocrino
exogène	exogenous	exógeno
exomphale	exomphalos	exónfalo, hernia umbilical
exophthalmie	exophthalmos	exoftalmía
exostose	exostosis	exostosis
exotoxine	exotoxin	exotoxina
expectorant (n)	expectorant (n)	expectorante (n)
expectorant (a)	expectorant (a)	expectorante (a)
expiration	expiration	espiración
exploration	exploration	exploración
expression	expression	expresión
exsudat	exudate	exudado
extenseur	extensor	extensor
extension	extension	extensión
extra-articulaire	extra-articular	extraarticular
extracellulaire	extracellular	extracelular
extraction	extraction	extracción
extraction par ventouse	ventouse extraction	extracción con ventosa
extradural	extradural	extradural

essenza	Essenz	essence
respiro affannoso	Kurzatmigkeit	essoufflement
stomaco	Magen	estomac
menarca	Menarche	établissement de la menstruation
starnuto	Niesen	éternuement
starnutire	niesen	éternuer
etmoide	Ethmoid, Siebbein	ethmoïde
etnico	ethnisch, rassisch	ethnique
eziologia	Ätiologie	étiologie
stordimento, capogiro, vertigini	Schwindel	étourdissement
staffa	Stapes, Steigbügel	étrier
euforia	Euphorie	euphorie
eutanasia	Euthanasie, Sterbehilfe	euthanasie
evacuazione	Ausleerung, Stuhlgang	évacuation
evaporare	verdampfen, verdunsten	évaporer
eversione, estrofia	Auswärtskehrung, Umstülpung	éversion
memoria	Errinerung, Errinerungsvermögen	évocation
ricordare	(sich) erinnern	évoquer
esacerbazione	Verschlimmerung	exacerbation
escissione	Exzision	excision
eccitabilità	Reizbarkeit, Erregbarkeit	excitabilité
eccitazione	Reizung, Erregung	excitation
escoriazione	Exkoriation, Abschürfung	excoriation
escrezione	Exkretion, Ausscheidung	excrétion
mastectomia parziale	Lumpektomie	exérèse locale d'une tumeur du sein
esfoliazione	Exfoliation	exfoliation
esibizionismo	Exhibitionismus	exhibitionnisme
esocrino	exokrin	exocrine
esogeno	exogen	exogène
ernia ombelicale, protrusione dell'ombelico	Exomphalos, Nabelbruch	exomphale
esoftalmo	Exophthalmus	exophthalmie
esostosi	Exostose	exostose
esotossina	Exotoxin	exotoxine
espettorante (n)	Expektorans (n), Sekretolytikum (n)	expectorant (n)
espettorante (a)	schleimlösend (a)	expectorant (a)
espirazione, termine	Exspiration, Ausatmen	expiration
esplorazione	Exploration	exploration
espressione	Expressio	expression
essudato	Exsudat	exsudat
estensore	Extensor, Streckmuskel	extenseur
estensione	Extension, Streck-	extension
extraartieolare	extraartikulär	extra-articulaire
extracellulare	extrazellulär	extracellulaire
estrazione	Extraktion	extraction
estrazione con ventosa ostetrica	Schröpfkopf	extraction par ventouse
extradurale	extradural	extradural

FRENCH	ENGLISH	SPANISH
extramural	extramural	extramural
extrasystole	extrasystole	extrasístole
extra-utérin	extrauterine	extrauterino
extravasation	extravasation	extravasación
extrinsèque	extrinsic	extrínseco

ITALIAN	GERMAN	FRENCH
extramurale	extramural	**extramural**
extrasistole	Extrasystole	**extrasystole**
extrauterino	extrauterin	**extra-utérin**
stravaso	Extravasat	**extravasation**
estrinseco	exogen	**extrinsèque**

F

FRENCH	ENGLISH	SPANISH
facette	facet	faceta
facial	facial	facial
faciès	facies	facies
facteur Rhésus	Rhesus factor	factor Rhesus
facultatif	facultative	facultativo
faiblesse	weakness	debilidad
faim	hunger	hambre
falciforme	falciform	falciforme
familial	familial	familiar
fascia	fascia	fascia, aponeurosis
fasciculation	fasciculation	fasciculación
fatigue	fatigue	fatiga, cansancio
fausse couche	miscarriage	aborto
fausse grossesse	phantom pregnancy	embarazo fantasma
faute professionnelle	malpractice	malpraxis
fébrile	febrile	febril
fécal	faecal (Eng), fecal (Am)	fecal
fèces	faeces (Eng), feces (Am)	heces
femelle	female	hembra
fémur	femur	fémur
fenestration	fenestration	fenestración
fente palatine	cleft palate	paladar hendido
ferreux	ferrous (Eng), ferrus (Am)	ferroso
fertilisation	fertilization	fertilización
fertilisation in vitro	in vitro fertilization (IVF)	fertilización in vitro (FIV)
fesse	buttock	nalga
fessier	gluteal	glúteo
fétoscopie	fetoscopy	fetoscopia
fibre	fiber (Am), fibre (Eng)	fibra
fibre alimentaire	dietary fiber (Am), dietary fibre (Eng)	fibra dietética
fibrillation	fibrillation	fibrilación
fibrillation auriculaire	atrial fibrillation	fibrilación auricular
fibrille	fibril	fibrilla
fibrine	fibrin	fibrina
fibrinogène	fibrinogen	fibrinógeno
fibroadénome	fibroadenoma	fibroadenoma
fibroblaste	fibroblast	fibroblasto
fibrokystique	fibrocystic	fibrocístico
fibrome	fibroma	fibroma
fibromyome	fibromyoma	fibromioma
fibroplasie rétrolentale	retrolental fibroplasia	fibroplasia retrolental
fibrosarcome	fibrosarcoma	fibrosarcoma
fibrose	fibrosis	fibrosis
fibrose cystique	cystic fibrosis (CF)	fibrosis quística

ITALIAN	GERMAN	FRENCH
faccetta	Facette	facette
facciale	Gesichts-	facial
facies	Facies, Gesicht	faciès
fattore Rh	Rhesusfaktor	facteur Rhésus
facoltativo	fakultativ	facultatif
debolezza	Schwäche	faiblesse
fame	Hunger	faim
falciforme	falciformis	falciforme
familiare	familiär	familial
fascia	Faszie	fascia
fascicolazione	Faszikulation	fasciculation
stanchezza, astenia	Ermüdung	fatigue
aborto	Fehlgeburt	fausse couche
pseudociesi	Scheinschwangerschaft, hysterische Schwangerschaft	fausse grossesse
pratica errata o disonesta	Kunstfehler	faute professionnelle
febbrile	Fieber-, fieberhaft	fébrile
fecale	fäkal, kotig	fécal
feci	Fäzes, Kot	fèces
femmina	weiblich	femelle
femore	Femur	fémur
fenestrazione	Fensterung	fenestration
palatoschisi	Gaumenspalte	fente palatine
ferroso	Eisen-	ferreux
fertilizzazione	Befruchtung	fertilisation
fertilizzazione in vitro	In-vitro-Fertilisation	fertilisation in vitro
natica	Gesäßbacke	fesse
gluteo	gluteal	fessier
fetoscopia	Fetoskopie	fétoscopie
fibra	Faser	fibre
fibra dietetica	Ballaststoff	fibre alimentaire
fibrillazione	Fibrillieren	fibrillation
fibrillazione atriale	Vorhofflimmern	fibrillation auriculaire
fibrilla	Fibrille, Fäserchen	fibrille
fibrina	Fibrin	fibrine
fibrinogeno	Fibrinogen	fibrinogène
fibroadenoma	Fibroadenom	fibroadénome
fibroblasto	Fibroblast	fibroblaste
fibrocistico	fibrozystisch	fibrokystique
fibroma	Fibrom	fibrome
fibromioma	Fibromyom	fibromyome
fibroplasia retrolenticolare	retrolentale Fibroplasie	fibroplasie rétrolentale
fibrosarcoma	Fibrosarkom	fibrosarcome
fibrosi	Fibrose	fibrose
mucoviscidosi, malattia fibrocistica del pancreas	Mukoviszidose	fibrose cystique

fibrosite	fibrositis	fibrositis
fibula	fibula	peroné
fièvre	fever	fiebre
fièvre de Lassa	Lassa fever	fiebre de Lassa
fièvre d'origine inconnue	pyrexia of unknown origin (PUO, FUO)	fiebre de origen desconocido
fièvre glandulaire	glandular fever	fiebre glandular
fièvre jaune	yellow fever	fiebre amarilla
fièvre paratyphoïde	paratyphoid fever	fiebre paratifoidea
fièvre pourprée des montagnes Rocheuses	Rocky Mountain spotted fever	fiebre manchada de las Montañas Rocosas
fièvre Q	Q fever	fiebre Q
fièvre typhoïde	typhoid fever	fiebre tifoidea
filariose	filariasis	filariasis
filtrat	filtrate	filtrado
filtration	filtration	filtración
fimbria	fimbria	fimbria, franja
fission	fission	fisión
fistule	fistula	fístula
fixation	fixation	fijación
flagellé	whipworm	trichuris trichiura
flatulence	flatulence	flatulencia
flatuosité	flatus	flato
fléchir	flex	flexionar
fléchisseur	flexor	flexor
flexion	flexion	flexión
flore	flora	flora
flottants	floaters	flotadores
fluide synovial	synovial fluid	líquido sinovial
fluorescéine	fluorescein	fluoresceína
fluorure	fluoride	flúor
flutter auriculaire	atrial flutter	aleteo auricular
foetus	fetus	feto
foie	liver	hígado
follicule	follicle	folículo
follicule de De Graaf	Graafian follicle	folículo de De Graaf
folliculite	folliculitis	foliculitis
fonction	function	función
fonctionnel	functional disorder	trastorno funcional
fonctionner	function	funcionar
fond	fundus	fundus
fontanelle	fontanelle	fontanela
forceps	forceps	fórceps
formation de godet	pitting	cavitación
former une croûte	scab	formar una costra
formulaire	formulary	formulario

ITALIAN	GERMAN	FRENCH
fibrosite	Fibrositis, Bindegewebsentzündung	fibrosite
fibula	Fibula, Wadenbein	fibula
febbre	Fieber	fièvre
febbre di Lassa	Lassafieber	fièvre de Lassa
piressia di origine sconosciuta (POS)	Fieber unklarer Genese	fièvre d'origine inconnue
mononucleosi infettiva	Mononukleose, Pfeiffersches Drüsenfieber	fièvre glandulaire
febbre gialla	Gelbfieber	fièvre jaune
febbre paratifoide	Paratyphus	fièvre paratyphoïde
febbre purpurica delle Montagne Rocciose	Rocky Mountain spotted fever	fièvre pourprée des montagnes Rocheuses
febbre Q	Q-Fieber	fièvre Q
febbre tifoide, tifo addominale, ileotifo	Typhus	fièvre typhoïde
filariasi	Filariasis, Fadenwurmbefall	filariose
filtrato	Filtrat	filtrat
filtrazione	Filtrieren, Filtration	filtration
fimbria	Fimbrie	fimbria
fissione	Spaltung	fission
fistola	Fistel	fistule
fissazione	Fixation, Fixierung	fixation
verme a frusta, tricocefalo	Oxyuris, Peitschenwurm	flagellé
flatulenza	Flatulenz, Blähung	flatulence
flatulenza, gas intestinale	Flatus, Wind	flatuosité
flettere	beugen, flektieren	fléchir
flessore	Flexor, Beugemuskel	fléchisseur
flessione	Flexion, Beugung	flexion
flora	Flora	flore
corpuscoli vitreali sospesi visibili	Mouches volantes	flottants
liquido sinoviale	Synovialflüssigkeit	fluide synovial
fluoresceina	Fluorescin	fluorescéine
fluoruro	Fluorid	fluorure
flutter atriale	Vorhofflattern	flutter auriculaire
feto	Fetus	foetus
fegato	Leber	foie
follicolo	Follikel	follicule
follicolo di Graaf	Graaf-Follikel	follicule de De Graaf
follicolite	Follikulitis	folliculite
funzione	Funktion	fonction
disturbo funzionale	funktionelle Störung	fonctionnel
funzionare	funktionieren	fonctionner
fondo	Fundus, Augenhintergrund	fond
fontanella	Fontanelle	fontanelle
forcipe	Zange, Pinzette, Klemme	forceps
depressioni puntiformi, fovea	Dellenbildung	formation de godet
ricoprirsi di croste	verkrusten	former une croûte
formulario	Formelbuch	formulaire

FRENCH	ENGLISH	SPANISH
formule	formula	fórmula, receta
formule leucocytaire	differential blood count	fórmula leucocitaria
fornix	fornix	fórnix, bóveda
fosse gutturale	fauces	fauces
foulure	sprain	esguince
fourchette	fourchette	horquilla, frenillo pudendo
fovea	fovea	fóvea
foyer morbide	nidus	nido
fracture	fracture	fractura
fracture de Pott	Pott's fracture	fractura de Pott
fracture de Pouteau-Colles	Colles' fracture	fractura de Colles
fracture esquilleuse	comminuted fracture	fractura conminuta
fracture incomplète	greenstick fracture	fractura en tallo verde
fracturer	fracture	fracturar
fracture spontanée	pathological fracture	fractura patológica
frein	frenum	frenillo
frénotomie	frenotomy	frenotomía
fréquence	incidence	incidencia
fréquence cardiaque foetale	fetal heart rate (FHR)	frecuencia cardíaca fetal (FCF)
frère ou soeur	sibling	hermano no gemelo
friable	friable	friable
friction	friction	fricción
frigidité	frigidity	frigidez
froid	cold	frío
front	brow, forehead	ceja, frente
frontal	frontal	frontal
frottis	smear	frotis
fugue	fugue	fuga
fuite des idées	flight of ideas	fuga de ideas
fulguration	fulguration	fulguración
fulminant	fulminant	fulminante
fundoplication	fundoplication	fundoplicatura
furoncle	boil, furuncle	forúnculo

ITALIAN	GERMAN	FRENCH
formula	Formel, Milchzusammensetzung	formule
formula leucocitaria	Differentialblutbild	formule leucocytaire
fornice	Fornix	fornix
fauci	Rachen, Schlund	fosse gutturale
distorsione	Verstauchung	foulure
forchetta	hintere Schamlippenkommissur	fourchette
fovea	Fovea	fovea
nido	Nidus	foyer morbide
frattura	Fraktur, Knochenbruch	fracture
frattura di Pott	Pott-Fraktur	fracture de Pott
frattura di Colles	distale Radiusfraktur	fracture de Pouteau-Colles
frattura comminuta	Splitterbruch	fracture esquilleuse
frattura a legno verde	Grünholzfraktur	fracture incomplète
fratturare	frakturieren, brechen	fracturer
frattura patologica	pathologische Fraktur	fracture spontanée
freno	Frenulum	frein
frenulotomia	Frenotomie, Zungenbändchendurchtrennung	frénotomie
incidenza	Inzidenz	fréquence
battito cardiaco fetale	fetale Herzfrequenz	fréquence cardiaque foetale
fratello germano	Geschwister	frère ou soeur
friabile	bröckelig, brüchig	friable
attrito, frizione	Friktion, Reibung	friction
frigidità	Frigidität, Kälte	frigidité
freddo	kalt	froid
arcata sopracciliare, sopracciglio, fronte	Augenbraue, Stirn	front
frontale	Stirn-, frontal	frontal
striscio	Belag, Abstrich	frottis
fuga	Fugue	fugue
fuga delle idee	Ideenflucht	fuite des idées
folgorazione	Fulguration	fulguration
fulminante	fulminant	fulminant
fundoplicazione	Fundoplikatio(n)	fundoplication
foruncolo	Furunkel, Eiterbeule	furoncle

FRENCH	ENGLISH	SPANISH

G

FRENCH	ENGLISH	SPANISH
galactagogue	galactagogue	galactogogo
galactorrhée	galactorrhea (Am), galactorrhoea (Eng)	galactorrea
galactose	galactose	galactosa
galactosémie	galactosaemia (Eng), galactosemia (Am)	galactosemia
gale	scabies	sarna
gamète	gamete	gameto
gamma-globuline	gammaglobulin	gammaglobulina
gamma-globuline humaine (GGH)	human gamma globulin (HGG)	gammaglobulina humana
gamma-glutamyl-transférase (GGT)	gamma glutamyl transferase (GGT)	gamma glutamil transferasa (GGT)
ganglion	ganglion	ganglio
ganglion lymphatique	lymph node	ganglio linfático
gangrène	gangrene	gangrena
gargarisme	gargle	gárgara, colutorio
gastrectomie	gastrectomy	gastrectomía
gastrine	gastrin	gastrina
gastrique	gastric	gástrico
gastrite	gastritis	gastritis
gastrocnémien	gastrocnemius	gastrocnemio, gemelos
gastrocolique	gastrocolic	gastrocólico
gastrodynie	gastrodynia	gastrodinia
gastro-entérite	gastroenteritis	gastroenteritis
gastro-entérologie	gastroenterology	gastroenterología
gastro-entéropathie	gastroenteropathy	gastroenteropatía
gastro-entérostomie	gastroenterostomy	gastroenterostomía
gastro-intestinal	gastrointestinal	gastrointestinal
gastrojéjunostomie	gastrojejunostomy	gastroyeyunostomía
gastro-oesophagien	gastroesophageal (Am), gastro-oesophageal (Eng)	gastroesofágico
gastroschisis	gastroschisis	gastrosquisis
gastroscope	gastroscope	gastroscopio
gastrostomie	gastrostomy	gastrotomía
gaucher	left-handed	zurdo
gaz	gas, wind	gas, flatulencia, ventosidad
gaze	gauze	gasa
gélatine	gelatine (Eng), gelatin (Am)	gelatina
gelure	frostbite	congelación, sabañón
gencive	gingiva	encía
gène	gene	gen
génératif	generative	generador
générique	generic	genérico
génétique	genetic, genetics	genético, genética
génital	genital	genital
génito-urinaire (GT)	genitourinary (GU)	genitourinario
génome	genome	genoma
génotype	genotype	genotipo

ITALIAN	GERMAN	FRENCH
galattagogo	Galaktagogum	galactagogue
galattorrea	Galaktorrhoe	galactorrhée
galattosio	Galaktose	galactose
galattosemia	Galaktosämie	galactosémie
scabbia	Skabies, Krätze	gale
gamete	Gamete	gamète
gammaglobulina	Gammaglobulin	gamma-globuline
gammaglobulina umana	Human-Gammaglobulin	gamma-globuline humaine (GGH)
transaminasi, transferasi glutammica	Gammaglutamyltransferase (gGT)	gamma-glutamyl-transférase (GGT)
ganglio	Ganglion, Überbein	ganglion
linfonodo	Lymphknoten	ganglion lymphatique
gangrena	Gangrän	gangrène
gargarismi	Gurgelmittel	gargarisme
gastrectomia	Magenresektion	gastrectomie
gastrina	Gastrin	gastrine
gastrico	gastrisch, Magen-	gastrique
gastrite	Gastritis, Magenschleim-hautentzündung	gastrite
gastrocnemio	gastrocnemius	gastrocnémien
gastrocolico	gastrokolisch	gastrocolique
gastrodinia	Magenschmerz	gastrodynie
gastroenterite	Gastroenteritis	gastro-entérite
gastroenterologia	Gastroenterologie	gastro-entérologie
gastroenteropatia	Gastroenteropathie	gastro-entéropathie
gastroenterostomia	Gastroenterostomie	gastro-entérostomie
gastrointestinale	gastrointestinal, Magendarm-	gastro-intestinal
gastrodigiunostomia	Gastrojejunostomie	gastrojéjunostomie
gastroesofageo	gastroösophageal	gastro-oesophagien
gastroschisi	Gastroschisis	gastroschisis
gastroscopio	Gastroskop, Magenspiegel	gastroscope
gastrostomia	Gastrostomie	gastrostomie
mancino	linkshändig	gaucher
gas, flatulenza, ventosità	Gas, Wind, Blähung	gaz
garza	Gaze, Mull	gaze
gelatina	Gelatine, Gallerte	gélatine
congelamento	Erfrierung	gelure
gengiva	Gingiva, Zahnfleisch	gencive
gene	Gen	gène
riproduttivo	fertil, Fortpflanzungs-	génératif
generico	generisch	générique
genetico, genetica	genetisch, Genetik	génétique
genitale	genital, Geschlechts-	génital
genito-urinario	urogenital	génito-urinaire (GT)
genoma	Genom	génome
genotipo	Genotyp	génotype

genou	knee	rodilla
genou cagneux	knock-knee	genu valgum
genre	genus	género
genu valgum	genu valgum	genu valgum
genu varum	genu varum	genu varum
gériatre	geriatrician	geriatra
gériatrie	geriatrics	geriatría
gériatrique	geriatric	geriátrico
germe	germ	gérmen
gestation	gestation	gestación
giardiase	giardiasis	giardiasis
gingivite	gingivitis	gingivitis
glande	gland	glándula
glande apocrine	apocrine gland	glándula apocrina
glande parathyroïde	parathyroid gland	glándula paratiroidea
glande parotide	parotid gland	glándula parótida
glande pinéale	pineal body	cuerpo pineal
glande salivaire	salivary gland	glándula salivar
glandes de Bartholin	Bartholin's glands	glándulas de Bartolino
glaucome	glaucoma	glaucoma
gléno-huméral	glenohumeral	glenohumeral
glénoïde	glenoid	glenoide
gliome	glioma	glioma
globule rouge	red blood cell (RBC)	eritrocito, glóbulo rojo
globuline humaine	human gamma globulin (HGG)	gammaglobulina humana
glomérule	glomerulus	glomérulo
glomérulite	glomerulitis	glomerulitis
glomérulonéphrite	glomerulonephritis	glomerulonefritis
glomérulosclérose	glomerulosclerosis	glomerulosclerosis
glossite	glossitis	glositis
glossodynie	glossodynia	glosodinia
glossopharyngien	glossopharyngeal	glosofaríngeo
glotte	glottis	glotis
glucagon	glucagon	glucagón
glucide	carbohydrate (CHO)	hidrato de carbono
glucocorticoïde	glucocorticoid	glucocorticoide
glucogenèse	glucogenesis	glucogénesis
gluconéogenèse	gluconeogenesis	gluconeogénesis
glucose	glucose	glucosa
gluten	gluten	gluten
glycémie	blood sugar	glucemia
glycémie à jeun	fasting blood sugar (FBS)	glucemia en ayunas
glycogenèse	glycogenesis	glucogénesis
glycolyse	glycolysis	glucolisis
glycosurie	glycosuria	glucosuria
goitre	goiter (Am), goitre (Eng)	bocio

ITALIAN	GERMAN	FRENCH
ginocchio	Knie	genou
ginocchio valgo	Genu valgum, X-Bein	genou cagneux
genere	Genus, Gattung	genre
ginocchio valgo	Genu valgum, X-Bein	genu valgum
ginocchio varo	Genu varum, O-Bein	genu varum
geriatra	Geriater	gériatre
geriatria	Geriatrie	gériatrie
geriatrico	geriatrisch	gériatrique
germe	Erreger, Keim, Bazillus	germe
gestazione	Gestation, Schwangerschaft	gestation
giardiasi	Lambliasis	giardiase
gengivite	Gingivitis, Zahnfleischentzündung	gingivite
ghiandola	Glandula, Drüse	glande
ghiandola apocrina	apokrine Drüse	glande apocrine
ghiandola paratiroide	Nebenschilddrüse, Parathyreoidea	glande parathyroïde
ghiandola parotide	Parotis, Ohrspeicheldrüse	glande parotide
ghiandola pineale	Epiphyse	glande pinéale
ghiandola salivare	Speicheldrüse	glande salivaire
ghiandole di Bartolini	Bartholini-Drüsen	glandes de Bartholin
glaucoma	Glaukom, grüner Star	glaucome
gleno-omerale	glenohumeral	gléno-huméral
glenoide	Schultergelenk-	glénoïde
glioma	Gliom	gliome
eritrocito, globulo rosso (RBC)	Erythrozyt	globule rouge
gammaglobulina umana	Human-Gammaglobulin	globuline humaine
glomerulo	Glomerulus	glomérule
glomerulite	Glomerulitis	glomérulite
glomerulonefrite	Glomerulonephritis	glomérulonéphrite
glomerulosclerosi	Glomerulosklerose	glomérulosclérose
glossite	Glossitis	glossite
glossodinia	Glossodynie, Zungenschmerz	glossodynie
glossofaringeo	glossopharyngeal	glossopharyngien
glottide	Glottis, Stimmritze	glotte
glucagone	Glukagon	glucagon
carboidrato	Kohlenhydrat, Kohlenwasserstoff	glucide
glicocorticoide	Glukokortikoid	glucocorticoïde
glucogenesi	Glukogenese	glucogenèse
gluconeogenesi	Glukoneogenese	gluconéogenèse
glucosio	Glukose, Traubenzucker	glucose
glutine	Gluten	gluten
glicemia	Blutzucker	glycémie
glicemia a digiuno	Nüchternblutzucker (NBZ)	glycémie à jeun
glicogenesi	Glykogenese	glycogenèse
glicolisi	Glykolyse, Glukoseabbau	glycolyse
glicosuria	Glykosurie, Glukoseausscheidung im Urin	glycosurie
gozzo	Struma, Kropf	goitre

FRENCH	ENGLISH	SPANISH
goitre exophtalmique	Graves' disease	enfermedad de Graves
gomme	gumma	goma
gonade	gonad	gónada
gonadotrophine	gonadotrophin (Eng), gonadotropin (Am)	gonadotropina
gonadotrophine A	follicle stimulating hormone (FSH)	hormona estimulante del folículo (FSH)
gonadotrophine chorionique humaine (GCH)	human chorionic gonadotrophin (HCG) (Eng), human chorionic gonadotropin (HCG) (Am)	gonadotropina coriónica humana (GCH)
gonorrhée	gonorrhea (Am), gonorrhoea (Eng)	gonorrea
goutte	gout	gota
gouttière	sulcus	surco
graisse	fat	grasa
grand mal	grand mal	gran mal
granulation	granulation	granulación
granulocyte	granulocyte	granulocito
granulome	granuloma	granuloma
gras	fat	graso
gravitationnel	gravitational	gestacional
gravité	gravity	gravedad
greffe	graft	injerto
greffe de la cornée	corneal graft	injerto corneal
greffe osseuse	bone graft	injerto óseo, osteoplastia
greffer	graft	injertar
grippe	influenza	influenza
grommet	grommet	cánula ótica
grossesse	cyesis, pregnancy	ciesis, embarazo
grossesse ectopique	ectopic pregnancy	embarazo ectópico
groupe sanguin	blood group	grupo sanguíneo
groupes de streptocoques suivant la classification de Lancefield	Lancefield's groups	grupos de Lancefield
gynécologie	gynaecology (Eng), gynecology (Am)	ginecología
gynécomastie	gynaecomastia (Eng), gynecomastia (Am)	ginecomastia
gypse	gypsum	yeso

ITALIAN	GERMAN	FRENCH
morbo di Graves	Basedow-Krankheit	goitre exophtalmique
gomma	Gumma	gomme
gonade	Gonade	gonade
gonadotropina	Gonadotropin	gonadotrophine
ormone follicolostimolante (FSH)	follikelstimulierendes Hormon (FSH)	gonadotrophine A
gonadotropina corionica umana (GCU)	Choriongonadotropin (HCG)	gonadotrophine chorionique humaine (GCH)
gonorrea	Gonorrhoe, Tripper	gonorrhée
gotta	Gicht	goutte
solco	Sulcus, Furche	gouttière
adipe	Fett	graisse
grande male	Grand mal	grand mal
granulazione	Granulation	granulation
granulocita	Granulozyt	granulocyte
granuloma	Granulom, Granulationsgeschwulst	granulome
grasso	fett, fetthaltig	gras
gravitazionale	Gravitations-	gravitationnel
gravità	Schwere (der Erkrankung)	gravité
trapianto, innesto	Transplantat, Transplantation, Plastik	greffe
trapianto corneale	Korneaplastik	greffe de la cornée
trapianto osseo	Osteoplastik, Knochentransplantation	greffe osseuse
trapiantare	transplantieren, übertragen	greffer
influenza	Influenza, Grippe	grippe
catetere per drenaggio auricolare	Öse	grommet
gravidanza	Schwangerschaft, Gravidität	grossesse
gravidanza ectopica	ektope Schwangerschaft	grossesse ectopique
gruppo sanguigno	Blutgruppe	groupe sanguin
gruppi di Lancefield	Lancefield-Gruppen	groupes de streptocoques suivant la classification de Lancefield
ginecologia	Gynäkologie, Frauenheilkunde	gynécologie
ginecomastia	Gynäkomastie	gynécomastie
gesso, solfato di calcio	Gips	gypse

H

FRENCH	ENGLISH	SPANISH
habitude	habit	hábito
haleine	breath	aliento
halitose	halitosis	halitosis
hallucination	hallucination, delusion	alucinación, idea delusiva, delirio
hallux	hallux	dedo gordo del pie
hallux valgus	bunion	juanete
hanche	hip	cadera
handicapé	handicap	disminución, minusvalía
haut-le-coeur	retching	arcadas
hébéphrénie	hebephrenia	hebefrenia
hémangiome	haemangioma (Eng), hemangioma (Am)	hemangioma
hémarthrose	haemarthrosis (Eng), hemarthrosis (Am)	hemartrosis
hématémèse	haematemesis (Eng), hematemesis (Am)	hematemesis
hématocolpos	haematocolpos (Eng), hematocolpos (Am)	hematocolpos
hématocrite	haematocrit (Eng), hematocrit (Am), packed cell volume (PCV)	hematócrito, volumen de células agregadas
hématologie	haematology (Eng), hematology (Am)	hematología
hématome	haematoma (Eng), hematoma (Am)	hematoma
hématurie	blackwater fever, haematuria (Eng), hematuria (Am)	fiebre hemoglobinúrica, hematuria
hémicolectomie	hemicolectomy	hemocolectomía
hémiparésie	hemiparesis	hemiparesia
hémiplégie	hemiplegia	hemiplejía
hémochromatose	haemochromatosis (Eng), hemochromatosis (Am)	hemocromatosis
hémoculture	blood culture	hemocultivo
hémodialyse	haemodialysis (Eng), hemodialysis (Am)	hemodiálisis
hémoglobine (Hb) (Hg)	haemoglobin (Hb) (Hg) (Eng), hemoglobin (Hb) (Hg) (Am)	hemoglobina (Hb)
hémoglobinopathie	haemoglobinopathy (Eng), hemoglobinopathy (Am)	hemoglobinopatía
hémoglobinurie	haemoglobinuria (Eng), hemoglobinuria (Am)	hemoglobinuria
hémolyse	haemolysis (Eng), hemolysis (Am)	hemólisis
hémolyse des nouveau-nés	haemolytic disease of the newborn (HDN) (Eng), hemolytic disease of the newborn (HDN) (Am)	enfermedad hemolítica del recién nacido
hémolyse urémique des nouveau-nés	haemolytic uraemic syndrome (HUS) (Eng), hemolytic uremic syndrome (HUS) (Am)	síndrome hemolítico urémico

ITALIAN	GERMAN	FRENCH
abitudine	Gewohnheit	**habitude**
respiro	Atem, Atemzug	**haleine**
alitosi	Foetor ex ore, Mundgeruch	**halitose**
allucinazione, fissazione	Halluzination, Wahn, Wahnvorstellung	**hallucination**
alluce	Hallux, Großzeh	**hallux**
borsite dell'alluce	entzündeter Fußballen	**hallux valgus**
anca	Hüfte	**hanche**
handicappato, minorato	Behinderung	**handicapé**
conati di vomito	Würgen, Brechreiz	**haut-le-coeur**
ebefrenia	Hebephrenie	**hébéphrénie**
emangioma	Hämangiom	**hémangiome**
emartrosi	Hämarthros	**hémarthrose**
ematemesi	Hämatemesis, Bluterbrechen	**hématémèse**
ematocolpo	Hämatokolpos	**hématocolpos**
ematrocrito, volume cellulare (VC)	Hämatokrit (HKT)	**hématocrite**
ematologia	Hämatologie	**hématologie**
ematoma	Hämatom, Bluterguß	**hématome**
febbre emoglobinurica da Plasmodium falciparum, ematuria	Schwarzwasserfieber, Hämaturie, Blut im Urin	**hématurie**
emicolectomia	Hemikolektomie	**hémicolectomie**
emiparesi	Hemiparese, unvollständige Halbseitenlähmung	**hémiparésie**
emiplegia	Hemiplegie, Halbseitenlähmung	**hémiplégie**
emocromatosi	Hämochromatose, Bronzediabetes	**hémochromatose**
emocoltura	Blutkultur	**hémoculture**
emodialisi	Hämodialyse	**hémodialyse**
emoglobina (E)	Hämoglobin	**hémoglobine (Hb) (Hg)**
emoglobinopatia	Hämoglobinopathie	**hémoglobinopathie**
emoglobinuria	Hämoglobinurie	**hémoglobinurie**
emolisi	Hämolyse	**hémolyse**
ittero dei neonati, eritroblastosi fetale (da incompatibilità Rh)	Morbus haemolyticus neonatorum	**hémolyse des nouveau-nés**
sindrome emolitico-uremica	hämolytisch-urämisches Syndrom	**hémolyse urémique des nouveau-nés**

FRENCH	ENGLISH	SPANISH
hémopéricarde	haemopericardium (Eng), hemopericardium (Am)	hemopericardio
hémopéritoine	haemoperitoneum (Eng), hemoperitoneum (Am)	hemoperitoneo
hémophilie	haemophilia (Eng), hemophilia (Am)	hemofilia
hémopneumothorax	haemopneumothorax (Eng), hemopneumothorax (Am)	hemoneumotórax
hémopoïèse	haemopoiesis (Eng), hemopoiesis (Am)	hemopoyesis
hémoptysie	haemoptysis (Eng), hemoptysis (Am)	hemoptisis
hémorragie	haemorrhage (Eng), hemorrhage (Am)	hemorragia
hémorragies des nouveau-nés	haemorrhagic disease of the newborn (Eng), hemorrhagic disease of the newborn (Am)	enfermedad hemorrágica neonatal
hémorragie sous-arachnoïdienne	subarachnoid haemorrhage (Eng), subarachnoid hemorrhage (Am)	hemorragia subaracnoidea
hémorroïde	haemorrhoid (Eng), hemorrhoid (Am)	hemorroide
hémorroïdectomie	haemorrhoidectomy (Eng), hemorrhoidectomy (Am)	hemorroidectomía
hémorroïdes	piles	hemorroides
hémostase	haemostasis (Eng), hemostasis (Am)	hemostasis
hémothorax	haemothorax (Eng), hemothorax (Am)	hemotórax
hépatique	hepatic	hepático
hépatite	hepatitis	hepatitis
hépatite virale	viral hepatitis	hepatitis vírica
hépatocellulaire	hepatocellular	hepatocelular
hépatome	hepatoma	hepatoma
hépatomégalie	hepatomegaly	hepatomegalia
hépatosplénomégalie	hepatosplenomegaly	hepatosplenomegalia
hépatotoxique	hepatotoxic	hepatotóxico
héréditaire	hereditary	hereditario
hérédité	heredity	herencia
hermaphrodite	hermaphrodite	hermafrodita
hernie	hernia, rupture	hernia, ruptura
hernie discale	slipped disc	hernia de disco
hernie étranglée	strangulated hernia	hernia estrangulada
hernie intestinale	enterocele	enterocele
hernie ombilicale	umbilical hernia	hernia umbilical
herniorrhaphie	herniorraphy	herniorrafia
herniotomie	herniotomy	herniotomía
herpès	cold sore, herpes	herpes labial, herpes
hétérogène	heterogenous	heterogéneo
hétérosexuel	heterosexual	heterosexual
hile	hilum	hilio
hippocratisme digital	clubbing	dedos en palillo de tambor, dedos hipocráticos
hirsutisme	hirsuties, hirsutism	hirsutismo
histiocyte	histiocyte	histiocito
histiocytome	histiocytoma	histiocitoma
histologie	histology	histología
histolyse	histolysis	histólisis

ITALIAN	GERMAN	FRENCH
emopericardio	Hämatoperikard	hémopéricarde
emoperitoneo	Hämatoperitoneum	hémopéritoine
emofilia	Hämophilie, Bluterkrankheit	hémophilie
emopneumotorace	Hämatopneumothorax	hémopneumothorax
ematopoiesi	Hämatopoese	hémopoïèse
cartilagine costale	Hämoptoe, Bluthusten	hémoptysie
emorragia	Hämorrhagie, Blutung	hémorragie
malattia emorragica del neonato	Morbus haemorrhagicus neonatorum	hémorragies des nouveau-nés
emorragia subaracnoidea	Subarachnoidalblutung	hémorragie sous-arachnoïdienne
emorroide	Hämorrhoide	hémorroïde
emorroidectomia	Hämorrhoidektomie, Hämorrhoidenoperation	hémorroïdectomie
emorroidi	Hämorrhoiden	hémorroïdes
emostasi	Hämostase, Blutgerinnung	hémostase
emotorace	Hämatothorax	hémothorax
epatico	hepatisch, Leber-	hépatique
epatite	Hepatitis	hépatite
epatite virale	Virushepatitis	hépatite virale
epatocellulare	hepatozellulär	hépatocellulaire
epatoma	Hepatom	hépatome
epatomegalia	Hepatomegalie	hépatomégalie
epatosplenomegalia	Hepatosplenomegalie	hépatosplénomégalie
epatotossico	leberschädigend	hépatotoxique
ereditario	hereditär, erblich	héréditaire
eredità	Erblichkeit, Vererbung	hérédité
ermafrodito	Hermaphrodit, Zwitter	hermaphrodite
ernia, rottura	Hernie, Bruch, Riß	hernie
ernia discale	Bandscheibenvorfall	hernie discale
ernia strozzata	inkarzerierte Hernie	hernie étranglée
enterocele	Enterozele	hernie intestinale
ernia ombelicale	Nabelbruch	hernie ombilicale
erniorrafia	Bruchoperation	herniorrhaphie
erniotomia	Herniotomie	herniotomie
labialis, herpes	Herpes, Bläschenausschlag	herpès
eterogenico	heterogen	hétérogène
eterosessuale	heterosexuell	hétérosexuel
ilo	Hilus	hile
dita a clava, ippocratismo	Trommelschlegelfinger	hippocratisme digital
irsutismo	Hirsutismus	hirsutisme
istiocito	Histiozyt	histiocyte
istiocitoma	Histiozytom	histiocytome
istologia	Histologie	histologie
istolisi	Histolyse	histolyse

FRENCH	ENGLISH	SPANISH
homéopathie	homeopathy (Am), homoeopathy (Eng)	homeopatía
homéostasie	homeostasis	homeostasis
homicide	homicide	homicidio
homogène	homogeneous (Eng), homogenous (Am)	homogéneo
homologue	homologous	homólogo
homonyme	homonymous	homónimo
homosexuel (n)	homosexual (n)	homosexual (n)
homosexuel (a)	homosexual (a)	homosexual (a)
homozygote	homozygous	homocigoto
hôpital	hospital	hospital
hôpital de jour	day hospital	hospital de día
hoquet	hiccup	hipo
hormone	hormone	hormona
hormone adrénocorticotrope (ACTH)	adrenocorticotrophic hormone (ACTH)	hormona adrenocorticotropa (ACTH)
hormone cortico-surrénale	adrenal cortical hormone (ACH)	hormona corticosuprarrenal (HCS)
hormone de croissance (HGH)	growth hormone (GH)	hormona del crecimiento (HC)
hormone folliculo-stimulante	follicle stimulating hormone (FSH)	hormona estimulante del folículo (FSH)
hormone lipotrope hypophysaire	lipotrophic	lipotrófico
hormone lutéinisante (HL)	luteinizing hormone (LH)	hormona luteinizante (LH)
hormonothérapie supplétive	hormone replacement therapy (HRT)	terapéutica de reposición de hormonas
hospice	hospice	hospicio
hôte	host	huésped
humérus	humerus	húmero
hyalite	hyalitis	hialitis
hyaloïde	hyaloid	hialoide
hydatidiforme	hydatidiform mole	mola hidatidiforme
hydramnios	hydramnios	hidramnios
hydrate	hydrate	hidrato
hydrater	hydrate	hidratar
hydrocèle	hydrocele	hidrocele
hydrocéphale	hydrocephalus	hidrocéfalo
hydrolyse	hydrolysis	hidrólisis
hydronéphrose	hydronephrosis	hidronefrosis
hydrosalpinx	hydrosalpinx	hidrosálpinx
hygiène	hygiene	higiene
hygiène du travail	occupational health	higiene profesional
hygroma	hygroma	higroma
hymen	hymen	himen
hymenectomie	hymenectomy	himenectomía
hyoïde	hyoid	hioides
hyperacidité	hyperacidity	hiperacidez
hyperactivité	hyperactivity	hiperactividad
hyperalgésie	hyperalgesia	hiperalgesia
hyperalgie	hyperalgesia	hiperalgesia

ITALIAN	GERMAN	FRENCH
omeopatia	Homöopathie	homéopathie
omeostasi	Homöostase	homéostasie
omicidio	Totschlag, Mord	homicide
omogeneo	homogen	homogène
omologo	homolog	homologue
omonimo	homonym	homonyme
omosessuale (n)	Homosexueller (n)	homosexuel (n)
omosessuale (a)	homosexuell (a)	homosexuel (a)
omozigote	homozygot	homozygote
ospedale	Krankenhaus, Hospital	hôpital
ospedale diurno	Tagesklinik	hôpital de jour
singhiozzo	Schluckauf	hoquet
ormone	Hormon	hormone
ormone corticotropo (ACTH)	adrenokortikotropes Hormon (ACTH)	hormone adrénocorticotrope (ACTH)
ormone corticosurrenale	Nebennierenrindenhormon (ACH)	hormone cortico-surrénale
ormone della crescita (GH)	Wachstumshormon	hormone de croissance (HGH)
ormone follicolostimolante (FSH)	follikelstimulierendes Hormon (FSH)	hormone folliculo-stimulante
lipotrofico	lipotroph	hormone lipotrope hypophysaire
ormone luteinizzante (LH)	luteinisierendes Hormon	hormone lutéinisante (HL)
terapia sostitutiva ormonale	Hormonsubstitutionstherapie	hormonothérapie supplétive
ricovero	Hospiz	hospice
ospite	Wirt	hôte
omero	Humerus, Oberarmknochen	humérus
ialinite	Hyalitis	hyalite
ialoideo	Glaskörper-	hyaloïde
idatiforme	Blasenmole	hydatidiforme
idramnios	Hydramnion	hydramnios
idrato	Hydrat	hydrate
idratare	hydrieren, hydratisieren	hydrater
idrocele	Hydrozele, Wasserbruch	hydrocèle
idrocefalo	Hydrozephalus	hydrocéphale
idrolisi	Hydrolyse	hydrolyse
idronefrosi	Hydronephrose	hydronéphrose
idrosalpinge	Hydrosalpinx	hydrosalpinx
igiene	Hygiene	hygiène
medicina del lavoro	Gewerbehygiene	hygiène du travail
igroma	Hygrom	hygroma
imene	Hymen	hymen
imenectomia	Hymenektomie	hymenectomie
ioide	Os hyeoideum	hyoïde
iperacidità	Hyperazidität	hyperacidité
iperattività	Überaktivität	hyperactivité
iperalgesia	Hyperalgesie	hyperalgésie
iperalgesia	Hyperalgesie	hyperalgie

hyperbilirubinémie	hyperbilirubinaemia (Eng), hyperbilirubinemia (Am)	hiperbilirrubinemia
hypercalcémie	hypercalcaemia (Eng), hypercalcemia (Am)	hipercalcemia
hypercalciurie	hypercalciuria	hipercalciuria
hypercapnie	hypercapnia	hipercapnia
hypercholestérolémie	hypercholesterolaemia (Eng), hypercholesterolemia (Am)	hipercolesterolemia
hyperémèse	hyperemesis	hiperemesis
hyperémie	hyperaemia (Eng), hyperemia (Am)	hiperemia
hyperesthésie	hyperaesthesia (Eng), hyperesthesia (Am)	hiperestesia
hyperextension	hyperextension	hiperextensión
hyperflexion	hyperflexion	hiperflexión
hyperglycémie	hyperglycaemia (Eng), hyperglycemia (Am)	hiperglucemia
hyperhidrose	hyperidrosis	hiperhidrosis
hyperkaliémie	hyperkalaemia (Eng), hyperkalemia (Am)	hipercaliemia
hyperlipémie	hyperlipaemia (Eng), hyperlipemia (Am)	hiperlipemia
hyperlipoprotéinémie	hyperlipoproteinaemia (Eng), hyperlipoproteinemia (Am)	hiperlipoproteinemia
hypermétropie	hypermetropia	hipermetropía
hypernéphrome	hypernephroma	hipernefroma
hyperparathyroïdisme	hyperparathyroidism	hiperparatiroidismo
hyperplasie	hyperplasia	hiperplasia
hyperpnoïa	hyperpnea (Am), hyperpnoea (Eng)	hiperpnea
hyperpyrexie	hyperpyrexia	hiperpirexia
hypersensibilité	hypersensitive	hipersensibilidad
hypertélorisme	hypertelorism	hipertelorismo
hypertension	hypertension	hipertensión
hypertension porte	portal circulation	circulación portal
hyperthermie	hyperthermia	hipertermia
hyperthyroïdisme	hyperthyroidism	hipertiroidismo
hypertonie	hypertonia	hipertonía
hypertonique	hypertonic	hipertónico
hypertrophie	hypertrophy	hipertrofia
hyperventilation	hyperventilation	hiperventilación
hypervolémie	hypervolaemia (Eng), hypervolemia (Am)	hipervolemia
hypesthésie	hypoaesthesia (Eng), hypoesthesia (Am)	hipoestesia
hyphéma	hyphaema (Eng), hyphema (Am)	hipema
hypnose	hypnosis	hipnosis
hypnothérapie	hypnotherapy	hipnoterapia
hypnotique (n)	hypnotic (n)	hipnótico (n)
hypnotique (a)	hypnotic (a)	hipnótico (a)
hypocalcémie	hypocalcaemia (Eng), hypocalcemia (Am)	hipocalcemia

ITALIAN	GERMAN	FRENCH
iperbilirubinemia	Hyperbilirubinämie	hyperbilirubinémie
ipercalcemia	Hyperkalzämie	hypercalcémie
ipercalciuria	Hyperkalziurie	hypercalciurie
ipercapnia	Hyperkapnie	hypercapnie
ipercolesterolemia	Hypercholesterinämie	hypercholestérolémie
iperemesi	Hyperemesis	hyperémèse
iperemia	Hyperämie	hyperémie
iperestesia	Hyperästhesie	hyperesthésie
iperestensione	Überdehnung, Überstreckung	hyperextension
iperflessione	Hyperflexion	hyperflexion
iperglicemia	Hyperglykämie	hyperglycémie
iperidrosi	Hyperhidrosis	hyperhidrose
iperkaliemia, iperpotassiemia	Hyperkaliämie	hyperkaliémie
iperlipemia	Hyperlipämie	hyperlipémie
iperlipoproteinemia	Hyperlipoproteinämie	hyperlipoprotéinémie
ipermetropia	Hypermetropie, Weitsichtigkeit	hypermétropie
ipernefroma	Hypernephrom	hypernéphrome
iperparatiroidismo	Hyperparathyreoidismus	hyperparathyroïdisme
iperplasia	Hyperplasie	hyperplasie
iperpnea	Hyperpnoe	hyperpnoïa
iperpiressia	Hyperpyrexie	hyperpyrexie
ipersensitività, ipersensibilità	Hypersensibilität, Überempfindlichkeit	hypersensibilité
ipertelorismo	Hypertelorismus	hypertélorisme
ipertensione	Hypertonie	hypertension
circolazione portale	Portalkreislauf, Pfortaderkreislauf	hypertension porte
ipertermia	Hyperthermie	hyperthermie
ipertiroidismo	Hyperthyreoidismus, Schilddrüsenüberfunktion	hyperthyroïdisme
ipertonia	Hypertension, Hypertonus	hypertonie
ipertonico	hyperton	hypertonique
ipertrofia	Hypertrophie	hypertrophie
iperventilazione	Hyperventilation	hyperventilation
ipervolemia	Hypervolämie	hypervolémie
ipoestesia	Hypästhesie	hypesthésie
ifema	Hyphaema	hyphéma
ipnosi	Hypnose	hypnose
ipnoterapia	Hypnotherapie	hypnothérapie
ipnotico (n)	Schlafmittel (n), Hypnotikum (n)	hypnotique (n)
ipnotico (a)	hypnotisch (a)	hypnotique (a)
ipocalcemia	Hypokalzämie	hypocalcémie

FRENCH	ENGLISH	SPANISH
hypocapnie	hypocapnia	hipocapnia
hypochromique	hypochromic	hipocrómico
hypocondre	hypochondrium	hipocondrio
hypocondrie	hypochondria	hipocondría
hypodermique	hypodermic	hipodérmico
hypoesthésie	hypoaesthesia (Eng), hypoesthesia (Am)	hipoestesia
hypofonction	hypofunction	hipofunción
hypogastre	hypogastrium	hipogastrio
hypoglosse	hypoglossal nerve	hipogloso
hypoglycémie	hypoglycaemia (Eng), hypoglycemia (Am)	hipoglucemia
hypohidrose	hypoidrosis	hipohidrosis
hypokalémie	hypokalaemia (Eng), hypokalemia (Am)	hipocaliemia
hypomanie	hypomania	hipomanía
hypoparathyroïdisme	hypoparathyroidism	hipoparatiroidismo
hypopharynx	hypopharynx	hipofaringe
hypophyse	pituitary gland	hipófisis
hypopituitarisme	hypopituitarism	hipopituitarismo
hypoplasie	hypoplasia	hipoplasia
hypopnée	hypopnea (Am), hypopnoea (Eng)	hipopnea
hypoprotéinémie	hypoproteinaemia (Eng), hypoproteinemia (Am)	hipoproteinemia
hypopyon	hypopyon	hipopión
hyposécrétion	hyposecretion	hiposecreción
hyposensibilité	hyposensitive	hiposensibilidad
hypospadias	hypospadias	hipospadias
hypostase	hypostasis	hipostasis
hypotension	hypotension	hipotensión
hypothalamus	hypothalamus	hipotálamo
hypothermie	hypothermia	hipotermia
hypothyroïdisme	hypothyroidism	hipotiroidismo
hypotonie	hypotonia	hipotonía
hypotonique	hypotonic	hipotónico
hypotrophie	low birth weight (LBW)	bajo peso al nacer
hypoventilation	hypoventilation	hipoventilación
hypovolémie	hypovolaemia (Eng), hypovolemia (Am), oligaemia (Eng), oligemia (Am)	hipovolemia, oligohemia
hypoxémie	hypoxaemia (Eng), hypoxemia (Am)	hipoxemia
hypoxie	hypoxia	hipoxia
hystérectomie	hysterectomy	histerectomía
hystérie	hysteria	histeria
hystéropexie abdominale	ventrofixation	ventrofijación
hystérosalpingectomie	hysterosalpingectomy	histerosalpingectomía
hystérosalpingographie	hysterosalpingography	histerosalpingografía
hystérotomie	hysterotomy	histerotomía

ITALIAN	GERMAN	FRENCH
ipocapnia	Hypokapnie	hypocapnie
ipocromico	hypochrom, farbarm	hypochromique
ipocondrio	Hypochondrium	hypocondre
ipocondria	Hypochondrie	hypocondrie
ipodermico	subkutan	hypodermique
ipoestesia	Hypästhesie	hypoesthésie
ipofunzione	Unterfunktion	hypofonction
ipogastrio	Hypogastrium	hypogastre
ipoglosso	Nervus hypoglossus	hypoglosse
ipoglicemia	Hypoglykämie	hypoglycémie
ipoidrosi	Hypohidrosis, Schweißmangel	hypohidrose
ipokalemia	Hypokaliämie	hypokalémie
ipomania	Hypomanie	hypomanie
ipoparatiroidismo	Hypoparathyreoidismus	hypoparathyroïdisme
ipofaringe	Hypopharynx	hypopharynx
ghiandola pituitaria, ipofisi	Hypophyse	hypophyse
ipopituitarismo	Hypopituitarismus	hypopituitarisme
ipoplasia	Hypoplasie	hypoplasie
ipopnea	flache Atmung	hypopnée
ipoproteinemia	Hypoproteinämie	hypoprotéinémie
ipopion	Hypopyon	hypopyon
iposecrezione	Sekretionsmangel, Sekretionsschwäche	hyposécrétion
iposensitività, iposensibilità	hyposensibel, unterempfindlich	hyposensibilité
ipospadia	Hypospadie	hypospadias
ipostasi	Hypostase	hypostase
ipotensione	Hypotonie	hypotension
ipotalamo	Hypothalamus	hypothalamus
ipotermia	Hypothermie	hypothermie
ipotiroidismo	Hypothyreose	hypothyroïdisme
ipotonia	Hypotonie	hypotonie
ipotonico	hypoton	hypotonique
basso peso alla nascita	niedriges Geburtsgewicht	hypotrophie
ipoventilazione	Hypoventilation	hypoventilation
ipovolemia, oligoemia	Hypovolämie, Oligämie, Blutmangel	hypovolémie
ipossiemia	Hypoxämie	hypoxémie
ipossia	Hypoxie	hypoxie
isterectomia	Hysterektomie	hystérectomie
isteria	Hysterie	hystérie
ventro-fissazione	Hysteropexie	hystéropexie abdominale
isterosalpingectomia	Hysterosalpingektomie	hystérosalpingectomie
isterosalpingografia	Hysterosalpingographie	hystérosalpingographie
isterotomia	Hysterotomie	hystérotomie

I

iatrogène	iatrogenic	yatrógeno
ichthyose	ichthyosis	ictiosis
ictère	icterus	ictericia
ictère cérébral	kernicterus	ictericia nuclear
idée	idea	idea
identification	identification	identificación
idiopathique	idiopathic	idiopático
idiosyncrasie	idiosyncrasy	idiosincrasia
iléite	ileitis	ileítis
iléite régionale	regional ileitis	ileítis regional
iléocaecal	ileocaecal (Eng), ileocecal (Am)	ileocecal
iléoctomie	ileectomy	ileoctomía
iléon	ileum	ileón
iléostomie	ileostomy	ileostomía
iléus	ileus	íleo
iliaque	iliac	ilíaco
ilion	ilium	ilion
illusion	illusion	ilusión
îlots de Langerhans	islets of Langerhans, pancreatic islets	islotes de Langerhans, islotes pancreáticos
îlots pancréatiques	islets of Langerhans, pancreatic islets	islotes de Langerhans, islotes pancreáticos
imagerie par résonance magnétique	magnetic resonance imaging (MRI)	formación de imágenes por resonancia magnética
immédiatement après le début	immediately after onset (IAO)	inmediatamente después del comienzo
immun	immune	inmune
immunisation	immunization	inmunización
immunité	immunity	inmunidad
immunodéficience	immunodeficiency	inmunodeficiencia
immunodosage	immunoassay	inmunoensayo
immunofluorescence	immunofluorescence	inmunofluorescencia
immunoglobuline (Ig)	immunoglobulin (Ig)	inmunoglobulina (Ig)
immunologie	immunology	inmunología
immunosuppression	immunosuppression	inmunosupresión
imperforé	imperforate	imperforado
impétigo	impetigo	impétigo
implant	implant	implante
implantation	implantation	implantación
implanter	implant	implantar
impotence	impotence	impotencia
impulsion	impulse	impulso
inadaptation	maladjustment	inadaptación
incarcéré	incarcerated	incarcerado
inceste	incest	incesto
incision	incision	incisión

ITALIAN	GERMAN	FRENCH
iatrogeno	iatrogen	**iatrogène**
ittiosi	Ichthyosis	**ichthyose**
ittero	Ikterus, Gelbsucht	**ictère**
ittero nucleare	Kernikterus	**ictère cérébral**
idea	Gedanke, Vorstellung	**idée**
indentificazione	Identifizierung	**identification**
idiopatico	idiopathisch, essentiell	**idiopathique**
idiosincrasia	Idiosynkrasie	**idiosyncrasie**
ileite	Ileitis	**iléite**
ileite regionale	Ileitis regionalis	**iléite régionale**
ileocecale	ileozäkal	**iléocaecal**
ileectomia	Ileumresektion	**iléoctomie**
ileo	Ileum	**iléon**
ileostomia	Ileostomie	**iléostomie**
ileo, occlusione intestinale acuta	Ileus, Darmverschluß	**iléus**
iliaco	ileo-	**Iliaque**
ilio, osso dell'anca	Os ilium	**ilion**
illusione	Illusion	**illusion**
isole di Langerhans, isolotti pancreatici	Langerhans-Inseln	**îlots de Langerhans**
isole di Langerhans, isolotti pancreatici	Langerhans-Inseln	**îlots pancréatiques**
indagine morfologica con risonanza magnetica	Kernspintomographie (NMR)	**imagerie par résonance magnétique**
immediatamente dopo l'attacco	unmittelbar nach Krankheitsausbruch	**immédiatement après le début**
immune	immun	**immun**
immunizzazione	Immunisierung, Schutzimpfung	**immunisation**
immunità	Immunität	**immunité**
immunodeficienza	Immundefekt	**immunodéficience**
dosaggio immunologico	Immunoassay	**immunodosage**
immunofluorescenza	Immunfluoreszenz	**immunofluorescence**
immunoglobulina (Ig)	Immunglobulin	**immunoglobuline (Ig)**
immunologia	Immunologie	**immunologie**
immunosoppressione	Immunsuppression	**immunosuppression**
imperforato	nicht perforiert	**imperforé**
impetigine	Impetigo	**impétigo**
impianto chirurgico sottocutaneo di farmaci	Implantat	**implant**
impianto	Implantation	**implantation**
impiantare	Implantieren	**implanter**
impotenza	Impotenz	**impotence**
impulso	Impuls, Reiz	**impulsion**
assestamento difettoso	Fehlanpassung	**inadaptation**
incarcerato	inkarzeriert, eingeklemmt	**incarcéré**
incesto	Inzest	**inceste**
incisione	Inzision, Einschnitt	**incision**

FRENCH	ENGLISH	SPANISH
incisive	incisor	incisivo
incompatibilité	incompatibility	incompatibilidad
incompatibilité Rhésus	Rhesus incompatibility	incompatibilidad Rhesus
incompétence	incompetence	incompetencia
incontinence	incontinence	incontinencia
incontinence nocturne	bedwetting	enuresis nocturna
incoordination	incoordination	incoordinación
incubateur	incubator	incubadora
incubation	incubation	incubación
index	trigger finger	dedo en gatillo
index de thyroxine libre	free thyroxine index (FTI)	indice de tiroxina libre
indicateur	indicator	indicador
indice d'Apgar	Apgar score	índice de Apgar
indice de masse corporelle (IMC)	body mass index (BMI)	índice de masa corporal (IMC)
indifférence	'belle indifference'	la belle indifférence
indigène	indigenous	indígena
indigeste	queasy	nauseabundo
indigestion	indigestion	indigestión
induction	induction	inducción
induration	induration	induración
inertie	inertia	inercia
infantile	infantile	infantil
infarcissement	infarction	infarto
infarctus du myocarde	myocardial infarction (MI)	infarto de miocardio (IM)
infectieux	infective	infeccioso
infection	infection	infección
infection des voies respiratoires supérieures	upper respiratory tract infection (URTI)	infección de las vías respiratorias altas
infection des voies urinaires	urinary tract infection (UTI)	infección de las vías urinarias (IVU)
infection du poumon profond	lower respiratory tract infection (LRTI)	infección de las vías respiratorias bajas
infection opportuniste	opportunistic infection	infección oportunista
inférieur	inferior	inferior
infertilité	infertility	infertilidad
infestation	infestation	infestación
infiltration	infiltration	infiltración
infirmière	nurse	enfermera
infirmité motrice cérébrale	cerebral palsy	parálisis cerebral
inflammation	inflammation	inflamación
infusion	infusion	infusión
ingestion	ingestion	ingestión
inguinal	inguinal	inguinal
inhalation	inhalation	inhalación
inhaler	inhale	inhalar
inhérent	inherent	inherente
inhibiteur de la monoamine-oxydase (IMAO)	monoamine oxidase inhibitor (MAOI)	inhibidor de la monoaminooxidasa (IMAO)

ITALIAN	GERMAN	FRENCH
incisore	Schneidezahn	incisive
incompatibilità	Inkompatibilität, Unverträglichkeit	incompatibilité
incompatibilità Rh	Rh-Unverträglichkeit	incompatibilité Rhésus
incompetenza	Insuffizienz	incompétence
incontinenza	Inkontinenz	incontinence
enuresi notturna	Bettnässen	incontinence nocturne
incoordinazione	Inkoordination	incoordination
incubatore	Inkubator, Brutkasten	incubateur
incubazione	Inkubation	incubation
dito a scatto	schnellender Finger	index
indice di tiroxina libera	freier Thyroxinindex (FTi)	index de thyroxine libre
indicatore	Indikator	indicateur
indice di Apgar	Apgar-Index	indice d'Apgar
indice di massa corporea (IMC)	Körpermassenindex	indice de masse corporelle (IMC)
'belle indifference'	belle indifference	indifférence
indigeno	eingeboren, einheimisch	indigène
nauseabondo, nauseato, a disagio	unwohl, übel	indigeste
indigestione	Verdauungsstörung, Magenverstimmung	indigestion
induzione	Induktion, Einleitung	induction
indurimento	Induration, Verhärtung	induration
inerzia	Trägheitsmoment, Untätigkeit	inertie
infantile	infantil, kindlich	infantile
infarto	Infarzierung	infarcissement
infarto miocardico	Myokardinfarkt, Herzinfarkt	infarctus du myocarde
infettivo	infektiös, ansteckend	infectieux
infezione	Infektion	infection
infezione del tratto respiratorio superiore (URTI)	Atemwegsinfekt	infection des voies respiratoires supérieures
infezione delle vie urinarie (IVU)	Harnwegsinfekt	infection des voies urinaires
infezione del tratto respiratorio inferiore (LRTI)	Atemwegsinfekt (untere)	infection du poumon profond
infezione opportunista	opportunistische Infektion	infection opportuniste
inferiore	tiefer gelegen, minderwertig	inférieur
infertilità	Infertilität	infertilité
infestazione	Befall	infestation
infiltrazione	Infiltration	infiltration
infermiere	Krankenschwester, Schwester, Pflegerin	infirmière
paralisi cerebrale	Zerebralparese	infirmité motrice cérébrale
infiammazione	Entzündung	inflammation
infusione	Infusion	infusion
ingestione	Einnahme, Aufnahme	ingestion
inguinale	inguinal, Leisten-	inguinal
inalazione	Inhalation, Einatmen	inhalation
inalare	inhalieren, einatmen	inhaler
inerente	eigen, angeboren	inhérent
inibitore monoaminoossidasi (IMAO)	Monoaminoxydase-Hemmer	inhibiteur de la monoamine-oxydase (IMAO)

FRENCH	ENGLISH	SPANISH
inhibition	inhibition	inhibición
injecter	inject	inyectar
injection	injection	inyección
innervation	innervation	inervación
innocent	innocent	inocente
inoculation	inoculation	inoculación
inoffensif	innocuous	inocuo
inorganique	inorganic	inorgánico
inotrope	inotropic	inotrópico
insémination	insemination	inseminación
insémination artificielle (IA)	artificial insemination (AI)	inseminación artificial
insémination hétérologue	artificial insemination by donor (AID)	inseminación artificial por donante (AID)
insensible	insensible	insensible
insertion	insertion	inserción
insidieux	insidious	insidioso
in situ	in situ	in situ
insolation	sunstroke	insolación
insomnie	insomnia	insomnio
inspiration	inspiration	inspiración
instillation	instillation	instilación
instinct	instinct	instinto
institutionalisation	institutionalization	institucionalización
insuffisance basilaire vertébrale	basilar-vertebral insufficiency	insuficiencia vértebrobasilar
insuffisance cardiaque	heart disease	cardiopatía
insuffisance cardiaque globale	congestive cardiac failure (CCF), congestive heart failure (CHF)	insuficiencia cardíaca congestiva (ICC)
insuffisance coronarienne cardiaque	coronary heart disease (CHD), coronary heart failure (CHF)	enfermedad coronaria, cardiopatía isquémica, insuficiencia coronaria
insuffisance coronarienne chronique	chronic coronary insufficiency (CCI)	insuficiencia coronaria crónico
insuffisance coronarienne globale	coronary artery disease (CAD)	enfermedad arterial coronaria, cardiopatía isquémica
insuffisance placentaire	placental insufficiency	insuficiencia placentaria
insuffisance respiratoire	respiratory failure	insuficiencia respiratoria
insuffisance vertébro-basilaire	vertebrobasilar insufficiency (VBI)	insuficiencia vertebrobasilar
insufflation	insufflation	insuflación
insuline	insulin	insulina
intellect	intellect	intelecto
intelligence	intelligence	inteligencia
interaction	interaction	interacción
interarticulaire	interarticular	interarticular
intercostal	intercostal	intercostal
intercurrent	intercurrent	intercurrente
interépineux	interspinous	interespinoso
interleukine	interleukin	interleucina
intermenstruel	intermenstrual	intermenstrual
intermittent	intermittent	intermitente
interne	internal, medial	interno, medial

ITALIAN	GERMAN	FRENCH
inibizione	Inhibierung, Hemmung	**inhibition**
iniettare	injizieren, spritzen	**injecter**
iniezione	Injektion, Spritze	**injection**
innervazione	Innervation	**innervation**
innocente	unschuldig, unschädlich	**innocent**
inoculazione	Impfung	**inoculation**
innocuo	unschädlich, harmlos	**inoffensif**
inorganico	anorganisch	**inorganique**
inotropo	inotrop	**inotrope**
inseminazione	Befruchtung	**insémination**
inseminazione artificiale	künstliche Befruchtung	**insémination artificielle (IA)**
fecondazione artificiale tramite donatore	heterologe Insemination	**insémination hétérologue**
insensibile	bewußtlos, unempfindlich	**insensible**
inserzione	Insertion	**insertion**
insidioso	heimtückisch, schleichend	**insidieux**
in situ	in situ	**in situ**
colpo di sole	Sonnenstich	**insolation**
insonnia	Schlaflosigkeit	**insomnie**
inspirazione	Inspiration, Einatmung	**inspiration**
istillazione	Einträufelung, Einflößung	**instillation**
istinto	Instinkt	**instinct**
istituzionalizzazione	Institutionalisierung	**institutionalisation**
insufficienza vertebrobasilare	Basilarvertebralinsuffizienz	**insuffisance basilaire vertébrale**
malattia cardiaca	Herzerkrankung, Herzleiden	**insuffisance cardiaque**
insufficienza cardiaca congestizia, scompenso cardiaco congestizio	Stauungsherz, Herzinsuffizienz mit Stauungszeichen	**insuffisance cardiaque globale**
malattia cardiaca coronarica (MCC), insufficienza cardiaca coronarica	koronare Herzkrankheit (KHK), Herzinfarkt	**insuffisance coronarienne cardiaque**
insufficienza coronarica cronica	chronische Koronarinsuffizienz	**insuffisance coronarienne chronique**
malattia delle arterie coronarica (MAC)	Koronaropathie	**insuffisance coronarienne globale**
insufficienza placentare	Plazentainsuffizienz	**insuffisance placentaire**
insufficienza respiratoria	respiratorische Insuffizienz	**insuffisance respiratoire**
insufficienza vertebrobasilare	vertebrobasiläre Insuffizienz	**insuffisance vertébro-basilaire**
insufflazione	Insufflation	**insufflation**
insulina	Insulin	**insuline**
intelletto	Intellekt	**intellect**
intelligenza	Intelligenz	**intelligence**
interazione	Wechselwirkung	**interaction**
interarticolare	interartikulär	**interarticulaire**
intercostale	interkostal	**intercostal**
intercorrente	interkurrent	**intercurrent**
interspinoso	interspinal	**interépineux**
interleuchina	Interleukin	**interleukine**
intermestruale	intermenstruel	**intermenstruel**
intermittente	intermittierend	**intermittent**
interno, mediale	intern, innerlich, medial	**interne**

FRENCH	ENGLISH	SPANISH
interosseux	interosseous	interóseo
interruption de grossesse (IG)	termination of pregnancy (TOP)	interrupción del embarazo
interstitiel	interstitial	intersticial
intertrigo	intertrigo	intertrigo
intertrochantérien	intertrochanteric	intertrocantéreo
intervertébral	intervertebral	intervertebral
intestin	bowel, gut, intestine	intestino
intima	intima	íntima
intolérance	intolerance	intolerancia
intoxication alimentaire	food poisoning	intoxicación alimentaria
intoxication par inhalation de solvant	glue sniffing	inhalación de pegamento
intoxication volontaire	self-poisoning	autointoxicación
intra-abdominal	intra-abdominal	intraabdominal
intra-artériel	intra-arterial	intraarterial
intracapsulaire	intracapsular	intracapsular
intracellulaire	intracellular	intracelular
intradermique	intradermal	intradérmico
intramural	intramural	intramural
intramusculaire (IM)	intramuscular (IM)	intramuscular (im)
intranasal	intranasal	intranasal
intra-oculaire	intraocular	intraocular
intra-oral	intraoral	intraoral
intrapartum	intrapartum	intra partum
intrapéritonéal	intraperitoneal	intraperitoneal
intrathécal	intrathecal	intratecal
intra-utérin	intrauterine	intrauterino
intravaginal	intravaginal	intravaginal
intraveineux (IV)	intravenous (IV)	intravenoso (IV)
intrinsèque	intrinsic	intrínseco
introspection	introspection	introspección
introversion	introversion	introversión
introverti	introvert	introvertido
intubation	airway breathing and circulation (ABC), intubation	vías respiratorias y circulación, intubación
intussusception	intussusception	intususcepción
invagination	invagination	invaginación
invasion	invasion	invasión
inversion	inversion	inversión
in vitro	in vitro	in vitro
in vivo	in vivo	in vivo
involontaire	involuntary	involuntario
involution	involution	involución
iode	iodine	yodo
ion	ion	ión
ipsilatéral	ipsilateral	ipsilateral
iris	iris	iris
iritis	iritis	iritis

ITALIAN	GERMAN	FRENCH
interosseo	interossär	interosseux
interruzione di gravidanza (IG)	Schwangerschaftsabbruch	interruption de grossesse (IG)
interstiziale	interstitiell	interstitiel
intertrigine	Intertrigo	intertrigo
intertrocanterico	intertrochantär	intertrochantérien
intervertebrale	intervertebral, Zwischenwirbel-	intervertébral
intestino	Darm	intestin
intima	Intima	intima
intolleranza	Intoleranz, Unverträglichkeit	intolérance
avvelenamento alimentare	Nahrungsmittelvergiftung	intoxication alimentaire
inalazione di toluene o collanti	Schnüffeln, Leimschnüffeln	intoxication par inhalation de solvant
autoavvelenamento	Selbstvergiftung	intoxication volontaire
intra-addominale	intraabdominal	intra-abdominal
intra-arterioso	intraarteriell	intra-artériel
intracapsulare	intrakapsulär	intracapsulaire
intracellulare	intrazellulär	intracellulaire
intradermico	intradermal, intrakutan	intradermique
intramurale	intramural	intramural
intramuscolare (IM)	intramuskulär	intramusculaire (IM)
intranasale	intranasal	intranasal
intraoculare	intraokulär	intra-oculaire
intraorale	intraoral	intra-oral
intraparto	intra partum	intrapartum
intraperitoneale	intraperitoneal	intrapéritonéal
intratecale	intrathekal	intrathécal
intrauterino	intrauterin	intra-utérin
intravaginale	intravaginal	intravaginal
endovenoso (EV)	intravenös, endovenös	intraveineux (IV)
intrinseco	intrinsisch, endogen	intrinsèque
introspezione	Introspektion	introspection
introversione	Introversion	introversion
introverso	Introvertierter	introverti
ventilazione e respirazione nelle vie respiratorie, intubazione	Luftwege Atmung und Kreislauf (ABC-Regel), Intubation	intubation
intussuscezione	Intussuszeption	intussusception
invaginazione	Invagination	invagination
invasione	Invasion	invasion
inversione	Inversion, Umkehrung	inversion
in vitro	in vitro	in vitro
in vivo	in vivo	in vivo
involontario	unabsichtlich, unwillkürlich	involontaire
involuzione	Involution, Rückbildung	involution
iodio	Jod	iode
ione	Ion	ion
ipsilaterale, omolaterale	ipsilateral	ipsilatéral
iride	Iris	iris
irite	Iritis	iritis

FRENCH	ENGLISH	SPANISH
irradiation	irradiation	irradiación
irréductible	irreducible	irreductible
irrigation	irrigation	irrigación
irritable	irritable	irritable
irritant	irritant	irritante
ischémie	ischaemia (Eng), ischemia (Am)	isquemia
ischion	ischium	isquión
ischio-rectal	ischiorectal	isquiorrectal
iso-immunisation	isoimmunization	isoinmunización
isolement	isolation	aislamiento
isométrique	isometric	isométrico
isotonique	isotonic	isotónico
isthme	isthmus	istmo

ITALIAN	GERMAN	FRENCH
irradiazione	Bestrahlung	irradiation
irriducibile	unreduzierbar	irréductible
irrigazione	Spülung	irrigation
irritabile	reizbar, erregbar	irritable
irritante	reizend	irritant
ischemia	Ischämie	ischémie
ischio	Ischium, Sitzbein	ischion
ischiorettale	ischiorektal	ischio-rectal
isoimmunizzazione	Isoimmunisierung	iso-immunisation
isolamento	Isolierung	isolement
isometrico	isometrisch	isométrique
isotonico	isotonisch	isotonique
istmo	Isthmus, Verengung	isthme

FRENCH	ENGLISH	SPANISH

J

jambe	leg	pierna
jaunisse	jaundice	ictericia
jéjunum	jejunum	yeyuno
jointure	knuckle	nudillo
joue	cheek	mejilla
jumeau	twin	mellizo
jumeaux univitellins	identical twins	gemelos idénticos

K

kala-azar	kala-azar	kala-azar
karyotype	karyotype	cariotipo
kératine	keratin	queratina
kératinisation	keratinization	queratinización
kératite	keratitis	queratitis
kératocèle	keratocele	queratocele
kératoconjonctivite	keratoconjunctivitis	queratoconjuntivitis
kératomalacie	keratomalacia	queratomalacia
kératome	keratome	queratoma
kératose	keratosis	queratosis
kinase	kinase	cinasa
koïlonychie	koilonychia	coiloniquia
kraurosis de la vulve	kraurosis vulvae	craurosis vulvar
kwashiorkor	kwashiorkor	kwashiorkor
kyste	cyst	quiste
kyste chocolat	chocolate cyst	quiste de chocolate
kyste hydatique	hydatid	quiste hidatídico

ITALIAN	GERMAN	FRENCH
arto, gamba, membro	Bein	**jambe**
ittero	Ikterus, Gelbsucht	**jaunisse**
digiuno	Jejunum	**jéjunum**
articolazione interfalangea	Knöchel	**jointure**
guancia	Wange, Backe	**joue**
gemello	Zwilling	**jumeau**
gemelli omozigoti	eineiige Zwillinge	**jumeaux univitellins**
kala-azar	Kala-Azar	**kala-azar**
cariotipo	Karyotyp	**karyotype**
cheratina	Keratin	**kératine**
cheratinizzazione	Keratinisation, Verhornung	**kératinisation**
cheratite	Keratitis, Hornhautentzündung	**kératite**
cheratocele	Keratozele	**kératocèle**
cheratocongiuntivite	Keratokonjunktivitis	**kératoconjonctivite**
cheratomalacia	Keratomalazie	**kératomalacie**
cheratomo	Keratotom	**kératome**
cheratosi	Keratose	**kératose**
chinasi	Kinase	**kinase**
coilonichia	Koilonychie, Löffelnagel	**koïlonychie**
craurosi vulvare	Craurosis vulvae	**kraurosis de la vulve**
kwashiorkor	Kwashiorkor	**kwashiorkor**
cisti	Zyste	**kyste**
cisti cioccolato (c. emosiderinica dell'endometriosi)	Schokoladenzyste, Teerzyste	**kyste chocolat**
cisti idatidea	Hydatide	**kyste hydatique**

L

FRENCH	ENGLISH	SPANISH
labile	labile	lábil
labilité	lability	labilidad
labyrinthe	labyrinth	laberinto
labyrinthite	labyrinthitis	laberintitis
lacéré	lacerated	lacerado
lacrymal	lacrimal	lagrimal
lactase	lactase	lactasa
lactate	lactate	lactato
lactation	lactation	lactación
lactose	lactose	lactosa
lactulose	lactulose	lactulosa
lait	milk	leche
lambeau	flap	colgajo, injerto
lame	lamina	lámina
laminectomie	laminectomy	laminectomía
langue	glossa, tongue	lengua
lanière	lash	pestaña
lanugo	lanugo	lanugo
laparotomie	laparotomy	laparotomía
larmes	tears	lágrimas
laryngien	laryngeal	laríngeo
laryngite	laryngitis	laringitis
laryngologie	laryngology	laringología
laryngoscope	laryngoscope	laringoscopio
laryngospasme	laryngospasm	laringospasmo
laryngotrachéobronchite	laryngotracheobronchitis	laringotraqueobronquitis
larynx	larynx	laringe
laser	laser	láser
latéral	lateral	lateral
lavage	lavage	lavado
lavement	enema	enema
lavement au baryte	barium enema	enema de bario
laxatif (n)	aperient (n), laxative (n)	laxante (n)
laxatif (a)	aperient (a), laxative (a)	laxante (a), laxativo (a)
lécithine	lecithin	lecitina
Leishmania donovani	Leishman-Donovan body	cuerpo de Leishman-Donovan
leishmaniose	leishmaniasis	leishmaniasis
lente	nit	liendre
lentigo	lentigo	lentigo
lentille	lens	cristalino
lèpre	leprosy	lepra
leptospirose	leptospirosis	leptospirosis
lesbien	lesbian	lesbiana
lésion	lesion	lesión
létal	lethal	letal

ITALIAN	GERMAN	FRENCH
labile	labil	labile
labilità	Labilität	labilité
labirinto	Labyrinth	labyrinthe
labirintite	Labyrinthitis	labyrinthite
lacerato	eingerissen, zerrissen	lacéré
lacrimale	Tränen-, Tränengangs-	lacrymal
lattasi	Laktase	lactase
lattato	Laktat	lactate
lattazione	Laktation, Milchbildung, Stillen	lactation
lattosio	Laktose, Milchzucker	lactose
lattulosio	Laktulose	lactulose
latte	Milch	lait
lembo, innesto	Lappen, Hautlappen	lambeau
lamina	Lamina	lame
laminectomia	Laminektomie, Wirbelbogenresektion	laminectomie
lingua	Zunge	langue
ciglio	Wimper	lanière
lanugine	Lanugo	lanugo
laparotomia	Laparotomie	laparotomie
lacrime	Tränen	larmes
laringeo	laryngeal, Kehlkopf-	laryngien
laringite	Laryngitis	laryngite
laringologia	Laryngologie	laryngologie
laringoscopio	Laryngoskop, Kehlkopfspiegel	laryngoscope
laringospasmo	Laryngospasmus	laryngospasme
laringotracheobronchite	Laryngo-Tracheobronchitis	laryngotrachéobronchite
laringe	Larynx, Kehlkopf	larynx
laser	Laser	laser
laterale	lateral, seitlich	latéral
lavaggio	Spülung	lavage
clistere	Klistier, Einlauf	lavement
clisma opaco	Bariumeinlauf	lavement au baryte
lassativo (n)	Abführmittel (n), Laxans (n)	laxatif (n)
lassativo (a),	abführend (a), laxierend (a)	laxatif (a)
lecitina	Lezithin	lécithine
corpi di Leishman-Donovan	Leishman-Donovan-Körper	Leishmania donovani
leishmaniosi	Leishmaniose	leishmaniose
lendine	Nisse	lente
lentiggine	Lentigo	lentigo
lente	Linse	lentille
lebbra	Lepra, Aussatz	lèpre
leptospirosi	Leptospirose	leptospirose
lesbismo	lesbisch	lesbien
lesione	Läsion, Verletzung	lésion
letale	letal, tödlich	létal

FRENCH	ENGLISH	SPANISH
léthal	lethal	letal
léthargie	lethargy	letargo
leucémie	leukaemia (Eng), leukemia (Am)	leucemia
leucémie humaine à lymphocytes T	human T-cell leukaemia virus (HTLV) (Eng), human T-cell leukemia virus (HTLV) (Am)	leucemia por virus humano de las células T
leucocyte	leucocyte (Eng), leukocyte (Am)	leucocito
leucocytose	leucocytosis (Eng), leukocytosis (Am)	leucocitosis
leucopénie	leucopenia (Eng), leukopenia (Am)	leucopenia
leucoplasie	leucoplakia (Eng), leukoplakia (Am)	leucoplasia
leucorrhée	leucorrhea (Eng), leukorrhea (Am)	leucorrea
leucotomie	leucotomy (Eng), leukotomy (Am)	leucotomía
lèvre	lip	labio
lèvres	labia	labios
levure	yeast	levadura
libido	libido	líbido
libre	patent	permeable
lichen	lichen	líquen
lichénification	lichenification	liquenificación
lié au sexe	sex-linked	vinculado al sexo
ligament	ligament	ligamento
ligaments larges	broad ligament	ligamento ancho
ligature	ligature	ligadura
ligaturer	ligate	ligar
ligne	linea	línea
limaçon osseux	cochlea	cóclea
linctus	linctus	linctus
liniment	liniment	linimento
lipase	lipase	lipasa
lipémie	lipaemia (Eng), lipemia (Am)	lipemia
lipide	lipid	lípido
lipidose	lipidosis	lipidosis
lipochondrodystrophie	lipochondrodystrophy	lipocondrodistrofia
lipodystrophie	lipodystrophy	lipodistrofia
lipolyse	lipolysis	lipolisis
lipome	lipoma	lipoma
lipoprotéine	lipoprotein	lipoproteína
lipoprotéine de basse densité (LBD)	low density lipoprotein (LDL)	lipoproteína de baja densidad (LDL)
lipoprotéine de haute densité (LHD)	high density lipoprotein (HDL)	lipoproteína de alta densidad (HDL)
lipoprotéine de très faible densité	very low density lipoprotein (VLDL)	lipoproteína de muy baja densidad (VLDL)
liquide	liquor	licor
liquide amniotique	amniotic fluid	líquido amniótico
liquide céphalo-rachidien	cerebrospinal fluid (CSF)	líquido cefalorraquídeo (LCR)
liquide de Brompton	Brompton's mixture	mezcla de Brompton
liquide de Hartmann	Hartmann's solution	solución de Hartmann

ITALIAN	GERMAN	FRENCH
letale	letal, tödlich	**léthal**
letargia	Lethargie	**léthargie**
leucemia	Leukämie	**leucémie**
virus della leucemia a cellule T	human T-cell leukemia virus (HTLV)	**leucémie humaine à lymphocytes T**
leucocito	Leukozyt	**leucocyte**
leucocitosi	Leukozytose	**leucocytose**
leucopenia	Leukopenie	**leucopénie**
leucoplachia	Leukoplakie	**leucoplasie**
leucorrea	Leukorrhoe	**leucorrhée**
leucotomia	Leukotomie	**leucotomie**
labbro	Lippe	**lèvre**
labbra	Labia	**lèvres**
lievito	Hefe, Hefepilz	**levure**
desiderio sessuale	Libido	**libido**
aperto, esposto	offen, durchgängig	**libre**
lichene	Lichen	**lichen**
lichenificazione	Lichenifikation	**lichénification**
legato al sesso	geschlechtsgebunden	**lié au sexe**
ligamento	Ligament, Band	**ligament**
legamento largo	ligamentum latum uteri	**ligaments larges**
legatura	Ligatur, Gefäßunterbindung	**ligature**
legare	abbinden	**ligaturer**
linea	Linea, Linie	**ligne**
coclea	Cochlea, Schnecke	**limaçon osseux**
sciroppo	Linctus	**linctus**
linimento	Liniment, Einreibemittel	**liniment**
lipasi	Lipase	**lipase**
lipemia	Lipämie	**lipémie**
lipide	Lipid	**lipide**
lipoidosi	Lipidose	**lipidose**
lipocondrodistrofia	Lipochondrodystrophie	**lipochondrodystrophie**
lipodistrofia	Lipodystrophie	**lipodystrophie**
lipolisi	Lipolyse	**lipolyse**
lipoma	Lipom	**lipome**
lipoproteina	Lipoprotein	**lipoprotéine**
lipoproteina a bassa densità (LBD)	low density lipoprotein (LDL)	**lipoprotéine de basse densité (LBD)**
lipoproteina ad alta densità (LAD)	high density lipoprotein (HDL)	**lipoprotéine de haute densité (LHD)**
lipoproteina a bassissima densità	Lipoprotein sehr geringer Dichte	**lipoprotéine de très faible densité**
liquido	Liquor, Flüssigkeit	**liquide**
fluido amniotico	Amnionflüssigkeit, Fruchtwasser	**liquide amniotique**
liquido cerebrospinale (LCS)	Liquor	**liquide céphalo-rachidien**
soluzione di Brompton	Brompton-Lösung (Alkohol, Morphin, Kokain)	**liquide de Brompton**
soluzione di Hartmann	Hartmann-Lösung	**liquide de Hartmann**

FRENCH	ENGLISH	SPANISH
liste d'attente	waiting list	lista de espera
lithonéphrotomie	lithonephrotomy	litonefrotomía
lithotomie	lithotomy	litotomía
lithotripsie	lithotripsy	litotripsia
lithotriteur	lithotriptor, lithotrite	litotriptor, litotritor
lithotritie	lithotripsy	litotripsia
livide	livid	lívido
livraison	delivery	parto
livres par pouce carré (psi)	pounds per square inch (psi)	libras por pulgada cuadrada (psi)
lobe	lobe	lóbulo
lobectomie	lobectomy	lobectomía
lobotomie	lobotomy	lobotomía
lobule	lobule	lóbulo
localiser	localize	localizar
lochies	lochia	loquios
locomoteur	locomotor	locomotor
loculé	loculated	loculado
lombaire	lumbar	lumbar
lombo-sacré	lumbosacral	lumbosacro
lordose	lordosis	lordosis
lucide	lucid	lúcido
lumbago	lumbago	lumbago
lumière	lumen	luz
lupus	lupus	lupus
lupus érythémateux	lupus erythematosus	lupus eritematoso
lupus érythémateux systémique	systemic lupus erythematosus (SLE)	lupus eritematoso sistémico (LES)
lymphadénectomie	lymphadenectomy	linfadenectomía
lymphadénite	lymphadenitis	linfadenitis
lymphadénopathie	lymphadenopathy	linfadenopatía
lymphangite	lymphangitis	linfangitis
lymphatique	lymphatic	linfático
lymphe	lymph	linfa
lymphoblaste	lymphoblast	linfoblasto
lymphocyte	lymphocyte	linfocito
lymphocytose	lymphocytosis	linfocitosis
lymphoedème	lymphedema (Am), lymphoedema (Eng)	linfedema
lymphogranulome vénérien	lymphogranuloma inguinale	linfogranuloma inguinal
lymphokine	lymphokine	linfocinesis
lymphome	lymphoma	linfoma
lymphosarcome	lymphosarcoma	linfosarcoma
lyse	lysis	lisis
lysosome	lysosome	lisosoma
lysozyme	lysozyme	lisozima

ITALIAN	GERMAN	FRENCH
lista d'attesa	Warteliste	**liste d'attente**
litonefrotomia	Nephrolithotomie	**lithonéphrotomie**
litotomia	Lithotomie	**lithotomie**
litotripsia	Lithotripsie	**lithotripsie**
litotritore	Lithotriptor	**lithotriteur**
litotripsia	Lithotripsie	**lithotritie**
livido	livide, bleich	**livide**
parto	Entbindung, Geburt	**livraison**
libbre per pollici quadrati	pounds per square inch (psi)	**livres par pouce carré (psi)**
lobo	Lappen (Organ-)	**lobe**
lobectomia	Lobektomie, Lungenlappenresektion	**lobectomie**
lobotomia	Lobotomie, Leukotomie	**lobotomie**
lobulo	Lobulus, Läppchen	**lobule**
localizzare	lokalisieren	**localiser**
lochi puerperali	Lochien, Wochenfluß	**lochies**
locomotore	fortbewegend, Bewegungs-	**locomoteur**
loculato	gekammert	**loculé**
lombare	Lumbal-, Lenden-	**lombaire**
lombosacrale	lumbosakral	**lombo-sacré**
lordosi	Lordose	**lordose**
lucido	glänzend, bei Bewußtsein	**lucide**
lombaggine	Lumbago, Hexenschuß	**lumbago**
lume	Lumen, Durchmesser	**lumière**
lupus	Lupus	**lupus**
lupus eritematoso	Lupus erythematodes	**lupus érythémateux**
lupus eritematoso sistemico (LES)	systemischer Lupus erythematodes, Lupus erythematodes visceralis (SLE)	**lupus érythémateux systémique**
linfoadenectomia	Lymphadenektomie	**lymphadénectomie**
linfadenite	Lymphadenitis	**lymphadénite**
linfadenopatia	Lymphadenopathie	**lymphadénopathie**
linfangite	Lymphangitis	**lymphangite**
linfatico	lymphatisch, Lymph-	**lymphatique**
linfa	Lymphe	**lymphe**
linfoblasto	Lymphoblast	**lymphoblaste**
linfocito	Lymphozyt	**lymphocyte**
linfocitosi	Lymphozytose	**lymphocytose**
linfedema	Lymphödem	**lymphoedème**
linfogranuloma inguinale	Lymphogranuloma inguinale	**lymphogranulome vénérien**
linfochina	Lymphokine	**lymphokine**
linfoma	Lymphom	**lymphome**
linfosarcoma	Lymphosarkom	**lymphosarcome**
lisi	Lysis	**lyse**
lisosoma	Lysosom	**lysosome**
lisozima	Lysozym	**lysozyme**

M

FRENCH	ENGLISH	SPANISH
macération	maceration	maceración
mâchoire	jaw-bone	mandíbula
macrocéphalie	macrocephaly	macrocefalia
macrocyte	macrocyte	macrocito
macrophage	macrophage	macrófago
macroscopique	macroscopic	macroscópico
macule	macula, macule	mácula
maculopapuleux	maculopapular	maculopapular
main	hand	mano
mal	mal	mal
malabsorption	malabsorption	malabsorción
malacie	malacia	malacia
malade à déficit immunitaire	immunocompromised patient	paciente inmunocomprometido
malade à suppression immunitaire	immunosuppressed patient	paciente inmunosuprimido
maladie	illness, disease	enfermedad
maladie à déclaration obligatoire	notifiable disease	enfermedad declarable
maladie auto-immune	autoimmune disease	enfermedad autoinmune
maladie coeliaque	gluten-induced enteropathy	enteropatía provocada por glúten
maladie d'Addison	Addison's disease	enfermedad de Addison
maladie d'Alzheimer	Alzheimer's disease	enfermedad de Alzheimer
maladie de Bornholm	Bornholm disease	enfermedad de Bornholm
maladie de Friedreich	Friedreich's ataxia	ataxia de Friedreich
maladie de Hirschsprung	Hirschsprung's disease	enfermedad de Hirschsprung
maladie de Hodgkin	Hodgkin's disease	enfermedad de Hodgkin
maladie de Hurler	lipochondrodystrophy	lipocondrodistrofia
maladie de La Peyronie	Peyronie's disease	enfermedad de Peyronie
maladie de Lyme	Lyme disease	enfermedad de Lyme
maladie de Paget	Paget's disease	enfermedad de Paget
maladie de Ramsay Hunt	Ramsay Hunt syndrome	síndrome de Ramsay-Hunt
maladie de Raynaud	Raynaud's disease	enfermedad de Raynaud
maladie des légionnaires	legionnaires' disease	enfermedad del legionario
maladie des membranes hyalines	hyaline membrane disease	enfermedad de la membrana hialina
maladie de Still	Still's disease	enfermedad de Still
maladie de Tay-Sachs	Tay-Sachs disease	enfermedad de Tay-Sachs
maladie de von Recklinghausen	von Recklinghausen's disease	enfermedad de von Recklinghausen
maladie de von Willebrand	von Willebrand's disease	enfermedad de von Willebrand
maladie de Weil	Weil's disease	enfermedad de Weil
maladie de Wilson	Wilson's disease	enfermedad de Wilson
maladie d'Hashimoto	Hashimoto's disease	enfermedad de Hashimoto
maladie d'Osgood-Schlatter	Osgood-Schlatter disease, Schlatter's disease	enfermedad de Osgood-Schlatter, enfermedad de Schlatter
maladie du coeur	heart failure	insuficiencia cardíaca
maladie infectieuse	infectious disease	enfermedad infecciosa

macerazione	Mazeration	**macération**
osso mandibolare	Kieferknochen	**mâchoire**
macrocefalia	Makrozephalie	**macrocéphalie**
macrocito	Makrozyt	**macrocyte**
macrofago	Phagozyt	**macrophage**
macroscopico	makroskopisch	**macroscopique**
macula	Makula, Fleck	**macule**
maculopapulare	makulopapulär	**maculopapuleux**
mano	Hand	**main**
male, malattia	Übel, Leiden	**mal**
malassorbimento	Malabsorption	**malabsorption**
malacia	Malazie, Erweichung	**malacie**
paziente immunocompromesso	immungestörter Patient	**malade à déficit immunitaire**
paziente immunosoppresso	immunsupprimierter Patient	**malade à suppression immunitaire**
malattia, affezione, infermità	Krankheit, Leiden	**maladie**
malattia da denunciare alle autorità sanitarie	meldepflichtige Erkrankung	**maladie à déclaration obligatoire**
malattia autoimmune	Autoimmunerkrankung	**maladie auto-immune**
enteropatia da glutine	Zöliakie	**maladie coeliaque**
morbo di Addison	Addison Krankheit	**maladie d'Addison**
morbo di Alzheimer	Alzheimer Krankheit	**maladie d'Alzheimer**
malattia di Bornholm, mialgia epidemica	Bornholm-Krankheit	**maladie de Bornholm**
malattia di Friedreich	Friedreich Ataxie	**maladie de Friedreich**
malattia di Hirschsprung	Hirschsprung-Krankheit	**maladie de Hirschsprung**
malattia di Hodgkin	Morbus Hodgkin	**maladie de Hodgkin**
lipocondrodistrofia	Lipochondrodystrophie	**maladie de Hurler**
malattia di Peyronie	Induratio penis plastica	**maladie de La Peyronie**
malattia di Lyme	Lyme-Arthritis, Lyme-Borreliose	**maladie de Lyme**
malattia di Paget	Morbus Paget	**maladie de Paget**
sindrome di Ramsay Hunt	Ramsay-Hunt-Syndrom	**maladie de Ramsay Hunt**
malattia di Raynaud	Raynaud-Krankheit	**maladie de Raynaud**
malattia dei legionari	Legionärskrankheit	**maladie des légionnaires**
malattia delle membrane ialine	Hyalinmembrankrankheit	**maladie des membranes hyalines**
malattia di Still	Still-Krankheit	**maladie de Still**
malattia di Tay-Sachs	Tay-Sachs-Krankheit	**maladie de Tay-Sachs**
malattia di von Recklinghausen, neurofibromatosi	Morbus von Recklinghausen	**maladie de von Recklinghausen**
malattia di von Willebrand	Willebrand-Krankheit	**maladie de von Willebrand**
malattia di Weil	Weil Krankheit	**maladie de Weil**
malattia di Wilson	Wilson-Krankheit	**maladie de Wilson**
tiroidite di Hashimoto	Hashimoto-Struma	**maladie d'Hashimoto**
malattia di Osgood-Schlatter, malattia di Schlatter	Osgood-Schlatter-Krankheit, Schlatter-Krankheit	**maladie d'Osgood-Schlatter**
scompenso cardiaco	Herzinsuffizienz, Herzversagen	**maladie du coeur**
malattia infettiva	Infektionskrankheit	**maladie infectieuse**

FRENCH	ENGLISH	SPANISH
maladie professionnelle	industrial disease, occupational disease	enfermedad industrial, enfermedad profesional
maladie sexuellement transmissible (MST)	sexually transmitted disease (STD)	enfermedad de transmisión sexual (ETS)
maladie tropicale	tropical disease	enfermedad tropical
maladie vénérienne (MV)	venereal disease (VD)	enfermedad venérea
malaire	malar	malar
malaise	malaise	destemplanza, malestar
malaise vasovagal	vasovagal attack	ataque vasovagal
malathion	malathion	malathion
mal d'altitude	altitude sickness	mal de altura
mal de Crohn	Crohn's disease	enfermedad de Crohn
mal de Pott	Pott's disease	enfermedad de Pott
mal des montagnes	altitude sickness	mal de altura
mal de tête	headache	cefalea
malformation	malformation	malformación
malformation d'Arnold Chiari	Arnold-Chiari malformation	malformación de Arnold-Chiari
malignité	malignancy	malignidad
malin	malignant	maligno
malléole	malleolus	maléolo
malnutrition	malnutrition	desnutrición
malocclusion	malocclusion	maloclusión
malposition	malposition	malposición
maltose	maltose	maltosa
mamelon	nipple	pezón
mammalgie	mastalgia	mastalgia
mammographie	mammography	mamografía
mammoplastie	mammoplasty	mamoplastia
mandibule	mandible	mandíbula
manie	mania	manía
manipulation	manipulation	manipulación
manubrium	manubrium	manubrio
marque	weal	verdugón
marsupialisation	marsupialization	marsupialización
marteau	malleus	martillo
martyre d'enfants	child abuse	abuso de menores
massage	massage	masaje
masse sanguine	blood volume (BV)	volumen hemático
mastalgie	mastalgia	mastalgia
mastectomie	mastectomy	mastectomía
mastication	mastication	masticación
mastite	mastitis	mastitis
mastoïde	mastoid	mastoideo
mastoïdectomie	mastoidectomy	mastoidectomía
mastoïdite	mastoiditis	mastoiditis
masturbation	masturbation	masturbación
matrice	matrix	matriz
maxillaire	maxilla	maxilar

malattia industriale, malattia professionale	Berufskrankheit	maladie professionnelle
malattia a trasmissione sessuale (STD)	Geschlechtskrankheit	maladie sexuellement transmissible (MST)
malattia tropicale	Tropenkrankheit	maladie tropicale
malattia venerea (MV)	Geschlechtskrankheit	maladie vénérienne (MV)
malare	Backe betr, Backen-	malaire
indisposizione, malessere	Unwohlsein	malaise
crisi vagale	vasovagale Synkope	malaise vasovagal
malathion	Malathion	malathion
mal di montagna	Höhenkrankheit	mal d'altitude
malattia di Crohn	Morbus Crohn	mal de Crohn
malattia di Pott	Malum Potti	mal de Pott
mal di montagna	Höhenkrankheit	mal des montagnes
mal di testa	Kopfschmerzen	mal de tête
malformazione	Mißbildung	malformation
sindrome di Arnold Chiari	Arnold-Chiari-Mißbildung	malformation d'Arnold Chiari
neoplasia maligna	Malignität, Bösartigkeit	malignité
maligno	maligne, bösartig	malin
malleolo	Malleolus, Knöchel	malléole
malnutrizione	Unterernährung, Fehlernährung	malnutrition
malocclusione	Malokklusion	malocclusion
malposizione	Lageanomalie	malposition
maltosio	Maltose	maltose
capezzolo	Brustwarze, Mamille	mamelon
mastalgia	Mastodynie	mammalgie
mammografia	Mammographie	mammographie
mammoplastica	Mammaplastik	mammoplastie
mandibola	Mandibula, Unterkiefer	mandibule
mania	Manie	manie
manipolazione	Manipulation, Handhabung	manipulation
manubrio	Manubrium	manubrium
pomfo	Schwiele, Striemen	marque
marsupializzazione	Marsupialisation	marsupialisation
martello	Malleus, Hammer	marteau
maltrattamento a bambini	Kindesmißhandlung	martyre d'enfants
massaggio	Massage	massage
volume sanguigno	Blutvolumen	masse sanguine
mastalgia	Mastodynie	mastalgie
mastectomia	Mastektomie, Brustamputation	mastectomie
masticazione	Kauen, Kauvermögen	mastication
mastite	Mastitis, Brustdrüsenentzündung	mastite
mastoide, mastoideo	mastoideus	mastoïde
mastoidectomia	Mastoidektomie	mastoïdectomie
mastoidite	Mastoiditis	mastoïdite
masturbazione	Masturbation, Selbstbefriedigung	masturbation
matrice	Matrix	matrice
mascella superiore	Maxilla, Oberkieferknochen	maxillaire

FRENCH	ENGLISH	SPANISH
maxillofacial	maxillofacial	maxilofacial
mèche	lash	pestaña
méconium	meconium	meconio
médecin	physician, doctor	facultativo, médico
médecine	medicine	medicina
médecine complémentaire	alternative medicine	medicina alternativa
médecine dentaire	dentistry	odontologia
médecine légale	forensic medicine	medicina forense
médecin légiste	coroner	médico forense
médian	median	mediana
médiastin	mediastinum	mediastino
médiastinite	mediastinitis	mediastinitis
médicament	medicament, drug	medicamento, fármaco
médicament contrôlé	controlled drug	fármaco controlado
médicamenté	medicated	medicado
médicament retard	slow release drug	medicamento de liberación lenta
médicaments contre la maladie de Parkinson	antiparkinson(ism) drugs	farmacos antiparkinsonianos
médico-légal	medicolegal	médicolegal
médico-social	medicosocial	médicosocial
médulloblastome	medulloblastoma	meduloblastoma
mégacôlon	megacolon	megacolon
mégaloblaste	megaloblast	megaloblasto
méiose	meiosis	meiossis
mélancolie	melancholia	melancolía
mélanine	melanin	melanina
mélanome	melanoma	melanoma
méléna	melaena (Eng), melena (Am)	melena
membrane	membrane	membrana
membrane cellulaire	cell membrane	membrana celular
membrane synoviale	synovial membrane	membrana sinovial
membre	limb	extremidad
mémoire	memory	memoria
méninges	meninges	meninges
méningiome	meningioma	meningioma
méningisme	meningism	meningismo
méningite	meningitis	meningitis
méningocèle	meningocele	meningocele
méningo-encéphalite	meningoencephalitis	meningoencefalitis
méningomyélocèle	meningomyelocele	mielomeningocele
méniscectomie	meniscectomy	meniscectomía
ménisque	meniscus	menisco
ménométrorragies fonctionnelles	dysfunctional uterine bleeding (DUB)	hemorragia uterina funcional
ménopause	menopause	menopausia
ménorrhagie	menorrhagia	menorragia
ménorrhée	menorrhea (Am), menorrhoea (Eng)	menorrea

ITALIAN	GERMAN	FRENCH
maxillofacciale	maxillofazial	maxillofacial
ciglio	Wimper	mèche
meconio	Mekonium	méconium
dottore, medico	Arzt	médecin
medicina	Medizin, Arznei	médecine
medicina alternativa	Alternativmedizin	médecine complémentaire
odontoiatria	Zahnheilkunde, Zahntechnik	médecine dentaire
medicina forense	Gerichtsmedizin, Rechtsmedizin	médecine légale
medico legale	Leichenbeschauer	médecin légiste
mediano	Median-	médian
mediastino	Mediastinum	médiastin
mediastinite	Mediastinitis	médiastinite
medicamento, farmaco, medicinale, droga	Medikament, Arzneimittel, Rauschgift	médicament
farmaco sottoposto a controllo	Betäubungsmittel (gemäß BTM)	médicament contrôlé
medicato, medicamentoso	medizinisch	médicamenté
farmaco a lenta dismissione	Retardmittel	médicament retard
farmaci antiparkinsoniani	Antiparkinsonmittel	médicaments contre la maladie de Parkinson
medicolegale	rechtsmedizinisch	médico-légal
medicosociale	sozialmedizinisch	médico-social
medulloblastoma	Medulloblastom	médulloblastome
megacolon	Megacoloncongenitum, Hirschsprung-Krankheit	mégacôlon
megaloblasto	Megaloblast	mégaloblaste
meiosi	Meiose	méiose
melanconia	Melancholie	mélancolie
melanina	Melanin	mélanine
melanoma	Melanom	mélanome
melena	Meläna, Blutstuhl	méléna
membrana	Membran	membrane
membrana cellulare	Zellmembran	membrane cellulaire
membrana sinoviale	Synovia	membrane synoviale
braccio	Glied, Extremität	membre
memoria	Gedächtnis, Erinnerungsvermögen	mémoire
meningi	Meningen, Hirnhäute	méninges
meningioma	Meningiom	méningiome
meningismo	Meningismus	méningisme
meningite	Meningitis, Gehirnhautentzündung	méningite
meningocele	Meningozele	méningocèle
meningoencefalite	Meningoenzephalitis	méningo-encéphalite
meningomielocele	Meningomyelozele	méningomyélocèle
meniscectomia	Meniskusentfernung	méniscectomie
menisco	Meniskus	ménisque
sanguinamento uterino funzionale	dysfunktionale Uterusblutung	ménométrorragies fonctionnelles
menopausa	Menopause, Wechseljahre	ménopause
menorragia	Menorrhagie	ménorrhagie
menorrea	Monatsblutung, Menstruation	ménorrhée

FRENCH	ENGLISH	SPANISH
menstruation	menstruation	menstruación
menstruel	menstrual	menstrual
mental	mental	mental
menton	chin, mentum	barbilla, mentón
mercure	mercury	mercurio
mésencéphale	midbrain	mesencéfalo
mésentère	mesentery	mesenterio
mésothéliome	mesothelioma	mesotelioma
métabolique	metabolic	metabólico
métabolisme	metabolism	metabolismo
métabolite	metabolite	metabolito
métacarpe	metacarpus	metacarpo
métacarpophalangien	metacarpophalangeal	metacarpofalángico
métastase	metastasis	metástasis
métatarsalgie	metatarsalgia	metatarsalgia
métatarse	metatarsus	metatarso
métatarsophalangien	metatarsophalangeal	metatarsofalángico
méthémoglobine	methaemoglobin (Eng), methemoglobin (Am)	metahemoglobina
méthémoglobinémie	methaemoglobinaemia (Eng), methemoglobinemia (Am)	metahemoglobinemia
méthylcellulose	methylcellulose	metilcelulosa
métropathie hémorragique	metropathia haemorrhagica (Eng), metropathia hemorrhagica (Am)	metropatía hemorrágica
métrorragie	metrorrhagia	metrorragia
mettre en pronation	pronate	pronar
microbiologie	microbiology	microbiología
microcéphalie	microcephaly	microcefalia
microchirurgie	microsurgery	microcirugía
microcirculation	microcirculation	microcirculación
microcyte	microcyte	microcito
microfilaire	microfilaria	microfilaria
micro-organisme	microorganism	microorganismo
micropoils	microvilli	microvellosidad
microscope	microscope	microscopio
microscope opératoire	operating microscope	microscopio quirúrgico
microscopique	microscopic	microscópico
micturition	micturition	micción
migraine	migraine	migraña
miliaire (n)	miliaria (n)	miliaria (n)
miliaire (a)	miliary (a)	miliar (a)
milieu	environment, medium	ambiente, medio
milliéquivalent (mEq)	milliequivalent (mEq)	miliequivalente (mEq)
minéralocorticoïde	mineralocorticoid	mineralocorticoide
mitochondrie	mitochondrion	mitocondria
mitose	mitosis	mitosis
mitral	mitral	mitral
mobile	motile	móvil

ITALIAN	GERMAN	FRENCH
mestruazione	Menstruation, Monatsblutung	menstruation
mestruale	menstruell	menstruel
mentale	geistig, seelisch	mental
mento	Kinn	menton
mercurio	Quecksilber	mercure
mesencefelo	Mittelhirn	mésencéphale
mesentere	Mesenterium	mésentère
mesotelioma	Mesotheliom	mésothéliome
metabolico	metabolisch, Stoffwechsel-	métabolique
metabolismo	Metabolismus, Stoffwechsel	métabolisme
metabolita	Metabolit, Stoffwechselprodukt	métabolite
metacarpo	Metakarpus, Mittelhand	métacarpe
metacarpofalangeo	metakarpophalangeal	métacarpophalangien
metastasi	Metastase	métastase
metatarsalgia	Metatarsalgie	métatarsalgie
metatarso	Metatarsus, Mittelfuß	métatarse
metatarsofalangeo	metatarsophalangeal	métatarsophalangien
metemoglobina	Methämoglobin	méthémoglobine
metemoglobinemia	Methämoglobinämie	méthémoglobinémie
metilcellulosa	Methylzellulose	méthylcellulose
metropatia emorragica	Metropathia haemorrhagica	métropathie hémorragique
metrorragia	Metrorrhagie, Zwischenblutung	métrorragie
pronare	pronieren	mettre en pronation
microbiologia	Mikrobiologie	microbiologie
microcefalia	Mikrozephalie	microcéphalie
microchirurgia	Mikrochirurgie	microchirurgie
microcircolazione	Mikrozirkulation	microcirculation
microcita	Mikrozyt	microcyte
microfilaria	Mikrofilarie	microfilaire
microoganismo	Mikroorganismus	micro-organisme
microvilli	Mikrovilli	micropolis
microscopio	Mikroskop	microscope
microscopio chirurgico	Operationsmikroskop	microscope opératoire
microscopico	mikroskopisch	microscopique
minzione	Wasserlassen, Blasenentleerung	micturition
emicrania	Migräne	migraine
miliaria (n), esantema miliare (n)	Miliaria (n)	miliaire (n)
miliare (a)	miliar (a)	miliaire (a)
ambiente, mezzo	Umgebung, Umwelt, Medium	milieu
milliequivalente (mEq)	Milli-Äquivalent	milliéquivalent (mEq)
mineralcorticoide	Mineralokortikoid	minéralocorticoïde
mitocondrio	Mitochondrium	mitochondrie
mitosi	Mitose	mitose
mitrale, mitralico	mitral	mitral
mobile	bewegungsfähig, beweglich	mobile

FRENCH	ENGLISH	SPANISH
moelle	medulla	médula
moelle osseuse	bone marrow	médula ósea
molaire	molar	molar
molécule	molecule	molécula
mollet	calf	pantorrilla
molluscum	molluscum	molusco
monochromat	monochromat	monocromato
mononucléaire	mononuclear	mononuclear
mononucléose	mononucleosis	mononucleosis
mononucléose infectieuse	infectious mononucleosis	mononucleosis infecciosa
monoplégie	monoplegia	monoplegia
morbidité	morbidity	morbilidad
morbilliforme	morbilliform	morbiliforme
moribond	moribund	moribundo
morphologie	morphology	morfología
mort (n)	death (n)	muerte (n)
mort (a)	dead (a)	muerto (a)
mort à l'arrivée	dead on arrival (DOA)	muerto al llegar
mortalité	mortality	mortalidad
mort-né	stillborn	mortinato, nacido muerto
mort subite de nourrisson	cot death	muerte en la cuna, muerte súbita infantil
moteur	motor	motor
mou	flaccid	fláccido
mouche tsé-tsé	tsetse	mosca tsetsé
mouvement	motion	movimiento
mucine	mucin	mucina
mucocèle	mucocele (Am), mucocoele (Eng)	mucocele
mucocutané	mucocutaneous	mucocutáneo
mucoïde	mucoid	mucoide
mucolytique	mucolytic	mucolítico
mucopolysaccharidose	mucopolysaccharidosis	mucopolisacaridosis
mucopurulent	mucopurulent	mucopurulento
multigeste	multigravida	multípara
multiloculaire	multilocular	multilocular
muqueuse	mucosa	mucosa
muqueux	mucous (Eng), mucus (Am)	moco
murmure	murmur	soplo
murmure respiratoire	thrill	frémito
murmure systolique	systolic murmur	soplo sistólico
muscle	muscle	músculo
muscles fessiers	gluteus muscles	músculos glúteos
muscles péroniers	peroneus muscles	músculos peroneos
muscle sternocléidomastoïdien	sternocleidomastoid muscle	músculo esternocleidomastoideo
muscles trapèzes	trapezius muscles	músculos trapecios

ITALIAN	GERMAN	FRENCH
midollo	Medulla, Mark	moelle
midollo osseo	Knochenmark	moelle osseuse
molare	molar	molaire
molecula	Molekül	molécule
polpaccio	Wade	mollet
mollusco	Molluscum	molluscum
monocromatico	Monochromat, monochrom Farbenblinder	monochromat
mononucleare	mononukleär	mononucléaire
mononucleosi	Mononukleose, Pfeiffersches Drüsenfieber	mononucléose
mononucleosi infettiva	Pfeiffersches Drüsenfieber, infektiöse Mononukleose	mononucléose infectieuse
monoplegia	Monoplegie	monoplégie
morbilità	Morbidität, Krankhaftigkeit	morbidité
morbilliforme	morbilliform, masernähnlich	morbilliforme
moribondo	moribund, sterbend	moribond
morfologia	Morphologie	morphologie
morte (n)	Tod (n), Todesfall (n)	mort (n)
morto (a)	tot (a)	mort (a)
deceduto all'arrivo in ospedale	tot bei Einlieferung	mort à l'arrivée
mortalità	Mortalität, Sterblichkeit	mortalité
nato morto	totgeboren	mort-né
sindrome da morte improvvisa del lattante	plötzlicher Säuglingstod	mort subite de nourrisson
motore	motorisch	moteur
flaccido	schlaff	mou
tse-tse	Tsetsefliege	mouche tsé-tsé
movimento	Bewegung, Stuhlgang	mouvement
mucina	Muzin	mucine
mucocele	Mukozele	mucocèle
mucocutaneo	mukokutan	mucocutané
mucoide	mukoid	mucoïde
mucolitico	schleimlösendes Mittel	mucolytique
mucopolisaccaridosi	Mukopolysaccharidose	mucopolysaccharidose
mucopurulento	mukopurulent, schleimig-eitrig	mucopurulent
plurigravida	Multigravida	multigeste
multiloculare	multilokulär	multiloculaire
mucosa	Mukosa, Schleimhaut	muqueuse
mucoso	mukös, schleimig	muqueux
soffio, rullio	Herzgeräusch, Geräusch	murmure
fremito	Vibrieren, Schwirren	murmure respiratoire
soffio sistolico	systolisches Geräusch, Systolikum	murmure systolique
muscolo	Muskel	muscle
muscoli glutei	Glutealmuskulatur, Gesäßmuskulatur	muscles fessiers
muscoli peronei	Musculi peronei	muscles péroniers
muscolo sternocleidomastoideo	Musculus sternocleidomastoideus	muscle sternocléidomastoïdien
muscoli trapezi	Musculi trapezii	muscles trapèzes

| --- | --- | --- |
musculo-cutané	musculocutaneous	musculocutáneo
musculo-squelettique	musculoskeletal	musculoesquelético
mutagène	mutagen	mutágeno
mutant	mutant	mutante
mutation	mutation	mutación
mutilation	mutilation	mutilación
mutisme	mutism	mutismo
myalgie	myalgia	mialgia
myasthénie	myasthenia	miastenia
mycète	fungus	hongo
mycose	mycosis	micosis
mydriase	mydriasis	midriasis
mydriatique (n)	mydriatic (n)	midriático (n)
mydriatique (a)	mydriatic (a)	midriático (a)
myéline	myelin	mielina
myélite	myelitis	mielitis
myélofibrose	myelofibrosis	mielofibrosis
myélographie	myelography	mielografía
myéloïde	myeloid	mieloide
myélomatose	myelomatosis	mielomatosis
myélome	myeloma	mieloma
myélopathie	myelopathy	mielopatía
myocarde	myocardium	miocardio
myocardite	myocarditis	miocarditis
myofibrose	myofibrosis	miofibrosis
myome	myoma	mioma
myomectomie	myomectomy	miomectomía
myomètre	myometrium	miometrio
myopathie	myopathy	miopatía
myope	myope	miope
myopie	myopia	miopía
myosis	miosis	miosis
myosite	myositis	miositis
myringotomie	myringotomy	miringotomía
myxoedème	myxedema (Am), myxoedema (Eng)	mixedema
myxome	myxoma	mixoma
myxovirus	myxovirus	mixovirus

ITALIAN	GERMAN	FRENCH
muscolocutaneo	muskulokutan	musculo-cutané
muscoloscheletrico	Skelettmuskulatur betr	musculo-squelettique
mutageno	Mutagen	mutagène
mutante	Mutante	mutant
mutazione	Mutation	mutation
mutilazione	Verstümmelung	mutilation
mutismo	Mutismus, Stummheit	mutisme
mialgia	Myalgie, Muskelschmerz	myalgie
miastenia	Myasthenie, Muskelschwäche	myasthénie
fungo	Pilz	mycète
micosi	Mykose, Pilzinfektion	mycose
midriasi	Mydriasis, Pupillenerweiterung	mydriase
midriatico *(n)*	Mydriatikum *(n)*	mydriatique *(n)*
midriatico *(a)*	mydriatisch *(a)*, pupillenerweiternd *(a)*	mydriatique *(a)*
mielina	Myelin	myéline
mielite	Myelitis	myélite
mielofibrosi	Myelofibrose	myélofibrose
mielografia	Myelographie	myélographie
mieloide	myeloisch	myéloïde
mielomatosi	Myelomatose	myélomatose
mieloma, plasmacitoma maligno	Myelom	myélome
mielopatia	Myelopathie	myélopathie
miocardio	Myokard, Herzmuskel	myocarde
miocardite	Myokarditis, Herzmuskelentzündung	myocardite
miosite	Myofibrose	myofibrose
leiomioma dell'utero, mioma	Myom	myome
miomectomia	Myomektomie	myomectomie
miometrio	Myometrium	myomètre
miopatia	Myopathie, Muskelerkrankung	myopathie
miope	Myoper, Kurzsichtiger	myope
miopia	Myopie, Kurzsichtigkeit	myopie
miosi	Miosis, Pupillenverengung	myosis
miosite	Myositis	myosite
miringotomia	Parazentese	myringotomie
mixedema	Myxödem	myxoedème
mixoma	Myxom	myxome
myxovirus	Myxovirus	myxovirus

FRENCH	ENGLISH	SPANISH

N

naevi	spider naevus (Eng), spider nevus (Am)	araña vascular
naevus	birthmark, mole, naevus (Eng), nevus (Am)	mancha de nacimiento, nevo
naissance	birth	nacimiento, parto
naissance par le siège	breech-birth presentation	presentación de nalgas
nanisme	dwarfism	enanismo
narcolepsie	narcolepsy	narcolepsia
narcose	narcosis	narcosis
narcotique (n)	narcotic (n)	narcótico (n)
narcotique (a)	narcotic (a)	narcótico (a)
narine	nostril	fosa nasale
nasal	nasal	nasal
nasogastrique	nasogastric	nasogástrico
nasolacrymal	nasolacrimal	nasolacrimal
nausée	nausea	náusea
nausées matinales	morning sickness	náuseas matinales
nébuliseur	nebulizer	nebulizador
nécrose	necrosis	necrosis
nécrose tubulaire	tubular necrosis	necrosis tubular
négligence	negligence	negligencia
nématode	nematode	nematodo
néoplasie	neoplasia	neoplasia
néoplasie intra-épithéliale cervicale	cervical intraepithelial neoplasia (CIN)	neoplasia intraepitelial cervical
néoplasme	neoplasm	neoplasma
néphralgie	nephralgia	nefralgia
néphrectomie	nephrectomy	nefrectomía
néphrite	nephritis	nefritis
néphrologie	nephrology	nefrología
néphron	nephron	nefrona
néphrose	nephrosis	nefrosis
néphrostomie	nephrostomy	nefrostomía
néphrotoxique	nephrotoxic	nefrotóxico
nerf	nerve	nervio
nerf crânien	cranial nerve	nervio craneal
nerf grand sciatique	sciatic nerve	nervio ciático
nerf moteur	motor nerve	nervio motor
nerf péronier	peroneal nerve	nervio peroneo
nerfs vasomoteurs	vasomotor nerves	nervios vasomotores
neural	neural	nervioso
neurapraxie	neurapraxia	neuropraxia
neurasthénie	neurasthenia	neurastenia
neurilemme	neurolemma	neurolema
neuroblastome	neuroblastoma	neuroblastoma

angioma stellare	Spider naevus, Naevus arachnoideus	**naevi**
nevo congenito, neo, nevo	Muttermal, Storchenbiß, Mole, Nävus	**naevus**
nascita	Geburt	**naissance**
presentazione podalica	Steißlage	**naissance par le siège**
nanismo	Zwergwuchs	**nanisme**
narcolessia	Narkolepsie	**narcolepsie**
narcosi	Narkose, Anästhesie	**narcose**
narcotico (n)	Narkosemittel (n), Betäubungsmittel (n), Rauschgift (n)	**narcotique (n)**
narcotico (a)	narkotisch (a)	**narcotique (a)**
narice	Nasenloch	**narine**
nasale	nasal	**nasal**
nasogastrico	nasogastrisch	**nasogastrique**
nasolacrimale	nasolakrimal	**nasolacrymal**
nausea	Nausea, Übelkeit, Brechreiz	**nausée**
malessere mattutino	morgendliche Übelkeit der Schwangeren	**nausées matinales**
nebulizzatore, atomizzatore	Zerstäuber, Vernebler	**nébuliseur**
necrosi	Nekrose	**nécrose**
necrosi tubulare	Tubulusnekrose	**nécrose tubulaire**
negligenza	Nachlässigkeit	**négligence**
nematode	Nematode, Fadenwurm	**nématode**
neoplasia	Neoplasie	**néoplasie**
neoplasia intraepiteliale della cervice uterina (CIN)	zervikale intraepitheliale Neoplasie (CIN)	**néoplasie intra-épithéliale cervicale**
neoplasma	Neoplasma, Tumor	**néoplasme**
nevralgia	Nephralgie	**néphralgie**
nefrectomia	Nephrektomie	**néphrectomie**
nefrite	Nephritis, Nierenentzündung	**néphrite**
nefrologia	Nephrologie	**néphrologie**
nefrone	Nephron	**néphron**
nefrosi, nefropatia	Nephrose	**néphrose**
nefrostomia	Nephrostomie	**néphrostomie**
nefrotossico	nephrotoxisch, nierenschädigend	**néphrotoxique**
nervo	Nerv	**nerf**
nervo craniale	Hirnnerv	**nerf crânien**
nervo sciatico	Ischiasnerv, Nervus ischiadicus	**nerf grand sciatique**
nervo motore	motorischer Nerv	**nerf moteur**
nervo peroneo	Nervus peroneus	**nerf péronier**
nervi vasomotori	vasomotorische Nerven	**nerfs vasomoteurs**
neurale	neural	**neural**
neuroaprassia	Neurapraxie	**neurapraxie**
neuroastenia	Neurasthenie	**neurasthénie**
neurilemma	Neurolemm	**neurilemme**
neuroblastoma	Neuroblastom	**neuroblastome**

FRENCH	ENGLISH	SPANISH
neurochirurgie	neurosurgery	neurocirugía
neurofibromatose	neurofibromatosis	neurofibromatosis
neurogène	neurogenic	neurógeno
neuroleptique (n)	neuroleptic (n)	neuroléptico (n)
neuroleptique (a)	neuroleptic (a)	neuroléptico (a)
neurologie	neurology	neurología
neuromusculaire	neuromuscular	neuromuscular
neurone	neuron	neurona
neurone moteur	motor neurone	neurona motora
neuropathie	neuropathy	neuropatia
neuropharmacologie	neuropharmacology	neurofarmacología
neuropsychiatrie	neuropsychiatry	neuropsiquiatría
neurosyphilis	neurosyphilis	neurosífilis
neurotrope	neurotropic	neurotrópico
neutropénie	neutropenia	neutropenia
neutrophile	neutrophil	neutrófilo
névralgie	neuralgia	neuralgia
névrite	neuritis	neuritis
névrose	neurosis	neurosis
névrose obsessionnelle	obsessional neurosis	neurosis obsesiva
nez	nose	nariz
nicotine	nicotine	nicotina
nocturne	nocturnal	nocturno
nodule	nodule	nódulo
nodules d'Osler	Osler's nodes	nódulos de Osler
noeud	node	nodo
noeud sinusal de Keith et Flack	sinoatrial node	nodo sinoauricular
nombre de globules blancs (NGB)	white blood cell count (WBC)	recuento de leucocitos
nombril	navel, umbilicus	ombligo
nom de marque	proprietary name	nombre de patente
non encore diagnostiqué	not yet diagnosed (NYD)	todavía no diagnosticado
non invasif	non-invasive	no invasivo
non observance	noncompliance	incumplimiento
noradrénaline	noradrenaline, norepinephrine	noradrenalina, norepinefrina
norépinéphrine	norepinephrine	norepinefrina
normoblaste	normoblast	normoblasto
normocyte	normocyte	normocito
normoglycémique	normoglycaemic (Eng), normoglycemic (Am)	normoglucémico
normotonique	normotonic	normotónico
nourricier	nutrient	nutriente
nourrisson	infant	lactante
nouveau-né (n)	neonate (n), newborn (n)	neonato (n)
nouveau-né (a)	neonate (a), newborn (a)	neonato (a)
noyau	nucleus	núcleo

ITALIAN	GERMAN	FRENCH
neurochirurgia	Neurochirurgie	neurochirurgie
neurofibromatosi	Neurofibromatose	neurofibromatose
neurogenico	neurogen	neurogène
neurolettico (n)	Neuroleptikum (n)	neuroleptique (n)
neurolettico (a)	neuroleptisch (a)	neuroleptique (a)
neurologia	Neurologie	neurologie
neuromuscolare	neuromuskulär	neuromusculaire
neurone	Neuron	neurone
neurone motore	Motoneuron	neurone moteur
neuropatia	Neuropathie	neuropathie
neurofarmacologia	Neuropharmakologie	neuropharmacologie
neuropsichiatria	Neuropsychiatrie	neuropsychiatrie
neurosifilide	Neurosyphilis	neurosyphilis
neurotropo	neurotrop	neurotrope
neutropenia	Neutropenie	neutropénie
neutrofilo	neutrophil	neutrophile
nevralgia	Neuralgie	névralgie
neurite	Neuritis, Nervenentzündung	névrite
nevrosi	Neurose	névrose
nevrosi ossessiva	Zwangsneurose	névrose obsessionnelle
naso	Nase	nez
nicotina	Nikotin	nicotine
notturno	nächtlich, Nacht-	nocturne
nodulo	Nodulus, Knötchen	nodule
noduli di Osler	Osler-Knötchen	nodules d'Osler
nodo	Knoten	noeud
nodo sinoatriale	Sinusknoten	noeud sinusal de Keith et Flack
conteggio dei globuli bianchi (CGB, WBC)	weißes Blutbild	nombre de globules blancs (NGB)
ombelico	Nabel	nombril
marchio depositato	Markenname	nom de marque
non ancora diagnosticato	noch nicht diagnostiziert	non encore diagnostiqué
non invasivo	nichtinvasiv	non invasif
inadempienza a prescrizioni	Noncompliance	non observance
noradrenalina, norepinefrina	Noradrenalin, Norepinephrin, Noradrenalin	noradrénaline
norepinefrina	Norepinephrin, Noradrenalin	norépinéphrine
normoblasto	Normoblast	normoblaste
normocito	Normozyt	normocyte
normoglicemico	Normoglykämie	normoglycémique
normotonico	normoton	normotonique
nutriente	nahrhaft	nourricier
infante	Kleinkind, Säugling	nourrisson
neonato (n)	Neugeborenes (n)	nouveau-né (n)
neonato (a)	neugeboren (a)	nouveau-né (a)
nucleo	Nukleus, Kern	noyau

FRENCH	ENGLISH	SPANISH
noyau caudé, noyau lenticulaire, avant mur et noyau amygdalien	basal ganglia	ganglios basales
nullipare	nullipara	nulípara
numération érythrocytaire	red blood cell count (RBC)	recuento de glóbulos rojos
numération globulaire	complete blood count (CBC)	hemograma completo
nuque	nape	nuca
nursage de protection	barrier nursing	enfermería por aislamiento
nutriment	nutrient	nutriente
nutrition	nutrition	nutrición
nyctalgie	nyctalgia	nictalgia
nycturie	nocturia, nycturia	nicturia
nystagmus	nystagmus	nistagmo

ITALIAN	GERMAN	FRENCH
gangli basali	Basalganglien	**noyau caudé, noyau lenticulaire, avant mur et noyau amygdalien**
nullipara	Nullipara	**nullipare**
conteggio dei globuli rossi (CGR)	rotes Blutbild	**numération érythrocytaire**
esame emocromocitometrico	großes Blutbild	**numération globulaire**
nuca	Nacken	**nuque**
isolamento	Isolierung (auf Isolierstation)	**nursage de protection**
sostanza nutritiva	Nahrungsmittel	**nutriment**
nutrizione	Ernährung	**nutrition**
nictalgia	Nyktalgie	**nyctalgie**
nicturia	Nykturie	**nycturie**
nistagmo	Nystagmus	**nystagmus**

O

FRENCH	ENGLISH	SPANISH
obèse	fat	graso
obésité	obesity	obesidad
observance du patient	patient compliance	cumplimiento del paciente
obstétrique	obstetrics	obstetricia
obstructif	obstructive	obstructivo
obturateur	obturator	obturador
occipital	occipital	occipital
occipito-antérieur	occipitoanterior	occipitoanterior
occipito-antérieur gauche	left occipito-anterior (LOA)	occipito anterior izquierdo
occipito-frontal	occipitofrontal	occipitofrontal
occipito-postérieur	occipitoposterior	occipitoposterior
occiput	occiput	occipucio
occlusion	occlusion	oclusión
occulte	occult	oculta
oculaire	ocular	ocular
oculogyre	oculogyric	oculógiro
oculomoteur	oculomotor	oculomotor
odontoïde	odontoid	odontoides
oedème	edema (Am), oedema (Eng)	edema
oedème angioneurotique	angioneurotic edema (solidus) (Am), angioneurotic oedema (solidus) (Eng)	edema angioneurótico (sólido)
oedème papillaire	papilledema (Am), papilloedema (Eng)	papiledema
oeil	eye	ojo
oesophage	esophagus (Am), gullet, oesophagus (Eng)	esófago, gaznate
oesophagien	esophageal (Am), oesophageal (Eng)	esofágico
oesophagite	esophagitis (Am), oesophagitis (Eng)	esofagitis
oestradiol	estradiol (Am), oestradiol (Eng)	estradiol
oestriol	estriol (Am), oestriol (Eng)	estriol
oestrogène	estrogen (Am), oestrogen (Eng)	estrógeno
oeuf	egg, ovum	huevo, óvulo
oeufs de Naboth	nabothian follicles	folículos de Naboth
olécrane	olecranon (process)	olécranon
olfactif	olfactory	olfatorio
oligurie	oliguria	oliguria
omoplate	scapula	omoplato
onchocercose	onchocerciasis	oncocerciasis
oncogène	oncogene	oncogén
oncologie	oncology	oncología
ongle	nail	uña
onychogryphose	onychogryphosis	onicogriposis
onycholyse	onycholysis	onicólisis

grasso	fett, fetthaltig	**obèse**
obesità	Adipositas, Obesitas	**obésité**
acquiescenza lle prescrizioni	Compliance	**observance du patient**
ostetricia	Geburtshilfe	**obstétrique**
ostruttivo	obstruktiv	**obstructif**
otturatorio	Obturator, Gaumenverschlußplatte	**obturateur**
occipitale	okzipital	**occipital**
occipitoanteriore	vordere Hinterhauptslage	**occipito-antérieur**
occipitoanteriore sinistro (OAS)	linke vordere Hinterhauptslage	**occipito-antérieur gauche**
occipitofrontale	okzipitofrontal	**occipito-frontal**
occipitoposteriore	hintere Hinterhauptslage	**occipito-postérieur**
occipite	Okziput, Hinterkopf	**occiput**
occlusione	Okklusion, Verschluß	**occlusion**
occulto	okkult	**occulte**
oculare	okular	**oculaire**
oculogiro	Bewegung der Augen betr	**oculogyre**
oculomotore	Oculomotorius-	**oculomoteur**
odontoide	odontoid	**odontoïde**
edema	Ödem, Flüssigkeitsansammlung	**oedème**
edema angioneurotico	Quincke-Ödem	**oedème angioneurotique**
papilledema	Papillenödem	**oedème papillaire**
occhio	Auge	**oeil**
esofago (gola)	Ösophagus, Speiseröhre	**oesophage**
esofageo	ösophageal	**oesophagien**
esofagite	Ösophagitis	**oesophagite**
estradiolo	Östradiol	**oestradiol**
estriolo	Östriol	**oestriol**
estrogeno	Östrogen	**oestrogène**
uovo, gamete femminile	Ei, Ovum	**oeuf**
follicoli di Naboth	Naboth-Eier	**oeufs de Naboth**
olecrano	Olekranon, Ellenbozen	**olécrane**
olfattorio	olfaktorisch	**olfactif**
oliguria	Oligurie	**oligurie**
scapola	Skapula, Schulterblatt	**omoplate**
oncocerchiasi	Onchozerkose	**onchocercose**
oncogene	Onkogen	**oncogène**
oncologia	Onkologie	**oncologie**
unghia	Nagel	**ongle**
onicogrifosi	Onychogryposis	**onychogryphose**
onicolisi	Onycholyse, Nagelablösung	**onycholyse**

FRENCH	ENGLISH	SPANISH
opacité	opacity	opacidad
opaque	opaque	opaco
opération	operation	intervención quirúrgica
opération de Billroth	Billroth's operation	operación de Billroth
opération de Caldwell-Luc	Caldwell-Luc operation	operación de Caldwell-Luc
opération de Ramstedt	Ramstedt's operation	operación de Ramstedt
opération de Shirodkar	Shirodkar's operation	operación de Shirodkar
ophtalmie	ophthalmia	oftalmía
ophtalmique	ophthalmic	oftálmico
ophtalmologie	ophthalmology	oftalmología
ophtalmoplégie	ophthalmoplegia	oftalmoplejía
ophtalmoscope	ophthalmoscope	oftalmoscopio
opticien	optician	óptico
optimum	optimum	óptimo
optique	optic	óptico
oral	oral	oral
orbite	orbit	órbita
orchidectomie	orchidectomy	orquidectomía
orchidopexie	orchidopexy, orchiopexy	orquidopexia, orquiopexia
orchi-épididymite	epididymo-orchitis	epididimoorquitis
orchite	orchitis	orquitis
orchodotomie	orchidotomy	orquidotomía
ordonnance	prescription	receta
oreille	ear	oído
oreillette	atrium	aurícula
oreillons	mumps	paperas
oreillons rougeole et rubéole	measles mumps and rubella (MMR)	sarampión parotiditis y rubeola
organes génitaux	genitalia	genitales
organique	organic	orgánico
organisme	organism	organismo
orgasme	orgasm	orgasmo
orgelet	stye	orzuelo
orientation	orientation	orientación
orifice	foramen, introitus, orifice	foramen, introito, orificio
origine	origin	origen
oropharynx	oropharynx	orofaringe
orteil	toe	dedo del pie
orthèse	orthosis	ortosis
orthodontie	orthodontics	ortodoncia
orthopédique	orthopaedic (Eng), orthopedic (Am)	ortopedia
orthophonie	speech therapy	logopedia
orthopnée	orthopnea (Am), orthopnoea (Eng)	ortopnea
orthoptique	orthoptics	ortóptica
orthostatique	orthostatic	ortostático

ITALIAN	GERMAN	FRENCH
opacità	Opazität	opacité
opaco	undurchsichtig, verschattet (radiolog)	opaque
operazione	Operation, Einwirkung, Eingriff	opération
operazione di Billroth	Billroth-Magenresektion	opération de Billroth
operazione di Caldwell-Luc	Caldwell-Luc-Operation	opération de Caldwell-Luc
intervento di Ramstedt, piloromiotomia	Weber-Ramstedt-Operation, Ramstedt-(Weber)-Operation	opération de Ramstedt
intervento di Shirodkar	Shirodkar-Operation	opération de Shirodkar
oftalmia	Ophthalmie	ophtalmie
oftalmico	Augen-	ophtalmique
oftalmologia	Ophthalmologie, Augenheilkunde	ophtalmologie
oftalmoplegia	Ophthalmoplegie, Augenmuskellähmung	ophtalmoplégie
oftalmoscopio	Ophthalmoskop, Augenspiegel	ophtalmoscope
ottico	Optiker	opticien
optimum	optimal	optimum
ottico	optisch, Seh-	optique
orale	oral	oral
orbita	Orbita, Augenhöhle	orbite
orchidectomia	Orchidektomie	orchidectomie
orchidopessia	Orchidopexie, Orchipexie	orchidopexie
epididimo-orchite	Epididymoorchitis	orchi-épididymite
orchite	Orchitis	orchite
orchidectomia	Orchidotomie	orchodotomie
prescrizione, ricetta	Rezept, Verschreibung	ordonnance
orecchio	Ohr	oreille
atrio	Atrium, Vorhof	oreillette
parotite epidemica	Mumps, Ziegenpeter	oreillons
parotide epidemica morbillo e rosolia	Masern Mumps und Röteln	oreillons rougeole et rubéole
organi genitali	Genitalien	organes génitaux
organico	organisch	organique
organismo	Organismus, Keim	organisme
orgasmo	Orgasmus	orgasme
orzaiolo	Hordeolum, Gerstenkorn	orgelet
orientamento	Orientierung	orientation
foramen, introito, orifizio	Foramen, Introitus, Öffnung	orifice
origine	Ursprung	origine
orofaringe	Mundrachenhöhle	oropharynx
dito del piede	Zehe	orteil
raddrizzamento, correzione di una deformità	Orthose	orthèse
ortodonzia	Kieferorthopädie	orthodontie
ortopedia	orthopädisch	orthopédique
terapia del linguaggio	Sprachtherapie	orthophonie
ortopnea	Orthopnoe	orthopnée
ortottica	Orthoptik	orthoptique
ortostatico	orthostatisch	orthostatique

FRENCH	ENGLISH	SPANISH
os	bone	hueso
oscillation	oscillation	oscilación
os coxal	hip bone	hueso coxal o ilíaco
osmolalité	osmolality	osmolalidad
osmolarité	osmolarity	osmolaridad
osmose	osmosis	osmosis
osselet	ossicle	huesecillos
osseux	osseous	óseo
ostéite	osteitis	osteítis
ostéo-arthrite	osteoarthritis (OA)	osteoartritis
ostéo-arthropathie	osteoarthropathy	osteoartropatía
ostéoblaste	osteoblast	osteoblasto
ostéochondrite	osteochondritis	osteocondritis
ostéochondrome	osteochondroma	osteocondroma
ostéochondrose	osteochondrosis	osteocondrosis
ostéoclaste	osteoclast	osteoclasto
ostéocyte	osteocyte	osteocito
ostéodystrophie	osteodystrophy	osteodistrofia
ostéogène	osteogenic	osteogénico
ostéolytique	osteolytic	osteolítico
ostéomalacie	osteomalacia	osteomalacia
ostéome	osteoma	osteoma
ostéomyélite	osteomyelitis	osteomielitis
ostéopathie	osteopathy	osteopatía
ostéopétrose	osteopetrosis	osteopetrosis
ostéophyte	osteophyte	osteofito
ostéoporose	osteoporosis	osteoporosis
ostéosarcome	osteosarcoma	osteosarcoma
ostéosclérose	osteosclerosis	osteosclerosis
ostéotomie	osteotomy, ostomy	osteotomía, ostomía
otalgie	otalgia	otalgia
otite	otitis	otitis
otite moyenne adhésive	glue ear	otitis media exudativa crónica, tapon de oído
otolaryngologie	otolaryngology	otolaringología
otologie	otology	otología
oto-rhino-laryngologie (ORL)	ear nose and throat (ENT)	otorrinolaringología (ORL)
otorrhée	otorrhea (Am), otorrhoea (Eng)	otorrea
otoscope	otoscope	otoscopio
otospongiose	otosclerosis	otosclerosis
ototoxique	ototoxic	ototóxico
ovaire	ovary	ovario
ovariectomie	oophorectomy	ooforectomía
ovarien	ovarian	ovárico
ovocyte de premier ordre	ovum	óvulo

ITALIAN	GERMAN	FRENCH
osso	Knochen, Gräte	os
oscillazione	Oszillation, Schwankung	oscillation
osso iliaco	Hüftknochen	os coxal
osmolalità	Osmolalität	osmolalité
osmolarità	Osmolarität	osmolarité
osmosi	Osmose	osmose
ossicino	Gehörknöchelchen, Ossikel	osselet
osseo	knöchern, Knochen-	osseux
osteite	Ostitis, Knochenentzündung	ostéite
osteoartrosi (OA)	Osteoarthritis	ostéo-arthrite
osteoartropatia	Osteoarthrose	ostéo-arthropathie
osteoblasto	Osteoblast	ostéoblaste
osteocondrite	Osteochondritis	ostéochondrite
osteocondroma	Osteochondrom	ostéochondrome
osteocondrosi	Osteochondrose	ostéochondrose
osteoclasto	Osteoklast	ostéoclaste
osteocito	Osteozyt	ostéocyte
osteodistrofia	Osteodystrophie	ostéodystrophie
osteogenico	osteogen	ostéogène
osteolitico	osteolytisch	ostéolytique
osteomalacia	Osteomalazie	ostéomalacie
osteoma	Osteom	ostéome
osteomielite	Osteomyelitis, Knochenmarksentzündung	ostéomyélite
osteopatia	Osteopathie	ostéopathie
osteoporosi	Osteopetrose	ostéopétrose
osteofito	Osteophyt	ostéophyte
osteoporosi	Osteoporose	ostéoporose
sarcoma osteogenico	Osteosarkom, Knochensarkom	ostéosarcome
osteosclerosi	Osteosklerose, Eburnifikation	ostéosclérose
osteotomia, otalgia	Osteotomie	ostéotomie
otite	Otalgie, Ohrenschmerz	otalgie
otite	Otitis, Mittelohrentzündung	otite
cerume nell orecchio	glue ear	otite moyenne adhésive
otolaringologia	Otolaryngologie	otolaryngologie
otologia	Otologie, Ohrenheilkunde	otologie
orecchio naso e gola, otorinolaringoiatria	Hals- Nasen- Ohren-	oto-rhino-laryngologie (ORL)
otorrea	Otorrhoe, Ohrenfluß	otorrhée
otoscopio	Otoskop, Ohrenspiegel	otoscope
otosclerosi	Otosklerose	otospongiose
ototossico	ototoxisch	ototoxique
ovaio	Ovarium, Eierstock	ovaire
ovariectomia, ooforectomia	Oophorektomie	ovariectomie
ovarico	ovarial, Eierstock-	ovarien
uovo, gamete femminile	Ovum, Ei	ovocyte de premier ordre

FRENCH	ENGLISH	SPANISH
ovulation	ovulation	ovulación
ovule	ovum	óvulo
oxydation	oxidation	oxidación
oxygénation	oxygenation	oxigenación
oxygénothérapie hyperbase	hyperbaric oxygen treatment	tratamiento con oxígeno hiperbárico
oxytocine	oxytocin	oxitocina

ITALIAN	GERMAN	FRENCH
ovulazione	Ovulation, Eisprung	**ovulation**
uovo, gamete femminile	Ovum, Ei	**ovule**
ossidazione	Oxydation	**oxydation**
ossigenazione	Sauerstoffsättigung, Oxygenierung	**oxygénation**
ossigenoterapia iperbarica	hyperbare Sauerstoffbehandlung	**oxygénothérapie hyperbase**
ossitocina	Oxytozin	**oxytocine**

P

FRENCH	ENGLISH	SPANISH
palais	palate	paladar
palatin	palatine	palatino
pâleur	pallor	palidez
palliatif (n)	palliative (n)	paliativo (n)
palliatif (a)	palliative (a)	paliativo (a)
palmaire	palmar	palmar
palpable	palpable	palpable
palpation	palpation	palpación
palpitation	palpitation	palpitación
paludisme	malaria	paludismo
panaris	whitlow	panadizo
panaris superficiel	paronychia	paroniquia
pancréas	pancreas	páncreas
pancréatite	pancreatitis	pancreatitis
pancytopénie	pancytopenia	pancitopenia
pandémie	pandemic	pandémico
pandémique	pandemic	pandémico
pansement	dressing	cura, vendaje
pansements	wound dressing	curas para heridas
papillaire	papillary	papilar
papillome	papilloma	papiloma
papule	papule	pápula
paradontolyse	periodontal disease	enfermedad periodontal
paralysie	palsy, paralysis	parálisis
paralysie de Bell	Bell's palsy	parálisis de Bell
paralysie générale des aliénés	general paralysis of the insane	parálisis cerebral
paralytique	paralytic	paralítico
paramédical	paramedical	paramédico
paranoïa	paranoia	paranoia
paraphimosis	paraphimosis	parafimosis
paraphrénie	paraphrenia	parafrenia
paraplégie	paraplegia	paraplejía
para-SIDA	AIDS-related complex	complejo relacionado con SIDA
parasite	parasite	parásito
parasuicide	parasuicide	parasuicidio
parasympathique	parasympathetic	parasimpático
parathormone	parathormone	parathormona
parathyroïdectomie	parathyroidectomy	paratiroidectomía
paravertébral	paravertebral	paravertebral
parenchyme	parenchyma	parénquima
parentéral	parenteral	parenteral
parésie	paresis	paresia
paresthésie	paraesthesia (Eng), paresthesia (Am)	parestesia
pariétal	mural, parietal	mural, parietal

ITALIAN	GERMAN	FRENCH
palato	Gaumen	palais
palatale, palatino	palatal	palatin
pallore	Blässe	pâleur
palliativo (n)	Palliativum (n)	palliatif (n)
palliativo (a)	palliativ (a)	palliatif (a)
palmare	palmar	palmaire
palpabile	palpabel, tastbar	palpable
palpazione	Palpation	palpation
palpitazione	Palpitation, Herzklopfen	palpitation
malaria	Malaria	paludisme
patereccio	Panaritium	panaris
paronichia	Paronychie	panaris superficiel
pancreas	Pankreas, Bauchspeicheldrüse	pancréas
pancreatite	Pankreatitis, Bauchspeicheldrüsenentzündung	pancréatite
pancitopenia	Panzytopenie	pancytopénie
pandemia	Pandemie	pandémie
pandemico	pandemisch	pandémique
medicazione	Verband, Umschlag	pansement
medicazione di ferita	Verbandmaterial	pansements
papillare	papillär	papillaire
papilloma	Papillom	papillome
papula	Papel, Knötchen	papule
periodontopatia	Periodontitis, Wurzelhautentzündung	paradontolyse
paralisi	Paralyse, Lähmung	paralysie
paralisi di Bell	Bell-Fazialisparese	paralysie de Bell
paralisi progressiva luetica	progressive Paralyse	paralysie générale des aliénés
paralitico	paralytisch, gelähmt	paralytique
paramedico	paramedizinisch	paramédical
paranoia	Paranoia	paranoïa
parafimosi	Paraphimose	paraphimosis
parafrenia	Paraphrenie	paraphrénie
paraplegia	Paraplegie, Querschnittslähmung	paraplégie
complesso AIDS-correlato	AIDS-related complex	para-SIDA
parassita	Parasit, Schmarotzer	parasite
suicidio figurato	parasuizidale Handlung	parasuicide
parasimpatico	parasympathisch	parasympathique
paratormone	Parathormon	parathormone
paratiroidectomia	Parathyreoidektomie	parathyroïdectomie
paravertebrale	paravertebral	paravertébral
parenchima	Parenchym	parenchyme
parenterale	parenteral	parentéral
paresi	Parese, Lähmung	parésie
parestesia	Parästhesie	paresthésie
murale, parietale	mural, parietal, wandständig	pariétal

FRENCH	ENGLISH	SPANISH
parité	parity	paridad
parkinsonisme	parkinsonism	parkinsonismo
parotite	parotitis	parotiditis
paroxysmal	paroxysmal	paroxístico
partiellement soluble	partly soluble (p.sol)	semisoluble
parties par million (ppm)	parts per million (ppm)	partes por millón (ppm)
parturient	parturient	parturienta
parturition	parturition	parturición, parto
passif	passive	pasivo
pasteurisation	pasteurization	pasteurización
pastille	lozenge	pastilla
pâte	paste	pasta
pathogène	pathogen	patógeno
pathogenèse	pathogenesis	patogenia
pathognomonique	pathognomonic	patognomónico
pathologie	pathology	patología
paume	palm	palma
paupière	palpebra	párpado
pavillon de l'oreille	pinna	pabellón de la oreja
pavillon de soins spéciaux aux nouveau-nés	special care baby unit (SCBU)	unidad para cuidados especiales neonatales
peau	skin	piel
peau d'orange	peau d'orange	piel de naranja
pectoral	pectoral	pectoral
pédiatrie	paediatrics (Eng), pediatrics (Am)	pediatría
pédiculose	pediculosis	pediculosis
pédicure	chiropodist	callista, podólogo
pédieux	pedal	pedal
pédoncule	peduncle	pedúnculo
pellagre	pellagra	pelagra
pellicules	dandruff	caspa
pelvimétrie	pelvimetry	pelvimetría
pelvipéritonite	pelvic inflammatory disease (PID)	enfermedad inflamatoria de la pelvis
pelvis	pelvis	pelvis
pemphigoïde	pemphigoid	penfigoide
pemphigus	pemphigus	pénfigo
pendant	pendulous	péndulo
pénis	penis	pene
pepsine	pepsin	pepsina
peptide	peptide	péptido
peptique	peptic	péptico
perception	perception	percepción
percussion	percussion	percusión
percutané	percutaneous	percutáneo
perforation	perforation	perforación
perfuser	drip	infundir

ITALIAN	GERMAN	FRENCH
parità, numero di gravidanze pregresse	Gebärfähigkeit, Ähnlichkeit	parité
parkinsonismo	Parkinsonismus	parkinsonisme
parotite	Parotitis	parotite
parossistico	paroxysmal, krampfartig	paroxysmal
parzialmente solubile	teilweise löslich	partiellement soluble
parti per milione (ppm)	ppm, mg/l	parties par million (ppm)
partoriente	gebärend	parturient
parto	Gebären, Geburt	parturition
passivo	passiv, teilnahmslos	passif
pastorizzazione	Pasteurisierung	pasteurisation
pastiglia	Pastille	pastille
pasta, pasta gelificante	Paste, Salbe	pâte
patogeno	Krankheitserreger, Erreger	pathogène
patogenesi	Pathogenese	pathogenèse
patognomonico	pathognomonisch	pathognomonique
patologia	Pathologie	pathologie
palmo	Handinnenfläche	paume
palpebra	Palpebra, Lid	paupière
padiglione auricolare	Ohrmuschel	pavillon de l'oreille
unità di cure speciali pediatriche	Säuglings-Intensivstation	pavillon de soins spéciaux aux nouveau-nés
pelle	Haut	peau
buccia d'arancia	Orangenhaut	peau d'orange
pettorale	pektoral, Brust-	pectoral
pediatria	Pädiatrie, Kinderheilkunde	pédiatrie
pediculosi	Pedikulose, Läusebefall	pédiculose
callista	Fußpfleger	pédicure
del piede	Fuß-	pédieux
peduncolo	Stiel	pédoncule
pellagra	Pellagra	pellagre
forfora	Schuppen	pellicules
pelvimetria	Pelvimetrie	pelvimétrie
malattia infiammatoria della pelvi (PID)	Salpingitis	pelvipéritonite
pelvi	Pelvis, Becken	pelvis
pemfigoide	pemphigoid	pemphigoïde
pemfigo	Pemphigus	pemphigus
pendulo	hängend, gestielt	pendant
pene	Penis	pénis
pepsina	Pepsin	pepsine
peptide	Peptide	peptide
peptico	peptisch	peptique
percezione	Perzeption, Wahrnehmung	perception
percussione	Perkussion	percussion
percutaneo	perkutan	percutané
perforazione	Perforation	perforation
gocciolare, far gocciolare	tröpfeln, tropfen	perfuser

333

perfusion	perfusion, drip	perfusión, gota a gota intravenoso
périanal	perianal	perianal
péribuccal	circumoral	circumoral, peroral
péricarde	pericardium	pericardio
péricardite	pericarditis	pericarditis
périchondre	perichondrium	pericondrio
périnatal	perinatal	perinatal
périnée	perineum	perineo
période des mouvements oculaires	rapid eye movement (REM)	movimiento rápido de los ojos (REM)
période néonatale	neonatal period	período neonatal
périombilical	periumbilical	periumbilical
périopératoire	perioperative	perioperatorio
périoral	perioral	perioral
périoste	periosteum	periostio
périphérique	peripheral	periférico
péristaltisme	peristalsis	peristalsis
péritoine	peritoneum	peritoneo
péritonite	peritonitis	peritonitis
perméable	permeable	permeable
peroral	peroral	peroral
persévération	perseveration	perseverancia
personnalité	personality	personalidad
personnalité psychopathique	antisocial personality, psychopathic personality	personalidad antisocial, personalidad psicopática
personnalité schizoïde	schizoid personality	personalidad esquizoide
perspiration	perspiration	sudor
perte de poids	weight loss	pérdida de peso
pertussis	pertussis	tos ferina
pessaire	pessary	pesario
peste	plague	peste, plaga
pétéchie	petechia	petequia
petit mal	petit mal	petit mal
petit pot	gallipot	bote
phagocyte	phagocyte	fagocito
phagocytose	phagocytosis	fagocitosis
phalanges	phalanges	falanges
phallus	phallus	falo
pharmaceutique	pharmaceutical	farmacéutico
pharmacien	pharmacist	farmacéutico
pharmacocinétique	pharmacokinetics	farmacocinética
pharmacogénétique	pharmacogenetics	farmacogenético
pharmacologie	pharmacology	farmacología
pharyngite	pharyngitis	faringitis
pharyngotomie	pharyngotomy	faringotomía
pharynx	pharynx	faringe
phénotype	phenotype	fenotipo

perfusione, fleboclisi	Durchblutung, Tropfinfusion	**perfusion**
perianale	perianal	**périanal**
circumorale	zirkumoral	**péribuccal**
pericardio	Perikard, Herzbeutel	**péricarde**
pericardite	Perikarditis	**péricardite**
pericondrio	Perichondrium, Knorpelhaut	**périchondre**
perinatale	perinatal	**périnatal**
perineo	Perineum, Damm	**périnée**
fase REM del sonno, movimento oculare rapido	rapid eye movement (REM)	**période des mouvements oculaires**
periodo neonatale	Neonatalperiode, Neugeborenenperiode	**période néonatale**
periombelicale	periumbilikal	**périombilical**
perioperatorio	perioperativ	**périopératoire**
periorale	perioral	**périoral**
periostio	Periost, Knochenhaut	**périoste**
periferico	peripher	**périphérique**
peristalsi	Peristaltik	**péristaltisme**
peritoneo	Peritoneum, Bauchfell	**péritoine**
peritonite	Peritonitis	**péritonite**
permeabile	permeabel, durchlässig	**perméable**
perorale	peroral	**peroral**
perseverazione	Perseveration	**persévération**
personalità	Persönlichkeit	**personnalité**
personalità antisociale, personalità psicopatica	asoziale Persönlichkeit, psychopathische Persönlichkeit	**personnalité psychopathique**
personalità schizoide	schizoide Persönlichkeit	**personnalité schizoïde**
perspirazione	Schweiß	**perspiration**
perdita di peso	Gewichtsverlust	**perte de poids**
pertosse	Pertussis, Keuchhusten	**pertussis**
pessario	Pessar	**pessaire**
peste	Pest, Seuche	**peste**
petecchia	Petechie	**pétéchie**
piccolo male	Petit mal	**petit mal**
ampolla o vasetto unguentario	Salbentopf	**petit pot**
fagocito	Phagozyt	**phagocyte**
fagocitosi	Phagozytose	**phagocytose**
falangi	Fingerglieder, Zehenglieder	**phalanges**
fallo	Phallus, Penis	**phallus**
farmaceutico	pharmazeutisch, Apotheker-	**pharmaceutique**
farmacista	Apotheker, Pharmazeut	**pharmacien**
farmacocinetica	Pharmakokinetik	**pharmacocinétique**
farmacogenetica	Pharmakogenetik	**pharmacogénétique**
farmacologia	Pharmakologie	**pharmacologie**
faringite	Pharyngitis	**pharyngite**
faringotomia	Pharyngotomie	**pharyngotomie**
faringe	Pharynx, Rachen	**pharynx**
fenotipo	Phänotyp	**phénotype**

FRENCH	ENGLISH	SPANISH
phénylcétonurie	phenylketonuria (PKU)	fenilcetonuria
phéochromocytome	phaeochromocytoma (Eng), pheochromocytoma (Am)	feocromocitoma
phimosis	phimosis	fimosis
phlébectomie	phlebectomy	flebectomía
phlébite	phlebitis	flebitis
phlébographie	venography	venografía
phlébolithe	phlebolith	flebolito
phlébotomie	phlebotomy, venesection	flebotomía, venisección
phlegme	phlegm	flema
phlegmon amygdalien ou périamygdalien	quinsy	absceso periamigdalino, angina
phlyctène	bleb	vesícula, bulla, ampolla
phobie	phobia	fobia
phocomélie	phocomelia	focomelia
photophobie	photophobia	fotofobia
photosensible	photosensitive	fotosensible
photothérapie	phototherapy	fototerapia
physiologique	physiological	fisiológico
pian	yaws	yaws, pian
pica	pica	pica
pièce	patch test	prueba del parche
pied	foot	pie
pied bot	club-foot, talipes	pie zambo, talipes
pied d'athlète	athlete's foot	pie de atleta
pied gelé	trench foot	pie de trinchera
pied plat	flat-foot	pie plano
pigment	pigment	pigmento
pigmentation	pigmentation	pigmentación
pilonidal	pilonidal	pilonidal
pilule	pill	píldora
pinguécula	pinguecula	pinguécula
pinta	pinta	mal de pinto
piqûre	sting	picadura
pityriasis	pityriasis	pitiriasis
placebo	placebo	placebo
placenta	placenta	placenta
plaie	wound	herida
plaie de décubitus	pressure sore	úlcera de decúbito
plaie par pénétration	penetrating wound	herida penetrante
plancher pelvien	pelvic floor	suelo de la pelvis
plantaire	plantar	plantar
plaque	patch test, plaque	prueba del parche, placa
plaques de Peyer	Peyer's patches	placas de Peyer
plaquette	platelet	plaqueta
plasma	plasma	plasma
plasmaphérèse	plasmapheresis	plasmaféresis

ITALIAN	GERMAN	FRENCH
fenilchetonuria	Phenylketonurie (PKU)	**phénylcétonurie**
feocromocitoma	Phäochromozytom	**phéochromocytome**
fimosi	Phimose	**phimosis**
flebectomia	Phlebektomie	**phlébectomie**
flebite	Phlebitis, Venenentzündung	**phlébite**
flebografia	Phlebographie	**phlébographie**
flebolito	Phlebolith	**phlébolithe**
flebotomia	Venae sectio	**phlébotomie**
flemma	Phlegma	**phlegme**
ascesso peritonsillare	Peritonsillarabszeß	**phlegmon amygdalien ou périamygdalien**
vescichetta, flittena	Bläschen	**phlyctène**
fobia	Phobie	**phobie**
focomelia	Phokomelie	**phocomélie**
fotofobia	Photophobie, Lichtscheue	**photophobie**
fotosensibile	lichtempfindlich	**photosensible**
fototerapia	Phototherapie	**photothérapie**
fisiologico	physiologisch	**physiologique**
framboesia, pian	Frambösie	**pian**
picacismo	Pica	**pica**
test epicutaneo	Läppchenprobe, Einreibeprobe	**pièce**
piede	Fuß	**pied**
piede torto, piede talo	Klumpfuß, pes equinovarus	**pied bot**
piede di atleta	Fußpilz	**pied d'athlète**
piede da trincea	Schützengrabenfuß	**pied gelé**
piede piatto	Plattfuß	**pied plat**
pigmento	Pigment, Farbstoff	**pigment**
pigmentazione	Pigmentierung, Färbung	**pigmentation**
pilonidale	pilonidal	**pilonidal**
pillola	Pille	**pilule**
pinguecula	Pinguekula	**pinguécula**
pinta, spirochetosi discromica	Pinta	**pinta**
dolore acuto, puntura	Stachel, Stich	**piqûre**
pitiriasi	Pityriasis	**pityriasis**
placebo	Plazebo	**placebo**
placenta	Plazenta, Nachgeburt	**placenta**
ferita	Wunde, Verletzung	**plaie**
ulcera da decubito	Druckgeschwür, Dekubitus	**plaie de décubitus**
ferita penetrante	penetrierende Verletzung	**plaie par pénétration**
pavimento pelvico	Beckenboden	**plancher pelvien**
plantare	plantar	**plantaire**
test epicutaneo, placca	Läppchenprobe, Einreibeprobe, Plaque, Zahnbelag	**plaque**
placche di Peyer	Peyer Plaques	**plaques de Peyer**
piastrina	Thrombozyt, Blutplättchen	**plaquette**
plasma	Plasma	**plasma**
plasmaferesi	Plasmapherese	**plasmaphérèse**

FRENCH	ENGLISH	SPANISH
plâtre	cast, plaster, plaster of Paris	enyesado, vendaje de yeso, yeso, escayola
pléthore	plethora	plétora
pleurésie	pleurisy (pleuritis)	pleuresia, pleuritis
pleurodèse	pleurodesis	pleurodesis
pleurodynie	pleurodynia	pleurodinia
plèvre	pleura	pleura
plexus	plexus	plexo
plexus solaire	solar plexus	plexo solar
plicature	plication	plicatura
plomb	lead	plomo
pneumaturie	pneumaturia	neumaturia
pneumocéphale	pneumocephalus	neumocéfalo
pneumoconiose	pneumoconiosis	neumoconiosis
pneumo-encéphale	pneumocephalus	neumocéfalo
pneumonectomie	pneumonectomy	neumonectomía
pneumonie	pneumonia	neumonía
pneumonite	pneumonitis	neumonitis
pneumopathie vasculaire	pulmonary vascular disease (PVD)	vasculopatia pulmonar
pneumopéritoine	pneumoperitoneum	neumoperitoneo
pneumothorax	pneumothorax	neumotórax
poche	pouch	bolsa
poche ectobranchiale et entobranchiale	pharyngeal pouch	bolsa faringea
poids atomique	atomic weight (at wt)	peso atómico
poids corporel total	total body weight (TBW)	peso corporal total
poignet	wrist	muñeca
poil	hair	pelo
point de McBurney	McBurney's point	punto de McBurney
point de suture	stitch	punto de sutura
point particulièrement sensible	pressure point	punto de presión
points de Koplik	Koplik's spots	manchas de Koplik
poison	poison	veneno
poliomyélite	poliomyelitis	poliomielitis
poliovirus	poliovirus	poliovirus
polyartérite	polyarteritis	poliarteritis
polyarthralgie	polyarthralgia	poliartralgia
polyarthrite	polyarthritis	poliartritis
polyarthrite chronique évolutive (PCE)	rheumatoid arthritis (RA)	artritis reumatoide (AR)
polyarthrite rhumatoïde (PR)	rheumatoid arthritis (RA)	artritis reumatoide (AR)
polycythémie	polycythaemia (Eng), polycythemia (Am)	policitemia
polydipsie	polydipsia	polidipsia
polykystique	polycystic	poliquístico
polymyalgie rhumatismale	polymyalgia rheumatica	polimialgia reumática
polymyosite	polymyositis	polimiositis

ingessatura, steccatura, gesso, gesso di Parigi (calcio solfato diidrato)	Abdruck, Gipsverband, Gips, Pflaster	plâtre
pletora	Plethora	pléthore
pleurite	Pleuritis, Rippenfellentzündung	pleurésie
pleurodesi	Pleurodese	pleurodèse
pleurodinia	Pleuralgie	pleurodynie
pleura	Pleura	plèvre
plesso	Plexus	plexus
plesso solare, plesso celiaco	Solarplexus	plexus solaire
plicazione, piegatura	Faltenbildung	plicature
piombo derivazione	Ableitung	plomb
pneumaturia	Pneumaturie	pneumaturie
pneumocefalo	Pneumozephalus	pneumocéphale
pneumoconiosi	Pneumokoniose, Staublunge	pneumoconiose
pneumocefalo	Pneumozephalus	pneumo-encéphale
pneumonectomia	Pneumonektomie, Lungenresektion	pneumonectomie
polmonite	Pneumonie, Lungenentzündung	pneumonie
polmonite	Pneumonitis	pneumonite
vasculopatia polmonare	Lungengefäßerkrankung	pneumopathie vasculaire
pneumoperitoneo	Pneumoperitoneum	pneumopéritoine
pneumotorace	Pneumothorax	pneumothorax
tasca	Beutel, Tasche	poche
tasca faringea	Schlundtasche	poche ectobranchiale et entobranchiale
peso atomico	Atomgewicht	poids atomique
peso corporeo totale	Körpergewicht	poids corporel total
polso	Handgelenk, Karpus	poignet
pelo, capello	Haar	poil
punto di McBurney	McBurney-Punkt	point de McBurney
punto	Stechen	point de suture
punto cutaneo sensibile alla pressione	Druckpunkt, Dekubitus	point particulièrement sensible
segni di Koplik	Koplik-Flecken	points de Koplik
veleno	Gift	poison
poliomielite	Poliomyelitis, Kinderlähmung	poliomyélite
virus della poliomielite	Poliovirus	poliovirus
poliarterite	Polyarteritis	polyartérite
poliartralgia	Polyarthralgie	polyarthralgie
poliartrite	Polyarthritis	polyarthrite
artrite reumatoide (AR)	Polyarthritis rheumatica (PCP), Rheumatoide Arthritis	polyarthrite chronique évolutive (PCE)
artrite reumatoide (AR)	Polyarthritis rheumatica (PCP), Rheumatoide Arthritis	polyarthrite rhumatoïde (PR)
policitemia	Polyzythämie	polycythémie
polidipsia	Polydipsie	polydipsie
policistico	polyzystisch	polykystique
polimialgia reumatica	Polymyalgia rheumatica	polymyalgie rhumatismale
polimiosite	Polymyositis	polymyosite

FRENCH	ENGLISH	SPANISH
polynévrite	polyneuritis	polineuritis
polynucléaire neutrophile	neutrophil	neutrófilo
polype	polyp	pólipo
polypectomie	polypectomy	polipectomía
polypharmacie	polypharmacy	polifarmacia
polypose	polyposis	poliposis
polysaccharide	polysaccharide	polisacárido
polyurie	polyuria	poliuria
pommade	ointment, salve	ungüento
pomme d'Adam	Adam's apple	huez de Adán
pompholyx	pompholyx	ponfólix
ponction	puncture, tapping	punción, paracentesis
ponction d'une veine	venepuncture, venipuncture	venopuntura, venipuntura
ponction lombaire	lumbar puncture (LP)	punción lumbar (PL)
ponctionner	puncture	pinchar
ponction sternale	sternal puncture	punción esternal
poplité	popliteal, popliteus	poplíteo
pore	pore	poro
poreux	parous	parir
porphyrie	porphyria	porfiria
porphyrine	porphyrin	porfirinas
porte	porta	porta
porteur	carrier	portador
porto-cave	portacaval	portocava
porto-hépatite	portahepatitis	portohepatitis
position de Sim	Sims' position	posición de Sim
postcure	aftercare	cuidados postoperatorios
postencéphalitique	postencephalitic	postencefalítico
postérieur	posterior	posterior
posthépatique	posthepatic	posthepático
postherpétique	postherpetic	postherpético
postmature	postmaturity	postmaduro
postménopausique	postmenopausal	postmenopáusico
post mortem	post-mortem	postmortem
postnatal	postnatal	postnatal
postopératoire	postoperative	postoperatorio
postpartum	postpartum	postpartum
postprandial	postprandial	postprandial
postural	postural	postural
posture antéromentonnière	mentoanterior	mentoanterior
posture postmentonnière	mentoposterior	mentoposterior
pou	louse	piojo
pouce	thumb	pulgar
pouls	pulse	pulso
pouls alternant	pulsus alternans	pulso alternante
pouls paradoxal	pulsus paradoxus	pulso paradójico

340

ITALIAN	GERMAN	FRENCH
polineurite	Polyneuritis	polynévrite
granulocito neutrofilo	Neutrophiler	polynucléaire neutrophile
polipo	Polyp	polype
polipectomia	Polypektomie	polypectomie
prescrizione multipla di farmaci, abuso di farmaci	Polypragmasie	polypharmacie
poliposi	Polyposis	polypose
polisaccaride	Polysaccharid	polysaccharide
poliuria	Polyurie	polyurie
unguento	Salbe	pommade
pomo di Adamo	Adamsapfel	pomme d'Adam
ponfolice (disidrosi vescicolare)	Pompholyx	pompholyx
puntura, aspirazione di fluido	Stich, Injektion, Abzapfen, Punktieren, Perkutieren	ponction
puntura di vena	Venenpunktion	ponction d'une veine
puntura lombare, rachicentesi	Lumbalpunktion	ponction lombaire
pungere	stechen, injizieren	ponctionner
puntura sternale	Sternalpunktion	ponction sternale
popliteo	popliteal, popliteus	poplité
poro	Pore	pore
che ha avuto figli	geboren habend	poreux
porfiria	Porphyrie	porphyrie
porfirina	Porphyrin	porphyrine
porta	Eingang	porte
portatore	Ausscheider, Trägerstoff	porteur
portocavale	portokaval	porto-cave
portaepatite	Porta hepatis, Leberpforte	porto-hépatite
posizione di Sim	Sims-Lage	position de Sim
assistenza post-operatoria	Nachbehandlung, Nachsorge	postcure
postencefalitico	postenzephalitisch	postencéphalitique
posteriore	posteriore, hintere, Gesäß-	postérieur
postepatico	posthepatisch	posthépatique
posterpetico	postherpetisch	postherpétique
postmaturo, ipermaturo	Überreife	postmature
postmenopausale	postmenopausal	postménopausique
post mortem	postmortal	post mortem
postnatale	postnatal	postnatal
postoperatorio	postoperativ	postopératoire
post partum	post partum	postpartum
postprandiale	postprandial	postprandial
posturale	Lage-	postural
mentoanteriore	mentoanterior	posture antéromentonnière
mentoposteriore	mentoposterior	posture postmentonnière
pidocchio	Laus	pou
pollice	Daumen	pouce
polso	Puls	pouls
polso alternante	Pulsus alternans	pouls alternant
polso paradosso	Pulsus paradoxus	pouls paradoxal

poumon	lung	pulmón
poumon d'acier	heart-lung machine	máquina de circulación extracorpórea
pouvoir pathogène	pathogenicity	patogenicidad
pouvoir sidéropexique	iron binding capacity (IBC)	capacidad de unión con el hierro
précancéreux	precancerous	precanceroso
préconceptuel	preconceptual	preconceptual
précordial	precordial	precordial
précurseur	precursor	precursor
précurseur de médicament	pro-drug	profármaco
prédisposition	predisposition	predisposición
prématuré	premature	prematuro
prémédication	premedication	premedicación
prémenstruel	premenstrual	premenstrual
premiers soins	first aid	primeros auxilios
prénatal	prenatal	prenatal
préopératoire	preoperative	preoperatorio
prépubertaire	prepubertal	prepubertal
prépuce	foreskin, prepuce	prepucio
prérénal	prerenal	prerrenal
présentant un retard de croissance	small-for-dates (SFD)	útero pequeño para la edad gestacional
présentation	breech-birth presentation, presentation	presentación de nalgas, presentación
présentation vicieuse	malpresentation	malpresentación
préservatif	condom	condón
pressif	pressor	presor
pression artérielle bloquée moyenne	pulmonary capillary pressure (PCP)	presión capilar pulmonar (PCP)
pression capillaire pulmonaire (PCP)	pulmonary capillary pressure (PCP)	presión capilar pulmonar (PCP)
pression intracrânienne	intracranial pressure (ICP)	presión intracraneal (PIC)
pression osmotique	osmotic pressure	presión osmótica
pression partielle	partial pressure	presión parcial
primigeste	primigravida	primigrávida
primipare	primipara	primípara
pris de vertige	giddy	mareado
prise en nourrice	fostering	adopción
procidence	procidentia	procidencia
proctalgie	proctalgia	proctalgia
proctocolectomie	proctocolectomy	proctocolectomia
prodromique	prodromal	prodrómico
produire l'abduction	abduct	abducir
produire l'adduction	adduct	aducir
prolapsus	prolapse	prolapso
proliférer	proliferate	proliferar
pronateur	pronator	pronador
pronostic	prognosis	pronóstico
prophylaxie	prophylaxis	profilaxis

ITALIAN	GERMAN	FRENCH
polmoni	Lunge	poumon
macchina cuore-polmone	Herzlungenmaschine	poumon d'acier
patogeneticità	Pathogenität	pouvoir pathogène
capacità di legame del ferro	Eisenbindungskapazität	pouvoir sidéropexique
precanceroso	präkanzerös	précancéreux
precedente il concepimento	vor Empfängnis	préconceptuel
precordiale, epigastrico	präkordial	précordial
precursore	Vorzeichen, Vorstufe, Präkursor	précurseur
profarmaco (precursore inattivo)	pro-drug (Pharmakon-Vorform)	précurseur de médicament
predisposizione	Prädisposition, Anfälligkeit	prédisposition
preamaturo	frühreif, vorzeitig	prématuré
premedicazione, preanestesia	Prämedikation	prémédication
premestruale	prämenstruell	prémenstruel
pronto soccorso	Erste Hilfe	premiers soins
prenatale	pränatal, vorgeburtlich	prénatal
preoperatorio	präoperativ	préopératoire
prepubertale	Präpubertäts-	prépubertaire
prepuzio	Präputium, Vorhaut	prépuce
prerenale	prärenal	prérénal
basso peso alla nascita	termingemäß klein	présentant un retard de croissance
presentazione podalica, presentazione	Steißlage, Lage, Kindslage	présentation
presentazione fetale anomala	anomale Kindslage	présentation vicieuse
profilattico maschile	Kondom, Präservativ	préservatif
pressorio	blutdruckerhöhend, vasopressorisch	pressif
pressione polmonare di incuneamento	Lungenkapillardruck	pression artérielle bloquée moyenne
pressione polmonare di incuneamento	Lungenkapillardruck	pression capillaire pulmonaire (PCP)
pressione intracranica	Hirndruck, intrakranieller Druck	pression intracrânienne
pressione osmotica	osmotischer Druck	pression osmotique
pressione parziale	Partialdruck	pression partielle
primigravida	Primigravida	primigeste
primipara	Primipara, Erstgebärende	primipare
stordito, affetto da vertigini o capogiro	schwindlig	pris de vertige
affido	Pflege	prise en nourrice
procidenza	Prolaps, Vorfall	procidence
proctalgia	Proktalgie	proctalgie
proctocolectomia, rettocolectomia	Proktokolektomie	proctocolectomie
prodromico	prodromal	prodromique
abdurre	abduzieren	produire l'abduction
addurre	adduzieren, zusammenziehen	produire l'adduction
prolasso	Prolaps, Vorfall	prolapsus
proliferare	proliferieren	proliférer
pronatore	Pronator	pronateur
prognosi	Prognose	pronostic
profilassi	Prophylaxe, Vorbeugung	prophylaxie

FRENCH	ENGLISH	SPANISH
proptose	proptosis	proptosis
prostaglandine	prostaglandin	prostaglandina
prostate	prostate	próstata
prostatectomie	prostatectomy	prostatectomía
prostatisme	prostatism	prostatismo
protéine	protein	proteína
protéine de Bence Jones (BJ)	Bence-Jones protein (BJ)	proteína de Bence-Jones
protéinurie	proteinuria	proteinuria
prothèse	prosthesis	prótesis
protozoaires	protozoa	protozoos
proximal	proximal	proximal
prurit	pruritus	prurito
pseudopolypose	pseudopolyposis	pseudopoliposis
psittacose	psittacosis	psitacosis
psoas	psoas	psoas
psoralène	psoralen	psoralen
psoriasis	psoriasis	psoriasis
psychanalyse	psychoanalysis	psicoanálisis
psychiatrie	psychiatry	psiquiatría
psychiatrique	psychiatric	psiquiátrico
psychique	phrenic, psychic	frénico, psíquico
psychodynamique	psychodynamics	psicodinámica
psychogène	psychogenic	psicógeno
psychogériatrique	psychogeriatric	psicogeriátrico
psychologie	psychology	psicología
psychomoteur	psychomotor	psicomotor
psychopathe	psychopath	psicópata
psychopathie	psychopathy	psicopatía
psychopathologie	psychopathology	psicopatología
psychose	psychosis	psicosis
psychose de Korsakoff	Korsakoff's psychosis	psicosis de Korsakoff
psychose maniacodépressive	manic-depressive psychosis	psicosis maniacodepresiva
psychosomatique	psychosomatic	psicosomático
psychothérapie	psychotherapy	psicoterapia
psychotrope	psychotropic	psicotrópico
ptérygion	pterygium	pterigión
ptose	ptosis	ptosis
puberté	puberty	pubertad
pubis	pubis	pubis
puce	flea	pulga
puerpéral	puerperal	puerperal
puerpérium	puerperium	puerperio
pulmonaire	pulmonary	pulmonar
pulsatile	pulsatile	pulsátil
pulsation	pulsation	pulsación
pulsation (de coeur)	heartbeat	patido cardíaco

ITALIAN	GERMAN	FRENCH
proptosi	Vorfall, Exophthalmus	proptose
prostaglandina	Prostaglandine	prostaglandine
prostata	Prostata	prostate
prostatectomia	Prostatektomie	prostatectomie
prostatismo	chronisches Prostataleiden	prostatisme
proteina	Protein	protéine
proteina di Bence-Jones	Bence-Jones-Proteine	protéine de Bence Jones (BJ)
proteinuria	Proteinurie	protéinurie
protesi	Prothese	prothèse
protozoi	Protozoe	protozoaires
prossimale	proximal	proximal
prurito	Pruritus, Jucken	prurit
pseudopoliposi	Pseudopolypse	pseudopolypose
psittacosi	Psittakose, Ornithose	psittacose
psoas	Psoas	psoas
psoralene	Psoralen	psoralène
psoriasi	Psoriasis, Schuppenflechte	psoriasis
psicoanalisi	Psychoanalyse	psychanalyse
psichiatria	Psychiatrie	psychiatrie
psichiatrico	psychiatrisch	psychiatrique
frenico (diaframmatico mentale), psichico	diaphragmatisch, Zwerchfell-, psychisch, seelisch	psychique
psicodinamica	Psychodynamik	psychodynamique
psicogenico	psychogen	psychogène
psicogeriatrico	gerontopsychiatrisch	psychogériatrique
psicologia	Psychologie	psychologie
psicomotorio	psychomotorisch	psychomoteur
psicopatico	Psychopath	psychopathe
psicopatia	Psychopathie	psychopathie
psicopatologia	Psychopathologie	psychopathologie
psicosi	Psychose	psychose
psicosi di Korsakoff	Korsakow-Psychose	psychose de Korsakoff
psicosi maniaco-depressiva	manisch-depressive Psychose	psychose maniacodépressive
psicosomatico	psychosomatisch, Leib-Seele-	psychosomatique
psicoterapia	Psychotherapie	psychothérapie
psicotropo	psychotrop	psychotrope
pterigio, eponichio	Pterygium	ptérygion
ptosi	Ptose	ptose
pubertà	Pubertät	puberté
pube	Os pubis, Schambein	pubis
pulce	Floh	puce
puerperale	puerperal, Kindbett-	puerpéral
puerperio	Wochenbett, Puerperium	puerpérium
polmonare	Lungen-	pulmonaire
pulsatile	pulsierend	pulsatile
pulsazione	Pulsieren, Pulsschlag	pulsation
battito cardiaco	Herzschlag	pulsation (de coeur)

FRENCH	ENGLISH	SPANISH
pupillaire	pupillary	pupilar
pupille	pupil	pupila
purgatif (n)	purgative (n)	purga (n)
purgatif (a)	purgative (a)	purgante (a)
purpura	purpura	púrpura
purpura rhumatoïde	Henoch-Schönlein purpura	púrpura de Schönlein-Henoch
purulent	purulent	purulento
pus	pus	pus
pustule	pustule	pústula
putréfaction	putrefaction	putrefacción
pyarthrose	pyarthrosis	piartrosis
pyélite	pyelitis	pielitis
pyélographie	pyelography	pielografía
pyélonéphrite	pyelonephritis	pielonefritis
pylore	pylorus	píloro
pyloroplastie	pyloroplasty	piloroplastia
pylorospasme	pylorospasm	pilorospasmo
pylorotomie	pyloromyotomy	piloromiotomía
pyodermie	pyoderma	pioderma
pyogène	pyogenic	piógeno
pyométrie	pyometra	piómetra
pyonéphrose	pyonephrosis	pionefrosis
pyosalpinx	pyosalpinx	piosalpinx
pyramidal	pyramidal	piramidal
pyrexie	pyrexia	pirexia, fiebre
pyrosis	pyrosis	pirosis
pyurie	pyuria	piuria

Q

quadriceps	quadriceps	cuádriceps
quadriplégie	quadriplegia	cuadriplejía
qualitatif	qualitative	cualitativo
quantitatif	quantitative	cuantitativo
quarantaine	quarantine	cuarentena
quarte	quartan	cuartana

ITALIAN	GERMAN	FRENCH
pupillare	pupillar, Pupillen-	pupillaire
pupilla	Pupille	pupille
lassativo (n)	Purgativum (n), Abführmittel (n)	purgatif (n)
purgante (a)	purgierend (a), abführend (a)	purgatif (a)
porpora	Purpura	purpura
porpora di Schönlein-Henoch	Purpura Schönlein-Henoch	purpura rhumatoïde
purulento	purulent, eitrig	purulent
pus	Eiter	pus
pustola	Pustel, Pickel	pustule
putrefazione	Verwesung, Fäulnis	putréfaction
pioartrosi, piartro	Pyarthrose, eitrige Gelenkentzündung	pyarthrose
pielite	Pyelitis, Nierenbeckenentzündung	pyélite
pielografia	Pyelographie	pyélographie
pielonefrite	Pyelonephritis	pyélonéphrite
piloro	Pylorus	pylore
piloroplastica	Pyloroplastik	pyloroplastie
pilorospasmo	Pylorospasmus	pylorospasme
piloromiotomia, intervento di Ramstedt	Pyloromyotomie	pylorotomie
piodermite, pioderma	Pyodermie	pyodermie
piogenico	pyogen	pyogène
piometra	Pyometra	pyométrie
pionefrosi	Pyonephrose	pyonéphrose
piosalpinge	Pyosalpinx	pyosalpinx
piramidale	pyramidal	pyramidal
piressia	Fieber	pyrexie
pirosi	Sodbrennen	pyrosis
piuria	Pyurie	pyurie

quadricipite	Quadrizeps	quadriceps
tetraplegia	Tetraplegie	quadriplégie
qualitativo	qualitativ	qualitatif
quantitativo	quantitativ	quantitatif
quarantena	Quarantäne	quarantaine
quartana	quartana (Malaria)	quarte

FRENCH	ENGLISH	SPANISH

R

rachitisme	rickets	raquitismo
radical	radical	radical
radioactif	radioactive	radiactivo
radiographe	radiograph	radiografía
radiographie	radiography	radiografía
radio-isotope	radioisotope	radioisótopo
radiologie	radiology	radiología
radio-opaque	radio-opaque	radiopaco
radiosensible	radiosensitive	radiosensible
radiothérapie	radiotherapy	radioterapia
radius	radius	radio
rage	rabies	rabia
rapports	intercourse	coito
rapports sexuels	sexual intercourse	coito
rash	rash	exantema
rate	spleen	bazo
rayons X	X-rays	rayos X
réactif	reagent	reactivo
réaction	reaction	reacción
réaction anaphylactique	anaphylactic reaction	reacción anafiláctica
réaction de Paul et Bunnell	Paul-Bunnell test	prueba de Paul-Bunnell
réaction de Schick	Schick test	prueba de Schick
réaction de Wassermann	Wassermann reaction	reacción de Wassermann
réaction de Widal	Widal reaction	reacción de Widal
réaction immunitaire	immune reaction	reacción inmunológica
réaction médicamenteuse indésirable	adverse drug reaction (ADR)	reacción adversa a un medicamento
réadaptation	rehabilitation	rehabilitación
réanimation au bouche-à-bouche	mouth to mouth resuscitation	respiración boca a boca
réanimation cardiorespiratoire	cardiopulmonary resuscitation (CPR)	resucitación cardiopulmonar
réapparition	recurrence	periódico
récepteur	receptor	receptor
récessif	recessive	recesivo
receveur	recipient	recipiente
rechute	relapse	recidiva
rechuter	relapse	recaer
rectite	proctitis	proctitis
rectocèle	rectocele	rectocele
rectocolite	proctocolitis	proctocolitis
rectoscope	proctoscope	proctoscopio
rectum	rectum	recto
réflexe	reflex	reflejo
réflexe conditionné	conditioned reflex	reflejo condicionado
réflexe de Babinski	Babinski's reflex	reflejo de Babinski

ITALIAN	GERMAN	FRENCH
rachitismo	Rachitis	rachitisme
radicale	radikal, Wurzel-	radical
radioattivo	radioaktiv	radioactif
immagine radiologica	Röntgenaufnahme	radiographe
radiografia	Röntgen	radiographie
radioisotopo	Radioisotop	radio-isotope
radiologia	Radiologie, Röntgenologie	radiologie
radioopaco	röntgendicht	radio-opaque
radiosensibile	strahlenempfindlich	radiosensible
radioterapia	Strahlentherapie, Radiotherapie	radiothérapie
radio	Radius, Halbmesser	radius
rabbia	Tollwut	rage
coito	Koitus, Geschlechtsverkehr	rapports
coito	Geschlechtsverkehr, Koitus	rapports sexuels
eruzione cutanea	Ausschlag, Hautausschlag	rash
milza	Milz	rate
raggi X	Röntgenstrahlen, Röntgenaufnahmen	rayons X
reagente	Reagens	réactif
reazione	Reaktion	réaction
reazione anafilattica	anaphylaktische Reaktion	réaction anaphylactique
test di Paul-Bunnell	Paul-Bunnell-Reaktion	réaction de Paul et Bunnell
test di Schick	Schick-Test	réaction de Schick
reazione di Wassermann	Wassermann-Reaktion	réaction de Wassermann
reazione di Widal	Widal-Reaktion	réaction de Widal
immunoreazione, reazione immune	Immunreaktion	réaction immunitaire
reazione dannosa (indesiderata) da farmaci	unerwünschte Arzneimittelreaktion	réaction médicamenteuse indésirable
riabilitazione	Rehabilitation	réadaptation
rianimazione bocca a bocca	Mund-zu-Mund-Wiederbelebung	réanimation au bouche-à-bouche
rianimazione cardiorespiratoria	Herz-Lungen-Wiederbelebung, Reanimation	réanimation cardiorespiratoire
recidiva	Rezidiv	réapparition
recettore	Rezeptor	récepteur
recessivo	rezessiv	récessif
ricevente	Empfänger	receveur
ricaduta, recidiva	Rückfall, Rezidiv	rechute
recidivare	rezidivieren, Rückfall erleiden	rechuter
proctite	Proktitis	rectite
rettocele	Rektozele	rectocèle
proctocolite	Proktokolitis	rectocolite
proctoscopio	Rektoskop	rectoscope
retto	Rektum	rectum
riflesso	Reflex	réflexe
riflesso condizionato	bedingter Reflex, konditionierter Reflex	réflexe conditionné
riflesso di Babinski	Babinski-Reflex	réflexe de Babinski

FRENCH	ENGLISH	SPANISH
réflexe de Moro	Moro reflex	reflejo de Moro
reflux	reflux	reflujo
réfractaire	refractory	refractario
réfraction	refraction	refracción
régénération	regeneration	regeneración
régime	regimen, diet	régimen
régime cétogène	ketogenic diet	dieta cetógena
région lombaire	loin	lomo
régression	regression	regresión
régurgitation	posseting, regurgitation	regurgitación láctea del neonato, regurgitación
rein	kidney	riñón
rejet	rejection	rechazo
relaxant (n)	relaxant (n)	relajante (n)
relaxant (a)	relaxant (a)	relajante (a)
releveur	levator	elevador
rémission	remission	remisión
rémittent	remittent	remitente
rénal	renal	renal
rénine	renin	renina
répétition	recurrence	periódico
répression	repression	represión
résection	resection	resección
résectoscope	resectoscope	resectoscopio
résiduel	residual	residual
résistant à l'alcool	alcohol-fast	resistente al alcohol
résistant à l'alcool et à l'acide	acid-alcohol-fast	ácido-alcohol-resistente
résolution	resolution	resolución
résonance	resonance	resonancia
résorption	resorption	resorción
respirateur	respirator	respirador
respiration	respiration	respiración
respiration anaérobie	anaerobic respiration (Eng), anerobic respiration (Am)	respiración anaerobia
ressuscitation	resuscitation	resucitación
retard	retardation	retraso
rétention	retention	retención
rétention foetale	missed abortion	aborto diferido
réticulaire	reticular	reticular
réticulocyte	reticulocyte	reticulocito
réticulocytose	reticulocytosis	reticulocitosis
rétine	retina	retina
rétine décollée	detached retina	desprendimiento de retina
rétinite	retinitis	retinitis
rétinoblastome	retinoblastoma	retinoblastoma
rétinopathie	retinopathy	retinopatía
rétracteur	retractor	retractor

ITALIAN	GERMAN	FRENCH
riflesso di Moro	Moro-Reflex	réflexe de Moro
reflusso	Reflux	reflux
refrattario	refraktär	réfractaire
rifrazione	Refraktion, Brechung	réfraction
rigenerazione	Regeneration	régénération
prescrizione dietetica, dieta, regime	Diät, Ernährung	régime
dieta chetogenica	ketogene Ernährung	régime cétogène
regione lombare	Lende	région lombaire
regressione	Regression, Rückbildung	régression
rigurgito, regurgito	Regurgitation bei Säuglingen, Regurgitieren	régurgitation
rene	Niere	rein
rigetto	Abstoßung	rejet
rilassante (n)	Relaxans (n)	relaxant (n)
rilassante (a)	entspannend (a), relaxierend (a)	relaxant (a)
muscolo elevatore	Levator	releveur
remissione	Remission	rémission
remittente	remittierend, abfallend	rémittent
renale	renal, Nieren-	rénal
renina	Renin	rénine
recidiva	Rezidiv	répétition
repressione	Unterdrückung, Verdrängung	répression
resezione	Resektion	résection
resettore endoscopico	Resektoskop, Resektionszystoskop	résectoscope
residuo	Residual-	résiduel
alcool-resistente	alkoholresistent	résistant à l'alcool
alcool-acido-resistente	säurealkoholbeständig	résistant à l'alcool et à l'acide
risoluzione	Auflösung, Rückgang	résolution
risonanza	Resonanz, Schall	résonance
riassorbimento	Resorption	résorption
respiratore	Respirator, Beatmungsgerät	respirateur
respirazione	Respiration, Atmung	respiration
respirazione anaerobica	anaerobe Respiration	respiration anaérobie
rianimazione	Reanimation, Wiederbelebung	ressuscitation
ritardo mentale, psicomotorio	Verzögerung, Hemmung	retard
ritenzione	Retention	rétention
aborto interno, aborto ritenuto	verhaltener Abort, missed abortion	rétention foetale
reticolare	retikulär	réticulaire
reticolocito	Retikulozyt	réticulocyte
reticolocitosi	Retikulozytose	réticulocytose
retina	Retina, Netzhaut	rétine
distacco di retina	abgelöste Netzhaut	rétine décollée
retinite	Retinitis, Netzhautentzündung	rétinite
retinoblastoma	Retinoblastom	rétinoblastome
retinopatia	Retinopathie	rétinopathie
divaricatore	Wundhaken, Spreizer, Retraktor	rétracteur

FRENCH	ENGLISH	SPANISH
rétractile	retractile	retráctil
retrait	withdrawal	supresión, abstinencia
retraité(e)	old age pensioner (OAP)	jubilado
rétrécissement	stricture	estrictura
rétrobulbaire	retrobulbar	retrobulbar
rétrocaecal	retrocaecal (Eng), retrocecal (Am)	retrocecal
rétrograde	retrograde	retrógrado
rétronasal	postnasal	postnasal
rétropéritonéal	retroperitoneal	retroperitoneal
rétropharyngien	retropharyngeal	retrofaríngeo
rétroplacentaire	retroplacental	retroplacentario
rétrosternal	retrosternal	retrosternal
rétroversion	retroversion	retroversión
revascularisation	revascularization	revascularización
rhésus négatif (Rh−)	rhesus negative (Rh−)	rhesus negativo (Rh−)
rhésus positif (Rh+)	rhesus positive (Rh+)	rhesus positivo (Rh+)
rhinite	rhinitis	rinitis
rhinopharynx	nasopharynx	nasofaringe
rhinophyma	rhinophyma	rinofima
rhinoplastie	rhinoplasty	rinoplastia
rhinorrhée	rhinorrhea (Am), rhinorrhoea (Eng)	rinorrea
rhinovirus	rhinovirus	rinovirus
rhumatisme	rheumatism	reumatismo
rhumatisme articulaire aigu	rheumatic fever	fiebre reumática
rhumatisme psoriasique	psoriatic arthritis	artritis psoriásica
rhumatoïde	rheumatoid	reumatoide
rhumatologie	rheumatology	reumatología
rhume	cold	resfriado
rhume des foins	hay fever	fiebre del heno
rigor	rigor	rigor
risque d'avortement	threatened abortion	amenaza de aborto
ronchus	rhonchus	roncus
ronflement	snore	ronquido
ronfler	snore	roncar
roséole	roseola	roséola
rotateur	rotator	rotatorio
rotavirus	rotavirus	rotavirus
rotule	patella	rótula
rougeole	measles	sarampión
rougeur	flush, rubor	rubor
rouleaux	rouleaux	rollos
rubéole	German measles, rubella	rubéola
rupture placentaire	placental abruption	desprendimiento prematuro de la placenta

ITALIAN	GERMAN	FRENCH
retrattile	retraktionsfähig	**rétractile**
ritiro, astinenza, sospensione	Entzug	**retrait**
anziano pensionato	Rentner	**retraité(e)**
stenosi, restringimento	Striktur	**rétrécissement**
retrobulbare	retrobulbär	**rétrobulbaire**
retrociecale	retrozökal	**rétrocaecal**
retrogrado	retrograd, rückläufig	**rétrograde**
retronasale	postnasal	**rétronasal**
retroperitoneale	retroperitoneal	**rétropéritonéal**
retrofaringeo	retropharyngeal	**rétropharyngien**
retroplacentare	retroplazental	**rétroplacentaire**
retrosternale	retrosternal	**rétrosternal**
retroversione	Retroversion	**rétroversion**
rivascolarizzazione	Revaskularisation	**revascularisation**
Rh negativo (Rh−)	Rh-negativ	**rhésus négatif (Rh−)**
Rh positivo (Rh+)	Rh-positiv	**rhésus positif (Rh+)**
rinite	Rhinitis	**rhinite**
nasofaringe	Nasopharynx, Nasenrachenraum	**rhinopharynx**
rinofima	Rhinophym	**rhinophyma**
rinoplastica	Rhinoplastik	**rhinoplastie**
rinorrea	Rhinorrhoe	**rhinorrhée**
rhinovirus	Rhinovirus	**rhinovirus**
reumatismo	Rheumatismus	**rhumatisme**
febbre reumatica	rheumatisches Fieber	**rhumatisme articulaire aigu**
artropatia psoriasica, psoriasi artropatica	Arthritis psoriatica	**rhumatisme psoriasique**
reumatoide	rheumatisch	**rhumatoïde**
reumatologia	Rheumatologie	**rhumatologie**
raffreddore	Kälte, Erkältung	**rhume**
febbre da fieno, raffreddore da fieno	Heuschnupfen	**rhume des foins**
rigor, ipertonia extrapiramidale	Rigor, Starre	**rigor**
minaccia d'aborto	drohender Abort	**risque d'avortement**
ronco	Rhonchus, Rasselgeräusch	**ronchus**
russo	Schnarchen	**ronflement**
russare	schnarchen	**ronfler**
roseola	Roseole	**roséole**
muscolo rotatore	Rotator	**rotateur**
rotavirus	Rotavirus	**rotavirus**
patella, rotula	Patella, Kniescheibe	**rotule**
morbillo	Masern	**rougeole**
eritema vasomotorio, arrossamento infiammatorio	Flush, Rubor, Rötung	**rougeur**
colonne di eritrociti	Geldrollenagglutination	**rouleaux**
rosolia	Rubella, Röteln	**rubéole**
distacco prematuro della placenta	Plazentaablösung	**rupture placentaire**

S

FRENCH	ENGLISH	SPANISH
sac	sac	saco
sacré	sacral	sacral
sacrococcygien	sacrococcygeal	sacrococcígeo
sacro-iliaque	sacroiliac	sacroílíaco
sacro-ilite	sacroiliitis	sacroileítis
sacrum	sacrum	sacro
s'affaisser	collapse	colapsar
sage-femme	midwife	comadrona
sagittal	sagittal	sagital
saignement de nez	nosebleed	epistaxis
saigner	bleed	sangrar
salin	saline	salino
salive	saliva, sputum	saliva, esputo
salpingectomie	salpingectomy	salpingectomía
salpingite	salpingitis	salpingitis
sang	blood	sangre
sang occulte	occult blood	sangre oculta
sang occulte fécal	faecal occult blood (FOB) (Eng), fecal occult blood (FOB) (Am)	sangre oculta fecal
sans connaissance	unconscious	inconsciente, sin sentido
santé	health	salud
santé mentale	sanity	cordura
saphène	saphenous	safeno
sarcoïde	sarcoid	sarcoideo
sarcoïdose	sarcoidosis	sarcoidosis
sarcome	sarcoma	sarcoma
sarcome de Kaposi	Kaposi's sarcoma	sarcoma de Kaposi
saturnisme	plumbism	plumbismo, saturnismo
scalpel	scalpel	escalpelo
scanographie	computerized tomography	tomografía computerizada
scaphoïde	scaphoid	escafoides
scarlatine	scarlet fever	escarlatina
schistosomiase	schistosomiasis	esquistosomiasis
schizophrénie	schizophrenia	esquizofrenia
schizophrénie paranoïaque	paranoid schizophrenia	esquizofrenia paranoica
sciatique (n)	sciatica (n)	ciática (n)
sciatique (a)	sciatic (a)	ciático (a)
scissure	sulcus	surco
sclérite	scleritis	escleritis
scléroderme	scleredema (Am), scleredoema (Eng), scleroderma	escleredema, escleroderma
sclérose	sclerosis	esclerosis
sclérose en plaques	multiple sclerosis (MS)	esclerosis múltiple
sclérose tubéreuse du cerveau	tuberous sclerosis	esclerosis tuberosa
sclérothérapie	sclerotherapy	escleroterapia
sclérotique (n)	sclera (n)	esclerótica (n)

ITALIAN	GERMAN	FRENCH
sacco, sacca	Sack, Beutel	sac
sacrale	sakral, Kreuzbein-	sacré
sacrococcigeo	sakrokokkygeal	sacrococcygien
sacroiliaco	Iliosakral-	sacro-iliaque
sacroiliite	Sakroiliitis	sacro-ilite
sacro	Sakrum, Kreuzbein	sacrum
collassarsi, crollare	kollabieren	s'affaisser
levatrice	Hebamme	sage-femme
sagittale	sagittal	sagittal
epistassi	Nasenbluten, Epistaxis	saignement de nez
sanguinare	bluten	saigner
salino	salinisch	salin
saliva, sputo, escreato	Speichel, Sputum, Auswurf	salive
salpingectomia	Salpingektomie	salpingectomie
salpingite	Salpingitis, Eileiterentzündung	salpingite
sangue	Blut	sang
sangue occulto	okkultes Blut	sang occulte
sangue occulto fecale	okkultes Blut (im Stuhl)	sang occulte fécal
inconscio	bewußtlos	sans connaissance
salute	Gesundheit	santé
sanità	geistige Gesundheit	santé mentale
safeno	saphenus	saphène
sarcoideo	fleischähnlich	sarcoïde
sarcoidosi	Sarkoidose, Morbus Boeck	sarcoïdose
sarcoma	Sarkom	sarcome
sarcoma di Kaposi	Kaposi-Sarkom	sarcome de Kaposi
intossicazione da piombo	Bleivergiftung	saturnisme
bisturi	Skalpell	scalpel
tomografia computerizzata	Computertomographie (CT)	scanographie
scafoide	Scaphoid	scaphoïde
scarlattina	Scharlach	scarlatine
schistosomiasi	Schistosomiasis, Bilharziose	schistosomiase
schizofrenia	Schizophrenie	schizophrénie
schizofrenia paranoide	paranoide Schizophrenie	schizophrénie paranoïaque
sciatica (n)	Ischias (n)	sciatique (n)
sciatico (a)	ischiadicus (a)	sciatique (a)
solco	Sulcus, Furche	scissure
sclerite	Skleritis	sclérite
scleredema, sclerodermia	Sklerödem, Sklerodermie	scléroderme
sclerosi	Sklerose	sclérose
sclerosi multipla	multiple Sklerose (MS)	sclérose en plaques
sclerosi tuberosa	tuberöse Sklerose	sclérose tubéreuse du cerveau
scleroterapia	Sklerotherapie	sclérothérapie
sclera (n), sclerotica (n)	Sklera (n)	sclérotique (n)

FRENCH	ENGLISH	SPANISH
sclérotique (a)	sclerotic (a)	esclerótico (a)
scoliose	scoliosis	escoliosis
scorbut	scurvy	escorbuto
scotome	scotoma	escotoma
scrofule	scrofula	escrófula
scrotum	scrotum	escroto
sébacé	sebaceous	sebáceo
séborrhée	seborrhea (Am), seborrhoea (Eng)	seborrea
sébum	sebum	sebo
se combiner	coalesce	coalescer
secourisme	first aid	primeros auxilios
secréteur	secretory	secretorio
sécrétion	secretion	secreción
sédatif (n)	sedative (n)	sedante (n)
sédatif (a)	sedative (a)	sedante (a)
sédation	sedation	sedación
sédentaire	sedentary	sedentario
se fouler	sprain	torcer
se gargariser	gargle	gargajear
segment	segment	segmento
sein	breast	mama, pecho
selle	stool	deposición
semi-lunaire	semilunar	semilunar
séminal	seminal	seminal
séminome	seminoma	seminoma
sémiologique	semeiotic	semiótica
semi-perméable	semipermeable	semipermeable
sénescence	senescence	senescencia
sénile	senile	senil
sens	sense	sentido
sensation	sensation	sensación
sensibilisation	sensitization	sensibilización
sensibilité	sensitivity	sensibilidad
sensible	sensitive	sensible
sensitif	sensory	sensorio
septicémie	sepsis, septicaemia (Eng), septicemia (Am)	sepsis, septicemia
septicopyohémie	pyaemia (Eng), pyemia (Am)	piemia
septum	septum	septo, tabique
séquelle	sequela	secuela
séquestre	sequestrum	secuestro
séreuse	serosa	serosa
séreux	serous	seroso
seringue	syringe	jeringuilla
sérologie	serology	serología
séropositif	seropositive	seropositivo
sérum	serum	suero

ITALIAN	GERMAN	FRENCH
sclerotico *(a)*	sklerotisch *(a)*, Sklera- *(a)*	sclérotique *(a)*
scoliosi	Skoliose	scoliose
scorbuto	Skorbut	scorbut
scotoma	Skotom, Gesichtsfeldausfall	scotome
scrofola, linfadenite tubercolare	Skrofula, Lymphknotentuberkulose	scrofule
scroto	Skrotum, Hodensack	scrotum
sebaceo	Talg-, talgig	sébacé
seborrea	Seborrhoe	séborrhée
sebo	Talg	sébum
aggregarsi	zusammenwachsen	se combiner
pronto soccorso	Erste Hilfe	secourisme
secretorio	sekretorisch	secréteur
secrezione	Sekretion	sécrétion
sedativo *(n)*	Sedativum *(n)*, Beruhigungsmittel *(n)*	sédatif *(n)*
sedativo *(a)*	sedierend *(a)*, beruhigend *(a)*	sédatif *(a)*
sedazione	Sedierung	sédation
sedentario	sitzend, seßhaft	sédentaire
distorcere	verstauchen	se fouler
gargarizzare	gurgeln	se gargariser
segmento	Segment	segment
mammella	Brust	sein
feci	Stuhl, Stuhlgang, Kot	selle
semilunare	semilunar, halbmondförmig	semi-lunaire
seminale	Samen-, Spermien-	séminal
seminoma	Seminom	séminome
semiotico	semiotisch	sémiologique
semipermeabile	semipermeabel	semi-perméable
senescenza	Seneszenz, Altern	sénescence
senile	senil, Alters-	sénile
sensi	Sinn	sens
sensazione, sensibilità	Sinneswahrnehmung, Gefühl	sensation
sensibilizzazione	Sensitivierung, Allergisierung	sensibilisation
sensibilità	Empfindlichkeit, Feingefühl	sensibilité
sensibile	sensitiv, empfindlich	sensible
sensoriale	sensorisch, Sinnes-	sensitif
sepsi, setticemia	Sepsis, Septikämie	septicémie
piemia	Pyämie	septicopyohémie
setto	Septum, Scheidewand	septum
sequela	Folgeerscheinung, Folgezustand	séquelle
sequestro	Sequester	séquestre
sierosa, membrana sierosa	Serosa	séreuse
sieroso	serös, Serum-	séreux
siringa	Spritze	seringue
sierologia	Serologie	sérologie
siero-positivo	seropositiv	séropositif
siero	Serum, Blutserum	sérum

FRENCH	ENGLISH	SPANISH
sérum antivenimeux	antivenin	antídoto
service de réanimation	intensive therapy unit (ITU)	unidad de cuidados intensivos (UCI)
service de soins intensifs néonatals	neonatal intensive care unit (NICU) (Am)	unidad de cuidados intensivos para recién nacidos
service des urgences/des traumatismes	emergency treatment/trauma unit (ETU)	servicio de urgencias/traumatologia
s'évanouir	faint	desmayar
sévices infligés aux enfants	child abuse	abuso de menores
sévices sexuels	sexual abuse	abuso sexual
sevrage	withdrawal	supresión, abstinencia
sidérophyline	iron binding protein (IBP)	proteína de unión con el hierro
siège	breech	nalgas
sigmoïde	sigmoid	sigmoideo
sigmoïdoscope	sigmoidoscope	sigmoidoscopio
sigmoïdostomie	sigmoidostomy	sigmoidostomía
signe	sign	signo
signe de Chvostek	Chvostek's sign	signo de Chvostek
signe de Kernig	Kernig's sign	signo de Kernig
signe de Trendelenburg	Trendelenburg sign	signo de Trendelenburg
silicose	silicosis	silicosis
sillon	sulcus	surco
simulation	malingering	simulación de síntomas
sinus	sinus	seno
sinusite	sinusitis	sinusitis
sociomédical	sociomedical	médico-social
soif	thirst	sed
soigner	nurse	cuidar
soins de santé primaires	primary care	asistencia primaria
soins pour malades en phase terminale	terminal care	cuidados terminales
solution	solution	solución
solution physiologique	saline	solución salina
solvant	solvent	disolvente
somatique	somatic	somático
somatomammotropine chorionique humaine (HCS)	human chorionic somatomammotrophin (HCS) (Eng), human chorionic somatomammotropin (HCS, HPL) (Am)	somatomamotropina corionica humana
somatoprolactine chorionique humaine	human chorionic somatomammotrophin (HCS) (Eng), human chorionic somatomammotropin (HCS, HPL) (Am)	somatomamotropina corionica humana
somatotrophine (STH)	growth hormone (GH)	hormona del crecimiento (HC)
sommeil	sleep	sueño
sommeil paradoxal	REM sleep	sueño REM
somnambulisme	somnambulism	sonambulismo
son	bran, sound	salvado, sonido
soporifique (n)	soporific (n)	soporífero (n)

ITALIAN	GERMAN	FRENCH
antiveleno, contravveleno	Schlangenserum	sérum antivenimeux
unità di terapia intensiva	Intensivstation	service de réanimation
reparto di terapia intensiva neonatale	Frühgeborenen-Intensivstation	service de soins intensifs néonatals
pronto soccorso	Notfallstation	service des urgences/des traumatismes
svenire	ohnmächtig werden	s'évanouir
maltrattamento a bambini	Kindesmißhandlung	sévices infligés aux enfants
violenza sessuale, violenza carnale	sexueller Mißbrauch	sévices sexuels
ritiro, astinenza, sospensione	Entzug	sevrage
proteina che lega il ferro	eisenbindendes Protein	sidérophylline
natica	Steiß, Gesäß	siège
sigmoide	sigmoid	sigmoïde
sigmoidoscopio	Sigmoidoskop	sigmoïdoscope
sigmoidostomia	Sigmoidostomie	sigmoïdostomie
segno	Zeichen, Symptom	signe
segno di Chvostek	Chvostek-Zeichen	signe de Chvostek
segno di Kernig	Kernig Zeichen	signe de Kernig
segno di Trendelenburg	Trendelenburg-Zeichen	signe de Trendelenburg
silicosi	Silikose	silicose
solco	Sulcus, Furche	sillon
simulazione di malattia	scheinkrank	simulation
seno, fistula suppurante	Sinus, Nebenhöhle	sinus
sinusite	Sinusitis	sinusite
sociosanitario	sozialmedizinisch	sociomédical
sete	Durst	soif
assistere	stillen, pflegen	soigner
primaria, neoplasia primitiva	Primärversorgung	soins de santé primaires
cura terminale	Pflege Sterbender	soins pour malades en phase terminale
soluzione	Lösung, Auflösung	solution
soluzione fisiologica	Kochsalzlösung	solution physiologique
solvente	Lösungsmittel	solvant
somatico	somatisch, körperlich	somatique
somatomammotropina corionica umana	human chorionic somatomammotropin (HCS)	somatomammotropine chorionique humaine (HCS)
somatomammotropina corionica umana	human chorionic somatomammotropin (HCS)	somatoprolactine chorionique humaine
ormone della crescita (GH)	Wachstumshormon	somatotrophine (STH)
sonno	Schlaf	sommeil
sonno REM, fase dei movimenti oculari rapidi	REM-Schlaf	sommeil paradoxal
sonnambulismo	Somnambulismus, Schlafwandeln	somnambulisme
crusca, suono	Kleie, Ton, Klang	son
ipnotico (n)	Schlafmittel (n)	soporifique (n)

soporifique *(a)*	soporific *(a)*	soporífero *(a)*
souffle	breath	aliento
sourcil	brow	ceja
sourd	deaf	sordo
sous-clavier	subclavian	subclavia
sous-clinique	subclinical	subclínico
sous-conjonctival	subconjunctival	subconjuntival
sous-costal	subcostal	subcostal
sous-cutané (SC)	subcutaneous (SC, SQ)	subcutáneo (SC)
sous-dural	subdural	subdural
sous-fertilité	subfertility	subfertilidad
sous-occipital	suboccipital	suboccipital
sous-phrénique	subphrenic	subfrénico
spanioménorrhée	oligomenorrhea (Am), oligomenorrhoea (Eng)	oligomenorrea
spasme	spasm	espasmo
spasme d'un vaisseau	vasospasm	vasospasmo
spastique	spastic	espástico
spatule	spatula	espátula
spécialités pharmaceutiques grand public	over the counter (OTC)	sin receta médica
spécifique	specific	específico
spéculum	speculum	espéculo
spéculum de Sim	Sims' speculum	espéculo de Sim
spermatique	seminal, spermatic	seminal, espermático
spermatocèle	spermatocele	espermatocele
sperme	semen, sperm	semen, esperma
spermicide	spermicide	espermicida
sphénoïde	sphenoid	esfenoides
sphérocytose	spherocytosis	esferocitosis
sphincter	sphincter	esfínter
sphygmomanomètre	sphygmomanometer	esfigmomanómetro
spica	spica	espica
spicule	spicule	espícula
spina bifida	spina bifida	espina bífida
spinal	spinal	espinal
spirochète	spirochaete (Eng), spirochete (Am)	espiroqueta
spirographe	spirograph	espirografía
spiromètre	spirometer	espirómetro
splanchnique	splanchnic	esplácnico
splénectomie	splenectomy	esplenectomía
splénomégalie	splenomegaly	esplenomegalia
spondylite	spondylitis	espondilitis
spondylolisthésis	spondylolisthesis	espondilolistesis
spongieux	cancellous	esponjoso, reticulado
sporadique	sporadic	esporádico
sprue	sprue	esprue
squameux	squamous	escamoso

ipnotico (a)	einschläfernd (a)	soporifique (a)
respiro	Atem, Atemzug	souffle
arcata sopracciliare, sopracciglio	Augenbraue	sourcil
sordo	taub, schwerhörig	sourd
succlavio, sottoclavicolare	Subklavia-	sous-clavier
subclinico	subklinisch	sous-clinique
sottocongiuntivale	subkonjunktival	sous-conjonctival
sottocostale	subkostal	sous-costal
sottocutaneo	subkutan	sous-cutané (SC)
subdurale, sottodurale	subdural	sous-dural
subfertilità	Subfertilität	sous-fertilité
suboccipitale	subokzipital	sous-occipital
subfrenico, sottodiaframmatico	subdiaphragmatisch	sous-phrénique
oligomenorrea	Oligomenorrhoe	spanioménorrhée
spasmo	Spasmus, Krampf	spasme
vasospasmo, angiospasmo	Vasospasmus	spasme d'un vaisseau
spastico	spastisch, krampfhaft	spastique
spatola	Spatel	spatule
(farmaco) ottenibile senza prescrizione medica	rezeptfrei	spécialités pharmaceutiques grand public
specifico	spezifisch, speziell	spécifique
speculum	Spekulum, Spiegel	spéculum
speculum di Sim	Sims-Spekulum	spéculum de Sim
seminale, spermatico	Samen-, Spermien-, Sperma-	spermatique
spermatocele	Spermatozele	spermatocèle
seme, sperma	Samen, Sperma	sperme
spermicida	Spermizid	spermicide
sfenoide	Sphenoid, Keilbein	sphénoïde
sferocitosi	Sphärozytose, Kugelzellanämie	sphérocytose
sfintere	Sphinkter, Schließmuskel	sphincter
sfigmomanometro	Blutdruckmeßgerät	sphygmomanomètre
spiga	Kornährenverband, Sporn	spica
spicola, picco	Spikulum	spicule
spina bifida	Spina bifida	spina bifida
spinale	spinal, Rückenmarks-, Wirbelsäulen-	spinal
spirocheta	Spirochäte	spirochète
spirografo	Spirograph	spirographe
spirometro	Spirometer	spiromètre
splancnico	viszeral, Eingeweide-	splanchnique
splenectomia	Splenektomie	splénectomie
splenomegalia	Splenomegalie	splénomégalie
spondilite	Spondylitis	spondylite
spondilolistesi	Spondylolisthesis	spondylolisthésis
spugnoso, trabecolare	spongiös, schwammartig	spongieux
sporadico	sporadisch	sporadique
sprue	Sprue	sprue
squamoso	squamös, schuppig	squameux

squelette	skeleton	esqueleto
stapédectomie	stapedectomy	estapedectomía
stase	stasis	estasis
statut	status	status
stéatorrhée	steatorrhea (Am), steatorrhoea (Eng)	esteatorrea
sténose	stenosis	estenosis
stérile	sterile	estéril
stérilet	intrauterine contraceptive device (IUD, IUCD)	dispositivo intrauterino anticonceptivo (DIU)
stérilisation	sterilization	esterilización
sternocostal	sternocostal	esternocostal
sternum	sternum	esternón
stéroïde	steroid	esteroide
stéthoscope	stethoscope	estetoscopio
stigmate	stigmata	estigmas
stilboestrol	stilbestrol (Am), stilboestrol (Eng)	estilbestrol
stimulant (n)	stimulant (n)	estimulante (n)
stimulant (a)	stimulant (a)	estimulante (a)
stimulateur cardiaque	pacemaker	marcapasos
stoma	stoma	estoma
stomatite	stomatitis	estomatitis
strabisme	squint, strabismus	estrabismo
strangulation	strangulation	estrangulación
strangurie	strangury	estranguria
stress	stress	stress, estrés
stridor	stridor	estridor
stries	striae	estrias
stupeur	stupor	estupor
styloïde	styloid	estiloides
subaigu	subacute	subagudo
subconscient	subconscious	subconsciente
subjectif	subjective	subjetivo
sublimé	sublimate	sublimado
subliminal	subliminal	subliminal
sublingual	sublingual	sublingual
subluxation	subluxation	subluxación
submandibulaire	submandibular	submandibular
subnormalité	subnormality	subnormalidad
substance libératrice de l'hormone lutéotrope	LH-releasing factor (LHRF)	factor liberador de la hormona luteinizante
succussion	succussion	sucusión
suer	sweat	sudar
sueur	sweat	sudor
sueurs nocturnes	night sweat	sudoración nocturna
suffocation	suffocation	asfixia
suggestion	suggestion	sugestión
suicide	suicide	suicidio

ITALIAN	GERMAN	FRENCH
scheletro	Skelett	squelette
stapedectomia	Stapedektomie	stapédectomie
stasi, ristagno	Stase	stase
stato	Status, Zustand	statut
steatorrea, seborrea	Steatorrhoe, Fettstuhl	stéatorrhée
stenosi	Stenose	sténose
sterile	steril, keimfrei, unfruchtbar	stérile
dispositivo anticoncezionale intrauterino (IUD)	Intrauterinpessar (IUP)	stérilet
sterilizzazione	Sterilisation, Sterilisierung	stérilisation
sternocostale	sternokostal	sternocostal
sterno	Sternum, Brustbein	sternum
steroide	Steroid	stéroïde
stetoscopio	Stethoskop	stéthoscope
stigmate	Stigmata, Kennzeichen	stigmate
stilbestrolo	Diäthylstilboestrol	stilboestrol
stimolante (n)	Stimulans (n)	stimulant (n)
stimolante (a)	stimulierend (a)	stimulant (a)
pacemaker	Schrittmacher	stimulateur cardiaque
stoma, orifizio	Stoma, Mund	stoma
stomatite	Stomatitis, Mundhöhlenentzündung	stomatite
strabismo	Schielen, Strabismus	strabisme
strangolamento	Strangulation, Einklemmung	strangulation
stranguria	Harnzwang	strangurie
stress	Belastung, Streß	stress
stridore	Stridor	stridor
stria	Striae, Streifen	stries
stupore	Stupor, Benommenheit	stupeur
stiloide, stiloideo	Styloid-	styloïde
subacuto	subakut	subaigu
subconscio	unterbewußt	subconscient
soggettivo	subjektiv	subjectif
sublimato	Sublimat, Quicksilberchlorid	sublimé
subliminale	unterschwellig	subliminal
sublinguale	sublingual	sublingual
sublussazione	Subluxation	subluxation
sottomandibolare	submandibulär	submandibulaire
subnormalità	Subnormalität	subnormalité
releasing factor dell'ormone LH	LH-luteinizing hormone releasing factor (LHRF)	substance libératrice de l'hormone lutéotrope
succussione, scuotimento	Erschutterung, Schütteln	succussion
sudare	schwitzen	suer
sudore	Schweiß	sueur
sudorazione notturna	Nachtschweiß	sueurs nocturnes
soffocamento	Ersticken, Erstickung	suffocation
suggestione	Vorschlag, Suggestion	suggestion
suicidio	Suizid, Selbstmord	suicide

sulfamide	sulfonamide (Am), sulphonamide (Eng)	sulfonamida
sulfate de calcium hydraté	plaster of Paris	escayola
sulfonylurée	sulfonylurea (Am), sulphonylurea (Eng)	sulfonilurea
supérieur	superior	superior
supinateur	supinator	supinador
supination	supination	supinar
suppositoire	suppository	supositorio
suppression	suppression, withdrawal	supresión, abstinencia
suppuration	suppuration	supuración
supraclaviculaire	supraclavicular	supraclavicular
supracondylaire	supracondylar	supracondilar
suprapubien	suprapubic	suprapúbico
suprasternal	suprasternal	supraesternal
surdité	deafness	sordera
surfactant	surfactant	tensoactivo
surrénale	adrenal	adrenal
susceptibilité	susceptibility	susceptibilidad
suture	suture	sutura
suturer	suture	suturar
symbiose	symbiosis	simbiosis
sympathectomie	sympathectomy	simpatectomía
sympathomimétique (n)	sympathomimetic (n)	simpaticomimético (n)
sympathomimétique (a)	sympathomimetic (a)	simpaticomimético (a)
symphyse	symphysis	sínfisis
symptôme	symptom	síntoma
synapse	synapse	sinapsis
syncope	syncope, faint	síncope, vahído
syndrome carcinoïde	carcinoid syndrome	síndrome carcinoide
syndrome chronique du cerveau	chronic brain syndrome (CBS)	síndrome cerebral crónico
syndrome d'alcoolisme	alcohol syndrome	síndrome alcohólico
syndrome d'alcoolisme foetal	fetal alcohol syndrome	síndrome alcohólico fetal
syndrome de Behçet	Behçet syndrome	síndrome de Behçet
syndrome de Bernard-Horner	Horner's syndrome	síndrome de Horner
syndrome de chasse	dumping syndrome	síndrome de dumping, síndrome del vaciamiento en gastrectomizados
syndrome de choc toxique staphylococcique	toxic shock syndrome	síndrome de shock tóxico
syndrome de Costen	temporomandibular joint syndrome	síndrome de la articulación temporomandibular
syndrome de Cushing	Cushing's syndrome	síndrome de Cushing
syndrome de Fiessinger-Leroy-Reiter	Reiter's syndrome	síndrome de Reiter
syndrome de Klinefelter	Klinefelter's syndrome	síndrome de Klinefelter
syndrome de l'anse borgne	blind loop syndrome	síndrome del asa ciega
syndrome de l'intestin irritable	irritable bowel syndrome	síndrome del intestino irritable

ITALIAN	GERMAN	FRENCH
sulfonammide	Sulfonamid	**sulfamide**
gesso di Parigi (calcio solfato diidrato)	Gips	**sulfate de calcium hydraté**
sulfonilurea	Sulfonylharnstoff	**sulfonylurée**
superiore	oben, überlegen	**supérieur**
supinatore	Supinator	**supinateur**
supinazione	Supination	**supination**
supposta	Suppositorium, Zäpfchen	**suppositoire**
soppressione, ritiro, astinenza, sospensione	Unterdrückung, Verdrängung, Entzug	**suppression**
suppurazione	Suppuration, Eiterung	**suppuration**
sopraclavicolare	supraklavikulär	**supraclaviculaire**
sopracondiloideo, epicondiloideo	suprakondylär	**supracondylaire**
soprapubico	suprapubisch	**suprapubien**
soprasternale	suprasternal	**suprasternal**
sordità	Taubheit, Schwerhörigkeit	**surdité**
tensioattivo, surfattante	Surfactant-Faktor	**surfactant**
surrenale	Nebennieren-	**surrénale**
suscettibilità	Anfälligkeit, Empfindlichkeit	**susceptibilité**
sutura	Naht	**suture**
suturare, cucire	nähen	**suturer**
simbiosi	Symbiose	**symblose**
simpatectomia, simpaticectomia	Sympathektomie	**sympathectomie**
simpaticomimetico *(n)*	Sympathomimetikum *(n)*	**sympathomimétique** *(n)*
simpaticomimetico *(a)*	sympathomimetisch *(a)*	**sympathomimétique** *(a)*
sinfisi	Symphyse	**symphyse**
sintomo	Symptom	**symptôme**
sinapsi, giunzione	Synapse	**synapse**
sincope, svenimento	Synkope, Ohnmacht	**syncope**
sindrome da carcinoide	Karzinoid-Syndrom	**syndrome carcinoïde**
sindrome cerebrale cronica	chronisches Gehirnsyndrom	**syndrome chronique du cerveau**
sindrome da alcool	Alkoholsyndrom	**syndrome d'alcoolisme**
sindrome da alcolismo materno	fetales Alkoholsyndrom	**syndrome d'alcoolisme foetal**
sindrome di Behçet	Behçet-Syndrom	**syndrome de Behçet**
sindrome di Horner	Horner-Syndrom	**syndrome de Bernard-Horner**
sindrome del gastroresecato	Dumping-Syndrom	**syndrome de chasse**
sindrome da shock tossico	toxisches Schocksyndrom (TSS)	**syndrome de choc toxique staphylococcique**
sindrome dell'articolazione temporomandibolare	Costen-Syndrom	**syndrome de Costen**
sindrome di Cushing	Cushing-Syndrom	**syndrome de Cushing**
sindrome di Reiter	Reiter-Syndrom	**syndrome de Fiessinger-Leroy-Reiter**
sindrome di Klinefelter	Klinefelter-Syndrom	**syndrome de Klinefelter**
sindrome dell'ansa cieca	Syndrom der blinden Schlinge	**syndrome de l'anse borgne**
sindrome dell'intestino irritabile	Reizdarm	**syndrome de l'intestin irritable**

FRENCH	ENGLISH	SPANISH
syndrome de membrane hyaline et de souffrance respiratoire	respiratory distress syndrome (RDS)	síndrome de distress respiratorio
syndrome de Mendelson	Mendelson's syndrome	síndrome de Mendelson
syndrome de Ménière	Ménière's disease	enfermedad de Ménière
syndrome de mort subite de nourrisson	sudden infant death syndrome (SIDS)	síndrome de muerte súbita infantil
syndrome de Münchhausen	Münchhausen's syndrome	síndrome de Münchhausen
syndrome de Reye	Reye's syndrome	síndrome de Reye
syndrome des enfants maltraités	battered baby syndrome	síndrome del niño apaleado
syndrome de Sjögren	Sjögren-Larsson syndrome	síndrome de Sjögren
syndrome de Stein-Leventhal	Stein-Leventhal syndrome	síndrome de Stein-Leventhal
syndrome de Stevens-Johnson	Stevens-Johnson syndrome	síndrome de Stevens-Johnson
syndrome de Stokes-Adams	Stokes-Adams syndrome	síndrome de Stokes-Adams
syndrome de 'surmenage'	burnout syndrome	surmenage, neurastenia
syndrome de Takayashu	pulseless disease	enfermedad sin pulso
syndrome de tension prémenstruelle	premenstrual tension (PMT)	tensión premenstrual
syndrome de Turner	Turner's syndrome	síndrome de Turner
syndrome de vibrations	vibration syndrome	síndrome de vibración
syndrome d'immuno-déficience acquise (SIDA)	acquired immune deficiency syndrome (AIDS)	síndrome de inmunodeficiencia adquirida (SIDA)
syndrome d'impatience musculaire	restless legs syndrome	síndrome de piernas inquietas
syndrome du canal carpien	carpal tunnel syndrome	síndrome del túnel carpiano
syndrome hyperkinétique	hyperkinetic syndrome	síndrome hipercinético
syndrome néphrotique	nephrotic syndrome	síndrome nefrótico
syndrome oculaire sympathique	Horner's syndrome	síndrome de Horner
syndrome respiratoire obstructif chronique	chronic obstructive airway disease (COAD)	enfermedad obstructiva crónica de las vias respiratorias
syndrome urétral	urethral syndrome	síndrome uretral
synéchie	synechia	sinequia
synergie	synergy	sinergia
syphilis	syphilis	sífilis
syringomyélie	syringomyelia	siringomielia
système digestif	digestive system	aparato digestivo
système nerveux central (CNS)	central nervous system (CNS)	sistema nervioso central (SNC)
système nerveux sympathique	sympathetic nervous system	sistema nervioso simpático
système reproducteur	reproductive system	aparato reproductor
système respiratoire	respiratory system	aparato respiratorio
système réticulo-endothélial	reticuloendothelial system (RES)	sistema reticuloendotelial (SRE)
systole	systole	sístole

ITALIAN	GERMAN	FRENCH
sindrome di sofferenza respiratoria	Respiratory-distress-Syndrom, Atemnotsyndrom	syndrome de membrane hyaline et de souffrance respiratoire
sindrome di Mendelson	Mendelson-Syndrom	syndrome de Mendelson
sindrome di Ménière	Morbus Ménière	syndrome de Ménière
sindrome della morte neonatale improvvisa (SIDS)	plötzlicher Säuglingstod, Sudden-infant-death-Syndrom (SIDS)	syndrome de mort subite de nourrisson
sindrome di Münchhausen	Münchhausen-Syndrom	syndrome de Münchhausen
sindrome di Reye	Reye-Syndrom	syndrome de Reye
sindrome del bambino maltrattato	Kindesmißhandlung (Folgen)	syndrome des enfants maltraités
sindrome di Sjögren-Larsson (eritrodermia ittiosiforme con oligofrenia spastica)	Sjögren-Syndrom	syndrome de Sjögren
sindrome di Stein-Leventhal	Stein-Leventhal-Syndrom	syndrome de Stein-Leventhal
sindrome di Stevens-Johnson	Stevens-Johnson-Syndrom	syndrome de Stevens-Johnson
sindrome di Stokes-Adams	Morgagni-Stokes-Adams-Syndrom	syndrome de Stokes-Adams
incapacità ad agire, sindrome di esaurimento professionale	Helfer-Syndrom	syndrome de 'surmenage'
sindrome dell'arco aortico	Pulsloskrankheit	syndrome de Takayashu
tensione premenstruale	prämenstruelles Syndrom	syndrome de tension prémenstruelle
sindrome di Turner, disgenesia gonadica	Turner-Syndrom	syndrome de Turner
sindrome vibratoria	Vibrationssyndrom	syndrome de vibrations
sindrome da immunodeficienza acquisita (AIDS)	erworbenes Immundefektsyndrom (AIDS)	syndrome d'immuno-déficience acquise (SIDA)
sindrome delle gambe irrequiete, sindrome di Ekbom	Wittmaack-Ekbom-Syndrom	syndrome d'impatience musculaire
sindrome del tunnel carpale	Karpaltunnelsyndrom	syndrome du canal carpien
sindrome ipercinetica	hyperkinetisches Syndrom	syndrome hyperkinétique
sindrome nefrosica	nephrotisches Syndrom	syndrome néphrotique
sindrome di Horner	Horner-Syndrom	syndrome oculaire sympathique
malattia ostruttiva cronica delle vie respiratorie	chronische obstruktive Lungenerkrankung	syndrome respiratoire obstructif chronique
sindrome uretrale	Urethralsyndrom	syndrome urétral
sinechia, aderenza	Synechie, Verwachsung	synéchie
sinergia	Synergie	synergie
sifilide	Syphilis, Lues	syphilis
siringomielia	Syringomyelie	syringomyélie
sistema digestivo	Verdauungsapparat	système digestif
sistema nervoso centrale	Zentralnervensystem (ZNS)	système nerveux central (CNS)
sistema nervoso simpatico	sympathisches Nervensystem	système nerveux sympathique
sistema riproduttivo	Fortpflanzungsapparat	système reproducteur
sistema respiratorio	Atmungsapparat, Atmungsorgane	système respiratoire
sistema reticoloendoteliale (RES)	retikuloendotheliales System	système réticulo-endothélial
sistole	Systole	systole

T

FRENCH	ENGLISH	SPANISH
tabès	tabes	tabes
tache	patch test	prueba del parche
tache aveugle	blind spot	mancha ciega
tache hépatique	liver spot	cloasma
tachycardie	tachycardia	taquicardia
tachypnée	tachypnea (Am), tachypnoea (Eng)	taquipnea
tacographie	computerized axial tomography (CAT)	tomografía axial computerizada (TAC)
tactile	tactile	táctil
talc	talc	talco
talon	heel	talón
tampon	swab	torunda
tamponnement	tamponade	taponamiento
tarsalgie	tarsalgia	tarsalgia
tarse	instep, tarsus	empeine, tarso
tarsorraphie	tarsorrhaphy	tarsorrafia
taux de filtration glomérulaire	glomerular filtration rate (GFR)	tasa de filtración glomerular (FG)
taux du métabolisme basal	basal metabolic rate (BMR)	tasa de metabolismo basal (MB)
taux quotidien recommandé	recommended daily allowance (RDA)	dosis diaria recomendada
technique aseptique	aseptic technique	técnica aséptica
technique du RAST	radioallergosorbent test (RAST)	prueba radioalergosorbente (RAST)
teigne	tinea	tiña
télangiectasie	telangiectasis	telangiectasia
tempe	temple	sien
tempérament	temperament	temperamento
temporal	temporal	temporal
temps de saignement	'bleeding time'	tiempo de sangría
tendinite	tendinitis (Am), tendonitis (Eng)	tendinitis
tendon	tendon	tendón
tendon d'Achille	Achilles tendon	tendón de Aquiles
tendon du jarret	hamstring	tendón del hueso poplíteo
ténesme	tenesmus	tenesmo
ténia	Taenia, tapeworm	tenia, tenia solitaria
'tennis elbow'	tennis elbow	codo del tenista
ténosynovite	tenosynovitis	tenosinovitis
ténotomie	tenotomy	tenotomía
tension artérielle (TA)	blood pressure (BP)	presión arterial (PA)
tension veineuse centrale	central venous pressure (CVP)	presión venosa central (PVC)
tératogène	teratogen	teratógeno
tératome	teratoma	teratoma
terminaison nerveuse	nerve ending	terminación nerviosa
tertiaire	tertiary	terciario

ITALIAN	GERMAN	FRENCH
tabe dorsale	Auszehrung, Schwindsucht	**tabès**
test epicutaneo	Läppchenprobe, Einreibeprobe	**tache**
punto cieco	blinder Fleck, Papille	**tache aveugle**
cloasma	Leberfleck	**tache hépatique**
tachicardia	Tachykardie	**tachycardie**
tachipnea	Tachypnoe	**tachypnée**
tomografia assiale computerizzata (TAC)	axiale Computertomographie	**tacographie**
tattile	taktil, tastbar	**tactile**
talco	Talkum	**talc**
tallone	Ferse	**talon**
tampone	Tupfer, Abstrichtupfer	**tampon**
tamponamento	Tamponade	**tamponnement**
tarsalgia	Tarsalgie	**tarsalgie**
dorso del piede, tarso	Fußrücken, Spann, Fußwurzel, Lidknorpel	**tarse**
tarsorrafia	Tarsorrhaphie	**tarsorraphie**
volume di filtrazione glomerulare (VFG)	glomeruläre Filtrationsrate (GFR)	**taux de filtration glomérulaire**
indice del metabolismo basale (MB)	Grundumsatz	**taux du métabolisme basal**
dose giornaliera raccomandata	empfohlene Tagesdosis	**taux quotidien recommandé**
tecnica asettica	aseptische Technik	**technique aseptique**
test di radioallergoassorbimento (RAST)	Radio-Allergo-Sorbent-Test (RAST)	**technique du RAST**
tigna	Tinea	**teigne**
telangectasia	Teleangiektasie	**télangiectasie**
tempia	Schläfe	**tempe**
temperamento	Temperament, Gemütsart	**tempérament**
temporale	temporal, Schläfen-	**temporal**
tempo di sanguinamento	Blutungszeit	**temps de saignement**
tendinite	Tendinitis, Sehnenentzündung	**tendinite**
tendine	Sehne	**tendon**
tendine di Achille	Achillessehne	**tendon d'Achille**
tendine del ginocchio	Kniesehne	**tendon du jarret**
tenesmo	Tenesmus	**ténesme**
Tenia, cestode	Bandwurm, Tänia,	**ténia**
epicondilite radio-omerale, gomito del tennista	Tennisellenbogen	**'tennis elbow'**
tenosinovite	Tendovaginitis, Tendosynovitis, Sehnenscheidenentzündung	**ténosynovite**
tenotomia	Tenotomie	**ténotomie**
pressione arteriosa	Blutdruck	**tension artérielle (TA)**
pressione venosa centrale	zentraler Venendruck (ZVD)	**tension veineuse centrale**
teratogeno	Teratogen	**tératogène**
teratoma	Teratom	**tératome**
terminazione nervosa	Nervenendigung	**terminaison nerveuse**
terziario	tertiär, dritten Grades	**tertiaire**

FRENCH	ENGLISH	SPANISH
test	test	prueba
test auditif	hearing test	prueba auditiva
test d'agrégation plaquettaire (PAT)	platelet aggregation test (PAT)	prueba de la agregación plaquetaria
test de Guthrie	Guthrie test	prueba de Guthrie
test de Kveim	Kveim test	prueba de Kveim
test de la fonction hépatique (TFH)	liver function test (LFT)	prueba de función hepática
test de la fonction respiratoire	respiratory function test	prueba de función respiratoria
test de Papanicolaou	Papanicolaou's stain test (Pap test)	prueba de tinción de Papanicolaou
test de protéine C-réactive	C-reactive protein (CRP)	proteína C-reactiva
test de sueur	sweat test	prueba del sudor
test d'immunofluorescence absorbée pour le diagnostic sérologique de la syphilis	fluorescent treponemal antibody (FTA)	anticuerpo anti-treponema fluorescente
tester	test	probar
testicule	orchis, testis	testículo
tétanie	tetany	tetania
tétanos	lock jaw, tetanus	trismo, tétanos
tête	head	cabeza
tétralogie de Fallot	tetralogy of Fallot	tetralogía de Fallot
tétraplégie	tetraplegia	tetraplejía
thalamus	thalamus	tálamo
thalassémie	thalassaemia (Eng), thalassemia (Am)	talasemia
thénar	thenar	tenar
thérapeutique	therapeutics	terapéutica
thérapie	therapy	terapéutica
thermique	thermal	termal
thermomètre	thermometer	termómetro
thoracique	thoracic	torácico
thoracoplastie	thoracoplasty	toracoplastia
thoracotomie	thoracotomy	toracotomía
thorax	thorax	tórax
thorax en carène	pigeon chest	tórax de pichón
thrombectomie	thrombectomy	trombectomía
thrombocyte	thrombocyte	trombocito
thrombocytémie	thrombocythaemia (Eng), thrombocythemia (Am)	trombocitemia
thrombocytose	thrombocytosis	trombocitosis
thrombo-embolique	thromboembolic	tromboembólico
thrombolytique	thrombolytic	trombolítico
thrombopénie	thrombocytopenia	trombocitopenia
thrombophlébite	thrombophlebitis	tromboflebitis
thrombose	thrombosis	trombosis
thrombose veineuse profonde (TVP)	deep vein thrombosis (DVT)	trombosis venosa profunda
thrombus	thrombus	trombo
thymus	thymus	timo
thyréostimuline	thyroid stimulating hormone (TSH)	hormona estimulante del tiroides (TSH)

ITALIAN	GERMAN	FRENCH
test, prova	Test, Untersuchung	test
test audiometrici	Hörtest	test auditif
test di aggregazione piastrinico	Plättchen-Aggregations-Test (PAT)	test d'agrégation plaquettaire (PAT)
test di Guthrie per la fenilchetonuria	Guthrie-Test	test de Guthrie
test di Kveim	Kveim-Test	test de Kveim
test di funzionalità epatica (TFE)	Leberfunktionstest	test de la fonction hépatique (TFH)
test di funzionalità respiratoria	Atemfunktionstest	test de la fonction respiratoire
test di Papanicolaou (Pap test)	Papanicolaou-Färbung (Pap)	test de Papanicolaou
proteina C reattiva	C-reaktives Protein (CRP)	test de protéine C-réactive
test del sudore, prova del sudore	Schweißtest	test de sueur
anticorpo immuno-fluorescente anti-treponema	Fluoreszenz-Treponemen-Antikörper	test d'immunofluorescence absorbée pour le diagnostic sérologique de la syphilis
valutare	testen, untersuchen	tester
testicolo	Hoden	testicule
tetania	Tetanie	tétanie
tetano, trisma	Kiefersperre, Tetanus, Wundstarrkrampf	tétanos
testa	Kopf	tête
tetralogia di Fallot	Fallot-Tetralogie	tétralogie de Fallot
tetraplegia	Tetraplegie	tétraplégie
talamo	Thalamus	thalamus
talassemia	Thalassämie, Mittelmeeranämie	thalassémie
pertinente al palmo della mano	Thenar-	thénar
terapia	Therapeutik, -therapie	thérapeutique
terapia	Therapie, Behandlung	thérapie
termale	thermal, Wärme-	thermique
termometro	Thermometer	thermomètre
toracico	thorakal, Brust-	thoracique
toracoplastica	Thorakoplastik	thoracoplastie
toracotomia	Thorakotomie	thoracotomie
torace	Thorax, Brustkorb	thorax
torace carenato	Hühnerbrust	thorax en carène
trombectomia	Thrombektomie	thrombectomie
trombocito	Thrombozyt, Blutplättchen	thrombocyte
trombocitemia	Thrombozythämie	thrombocytémie
trombocitosi	Thrombozytose	thrombocytose
tromboembolico	thromboembolisch	thrombo-embolique
trombolitico	thrombolytisch	thrombolytique
trombocitopenia	Thrombopenie	thrombopénie
tromboflebite	Thrombophlebitis	thrombophlébite
trombosi	Thrombose	thrombose
trombosi venosa profonda (TVP)	tiefe Venenthrombose	thrombose veineuse profonde (TVP)
trombo	Thrombus	thrombus
timo	Thymus	thymus
ormone tireotropo (TSH)	Thyreotropin	thyréostimuline

FRENCH	ENGLISH	SPANISH
thyroglossien	thyroglossal	tirogloso
thyroïde	thyroid	tiroides
thyroïdectomie	thyroidectomy	tiroidectomía
thyroïdite	thyroiditis	tiroiditis
thyrotoxicose	thyrotoxicosis	tirotoxicosis
thyrotrophine	thyroid stimulating hormone (TSH)	hormona estimulante del tiroides (TSH)
thyroxine libre (TL)	free thyroxine (FT)	tiroxina libre
tibia	shin bone, tibia	tibia
tibiofibulaire	tibiofibular	tibioperoneo
tic	tic	tic
tic douloureux	tic douloureux	tic doloroso
tige de Harrington	Harrington rod	varilla de Harrington
tintement	tinnitus	tinnitus
tique	tick	garrapata
tissu	tissue	tejido
tissu sous-muqueux	submucosa	submucosa
titrage	titration	titulación
titre	titer (Am), titre (Eng)	titulo
tolérance	tolerance	tolerancia
tomographie avec ordinateur	computerized tomography	tomografía computerizada
tonique	tonic	tónico
tonomètre	tonometer	tonómetro
tonus	tone	tono
tophus	tophus	tofo
topique	topical	tópico
torsion	torsion	torsión
torticolis	wry-neck	tortícolis
tournesol	litmus	tornasol
tourniquet	tourniquet	torniquete
tousser	cough	toser
toux	cough	tos
toxémie	toxaemia (Eng), toxemia (Am)	toxemia
toxicité	toxicity	toxicidad
toxicomanie	drug abuse	abuso de drogas
toxine	toxin	toxina
toxique	toxic	tóxico
toxoïde	toxoid	toxoide
toxoplasmose	toxoplasmosis	toxoplasmosis
traceur	tracer	trazador
trachée	trachea, windpipe	tráquea
trachéite	tracheitis	traqueitis
trachéo-oesophagien	tracheoesophageal (Am), tracheo-oesophageal (Eng)	traqueoesofágico
trachéostomie	tracheostomy	traqueostomía
trachéotomie	tracheotomy	traqueotomía

ITALIAN	GERMAN	FRENCH
tireoglosso	thyreoglossus	thyroglossien
tiroide	Thyreoidea, Schilddrüse	thyroïde
tiroidectomia	Thyreoidektomie	thyroïdectomie
tiroidite	Thyreoiditis	thyroïdite
tireotossicosi, ipertiroidismo	Thyreotoxikose	thyrotoxicose
ormone tireotropo (TSH)	Thyreotropin	thyrotrophine
tiroxina libera (FT)	freies Thyroxin (FT)	thyroxine libre (TL)
tibia	Schienbein, Tibia	tibia
tibiofibulare	tibiofibular	tibiofibulaire
tic	Tic	tic
tic doloroso, nevralgia del trigemino	Tic douloureux	tic douloureux
bastoncello retinico (per anestetizzare la dentina)	Harrington Stab	tige de Harrington
tinnito	Tinnitus	tintement
zecca	Zecke	tique
tessuto	Gewebe	tissu
sottomucosa	Submukosa	tissu sous-muqueux
titolazione	Titration	titrage
titolo	Titer	titre
tolleranza	Toleranz	tolérance
tomografia computerizzata	Computertomographie (CT)	tomographie avec ordinateur
tonico	Tonikum, Stärkungsmittel	tonique
tonometro	Tonometer	tonomètre
tono	Ton, Laut	tonus
tofo, concrezione tofacea	Tophus, Gichtknoten	tophus
topico, locale	topisch, örtlich	topique
torsione	Torsion	torsion
torcicollo	Tortikollis, (angeborener) Schiefhals	torticolis
tornasole	Lackmus	tournesol
laccio emostatico	Tourniquet	tourniquet
tossire	husten	tousser
tosse	Husten	toux
tossiemia	Toxämie, Toxikämie, Blutvergiftung	toxémie
tossicità	Toxizität	toxicité
abuso di droga, abuso di farmaci	Arzneimittelmißbrauch, Drogenmißbrauch	toxicomanie
tossina	Toxin	toxine
tossico	toxisch, giftig	toxique
tossoide	Toxoid	toxoïde
toxoplasmosi	Toxoplasmose	toxoplasmose
tracciante	Tracer	traceur
trachea	Trachea, Luftröhre	trachée
tracheite	Tracheitis	trachéite
tracheoesofageo	Tracheoösophageal-	trachéo-oesophagien
tracheostomia	Tracheostomie	trachéostomie
tracheotomia	Tracheotomie, Luftröhrenschnitt	trachéotomie

FRENCH	ENGLISH	SPANISH
trachome	trachoma	tracoma
traction	traction	tracción
trait	trait	rasgo
traitement complémentaire	complementary medicine	medicina complementaria
traitement hormonal substitutif	hormone replacement therapy (HRT)	terapéutica de reposición de hormonas
tranchées utérines	afterpains	entuertos
tranquillisant	tranquilizer	tranquilizante
transabdominal	transabdominal	transabdominal
transamniotique	transamniotic	transamniótico
transcutané	transcutaneous	transcutáneo
transfusion	transfusion	transfusión
translocation	translocation	translocación
translucide	translucent	translúcido
transmural	transmural	transmural
transplantation	transplant	trasplante
transplanter	transplant	trasplantar
transsection	transection	transección
transsudat	transudate	trasudado
transthoracique	transthoracic	transtorácico
transurétral	transurethral	transuretral
traumatisme	trauma	trauma
traumatisme non accidentel	non-accidental injury (NAI)	lesión no accidental
travail	labor (Am), labour (Eng)	parto
tremblement	tremor	temblor
tremblement fin	fine tremor	temblor fino
trépaner	trephine	trepanar
tréphine	trephine	trépano
triage	triage	triage
triceps	triceps	tríceps
trichotillomanie	trichotillomania	tricotilomanía
tricuspide	tricuspid	tricúspide
trigéminal	trigeminal	trigémino
trilogie de Fallot	Fallot's tetralogy	tetralogía de Fallot
trimestre	trimester	trimestre
triple antigène	triple antigen	antígeno triple
triple vaccin	triple vaccine	vacuna triple
trisomie	trisomy	trisomía
trisomie 21	Down's syndrome	síndrome de Down
trochanter	trochanter	trocánter
trompe de Fallope	Fallopian tube	trompa de Falopio
trompe d'Eustache	Eustachian tube	trompa de Eustaquio
trypanosomiase	trypanosomiasis	tripanosomiasis
tubaire	tubal	tubárico
tube	tubule	túbulo
tube à essai	test tube	tubo de ensayo
tubercule	tubercle	tubérculo

ITALIAN	GERMAN	FRENCH
tracoma	Trachom, ägyptische Augenkrankheit	trachome
trazione, attrazione	Traktion, Zug	traction
tratto, carattere ereditario	Zug, Charakterzug, Eigenschaft	trait
medicina complementare	komplementäre Medizin	traitement complémentaire
terapia sostitutiva ormonale	Hormonsubstitutionstherapie	traitement hormonal substitutif
contrazioni uterine post partum	Nachwehen	tranchées utérines
tranquillante	Tranquilizer, Beruhigungsmittel	tranquillisant
transaddominale	transabdominal	transabdominal
transamniotico	transamniotisch	transamniotique
percutaneo	transkutan	transcutané
trasfusione	Transfusion, Bluttransfusion	transfusion
traslocazione	Translokation	translocation
translucido	durchscheinend, durchsichtig	translucide
transmurale	transmural	transmural
trapianto	Transplantat, Transplantation	transplantation
trapiantare	transplantieren	transplanter
sezione trasversale	Querschnitt	transsection
trasudato	Transsudat	transsudat
transtoracico	transthorakal	transthoracique
transuretrale	transurethral	transurétral
trauma	Trauma	traumatisme
lesione non accidentale	nicht unfallbedingte Verletzung	traumatisme non accidentel
travaglio di parto	Wehen	travail
tremore	Tremor	tremblement
tremore fino	feinschlägiger Tremor	tremblement fin
trapanare	trepanieren	trépaner
trapano	Trepan	tréphine
selezione e distribuzione dei malati	Triage	triage
tricipite	Trizeps	triceps
tricotíllomania	Trichotillomanie	trichotillomanie
tricuspide	Trikuspidal	tricuspide
trigemino	Trigeminus-	trigéminal
tetralogia di Fallot	Fallot-Tetralogie	trilogie de Fallot
trimestre	Trimester	trimestre
antigene triplo	Dreifachantigen	triple antigène
triplo vaccino	Dreifachimpfstoff	triple vaccin
trisomia	Trisomie	trisomie
mongoloidismo, sindrome di Down	Down-Syndrom, Mongolismus	trisomie 21
trocantere	Trochanter	trochanter
tuba di Falloppio	Tube, Eileiter	trompe de Fallope
tuba d'Eustachio	Eustachische Röhre	trompe d'Eustache
tripanosomiasi	Trypanosomiasis	trypanosomiase
tubarico	Tuben-, Eileiter-	tubaire
tubulo	Tubulus, Röhrchen	tube
provetta	Reagenzglas	tube à essai
tubercolo	Tuberkel	tubercule

FRENCH	ENGLISH	SPANISH
tuberculoïde	tuberculoid	tuberculoide
tuberculose (TB)	tuberculosis (TB)	tuberculosis (TB)
tubérosité	tuberosity	tuberosidad
tumescence	tumescence	tumescencia
tumeur	tumor (Am), tumour (Eng)	tumor
tumeur de Wilms	Wilms' tumor (Am), Wilms' tumour (Eng)	tumor de Wilms
tumeur d'Ewing	Ewing's tumour	sarcoma de Ewing
turbo-inhalateur	spinhaler	inhalador spinhaler
tympan	eardrum, tympanum	tímpano
tympanique	tympanic	timpánico
tympanoplastie	tympanoplasty	timpanoplastia
type	type	tipo
typhus	typhus	tifus

tubercoloide	tuberkuloid	**tuberculoïde**
tubercolosi (TBC)	Tuberkulose	**tuberculose (TB)**
tuberosità	Tuberositas	**tubérosité**
tumefazione	Tumeszenz, diffuse Anschwellung	**tumescence**
tumore, tumefazione	Tumor	**tumeur**
tumore di Wilms	Wilms-Tumor	**tumeur de Wilms**
tumore di Ewing	Ewing-Sarkom	**tumeur d'Ewing**
nebulizzatore per farmaci	Drehinhaliergerät	**turbo-inhalateur**
timpano	Trommelfell, Tympanon	**tympan**
timpanico, risonante	Trommelfell	**tympanique**
timpanoplastica	Tympanoplastik	**tympanoplastie**
tipo	Typ, Art	**type**
tifo	Typhus, Fleckfieber	**typhus**

U

FRENCH	ENGLISH	SPANISH
ulcératif	ulcerative	ulcerativo
ulcère	ulcer	úlcera
ulcère dendritique	dendritic ulcer	úlcera dendrítica
ulcère duodénal	duodenal ulcer	úlcera duodenal
ulcère trophique	trophic ulcer	úlcera trófica
ulcus rodens	rodent ulcer	úlcera corrosiva
ultraviolet (UV)	ultraviolet (UV)	ultravioleta (UV)
unilatéral	unilateral	unilateral
unioculé	uniocular	uniocular
unité de soins intensifs	intensive care unit (ICU)	unidad de cuidados intensivos (UCI)
unité de soins intensifs coronaires	coronary care unit (CCU)	unidad de cuidados coronarios (UCC)
unité de soins spéciaux	special care unit (SCU)	unidad de cuidados especiales
urate	urate	urato
urée	urea	urea
urée du sang	blood urea	urea sérica
uréite	uveitis	uveitis
urémie	uraemia (Eng), uremia (Am)	uremia
uretère	ureter	uréter
urétérocolique	ureterocolic	ureterocólico
urètre	urethra	uretra
urétrite	urethritis	uretritis
urétrite aspécifique	non-specific urethritis (NSU)	uretritis inespecífica
urétrite non gonococcique	non-gonococcal urethritis (NGU)	uretritis no gonocócica
urétrocèle	urethrocele	uretrocele
uricémie	uricaemia (Eng), uricemia (Am)	uricemia
uricosurique	uricosuria	uricosúrico
urine	urine	orina
urine du milieu du jet	midstream urine specimen (MUS)	muestra de orina de la parte media de la micción
urographie	urography	urografía
urographie intraveineuse (UIV)	intravenous pyelogram (IVP)	pielograma intravenoso
urologie	urology	urología
urticaire	nettle rash, urticaria	urticaria
utéro-sacré	uterosacral	uterosacro
utéro-vésical	uterovesical	uterovesical
utérus	uterus, womb	útero, matriz
uvule	uvula	úvula
uvulite	uvulitis	uvulitis

ulcerativo, ulceroso	ulzerierend, geschwürig	ulcératif
ulcera	Ulkus, Geschwür	ulcère
ulcera dendritica	verzweigtes Geschwür	ulcère dendritique
ulcera duodenale	Duodenalulkus, Zwölffingerdarmgeschwür	ulcère duodénal
ulcera trofica	trophisches Ulkus	ulcère trophique
ulcus rodens, basalioma	Ulcus rodens	ulcus rodens
ultravioletto (UV)	ultraviolett	ultraviolet (UV)
unilaterale	einseitig	unilatéral
monoculare	einäugig	unioculé
unità di cura intensiva	Intensivstation	unité de soins intensifs
reparto coronarico	Infarktpflegestation	unité de soins intensifs coronaires
unità pediatrica di cure speciali	Intensivstation	unité de soins spéciaux
urato	Urat	urate
urea, carbammide	Urea, Harnstoff	urée
azotemia	Blutharnstoff	urée du sang
uveite	Uveitis	uréite
uremia	Urämie, Harnvergiftung	urémie
uretere	Ureter, Harnleiter	uretère
ureterocolico	Ureterkolik	urétérocolique
uretra	Urethra, Harnröhre	urètre
uretrite	Urethritis	urétrite
uretrite aspecifica	unspezifische Urethritis	urétrite aspécifique
uretrite non gonococcica	nicht durch Gonokokken bedingte Urethritis	urétrite non gonococcique
uretrocele	Urethrozele	urétrocèle
uricemia	Urikämie	uricémie
uricuria	Urikosurie	uricosurique
urina	Urin, Harn	urine
campione urinario del mitto intermedio (CUM)	Mittelstrahlurin	urine du milieu du jet
urografia	Urographie	urographie
pielografia endovenosa (PE)	i.v. – Pyelogramm	urographie intraveineuse (UIV)
urologia	Urologie	urologie
orticaria	Nesselfieber, Urtikaria, Nesselsucht	urticaire
uterosacrale	uterosakral	utéro-sacré
uterovescicale	uterovesikal	utéro-vésical
utero	Uterus, Gebärmutter	utérus
ugola	Uvula, Zäpfchen	uvule
stafilite	Uvulitis	uvulite

V

FRENCH	ENGLISH	SPANISH
vagin	vagina	vagina
vaginisme	vaginismus	vaginismo
vaginite	vaginitis	vaginitis
vagotomie	vagotomy	vagotomía
vague	vagal	vagal
vaisseau	vessel	vaso
valgus	valgus	valgus
valve	valve	válvula
valvulotomie	valvotomy	valvotomía
variation	fluctuation	fluctuación
varicelle	chickenpox, varicella	varicela
varices	varicose veins	varices
variole	smallpox	viruela
varus	varus	varus
vasculaire	vascular	vascular
vasculite	vasculitis	vasculitis
vasectomie	vasectomy	vasectomía
vasoconstricteur *(n)*	vasoconstrictor *(n)*	vasoconstrictor *(n)*
vasoconstricteur *(a)*	vasoconstrictor *(a)*	vasoconstrictor *(a)*
vasodilatateur *(n)*	vasodilator *(n)*	vasodilatador *(n)*
vasodilatateur *(a)*	vasodilator *(a)*	vasodilatador *(a)*
vasopresseur *(n)*	vasopressor *(n)*	vasopresor *(n)*
vasopresseur *(a)*	vasopressor *(a)*	vasopresor *(a)*
vecteur	vector	vector
végétations adénoïdes	adenoids	adenoides
veine	vein	vena
veine cave	vena cava	vena cava
veine de l'avant-bras	cubital vein	vena cubital
veine fémorale	femoral vein	vena femoral
veine jugulaire	jugular vein	vena yugular
veine porte	portal vein	vena porta
veine radiale	radial vein	vena radial
veinule	venule	vénula
vénéréologie	venereology	venereología
vénérien	venereal	venéreo
ventilation à pression positive	positive pressure ventilation	ventilación con presión positiva
ventilation et circulation	airway breathing and circulation (ABC)	vías respiratorias y circulación
ventilation spontanée en pression positive continue	continuous positive airway pressure (CPAP)	presión continua positiva de las vías respiratorias
ventouse obstétricale	vacuum extractor	extractor al vacío
ventral	ventral	ventral
ventre	belly	vientre
ventricule	ventricle	ventrículo
ventro-suspension	ventrosuspension	ventrosuspensión
ver	worm	lombriz

ITALIAN	GERMAN	FRENCH
vagina	Vagina, Scheide	vagin
vaginismo	Vaginismus	vaginisme
vaginite	Vaginitis	vaginite
vagotomia	Vagotomie	vagotomie
vagale	vagal, Vagus-	vague
vaso	Gefäß, Ader	vaisseau
valgo	valgus	valgus
valvola	Klappe, Ventil	valve
valvulotomia	Valvotomie	valvulotomie
fluttuazione	Fluktuation	variation
varicella	Varizellen, Windpocken	varicelle
vene varicose	Varizen, Krampfadern	varices
vaiolo	Variola, Pocken	variole
varo	varus	varus
vascolare	vaskulär, Gefäß-	vasculaire
vasculite	Vaskulitis	vasculite
vasectomia	Vasektomie, Vasoresektion	vasectomie
vasocostrittore (n)	Vasokonstriktor (n)	vasoconstricteur (n)
vasocostrittore (a)	vasokonstriktorisch (a)	vasoconstricteur (a)
vasodilatatore (n)	Vasodilatator (n)	vasodilatateur (n)
vasodilatatore (a)	vasodilatatorisch (a)	vasodilatateur (a)
vasopressore (n)	Vasopressor (n)	vasopresseur (n)
vasopressore (a)	vasopressorisch (a)	vasopresseur (a)
vettore	Überträger, Vektor	vecteur
adenoidi	Adenoide, Nasenpolypen	végétations adénoïdes
vena	Vene	veine
vena cava	Vena cava	veine cave
vena cubitale	Unterarmvene	veine de l'avant-bras
vena femorale	Vena femoralis	veine fémorale
vena giugulare	Vena jugularis	veine jugulaire
vena porta	Pfortader	veine porte
vena radiale	Vena radialis	veine radiale
venula	Venula	veinule
venereologia	Venerologie	vénéréologie
venereo	venerisch	vénérien
ventilazione a pressione positiva	Überdruckbeatmung	ventilation à pression positive
ventilazione e respirazione nelle vie respiratorie	Luftwege Atmung und Kreislauf (ABC-Regel)	ventilation et circulation
pressione continua positiva delle vie aeree	kontinuierlich positiver Atemwegsdruck	ventilation spontanée en pression positive continue
ventosa ostetrica, ventosa cefalica	Vakuumextraktor, Saugglocke	ventouse obstétricale
ventrale	ventral, Bauch-	ventral
addome, ventre	Bauch	ventre
ventricolo	Ventrikel, Kammer	ventricule
ventrosospensione, ventrofissazione	Ventrofixation, Ligamentopexie	ventro-suspension
verme	Wurm	ver

FRENCH	ENGLISH	SPANISH
verre de contact	contact lens	lente de contacto
verrue	verruca, wart	verruga
version	version	versión
version céphalique externe	external cephalic version (ECV)	versión cefálica externa
vertèbre	vertebra	vértebra
vertex	vertex	vértice
vertige	vertigo	vértigo
vésico-urétérique	vesicoureteric	vesicoureteral
vésico-vaginal	vesicovaginal	vesicovaginal
vésicule	vesicle	vesícula
vésicule biliaire	gall bladder	vesícula biliar
vessie	bladder	vejiga
vestibule	vestibule	vestíbulo
viable	viable	viable
vieillissement	ageing	envejecimiento
villosité	villus	vellosidad
villosités du chorion	chorionic villi	vellosidades coriónicas
virémie	viraemia (Eng), viremia (Am)	viremia
virilisme	virilism	virilismo
virologie	virology	virología
virulence	virulence	virulencia
virus	virus	virus
virus Coxsackie	Coxsackie virus	virus Coxsackie
virus de l'herpès simplex (HSV)	herpes simplex virus (HSV)	virus del herpes simple (VHS)
virus de l'immunodéficience humaine	human immunodeficiency virus (HIV)	virus de la inmunodeficiencia humana (VIH)
virus d'Epstein-Barr	Epstein-Barr virus (EBV)	virus de Epstein-Barr
virus de type herpétique (HLV)	herpes-like virus (HLV)	virus semejante al del herpes (HLV)
virus respiratoire syncytial	respiratory syncytial virus (RSV)	virus sincitial respiratorio (VSR)
viscères	viscera	visceras
vision binoculaire	binocular vision	visión binocular
visqueux	viscid	viscoso
visuel	visual	visual
vitamine	vitamin	vitamina
vitesse de sédimentation (VS)	sedimentation rate (SR)	velocidad de sedimentación globular (VSG)
vitesse de sédimentation globulaire	erythrocyte sedimentation rate (ESR)	velocidad de sedimentación globular (VSG)
vitesse de sédimentation sanguine	blood sedimentation rate (BSR)	velocidad de sedimentación globular (VSG)
vitiligo	vitiligo	vitfligo
vitré	vitreous body	vítreo
voile du palais	soft palate	paladar blando
volet thoracique	flail chest	volet torácico

ITALIAN	GERMAN	FRENCH
lente a contatto	Kontaktlinse	verre de contact
verruca, verruca volgare	Warze, Verruca	verrue
versione	Versio, Wendung	version
versione cefalica esterna	äußere Wendung auf den Kopf	version céphalique externe
vertebra	Wirbel	vertèbre
vertice	Vertex, Scheitel	vertex
vertigine	Schwindel, Vertigo	vertige
vescicoureterale	vesikoureteral	vésico-urétérique
vescicovaginale	vesikovaginal	vésico-vaginal
vescicola	Vesikula, Bläschen	vésicule
cistifellea	Gallenblase	vésicule biliaire
vescica	Blase, Harnblase	vessie
vestibolo	Vestibulum, Vorhof	vestibule
vitale, in grado di vivere	lebensfähig	viable
senescenza, invecchiamento	Altern	vieillissement
villo	Zotte	villosité
villi coriali	Chorionzotten	villosités du chorion
viremia	Virämie	virémie
virilismo	Virilismus	virilisme
virologia	Virologie	virologie
virulenza	Virulenz	virulence
virus	Virus	virus
virus Coxsackie	Coxsackie-Virus	virus Coxsackie
virus herpes simplex	Herpes simplex-Virus (HSV)	virus de l'herpès simplex (HSV)
virus dell'immunodeficienza umana (HIV)	human immunodeficiency virus (HIV), AIDS-Virus	virus de l'immunodéficience humaine
virus di Epstein Barr	Epstein-Barr-Virus (EBV)	virus d'Epstein-Barr
virus della famiglia dell'herpes	Herpes-ähnlicher Virus	virus de type herpétique (HLV)
virus respiratorio sinciziale (RSV)	RS-Virus	virus respiratoire syncytial
visceri	Eingeweide, Viszera	viscères
visione binoculare	binokulares Sehen, beidäugiges Sehen	vision binoculaire
viscido	zäh, klebrig	visqueux
visivo	visuell, Seh-	visuel
vitamina	Vitamin	vitamine
velocità di eritrosedimentazione (VES)	Blutkörperchen-Senkungsgeschwindigkeit (BSG, BKS)	vitesse de sédimentation (VS)
velocità di eritrosedimentazione (VES)	Blutkörperchen-Senkungsgeschwindigkeit (BSG, BKS)	vitesse de sédimentation globulaire
velocità di eritrosedimentazione (VES)	Blutkörperchen-Senkungsgeschwindigkeit (BSG, BKS)	vitesse de sédimentation sanguine
vitiligine	Vitiligo	vitiligo
corpo vitreo	Glaskörper	vitré
palato molle	weicher Gaumen	voile du palais
anomala motilità respiratoria della cassa toracica in conseguenza di fratture	Flatterbrust	volet thoracique

FRENCH	ENGLISH	SPANISH
volume expiratoire maximum (VEM)	peak expiratory velocity (PEV), forced expiratory volume (FEV)	velocidad espiratoria máxima (VEM), volumen espiratorio forzado (VEF)
volume globulaire moyen (VGM)	mean corpuscular volume (MCV)	volumen corpuscular medio (VCM)
volvulus	volvulus	vólvulo
vomir	vomit	vomitar
vomissement	emesis	emesis
vomissement cyclique	cyclical vomiting	vómito cíclico
vulve	pudendal block, vulva	bloqueo del pudendo, yulva
vulvite	vulvitis	vulvitis
vulvo-vaginal	vulvovaginal	vulvovaginal

ITALIAN	GERMAN	FRENCH
velocità espiratoria massima (VEM), volume espiratorio forzato	maximale exspiratorische Atemgeschwindigkeit, forciertes Exspirationsvolumen, Atemstoßwert	volume expiratoire maximum (VEM)
volume corpuscolare medio (VCM)	mittleres Erythrozytenvolumen (MCV)	volume globulaire moyen (VGM)
volvolo	Volvulus	volvulus
vomitare	sich übergeben, erbrechen	vomir
vomito, emesi	Erbrechen	vomissement
vomito ciclico	zyklisches Erbrechen	vomissement cyclique
anestesia della regione pubica, vulva	Pudendusblock, Vulva	vulve
vulvite	Vulvitis	vulvite
vulvovaginale	vulvovaginal	vulvo-vaginal

W

wheezing	wheeze	jadeo

X

xanthélasma	xanthelasma	xantelasma
xanthémie	xanthaemia (Eng), xanthemia (Am)	xantemia
xanthome	xanthoma	xantoma
xérodermie	xeroderma	xeroderma
xérophtalmie	xerophthalmia	xeroftalmia

Z

zona	shingles, zoster	herpes zóster, zóster
zone particulièrement sensible	pressure area	zona de decúbito
zoonose	zoonosis	zoonosis
zygoma	zygoma	cigoma
zygote	zygote	cigoto

ITALIAN	GERMAN	FRENCH
sibilo	Giemen	**wheezing**
xantelasma	Xanthelasma	**xanthélasma**
xantemia	Xanthämie	**xanthémie**
xantoma, malattia di Rayer	Xanthom	**xanthome**
xerodermia	Xerodermie	**xérodermie**
xeroftalmia	Xerophthalmie	**xérophtalmie**
herpes zoster	Herpes zoster, Gürtelrose	**zona**
area di pressione	Druckfläche	**zone particulièrement sensible**
zoonosi	Zoonose, Tierkrankheit	**zoonose**
zigomo, osso zigomatico	Zygoma, Jochbein	**zygoma**
zigote	Zygote	**zygote**

ABRÉVIATIONS FRANÇAISES
FRANZÖSISCHE ABKÜRZUNGEN
ABBREVIAZIONI FRANCESI
ABREVIATURAS FRANCESAS

ACTH	hormone adrénocorticotrope
ADN	acide désoxyribonucléique
BCG	bacille de Calmette-Guérin
BJ	(protéine) de Bence Jones
CID	coagulation intravasculaire disséminée
CNS	système nerveux central
CPRE	cholangio-pancréatographie rétrograde endoscopique
DIU	dispositif intra-utérin
ECG	électrocardiogramme
EEG	électroencéphalogramme
EP	embolie pulmonaire
GCH	gonadotrophine chorionique humaine
GGH	gamma-globuline humaine
GGT	gamma-glutamyl-transférase
GT	génito-urinaire
Hb	hémoglobine
HCS	somatomammotropine chorionique humaine
Hg	hémoglobine
HGH	hormone de croissance
HL	hormone lutéinisante
HLV	virus de type herpétique
HSV	virus de l'herpès simplex
IA	insémination artificielle
Ig	immunoglobuline
IG	interruption de grossesse
IM	intramusculaire
IMAO	inhibiteur de la monoamine-oxydase
IMC	indice de masse corporelle
IV	intraveineux
LBD	lipoprotéine de basse densité
LHD	lipoprotéine de haute densité
mEq	milliéquivalent
MST	maladie sexuellement transmissible
MV	maladie vénérienne
NE	numération érythrocytaire
NGB	nombre de globules blancs
ORL	oto-rhino-laryngologie
PAT	test d'agrégation plaquettaire
PCE	polyarthrite chronique évolutive
PCP	pression capillaire pulmonaire
ppm	parties par million
PR	polyarthrite rhumatoïde
psi	livres par pouce carré
Rh−	rhésus négatif
Rh+	rhésus positif
RNA	acide ribonucléique
sc	sous-cutané
SIDA	syndrome d'immuno-déficience acquise
SNC	système nerveux central

STH	somatotrophine
TA	tension artérielle
TB	tuberculose
TFH	test de la fonction hépatique
TL	thyroxine libre
TVP	thrombose veineuse profonde
UIV	urographie intraveineuse
UV	ultraviolet
VEM	volume expiratoire maximum
VGM	volume globulaire moyen
VS	vitesse de sédimentation

GERMAN
English
Spanish
French
Italian
GERMAN

GERMAN	ENGLISH	SPANISH

A

abartig	aberrant	aberrante, desviado
Abbaustoffwechsel	catabolism	catabolismo
abbinden	ligate	ligar
Abdomen	abdomen	abdomen
abdominal	abdominal, celiac (Am), coeliac (Eng)	abdominal, celíaco
abdominoperineal	abdomino-perineal	abdominoperineal
Abdruck	cast	enyesado, vendaje de yeso
Abduktion	abduction	abducción
Abduktor	abductor	abductor
abduzieren	abduct	abducir
aberrans	aberrant	aberrante, desviado
Aberration	aberration	aberración
abfallend	remittent	remitente
abführend	aperient, laxative, purgative	laxante, laxativo, purgante
Abführmittel	aperient, laxative, purgative	laxante, purga
Abhören	auscultation	auscultación
Ablatio	ablation	ablación, excisión
Ableitung	lead	plomo
abnormal	abnormal	anormal
Abort	abortion	aborto
Abort, drohender	threatened abortion	amenaza de aborto
Abort, indizierter	therapeutic abortion	aborto terapéutico
Abort, künstlicher	induced abortion	aborto inducido
Abort, verhaltener	missed abortion	aborto diferido
Abreaktion	abreaction	abreacción, catarsis
Abriß	avulsion	avulsión
Abschabung	abrasion	abrasión
Abschürfung	excoriation	excoriación
Abschwächung	attenuation	atenuación
Absetzung	ablation	ablación, excisión
Absorption	absorption	absorción
Abstoßung	rejection	rechazo
Abstrich	smear	frotis
Abstrichtupfer	swab	torunda
Abszeß	abscess	absceso
Abszeß, kalter	cold abscess	absceso frío
Abtreibung	induced abortion	aborto inducido
Abusus	abuse	abuso
Abweichung	aberration	aberración
Abzapfen	tapping	paracentesis
Achalasie	achalasia	acalasia
Achillessehne	Achilles tendon	tendón de Aquiles
Achondroplasie	achondroplasia	acondroplasia
Achse	axis	eje

FRENCH	ITALIAN	GERMAN
aberrant	aberrante	abartig
catabolisme	catabolismo	Abbaustoffwechsel
ligaturer	legare	abbinden
abdomen	addome	Abdomen
abdominal, coeliaque	addominale, celiaco	abdominal
abdomino-périnéal	addomino-perineale	abdominoperineal
plâtre	ingessatura, steccatura	Abdruck
abduction	abduzione	Abduktion
abducteur	abduttore	Abduktor
produire l'abduction	abdurre	abduzieren
aberrant	aberrante	aberrans
aberration	aberrazione	Aberration
rémittent	remittente	abfallend
laxatif, purgatif	lassativo, purgante	abführend
laxatif, purgatif	lassativo	Abführmittel
auscultation	auscultazione	Abhören
ablation	ablazione	Ablatio
plomb	piombo derivazione	Ableitung
anormal	anormale	abnormal
avortement	aborto	Abort
risque d'avortement	minaccia d'aborto	Abort, drohender
avortement thérapeutique	aborto terapeutico	Abort, indizierter
avortement provoqué	aborto procurato	Abort, künstlicher
rétention foetale	aborto interno, aborto ritenuto	Abort, verhaltener
abréaction	abreazione, catarsi	Abreaktion
avulsion	avulsione	Abriß
abrasion	abrasione	Abschabung
excoriation	escoriazione	Abschürfung
atténuation	attenuazione	Abschwächung
ablation	ablazione	Absetzung
absorption	assorbimento	Absorption
rejet	rigetto	Abstoßung
frottis	striscio	Abstrich
tampon	tampone	Abstrichtupfer
abcès	ascesso	Abszeß
abcès froid	ascesso freddo	Abszeß, kalter
avortement provoqué	aborto procurato	Abtreibung
abus	abuso	Abusus
aberration	aberrazione	Abweichung
ponction	aspirazione di fluido	Abzapfen
achalasie	acalasia	Achalasie
tendon d'Achille	tendine di Achille	Achillessehne
achondroplasie	acondroplasia	Achondroplasie
axe	asse, colonna vertebrale	Achse

GERMAN	ENGLISH	SPANISH
Achsel(höhle)	axilla	axila
Adamsapfel	Adam's apple	huez de Adán
Addison Krankheit	Addison's disease	enfermedad de Addison
Adduktion	adduction	aducción
Adduktor	adductor	aductor
adduzieren	adduct	aducir
Adenoide	adenoids	adenoides
Adenoidektomie	adenoidectomy	adenoidectomía
Adenokarzinom	adenocarcinoma	adenocarcinoma
Adenom	adenoma	adenoma
Adenomyom	adenomyoma	adenomioma
Adenotonsillektomie	adenotonsillectomy	amigdaloadenoidectomía
Adenovirus	adenovirus	adenovirus
Ader	vessel	vaso
Aderhaut	choroid	coroides
Adhäsion	adhesion	adherencia
adipös	adipose	adiposo, graso
Adipositas	obesity	obesidad
Adjuvans	adjuvant	coadyuvante
Adnexe	adnexa	anejos, anexos
Adoleszenz	adolescence	adolescencia
Adoption	adoption	adopción
Adrenalin	adrenaline, epinephrine	adrenalina, epinefrina
adrenerg	adrenergic	adrenérgico
adrenokortikotropes Hormon (ACTH)	adrenocorticotrophic hormone (ACTH)	hormona adrenocorticotropa (ACTH)
Adsorption	adsorption	adsorción
adstringierend	astringent	astringente
Aerobier	aerobe	aerobio, aeróbico
Aerophagie	aerophagia	aerofagia
Aerosol	aerosol	aerosol
Affekt	affect	afecto
affektiv	affective	afectivo
afferent	afferent	aferente
After	anus	ano
Agenesie	agenesis	agenesia
Agglutination	agglutination	aglutinación
Agglutinin	agglutinin	aglutinina
Aggression	aggression	agresión
Agnathie	agnathia	agnatia
Agnosie	agnosia	agnosia
Agonist	agonist	agonista
Agoraphobie	agoraphobia	agorafobia
Agranulozytose	agranulocytosis	agranulocitosis
ägyptische Augenkrankheit	trachoma	tracoma
Ähnlichkeit	parity	paridad

FRENCH	ITALIAN	GERMAN
aisselle	ascella	Achsel(höhle)
pomme d'Adam	pomo di Adamo	Adamsapfel
maladie d'Addison	morbo di Addison	Addison Krankheit
adduction	adduzione	Adduktion
adducteur	adduttore	Adduktor
produire l'adduction	addurre	adduzieren
végétations adénoïdes	adenoidi	Adenoide
adénoïdectomie	adenoidectomia	Adenoidektomie
adénocarcinome	adenocarcinoma	Adenokarzinom
adénome	adenoma	Adenom
adénomyome	adenomioma	Adenomyom
adéno-amygdalectomie	adenotonsillectomia	Adenotonsillektomie
adénovirus	adenovirus	Adenovirus
vaisseau	vaso	Ader
choroïde	coroide	Aderhaut
adhésion	adesione	Adhäsion
adipeux	adiposo	adipös
obésité	obesità	Adipositas
adjuvant	adiuvante	Adjuvans
annexes	annessi	Adnexe
adolescence	adolescenza	Adoleszenz
adoption	adozione	Adoption
adrénaline, épinéphrine	adrenalina	Adrenalin
adrénergique	adrenergico	adrenerg
hormone adrénocorticotrope (ACTH)	ormone corticotropo (ACTH)	adrenokortikotropes Hormon (ACTH)
adsorption	adsorbimento	Adsorption
astringent	astringente	adstringierend
aérobie	aerobio	Aerobier
aérophagie	aerofagia	Aerophagie
aérosol	aerosol	Aerosol
affect	emozione	Affekt
affectif	affettivo	affektiv
afférent	afferente	afferent
anus	ano	After
agénésic	agenesia	Agenesie
agglutination	agglutinazione	Agglutination
agglutinine	agglutinine	Agglutinin
agression	aggressività	Aggression
agnathie	agnazia	Agnathie
agnosie	agnosia	Agnosie
agoniste	agonista	Agonist
agoraphobie	agorafobia	Agoraphobie
agranulocytose	agranulocitosi	Agranulozytose
trachome	tracoma	ägyptische Augenkrankheit
parité	parità, numero di gravidanze pregresse	Ähnlichkeit

GERMAN	ENGLISH	SPANISH
AIDS-related complex	AIDS-related complex	complejo relacionado con SIDA
AIDS-Virus	human immunodeficiency virus (HIV)	virus de la inmunodeficiencia humana (VIH)
akinetisch	akinetic	acinético
Akkommodation	accommodation	acomodación
Akne	acne	acné
Akromegalie	acromegaly	acromegalia
akromioklavikular	acromioclavicular	acromioclavicular
Akromion	acromion	acromion
Aktinomykose	actinomycosis	actinomicosis
aktiv	active	activo
Akupunktur	acupuncture	acupuntura
akustisch	acoustic	acústico
Albumin	albumin	albúmina
Albuminurie	albuminuria	albuminuria
Alkali	alkali	álcali
alkalisch	alkaline	alcalino
Alkalose	alkalosis	alcalosis
Alkohol	alcohol	alcohol
Alkoholismus	alcoholism	alcoholismo
alkoholresistent	alcohol-fast	resistente al alcohol
Alkoholsyndrom	alcohol syndrome	síndrome alcohólico
Alkoholsyndrom, fetales	fetal alcohol syndrome	síndrome alcohólico fetal
Alkoholvergiftung	alcoholism	alcoholismo
Allergen	allergen	alérgeno
Allergie	allergy	alergia
Allergisierung	sensitization	sensibilización
Allopurinol	allopurinol	alopurinol
Alopezie	alopecia	alopecia, calvicie
Alpha-Fetoprotein	alpha-fetoprotein (AFP)	alfafetoproteína (AFP)
Altern	ageing, senescence	envejecimiento, senescencia
Alternativmedizin	alternative medicine	medicina alternativa
Alters-	senile	senil
Alveole	alveolus	alvéolo
Alveolitis	alveolitis	alveolitis
Alzheimer Krankheit	Alzheimer's disease	enfermedad de Alzheimer
Amaurose	amaurosis	amaurosis, ceguera
Amblyopie	amblyopia	ambliopía
Amboß	incus	incus, yunque
ambulant	ambulant, ambulatory	ambulante, ambulatorio
Amenorrhoe	amenorrhea (Am), amenorrhoea (Eng)	amenorrea
Aminosäure	amino acid	aminoácido
Aminosäure, essentielle	essential amino acid	aminoácido esenciale
Amnesie	amnesia	amnesia
Amnion	amnion	amnios
Amnionflüssigkeit	amniotic fluid	líquido amniótico
Amnionhöhle	amniotic cavity	cavidad amniótica

FRENCH	ITALIAN	GERMAN
para-SIDA	complesso AIDS-correlato	**AIDS-related complex**
virus de l'immunodéficience humaine	virus dell'immunodeficienza umana (HIV)	**AIDS-Virus**
acinétique	acinetico	**akinetisch**
accommodation	accomodazione	**Akkommodation**
acné	acne	**Akne**
acromégalie	acromegalia	**Akromegalie**
acromio-claviculaire	acromioclavicolare	**akromioklavikular**
acromion	acromion	**Akromion**
actinomycose	actinomicosi	**Aktinomykose**
actif	attivo	**aktiv**
acupuncture	agopuntura	**Akupunktur**
acoustique	acustico	**akustisch**
albumine	albumina	**Albumin**
albuminurie	albuminuria	**Albuminurie**
alcali	alcali	**Alkali**
alcalin	alcalino	**alkalisch**
alcalose	alcalosi	**Alkalose**
alcool	alcool	**Alkohol**
alcoolisme	alcolismo	**Alkoholismus**
résistant à l'alcool	alcool-resistente	**alkoholresistent**
syndrome d'alcoolisme	sindrome da alcool	**Alkoholsyndrom**
syndrome d'alcoolisme foetal	sindrome da alcolismo materno	**Alkoholsyndrom, fetales**
alcoolisme	alcolismo	**Alkoholvergiftung**
allergène	allergene	**Allergen**
allergie	allergia	**Allergie**
sensibilisation	sensibilizzazione	**Allergisierung**
allopurinol	allopurinolo	**Allopurinol**
alopécie	alopecia	**Alopezie**
alpha-foetoprotéine	alfafetoproteina	**Alpha-Fetoprotein**
vieillissement, sénescence	senescenza, invecchiamento	**Altern**
médecine complémentaire	medicina alternativa	**Alternativmedizin**
sénile	senile	**Alters-**
alvéole	alveolo	**Alveole**
alvéolite	alveolite	**Alveolitis**
maladie d'Alzheimer	morbo di Alzheimer	**Alzheimer Krankheit**
amaurose	amaurosi	**Amaurose**
amblyopie	ambliopia	**Amblyopie**
enclume	incudine	**Amboß**
ambulant, ambulatoire	ambulatorio, ambulatoriale	**ambulant**
aménorrhée	amenorrea	**Amenorrhoe**
acide aminé	aminoacido	**Aminosäure**
acide aminé essentiel	aminoacido essenziale	**Aminosäure, essentielle**
amnésie	amnesia	**Amnesie**
amnion	amnios	**Amnion**
liquide amniotique	fluido amniotico	**Amnionflüssigkeit**
cavité amniotique	cavità amniotica	**Amnionhöhle**

GERMAN	ENGLISH	SPANISH
Amnionpunktur	amniotomy	amniotomía
Amnioskopie	amnioscopy	amnioscopia
Amniozentese	amniocentesis	amniocentesis
Amöbe	ameba (Am), amoeba (Eng)	ameba
Amöbengranulom	ameboma (Am), amoeboma (Eng)	ameboma
Amöbenkrankheit	amebiasis (Am), amoebiasis (Eng)	amebiasis
Amöbiasis	amebiasis (Am), amoebiasis (Eng)	amebiasis
amorph	amorphous	amorfo
Ampulle	ampoule (Eng), ampule (Am), ampulla	ampolla, víal, ampolla
Amputation	amputation	amputación
Amputierter	amputee	amputado
Amyloid	amyloid	amiloide
amyloid	amyloid	amiloideo
Amyloidose	amyloidosis	amiloidosis
Anabolismus	anabolism	anabolismo
anaerobe Respiration	anaerobic respiration (Eng), anerobic respiration (Am)	respiración anaerobia
Anaerobier	anaerobe (Eng), anerobe (Am)	anaerobio
Analeptikum	analeptic	analéptico, estimulante
analeptisch	analeptic	analéptico, estimulante
Analgesie	analgesia	analgesia
Analgetikum	analgesic	analgésico
analgetisch	analgesic	analgésico
Analyse	analysis	análisis
Anämie	anaemia (Eng), anemia (Am)	anemia
anaphylaktische Reaktion	anaphylactic reaction	reacción anafiláctica
Anaphylaxie	anaphylaxis	anafilaxis
Anaplasie	anaplasia	anaplasia
Anarthrie	anarthria	anartria
Anästhesie	anaesthesia (Eng), anesthesia (Am) narcosis	anestesia, narcosis
Anästhetikum	anaesthetic (Eng), anesthetic (Am)	anestésico
anästhetisch	anaesthetic (Eng), anesthetic (Am)	anestésico
Anastomose	anastomosis	anastómosis
Anatomie	anatomy	anatomía
Androgene	androgens	andrógenos
Anenzephalie	anencephaly	anencefalia
Aneurysma	aneurysm	aneurisma
Anfall	attack, fit, seizure	ataque, acceso
Anfälligkeit	predisposition, susceptibility	predisposición, susceptibilidad
angeboren	congenital, inherent, innate	congénito, inherente, innato
Angina	angina	angina
Angioplastie	angioplasty	angioplastia
Angiotensin	angiotensin	angiotensina
Angst	anxiety	ansiedad
Anhaften	adhesion	adherencia
Anisozytose	anisocytosis	anisocitosis
Ankylose	ankylosis	anquilosis

FRENCH	ITALIAN	GERMAN
amniotomie	amniotomia	**Amnionpunktur**
amnioscopie	amnioscopia	**Amnioskopie**
amniocentèse	amniocentesi	**Amniozentese**
amibe	ameba	**Amöbe**
amibome	ameboma	**Amöbengranulom**
amibiase	amebiasi	**Amöbenkrankheit**
amibiase	amebiasi	**Amöbiasis**
amorphe	amorfo	**amorph**
ampoule	ampolla, fiala	**Ampulle**
amputation	amputazione	**Amputation**
amputé	amputato	**Amputierter**
amyloïde	amiloide	**Amyloid**
amyloïde	amiloide	**amyloid**
amylose	amiloidosi	**Amyloidose**
anabolisme	anabolismo	**Anabolismus**
respiration anaérobie	respirazione anaerobica	**anaerobe Respiration**
anaérobie	anaerobio	**Anaerobier**
analeptique	analettico	**Analeptikum**
analeptique	analettico	**analeptisch**
analgésie	analgesia	**Analgesie**
analgésique	analgesico	**Analgetikum**
analgésique	analgesico	**analgetisch**
analyse	analisi	**Analyse**
anémie	anemia	**Anämie**
réaction anaphylactique	reazione anafilattica	**anaphylaktische Reaktion**
anaphylaxie	anafilassi	**Anaphylaxie**
anaplasie	anaplasia	**Anaplasie**
anarthrie	anartria	**Anarthrie**
anesthésie, narcose	anestesia, narcosi	**Anästhesie**
anesthésique	anestetico	**Anästhetikum**
anesthésique	anestetico	**anästhetisch**
anastomose	anastomosi	**Anastomose**
anatomie	anatomia	**Anatomie**
androgènes	androgeni	**Androgene**
anencéphalic	anencefalia	**Anenzephalie**
anévrisme	aneurisma	**Aneurysma**
attaque, accès	attacco, convulsione	**Anfall**
prédisposition, susceptibilité	predisposizione, suscettibilità	**Anfälligkeit**
congénital, inhérent, endogène	congenito, inerente, innato	**angeboren**
angor	angina	**Angina**
angioplastie	angioplastica	**Angioplastie**
angiotensine	angiotensina	**Angiotensin**
anxiété	ansietà	**Angst**
adhésion	adesione	**Anhaften**
anisocytose	anisocitosi	**Anisozytose**
ankylose	anchilosi	**Ankylose**

GERMAN	ENGLISH	SPANISH
anogenital	anogenital	anogenital
Anomalie	anomaly	anomalía
anorektal	anorectal	anorrectal
Anorektiker(in)	anorectic	anoréxico
anorektisch	anorectic	anoréxico
Anorexie	anorexia	anorexia
anorganisch	inorganic	inorgánico
Anosmie	anosmia	anosmia
anovulatorisch	anovular	anovular
Anoxie	anoxia	anoxia
Anschoppung	engorgement	estancamiento
Anschwellung, diffuse	tumescence	tumescencia
ansteckend	contagious, infective	contagioso, trasmisible, infeccioso
Anstrengung	strain	cepa
Antagonismus	antagonism	antagonismo
Antagonist	antagonist	antagonista
Antazidum	antacid	antiácido
ante partum	ante-partum	ante partum, preparto
anterior	anterior	anterior
anterograd	anterograde	anterógrado
Anteversion	anteversion	anteversión
Anthrax	anthrax	carbunco
anthropoid	anthropoid	antropoide
Anthropologie	anthropology	antropología
antiarrhythmisch	anti-arrhythmic	antiarrítmico
antibakteriell	antibacterial	antibacteriano
Antibiotika	antibiotics	antibióticos
anticholinerg	anticholinergic	anticolinérgico
Antidepressivum	antidepressant	antidepresivo
Anti-D-Immununglobulin	anti-D	anti-D
Antidot	antidote	antídoto
Antiemetikum	antiemetic	antiemético
antiemetisch	antiemetic	antiemético
Antiepileptikum	anticonvulsant, anti-epileptic	anticonvulsivo, antiepiléptico
antiepileptisch	anticonvulsant, anti-epileptic	anticonvulsivo, antiepiléptico
Antigen	antigen	antígeno
Antigen-Bindungskapazität	antigen binding capacity (ABC)	capacidad de unión con antígenos
Antihistamine	antihistamine	antihistamínico
antihypertensiv	antihypertensive	hipotensor
Antihypertensivum	antihypertensive	hipotensor
Antihypertonikum	antihypertensive	hipotensor
Antikoagulans	anticoagulant	anticoagulante
antikonvulsiv	anticonvulsant, anti-epileptic	anticonvulsivo, antiepiléptico
Antikonvulsivum	anticonvulsant, anti-epileptic	anticonvulsivo, antiepiléptico
Antikörper	antibodies (Ab)	anticuerpos
Antimalaria-	antimalarial	antipalúdico

FRENCH	ITALIAN	GERMAN
anogénital	anogenitale	anogenital
anomalie	anomalia	Anomalie
anorectal	anorettale	anorektal
anorexique	anoressico	Anorektiker(in)
anorexique	anoressico	anorektisch
anorexie	anoressia	Anorexie
inorganique	inorganico	anorganisch
anosmie	anosmia	Anosmie
anovulaire	anovulare	anovulatorisch
anoxie	anossia	Anoxie
engorgement	congestione	Anschoppung
tumescence	tumefazione	Anschwellung, diffuse
contagieux, infectieux	contagioso, infettivo	ansteckend
entorse	tensione	Anstrengung
antagonisme	antagonismo	Antagonismus
antagoniste	antagonista	Antagonist
antiacide	antiacido	Antazidum
ante partum	preparto	ante partum
antérieur	anteriore	anterior
antérograde	anterogrado	anterograd
antéversion	antiversione	Anteversion
anthrax	antrace, carbonchio	Anthrax
anthropoïde	antropoide	anthropoid
anthropologie	antropologia	Anthropologie
antiarythmique	anti-aritmico	antiarrhythmisch
antibactérien	antibatterico	antibakteriell
antibiotiques	antibiotici	Antibiotika
anticholinergique	anticolinergico	anticholinerg
antidépresseur	antidepressivo	Antidepressivum
anti-D	anti-D	Anti-D-Immununglobulin
antidote	antidoto	Antidot
antiémétique	anti-emetico	Antiemetikum
antiémétique	anti-emetico	antiemetisch
anticonvulsant, antiépileptique	anticonvulsivante, anticomiziale	Antiepileptikum
anticonvulsant, antiépileptique	anticonvulsivante, anticomiziale	antiepileptisch
antigène	antigene	Antigen
capacité de liaison d'un antigène, capacité de fixation d'un antigène	capacità di legame dell'antigene	Antigen-Bindungskapazität
antihistamine	anti-istaminico	Antihistamine
antihypertensif	anti-ipertensivo	antihypertensiv
antihypertenseur	anti-ipertensivo	Antihypertensivum
antihypertenseur	anti-ipertensivo	Antihypertonikum
anticoagulant	anticoagulante	Antikoagulans
anticonvulsant, antiépileptique	anticonvulsivante, anticomiziale	antikonvulsiv
anticonvulsant, antiépileptique	anticonvulsivante, anticomiziale	Antikonvulsivum
anticorps	anticorpi (Ac)	Antikörper
antipaludique	antimalarico	Antimalaria-

Antimalariamittel	antimalarial	antipalúdico
Antimetabolit	antimetabolite	antimetabolito
antimikrobiell	antimicrobial	antimicrobiano
Antimykotikum	antimycotic	antimicótico
antimykotisch	antimycotic	antimicótico
Antiparkinsonmittel	antiparkinson(ism) drugs	farmacos antiparkinsonianos
Antiphlogistikum, nicht steroidales	non-steroidal anti-inflammatory drug (NSAID)	fármaco antiinflamatorio no esteroide (AINE)
antipruriginös	antipruritic	antipruriginoso
Antipruriginosum	antipruritic	antipruriginoso
Antipsychotikum	antipsychotic	antipsicótico
antipsychotisch	antipsychotic	antipsicótico
Antipyretikum	antipyretic	antipirético
antipyretisch	antipyretic	antipirético
Antisepsis	antisepsis	antisepsia
Antiseptikum	antiseptic	antiséptico
antiseptisch	antiseptic	antiséptico
Antiserum	antiserum	antisuero
Antithenar	hypothenar eminence	eminencia hipotenar
Antitoxin	antitoxin	antitoxina
antitussiv	antitussive	antitusígeno
Antitussivum	antitussive	antitusígeno
Antrum	antrum	antro
Antrumeröffnung	antrostomy	antrostomía
Anurie	anuria	anuria
Anus	anus	ano
Anxiolytikum	anxiolytic	ansiolítico
anxiolytisch	anxiolytic	ansiolítico
Aorta	aorta	aorta
Apathie	apathy	apatía
Apettitzügler	anorectic	anoréxico
Apex	apex	ápex
Apgar-Index	Apgar score	índice de Apgar
Aphasie	aphasia	afasia
Aphthe	aphthae	aftas
Apnoe	apnea (Am), apnoea (Eng)	apnea
apokrine Drüse	apocrine gland	glándula apocrina
Apoplex	cerebrovascular accident (CVA)	accidente vascular cerebral (ACV)
Apotheker	pharmacist	farmacéutico
Apotheker-	pharmaceutical	farmacéutico
Appendektomie	appendectomy, appendicectomy	apendicectomía
Appendix	appendix	apéndice
Appendizitis	appendicitis	apendicitis
Applikator	applicator	aplicador
Apposition	apposition	aposición
Apraxie	apraxia	apraxia

antipaludique	antimalarico	**Antimalariamittel**
antimétabolite	antimetabolita	**Antimetabolit**
antimicrobien	antimicrobico	**antimikrobiell**
antimycotique	antimicotico	**Antimykotikum**
antimycotique	antimicotico	**antimykotisch**
médicaments contre la maladie de Parkinson	farmaci antiparkinsoniani	**Antiparkinsonmittel**
anti-inflammatoire non stéroïdien	farmaco antinfiammatorio non steroideo (FANS)	**Antiphlogistikum, nicht steroidales**
antiprurigineux	antipruriginoso	**antipruriginös**
antiprurigineux	antipruriginoso	**Antipruriginosum**
antipsychotique	antipsicotico	**Antipsychotikum**
antipsychotique	antipsicotico	**antipsychotisch**
antipyrétique	anti-piretico	**Antipyretikum**
antipyrétique	anti-piretico	**antipyretisch**
antisepsie	antisepsi	**Antisepsis**
antiseptique	antisettico	**Antiseptikum**
antiseptique	antisettico	**antiseptisch**
anti-serum	anti-siero	**Antiserum**
éminence hypothénar	eminenza ipotenar	**Antithenar**
antitoxine	antitossina	**Antitoxin**
antitussif	antibechico	**antitussiv**
antitussif	antibechico	**Antitussivum**
antre	antro	**Antrum**
antrostomie	antrostomia	**Antrumeröffnung**
anurie	anuria	**Anurie**
anus	ano	**Anus**
anxiolytique	ansiolitico	**Anxiolytikum**
anxiolytique	ansiolitico	**anxiolytisch**
aorte	aorta	**Aorta**
apathie	apatia	**Apathie**
anorexique	anoressico	**Apettitzügler**
apex	apice	**Apex**
indice d'Apgar	indice di Apgar	**Apgar-Index**
aphasie	afasia	**Aphasie**
aphtes	afte	**Aphthe**
apnée	apnea	**Apnoe**
glande apocrine	ghiandola apocrina	**apokrine Drüse**
accident cérébrovasculaire	ictus, accidente cerebrovascolare (ACV)	**Apoplex**
pharmacien	farmacista	**Apotheker**
pharmaceutique	farmaceutico	**Apotheker-**
appendicectomie	appendicectomia	**Appendektomie**
appendice	appendice	**Appendix**
appendicite	appendicite	**Appendizitis**
applicateur	applicatore	**Applikator**
apposition	apposizione	**Apposition**
apraxie	aprassia	**Apraxie**

GERMAN	ENGLISH	SPANISH
Apyrexie	apyrexia	apirexia
Aquädukt	aqueduct	acueducto
arachnoid	arachnoid	aracnoideo
ARBO-Virus	arbovirus	arbovirus
Areola	areola	areola
Arm	arm	brazo
Arm-	brachial	braquial
Arnold-Chiari-Mißbildung	Arnold-Chiari malformation	malformación de Arnold-Chiari
Arrhythmie	arrhythmia	arritmia
Art	species, type	especie, tipo
Artefakt	artefact (Eng), artifact (Am)	artefacto
Arteria femoralis	femoral artery	arteria femoral
Arteria radialis	radial artery	arteria radial
Arterie	artery	arteria
Arterienerkrankung	arteriopathy	arteriopatía
Arterienverkalkung	arteriosclerosis	arteriosclerosis
Arteriitis	arteritis	arteritis
Arteriole	arteriole	arteriola
Arteriopathie	arteriopathy	arteriopatía
Arteriosklerose	arteriosclerosis	arteriosclerosis
arteriovenös	arteriovenous	arteriovenoso
Arthralgie	arthralgia	artralgia
Arthritis	arthritis	artritis
Arthritis psoriatica	psoriatic arthritis	artritis psoriásica
Arthrodese	arthrodesis	artrodesis
Arthrographie	arthrography	artrografía
Arthropathie	arthropathy	artropatía
Arthroplastik	arthroplasty	artroplastia
Arthroskopie	arthroscopy	artroscopia
Artikulation	articulation	articulación
Arznei	medicine	medicina
Arzneimittel	drug, medicament	fármaco, medicamento
Arzneimittelmißbrauch	drug abuse	abuso de drogas
Arzneimittelreaktion, unerwünschte	adverse drug reaction (ADR)	reacción adversa a un medicamento
Arzt	doctor, physician	médico, facultativo
Asbest	asbestos	asbesto
Asbestose	asbestosis	asbestosis
Asepsis	asepsis	asepsia
aseptische Technik	aseptic technique	técnica aséptica
Aspergillose	aspergillosis	aspergilosis
Asphyxie	asphyxia	asfixia
Aspiration	aspiration	aspiración
Assimilation	assimilation	asimilación
Assoziation	association	asociación
Astereognosie	astereognosis	astereognosia

404

FRENCH	ITALIAN	GERMAN
apyrexie	apiressia	**Apyrexie**
aqueduc	acquedotto	**Aquädukt**
arachnoïde	aracnoidea	**arachnoid**
arbovirus	arbovirus	**ARBO-Virus**
aréole	areola	**Areola**
bras	braccio	**Arm**
brachial	brachiale	**Arm-**
malformation d'Arnold Chiari	sindrome di Arnold Chiari	**Arnold-Chiari-Mißbildung**
arythmie	aritmia	**Arrhythmie**
espèce, type	specie, tipo	**Art**
artefact	artefatto	**Artefakt**
artère fémorale	arteria femorale	**Arteria femoralis**
artère radiale	arteria radiale	**Arteria radialis**
artère	arteria	**Arterie**
artériopathie	arteriopatia	**Arterienerkrankung**
artériosclérose	arteriosclerosi	**Arterienverkalkung**
artérite	arterite	**Arteriitis**
artériole	arteriola	**Arteriole**
artériopathie	arteriopatia	**Arteriopathie**
artériosclérose	arteriosclerosi	**Arteriosklerose**
artérioveineux	arterovenosa	**arteriovenös**
arthralgie	artralgia	**Arthralgie**
arthrite	artrite	**Arthritis**
rhumatisme psoriasique	artropatia psoriasica, psoriasi artropatica	**Arthritis psoriatica**
arthrodèse	artrodesi	**Arthrodese**
arthrographie	artrografia	**Arthrographie**
arthropathie	artropatia	**Arthropathie**
arthroplastie	artroplastica	**Arthroplastik**
arthroscopie	artroscopia	**Arthroskopie**
articulation	articolazione	**Artikulation**
médecine	medicina	**Arznei**
médicament	farmaco, medicinale, droga, medicamento	**Arzneimittel**
toxicomanie	abuso di droga, abuso di farmaci	**Arzneimittelmißbrauch**
réaction médicamenteuse indésirable	reazione dannosa (indesiderata) da farmaci	**Arzneimittelreaktion, unerwünschte**
médecin	dottore, medico	**Arzt**
asbeste	asbesto	**Asbest**
asbestose	asbestosi	**Asbestose**
asepsie	asepsi	**Asepsis**
technique aseptique	tecnica asettica	**aseptische Technik**
aspergillose	aspergillosi	**Aspergillose**
asphyxie	asfissia	**Asphyxie**
aspiration	aspirazione	**Aspiration**
assimilation	assimilazione	**Assimilation**
association	associazione	**Assoziation**
astéréognosie	astereognosia	**Astereognosie**

GERMAN	ENGLISH	SPANISH
Asthma	asthma	asma
Asthma bronchiale	bronchial asthma	asma bronquial
Astigmatismus	astigmatism	astigmatismo
Asymmetrie	asymmetry	asimetría
asymptomatisch	asymptomatic	asintomático
Aszites	ascites	ascitis
Ataxie	ataxia	ataxia
Atelektase	atelectasis	atelectasia
Atem	breath	aliento
Atemfunktionstest	respiratory function test	prueba de función respiratoria
Atemnot	dyspnea (Am), dyspnoea (Eng)	disnea
Atemnotsyndrom	respiratory distress syndrome (RDS)	síndrome de distress respiratorio
Atemstillstand	apnea (Am), apnoea (Eng)	apnea
Atemstoßwert	forced expiratory volume (FEV)	volumen espiratorio forzado (VEF)
Atemwegsdruck, kontinuierlich positiver	continuous positive airway pressure (CPAP)	presión continua positiva de las vías respiratorias
Atemwegsinfekt	upper respiratory tract infection (URTI)	infección de las vías respiratorias altas
Atemwegsinfekt (akut fieberhaft)	acute febrile respiratory disease/illness (AFRD/I)	enfermedad respiratoria febril aguda
Atemwegsinfekt (untere)	lower respiratory tract infection (LRTI)	infección de las vías respiratorias bajas
Atemzug	breath	aliento
atherogen	atherogenic	aterogénico
Atherom	atheroma	ateroma
Atherosklerose	atherosclerosis	aterosclerosis
Athetose	athetosis	atetosis
Ätiologie	aetiology	etiología
Atmung	respiration	respiración
Atmungsapparat	respiratory system	aparato respiratorio
Atmungsorgane	respiratory system	aparato respiratorio
Atom	atom	átomo
Atomgewicht	atomic weight (at wt)	peso atómico
atonisch	atonic	atono
Atresie	atresia	atresia
atrioventrikulär	atrioventricular (AV)	atrioventricular, aurículo-ventricular (AV)
Atrium	atrium	aurícula
Atrophie	atrophy	atrofia
Atropin	atropine	atropina
Attacke	attack	ataque
atypisch	atypical	atípico
ätzen	cauterize	cauterizar
ätzend	caustic	cáustico
Ätzmittel	caustic	cáustico
Audiogramm	audiogram	audiograma
Audiologie	audiology	audiología
Aufbaustoffwechsel	anabolism	anabolismo

FRENCH	ITALIAN	GERMAN
asthme	asma	**Asthma**
asthme bronchique	asma bronchiale	**Asthma bronchiale**
astigmatisme	astigmatismo	**Astigmatismus**
asymétrie	asimmetria	**Asymmetrie**
asymptomatique	asintomatico	**asymptomatisch**
ascite	ascite	**Aszites**
ataxie	atassia	**Ataxie**
atélectasie	atelettasia	**Atelektase**
haleine, souffle	respiro	**Atem**
test de la fonction respiratoire	test di funzionalità respiratoria	**Atemfunktionstest**
dyspnée	dispnea	**Atemnot**
syndrome de membrane hyaline et de souffrance respiratoire	sindrome di sofferenza respiratoria	**Atemnotsyndrom**
apnée	apnea	**Atemstillstand**
volume expiratoire maximum (VEM)	volume espiratorio forzato	**Atemstoßwert**
ventilation spontanée en pression positive continue	pressione continua positiva delle vie aeree	**Atemwegsdruck, kontinuierlich positiver**
infection des voies respiratoires supérieures	infezione del tratto respiratorio superiore (URTI)	**Atemwegsinfekt**
affection/maladie respiratoire fébrile aiguë	malattia respiratoria acuta febbrile	**Atemwegsinfekt (akut fieberhaft)**
infection du poumon profond	infezione del tratto respiratorio inferiore (LRTI)	**Atemwegsinfekt (untere)**
haleine, souffle	respiro	**Atemzug**
athérogène	aterogenico	**atherogen**
athérome	ateroma	**Atherom**
athérosclérose	aterosclerosi	**Atherosklerose**
athétose	atetosi	**Athetose**
étiologie	eziologia	**Ätiologie**
respiration	respirazione	**Atmung**
système respiratoire	sistema respiratorio	**Atmungsapparat**
système respiratoire	sistema respiratorio	**Atmungsorgane**
atome	atomo	**Atom**
poids atomique	peso atomico	**Atomgewicht**
atonique	atonico	**atonisch**
atrésie	atresia	**Atresie**
atrio-ventriculaire	atrioventricolare	**atrioventrikulär**
oreillette	atrio	**Atrium**
atrophie	atrofia	**Atrophie**
atropine	atropina	**Atropin**
attaque	attacco	**Attacke**
atypique	atipico	**atypisch**
cautériser	cauterizzare	**ätzen**
caustique	caustico	**ätzend**
caustique	caustico	**Ätzmittel**
audiogramme	audiogramma	**Audiogramm**
audiologie	audiologia	**Audiologie**
anabolisme	anabolismo	**Aufbaustoffwechsel**

GERMAN	ENGLISH	SPANISH
Auflösung	resolution, solution	resolución, solución
Aufnahme	ingestion	ingestión
Aufstoßen	belching	eructo
Auge	eye	ojo
Augen-	ophthalmic	oftálmico
Augenbraue	brow	ceja
Augenheilkunde	ophthalmology	oftalmología
Augenhintergrund	fundus	fundus
Augenhöhle	orbit	órbita
Augenmuskellähmung	ophthalmoplegia	oftalmoplejía
Augenspiegel	ophthalmoscope	oftalmoscopio
Aura	aura	aura
Aura-	aural	aural
Ausatmen	expiration	espiración
Ausbruch	eruption	erupción
ausgetragen	full-term	embarazo a término
Auskultation	auscultation	auscultación
Ausleerung	evacuation	evacuación
Ausreißen	avulsion	avulsión
Aussatz	leprosy	lepra
Ausschabung	abrasion, curettage, curetting	abrasión, raspado, legrado, curetaje, raspados, material de legrado
Ausschälung	enucleation	enucleación
Ausscheider	carrier	portador
Ausscheidung	elimination, excretion	eliminación, excreción
Ausschlag	eruption, hives, rash	erupción, urticaria, exantema
Australia-Antigen (HBsAG)	Australian antigen	antígeno Australia
Auswärtskehrung	eversion	eversión
Auswurf	sputum	esputo
Auszehrung	emaciation, tabes	emaciación, tabes
Autismus	autism	autismo
autistisch	autistic	persona autística
Autoantigen	autoantigen	autoantígeno
Autoantikörper	autoantibody	autoanticuerpo
Autoimmunerkrankung	autoimmune disease	enfermedad autoinmune
Autoimmunität	autoimmunity	autoinmunización
Autoklav	autoclave	autoclave
autolog	autologous	autólogo
Autolyse	autolysis	autólisis
autonom	autonomic	autónomo
Autoplastik	autograft	autoinjerto
Autopsie	autopsy	autopsia
Aversionstherapie	aversion therapy	tratamiento por aversión
Axilla	axilla	axila
Axon	axon	axón
Axonotmesis	axonotmesis	axonotmesis

FRENCH	ITALIAN	GERMAN
résolution, solution	risoluzione, soluzione	**Auflösung**
ingestion	ingestione	**Aufnahme**
éructation	eruttazione	**Aufstoßen**
oeil	occhio	**Auge**
ophtalmique	oftalmico	**Augen-**
front, sourcil	arcata sopracciliare, sopracciglio	**Augenbraue**
ophtalmologie	oftalmologia	**Augenheilkunde**
fond	fondo	**Augenhintergrund**
orbite	orbita	**Augenhöhle**
ophtalmoplégie	oftalmoplegia	**Augenmuskellähmung**
ophtalmoscope	oftalmoscopio	**Augenspiegel**
aura	aura	**Aura**
aural	auricolare	**Aura-**
expiration	espirazione, termine	**Ausatmen**
éruption	eruzione	**Ausbruch**
à terme	gravidanza a termine	**ausgetragen**
auscultation	auscultazione	**Auskultation**
évacuation	evacuazione	**Ausleerung**
avulsion	avulsione	**Ausreißen**
lèpre	lebbra	**Aussatz**
abrasion, curetage, curetages	abrasione, curettage, raschiamento	**Ausschabung**
énucléation	enucleazione	**Ausschälung**
porteur	portatore	**Ausscheider**
élimination, excrétion	eliminazione, escrezione	**Ausscheidung**
éruption, rash	eruzione, orticaria, eruzione cutanea	**Ausschlag**
antigène australien	antigene Australia	**Australia-Antigen (HBsAG)**
éversion	eversione, estrofia	**Auswärtskehrung**
salive	sputo, escreato	**Auswurf**
émaciation, tabès	emaciazione, tabe dorsale	**Auszehrung**
autisme	autismo	**Autismus**
autiste	autistico	**autistisch**
auto-antigène	autoantigene	**Autoantigen**
auto-anticorps	autoanticorpo	**Autoantikörper**
maladie auto-immune	malattia autoimmune	**Autoimmunerkrankung**
auto-immunisation	autoimmunizzazione	**Autoimmunität**
autoclave	autoclave	**Autoklav**
autologue	autologo	**autolog**
autolyse	autolisi	**Autolyse**
autonome	autonomo	**autonom**
autogreffe	autoinnesto	**Autoplastik**
autopsie	autopsia	**Autopsie**
cure de dégoût	decondizionamento	**Aversionstherapie**
aisselle	ascella	**Axilla**
axone	cilindrasse, assone	**Axon**
axonotmésis	degenerazione del cilindrasse, con possibile rigenerazione	**Axonotmesis**

GERMAN	ENGLISH	SPANISH
Azetabulum	acetabulum	acetábulo
Azidose	acidosis	acidosis
azygos	azygous	ácigos

FRENCH	ITALIAN	ENGLISH	GERMAN
acétabule	acetabolo		**Azetabulum**
acidose	acidosi		**Azidose**
azygos	azygos		**azygos**

B

German	English	Spanish
Babinski-Reflex	Babinski's reflex	reflejo de Babinski
Bacillus Calmette-Guérin (BCG)	bacille Calmette-Guérin (BCG)	bacilo de Calmette-Guérin (BCG)
Backe	cheek	mejilla
Backe betr	malar	malar
Backen-	malar	malar
Bad	bath	baño
Bakteriämie	bacteraemia (Eng), bacteremia (Am)	bacteriemia
Bakterien	bacteria	bacteria
Bakterienkultur	culture	cultivo
Bakteriologie	bacteriology	bacteriología
Bakteriostase	bacteriostasis	bacteriostasis
Bakteriurie	bacteriuria	bacteriuria
Bakterizid	bactericide	bactericida
Balanitis	balanitis	balanitis
Balanoposthitis	balanoposthitis	balanopostitis
Ballaststoff	dietary fiber (Am), dietary fibre (Eng), roughage	fibra dietética, fibra alimentaria
Ballottement	ballottement	peloteo
Band	ligament	ligamento
Bandscheibenvorfall	slipped disc	hernia de disco
Bandwurm	Taenia, tapeworm	tenia, tenia solitaria
Bariumeinlauf	barium enema	enema de bario
Bartholini-Drüsen	Bartholin's glands	glándulas de Bartolino
Basalganglien	basal ganglia	ganglios basales
Base	alkali	álcali
Basedow-Krankheit	Graves' disease	enfermedad de Graves
Basilarvertebralinsuffizienz	basilar-vertebral insufficiency	insuficiencia vertebrobasilar
basisch	alkaline	alcalino
Bauch	belly	vientre
Bauch-	ventral	ventral
Bauchfell	peritoneum	peritoneo
Bauchschmerzen	gripe	cólico intestinal
Bauchspeicheldrüse	pancreas	páncreas
Bauchspeicheldrüsenentzündung	pancreatitis	pancreatitis
Bauchspiegelung	laparoscopy	laparoscopia
Bazillus	bacillus	bacilo
Beatmungsgerät	respirator	respirador
Becken	pelvis	pelvis
Beckenboden	pelvic floor	suelo de la pelvis
Beckendurchmesser	conjugate	conjugado
Beckengürtel	pelvic girdle	cintura pélvica
Befall	infestation	infestación
befallen	affect	afectar
Befruchtung	fertilization, insemination	fertilización, inseminación
beginnend	incipient	incipiente

réflexe de Babinski	riflesso di Babinski	**Babinski-Reflex**
bacille de Calmette-Guérin (BCG)	bacillo di Calmette e Guérin	**Bacillus Calmette-Guérin (BCG)**
joue	guancia	**Backe**
malaire	malare	**Backe betr**
malaire	malare	**Backen-**
bain	bagno	**Bad**
bactériémie	batteriemia	**Bakteriämie**
bactérie	batteri	**Bakterien**
culture	coltura	**Bakterienkultur**
bactériologie	batteriologia	**Bakteriologie**
bactériostase	batteriostasi	**Bakteriostase**
bactériurie	batteriuria	**Bakteriurie**
bactéricide	battericida	**Bakterizid**
balanite	balanite	**Balanitis**
balanoposthite	balanopostite	**Balanoposthitis**
fibre alimentaire, ballant intestinal	fibra dietetica, alimento ricco di fibre	**Ballaststoff**
ballottement	ballottamento	**Ballottement**
ligament	ligamento	**Band**
hernie discale	ernia discale	**Bandscheibenvorfall**
ténia	Tenia, cestode	**Bandwurm**
lavement au baryte	clisma opaco	**Bariumeinlauf**
glandes de Bartholin	ghiandole di Bartolini	**Bartholini-Drüsen**
noyau lenticulaire, noyau caudé, avant-mur et noyau amygdalien	gangli basali	**Basalganglien**
alcali	alcali	**Base**
goitre exophtalmique	morbo di Graves	**Basedow-Krankheit**
insuffisance basilaire vertébrale	insufficienza vertebrobasilare	**Basilarvertebralinsuffizienz**
alcalin	alcalino	**basisch**
ventre	addome, ventre	**Bauch**
ventral	ventrale	**Bauch-**
péritoine	peritoneo	**Bauchfell**
colique	colica addominale	**Bauchschmerzen**
pancréas	pancreas	**Bauchspeicheldrüse**
pancréatite	pancreatite	**Bauchspeicheldrüsenentzündung**
coelioscopie	laparoscopia	**Bauchspiegelung**
bacille	bacillo	**Bazillus**
respirateur	respiratore	**Beatmungsgerät**
pelvis	pelvi	**Becken**
plancher pelvien	pavimento pelvico	**Beckenboden**
diamètre conjugué	coniugata	**Beckendurchmesser**
ceinture pelvienne	cingolo pelvico	**Beckengürtel**
infestation	infestazione	**Befall**
affecter	attaccare , influenzare	**befallen**
fertilisation, insémination	fertilizzazione, inseminazione	**Befruchtung**
débutant	incipiente	**beginnend**

Behandlung	therapy	terapéutica
Behçet-Syndrom	Behçet syndrome	síndrome de Behçet
Behinderung	handicap	disminución, minusvalía
bei Bewußtsein	conscious, lucid	consciente, lúcido
beidäugiges Sehen	binocular vision	visión binocular
beidhändig	bimanual	bimanual
Bein	leg	pierna
Belag	smear	frotis
Belastung	strain, stress	cepa, stress, estrés
belle indifference	'belle indifference'	la belle indifférence
Bell-Fazialisparese	Bell's palsy	parálisis de Bell
Bence-Jones-Proteine	Bence-Jones protein (BJ)	proteína de Bence-Jones
benigne	benign	benigno
Benommenheit	stupor	estupor
Beratung	counselling	asesoramiento, consejo, consulta psicológica
Beriberi	beri-beri	beri-beri
Berufskrankheit	industrial disease, occupational disease	enfermedad industrial, enfermedad profesional
beruhigend	sedative	sedante
Beruhigungsmittel	tranquilizer, sedative	tranquilizante, sedante
Berührung	contact	contacto
Beschäftigungstherapie	occupational therapy	terapéutica ocupacional
Beschneidung	circumcision	circuncisión
Besserung	amelioration	mejoría
Bestrahlung	irradiation	irradiación
Betablocker	beta blocker	beta-bloqueador
betäubend	anaesthetic (Eng), anesthetic (Am)	anestésico
Betäubung	anaesthesia (Eng), anesthesia (Am)	anestesia
Betäubungsmittel	anaesthetic (Eng), anesthetic (Am), narcotic	anestésico, narcótico
Betäubungsmittel (gemäß BTM)	controlled drug	fármaco controlado
Bettnässen	bedwetting, enuresis	enuresis nocturna, enuresis
Beugemuskel	flexor	flexor
beugen	flex	flexionar
Beugung	flexion	flexión
Beutel	pouch, sac	bolsa, saco
beweglich	motile	móvil
Bewegung	motion	movimiento
Bewegung der Augen betr	oculogyric	oculógiro
Bewegungs-	locomotor	locomotor
bewegungsfähig	motile	móvil
bewußt	conscious	consciente
bewußtlos	insensible, unconscious	insensible, inconsciente, sin sentido
bicornis	bicornuate	bicornio
bicuspidal	bicuspid	bicúspide
bifidus	bifid	bífido

FRENCH	ITALIAN	GERMAN
thérapie	terapia	**Behandlung**
syndrome de Behçet	sindrome di Behçet	**Behçet-Syndrom**
handicapé	handicappato, minorato	**Behinderung**
conscient, lucide	conscio, lucido	**bei Bewußtsein**
vision binoculaire	visione binoculare	**beidäugiges Sehen**
bimanuel	bimanuale	**beidhändig**
jambe	arto, gamba, membro	**Bein**
frottis	striscio	**Belag**
entorse, stress	tensione, stress	**Belastung**
indifférence	'belle indifference'	**belle indifference**
paralysie de Bell	paralisi di Bell	**Bell-Fazialisparese**
protéine de Bence Jones (BJ)	proteina di Bence-Jones	**Bence-Jones-Proteine**
bénin (bénigne)	benigno	**benigne**
stupeur	stupore	**Benommenheit**
consultation	consulenza eugenetica	**Beratung**
béribéri	beri-beri	**Beriberi**
maladie professionnelle	malattia industriale, malattia professionale	**Berufskrankheit**
sédatif	sedativo	**beruhigend**
tranquillisant, sédatif	tranquillante, sedativo	**Beruhigungsmittel**
contact	contatto	**Berührung**
ergothérapie	ergoterapia	**Beschäftigungstherapie**
circoncision	circoncisione	**Beschneidung**
amélioration	miglioramento	**Besserung**
irradiation	irradiazione	**Bestrahlung**
bêtabloquant	beta-bloccante	**Betablocker**
anesthésique	anestetico	**betäubend**
anesthésie	anestesia	**Betäubung**
anesthésique, narcotique	anestetico, narcotico	**Betäubungsmittel**
médicament contrôlé	farmaco sottoposto a controllo	**Betäubungsmittel (gemäß BTM)**
incontinence nocturne, énurèse	enuresi notturna, enuresi	**Bettnässen**
fléchisseur	flessore	**Beugemuskel**
fléchir	flettere	**beugen**
flexion	flessione	**Beugung**
poche, sac	tasca, sacco, sacca	**Beutel**
mobile	mobile	**beweglich**
mouvement	movimento	**Bewegung**
oculogyre	oculogiro	**Bewegung der Augen betr**
locomoteur	locomotore	**Bewegungs-**
mobile	mobile	**bewegungsfähig**
conscient	conscio	**bewußt**
insensible, sans connaissance	insensibile, inconscio	**bewußtlos**
bicorne	bicorne	**bicornis**
bicuspide	bicuspide	**bicuspidal**
bifide	bifido	**bifidus**

GERMAN	ENGLISH	SPANISH
Bifurkation	bifurcation	bifurcación
Bilharziose	schistosomiasis	esquistosomiasis
biliär	biliary	biliar
biliös	bilious	bilioso
Bilirubin	bilirubin	bilirrubina
Bilirubinurie	biliuria	biliuria
Billroth-Magenresektion	Billroth's operation	operación de Billroth
bimanuell	bimanual	bimanual
Bindegewebsentzündung	fibrositis	fibrositis
Bindehaut	conjunctiva	conjuntiva
Bindehautentzündung	conjunctivitis	conjuntivitis
Bindung	bonding	vinculación
binokulares Sehen	binocular vision	visión binocular
biologisch	biological	biológico
Biopsie	biopsy	biopsia
Biorhythmus	biorhythm	biorritmo
bipolar	bipolar	bipolar
bisexuell	bisexual	bisexual
Bizeps	biceps	bíceps
Blähung	flatulence, wind	flatulencia, ventosidad
Bläschen	bleb, vesicle	vesícula, bulla, ampolla
Bläschenausschlag	herpes	herpes
Blase	bladder, blister, bulla	vejiga, vesícula, ampolla, flictena, bulla
Blasendruckmessung	cystometry	cistometría
Blasenentleerung	micturition	micción
Blasenentzündung	cystitis	cistitis
Blasenmole	hydatidiform mole	mola hidatidiforme
Blasenspiegel	cystoscope	citoscopio
Blasenspiegelung	cystoscopy	citoscopía
Blässe	pallor	palidez
bleich	livid	lívido
Bleivergiftung	plumbism	plumbismo, saturnismo
Blepharitis	blepharitis	blefaritis
Blepharospasmus	blepharospasm	blefarospasmo
Blinddarm	appendix	apéndice
Blinddarmentzündung	appendicitis	apendicitis
Blinddarmoperation	appendectomy, appendicectomy	apendicectomía
blinder Fleck	blind spot	mancha ciega
Blindheit	blindness	ceguera
Blut	blood	sangre
Blutbank	blood bank	banco de sangre
Blutbild	blood count	recuento sanguíneo
Blutbild, großes	complete blood count (CBC)	hemograma completo
Blutbild, rotes	red blood cell count (RBC)	recuento de glóbulos rojos
Blutbild, weißes	white blood cell count (WBC)	recuento de leucocitos
Blutdruck	blood pressure (BP)	presión arterial (PA)

FRENCH	ITALIAN	GERMAN
bifurcation	biforcazione	**Bifurkation**
schistosomiase	schistosomiasi	**Bilharzlose**
biliaire	biliare	**biliär**
bilieux	biliare	**biliös**
bilirubine	bilirubina	**Bilirubin**
biliurie	biliuria	**Bilirubinurie**
opération de Billroth	operazione di Billroth	**Billroth-Magenresektion**
bimanuel	bimanuale	**bimanuell**
fibrosite	fibrosite	**Bindegewebsentzündung**
conjonctive	congiuntiva	**Bindehaut**
conjonctivite	congiuntivite	**Bindehautentzündung**
attachement	legame	**Bindung**
vision binoculaire	visione binoculare	**binokulares Sehen**
biologique	biologico	**biologisch**
biopsie	biopsia	**Biopsie**
biorythme	bioritmo	**Biorhythmus**
bipolaire	bipolare	**bipolar**
bisexuel	bisessuale	**bisexuell**
biceps	bicipite	**Bizeps**
flatulence, gaz	flatulenza, ventosità	**Blähung**
phlyctène, vésicule	vescichetta, flittena, vescicola	**Bläschen**
herpès	herpes	**Bläschenausschlag**
vessie, ampoule, bulle	vescica, vescicola, bolla	**Blase**
cystométrie	cistometria	**Blasendruckmessung**
micturition	minzione	**Blasenentleerung**
cystite	cistite	**Blasenentzündung**
hydatidiforme	idatiforme	**Blasenmole**
cystoscope	cistoscopio	**Blasenspiegel**
cystoscopie	cistoscopia	**Blasenspiegelung**
pâleur	pallore	**Blässe**
livide	livido	**bleich**
saturnisme	intossicazione da piombo	**Bleivergiftung**
blépharite	blefarite	**Blepharitis**
blépharospasme	blefarospasmo	**Blepharospasmus**
appendice	appendice	**Blinddarm**
appendicite	appendicite	**Blinddarmentzündung**
appendicectomie	appendicectomia	**Blinddarmoperation**
tache aveugle	punto cieco	**blinder Fleck**
cécité	cecità	**Blindheit**
sang	sangue	**Blut**
banque de sang	banca del sangue	**Blutbank**
dénombrement des hématies	emocitometria	**Blutbild**
numération globulaire	esame emocromocitometrico	**Blutbild, großes**
numération érythrocytaire	conteggio dei globuli rossi (CGR)	**Blutbild, rotes**
nombre de globules blancs (NGB)	conteggio dei globuli bianchi (CGB, WBC)	**Blutbild, weißes**
tension artérielle (TA)	pressione arteriosa	**Blutdruck**

GERMAN	ENGLISH	SPANISH
blutdruckerhöhend	pressor	presor
Blutdruckmeßgerät	sphygmomanometer	esfigmomanómetro
blutdrucksenkend	antihypertensive	hipotensor
bluten	bleed	sangrar
Bluterbrechen	haematemesis (Eng), hematemesis (Am)	hematemesis
Bluterguß	haematoma (Eng), hematoma (Am)	hematoma
Bluterkrankheit	haemophilia (Eng), hemophilia (Am)	hemofilia
Blutgerinnsel	clot	coágulo
Blutgerinnung	blood clotting, blood coagulation, haemostasis (Eng), hemostasis (Am)	coagulación de la sangre, hemostasis
Blutgruppe	blood group	grupo sanguíneo
Blutharnstoff	blood urea	urea sérica
Blut-Hirn-Schranke	blood-brain barrier (BBB)	barrera hematoencefálica (BHE)
Bluthusten	haemoptysis (Eng), hemoptysis (Am)	hemoptisis
Blut im Urin	haematuria (Eng), hematuria (Am)	hematuria
Blutkörperchen-Senkungsgeschwindigkeit (BSG, BKS)	erythrocyte sedimentation rate (ESR), blood sedimentation rate (BSR), sedimentation rate (SR)	velocidad de sedimentación globular (VSG)
Blutkultur	blood culture	hemocultivo
Blutmangel	oligaemia (Eng), oligemia (Am)	oligohemia
Blutplättchen	platelet, thrombocyte	plaqueta, trombocito
Blutserum	serum	suero
Blutstuhl	melaena (Eng), melena (Am)	melena
Bluttransfusion	transfusion	transfusión
Blutung	haemorrhage (Eng), hemorrhage (Am)	hemorragia
Blutungszeit	'bleeding time'	tiempo de sangría
Blutvergiftung	toxaemia (Eng), toxemia (Am)	toxemia
Blutvolumen	blood volume (BV)	volumen hemático
Blutzucker	blood sugar	glucemia
Bogengang	semicircular canal	conducto semicircular
Bolus	bolus	bolo
Bornholm-Krankheit	Bornholm disease	enfermedad de Bornholm
Borreliose	borreliosis	borreliosis
bösartig	malignant	maligno
Bösartigkeit	malignancy	malignidad
Botulismus	botulism	botulismo
Bovine Spongiforme Enzephalitis (BSE)	bovine spongiform encephalitis (BSE)	encefalitis espongiforme bovina
Bradykardie	bradycardia	bradicardia
branchial-	branchial	branquial
Brandblase	blister	vesícula, ampolla, flictena
Brandschorf	eschar	escara, costra
Brandwunde	scald, burn	escaldadura, quemadura
Brechdurchfall	diarrhea and vomiting (D & V) (Am), diarrhoea and vomiting (D & V) (Eng)	diarrea y vómitos
brechen	fracture	fracturar

FRENCH	ITALIAN	GERMAN
pressif	pressorio	**blutdruckerhöhend**
sphygmomanomètre	sfigmomanometro	**Blutdruckmeßgerät**
antihypertensif	anti-ipertensivo	**blutdrucksenkend**
saigner	sanguinare	**bluten**
hématémèse	ematemesi	**Bluterbrechen**
hématome	ematoma	**Bluterguß**
hémophilie	emofilia	**Bluterkrankheit**
caillot	coagulo	**Blutgerinnsel**
coagulation du sang, coagulation sanguine, hémostase	coagulazione ematica, coagulazione del sangue, emostasi	**Blutgerinnung**
groupe sanguin	gruppo sanguigno	**Blutgruppe**
urée du sang	azotemia	**Blutharnstoff**
barrière hémato-encéphalique	barriera ematoencefalica	**Blut-Hirn-Schranke**
hémoptysie	cartilagine costale	**Bluthusten**
hématurie	ematuria	**Blut im Urin**
vitesse de sédimentation globulaire, vitesse de sédimentation (VS)	velocità di eritrosedimentazione (VES)	**Blutkörperchen-Senkungsgeschwindigkeit (BSG, BKS)**
hémoculture	emocoltura	**Blutkultur**
hypovolémie	oligoemia	**Blutmangel**
plaquette, thrombocyte	piastrina, trombocito	**Blutplättchen**
sérum	siero	**Blutserum**
méléna	melena	**Blutstuhl**
transfusion	trasfusione	**Bluttransfusion**
hémorragie	emorragia	**Blutung**
temps de saignement	tempo di sanguinamento	**Blutungszeit**
toxémie	tossiemia	**Blutvergiftung**
masse sanguine	volume sanguigno	**Blutvolumen**
glycémie	glicemia	**Blutzucker**
canal semi-circulaire	canale semicircolare	**Bogengang**
bol	bolo	**Bolus**
maladie de Bornholm	malattia di Bornholm, mialgia epidemica	**Bornholm-Krankheit**
borréliose	borreliosi	**Borreliose**
malin	maligno	**bösartig**
malignité	neoplasia maligna	**Bösartigkeit**
botulisme	botulismo	**Botulismus**
encéphalite spongiforme bovine	encefalite spongiforme bovina	**Bovine Spongiforme Enzephalitis (BSE)**
bradycardie	bradicardia	**Bradykardie**
branchial	branchiale	**branchial-**
ampoule	vescicola, bolla	**Brandblase**
escarre	escara	**Brandschorf**
échaudure, brûlure	scottatura, ustione	**Brandwunde**
diarrhées et vomissements	diarrea e vomito	**Brechdurchfall**
fracturer	fratturare	**brechen**

GERMAN	ENGLISH	SPANISH
Brechmittel	emetic	emético
Brechreiz	nausea, retching	náusea, arcadas
Brechung	refraction	refracción
brennen	burn, cauterize	quemar, cauterizar
brennend	caustic	cáustico
Broca-Sprachzentrum	Broca's area	área de Broca
bröckelig	friable	friable
Brompton-Lösung (Alkohol, Morphin, Kokain)	Brompton's mixture	mezcla de Brompton
Bronchiektase	bronchiectasis	bronquiectasia
Bronchien	bronchi	bronquios
Bronchiole	bronchiole	bronquiolo
Bronchiolitis	bronchiolitis	bronquiolitis
Bronchiolus	bronchiole	bronquiolo
Bronchitis	bronchitis	bronquitis
Bronchodilatator	bronchodilator	broncodilatador
Bronchokonstriktor	bronchoconstrictor	broncoconstrictor
Bronchopneumonie	bronchopneumonia	bronconeumonia
bronchopulmonal	bronchopulmonary	broncopulmonar
Bronchoskop	bronchoscope	broncoscopio
Bronchospasmus	bronchospasm	broncospasmo
Bronchus	bronchus	bronquio
Bronzediabetes	haemochromatosis (Eng), hemochromatosis (Am)	hemocromatosis
Brucellose	brucellosis	brucelosis
Bruch	hernia, rupture	hernia, ruptura
brüchig	friable	friable
Bruchoperation	herniorraphy	herniorrafia
Brust	breast	mama, pecho
Brust-	pectoral, thoracic	pectoral, torácico
Brustamputation	mastectomy	mastectomía
Brustbein	sternum	esternón
Brustdrüsenentzündung	mastitis	mastitis
Brustkorb	thorax	tórax
Brustwarze	nipple	pezón
Brustwarzenhof	areola	areola
Brutkasten	incubator	incubadora
bukkal	buccal	bucal
bulbär	bulbar	bulbar
Bulimie	bulimia	bulimia
Bulla	bulla	bulla
Bursa	bursa	bolsa
Bursitis	bursitis	bursitis

FRENCH	ITALIAN	GERMAN
émétique	emetico	Brechmittel
nausée, haut-le-coeur	nausea, conati di vomito	Brechreiz
réfraction	rifrazione	Brechung
brûler, cautériser	bruciare, cauterizzare	brennen
caustique	caustico	brennend
centre moteur de Broca	area di Broca	Broca-Sprachzentrum
friable	friabile	bröckelig
liquide de Brompton	soluzione di Brompton	Brompton-Lösung (Alkohol, Morphin, Kokain)
bronchectasie	bronchiettasia	Bronchicktase
bronches	bronchi	Bronchien
bronchiole	bronchiolo	Bronchiole
bronchiolite	bronchiolite	Bronchiolitis
bronchiole	bronchiolo	Bronchiolus
bronchite	bronchite	Bronchitis
bronchodilatateur	broncodilatatore	Bronchodilatator
bronchoconstricteur	broncocostrittore	Bronchokonstriktor
bronchopneumonie	broncopolmonite	Bronchopneumonie
bronchopulmonaire	broncopolmonare	bronchopulmonal
bronchoscope	broncoscopio	Bronchoskop
bronchospasme	broncospasmo	Bronchospasmus
bronche	bronco	Bronchus
hémochromatose	emocromatosi	Bronzediabetes
brucellose	brucellosi	Brucellose
hernie	ernia, rottura	Bruch
friable	friabile	brüchig
herniorrhaphie	erniorrafia	Bruchoperation
sein	mammella	Brust
pectoral, thoracique	pettorale, toracico	Brust-
mastectomie	mastectomia	Brustamputation
sternum	sterno	Brustbein
mastite	mastite	Brustdrüsenentzündung
thorax	torace	Brustkorb
mamelon	capezzolo	Brustwarze
aréole	areola	Brustwarzenhof
incubateur	incubatore	Brutkasten
buccal	buccale	bukkal
bulbaire	bulbare	bulbär
boulimie	bulimia	Bulimie
bulle	bolla	Bulla
bourse	borsa	Bursa
bursite	borsite	Bursitis

C

German	English	Spanish
Caldwell-Luc-Operation	Caldwell-Luc operation	operación de Caldwell-Luc
Candidiasis	candidiasis	candidiasis
Carboxyhämoglobin	carboxyhaemoglobin (Eng), carboxyhemoglobin (Am)	carboxihemoglobina
Carina	carina	carina
Catgut	catgut	catgut
Celsiusgrad	centigrade	centígrado
Cerebellum	cerebellum	cerebelo
Chalazion	chalazion	chalacio, orzuelo
Charakter	character	carácter
Charakterzug	trait	rasgo
Charcot-Gelenk	Charcot's joint	articulación de Charcot
Chelatbildner	chelating agent	quelantes
Chemoprophylaxe	chemoprophylaxis	quimioprofilaxis
Chemorezeptor	chemoreceptor	quimiorreceptor
Chemosis	chemosis	quemosis
Chemotaxis	chemotaxis	quimiotaxis
Chemotherapie	chemotherapy	quimioterapia
Cheyne-Stokes-Atmung	Cheyne-Stokes respiration	respiración de Cheyne-Stokes
Chiasma	chiasma	quiasma
Chiropraktik	chiropractic	quiropráctica
Chiropraktiker	chiropractor	quiropractor
Chirurg	surgeon	cirujano
Chirurgie	surgery	cirugía
Chloasma	chloasma	cloasma
Cholangiographie	cholangiography	colangiografía
Cholangitis	cholangitis	colangitis
Choledochographie	choledochography	coledocografía
Choledocholithiasis	choledocholithiasis	coledocolitiasis
Cholelithiasis	cholelithiasis	colelitiasis
Cholera	cholera	cólera
Cholestase	cholestasis	colestasis
Cholesteatom	cholesteatoma	colesteatoma
Cholesterin	cholesterol (chol)	colesterol
Cholezystektomie	cholecystectomy	colecistectomía
Cholezystitis	cholecystitis	colecistitis
Cholezystographie	cholecystography	colecistografía
cholinergisch	cholinergic	colinérgico
Chondritis	chondritis	condritis
Chondrom	chondroma	condroma
Chondromalazie	chondromalacia	condromalacia
Chorea	chorea	corea
Chorea Huntington	Huntington's chorea	corea de Huntington
Chorion	chorion	corion

opération de Caldwell-Luc	operazione di Caldwell-Luc	**Caldwell-Luc-Operation**
candidose	candidiasi	**Candidiasis**
carboxyhémoglobine	carbossiemoglobina	**Carboxyhämoglobin**
carène	carena tracheale	**Carina**
catgut	catgut	**Catgut**
centigrade	centigrado	**Celsiusgrad**
cervelet	cervelletto	**Cerebellum**
chalazion	calazion	**Chalazion**
caractère	carattere	**Charakter**
trait	tratto, carattere ereditario	**Charakterzug**
arthropathie neurogène	artropatia di Charcot	**Charcot-Gelenk**
agent chélateur	agente chelante	**Chelatbildner**
chimioprophylaxie	chemioprofilassi	**Chemoprophylaxe**
chimiorécepteur	chemorecettore	**Chemorezeptor**
chémosis	chemosi	**Chemosis**
chimiotaxie	chemiotassi	**Chemotaxis**
chimiothérapie	chemioterapia	**Chemotherapie**
dyspnée de Cheyne-Stokes	respiro di Cheyne-Stokes	**Cheyne-Stokes-Atmung**
chiasma	chiasma	**Chiasma**
chiropractique	chiropratica	**Chiropraktik**
chiropracteur	chiropratico	**Chiropraktiker**
chirurgien	chirurgo	**Chirurg**
chirurgie	chirurgia	**Chirurgie**
chloasma	cloasma	**Chloasma**
cholangiographie	colangiografia	**Cholangiographie**
cholangite	colangite	**Cholangitis**
cholédochographie	coledocografia	**Choledochographie**
cholédocholithiase	coledocolitiasi	**Choledocholithiasis**
cholélithiase	colelitiasi	**Cholelithiasis**
choléra	colera	**Cholera**
cholestase	colestasi	**Cholestase**
cholestéatome	colesteatoma	**Cholesteatom**
cholestérol	colesterolo	**Cholesterin**
cholécystectomie	colecistectomia	**Cholezystektomie**
cholécystite	colecistite	**Cholezystitis**
cholécystographie	colecistografia	**Cholezystographie**
cholinergique	colinergico	**cholinergisch**
chondrite	condrite	**Chondritis**
chondrome	condroma	**Chondrom**
chondromalacie	condromalacia	**Chondromalazie**
chorée	corea	**Chorea**
chorée de Huntington	corea di Huntington	**Chorea Huntington**
chorion	corion	**Chorion**

GERMAN	ENGLISH	SPANISH
Choriongonadotropin (HCG)	human chorionic gonadotrophin (HCG) (Eng), human chorionic gonadotropin (HCG) (Am)	gonadotropina coriónica humana (GCH)
Chorionzotten	chorionic villi	vellosidades coriónicas
Chorionzottenbiopsie	chorionic villus biopsy	biopsia de las vellosidades coriónicas
Choroidea	choroid	coroides
Choroiditis	choroiditis	coroiditis
Chromatographie	chromatography	cromatografía
Chromosom	chromosome	cromosoma
chronisch	chronic	crónico
Chron, Morbus	Crohn's disease	enfermedad de Crohn
Chvostek-Zeichen	Chvostek's sign	signo de Chvostek
Chylus	chyle	quilo
Claudicatio	claudication	claudicación
Coarctatio	coarctation	coartación
Cochlea	cochlea	cóclea
coliform	coliform	coliforme
Colon ascendens	ascending colon	colon ascendente
Colon descendens	descending colon	colon descendente
Colon transversum	transverse colon	colon transverso
Commotio	concussion	concusión, contusión violenta
Compliance	patient compliance	cumplimiento del paciente
Computertomographie (CT)	computerized tomography	tomografía computerizada
Computertomographie, axiale	computerized axial tomography (CAT)	tomografía axial computerizada (TAC)
contre coup	contrecoup	contragolpe
Cor pulmonale	cor pulmonale	cor pulmonale
Corpus	corpus	cuerpo
Corpusculum	corpuscle	corpúsculo
Cortex	cortex	corteza
Costen-Syndrom	temporomandibular joint syndrome	síndrome de la articulación temporomandibular
Coxsackie-Virus	Coxsackie virus	virus Coxsackie
Craurosis vulvae	kraurosis vulvae	craurosis vulvar
C-reaktives Protein (CRP)	C-reactive protein (CRP)	proteína C-reactiva
Cushing-Syndrom	Cushing's syndrome	síndrome de Cushing
Cuticula	cuticle	cutícula

FRENCH	ITALIAN	GERMAN
gonadotrophine chorionique humaine (GCH)	gonadotropina corionica umana (GCU)	**Choriongonadotropin (HCG)**
villosités du chorion	villi coriali	**Chorionzotten**
biopsie du villus chorionique	biopsia dei villi coriali	**Chorionzottenbiopsie**
choroïde	coroide	**Choroidea**
choroïdite	coroidite	**Choroiditis**
chromatographie	cromatografia	**Chromatographie**
chromosome	cromosoma	**Chromosom**
chronique	cronico	**chronisch**
mal de Crohn	malattia di Crohn	**Chron, Morbus**
signe de Chvostek	segno di Chvostek	**Chvostek-Zeichen**
chyle	chilo	**Chylus**
claudication	claudicazione	**Claudicatio**
coarctation	coartazione	**Coarctatio**
limaçon osseux	coclea	**Cochlea**
coliforme	coliforme	**coliform**
côlon ascendant	colon ascendente	**Colon ascendens**
côlon descendant	colon discendente	**Colon descendens**
côlon transversal	colon trasverso	**Colon transversum**
commotion	commozione	**Commotio**
observance du patient	acquiescenza alle prescrizioni	**Compliance**
tomographie avec ordinateur, scanographie	tomografia computerizzata	**Computertomographie (CT)**
tacographie	tomografia assiale computerizzata (TAC)	**Computertomographie, axiale**
contrecoup	contraccolpo	**contre coup**
coeur pulmonaire	cuore polmonare	**Cor pulmonale**
corps	corpo	**Corpus**
corpuscule	corpuscolo	**Corpusculum**
cortex	corteccia	**Cortex**
syndrome de Costen	sindrome dell'articolazione temporomandibolare	**Costen-Syndrom**
virus Coxsackie	virus coxsackie	**Coxsackie-Virus**
kraurosis de la vulve	craurosi vulvare	**Craurosis vulvae**
test de protéine C-réactive	proteina C reattiva	**C-reaktives Protein (CRP)**
syndrome de Cushing	sindrome di Cushing	**Cushing-Syndrom**
cuticule	cuticola	**Cuticula**

D

Dakryozystitis	dacryocystitis	dacriocistitis
Damm	perineum	perineo
Dammschnitt	episiotomy	episiotomía
Darm	bowel, gut, intestine	intestino
Darmentleerung	defaecation (Eng), defecation (Am)	defecación
Darmverschluß	ileus	íleo
Daumen	thumb	pulgar
Debridement	debridement	desbridamiento
Defäkation	defaecation (Eng), defecation (Am)	defecación
Defekt	defect	defecto
Defibrillator	defibrillator	desfibrilador
Defibrillierung	defibrillation	desfibrilación
Degeneration	degeneration	degeneración
Dehiszenz	dehiscence	dehiscencia
Dehydration	dehydration	deshidratación
Dekompensation	decompensation	descompensación
Dekompression	decompression	descompresión
Dekongestionsmittel	decongestant	descongestivo
Dekubitus	bedsore, pressure point, pressure sore	úlcera por decúbito, punto de presión, úlcera de decúbito
Delirium	delirium	delirio
Dellenbildung	pitting	cavitación
Deltamuskel	deltoid	deltoides
Deltoides	deltoid	deltoides
Demarkation	demarcation	demarcación
Demenz	dementia	demencia
Demenz, präsenile	presenile dementia	demencia presenil
Demographie	demography	demografia
Demyelinisierung	demyelination	desmielinización
Denervierung	denervation	denervación
Denguefieber	dengue	dengue
Dentition	dentition	dentición
Deodorant	deodorant	desodorante
Depression	depression	depresión
Depression, agitierte	agitated depression	depresión agitada
Derealisation	derealization	desrealización
Dermatitis	dermatitis	dermatitis
Dermatologe	dermatologist	dermatólogo
Dermatologie	dermatology	dermatología
Dermatom	dermatome	dermátomo
Dermatomyositis	dermatomyositis	dermatomiositis
Dermatose	dermatosis	dermatosis
Dermoid	dermoid	dermoide
Dermoidzyste	dermoid	dermoide

FRENCH	ITALIAN	GERMAN
dacryocystite	dacriocistite	Dakryozystitis
périnée	perineo	Damm
épisiotomie	episiotomia	Dammschnitt
intestin	intestino	Darm
défécation	defecazione	Darmentleerung
iléus	ileo, occlusione intestinale acuta	Darmverschluß
pouce	pollice	Daumen
débridement	sbrigliamento	Debridement
défécation	defecazione	Defäkation
anomalie, défaut	difetto	Defekt
défibrillateur	defibrillatore	Defibrillator
défibrillation	defibrillazione	Defibrillierung
dégénération	degenerazione	Degeneration
déhiscence	deiscenza	Dehiszenz
déshydratation	deidratazione	Dehydration
décompensation	decompensazione	Dekompensation
décompression	decompressione	Dekompression
décongestionnant	decongestionante	Dekongestionsmittel
escarre de décubitus, point particulièrement sensible, plaie de décubitus	piaga da decubito, punto cutaneo sensibile alla pressione, ulcera da decubito	Dekubitus
délire	delirio	Delirium
formation de godet	depressioni puntiformi, fovea	Dellenbildung
deltoïde	deltoide	Deltamuskel
deltoïde	deltoide	Deltoides
démarcation	demarcazione	Demarkation
démence	demenza	Demenz
démence présénile	demenza presenile	Demenz, präsenile
démographie	demografia	Demographie
démyélinisation	demielinizzazione	Demyelinisierung
énervation	denervazione	Denervierung
dengue	dengue, infezione da Flavivirus ('febbre rompiossa')	Denguefieber
dentition	dentizione	Dentition
déodorant	deodorante	Deodorant
dépression	depressione	Depression
dépression anxieuse	depressione agitata	Depression, agitierte
déréalisation	derealizzazione	Derealisation
dermatite	dermatite	Dermatitis
dermatologue	dermatologo	Dermatologe
dermatologie	dermatologia	Dermatologie
dermatome	dermatomo	Dermatom
dermatomyosite	dermatomiosite	Dermatomyositis
dermatose	dermatosi	Dermatose
dermoïde	dermoide	Dermoid
dermoïde	dermoide	Dermoidzyste

GERMAN	ENGLISH	SPANISH
Desensibilisierung	desensitization	desensibilización
Desinfektion	disinfection	desinfección
Desinfektionsmittel	disinfectant	desinfectante
desinfizieren	disinfect	desinfectar
Desobliteration	rebore	desobliteración, repermeabilización
desodorierend	deodorant	desodorante
Desorientiertheit	disorientation	desorientación
Desoxydation	deoxygenation	desoxigenación
Desoxyribonukleinsäure (DNS)	deoxyribonucleic acid (DNA)	ácido desoxirribonucléico (ADN)
Desquamation	desquamation	desescamación
Dextrokardie	dextrocardia	dextrocardia
dezerebriert	decerebrate	descerebrado
Dezidua	decidua	decidua
Diabetes	diabetes	diabetes
Diabetes insipidus	diabetes insipidus	diabetes insípida
Diabetes mellitus	diabetes mellitus (DM)	diabetes mellitus
Diabetes mellitus, insulinabhängiger	insulin dependent diabetes mellitus (IDDM)	diabetes mellitus insulinodependiente
Diabetes mellitus Typ II	non-insulin dependent diabetes mellitus (NIDDM)	diabetes mellitus no insulinodependiente
Diagnose	diagnosis	diagnóstico
diagnostisch	diagnostic	diagnóstico
Dialysat	dialysate	dializado
Dialysator	dialyser (Eng), dialyzer (Am)	dializador
Dialyse	dialysis	diálisis
Diaphorese	diaphoresis	diaforesis
Diaphragma	diaphragm, midriff	diafragma
diaphragmatisch	phrenic	frénico
Diaphyse	diaphysis	diáfisis
Diarrhoe	diarrhea (Am), diarrhoea (Eng)	diarrea
Diastase	diastasis	diastasis
Diastole	diastole	diástole
Diät	diet, regimen	régimen
Diathermie	diathermy	diatermia
Diäthylstilboestrol	stilbestrol (Am), stilboestrol (Eng)	estilbestrol
Diätlehre	dietetics	dietética
Diätspezialist	dietitian	dietista
Differentialblutbild	differential blood count	fórmula leucocitaria
Differentialdiagnose	differential diagnosis	diagnóstico diferencial
Digitalis	digitalis	digital
Digitalisierung	digitalization	digitalización
Dilatation	dilatation (Eng), dilation (Am)	dilatación
Dilatation und Kürettage	dilatation and curettage (D & C) (Eng), dilation and curettage (D & C) (Am)	dilatación y raspado/legrado,
Diphtherie	diphtheria	difteria
Diplegie	diplegia	diplejía, parálisis bilateral
Diplopie	diplopia, double vision	diplopia, visión doble

désensibilisation	desensibilizzazione	Desensibilisierung
désinfection	disinfezione	Desinfektion
désinfectant	disinfettante	Desinfektionsmittel
désinfecter	disinfettare	desinfizieren
désobstruction	disobliterazione	Desobliteration
déodorant	deodorante	desodorierend
désorientation	disorientamento	Desorientiertheit
désoxygénation	deossigenazione	Desoxydation
acide désoxyribonucléique (ADN)	acido deossiribonucleico	Desoxyribonukleinsäure (DNS)
desquamation	desquamazione	Desquamation
dextrocardie	destrocardia	Dextrokardie
décérébré	decerebrato	dezerebriert
caduque	decidua	Dezidua
diabète	diabete	Diabetes
diabète insipide	diabete insipido	Diabetes insipidus
diabète sucré	diabete mellito	Diabetes mellitus
diabète sucré insulinodépendant	diabete mellito insulinodipendente	Diabetes mellitus, insulinabhängiger
diabète sucré non insulinodépendant	diabete mellito non insulinodipendente	Diabetes mellitus Typ II
diagnostic	diagnosi	Diagnose
diagnostique	diagnostico	diagnostisch
dialysat	dialisato	Dialysat
dialyseur	dializzatore	Dialysator
dialyse	dialisi	Dialyse
diaphorèse	diaforesi	Diaphorese
diaphragme	diaframma, parte bassa del torace	Diaphragma
psychique	frenico (diaframmatico mentale)	diaphragmatisch
diaphyse	diafisi	Diaphyse
diarrhée	diarrea	Diarrhoe
diastasis	diastasi, amilasi	Diastase
diastole	diastole	Diastole
régime	regime, dieta, prescrizione dietetica	Diät
diathermie	diatermia	Diathermie
stilboestrol	stilbestrolo	Diäthylstilboestrol
diététique	dietetica	Diätlehre
diététicien	dietista, dietologo	Diätspezialist
formule leucocytaire	formula leucocitaria	Differentialblutbild
diagnostic différentiel	diagnosi differenziale	Differentialdiagnose
digitale	digitale	Digitalis
digitalisation	digitalizzazione	Digitalisierung
dilatation	dilatazione	Dilatation
dilatation et curetage	dilatazione e raschiamento	Dilatation und Kürettage
diphtérie	difterite	Diphtherie
diplégie	diplegia	Diplegie
diplopie, double vision	diplopia	Diplopie

GERMAN	ENGLISH	SPANISH
Diskektomie	discectomy (Eng), diskectomy (Am)	disquectomía
diskret	discrete	discreto
Dislokation	dislocation	dislocación
disseminiert	disseminated	diseminado
disseminierte intravasale Gerinnung (DIC)	disseminated intravascular coagulation (DIC)	coagulación intravascular diseminada (CID)
dissozial	antisocial	antisocial
Dissoziation	dissociation	disociación
distal	distal	distal
distale Radiusfraktur	Colles' fracture	fractura de Colles
Diurese	diuresis	diuresis
Diuretikum	diuretic	diurético
diuretisch	diuretic	diurético
Divertikel	diverticulum	divertículo
Divertikulitis	diverticulitis	diverticulitis
Divertikulose	diverticulosis	diverticulosis
dominant	dominant	dominante
Dopamin	dopamine	dopamina
Doppelsehen	diplopia, double vision	diplopia, visión doble
doppelseitige Lähmung	diplegia	diplejía, parálisis bilateral
Doppler-Sonographie	Doppler ultrasound technique	técnica de ultrasonidos Doppler
dorsal	dorsal	dorsal
Dorsalflexion	dorsiflexion	dorsiflexión
Down-Syndrom	Down's syndrome	síndrome de Down
Drain	drain	drenaje
drainieren	drain	drenar
Drehinhaliergerät	spinhaler	inhalador spinhaler
Dreifachantigen	triple antigen	antígeno triple
Dreifachimpfstoff	triple vaccine	vacuna triple
dritten Grades	tertiary	terciario
Drogenmißbrauch	drug abuse	abuso de drogas
Drop attack	drop attack	ataque isquémico transitorio (AIT), caida
Druckfläche	pressure area	zona de decúbito
Druckgeschwür	pressure sore	úlcera de decúbito
Druckpunkt	pressure point	punto de presión
Drucksenkung	decompression	descompresión
Drüse	gland	glándula
Ductus	duct	conducto
Ductus arteriosus	ductus arteriosus	ductus arteriosus
Dumping-Syndrom	dumping syndrome	síndrome de dumping, síndrome del vaciamiento en gastrectomizados
Duodenalulkus	duodenal ulcer	úlcera duodenal
Duodenitis	duodenitis	duodenitis
Duodenum	duodenum	duodeno
Durchblutung	circulation, perfusion	circulación, perfusión
Durchfall	diarrhea (Am), diarrhoea (Eng)	diarrea

FRENCH	ITALIAN	GERMAN
discectomie	discectomia, asportazione di disco intervertebrale	Diskektomie
discret	discreto	diskret
dislocation	dislocazione	Dislokation
disséminé	disseminato	disseminiert
coagulation intravasculaire disséminée (CID)	coagulazione intravascolare disseminata (CID)	disseminierte intravasale Gerinnung (DIC)
antisocial	antisociale	dissozial
dissociation	dissociazione	Dissoziation
distal	distale	distal
fracture de Pouteau-Colles	frattura di Colles	distale Radiusfraktur
diurèse	diuresi	Diurese
diurétique	diuretico	Diuretikum
diurétique	diuretico	diuretisch
diverticulum	diverticolo	Divertikel
diverticulite	diverticolite	Divertikulitis
diverticulose	diverticolosi	Divertikulose
dominant	dominante	dominant
dopamine	dopammina	Dopamin
diplopie, double vision	diplopia	Doppelsehen
diplégie	diplegia	doppelseitige Lähmung
échographie de Doppler	tecnica ultrasonografica Doppler	Doppler-Sonographie
dorsal	dorsale	dorsal
dorsiflexion	dorsiflessione	Dorsalflexion
trisomie 21	mongoloidismo, sindrome di Down	Down-Syndrom
drain	drenaggio	Drain
drainer	drenare	drainieren
turbo-inhalateur	nebulizzatore per farmaci	Drehinhaliergerät
triple antigène	antigene triplo	Dreifachantigen
triple vaccin	triplo vaccino	Dreifachimpfstoff
tertiaire	terziario	dritten Grades
toxicomanie	abuso di droga, abuso di farmaci	Drogenmißbrauch
chute brusque par dérobement des jambes	improvvisa perdita della postura ad insorgenza periodica	Drop attack
zone particulièrement sensible	area di pressione	Druckfläche
plaie de décubitus	ulcera da decubito	Druckgeschwür
point particulièrement sensible	punto cutaneo sensibile alla pressione	Druckpunkt
décompression	decompressione	Drucksenkung
glande	ghiandola	Drüse
conduit	dotto	Ductus
canal artériel	dotto arterioso	Ductus arteriosus
syndrome de chasse	sindrome del gastroresecato	Dumping-Syndrom
ulcère duodénal	ulcera duodenale	Duodenalulkus
duodénite	duodenite	Duodenitis
duodénum	duodeno	Duodenum
circulation, perfusion	circolazione, perfusione	Durchblutung
diarrhée	diarrea	Durchfall

durchgängig	patent	permeable
durchlässig	permeable	permeable
Durchliegen	bedsore	úlcera por decúbito
Durchmesser	lumen	luz
durchscheinend	translucent	translúcido
durchsichtig	translucent	translúcido
Durst	thirst	sed
Dusche	douche	ducha
Dysarthrie	dysarthria	disartria
Dysenterie	dysentery	disentería
Dysfunktion	dysfunction	disfunción
Dyskinesie	dyskinesia	discinesia
Dyskrasie	dyscrasia	discrasia
Dyslexie	dyslexia	dislexia
Dysmenorrhoe	dysmenorrhea (Am), dysmenorrhoea (Eng)	dismenorrea
Dyspareunie	dyspareunia	dispareunia
Dyspepsie	dyspepsia	dispepsia
Dysphagie	dysphagia	disfagia
Dysphasie	dysphasia	disfasia
Dysplasie	dyskaryosis, dysplasia	discariosis, displasia
Dyspnoe	dyspnea (Am), dyspnoea (Eng)	disnea
Dyspraxie	dyspraxia	dispraxia
Dysrhythmie	dysrhythmia	disritmia
Dystrophie	dystrophy	distrofia
Dysurie	dysuria	disuria

FRENCH	ITALIAN	GERMAN
libre	aperto, esposto	**durchgängig**
perméable	permeabile	**durchlässig**
escarre de décubitus	piaga da decubito	**Durchliegen**
lumière	lume	**Durchmesser**
translucide	translucido	**durchscheinend**
translucide	translucido	**durchsichtig**
soif	sete	**Durst**
douche	lavanda vaginale	**Dusche**
dysarthrie	disartria	**Dysarthrie**
dysenterie	dissenteria	**Dysenterie**
dysfonctionnement	disfunzione	**Dysfunktion**
dyskinésie	discinesia	**Dyskinesie**
dyscrasie	discrasia	**Dyskrasie**
dyslexie	dislessia	**Dyslexie**
dysménorrhée	dismenorrea	**Dysmenorrhoe**
dyspareunie	dispareunia	**Dyspareunie**
dyspepsie	dispepsia	**Dyspepsie**
dysphagie	disfagia	**Dysphagie**
dysphasie	disfasia	**Dysphasie**
dyskaryose, dysplasie	discariosi, displasia	**Dysplasie**
dyspnée	dispnea	**Dyspnoe**
dyspraxie	disprassia	**Dyspraxie**
dysrythmie	disritmia	**Dysrhythmie**
dystrophie	distrofia	**Dystrophie**
dysurie	disuria	**Dysurie**

E

German	English	Spanish
Eburnifikation	osteosclerosis	osteosclerosis
Echoenzephalographie	echoencephalography	ecoencefalografía
Echokardiographie	echocardiography	ecocardiografía
Echolalie	echolalia	ecolalia
ECHO-Virus	echovirus	virus ECHO
efferent	efferent	eferente
Ei	egg, ovum	huevo, óvulo
Eierstock	ovary	ovario
Eierstock-	ovarian	ovárico
eigen	inherent	inherente
Eigenschaft	trait	rasgo
Eileiter	Fallopian tube	trompa de Falopio
Eileiter-	tubal	tubárico
Eileiterentzündung	salpingitis	salpingitis
Einatmen	inhalation	inhalación
einatmen	inhale	inhalar
Einatmung	inspiration	inspiración
einäugig	uniocular	uniocular
Einengung	constriction	constricción
Einflößung	instillation	instilación
Einfühlungsvermögen	empathy	empatía
Eingang	porta	porta
eingeboren	indigenous	indígena
eingedickt	inspissated	espesado
eingeklemmt	incarcerated	incarcerado
eingerissen	lacerated	lacerado
Eingeweide	viscera	visceras
Eingeweide-	splanchnic	esplácnico
Eingriff	operation	intervención quirúrgica
einheimisch	indigenous	indígena
Einklemmung	strangulation	estrangulación
Einkoten	encopresis	encopresis
Einlauf	enema	enema
Einleitung	induction	inducción
Einnahme	ingestion	ingestión
Einreibemittel	liniment	linimento
Einreibeprobe	patch test	prueba del parche
einschläfernd	soporific	soporífero
Einschluß(körperchen)kon-junktivitis	trachoma inclusion conjunctivitis (TRIC)	conjuntivitis de inclusion por tracomas
Einschnitt	incision	incisión
einseitig	unilateral	unilateral
Einträufelung	instillation	instilación
Einwirkung	operation	intervención quirúrgica
Eisen-	ferrous (Eng), ferrus (Am)	ferroso

FRENCH	ITALIAN	GERMAN
ostéosclérose	osteosclerosi	**Eburnifikation**
écho-encéphalographie	ecoencefalografia	**Echoenzephalographie**
échocardiographie	ecocardiografia	**Echokardiographie**
écholalie	ecolalia	**Echolalie**
échovirus	echovirus	**ECHO-Virus**
efférent	efferente	**efferent**
oeuf, ovule, ovocyte de premier ordre	uovo, gamete femminile	**Ei**
ovaire	ovaio	**Eierstock**
ovarien	ovarico	**Eierstock-**
inhérent	inerente	**eigen**
trait	tratto, carattere ereditario	**Eigenschaft**
trompe de Fallope	tuba di Falloppio	**Eileiter**
tubaire	tubarico	**Eileiter-**
salpingite	salpingite	**Eileiterentzündung**
inhalation	inalazione	**Einatmen**
inhaler	inalare	**einatmen**
inspiration	inspirazione	**Einatmung**
unioculé	monoculare	**einäugig**
constriction	costrizione	**Einengung**
instillation	istillazione	**Einflößung**
empathie	immedesimazione, identificazione	**Einfühlungsvermögen**
porte	porta	**Eingang**
indigène	indigeno	**eingeboren**
épaissir	inspessito	**eingedickt**
incarcéré	incarcerato	**eingeklemmt**
lacéré	lacerato	**eingerissen**
viscères	visceri	**Eingeweide**
splanchnique	splancnico	**Eingeweide-**
opération	operazione	**Eingriff**
indigène	indigeno	**einheimisch**
strangulation	strangolamento	**Einklemmung**
encoprésie	encopresi	**Einkoten**
lavement	clistere	**Einlauf**
induction	induzione	**Einleitung**
ingestion	ingestione	**Einnahme**
liniment	linimento	**Einreibemittel**
tache, plaque, pièce	test epicutaneo	**Einzelprobe**
soporifique	ipnotico	**einschläfernd**
conjonctivite à inclusions trachomateuses	congiuntivite tracomatosa	**Einschluß(körperchen)konjunktivitis**
incision	incisione	**Einschnitt**
unilatéral	unilaterale	**einseitig**
instillation	istillazione	**Einträufelung**
opération	operazione	**Einwirkung**
ferreux	ferroso	**Eisen-**

GERMAN	ENGLISH	SPANISH
eisenbindendes Protein	iron binding protein (IBP)	proteína de unión con el hierro
Eisenbindungskapazität	iron binding capacity (IBC)	capacidad de unión con el hierro
Eisprung	ovulation	ovulación
Eiter	pus	pus
Eiterbeule	boil	forúnculo
Eiterung	suppuration	supuración
eitrig	purulent	purulento
Ejakulation	ejaculation	eyaculación
Ekchymose	ecchymosis	equímosis
Eklampsie	eclampsia	eclampsia
Eklampsiebereitschaft	pre-eclampsia	preeclampsia
Ektoderm	ectoderm	ectodermo
ektop	ectopic	ectópico
Ektoparasit	ectoparasite	ectoparásito
Ektropion	ectropion	ectropión
Ekzem	eczema	eccema
Ekzem, seborrhoisches	seborrheic dermatitis (Am), seborrhoeic dermatitis (Eng)	dermatitis seborréica
Elastin	elastin	elastina
Elektrode	electrode	electrodo
Elektroenzephalogramm (EEG)	electroencephalogram (EEG)	electroencefalograma (EEG)
Elektrokardiogramm (EKG)	electrocardiogram (ECG)	electrocardiograma (ECG)
Elektrolyse	electrolysis	electrólisis
Elektrolyt	electrolyte	electrólito
Elektromyographie	electromyography	electromiografía
Elektroschocktherapie	electroconvulsive therapy (ECT)	electrochoqueterapia (ECT)
Elephantiasis	elephantiasis	elefantiasis
Elimination	elimination	eliminación
Elixier	elixir	elixir
Elle	ulna	cúbito
Ellenbozen	olecranon (process)	olécranon
Elliptozytose	elliptocytosis	eliptocitosis
Emaille	enamel	esmalte
Embolie	embolism	embolia
embolisch	embolic	embólico
Embolus	embolus	émbolo
Embryo	embryo	embrión
Embryologie	embryology	embriología
Embryopathie	embryopathy	embriopatía
Emetikum	emetic	emético
emetisch	emetic	emético
Emollientium	emollient	emoliente
Emotion	emotion	emoción
emotional	emotional	emocional
Empathie	empathy	empatía
Empfänger	recipient	recipiente
empfänglich	prone	prono, inclinado

sidérophyline	proteina che lega il ferro	**eisenbindendes Protein**
pouvoir sidéropexique, capacité de fixation du fer	capacità di legame del ferro	**Eisenbindungskapazität**
ovulation	ovulazione	**Eisprung**
pus	pus	**Eiter**
furoncle	foruncolo	**Eiterbeule**
suppuration	suppurazione	**Eiterung**
purulent	purulento	**eitrig**
éjaculation	eiaculazione	**Ejakulation**
ecchymose	ecchimosi	**Ekchymose**
éclampsie	eclampsia	**Eklampsie**
éclampsisme	preeclampsia	**Eklampsiebereitschaft**
ectoderme	ectoderma	**Ektoderm**
ectopique	ectopico	**ektop**
ectoparasite	ectoparassita	**Ektoparasit**
ectropion	ectropion	**Ektropion**
eczéma	eczema	**Ekzem**
eczéma	dermatite seborroica	**Ekzem, seborrhoisches**
élastine	elastina	**Elastin**
électrode	elettrodo	**Elektrode**
électroencéphalogramme (EEG)	elettroencefalogramma (EEG)	**Elektroenzephalogramm (EEG)**
électrocardiogramme (ECG)	elettrocardiogramma (ECG)	**Elektrokardiogramm (EKG)**
électrolyse	elettrolisi	**Elektrolyse**
électrolyte	elettrolito	**Elektrolyt**
électromyographie	elettromiografia	**Elektromyographie**
électrochoc	terapia elettroconvulsiva, elettroshock	**Elektroschocktherapie**
éléphantiasis	elefantiasi	**Elephantiasis**
élimination	eliminazione	**Elimination**
élixir	elisir	**Elixier**
cubitus	ulna	**Elle**
olécrane	olecrano	**Ellenbozen**
elliptocytose	ellissocitosi	**Elliptozytose**
émail	smalto	**Emaille**
embolisme	embolia	**Embolie**
embolique	embolico	**embolisch**
embole	embolo	**Embolus**
embryon	embrione	**Embryo**
embryologie	embriologia	**Embryologie**
embryopathie	embriopatia	**Embryopathie**
émétique	emetico	**Emetikum**
émétique	emetico	**emetisch**
émollient	emoliente	**Emollientium**
émotion	emozione	**Emotion**
émotionnel	emotivo	**emotional**
empathie	immedesimazione, identificazione	**Empathie**
receveur	ricevente	**Empfänger**
en pronation	prono	**empfänglich**

GERMAN	ENGLISH	SPANISH
Empfängnis	conception	concepción
Empfängnisdatum	date of conception (DOC)	fecha de concepción
empfindlich	sensitive	sensible
Empfindlichkeit	sensitivity, susceptibility	sensibilidad, susceptibilidad
Emphysem	emphysema	enfisema
empirisch	empirical	empírico
Empyem	empyema	empiema
Emulsion	emulsion	emulsión
Endarteriektomie	endarterectomy	endarterectomía
Endarteriitis	endarteritis	endarteritis
Endemie	endemic	endémico
endemisch	endemic	endémico
Endocarditis lenta	subacute bacterial endocarditis (SBE)	endocarditis bacteriana subaguda
endogen	endogenous, intrinsic	endógeno, intrínseco
Endokarditis	endocarditis	endocarditis
endokrin	endocrine	endocrino
Endokrinologie	endocrinology	endocrinología
Endometriose	endometriosis	endometriosis
Endometritis	endometritis	endometritis
Endometrium	endometrium	endometrio
Endoneurium	endoneurium	endoneuro
Endoparasit	endoparasite	endoparásito
Endorphin	endorphin	endorfina
Endoskop	endoscope	endoscopio
Endoskopie	endoscopy	endoscopia
endoskopische retrograde Cholangiopankreatographie (ERCP)	endoscopic retrograde cholangiopancreatography (ERCP)	colangiopancreatografía endoscópica retrógrada
Endothel	endothelium	endotelio
Endotoxin	endotoxin	endotoxina
endotracheal	endotracheal	endotraqueal
endovenös	intravenous (IV)	intravenoso (IV)
endozervikal	endocervical	endocervical
Enkopresis	encopresis	encopresis
Enophtalmus	enophthalmos	enoftalmos
Entbindung	delivery	parto
entblähend	carminative	carminativo
enteral	enteral	enteral
enterisch	enteric	entérico
Enteritis	enteritis	enteritis
Enteroanastomose	enteroanastomosis	enteroanastómosis
Enterokolitis	enterocolitis	enterocolitis
Enterokolitis, nekrotisierende	necrotizing enterocolitis (NEC)	enterocolitis necrotizante
Enterostomie	enterostomy	enterostomía
Enterovirus	enterovirus	enterovirus
Enterozele	enterocele	enterocele
Entlausung	disinfestation	desinfestación
Entmarkung	demyelination	desmielinización

FRENCH	ITALIAN	GERMAN
conception	concepimento	**Empfängnis**
date du rapport fécondant	data del concepimento	**Empfängnisdatum**
sensible	sensibile	**empfindlich**
sensibilité, susceptibilité	sensibilità, suscettibilità	**Empfindlichkeit**
emphysème	enfisema	**Emphysem**
empirique	empirico	**empirisch**
empyème	empiema	**Empyem**
émulsion	emulsione	**Emulsion**
endartériectomie	endoarterectomia	**Endarteriektomie**
endartérite	endoarterite	**Endarteriitis**
endémie	endemia	**Endemie**
endémique	endemico	**endemisch**
endocardite lente	endocardite batterica subacuta	**Endocarditis lenta**
endogène, intrinsèque	endogeno, intrinseco	**endogen**
endocardite	endocardite	**Endokarditis**
endocrine	endocrino	**endokrin**
endocrinologie	endocrinologia	**Endokrinologie**
endométriose	endometriosi	**Endometriose**
endométrite	endometrite	**Endometritis**
endomètre	endometrio	**Endometrium**
endonèvre	endonevrio	**Endoneurium**
endoparasite	endoparassita	**Endoparasit**
endorphine	endorfina	**Endorphin**
endoscope	endoscopio	**Endoskop**
endoscopie	endoscopia	**Endoskopie**
cholangio-pancréatographie rétrograde endoscopique (CPRE)	colangio-pancreatografia retrograda endoscopica (ERCP)	**endoskopische retrograde Cholangiopankreatographie (ERCP)**
endothélium	endotelio	**Endothel**
endotoxine	endotossina	**Endotoxin**
endotrachéique	endotracheale	**endotracheal**
intraveineux (IV)	endovenoso (EV)	**endovenös**
endocervical	endocervicale	**endozervikal**
encoprésic	encopresi	**Enkopresis**
énophtalmie	enoftalmo	**Enophtalmus**
livraison, accouchement	parto	**Entbindung**
carminatif	carminativo	**entblähend**
entéral	enterale, intestinale	**enteral**
entérique	enterico	**enterisch**
entérite	enterite	**Enteritis**
entéro-anastomose	enteroanastomosi	**Enteroanastomose**
entérocolite	enterocolite	**Enterokolitis**
entérocolite nécrosante	enterocolite necrotizzante	**Enterokolitis, nekrotisierende**
entérostomie	enterostomia	**Enterostomie**
entérovirus	enterovirus	**Enterovirus**
entérocèle, hernie intestinale	enterocele	**Enterozele**
désinfestation	disinfestazione	**Entlausung**
démyélinisation	demielinizzazione	**Entmarkung**

GERMAN	ENGLISH	SPANISH
Entropion	entropion	entropión
Entschädigung	compensation	compensación
entspannend	relaxant	relajante
Entwesung	disinfestation	desinfestación
Entzug	withdrawal	supresión, abstinencia
Entzündung	inflammation	inflamación
entzündungshemmend	anti-inflammatory	antiinflamatorio
Enukleation	enucleation	enucleación
Enuresis	enuresis	enuresis
Enzephalin	encephalin (Eng), enkephalin (Am)	encefalina
Enzephalitis	encephalitis	encefalitis
Enzephalomyelitis	encephalomyelitis	encefalomielitis
Enzephalopathie	encephalopathy	encefalopatía
Enzym	enzyme	enzima
enzyme-linked immunosorbent assay (ELISA)	enzyme-linked immunosorbent assay (ELISA)	análisis enzimático por inmunoabsorción
Enzymologie	enzymology	enzimología
eosinophil	eosinophil	eosinófilo
Eosinophiler	eosinophil	eosinófilo
Eosinophilie	eosinophilia	eosinofilia
Ependymom	ependymoma	ependimoma
Ephedrin	ephedrine	efedrina
Epidemie	epidemic	epidemia
Epidemiologie	epidemiology	epidemiología
epidemisch	epidemic	epidémico
Epidermis	epidermis	epidermis
Epididymis	epididymis	epidídimo
Epididymitis	epididymitis	epididimitis
Epididymoorchitis	epididymo-orchitis	epididimoorquitis
epidural	epidural	epidural
Epigastrium	epigastrium	epigastrio
Epiglottis	epiglottis	epiglotis
Epiglottitis	epiglottitis	epiglotitis
Epikanthus	epicanthus	epicanto
Epikard	epicardium	epicardio
Epilepsie	epilepsy	epilepsia
epileptiform	epileptiform	epileptiforme
epileptisch	epileptic	epiléptico
epileptogen	epileptogenic	epileptógeno
Epiphyse	epiphysis, pineal body	epífisis, cuerpo pineal
Epiphyseolyse	slipped epiphysis	epífisis desplazada
Episiotomie	episiotomy	episiotomía
Episklera	episclera	episclera
Episkleritis	episcleritis	episcleritis
Epistaxis	epistaxis, nosebleed	epistaxis
Epithel	epithelium	epitelio
Epitheliom	epithelioma	epitelioma

FRENCH	ITALIAN	GERMAN
entropion	entropion	**Entropion**
compensation	compenso	**Entschädigung**
relaxant	rilassante	**entspannend**
désinfestation	disinfestazione	**Entwesung**
retrait, sevrage, suppression	ritiro, astinenza, sospensione	**Entzug**
inflammation	infiammazione	**Entzündung**
anti-inflammatoire	anti-infiammatorio	**entzündungshemmend**
énucléation	enucleazione	**Enukleation**
énurèse	enuresi	**Enuresis**
encéphaline	encefalina	**Enzephalin**
encéphalite	encefalite	**Enzephalitis**
encéphalomyélite	encefalomielite	**Enzephalomyelitis**
encéphalopathie	encefalopatia	**Enzephalopathie**
enzyme	enzima	**Enzym**
dosage par la méthode (ELISA)	test di immunoassorbimento enzimatico	**enzyme-linked immunosorbent assay (ELISA)**
enzymologie	enzimologia	**Enzymologie**
éosinophile	eosinofilo	**eosinophil**
éosinophile	eosinofilo	**Eosinophiler**
éosinophilie	eosinofilia	**Eosinophilie**
épendymome	ependimoma	**Ependymom**
éphédrine	efedrina	**Ephedrin**
épidémie	epidemia	**Epidemie**
épidémiologie	epidemiologia	**Epidemiologie**
épidémique	epidemico	**epidemisch**
épiderme	epidermide	**Epidermis**
épididyme	epididimo	**Epididymis**
épididymite	epididimite	**Epididymitis**
orchi-épididymite	epididimo-orchite	**Epididymoorchitis**
épidural	epidurale	**epidural**
épigastre	epigastrio	**Epigastrium**
épiglotte	epiglottide	**Epiglottis**
épiglottite	epiglottite	**Epiglottitis**
épicanthus	epicanto	**Epikanthus**
épicarde	epicardio	**Epikard**
épilepsie	epilessia	**Epilepsie**
épileptiforme	epilettiforme	**epileptiform**
épileptique	epilettico	**epileptisch**
épileptogène	epilettogeno	**epileptogen**
épiphyse, glande pinéale	epifisi, ghiandola pineale	**Epiphyse**
épiphysiolyse	distacco epifisario	**Epiphyseolyse**
épisiotomie	episiotomia	**Episiotomie**
épisclérotique	episclera	**Episklera**
épisclérite	episclerite	**Episkleritis**
épistaxis, saignement de nez	epistassi	**Epistaxis**
épithélium	epitelio	**Epithel**
épithélioma	epitelioma	**Epitheliom**

GERMAN	ENGLISH	SPANISH
Epstein-Barr-Virus (EBV)	Epstein-Barr virus (EBV)	virus de Epstein-Barr
erblich	hereditary	hereditario
Erblichkeit	heredity	herencia
Erbrechen	emesis	emesis
erbrechen	vomit	vomitar
Erbrechen, zyklisches	cyclical vomiting	vómito cíclico
erektil	erectile	eréctil
Erektion	erection	erección
Erfrierung	frostbite	congelación, sabañón
Erguß	effusion	derrame
Erinnerungsvermögen	memory	memoria
Erkältung	cold	resfriado
Erkennungsvermögen	cognition	cognición
Ermüdung	fatigue	fatiga, cansancio
Ernährung	alimentation, diet, nutrition	alimentación, régimen, nutrición
Ernährung, parenterale	total parenteral nutrition (TPN)	nutrición parenteral total
Ernährungskunde	dietetics	dietética
erregbar	irritable	irritable
Erregbarkeit	excitability	excitabilidad
Erreger	germ, pathogen	gérmen, patógeno
Erregung	excitation, affect	excitación, afecto
Errinerung	recall	recuerdo
Errinerungsvermögen	recall	recuerdo
Erschütterung	concussion, succussion	concusión, contusión violenta, sucusión
Erste Hilfe	first aid	primeros auxilios
Erstgebärende	primipara	primípara
Ersticken	suffocation	asfixia
Erstickung	suffocation	asfixia
erweichend	emollient	emoliente
Erweichung	malacia	malacia
Erweiterung	dilatation (Eng), dilation (Am)	dilatación
Erysipel	erysipelas	erisipela
Erythem	erythema	eritema
Erythroblast	erythroblast	eritroblasto
Erythrodermie	erythroderma	eritrodermia
Erythropoese	erythropoiesis	eritropoyesis
Erythropoetin	erythropoietin	eritropoyetina
erythropoetischer Faktor	erythropoietin	eritropoyetina
Erythrozyt	erythrocyte, red blood cell (RBC)	eritrocito, glóbulo rojo
Erythrozyten-Antigen, menschliches	human erythrocyte antigen (HEA)	antígeno eritrocitario humano
Es	id	id
essentiell	idiopathic	idiopático
Essenz	essence	esencia
Ethmoid	ethmoid	etmoides
ethnisch	ethnic	étnico
Euphorie	euphoria	euforia

FRENCH	ITALIAN	GERMAN
virus d'Epstein-Barr	virus di Epstein Barr	**Epstein-Barr-Virus (EBV)**
héréditaire	ereditario	**erblich**
hérédité	eredità	**Erblichkeit**
vomissement	vomito, emesi	**Erbrechen**
vomir	vomitare	**erbrechen**
vomissement cyclique	vomito ciclico	**Erbrechen, zyklisches**
érectile	erettile	**erektil**
érection	erezione	**Erektion**
gelure	congelamento	**Erfrierung**
effusion	effusione	**Erguß**
mémoire	memoria	**Erinnerungsvermögen**
rhume	raffreddore	**Erkältung**
cognition	cognizione	**Erkennungsvermögen**
fatigue	stanchezza, astenia	**Ermüdung**
alimentation, régime, nutrition	alimentazione, regime, dieta, nutrizione	**Ernährung**
alimentation parentérale totale	nutrizione parenterale totale	**Ernährung, parenterale**
diététique	dietetica	**Ernährungskunde**
irritable	irritabile	**erregbar**
excitabilité	eccitabilità	**Erregbarkeit**
germe, pathogène	germe, patogeno	**Erreger**
excitation, affect	eccitazione, emozione	**Erregung**
évocation	memoria	**Errinerung**
évocation	memoria	**Errinerungsvermögen**
commotion, succussion	commozione, succussione, scuotimento	**Erschütterung**
secourisme, premiers soins	pronto soccorso	**Erste Hilfe**
primipare	primipara	**Erstgebärende**
suffocation	soffocamento	**Ersticken**
suffocation	soffocamento	**Erstickung**
émollient	emoliente	**erweichend**
malacie	malacia	**Erweichung**
dilatation	dilatazione	**Erweiterung**
érysipèle	erisipela	**Erysipel**
érythème	eritema	**Erythem**
érythroblaste	eritroblasto	**Erythroblast**
érythroderme	eritrodermia	**Erythrodermie**
érythropoïèse	eritropoiesi	**Erythropoese**
érythropoïétine	eritropoietina	**Erythropoetin**
érythropoïétine	eritropoietina	**erythropoetischer Faktor**
érythrocyte, globule rouge	eritrocito, globulo rosso (RBC)	**Erythrozyt**
antigène humain des erythrocytes	antigene eritrocitico umano	**Erythrozyten-Antigen, menschliches**
ça	incoscio	**Es**
idiopathique	idiopatico	**essentiell**
essence	essenza	**Essenz**
ethmoïde	etmoide	**Ethmoid**
ethnique	etnico	**ethnisch**
euphorie	euforia	**Euphorie**

Eustachische Röhre	Eustachian tube	trompa de Eustaquio
Euthanasie	euthanasia	eutanasia
Ewing-Sarkom	Ewing's tumour	sarcoma de Ewing
Exartikulation	disarticulation	desarticulación
Exfoliation	exfoliation	exfoliación
Exhibitionismus	exhibitionism	exhibicionismo
Exkoriation	excoriation	excoriación
Exkretion	excretion	excreción
exogen	exogenous, extrinsic	exógeno, extrínseco
exokrin	exocrine	exocrino
Exomphalos	exomphalos	exónfalo, hernia umbilical
Exophthalmus	exophthalmos, proptosis	exoftalmía, proptosis
Exostose	exostosis	exostosis
Exotoxin	exotoxin	exotoxina
Expektorans	expectorant	expectorante
Exploration	exploration	exploración
Expressio	expression	expresión
Exspiration	expiration	espiración
Exsudat	exudate	exudado
Extension	extension	extensión
Extensor	extensor	extensor
extraartikulär	extra-articular	extraarticular
extradural	extradural	extradural
Extraktion	extraction	extracción
extramural	extramural	extramural
extrapyramidale Nebenwirkungen	extrapyramidal side effects	efectos secundarios extrapiramidales
Extrasystole	extrasystole	extrasístole
extrauterin	extrauterine	extrauterino
Extravasat	extravasation	extravasación
extrazellulär	extracellular	extracelular
Extremität	limb	extremidad
Exzision	excision	excisión

FRENCH	ITALIAN	GERMAN
trompe d'Eustache	tuba d'Eustachio	Eustachische Röhre
euthanasie	eutanasia	Euthanasie
tumeur d'Ewing	tumore di Ewing	Ewing-Sarkom
désarticulation	disarticolazione	Exartikulation
exfoliation	esfoliazione	Exfoliation
exhibitionnisme	esibizionismo	Exhibitionismus
excoriation	escoriazione	Exkoriation
excrétion	escrezione	Exkretion
exogène, extrinsèque	esogeno, estrinseco	exogen
exocrine	esocrino	exokrin
exomphale	ernia ombelicale, protrusione dell'ombelico	Exomphalos
exophthalmie, proptose	esoftalmo, proptosi	Exophthalmus
exostose	esostosi	Exostose
exotoxine	esotossina	Exotoxin
expectorant	espettorante	Expektorans
exploration	esplorazione	Exploration
expression	espressione	Expressio
expiration	espirazione, termine	Exspiration
exsudat	essudato	Exsudat
extension	estensione	Extension
extenseur	estensore	Extensor
extra-articulaire	extraarticolare	extraartikulär
extradural	extradurale	extradural
extraction	estrazione	Extraktion
extramural	extramurale	extramural
effets latéraux extrapyramidaux	reazioni collaterali extrapiramidali da farmaci	extrapyramidale Nebenwirkungen
extrasystole	extrasistole	Extrasystole
extra-utérin	extrauterino	extrauterin
extravasation	stravaso	Extravasat
extracellulaire	extracellulare	extrazellulär
membre	braccio	Extremität
excision	escissione	Exzision

F

GERMAN	ENGLISH	SPANISH
Facette	facet	faceta
Facies	facies	facies
Fadenpilzerkrankung	ringworm	tiña
Fadenwurm	nematode, threadworm	nematodo, enterobius vermincularis, oxiuros
Fadenwurmbefall	filariasis	filariasis
Fähigkeit	ability	habilidad, capacidad
fäkal	faecal (Eng), fecal (Am)	fecal
fakultativ	facultative	facultativo
falciformis	falciform	falciforme
Fallot-Tetralogie	Fallot's tetralogy, tetralogy of Fallot	tetralogía de Fallot
Faltenbildung	plication	plicatura
familiär	familial	familiar
Familienplanung	family planning	planificación familiar
farbarm	hypochromic	hipocrómico
Farbenblindheit	color blindness (Am), colour blindness (Eng)	daltonismo, ceguera de colores
Farbstoff	pigment	pigmento
Färbung	pigmentation	pigmentación
Faser	fiber (Am), fibre (Eng)	fibra
Fäserchen	fibril	fibrilla
Faszie	fascia	fascia, aponeurosis
Faszikulation	fasciculation	fasciculación
Fäulnis	putrefaction	putrefacción
Fäzes	faeces (Eng), feces (Am)	heces
Fehlanpassung	maladjustment	inadaptación
Fehlbildung	anomaly, dysplasia	anomalía, displasia
Fehlernährung	malnutrition	desnutrición
fehlgebären	abort	abortar
Fehlgeburt	abortion, miscarriage	aborto
Fehlstellung (Frakturenden)	malunion	unión defectuosa
Feingefühl	sensitivity	sensibilidad
Femur	femur	fémur
Fensterung	fenestration	fenestración
Ferse	heel	talón
fertil	generative	generador
Festigung	consolidation	consolidación
fetale Herzfrequenz	fetal heart rate (FHR)	frecuencia cardíaca fetal (FCF)
fetaler Kreislauf	fetal circulation	circulación fetal
Fetoskopie	fetoscopy	fetoscopia
Fett	fat	grasa
fett	fat	graso
fetthaltig	fat	graso
fettige Degeneration	fatty degeneration	degeneración grasa
fettleibig	adipose	adiposo, graso
Fettsäure	fatty acid	ácido graso

FRENCH	ITALIAN	GERMAN
facette	faccetta	**Facette**
faciès	facies	**Facies**
dermatophytose	tricofizia, tinea	**Fadenpilzerkrankung**
nématode, ascaride	nematode, ossiuro	**Fadenwurm**
filariose	filariasi	**Fadenwurmbefall**
capacité, aptitude, compétence	abilità, capacità	**Fähigkeit**
fécal	fecale	**fäkal**
facultatif	facoltativo	**fakultativ**
falciforme	falciforme	**falciformis**
trilogie de Fallot, tétralogie de Fallot	tetralogia di Fallot	**Fallot-Tetralogie**
plicature	plicazione, piegatura	**Faltenbildung**
familial	familiare	**familiär**
contrôle des naissances	controllo delle nascite	**Familienplanung**
hypochromique	ipocromico	**farbarm**
daltonisme	cecità ai colori, acromatopsia	**Farbenblindheit**
pigment	pigmento	**Farbstoff**
pigmentation	pigmentazione	**Färbung**
fibre	fibra	**Faser**
fibrille	fibrilla	**Fäserchen**
fascia	fascia	**Faszie**
fasciculation	fascicolazione	**Faszikulation**
putréfaction	putrefazione	**Fäulnis**
fèces	feci	**Fäzes**
inadaptation	assestamento difettoso	**Fehlanpassung**
anomalie, dysplasie	anomalia, displasia	**Fehlbildung**
malnutrition	malnutrizione	**Fehlernährung**
avorter	abortire	**fehlgebären**
avortement, fausse couche	aborto	**Fehlgeburt**
cal vicieux	unione difettosa	**Fehlstellung (Frakturenden)**
sensibilité	sensibilità	**Feingefühl**
fémur	femore	**Femur**
fenestration	fenestrazione	**Fensterung**
talon	tallone	**Ferse**
génératif	riproduttivo	**fertil**
consolidation	solidificazione, addensamento	**Festigung**
fréquence cardiaque foetale	battito cardiaco fetale	**fetale Herzfrequenz**
circulation foetale	circolazione fetale	**fetaler Kreislauf**
fétoscopie	fetoscopia	**Fetoskopie**
graisse	adipe	**Fett**
gras, obèse	grasso	**fett**
gras, obèse	grasso	**fetthaltig**
dégénérescence graisseuse	degenerazione grassa	**fettige Degeneration**
adipeux	adiposo	**fettleibig**
acide gras	acido grasso	**Fettsäure**

GERMAN	ENGLISH	SPANISH
Fettsäure, essentielle	essential fatty acid	ácido graso esenciale
Fettstuhl	steatorrhea (Am), steatorrhoea (Eng)	esteatorrea
Fetus	fetus	feto
Fibrille	fibril	fibrilla
Fibrillieren	fibrillation	fibrilación
Fibrin	fibrin	fibrina
Fibrinogen	fibrinogen	fibrinógeno
Fibroadenom	fibroadenoma	fibroadenoma
Fibroblast	fibroblast	fibroblasto
Fibrom	fibroma	fibroma
Fibromyom	fibromyoma	fibromioma
Fibrosarkom	fibrosarcoma	fibrosarcoma
Fibrose	fibrosis	fibrosis
Fibrositis	fibrositis	fibrositis
fibrozystisch	fibrocystic	fibrocístico
Fibula	fibula	peroné
Fieber	calor, fever, pyrexia	calor, fiebre, pirexia
Fieber-	febrile	febril
fieberfrei	afebrile	apirético, afebril
fieberhaft	febrile	febril
Fiebermittel	antipyretic	antipirético
fiebersenkend	antipyretic	antipirético
Fieber unklarer Genese	pyrexia of unknown origin (PUO, FUO)	fiebre de origen desconocido
Fieberwahn	delirium	delirio
Filariasis	filariasis	filariasis
Filtrat	filtrate	filtrado
Filtration	filtration	filtración
Filtrieren	filtration	filtración
Fimbrie	fimbria	fimbria, franja
Finger	finger	dedo de la mano
Fingerdruck	digital compression	compresión digital
Fingerglieder	phalanges	falanges
Fingerhut	digitalis	digital
Fistel	fistula	fístula
Fixation	fixation	fijación
Fixierung	fixation	fijación
flache Atmung	hypopnea (Am), hypopnoea (Eng)	hipopnea
Flatterbrust	flail chest	volet torácico
Flatulenz	flatulence	flatulencia
Flatus	flatus	flato
Fleck	macula	mácula
Flecken	spot	mancha
Fleckfieber	typhus	tifus
fleischähnlich	sarcoid	sarcoideo
flektieren	flex	flexionar

FRENCH	ITALIAN	GERMAN
acide gras essentiel	acido grasso essenziale	**Fettsäure, essentielle**
stéatorrhée	steatorrea, seborrea	**Fettstuhl**
foetus	feto	**Fetus**
fibrille	fibrilla	**Fibrille**
fibrillation	fibrillazione	**Fibrillieren**
fibrine	fibrina	**Fibrin**
fibrinogène	fibrinogeno	**Fibrinogen**
fibroadénome	fibroadenoma	**Fibroadenom**
fibroblaste	fibroblasto	**Fibroblast**
fibrome	fibroma	**Fibrom**
fibromyome	fibromioma	**Fibromyom**
fibrosarcome	fibrosarcoma	**Fibrosarkom**
fibrose	fibrosi	**Fibrose**
fibrosite	fibrosite	**Fibrositis**
fibrokystique	fibrocistico	**fibrozystisch**
fibula	fibula	**Fibula**
chaleur, fièvre, pyrexie	calore, febbre, piressia	**Fieber**
fébrile	febbrile	**Fieber-**
afébrile	afebbrile	**fieberfrei**
fébrile	febbrile	**fieberhaft**
antipyrétique	anti-piretico	**Fiebermittel**
antipyrétique	anti-piretico	**fiebersenkend**
fièvre d'origine inconnue	piressia di origine sconosciuta (POS)	**Fieber unklarer Genese**
délire	delirio	**Fieberwahn**
filariose	filariasi	**Filariasis**
filtrat	filtrato	**Filtrat**
filtration	filtrazione	**Filtration**
filtration	filtrazione	**Filtrieren**
fimbria	fimbria	**Fimbrie**
doigt	dito	**Finger**
compression digitale	compressione digitale	**Fingerdruck**
phalanges	falangi	**Fingerglieder**
digitale	digitale	**Fingerhut**
fistule	fistola	**Fistel**
fixation	fissazione	**Fixation**
fixation	fissazione	**Fixierung**
hypopnée	ipopnea	**flache Atmung**
volet thoracique	anomala motilità respiratoria della cassa toracica in conseguenza di fratture	**Flatterbrust**
flatulence	flatulenza	**Flatulenz**
flatuosité	flatulenza, gas intestinale	**Flatus**
macule	macula	**Fleck**
bouton	foruncolo	**Flecken**
typhus	tifo	**Fleckfieber**
sarcoïde	sarcoideo	**fleischähnlich**
fléchir	flettere	**flektieren**

GERMAN	ENGLISH	SPANISH
Flexion	flexion	flexión
Flexor	flexor	flexor
Flexur	flexure	flexura
Floh	flea	pulga
Flora	flora	flora
floride	florid	florido, bien desarrollado
Fluktuation	fluctuation	fluctuación
Fluorescin	fluorescein	fluoresceína
Fluoreszenz-Treponemen-Antikörper	fluorescent treponemal antibody (FTA)	anticuerpo anti-treponema fluorescente
Fluorid	fluoride	flúor
Flush	flush	rubor
Flußblindheit	river blindness	oncocerciasis ocular
Flüssigkeit	liquor	licor
Flüssigkeitsansammlung	edema (Am), oedema (Eng)	edema
Flüssigkeitsmangel	dehydration	deshidratación
Foetor ex ore	halitosis	halitosis
Folgeerscheinung	sequela	secuela
Folgezustand	sequela	secuela
Follikel	follicle	folículo
follikelstimulierendes Hormon (FSH)	follicle stimulating hormone (FSH)	hormona estimulante del folículo (FSH)
Follikulitis	folliculitis	foliculitis
Folsäure	folic acid	ácido fólico
Fontanelle	fontanelle	fontanela
Foramen	foramen	foramen
forciertes Exspirationsvolumen	forced expiratory volume (FEV)	volumen espiratorio forzado (VEF)
Formel	formula	fórmula, receta
Formelnbuch	formulary	formulario
Fornix	fornix	fórnix, bóveda
fortbewegend	locomotor	locomotor
Fortpflanzungs-	generative	generador
Fortpflanzungsapparat	reproductive system	aparato reproductor
Fovea	fovea	fóvea
Fragmentlösung	disimpaction	desimpactación
Fraktur	fracture	fractura
frakturieren	fracture	fracturar
Frambösie	yaws	yaws, pian
Frauenheilkunde	gynaecology (Eng), gynecology (Am)	ginecología
freier Thyroxinindex (FTi)	free thyroxine index (FTI)	indice de tiroxina libre
freies Thyroxin (FT)	free thyroxine (FT)	tiroxina libre
Frenotomie	frenotomy	frenotomía
Frenulum	frenum	frenillo
Friedreich Ataxie	Friedreich's ataxia	ataxia de Friedreich
Frigidität	frigidity	frigidez
Friktion	friction	fricción
frontal	frontal	frontal

FRENCH	ITALIAN	GERMAN
flexion	flessione	**Flexion**
fléchisseur	flessore	**Flexor**
angle	flessura	**Flexur**
puce	pulce	**Floh**
flore	flora	**Flora**
coloré	florido	**floride**
variation	fluttuazione	**Fluktuation**
fluorescéine	fluoresceina	**Fluorescin**
test d'immunofluorescence absorbée pour le diagnostic sérologique de la syphilis	anticorpo immuno-fluorescente anti-treponema	**Fluoreszenz-Treponemen-Antikörper**
fluorure	fluoruro	**Fluorid**
rougeur	eritema vasomotorio	**Flush**
cécité des rivières	oncocerchiasi, cecità fluviale	**Flußblindheit**
liquide	liquido	**Flüssigkeit**
oedème	edema	**Flüssigkeitsansammlung**
déshydratation	deidratazione	**Flüssigkeitsmangel**
halitose	alitosi	**Foetor ex ore**
séquelle	sequela	**Folgeerscheinung**
séquelle	sequela	**Folgezustand**
follicule	follicolo	**Follikel**
hormone folliculo-stimulante, gonadotrophine A	ormone follicolostimolante (FSH)	**follikelstimulierendes Hormon (FSH)**
folliculite	follicolite	**Follikulitis**
acide folique	acido folico	**Folsäure**
fontanelle	fontanella	**Fontanelle**
orifice	foramen	**Foramen**
volume expiratoire maximum (VEM)	volume espiratorio forzato	**forciertes Exspirationsvolumen**
formule	formula	**Formel**
formulaire	formulario	**Formelnbuch**
fornix	fornice	**Fornix**
locomoteur	locomotore	**fortbewegend**
génératif	riproduttivo	**Fortpflanzungs-**
système reproducteur	sistema riproduttivo	**Fortpflanzungsapparat**
fovea	fovea	**Fovea**
désimpaction	riduzione	**Fragmentlösung**
fracture	frattura	**Fraktur**
fracturer	fratturare	**frakturieren**
pian	framboesia, pian	**Frambösie**
gynécologie	ginecologia	**Frauenheilkunde**
index de thyroxine libre	indice di tiroxina libera	**freier Thyroxinindex (FTi)**
thyroxine libre (TL)	tiroxina libera (FT)	**freies Thyroxin (FT)**
frénotomie	frenulotomia	**Frenotomie**
frein	freno	**Frenulum**
maladie de Friedreich	malattia di Friedreich	**Friedreich Ataxie**
frigidité	frigidità	**Frigidität**
friction	attrito, frizione	**Friktion**
frontal	frontale	**frontal**

GERMAN	ENGLISH	SPANISH
Frostbeule	chilblain	sabañón
Frozen shoulder	frozen shoulder	hombro congelado/rígido
Fruchtwasser	amniotic fluid	líquido amniótico
Frühgeborenen-Intensivstation	neonatal intensive care unit (NICU) (Am)	unidad de cuidados intensivos para recién nacidos
frühreif	premature	prematuro
Fugue	fugue	fuga
Fulguration	fulguration	fulguración
fulminant	fulminant	fulminante
Fundoplikatio(n)	fundoplication	fundoplicatura
Fundus	fundus	fundus
Funktion	function	función
funktionelle Störung	functional disorder	trastorno funcional
funktionieren	function	funcionar
Funktionsstörung	dysfunction	disfunción
Furche	sulcus	surco
Furunkel	boil, furuncle	forúnculo
Fuß	foot	pie
Fuß-	pedal	pedal
Fußballen, entzündeter	bunion	juanete
Fußpflege	chiropody	podología
Fußpfleger	chiropodist	callista, podólogo
Fußpilz	athlete's foot	pie de atleta
Fußrücken	instep	empeine
Fußwurzel	tarsus	tarso

FRENCH	ITALIAN	GERMAN
engelure	gelone	**Frostbeule**
épaule ankylosée	'spalla congelata', periartrite scapoloomerale	**Frozen shoulder**
liquide amniotique	fluido amniotico	**Fruchtwasser**
service de soins intensifs néonatals	reparto di terapia intensiva neonatale	**Frühgeborenen-Intensivstation**
prématuré	preamaturo	**frühreif**
fugue	fuga	**Fugue**
fulguration	folgorazione	**Fulguration**
fulminant	fulminante	**fulminant**
fundoplication	fundoplicaziono	**Fundoplikatio(n)**
fond	fondo	**Fundus**
fonction	funzione	**Funktion**
fonctionnel	disturbo funzionale	**funktionelle Störung**
fonctionner	funzionare	**funktionieren**
dysfonctionnement	disfunzione	**Funktionsstörung**
sillon, gouttière, scissure	solco	**Furche**
furoncle	foruncolo	**Furunkel**
pied	piede	**Fuß**
pédieux	del piede	**Fuß-**
hallux valgus	borsite dell'alluce	**Fußballen, entzündeter**
chiropodie	chiropodia	**Fußpflege**
pédicure	callista	**Fußpfleger**
pied d'athlète	piede di atleta	**Fußpilz**
tarse	dorso del piede	**Fußrücken**
tarse	tarso	**Fußwurzel**

G

German	English	Spanish
Gähnen	yawn	bostezo
Galaktagogum	galactagogue	galactogogo
Galaktorrhoe	galactorrhea (Am), galactorrhoea (Eng)	galactorrea
Galaktosämie	galactosaemia (Eng), galactosemia (Am)	galactosemia
Galaktose	galactose	galactosa
Galle	bile	bilis
Gallenblase	gall bladder	vesícula biliar
Gallenstauung	cholestasis	colestasis
Gallensteine	gallstones	cálculos biliares
Gallensteinleiden	cholelithiasis	colelitiasis
Gallerte	gelatine (Eng), gelatin (Am)	gelatina
Gamete	gamete	gameto
Gammaglobulin	gammaglobulin	gammaglobulina
Gammaglutamyltransferase (gGT)	gamma glutamyl transferase (GGT)	gamma glutamil transferasa (GGT)
Gang	canal, duct, gait	canal, conducto, marcha
Ganglion	ganglion	ganglio
Gangrän	gangrene	gangrena
Gas	gas	gas
Gastrin	gastrin	gastrina
gastrisch	gastric	gástrico
Gastritis	gastritis	gastritis
gastrocnemius	gastrocnemius	gastrocnemio, gemelos
Gastroenteritis	gastroenteritis	gastroenteritis
Gastroenterologie	gastroenterology	gastroenterología
Gastroenteropathie	gastroenteropathy	gastroenteropatía
Gastroenterostomie	gastroenterostomy	gastroenterostomía
gastrointestinal	gastrointestinal	gastrointestinal
Gastrojejunostomie	gastrojejunostomy	gastroyeyunostomía
gastrokolisch	gastrocolic	gastrocólico
gastroösophageal	gastroesophageal (Am), gastro-oesophageal (Eng)	gastroesofágico
Gastroschisis	gastroschisis	gastrosquisis
Gastroskop	gastroscope	gastroscopio
Gastrostomie	gastrostomy	gastrotomía
Gattung	genus	género
Gaumen	palate	paladar
Gaumenspalte	cleft palate	paladar hendido
Gaumenverschlußplatte	obturator	obturador
Gaumen, weicher	soft palate	paladar blando
Gaze	gauze	gasa
Gebären	parturition	parturición, parto
gebärend	parturient	parturienta
Gebärfähigkeit	parity	paridad
Gebärmutter	uterus, womb	útero, matriz
Gebärmutterhals	cervix	cuello uterino

FRENCH	ITALIAN	GERMAN
bâillement	sbadiglio	**Gähnen**
galactagogue	galattagogo	**Galaktagogum**
galactorrhée	galattorrea	**Galaktorrhoe**
galactosémie	galattosemia	**Galaktosämie**
galactose	galattosio	**Galaktose**
bile	bile	**Galle**
vésicule biliaire	cistifellea	**Gallenblase**
cholestase	colestasi	**Gallenstauung**
calculs biliaires	calcoli biliari	**Gallensteine**
cholélithiase	colelitiasi	**Gallensteinleiden**
gélatine	gelatina	**Gallerte**
gamète	gamete	**Gamete**
gamma-globuline	gammaglobulina	**Gammaglobulin**
gamma-glutamyl-transférase (GGT)	transaminasi, transferasi glutammica	**Gammaglutamyltransferase (gGT)**
canal, conduit, démarche	canale, dotto, andatura	**Gang**
ganglion	ganglio	**Ganglion**
gangrène	gangrena	**Gangrän**
gaz	gas	**Gas**
gastrine	gastrina	**Gastrin**
gastrique	gastrico	**gastrisch**
gastrite	gastrite	**Gastritis**
gastrocnémien	gastrocnemio	**gastrocnemius**
gastro-entérite	gastroenterite	**Gastroenteritis**
gastro-entérologie	gastroenterologia	**Gastroenterologie**
gastro-entéropathie	gastroenteropatia	**Gastroenteropathie**
gastro-entérostomie	gastroenterostomia	**Gastroenterostomie**
gastro-intestinal	gastrointestinale	**gastrointestinal**
gastrojéjunostomie	gastrodigiunostomia	**Gastrojejunostomie**
gastrocolique	gastrocolico	**gastrokolisch**
gastro-oesophagien	gastroesofageo	**gastroösophageal**
gastroschisis	gastroschisi	**Gastroschisis**
gastroscope	gastroscopio	**Gastroskop**
gastrostomie	gastrostomia	**Gastrostomie**
genre	genere	**Gattung**
palais	palato	**Gaumen**
fente palatine	palatoschisi	**Gaumenspalte**
obturateur	otturatorio	**Gaumenverschlußplatte**
voile du palais	palato molle	**Gaumen, weicher**
gaze	garza	**Gaze**
parturition	parto	**Gebären**
parturient	partoriente	**gebärend**
parité	parità, numero di gravidanze pregresse	**Gebärfähigkeit**
utérus	utero	**Gebärmutter**
cou	cervice	**Gebärmutterhals**

GERMAN	ENGLISH	SPANISH
Gebiß	denture, teeth	dentadura, dientes
geboren habend	parous	parir
Geburt	birth, delivery, parturition	nacimiento, parto, parturición
Geburtsbeginn (Anzeichen)	'show'	'señal sanguinolenta menstrual'
Geburtsdatum	date of birth (DOB)	fecha de nacimiento
Geburtsgeschwulst	caput succedaneum	caput succedaneum
Geburtsgewicht, niedriges	low birth weight (LBW)	bajo peso al nacer
Geburtshilfe	obstetrics	obstetricia
Geburtstermin, errechneter	expected date of confinement (EDC), expected date of delivery (EDD)	fecha esperada del parto, fecha probable del parto (FPP)
Gedächtnis	memory	memoria
Gedanke	idea	idea
Gedeihstörung	failure to thrive (FTT)	desmedro, marasmo
Gefäß	vessel	vaso
Gefäß-	vascular	vascular
gefäßlos	avascular	avascular
Gefäßunterbindung	ligature	ligadura
Gefühl	emotion, sensation	emoción, sensación
gefühllos	anaesthetic (Eng), anesthetic (Am)	anestésico
Gegenanzeige	contraindication	contraindicación
Gegengift	antitoxin	antitoxina
Gehirn	brain, cerebrum	cerebro
Gehirn-	cerebral	cerebral
Gehirnhautentzündung	meningitis	meningitis
Gehirnsyndrom, chronisches	chronic brain syndrome (CBS)	síndrome cerebral crónico
Gehör	hearing	oído
Gehör-	auditory, acoustic, aural	auditorio, acústico, aural
Gehörknöchelchen	ossicle	huesecillos
Geisteskrankheit	insanity	locura, demencia
geistig	mental	mental
geistige Gesundheit	sanity	cordura
gekammert	loculated	loculado
gelähmt	paralytic	paralítico
Gelatine	gelatine (Eng), gelatin (Am)	gelatina
Gelbfieber	yellow fever	fiebre amarilla
Gelbsucht	icterus, jaundice	ictericia
Geldrollenagglutination	rouleaux	rollos
Gelenk	joint	articulación
Gelenk-	articular	articular
Gelenkendoskopie	arthroscopy	artroscopia
Gelenkentzündung	arthritis	artritis
Gelenkentzündung, eitrige	pyarthrosis	piartrosis
Gelenkleiden	arthropathy	artropatía
Gelenkplastik	arthroplasty	artroplastia
Gelenkschmerz	arthralgia	artralgia

FRENCH	ITALIAN	GERMAN
dentier, dents	dentiera, denti	**Gebiß**
poreux	che ha avuto figli	**geboren habend**
naissance, livraison, accouchement, parturition	nascita, parto	**Geburt**
eaux de l'amnios	perdita ematica che precede il parto o la mestruazione	**Geburtsbeginn (Anzeichen)**
date de naissance	data di nascita	**Geburtsdatum**
caput succedaneum	tumore da parto	**Geburtsgeschwulst**
hypotrophie	basso peso alla nascita	**Geburtsgewicht, niedriges**
obstétrique	ostetricia	**Geburtshilfe**
date présumée de l'accouchement	data presunta delle doglie, data prevista per il parto	**Geburtstermin, errechneter**
mémoire	memoria	**Gedächtnis**
idée	idea	**Gedanke**
absence de développement pondéro-statural normal	marasma infantile	**Gedeihstörung**
vaisseau	vaso	**Gefäß**
vasculaire	vascolare	**Gefäß-**
avasculaire	avascolare	**gefäßlos**
ligature	legatura	**Gefäßunterbindung**
émotion, sensation	emozione, sensazione, sensibilità	**Gefühl**
anesthésique	anestetico	**gefühllos**
contre-indication	controindicazione	**Gegenanzeige**
antitoxine	antitossina	**Gegengift**
cerveau	cervello	**Gehirn**
cérébral	cerebrale	**Gehirn-**
méningite	meningite	**Gehirnhautentzündung**
syndrome chronique du cerveau	sindrome cerebrale cronica	**Gehirnsyndrom, chronisches**
audition	udito	**Gehör**
auditif, acoustique, aural	auditivo, acustico, auricolare	**Gehör-**
osselet	ossicino	**Gehörknöchelchen**
aliénation	pazzia	**Geisteskrankheit**
mental	mentale	**geistig**
santé mentale	sanità	**geistige Gesundheit**
loculé	loculato	**gekammert**
paralytique	paralitico	**gelähmt**
gélatine	gelatina	**Gelatine**
fièvre jaune	febbre gialla	**Gelbfieber**
ictère, jaunisse	ittero	**Gelbsucht**
rouleaux	colonne di eritrociti	**Geldrollenagglutination**
articulation	articolazione	**Gelenk**
articulaire	articolare	**Gelenk-**
arthroscopie	artroscopia	**Gelenkendoskopie**
arthrite	artrite	**Gelenkentzündung**
pyarthrose	pioartrosi, piartro	**Gelenkentzündung, eitrige**
arthropathie	artropatia	**Gelenkleiden**
arthroplastie	artroplastica	**Gelenkplastik**
arthralgie	artralgia	**Gelenkschmerz**

GERMAN	ENGLISH	SPANISH
Gemütsart	temperament	temperamento
Gen	gene	gen
Generic	generic	genérico
generisch	generic	genérico
Genetik	genetics	genética
genetisch	genetic	genético
genital	genital	genital
Genitalien	genitalia	genitales
Genom	genome	genoma
Genotyp	genotype	genotipo
Genus	genus	género
Genu valgum	genu valgum, knock-knee	genu valgum
Genu varum	genu varum	genu varum
Geräusch	murmur	soplo
Geräusch, systolisches	systolic murmur	soplo sistólico
Geriater	geriatrician	geriatra
Geriatrie	geriatrics	geriatría
geriatrisch	geriatric	geriátrico
Gerichtsmedizin	forensic medicine	medicina forense
gerinnen	clot	coagular
Gerinnungshemmer	anticoagulant	anticoagulante
gerontopsychiatrisch	psychogeriatric	psicogeriátrico
Gerstenkorn	stye	orzuelo
Gesäß	breech	nalgas
Gesäß-	posterior	posterior
Gesäßbacke	buttock	nalga
Gesäßmuskulatur	gluteus muscles	músculos glúteos
Geschlechts-	genital	genital
geschlechtsgebunden	sex-linked	vinculado al sexo
Geschlechtskrankheit	sexually transmitted disease (STD), venereal disease (VD)	enfermedad de transmisión sexual (ETS), enfermedad venérea
Geschlechtsverkehr	coitus, intercourse, pareunia, sexual intercourse	coito, pareunia
Geschwister	sibling	hermano no gemelo
geschwollen	swollen, turgid	hinchado, túrgido
Geschwulst	growth	crecimiento
Geschwür	ulcer	úlcera
geschwürig	ulcerative	ulcerativo
Gesicht	facies	facies
Gesichts-	facial	facial
Gesichtsfeld	field of vision	campo de visión
Gesichtsfeldausfall	scotoma	escotoma
Gestation	gestation	gestación
gestielt	pendulous	péndulo
Gesundheit	health	salud
Gewebe	tissue	tejido
Gewerbehygiene	occupational health	higiene profesional

tempérament	temperamento	**Gemütsart**
gène	gene	**Gen**
dénomination commune d'un médicament	medico generico	**Generic**
générique	generico	**generisch**
génétique	genetica	**Genetik**
génétique	genetico	**genetisch**
génital	genitale	**genital**
organes génitaux	organi genitali	**Genitalien**
génome	genoma	**Genom**
génotype	genotipo	**Genotyp**
genre	genere	**Genus**
genu valgum, genou cagneux	ginocchio valgo	**Genu valgum**
genu varum	ginocchio varo	**Genu varum**
murmure	soffio, rullio	**Geräusch**
murmure systolique	soffio sistolico	**Geräusch, systolisches**
gériatre	geriatra	**Geriater**
gériatrie	geriatria	**Geriatrie**
gériatrique	geriatrico	**geriatrisch**
médccine légale	medicina forense	**Gerichtsmedizin**
coaguler	coagulare	**gerinnen**
anticoagulant	anticoagulante	**Gerinnungshemmer**
psychogériatrique	psicogeriatrico	**gerontopsychiatrisch**
orgelet	orzaiolo	**Gerstenkorn**
siège	natica	**Gesäß**
postérieur	posteriore	**Gesäß-**
fesse	natica	**Gesäßbacke**
muscles fessiers	muscoli glutei	**Gesäßmuskulatur**
génital	genitale	**Geschlechts-**
lié au sexe	legato al sesso	**geschlechtsgebunden**
maladie sexuellement transmissible (MST), maladie vénérienne (MV)	malattia a trasmissione sessuale (STD), malattia venerea (MV)	**Geschlechtskrankheit**
coït, rapports, rapports sexuels	coito	**Geschlechtsverkehr**
frère ou soeur	fratello germano	**Geschwister**
enflé	gonfio, tumefatto, turgido	**geschwollen**
croissance	crescìta	**Geschwulst**
ulcère	ulcera	**Geschwür**
ulcératif	ulcerativo, ulceroso	**geschwürig**
faciès	facies	**Gesicht**
facial	facciale	**Gesichts-**
champ de vision	campo visivo	**Gesichtsfeld**
scotome	scotoma	**Gesichtsfeldausfall**
gestation	gestazione	**Gestation**
pendant	pendulo	**gestielt**
santé	salute	**Gesundheit**
tissu	tessuto	**Gewebe**
hygiène du travail	medicina del lavoro	**Gewerbehygiene**

GERMAN	ENGLISH	SPANISH
Gewichtsverlust	weight loss	pérdida de peso
Gewohnheit	habit	hábito
Gewöhnung	addiction, habituation	adicción, toxicomanía, habituación
Gicht	gout	gota
Gichtknoten	tophus	tofo
Giemen	wheeze	jadeo
Gift	poison	veneno
giftig	toxic	tóxico
Gingiva	gingiva	encía
Gingivitis	gingivitis	gingivitis
Gips	gypsum, plaster, plaster of Paris	yeso, escayola
Gipsverband	cast	enyesado, vendaje de yeso
Glandula	gland	glándula
glänzend	lucid	lúcido
Glaskörper	vitreous body	vítreo
Glaskörper-	hyaloid	hialoide
Glaukom	glaucoma	glaucoma
Gleichgewichtsstörung	imbalance	desequilibrio
glenohumeral	glenohumeral	glenohumeral
Glied	limb	extremidad
Gliom	glioma	glioma
Globusgefühl	globus hystericus	globo histérico
Globus hystericus	globus hystericus	globo histérico
glomeruläre Filtrationsrate (GFR)	glomerular filtration rate (GFR)	tasa de filtración glomerular (FG)
Glomerulitis	glomerulitis	glomerulitis
Glomerulonephritis	glomerulonephritis	glomerulonefritis
Glomerulosklerose	glomerulosclerosis	glomerulosclerosis
Glomerulus	glomerulus	glomérulo
Glossitis	glossitis	glositis
Glossodynie	glossodynia	glosodinia
glossopharyngeal	glossopharyngeal	glosofaríngeo
Glottis	glottis	glotis
glue ear	glue ear	otitis media exudativa crónica, tapon de oído
Glukagon	glucagon	glucagón
Glukogenese	glucogenesis	glucogénesis
Glukokortikoid	glucocorticoid	glucocorticoide
Glukoneogenese	gluconeogenesis	gluconeogénesis
Glukose	glucose	glucosa
Glukoseabbau	glycolysis	glucolisis
Glukoseausscheidung im Urin	glycosuria	glucosuria
Glukose-Insulin-Toleranztest	glucose insulin tolerance test (GITT)	prueba de resistencia a la insulina
Glukose-Toleranztest	glucose tolerance test (GTT)	prueba de tolerancia a la glucosa
gluteal	gluteal	glúteo
Glutealmuskulatur	gluteus muscles	músculos glúteos

FRENCH	ITALIAN	GERMAN
perte de poids	perdita di peso	**Gewichtsverlust**
habitude	abitudine	**Gewohnheit**
accoutumance	tossicomania, assuefazione	**Gewöhnung**
goutte	gotta	**Gicht**
tophus	tofo, concrezione tofacea	**Gichtknoten**
wheezing	sibilo	**Giemen**
poison	veleno	**Gift**
toxique	tossico	**giftig**
gencive	gengiva	**Gingiva**
gingivite	gengivite	**Gingivitis**
gypse, plâtre, sulfate de calcium hydraté	gesso, solfato di calcio, gesso di Parigi (calcio solfato diidrato)	**Gips**
plâtre	ingessatura, steccatura	**Gipsverband**
glande	ghiandola	**Glandula**
lucide	lucido	**glänzend**
vitré	corpo vitreo	**Glaskörper**
hyaloïde	ialoideo	**Glaskörper-**
glaucome	glaucoma	**Glaukom**
déséquilibre	squilibrio	**Gleichgewichtsstörung**
gléno-huméral	gleno-omerale	**glenohumeral**
membre	braccio	**Glied**
gliome	glioma	**Gliom**
boule hystérique	bolo isterico	**Globusgefühl**
boule hystérique	bolo isterico	**Globus hystericus**
taux de filtration glomérulaire	volume di filtrazione glomerulare (VFG)	**glomeruläre Filtrationsrate (GFR)**
glomérulite	glomerulite	**Glomerulitis**
glomérulonéphrite	glomerulonefrite	**Glomerulonephritis**
glomérulosclérose	glomerulosclerosi	**Glomerulosklerose**
glomérule	glomerulo	**Glomerulus**
glossite	glossite	**Glossitis**
glossodynie	glossodinia	**Glossodynie**
glossopharyngien	glossofaringeo	**glossopharyngeal**
glotte	glottide	**Glottis**
otite moyenne adhésive	cerume nell orecchio	**glue ear**
glucagon	glucagone	**Glukagon**
glucogenèse	glucogenesi	**Glukogenese**
glucocorticoïde	glicocorticoide	**Glukokortikoid**
gluconéogenèse	gluconeogenesi	**Glukoneogenese**
glucose	glucosio	**Glukose**
glycolyse	glicolisi	**Glukoseabbau**
glycosurie	glicosuria	**Glukoseausscheidung im Urin**
épreuve de tolérance au glucose et à l'insuline	test insulinico di tolleranza al glucosio	**Glukose-Insulin-Toleranztest**
épreuve d'hyperglycémie provoquée	test di tolleranza al glucosio (TTG)	**Glukose-Toleranztest**
fessier	gluteo	**gluteal**
muscles fessiers	muscoli glutei	**Glutealmuskulatur**

GERMAN	ENGLISH	SPANISH
Gluten	gluten	gluten
Glykogenese	glycogenesis	glucogénesis
Glykolyse	glycolysis	glucolisis
Glykosurie	glycosuria	glucosuria
Gonade	gonad	gónada
Gonadotropin	gonadotrophin (Eng), gonadotropin (Am)	gonadotropina
Gonorrhoe	gonorrhea (Am), gonorrhoea (Eng)	gonorrea
Graaf-Follikel	Graafian follicle	folículo de De Graaf
Gramfärbung	Gram stain	tinción de Gram
Grand mal	grand mal	gran mal
Granulation	granulation	granulación
Granulationsgeschwulst	granuloma	granuloma
Granulom	granuloma	granuloma
Granulozyt	granulocyte	granulocito
Gräte	bone	hueso
grauer Star	cataract	catarata
Gravidität	pregnancy	embarazo
Gravitations-	gravitational	gestacional
Grippe	influenza	influenza
Großer Kreislauf	systemic circulation	circulación sistémica
Großhirn	cerebrum	cerebro
Großzeh	hallux	dedo gordo del pie
Grundumsatz	basal metabolic rate (BMR)	tasa de metabolismo basal (MB)
grüner Star	glaucoma	glaucoma
Grünholzfraktur	greenstick fracture	fractura en tallo verde
Grützbeutel	atheroma	ateroma
Gumma	gumma	goma
Gurgelmittel	gargle	gárgara, colutorio
gurgeln	gargle	gargajear
Gürtel	girdle	cintura
Gürtelrose	shingles, zoster	herpes zóster, zóster
gutartig	benign	benigno
Guthrie-Test	Guthrie test	prueba de Guthrie
Gynäkologie	gynaecology (Eng), gynecology (Am)	ginecología
Gynäkomastie	gynaecomastia (Eng), gynecomastia (Am)	ginecomastia

FRENCH	ITALIAN	GERMAN
gluten	glutine	**Gluten**
glycogenèse	glicogenesi	**Glykogenese**
glycolyse	glicolisi	**Glykolyse**
glycosurie	glicosuria	**Glykosurie**
gonade	gonade	**Gonade**
gonadotrophine	gonadotropina	**Gonadotropin**
gonorrhée	gonorrea	**Gonorrhoe**
follicule de De Graaf	follicolo di Graaf	**Graaf-Follikel**
coloration de Gram	colorazione di Gram	**Gramfärbung**
grand mal	grande male	**Grand mal**
granulation	granulazione	**Granulation**
granulome	granuloma	**Granulationsgeschwulst**
granulome	granuloma	**Granulom**
granulocyte	granulocita	**Granulozyt**
os	osso	**Gräte**
cataracte	cataratta	**grauer Star**
grossesse	gravidanza	**Gravidität**
gravitationnel	gravitazionale	**Gravitations-**
grippe	influenza	**Grippe**
circulation systémique	circolazione sistemica	**Großer Kreislauf**
cerveau	cervello	**Großhirn**
hallux	alluce	**Großzeh**
taux du métabolisme basal	indice del metabolismo basale (MB)	**Grundumsatz**
glaucome	glaucoma	**grüner Star**
fracture incomplète	frattura a legno verde	**Grünholzfraktur**
athérome	ateroma	**Grützbeutel**
gomme	gomma	**Gumma**
gargarisme	gargarismi	**Gurgelmittel**
se gargariser	gargarizzare	**gurgeln**
ceinture	cintura	**Gürtel**
zona	herpes zoster	**Gürtelrose**
bénin (bénigne)	benigno	**gutartig**
test de Guthrie	test di Guthrie per la fenilchetonuria	**Guthrie-Test**
gynécologie	ginecologia	**Gynäkologie**
gynécomastie	ginecomastia	**Gynäkomastie**

GERMAN	ENGLISH	SPANISH

H

H2-Antagonist	H2 antagonist	antagonista H2
Haar	hair	pelo
Haarausfall	alopecia	alopecia, calvicie
Habituation	habituation	habituación
Hagelkorn	chalazion	chalacio, orzuelo
Hakenwurm	hookworm	anquilostoma duodenal
Halbmesser	radius	radio
halbmondförmig	semilunar	semilunar
Halbseitenlähmung	hemiplegia	hemiplejía
Halbseitenlähmung, unvollständige	hemiparesis	hemiparesia
Hallux	hallux	dedo gordo del pie
Halluzination	hallucination	alucinación
Hals	neck	cuello
Hals- Nasen- Ohren-	ear nose and throat (ENT)	otorrinolaringología (ORL)
Hämangiom	haemangioma (Eng), hemangioma (Am)	hemangioma
Hämarthros	haemarthrosis (Eng), hemarthrosis (Am)	hemartrosis
Hämatemesis	haematemesis (Eng), hematemesis (Am)	hematemesis
Hämatokolpos	haematocolpos (Eng), hematocolpos (Am)	hematocolpos
Hämatokrit (HKT)	packed cell volume (PCV), haematocrit (Eng), hematocrit (Am)	volumen de células agregadas, hematócrito
Hämatologie	haematology (Eng), hematology (Am)	hematología
Hämatom	haematoma (Eng), hematoma (Am)	hematoma
Hämatoperikard	haemopericardium (Eng), hemopericardium (Am)	hemopericardio
Hämatoperitoneum	haemoperitoneum (Eng), hemoperitoneum (Am)	hemoperitoneo
Hämatopneumothorax	haemopneumothorax (Eng), hemopneumothorax (Am)	hemoneumotórax
Hämatopoese	haemopoiesis (Eng), hemopoiesis (Am)	hemopoyesis
Hämatothorax	haemothorax (Eng), hemothorax (Am)	hemotórax
Hämaturie	haematuria (Eng), hematuria (Am)	hematuria
Hammer	malleus	martillo
Hämochromatose	haemochromatosis (Eng), hemochromatosis (Am)	hemocromatosis
Hämodialyse	haemodialysis (Eng), hemodialysis (Am)	hemodiálisis
Hämoglobin	haemoglobin (Hb) (Hg) (Eng), hemoglobin (Hb) (Hg) (Am)	hemoglobina (Hb)
Hämoglobinopathie	haemoglobinopathy (Eng), hemoglobinopathy (Am)	hemoglobinopatía
Hämoglobinurie	haemoglobinuria (Eng), hemoglobinuria (Am)	hemoglobinuria
Hämolyse	haemolysis (Eng), hemolysis (Am)	hemólisis

464

antagoniste H2	antagonista H2	**H2-Antagonist**
poil	pelo, capello	**Haar**
alopécie	alopecia	**Haarausfall**
accoutumance	assuefazione	**Habituation**
chalazion	calazion	**Hagelkorn**
ankylostome	strongiloide	**Hakenwurm**
radius	radio	**Halbmesser**
semi-lunaire	semilunare	**halbmondförmig**
hémiplégie	emiplegia	**Halbseitenlähmung**
hémiparésie	emiparesi	**Halbseitenlähmung, unvollständige**
hallux	alluce	**Hallux**
hallucination	allucinazione	**Halluzination**
cou	collo	**Hals**
oto-rhino-laryngologie (ORL)	orecchio naso e gola, otorinolaringoiatria	**Hals- Nasen- Ohren-**
hémangiome	emangioma	**Hämangiom**
hémarthrose	emartrosi	**Hämarthros**
hématémèse	ematemesi	**Hämatemesis**
hématocolpos	ematocolpo	**Hämatokolpos**
hématocrite	volume cellulare (VC), ematrocrito	**Hämatokrit (HKT)**
hématologie	ematologia	**Hämatologie**
hématome	ematoma	**Hämatom**
hémopéricarde	emopericardio	**Hämatoperikard**
hémopéritoine	emoperitoneo	**Hämatoperitoneum**
hémopneumothorax	emopneumotorace	**Hämatopneumothorax**
hémopoïèse	ematopolesi	**Hämatopoese**
hémothorax	emotorace	**Hämatothorax**
hématurie	ematuria	**Hämaturie**
marteau	martello	**Hammer**
hémochromatose	emocromatosi	**Hämochromatose**
hémodialyse	emodialisi	**Hämodialyse**
hémoglobine (Hb) (Hg)	emoglobina (E)	**Hämoglobin**
hémoglobinopathie	emoglobinopatia	**Hämoglobinopathie**
hémoglobinurie	emoglobinuria	**Hämoglobinurie**
hémolyse	emolisi	**Hämolyse**

GERMAN	ENGLISH	SPANISH
hämolytisch-urämisches Syndrom	haemolytic uraemic syndrome (HUS) (Eng), hemolytic uremic syndrome (HUS) (Am)	síndrome hemolítico urémico
Hämophilie	haemophilia (Eng), hemophilia (Am)	hemofilia
Hämoptoe	haemoptysis (Eng), hemoptysis (Am)	hemoptisis
Hämorrhagie	haemorrhage (Eng), hemorrhage (Am)	hemorragia
Hämorrhoide	haemorrhoid (Eng), hemorrhoid (Am)	hemorroide
Hämorrhoidektomie	haemorrhoidectomy (Eng), hemorrhoidectomy (Am)	hemorroidectomía
Hämorrhoiden	piles	hemorroides
Hämorrhoidenoperation	haemorrhoidectomy (Eng), hemorrhoidectomy (Am)	hemorroidectomía
Hämostase	haemostasis (Eng), hemostasis (Am)	hemostasis
Hand	hand	mano
Handgelenk	wrist	muñeca
Handhabung	manipulation	manipulación
Handinnenfläche	palm	palma
hängend	pendulous	péndulo
harmlos	innocuous	inocuo
Harn	urine	orina
Harnblase	bladder	vejiga
Harnleiter	ureter	uréter
Harnröhre	urethra	uretra
Harnsäure	uric acid	ácido úrico
Harnstoff	urea	urea
Harnvergiftung	uraemia (Eng)	uremia
Harnverhaltung	anuria	anuria
Harnwegsinfekt	urinary tract infection (UTI)	infección de las vías urinarias (IVU)
Harnzwang	strangury	estranguria
Harrington Stab	Harrington rod	varilla de Harrington
Hartmann-Lösung	Hartmann's solution	solución de Hartmann
Hasenscharte	harelip	labio leporino
Hashimoto-Struma	Hashimoto's disease	enfermedad de Hashimoto
Hauptschlagader	aorta	aorta
Haut	dermis, skin	dermis, piel
Haut-	cutaneous	cutáneo
Hautausschlag	rash	exantema
Hautblase	blister	vesícula, ampolla, flictena
Häutchen	cuticle	cutícula
Hauterkrankung	dermatosis	dermatosis
Hautlappen	flap	colgajo, injerto
Hautmesser	dermatome	dermátomo
Heaf-Test	Heaf test	prueba de Heaf
Hebamme	midwife	comadrona
Hebephrenie	hebephrenia	hebefrenia
Hefe	yeast	levadura
Hefepilz	yeast	levadura
Heilung	healing	curación

466

FRENCH	ITALIAN	GERMAN
hémolyse urémique des nouveau-nés	sindrome emolitico-uremica	**hämolytisch-urämisches Syndrom**
hémophilie	emofilia	**Hämophilie**
hémoptysie	cartilagine costale	**Hämoptoe**
hémorragie	emorragia	**Hämorrhagie**
hémorroïde	emorroide	**Hämorrhoide**
hémorroïdectomie	emorroidectomia	**Hämorrhoidektomie**
hémorroïdes	emorroidi	**Hämorrhoiden**
hémorroïdectomie	emorroidectomia	**Hämorrhoidenoperation**
hémostase	emostasi	**Hämostase**
main	mano	**Hand**
poignet	polso	**Handgelenk**
manipulation	manipolazione	**Handhabung**
paume	palmo	**Handinnenfläche**
pendant	pendulo	**hängend**
inoffensif	innocuo	**harmlos**
urine	urina	**Harn**
vessie	vescica	**Harnblase**
uretère	uretere	**Harnleiter**
urètre	uretra	**Harnröhre**
acide urique	acido urico	**Harnsäure**
urée	urea, carbammide	**Harnstoff**
urémie	uremia	**Harnvergiftung**
anurie	anuria	**Harnverhaltung**
infection des voies urinaires	infezione delle vie urinarie (IVU)	**Harnwegsinfekt**
strangurie	stranguria	**Harnzwang**
tige de Harrington	bastoncello retinico (per anestetizzare la dentina)	**Harrington Stab**
liquide de Hartmann	soluzione di Hartmann	**Hartmann-Lösung**
bec-de-lièvre	labbro leporino	**Hasenscharte**
maladie d'Hashimoto	tiroidite di Hashimoto	**Hashimoto-Struma**
aorte	aorta	**Hauptschlagader**
derme, peau	derma, pelle	**Haut**
cutané	cutaneo	**Haut-**
rash	eruzione cutanea	**Hautausschlag**
ampoule	vescicola, bolla	**Hautblase**
cuticule	cuticola	**Häutchen**
dermatose	dermatosi	**Hauterkrankung**
lambeau	lembo, innesto	**Hautlappen**
dermatome	dermatomo	**Hautmesser**
cuti-réaction de Heaf	test alla tubercolina	**Heaf-Test**
sage-femme	levatrice	**Hebamme**
hébéphrénie	ebefrenia	**Hebephrenie**
levure	lievito	**Hefe**
levure	lievito	**Hefepilz**
curatif	cicatrizzazione, guarigione	**Heilung**

German	English	Spanish
heimtückisch	insidious	insidioso
Helfer-Syndrom	burnout syndrome	surmenage, neurastenia
Hemikolektomie	hemicolectomy	hemocolectomía
Hemiparese	hemiparesis	hemiparesia
Hemiplegie	hemiplegia	hemiplejía
Hemmung	inhibition, retardation	inhibición, retraso
hepatisch	hepatic	hepático
Hepatitis	hepatitis	hepatitis
Hepatom	hepatoma	hepatoma
Hepatomegalie	hepatomegaly	hepatomegalia
Hepatosplenomegalie	hepatosplenomegaly	hepatosplenomegalia
hepatozellulär	hepatocellular	hepatocelular
hereditär	hereditary	hereditario
Hermaphrodit	hermaphrodite	hermafrodita
Hernie	hernia	hernia
Hernie, inkarzerierte	strangulated hernia	hernia estrangulada
Herniotomie	herniotomy	herniotomía
Herpes	cold sore, herpes	herpes labial, herpes
Herpes-ähnlicher Virus	herpes-like virus (HLV)	virus semejante al del herpes (HLV)
Herpes simplex-Virus (HSV)	herpes simplex virus (HSV)	virus del herpes simple (VHS)
Herpes zoster	shingles, zoster	herpes zóster, zóster
Herz	heart	corazón
Herz-	cardiac	cardíaco
Herzbeutel	pericardium	pericardio
Herzerkrankung	heart disease	cardiopatía
Herzgeräusch	murmur	soplo
Herzinfarkt	coronary heart failure (CHF), myocardial infarction (MI)	insuficiencia coronaria, infarto de miocardio (IM)
Herzinsuffizienz	heart failure	insuficiencia cardíaca
Herzinsuffizienz mit Stauungszeichen	congestive cardiac failure (CCF), congestive heart failure (CHF)	insuficiencia cardíaca congestiva (ICC)
Herzklopfen	palpitation	palpitación
Herzleiden	heart disease	cardiopatía
Herz-Lungen-	cardiopulmonary	cardiopulmonar
Herzlungenmaschine	heart-lung machine	máquina de circulación extracorpórea
Herz-Lungen-Wiederbelebung	cardiopulmonary resuscitation (CPR)	resucitación cardiopulmonar
Herzmuskel	myocardium	miocardio
Herzmuskelentzündung	myocarditis	miocarditis
herzschädigend	cardiotoxic	cardiotóxico
Herzschlag	heartbeat	patido cardíaco
Herzversagen	heart failure	insuficiencia cardíaca
heterogen	heterogenous	heterogéneo
heterolog	atypical	atípico
heterosexuell	heterosexual	heterosexual
Heuschnupfen	hay fever	fiebre del heno
Hexenschuß	lumbago	lumbago

FRENCH	ITALIAN	GERMAN
insidieux	insidioso	heimtückisch
syndrome de 'surmenage'	incapacità ad agire, sindrome di esaurimento professionale	Helfer-Syndrom
hémicolectomie	emicolectomia	Hemikolektomie
hémiparésie	emiparesi	Hemiparese
hémiplégie	emiplegia	Hemiplegie
inhibition, retard	inibizione, ritardo mentale, psicomotorio	Hemmung
hépatique	epatico	hepatisch
hépatite	epatite	Hepatitis
hépatome	epatoma	Hepatom
hépatomégalie	epatomegalia	Hepatomegalie
hépatosplénomégalie	epatosplenomegalia	Hepatosplenomegalie
hépatocellulaire	epatocellulare	hepatozellulär
héréditaire	ereditario	hereditär
hermaphrodite	ermafrodito	Hermaphrodit
hernie	ernia	Hernie
hernie étranglée	ernia strozzata	Hernie, inkarzerierte
herniotomie	erniotomia	Herniotomie
herpès	herpes, labialis	Herpes
virus de type herpétique (HLV)	virus della famiglia dell'herpes	Herpes-ähnlicher Virus
virus de l'herpès simplex (HSV)	virus herpes simplex	Herpes simplex-Virus (HSV)
zona	herpes zoster	Herpes zoster
coeur	cuore	Herz
cardiaque	cardiaco	Herz-
péricarde	pericardio	Herzbeutel
insuffisance cardiaque	malattia cardiaca	Herzerkrankung
murmure	soffio, rullio	Herzgeräusch
insuffisance coronarienne cardiaque, infarctus du myocarde	insufficienza cardiaca coronarica, infarto miocardico	Herzinfarkt
cardiopathie, maladie du coeur	scompenso cardiaco	Herzinsuffizienz
insuffisance cardiaque globale	insufficienza cardiaca congestizia, scompenso cardiaco congestizio	Herzinsuffizienz mit Stauungszeichen
palpitation	palpitazione	Herzklopfen
insuffisance cardiaque	malattia cardiaca	Herzleiden
cardiopulmonaire	cardiopolmonare	Herz-Lungen-
poumon d'acier	macchina cuore-polmone	Herzlungenmaschine
réanimation cardiorespiratoire	rianimazione cardiorespiratoria	Herz-Lungen-Wiederbelebung
myocarde	miocardio	Herzmuskel
myocardite	miocardite	Herzmuskelentzündung
cardiotoxique	cardiotossico	herzschädigend
pulsation (de coeur)	battito cardiaco	Herzschlag
cardiopathie, maladie du coeur	scompenso cardiaco	Herzversagen
hétérogène	eterogenico	heterogen
atypique	atipico	heterolog
hétérosexuel	eterosessuale	heterosexuell
rhume des foins	febbre da fieno, raffreddore da fieno	Heuschnupfen
lumbago	lombaggine	Hexenschuß

GERMAN	ENGLISH	SPANISH
Hidrosis	hidrosis	hidrosis
high density lipoprotein (HDL)	high density lipoprotein (HDL)	lipoproteína de alta densidad (HDL)
high density lipoprotein-cholesterol (HDL-Cholesterol)	high density lipoprotein cholesterol (HDLC)	colesterol unido a las lipoproteínas de alta densidad (HDLC)
Hilus	hilum	hilio
Hinken	claudication	claudicación
hintere	posterior	posterior
Hinterhauptslage, hintere	occipitoposterior	occipitoposterior
Hinterhauptslage, linke vordere	left occipito-anterior (LOA)	occipito anterior izquierdo
Hinterhauptslage, vordere	occipitoanterior	occipitoanterior
Hinterkopf	occiput	occipucio
Hirndruck	intracranial pressure (ICP)	presión intracraneal (PIC)
Hirnhäute	meninges	meninges
Hirnnerv	cranial nerve	nervio craneal
Hirschsprung-Krankheit	Hirschsprung's disease, megacolon	enfermedad de Hirschsprung, megacolon
Hirsutismus	hirsuties, hirsutism	hirsutismo
Histiozyt	histiocyte	histiocito
Histiozytom	histiocytoma	histiocitoma
Histokompatibilitäts-Antigen	histocompatibility antigen	antígeno de histocompatibilidad
Histologie	histology	histología
Histolyse	histolysis	histólisis
Hitze	calor	calor
Hitzschlag	heat exhaustion, heatstroke	agotamiento por calor, insolación
Hoden	orchis, testis	testículo
Hodensack	scrotum	escroto
Höhenkrankheit	altitude sickness	mal de altura
Höhle	cavity	cavidad
Holzkohle	charcoal	carbón vegetal
homogen	homogeneous (Eng), homogenous (Am)	homogéneo
homolog	homologous	homólogo
homonym	homonymous	homónimo
Homöopathie	homeopathy (Am), homoeopathy (Eng)	homeopatía
Homöostase	homeostasis	homeostasis
homosexuell	homosexual	homosexual
Homosexueller	homosexual	homosexual
Homovanillinsäure	homovanillic acid (HVA)	ácido homovaníllico
homozygot	homozygous	homocigoto
Hör-	auditory, acoustic, aural	auditorio, acústico, aural
Hordeolum	stye	orzuelo
Hören	hearing	oído
Hörkurve	audiogram	audiograma
Hormon	hormone	hormona
Hormonsubstitutionstherapie	hormone replacement therapy (HRT)	terapéutica de reposición de hormonas

FRENCH	ITALIAN	GERMAN
transpiration	idrosi, sudorazione	**Hidrosis**
lipoprotéine de haute densité (LHD)	lipoproteina ad alta densità (LAD)	**high density lipoprotein (HDL)**
cholestérol composé de lipoprotéines de haute densité	colesterolo legato a lipoproteina ad alta densità	**high density lipoprotein-cholesterol (HDL-Cholesterol)**
hile	ilo	**Hilus**
claudication	claudicazione	**Hinken**
postérieur	posteriore	**hintere**
occipito-postérieur	occipitoposteriore	**Hinterhauptslage, hintere**
occipito-antérieur gauche	occipitoanteriore sinistro (OAS)	**Hinterhauptslage, linke vordere**
occipito-antérieur	occipitoanteriore	**Hinterhauptslage, vordere**
occiput	occipite	**Hinterkopf**
pression intracrânienne	pressione intracranica	**Hirndruck**
méninges	meningi	**Hirnhäute**
nerf crânien	nervo craniale	**Hirnnerv**
maladie de Hirschsprung, mégacôlon	malattia di Hirschsprung, megacolon	**Hirschsprung-Krankheit**
hirsutisme	irsutismo	**Hirsutismus**
histiocyte	istiocito	**Histiozyt**
histiocytome	istiocitoma	**Histiozytom**
antigène d'histocompatibilité	antigene di istocompatibilità	**Histokompatibilitäts-Antigen**
histologie	istologia	**Histologie**
histolyse	istolisi	**Histolyse**
chaleur	calore	**Hitze**
échauffement, coup de chaleur	collasso da colpo di calore, colpo di calore	**Hitzschlag**
testicule	testicolo	**Hoden**
scrotum	scroto	**Hodensack**
mal d'altitude, mal des montagnes	mal di montagna	**Höhenkrankheit**
cavité	cavità	**Höhle**
charbon	carbone vegetale	**Holzkohle**
homogène	omogeneo	**homogen**
homologue	omologo	**homolog**
homonyme	omonimo	**homonym**
homéopathie	omeopatia	**Homöopathie**
homéostasie	omeostasi	**Homöostase**
homosexuel	omosessuale	**homosexuell**
homosexuel	omosessuale	**Homosexueller**
acide homovanillique	acido omovanillico	**Homovanillinsäure**
homozygote	omozigote	**homozygot**
auditif, acoustique, aural	auditivo, acustico, auricolare	**Hör-**
orgelet	orzaiolo	**Hordeolum**
audition	udito	**Hören**
audiogramme	audiogramma	**Hörkurve**
hormone	ormone	**Hormon**
traitement hormonal substitutif, hormonothérapie supplétive	terapia sostitutiva ormonale	**Hormonsubstitutionstherapie**

GERMAN	ENGLISH	SPANISH
Horner-Syndrom	Horner's syndrome	síndrome de Horner
Hornhaut	callosity	callosidad
Hornhaut (des Auges)	cornea	córnea
Hornhautentzündung	keratitis	queratitis
Hörtest	hearing test	prueba auditiva
Hospital	hospital	hospital
Hospiz	hospice	hospicio
Hüfte	hip	cadera
Hüftgelenkspfanne	acetabulum	acetábulo
Hüftknochen	hip bone	hueso coxal o ilíaco
Hühnerauge	corn	callo, papiloma
Hühnerbrust	pigeon chest	tórax de pichón
human chorionic somatomammotropin (HCS)	human chorionic somatomammotrophin (HCS) (Eng), human chorionic somatomammotropin (HCS, HPL) (Am)	somatomamotropina corionica humana
Human-Gammaglobulin	human gamma globulin (HGG)	gammaglobulina humana
human immunodeficiency virus (HIV)	human immunodeficiency virus (HIV)	virus de la inmunodeficiencia humana (VIH)
human lymphocytic antigen (HLA)	human lymphocytic antigen (HLA)	antígeno linfocitario humano (HLA)
human T-cell leukemia virus (HTLV)	human T-cell leukaemia virus (HTLV) (Eng), human T-cell leukemia virus (HTLV) (Am)	leucemia por virus humano de las células T
Humerus	humerus	húmero
Hunde-	canine	canino
Hunger	hunger	hambre
Husten	cough	tos
husten	cough	toser
Hustenmittel	antitussive	antitusígeno
Hyalinmembrankrankheit	hyaline membrane disease	enfermedad de la membrana hialina
Hyalitis	hyalitis	hialitis
Hydatide	hydatid	quiste hidatídico
Hydramnion	hydramnios	hidramnios
Hydrat	hydrate	hidrato
hydratisieren	hydrate	hidratar
hydrieren	hydrate	hidratar
Hydrolyse	hydrolysis	hidrólisis
Hydronephrose	hydronephrosis	hidronefrosis
Hydrops fetalis	hydrops fetalis	hydrops fetal
Hydrosalpinx	hydrosalpinx	hidrosálpinx
Hydrozele	hydrocele	hidrocele
Hydrozephalus	hydrocephalus	hidrocéfalo
Hygiene	hygiene	higiene
Hygrom	hygroma	higroma
Hymen	hymen	himen
Hypästhesie	hypoaesthesia (Eng), hypoesthesia (Am)	hipoestesia

472

FRENCH	ITALIAN	GERMAN
syndrome de Bernard-Horner, syndrome oculaire sympathique	sindrome di Horner	**Horner-Syndrom**
callosité	callosità	**Hornhaut**
cornée	cornea	**Hornhaut (des Auges)**
kératite	cheratite	**Hornhautentzündung**
test auditif	test audiometrici	**Hörtest**
hôpital	ospedale	**Hospital**
hospice, asile	ricovero	**Hospiz**
hanche	anca	**Hüfte**
acétabule	acetabolo	**Hüftgelenkspfanne**
os coxal	osso iliaco	**Hüftknochen**
cor	callo	**Hühnerauge**
thorax en carène	torace carenato	**Hühnerbrust**
somatomammotropine chorionique humaine (HCS), somatoprolactine chorionique humain	somatomammotropina corionica umana	**human chorionic somatomammotropin (HCS)**
gamma-globuline humaine (GGH), globuline humaine	gammaglobulina umana	**Human-Gammaglobulin**
virus de l'immunodéficience humaine	virus dell'immunodeficienza umana (HIV)	**human immunodeficiency virus (HIV)**
antigène lymphocytaire humain	antigene linfocitario umano	**human lymphocytic antigen (HLA)**
leucémie humaine à lymphocytes T	virus della leucemia a cellule T	**human T-cell leukemia virus (HTLV)**
humérus	omero	**Humerus**
canin	canino	**Hunde-**
faim	fame	**Hunger**
toux	tosse	**Husten**
tousser	tossire	**husten**
antitussif	antibechico	**Hustenmittel**
maladie des membranes hyalines	malattia delle membrane ialine	**Hyalinmembrankrankheit**
hyalite	ialinite	**Hyalitis**
kyste hydatique	cisti idatidea	**Hydatide**
hydramnios	idramnios	**Hydramnion**
hydrate	idrato	**Hydrat**
hydrater	idratare	**hydratisieren**
hydrater	idratare	**hydrieren**
hydrolyse	idrolisi	**Hydrolyse**
hydronéphrose	idronefrosi	**Hydronephrose**
anasarque foeto-placentaire	idrope fetale	**Hydrops fetalis**
hydrosalpinx	idrosalpinge	**Hydrosalpinx**
hydrocèle	idrocele	**Hydrozele**
hydrocéphale	idrocefalo	**Hydrocephalus**
hygiène	igiene	**Hygiene**
hygroma	igroma	**Hygrom**
hymen	imene	**Hymen**
hypoesthésie, hypesthésie	ipoestesia	**Hypästhesie**

GERMAN	ENGLISH	SPANISH
Hymenektomie	hymenectomy	himenectomía
Hyperalgesie	hyperalgesia	hiperalgesia
Hyperämie	hyperaemia (Eng), hyperemia (Am)	hiperemia
Hyperästhesie	hyperaesthesia (Eng), hyperesthesia (Am)	hiperestesia
Hyperazidität	hyperacidity	hiperacidez
hyperbare Sauerstoffbehandlung	hyperbaric oxygen treatment	tratamiento con oxígeno hiperbárico
Hyperbilirubinämie	hyperbilirubinaemia (Eng), hyperbilirubinemia (Am)	hiperbilirrubinemia
Hypercholesterinämie	hypercholesterolaemia (Eng), hypercholesterolemia (Am)	hipercolesterolemia
Hyperemesis	hyperemesis	hiperemesis
Hyperflexion	hyperflexion	hiperflexión
Hyperglykämie	hyperglycaemia (Eng), hyperglycemia (Am)	hiperglucemia
Hyperhidrosis	hyperidrosis	hiperhidrosis
Hyperkaliämie	hyperkalaemia (Eng), hyperkalemia (Am)	hipercaliemia
Hyperkalzämie	hypercalcaemia (Eng), hypercalcemia (Am)	hipercalcemia
Hyperkalziurie	hypercalciuria	hipercalciuria
Hyperkapnie	hypercapnia	hipercapnia
hyperkinetisches Syndrom	hyperkinetic syndrome	síndrome hipercinético
Hyperlipämie	hyperlipaemia (Eng), hyperlipemia (Am)	hiperlipemia
Hyperlipoproteinämie	hyperlipoproteinaemia (Eng), hyperlipoproteinemia (Am)	hiperlipoproteinemia
Hypermetropie	hypermetropia	hipermetropía
Hypernephrom	hypernephroma	hipernefroma
Hyperparathyreoidismus	hyperparathyroidism	hiperparatiroidismo
Hyperpigmentierung	chloasma	cloasma
Hyperplasie	hyperplasia	hiperplasia
Hyperpnoe	hyperpnea (Am), hyperpnoea (Eng)	hiperpnea
Hyperpyrexie	hyperpyrexia	hiperpirexia
Hypersensibilität	hypersensitive	hipersensibilidad
Hypertelorismus	hypertelorism	hipertelorismo
Hypertension	hypertonia	hipertonía
Hyperthermie	hyperthermia	hipertermia
Hyperthyreoidismus	hyperthyroidism	hipertiroidismo
hyperton	hypertonic	hipertónico
Hypertonie	hypertension	hipertensión
Hypertonus	hypertonia	hipertonía
Hypertrophie	hypertrophy	hipertrofia
Hyperventilation	hyperventilation	hiperventilación
Hypervolämie	hypervolaemia (Eng), hypervolemia (Am)	hipervolemia
Hyphaema	hyphaema (Eng), hyphema (Am)	hipema
Hypnose	hypnosis	hipnosis
Hypnotherapie	hypnotherapy	hipnoterapia
Hypnotikum	hypnotic	hipnótico

hymenectomie	imenectomia	**Hymenektomie**
hyperalgie, hyperalgésie	iperalgesia	**Hyperalgesie**
hyperémie	iperemia	**Hyperämie**
hyperesthésie	iperestesia	**Hyperästhesie**
hyperacidité	iperacidità	**Hyperazidität**
oxygénothérapie hyperbase	ossigenoterapia iperbarica	hyperbare Sauerstoffbehandlung
hyperbilirubinémie	iperbilirubinemia	**Hyperbilirubinämie**
hypercholestérolémie	ipercolesterolemia	**Hypercholesterinämie**
hyperémèse	iperemesi	**Hyperemesis**
hyperflexion	iperflessione	**Hyperflexion**
hyperglycémie	iperglicemia	**Hyperglykämie**
hyperhidrose	iperidrosi	**Hyperhidrosis**
hyperkaliémie	iperkaliemia, iperpotassiemia	**Hyperkaliämie**
hypercalcémie	ipercalcemia	**Hyperkalzämie**
hypercalciurie	ipercalciuria	**Hyperkalziurie**
hypercapnie	ipercapnia	**Hyperkapnie**
syndrome hyperkinétique	sindrome ipercinetica	hyperkinetisches Syndrom
hyperlipémie	iperlipemia	**Hyperlipämie**
hyperlipoprotéinémie	iperlipoproteinemia	**Hyperlipoproteinämie**
hypermétropie	ipermetropia	**Hypermetropie**
hypernéphrome	ipernefroma	**Hypernephrom**
hyperparathyroïdisme	iperparatiroidismo	**Hyperparathyreoidismus**
chloasma	cloasma	**Hyperpigmentierung**
hyperplasie	iperplasia	**Hyperplasie**
hyperpnoïa	iperpnea	**Hyperpnoe**
hyperpyrexie	iperpiressia	**Hyperpyrexie**
hypersensibilité	ipersensitività, ipersensibilità	**Hypersensibilität**
hypertélorisme	ipertelorismo	**Hypertelorismus**
hypertonie	ipertonia	**Hypertension**
hyperthermie	ipertermia	**Hyperthermie**
hyperthyroïdisme	ipertiroidismo	**Hyperthyreoidismus**
hypertonique	ipertonico	**hyperton**
hypertension	ipertensione	**Hypertonie**
hypertonie	ipertonia	**Hypertonus**
hypertrophie	ipertrofia	**Hypertrophie**
hyperventilation	iperventilazione	**Hyperventilation**
hypervolémie	ipervolemia	**Hypervolämie**
hyphèma	ifema	**Hyphaema**
hypnose	ipnosi	**Hypnose**
hypnothérapie	ipnoterapia	**Hypnotherapie**
hypnotique	ipnotico	**Hypnotikum**

hypnotisch	hypnotic	hipnótico
Hypochondrie	hypochondria	hipocondría
Hypochondrium	hypochondrium	hipocondrio
hypochrom	hypochromic	hipocrómico
Hypogastrium	hypogastrium	hipogastrio
Hypoglykämie	hypoglycaemia (Eng), hypoglycemia (Am)	hipoglucemia
Hypohidrosis	hypoidrosis	hipohidrosis
Hypokaliämie	hypokalaemia (Eng), hypokalemia (Am)	hipocaliemia
Hypokalzämie	hypocalcaemia (Eng), hypocalcemia (Am)	hipocalcemia
Hypokapnie	hypocapnia	hipocapnia
Hypomanie	hypomania	hipomanía
Hypoparathyreoidismus	hypoparathyroidism	hipoparatiroidismo
Hypopharynx	hypopharynx	hipofaringe
Hypophyse	pituitary gland	hipófisis
Hypopituitarismus	hypopituitarism	hipopituitarismo
Hypoplasie	hypoplasia	hipoplasia
Hypoproteinämie	hypoproteinaemia (Eng), hypoproteinemia (Am)	hipoproteinemia
Hypopyon	hypopyon	hipopión
hyposensibel	hyposensitive	hiposensibilidad
Hypospadie	hypospadias	hipospadias
Hypostase	hypostasis	hipostasis
Hypothalamus	hypothalamus	hipotálamo
Hypothermie	hypothermia	hipotermia
Hypothyreose	hypothyroidism	hipotiroidismo
hypoton	hypotonic	hipotónico
Hypotonie	hypotension, hypotonia	hipotensión, hipotonía
Hypoventilation	hypoventilation	hipoventilación
Hypovolämie	hypovolaemia (Eng), hypovolemia (Am)	hipovolemia
Hypoxämie	hypoxaemia (Eng), hypoxemia (Am)	hipoxemia
Hypoxie	hypoxia	hipoxia
Hysterektomie	hysterectomy	histerectomía
Hysterie	hysteria	histeria
Hysteropexie	ventrofixation	ventrofijación
Hysterosalpingektomie	hysterosalpingectomy	histerosalpingectomía
Hysterosalpingographie	hysterosalpingography	histerosalpingografía
Hysterotomie	hysterotomy	histerotomía

FRENCH	ITALIAN	GERMAN
hypnotique	ipnotico	hypnotisch
hypocondrie	ipocondria	Hypochondrie
hypocondre	ipocondrio	Hypochondrium
hypochromique	ipocromico	hypochrom
hypogastre	ipogastrio	Hypogastrium
hypoglycémie	ipoglicemia	Hypoglykämie
hypohidrose	ipoidrosi	Hypohidrosis
hypokalémie	ipokalemia	Hypokaliämie
hypocalcémie	ipocalcemia	Hypokalzämie
hypocapnie	ipocapnia	Hypokapnie
hypomanie	ipomania	Hypomanie
hypoparathyroïdisme	ipoparatiroidismo	Hypoparathyreoidismus
hypopharynx	ipofaringe	Hypopharynx
hypophyse	ghiandola pituitaria, ipofisi	Hypophyse
hypopituitarisme	ipopituitarismo	Hypopituitarismus
hypoplasie	ipoplasia	Hypoplasie
hypoprotéinémie	ipoproteinemia	Hypoproteinämie
hypopyon	ipopion	Hypopyon
hyposensibilité	iposensitività, iposensibilità	hyposensibel
hypospadias	ipospadia	Hypospadie
hypostase	ipostasi	Hypostase
hypothalamus	ipotalamo	Hypothalamus
hypothermie	ipotermia	Hypothermie
hypothyroïdisme	ipotiroidismo	Hypothyreose
hypotonique	ipotonico	hypoton
hypotension, hypotonie	ipotensione, ipotonia	Hypotonie
hypoventilation	ipoventilazione	Hypoventilation
hypovolémie	ipovolemia	Hypovolämie
hypoxémie	ipossiemia	Hypoxämie
hypoxie	ipossia	Hypoxie
hystérectomie	isterectomia	Hysterektomie
hystérie	isteria	Hysterie
hystéropexie abdominale	ventro-fissazione	Hysteropexie
hystérosalpingectomie	isterosalpingectomia	Hysterosalpingektomie
hystérosalpingographie	isterosalpingografia	Hysterosalpingographie
hystérotomie	isterotomia	Hysterotomie

I

German	English	Spanish
iatrogen	iatrogenic	yatrógeno
Ichthyosis	ichthyosis	ictiosis
Ideenflucht	flight of ideas	fuga de ideas
Identifizierung	identification	identificación
idiopathisch	idiopathic	idiopático
Idiosynkrasie	idiosyncrasy	idiosincrasia
Ikterus	icterus, jaundice	ictericia
Ileitis	ileitis	ileítis
Ileitis regionalis	regional ileitis	ileítis regional
ileo-	iliac	ilíaco
Ileostomie	ileostomy	ileostomía
ileozäkal	ileocaecal (Eng), ileocecal (Am)	ileocecal
Ileum	ileum	ileón
Ileumconduit	ileal conduit	conducto ileal
Ileumresektion	ileectomy	ileoctomía
Ileus	ileus	íleo
Iliosakral-	sacroiliac	sacroíliaco
Illusion	illusion	ilusión
immun	immune	inmune
Immundefekt	immunodeficiency	inmunodeficiencia
Immundefektsyndrom, erworbenes (AIDS)	acquired immune deficiency syndrome (AIDS)	síndrome de inmunodeficiencia adquirida (SIDA)
Immunfluoreszenz	immunofluorescence	inmunofluorescencia
immungestörter Patient	immunocompromised patient	paciente inmunocomprometido
Immunglobulin	immunoglobulin (Ig)	inmunoglobulina (Ig)
Immunisierung	immunization	inmunización
Immunität	immunity	inmunidad
Immunoassay	immunoassay	inmunoensayo
Immunologie	immunology	inmunología
Immunreaktion	immune reaction	reacción inmunológica
Immunserum	antiserum	antisuero
Immunsuppression	immunosuppression	inmunosupresión
immunsupprimierter Patient	immunosuppressed patient	paciente inmunosuprimido
impaktiert	impacted	impactado
Impetigo	impetigo	impétigo
Impfstoff	vaccine	vacuna
Impfung	inoculation, vaccination	inoculación, vacunación
Implantat	implant	implante
Implantation	implantation	implantación
implantieren	implant	implantar
Impotenz	impotence	impotencia
Impressionsfraktur	depressed fracture	fractura con hundimiento
Impuls	impulse	impulso

FRENCH	ITALIAN	GERMAN
iatrogène	iatrogeno	**iatrogen**
ichthyose	ittiosi	**Ichthyosis**
fuite des idées	fuga delle idee	**Ideenflucht**
identification	indentificazione	**Identifizierung**
idiopathique	idiopatico	**idiopathisch**
idiosyncrasie	idiosincrasia	**Idiosynkrasie**
ictère, jaunisse	ittero	**Ikterus**
iléite	ileite	**Ileitis**
iléite régionale	ileite regionale	**Ileitis regionalis**
iliaque	iliaco	**ileo-**
iléostomie	ileostomia	**Ileostomie**
iléocaecal	ileocecale	**ileozäkal**
iléon	ileo	**Ileum**
conduit iléal	vescica ileale (protesi mediante segmento ileale)	**Ileumconduit**
iléoctomie	ileectomia	**Ileumresektion**
iléus	ileo, occlusione intestinale acuta	**Ileus**
sacro-iliaque	sacroiliaco	**Iliosakral-**
illusion	illusione	**Illusion**
immun	immune	**immun**
immunodéficience	immunodeficienza	**Immundefekt**
syndrome d'immuno-déficience acquise (SIDA)	sindrome da immunodeficienza acquisita (AIDS)	**Immundefektsyndrom, erworbenes (AIDS)**
immunofluorescence	immunofluorescenza	**Immunfluoreszenz**
malade à déficit immunitaire	paziente immunocompromesso	**immungestörter Patient**
immunoglobuline (lg)	immunoglobulina (Ig)	**Immunglobulin**
immunisation	immunizzazione	**Immunisierung**
immunité	immunità	**Immunität**
dosage immunologique, immunodosage	dosaggio immunologico	**Immunoassay**
immunologie	immunologia	**Immunologie**
réaction immunitaire	immunoreazione, reazione immune	**Immunreaktion**
anti-serum	anti-siero	**Immunserum**
immunosuppression	immunosoppressione	**Immunsuppression**
malade à suppression immunitaire	paziente immunosoppresso	**immunsupprimierter Patient**
enclavé	impatto, compresso, incuneato	**impaktiert**
impétigo	impetigine	**Impetigo**
vaccin	vaccino	**Impfstoff**
inoculation, vaccination	inoculazione, vaccinazione	**Impfung**
implant	impianto chirurgico sottocutaneo di farmaci	**Implantat**
implantation	impianto	**Implantation**
implanter	impiantare	**implantieren**
impotence	impotenza	**Impotenz**
enfoncement localisé	frattura con infossamento dei frammenti	**Impressionsfraktur**
impulsion	impulso	**Impuls**

German	English	Spanish
Incus	incus	incus, yunque
Indikator	indicator	indicador
Induktion	induction	inducción
Induration	induration	induración
Induratio penis plastica	Peyronie's disease	enfermedad de Peyronie
infantil	infantile	infantil
Infarktpflegestation	coronary care unit (CCU)	unidad de cuidados coronarios (UCC)
Infarzierung	infarction	infarto
Infektion	infection	infección
Infektion, opportunistische	opportunistic infection	infección oportunista
Infektionskrankheit	infectious disease	enfermedad infecciosa
infektiös	infective	infeccioso
Infertilität	infertility	infertilidad
Infiltration	infiltration	infiltración
Influenza	influenza	influenza
Infusion	infusion	infusión
inguinal	inguinal	inguinal
Inhalation	inhalation	inhalación
inhalieren	inhale	inhalar
Inhibierung	inhibition	inhibición
Injektion	injection, puncture	inyección, punción
injizieren	inject, puncture	inyectar, pinchar
inkarzeriert	incarcerated	incarcerado
Inkompatibilität	incompatibility	incompatibilidad
Inkontinenz	incontinence	incontinencia
Inkoordination	incoordination	incoordinación
Inkubation	incubation	incubación
Inkubator	incubator	incubadora
innerlich	internal	interno
Innervation	innervation	inervación
inotrop	inotropic	inotrópico
Insemination, heterologe	artificial insemination by donor (AID)	inseminación artificial por donante (AID)
Insertion	insertion	inserción
in situ	in situ	in situ
Inspiration	inspiration	inspiración
Instinkt	instinct	instinto
Institutionalisierung	institutionalization	institucionalización
Insuffizienz	decompensation, incompetence	descompensación, incompetencia
Insufflation	insufflation	insuflación
Insulin	insulin	insulina
Insulintoleranztest	insulin tolerance test (ITT)	prueba de la tolerancia a la insulina
Intellekt	intellect	intelecto
Intelligenz	intelligence	inteligencia
Intensivstation	intensive care unit (ICU), intensive therapy unit (ITU), special care unit (SCU)	unidad de cuidados intensivos (UCI), unidad de cuidados especiales
interartikulär	interarticular	interarticular

FRENCH	ITALIAN	GERMAN
enclume	incudine	**Incus**
indicateur	indicatore	**Indikator**
induction	induzione	**Induktion**
induration	indurimento	**Induration**
maladie de La Peyronie	malattia di Peyronie	**Induratio penis plastica**
infantile	infantile	**infantil**
unité de soins intensifs coronaires	reparto coronarico	**Infarktpflegestation**
infarcissement	infarto	**Infarzierung**
infection	infezione	**Infektion**
infection opportuniste	infezione opportunista	**Infektion, opportunistische**
maladie infectieuse	malattia infettiva	**Infektionskrankheit**
infectieux	infettivo	**infektiös**
infertilité	infertilità	**Infertilität**
infiltration	infiltrazione	**Infiltration**
grippe	influenza	**Influenza**
infusion	infusione	**Infusion**
inguinal	inguinale	**inguinal**
inhalation	inalazione	**Inhalation**
inhaler	inalare	**inhalieren**
inhibition	inibizione	**Inhibierung**
injection, ponction	iniezione, puntura	**Injektion**
injecter, ponctionner	iniettare, pungere	**injizieren**
incarcéré	incarcerato	**inkarzeriert**
incompatibilité	incompatibilità	**Inkompatibilität**
incontinence	incontinenza	**Inkontinenz**
incoordination	incoordinazione	**Inkoordination**
incubation	incubazione	**Inkubation**
incubateur	incubatore	**Inkubator**
interne	interno	**innerlich**
innervation	innervazione	**Innervation**
inotrope	inotropo	**inotrop**
insémination hétérologue	fecondazione artificiale tramite donatore	**Insemination, heterologe**
insertion	inserzione	**Insertion**
in situ	in situ	**in situ**
inspiration	inspirazione	**Inspiration**
instinct	istinto	**Instinkt**
institutionalisation	istituzionalizzazione	**Institutionalisierung**
décompensation, incompétence	decompensazione, incompetenza	**Insuffizienz**
insufflation	insufflazione	**Insufflation**
insuline	insulina	**Insulin**
épreuve de tolérance à l'insuline	test di tolleranza all' insulina	**Insulintoleranztest**
intellect	intelletto	**Intellekt**
intelligence	intelligenza	**Intelligenz**
unité de soins intensifs, service de réanimation, unité de soins spéciaux	unità di cura intensiva, unità di terapia intensiva, unità pediatrica di cure speciali	**Intensivstation**
interarticulaire	interarticolare	**interartikulär**

GERMAN	ENGLISH	SPANISH
interkostal	intercostal	intercostal
interkurrent	intercurrent	intercurrente
Interleukin	interleukin	interleucina
intermenstruel	intermenstrual	intermenstrual
intermittierend	intermittent	intermitente
intern	internal	interno
interossär	interosseous	interóseo
interspinal	interspinous	interespinoso
interstitiell	interstitial	intersticial
Intertrigo	intertrigo	intertrigo
intertrochantär	intertrochanteric	intertrocantéreo
intervertebral	intervertebral	intervertebral
Intima	intima	íntima
Intoleranz	intolerance	intolerancia
intraabdominal	intra-abdominal	intraabdominal
intraarteriell	intra-arterial	intraarterial
intradermal	intradermal	intradérmico
intrakapsulär	intracapsular	intracapsular
intrakranieller Druck	intracranial pressure (ICP)	presión intracraneal (PIC)
intrakutan	intradermal	intradérmico
intramural	intramural	intramural
intramuskulär	intramuscular (IM)	intramuscular (im)
intranasal	intranasal	intranasal
intraokulär	intraocular	intraocular
intraoral	intraoral	intraoral
intra partum	intrapartum	intra partum
intraperitoneal	intraperitoneal	intraperitoneal
intrathekal	intrathecal	intratecal
intrauterin	intrauterine	intrauterino
Intrauterinpessar (IUP)	intrauterine contraceptive device (IUD, IUCD)	dispositivo intrauterino anticonceptivo (DIU)
intravaginal	intravaginal	intravaginal
intravenös	intravenous (IV)	intravenoso (IV)
intrazellulär	intracellular	intracelular
intrinsisch	intrinsic	intrínseco
Introitus	introitus	introito
Introspektion	introspection	introspección
Introversion	introversion	introversión
Introvertierter	introvert	introvertido
Intubation	intubation	intubación
Intussuszeption	intussusception	intususcepción
Invagination	invagination	invaginación
Invasion	invasion	invasión
Inversion	inversion	inversión
in vitro	in vitro	in vitro
In-vitro-Fertilisation	in vitro fertilization (IVF)	fertilización in vitro (FIV)
in vivo	in vivo	in vivo

intercostal	intercostale	**interkostal**
intercurrent	intercorrente	**interkurrent**
interleukine	interleuchina	**Interleukin**
intermenstruel	intermestruale	**intermenstruel**
intermittent	intermittente	**intermittierend**
interne	interno	**intern**
interosseux	interosseo	**interossär**
interépineux	interspinoso	**interspinal**
interstitiel	interstiziale	**interstitiell**
intertrigo	intertrigine	**Intertrigo**
intertrochantérien	intertrocanterico	**intertrochantär**
intervertébral	intervertebrale	**intervertebral**
intima	intima	**Intima**
intolérance	intolleranza	**Intoleranz**
intra-abdominal	intra-addominale	**intraabdominal**
intra-artériel	intra-arterioso	**intraarteriell**
intradermique	intradermico	**intradermal**
intracapsulaire	intracapsulare	**intrakapsulär**
pression intracrânienne	pressione intracranica	**intrakranieller Druck**
intradermique	intradermico	**intrakutan**
intramural	intramurale	**intramural**
intramusculaire (IM)	intramuscolare (IM)	**intramuskulär**
intranasal	intranasale	**intranasal**
intra-oculaire	intraoculare	**intraokulär**
intra-oral	intraorale	**intraoral**
intrapartum	intraparto	**intra partum**
intrapéritonéal	intraperitoneale	**intraperitoneal**
intrathécal	intratecale	**intrathekal**
intra-utérin	intrauterino	**intrauterin**
dispositif intra-utérin (DIU), stérilet	dispositivo anticoncezionale intrauterino (IUD)	**Intrauterinpessar (IUP)**
intravaginal	intravaginale	**intravaginal**
intraveineux (IV)	endovenoso (EV)	**Intravenös**
intracellulaire	intracellulare	**intrazellulär**
intrinsèque	intrinseco	**intrinsisch**
orifice	introito	**Introitus**
introspection	introspezione	**Introspektion**
introversion	introversione	**Introversion**
introverti	introverso	**Introvertierter**
intubation	intubazione	**Intubation**
intussusception	intussuscezione	**Intussuszeption**
invagination	invaginazione	**Invagination**
invasion	invasione	**Invasion**
inversion	inversione	**Inversion**
in vitro	in vitro	**in vitro**
fertilisation in vitro	fertilizzazione in vitro	**In-vitro-Fertilisation**
in vivo	in vivo	**in vivo**

GERMAN	ENGLISH	SPANISH
Involution	involution	involución
Inzest	incest	incesto
Inzidenz	incidence	incidencia
Inzision	incision	incisión
Ion	ion	ión
ipsilateral	ipsilateral	ipsilateral
Iris	iris	iris
Iritis	iritis	iritis
Ischämie	ischaemia (Eng), ischemia (Am)	isquemia
ischämische Herzkrankheit (IHK)	ischaemic heart disease (IHD) (Eng), ischemic heart disease (IHD) (Am)	cardiopatía isquémica
ischiadicus	sciatic	ciático
Ischias	sciatica	ciática
Ischiasnerv	sciatic nerve	nervio ciático
ischiorektal	ischiorectal	isquiorrectal
Ischium	ischium	isquión
Isoimmunisierung	isoimmunization	isoinmunización
Isolierung	isolation	aislamiento
Isolierung (auf Isolierstation)	barrier nursing	enfermería por aislamiento
isometrisch	isometric	isométrico
isotonisch	isotonic	isotónico
Isthmus	isthmus	istmo
i.v. – Pyelogramm	intravenous pyelogram (IVP)	pielograma intravenoso

J

Jejunum	jejunum	yeyuno
Jejunumbiopsie	jejunal biopsy	biopsia del yeyuno
Jochbein	zygoma	cigoma
Jod	iodine	yodo
Jucken	itch, pruritus	picor, prurito
juckreizlindernd	antipruritic	antipruriginoso
Jugendalter	adolescence	adolescencia

FRENCH	ITALIAN	GERMAN
involution	involuzione	**Involution**
inceste	incesto	**Inzest**
fréquence	incidenza	**Inzidenz**
incision	incisione	**Inzision**
ion	ione	**Ion**
ipsilatéral	ipsilaterale, omolaterale	**ipsilateral**
iris	iride	**Iris**
iritis	irite	**Iritis**
ischémie	ischemia	**Ischämie**
cardiopathie ischémique	cardiopatia ischemica	**ischämische Herzkrankheit (IHK)**
sciatique	sciatico	**ischiadicus**
sciatique	sciatica	**Ischias**
nerf grand sciatique	nervo sciatico	**Ischiasnerv**
ischio-rectal	ischiorettale	**ischiorektal**
ischion	ischio	**Ischium**
iso-immunisation	isoimmunizzazione	**Isoimmunisierung**
isolement	isolamento	**Isolierung**
nursage de protection	isolamento	**Isolierung (auf Isolierstation)**
isométrique	isometrico	**isometrisch**
isotonique	isotonico	**isotonisch**
isthme	istmo	**Isthmus**
urographie intraveineuse (UIV)	pielografia endovenosa (PE)	**i.v. – Pyelogramm**
jéjunum	digiuno	**Jejunum**
biopsie jéjunale	biopsia digiunale	**Jejunumbiopsie**
zygoma	zigomo, osso zigomatico	**Jochbein**
iode	iodio	**Jod**
démangeaison, prurit	prurito	**Jucken**
antiprurigineux	antipruriginoso	**juckreizlindernd**
adolescence	adolescenza	**Jugendalter**

K

Kachexie	cachexia	caquexia
Kadaver	cadaver	cadáver
Kaiserschnitt	caesarean section (Eng), cesarean section (Am)	cesárea
Kala-Azar	kala-azar	kala-azar
Kallus	callus	callo
Kalorie	calorie	caloría
kalorische Prüfung	caloric test	prueba calórica
kalt	cold	frío
Kälte	cold, frigidity	resfriado, frigidez
Kalzifikation	calcification	calcificación
Kalzium	calcium	calcio
Kammer	ventricle	ventrículo
Kanal	canal	canal
Kanüle	cannula, needle	cánula, aguja
Kapillare	capillary	capilar
Kaposi-Sarkom	Kaposi's sarcoma	sarcoma de Kaposi
Kapsel	capsule	cápsula
Kapselentzündung	capsulitis	capsulitis
Karbunkel	carbuncle	ántrax
Kardia	cardia	cardias
kardiogen	cardiogenic	cardiógenico
Kardiologie	cardiology	cardiología
Kardiomegalie	cardiomegaly	cardiomegalia
Kardiomyopathie	cardiomyopathy	cardiomiopatía, miocardiopatía
kardiopulmonal	cardiopulmonary	cardiopulmonar
kardiorespiratorisch	cardiorespiratory	cardiorespiratorio
Kardiospasmus	cardiospasm	cardiospasmo
kardiothorakal	cardiothoracic	cardiotorácico
Kardiotokograph	cardiotocograph	tococardiógrafo
kardiotoxisch	cardiotoxic	cardiotóxico
kardiovaskulär	cardiovascular	cardiovascular
Kardioversion	cardioversion	cardioversión
Karies	caries	caries
karminativ	carminative	carminativo
Karminativum	carminative	carminativo
Karotin	carotene	carotenos
Karotis-	carotid	carótida
Karpaltunnelsyndrom	carpal tunnel syndrome	síndrome del túnel carpiano
karpometakarpal	carpometacarpal	carpometacarpiano
karpopedal	carpopedal	carpopedal
Karpus	wrist	muñeca
Karunkel	caruncle	carúncula
Karyotyp	karyotype	cariotipo
Karzinogen	carcinogen	carcinogénico

FRENCH	ITALIAN	GERMAN
cachexie	cachessia	Kachexie
cadavre	cadavere	Kadaver
césarienne	taglio cesareo	Kaiserschnitt
kala-azar	kala-azar	Kala-Azar
cal	callo	Kallus
calorie	caloria	Kalorie
essai calorique	test calorico	kalorische Prüfung
froid	freddo	kalt
rhume, frigidité	raffreddore, frigidità	Kälte
calcification	calcificazione	Kalzifikation
calcium	calcio	Kalzium
ventricule	ventricolo	Kammer
canal	canale	Kanal
canule, aiguille	cannula, ago	Kanüle
capillaire	capillare	Kapillare
sarcome de Kaposi	sarcoma di Kaposi	Kaposi-Sarkom
capsule	capsula	Kapsel
capsulite	capsulite	Kapselentzündung
charbon	carbonchio, antrace, favo	Karbunkel
cardia	cardias	Kardia
cardiogène	cardiogeno	kardiogen
cardiologie	cardiologia	Kardiologie
cardiomégalie	cardiomegalia	Kardiomegalie
cardiomyopathie	cardiomiopatia	Kardiomyopathie
cardiopulmonaire	cardiopolmonare	kardiopulmonal
cardiorespiratoire	cardiorespiratorio	kardiorespiratorisch
cardiospasme	spasmo cardiale, acalasia esofagea	Kardiospasmus
cardiothoracique	cardiotoracico	kardiothorakal
cardiotocographe	cardiotocografia	Kardiotokograph
cardiotoxique	cardiotossico	kardiotoxisch
cardiovasculaire	cardiovascolare	kardiovaskulär
cardioversion	cardioversione	Kardioversion
carie	carie	Karies
carminatif	carminativo	karminativ
carminatif	carminativo	Karminativum
carotène	carotene	Karotin
carotide	carotide	Karotis-
syndrome du canal carpien	sindrome del tunnel carpale	Karpaltunnelsyndrom
carpo-métarcarpien	carpometacarpale	karpometakarpal
carpo-pédal	carpopedalico	karpopedal
poignet	polso	Karpus
caroncule	caruncola	Karunkel
karyotype	cariotipo	Karyotyp
carcinogène	carcinogeno	Karzinogen

GERMAN	ENGLISH	SPANISH
Karzinogenese	carcinogenesis	carcinogénesis
Karzinoid-Syndrom	carcinoid syndrome	síndrome carcinoide
Karzinom	cancer, carcinoma	cáncer, carcinoma
Karzinomatose	carcinomatosis	carcinomatosis
Karzinose	carcinomatosis	carcinomatosis
Kastration	castration	castración
Katabolismus	catabolism	catabolismo
Katalysator	catalyst	catalizador
Katarakt	cataract	catarata
Katarrh	catarrh	catarro
kataton	catatonic	catatónico
Katheter	catheter	catéter
Katheterisierung	catheterization	cateterismo
Kauen	mastication	masticación
Kausalgie	causalgia	causalgia
Kaustikum	caustic	cáustico
kauterisieren	cauterize	cauterizar
Kauvermögen	mastication	masticación
kavernös	cavernous	cavernoso
Kehlkopf	larynx	laringe
Kehlkopf-	laryngeal	laríngeo
Kehlkopfspiegel	laryngoscope	laringoscopio
Keilbein	sphenoid	esfenoides
Keim	germ, organism	gérmen, organismo
keimfrei	sterile	estéril
Keloid	keloid	queloide
Kennzeichen	stigmata	estigmas
Kephalhämatom	cephalhaematoma (Eng), cephalhematoma (Am)	hematoma cefálico
Kephalometrie	cephalometry	cefalometría
Keratin	keratin	queratina
Keratinisation	keratinization	queratinización
Keratitis	keratitis	queratitis
Keratokonjunktivitis	keratoconjunctivitis	queratoconjuntivitis
Keratomalazie	keratomalacia	queratomalacia
Keratose	keratosis	queratosis
Keratotom	keratome	queratoma
Keratozele	keratocele	queratocele
Kern	nucleus	núcleo
Kernanomalie	dyskaryosis	discariosis
Kernig Zeichen	Kernig's sign	signo de Kernig
Kernikterus	kernicterus	ictericia nuclear
Kernspintomographie (NMR)	magnetic resonance imaging (MRI)	formación de imágenes por resonancia magnética
Ketoazidose	ketoacidosis	cetoacidosis
ketogene Ernährung	ketogenic diet	dieta cetógena
Ketogenese	ketogenesis	cetogénesis
Keton	ketone	acetona

FRENCH	ITALIAN	GERMAN
carcinogenèse	carcinogenesi	**Karzinogenese**
syndrome carcinoïde	sindrome da carcinoide	**Karzinoid-Syndrom**
cancer, carcinome	cancro, carcinoma	**Karzinom**
carcinomatose	carcinomatosi	**Karzinomatose**
carcinomatose	carcinomatosi	**Karzinose**
castration	castrazione	**Kastration**
catabolisme	catabolismo	**Katabolismus**
catalyseur	catalizzatore	**Katalysator**
cataracte	cataratta	**Katarakt**
catarrhe	catarro	**Katarrh**
catatonique	catatonico	**kataton**
cathéter	catetere	**Katheter**
cathétérisme	cateterizzazione	**Katheterisierung**
mastication	masticazione	**Kauen**
causalgie	causalgia	**Kausalgie**
caustique	caustico	**Kaustikum**
cautériser	cauterizzare	**kauterisieren**
mastication	masticazione	**Kauvermögen**
caverneux	cavernoso	**kavernös**
larynx	laringe	**Kehlkopf**
laryngien	laringeo	**Kehlkopf-**
laryngoscope	laringoscopio	**Kehlkopfspiegel**
sphénoïde	sfenoide	**Keilbein**
germe, organisme	germe, organismo	**Keim**
stérile	sterile	**keimfrei**
chéloïde	cheloide	**Keloid**
stigmate	stigmate	**Kennzeichen**
céphalhématome	cefaloematoma	**Kephalhämatom**
céphalométrie	cefalometria	**Kephalometrie**
kératine	cheratina	**Keratin**
kératinisation	cheratinizzazione	**Keratinisation**
kératite	cheratite	**Keratitis**
kératoconjonctivite	cheratocongiuntivite	**Keratokonjunktivitis**
kératomalacie	cheratomalacia	**Keratomalazie**
kératose	cheratosi	**Keratose**
kératome	cheratomo	**Keratotom**
kératocèle	cheratocele	**Keratozele**
noyau	nucleo	**Kern**
dyskaryose	discariosi	**Kernanomalie**
signe de Kernig	segno di Kernig	**Kernig Zeichen**
ictère cérébral	ittero nucleare	**Kernikterus**
imagerie par résonance magnétique	indagine morfologica con risonanza magnetica	**Kernspintomographie (NMR)**
céto-acidose	chetoacidosi	**Ketoazidose**
régime cétogène	dieta chetogenica	**ketogene Ernährung**
cétogenèse	chetogenesi	**Ketogenese**
cétone	chetoni	**Keton**

GERMAN	ENGLISH	SPANISH
Ketonkörper	ketone	acetona
Ketonurie	ketonuria	cetonuria
Ketose	ketosis	cetosis
Keuchhusten	pertussis, whooping cough	tos ferina
Kieferknochen	jaw-bone	mandíbula
Kieferorthopädie	orthodontics	ortodoncia
Kiefersperre	lock jaw	trismo
Kinase	kinase	cinasa
Kindbett-	puerperal	puerperal
Kinderheilkunde	paediatrics (Eng), pediatrics (Am)	pediatría
Kinderlähmung	poliomyelitis	poliomielitis
Kindesmißhandlung	child abuse	abuso de menores
Kindesmißhandlung (Folgen)	battered baby syndrome	síndrome del niño apaleado
kindlich	infantile	infantil
Kindslage	presentation	presentación
Kindslage, anomale	malpresentation	malpresentación
Kinn	chin, mentum	barbilla, mentón
Klang	sound	sonido
Klappe	valve	válvula
Klaustrophobie	claustrophobia	claustrofobia
Klavus	corn	callo, papiloma
klebrig	viscid	viscoso
Kleie	bran	salvado
Kleinhirn	cerebellum	cerebelo
Kleinkind	infant	lactante
kleinzelliges Bronchialkarzinom	oat cell cancer	carcinoma de células de avena
Klemme	forceps	fórceps
Klimakterium	climacteric	climatérico
Klinefelter-Syndrom	Klinefelter's syndrome	síndrome de Klinefelter
klinisch	clinical	clínico
Klistier	enema	enema
Klitoris	clitoris	clítoris
Klonus	clone, clonus	clono, clonus
Klumpfuß	club-foot, talipes	pie zambo, talipes
Knie	knee	rodilla
Kniescheibe	patella	rótula
Kniesehne	hamstring	tendón del hueso poplíteo
Knöchel	ankle	tobillo
Knochen	bone	hueso
Knochen-	osseous	óseo
Knochenbruch	fracture	fractura
Knochenentzündung	osteitis	osteítis
Knochenhaut	periosteum	periostio
Knochenmark	bone marrow	médula ósea
Knochenmarksentzündung	osteomyelitis	osteomielitis

FRENCH	ITALIAN	GERMAN
cétone	chetoni	**Ketonkörper**
cétonurie	chetonuria	**Ketonurie**
cétose	chetosi	**Ketose**
pertussis, coqueluche	pertosse	**Keuchhusten**
mâchoire	osso mandibolare	**Kieferknochen**
orthodontie	ortodonzia	**Kieferorthopädie**
tétanos	tetano, trisma	**Kiefersperre**
kinase	chinasi	**Kinase**
puerpéral	puerperale	**Kindbett-**
pédiatrie	pediatria	**Kinderheilkunde**
poliomyélite	poliomielite	**Kinderlähmung**
sévices infligés aux enfants, martyre d'enfants	maltrattamento a bambini	**Kindesmißhandlung**
syndrome des enfants maltraités	sindrome del bambino maltrattato	**Kindesmißhandlung (Folgen)**
infantile	infantile	**kindlich**
présentation	presentazione	**Kindslage**
présentation vicieuse	presentazione fetale anomala	**Kindslage, anomale**
menton	mento	**Kinn**
son	suono	**Klang**
valve	valvola	**Klappe**
claustrophobie	claustrofobia	**Klaustrophobie**
cor	callo	**Klavus**
visqueux	viscido	**klebrig**
son	crusca	**Kleie**
cervelet	cervelletto	**Kleinhirn**
enfant, nourrisson	infante	**Kleinkind**
épithélioma à petites cellules	microcitoma, carcinoma a piccole cellule	**kleinzelliges Bronchialkarzinom**
forceps	forcipe	**Klemme**
climatérique	climaterio	**Klimakterium**
syndrome de Klinefelter	sindrome di Klinefelter	**Klinefelter-Syndrom**
clinique	clinico	**klinisch**
lavement	clistere	**Klistier**
clitoris	clitoride	**Klitoris**
clone, clonus	clone, clono	**Klonus**
pied bot	piede torto, piede talo	**Klumpfuß**
genou	ginocchio	**Knie**
rotule	patella, rotula	**Kniescheibe**
tendon du jarret	tendine del ginocchio	**Kniesehne**
cheville	caviglia	**Knöchel**
os	osso	**Knochen**
osseux	osseo	**Knochen-**
fracture	frattura	**Knochenbruch**
ostéite	osteite	**Knochenentzündung**
périoste	periostio	**Knochenhaut**
moelle osseuse	midollo osseo	**Knochenmark**
ostéomyélite	osteomielite	**Knochenmarksentzündung**

GERMAN	ENGLISH	SPANISH
Knochensarkom	osteosarcoma	osteosarcoma
Knochenschaft	diaphysis	diáfisis
Knochentransplantation	bone graft	injerto óseo, osteoplastia
knöchern	osseous	óseo
Knorpel	cartilage	cartílago
Knorpelhaut	perichondrium	pericondrio
Knötchen	nodule, papule	nódulo, pápula
Knoten	node, knuckle, malleolus	nodo, nudillo, maléolo
Koagel	clot	coágulo
koagulieren	clot	coagular
Kochsalzlösung	saline	solución salina
Koffein	caffeine	cafeína
Kohlenhydrat	carbohydrate (CHO)	hidrato de carbono
Kohlenwasserstoff	carbohydrate (CHO)	hidrato de carbono
Koilonychie	koilonychia	coiloniquia
Koitus	coitus, intercourse, pareunia, sexual intercourse	coito, pareunia
Kolektomie	colectomy	colectomía
Kolik	colic, gripe	cólico, cólico intestinal
Kolitis	colitis	colitis
kollabieren	collapse	colapsar
Kollagen	collagen	colágeno
Kollaps	collapse	colapso
Kollateralkreislauf	collateral circulation	circulación colateral
Kolloid	colloid	coloide
Kolobom	coloboma	coloboma
Kolon	colon	colon
kolonisieren	colonize	colonizar
Kolonresektion	colectomy	colectomía
kolorektal	colorectal	colorrectal
Koloskopie	colonoscopy	colonoscopia
Kolostomie	colostomy	colostomía
Kolostrum	colostrum	calostro
Kolporrhaphie	colporrhaphy	colporrafia
Kolposkop	colposcope	colposcopio
Koma	coma	coma
komatös	comatose	comatoso
Kommissur	commissure	comisura
Kompatibilität	compatibility	compatibilidad
Kompensation	compensation	compensación
Komplement	complement	complemento
komplementäre Medizin	complementary medicine	medicina complementaria
Kompression	compression	compresión
kondensiert	inspissated	espesado
Kondom	condom	condón
kongenital	innate	innato
konjugiert	conjugate	conjugado

FRENCH	ITALIAN	GERMAN
ostéosarcome	sarcoma osteogenico	Knochensarkom
diaphyse	diafisi	Knochenschaft
greffe osseuse	trapianto osseo	Knochentransplantation
osseux	osseo	knöchern
cartilage	cartilagine	Knorpel
périchondre	pericondrio	Knorpelhaut
nodule, papule	nodulo, papula	Knötchen
noeud, jointure, malléole	nodo, articolazione interfalangea, malleolo	Knoten
caillot	coagulo	Koagel
coaguler	coagulare	koagulieren
solution physiologique	soluzione fisiologica	Kochsalzlösung
caféine	caffeina	Koffein
glucide	carboidrato	Kohlenhydrat
glucide	carboidrato	Kohlenwasserstoff
koilonychie	coilonichia	Koilonychie
coït, rapports, rapports sexuels	coito	Koitus
colectomie	colectomia	Kolektomie
colique	colica, colica addominale	Kolik
colite	colite	Kolitis
s'affaisser	collassarsi, crollare	kollabieren
collagène	collageno	Kollagen
affaissement	collasso	Kollaps
circulation collatérale	circolazione collaterale	Kollateralkreislauf
colloïde	colloide	Kolloid
colobome, coloboma	coloboma	Kolobom
côlon	colon	Kolon
coloniser	colonizzare	kolonisieren
colectomie	colectomia	Kolonresektion
colorectal	colorettale	kolorektal
coloscopie	colonscopia	Koloskopie
colostomie	colostomia	Kolostomie
colostrum	colostro	Kolostrum
colporraphie	colporrafia	Kolporrhaphie
colposcope	colposcopio	Kolposkop
coma	coma	Koma
comateux	comatoso	komatös
commissure	commessura	Kommissur
compatibilité	compatibilità	Kompatibilität
compensation	compenso	Kompensation
complément	complemento	Komplement
traitement complémentaire	medicina complementare	komplementäre Medizin
compression	compressione	Kompression
épaissir	inspessito	kondensiert
préservatif	profilattico maschile	Kondom
endogène	innato	kongenital
conjugué	coniugato	konjugiert

GERMAN	ENGLISH	SPANISH
Konjunktiva	conjunctiva	conjuntiva
Konjunktivitis	conjunctivitis	conjuntivitis
Konjunktivitis, epidemische	pinkeye	conjuntivitis
Konsolidierung	consolidation	consolidación
Konstriktion	constriction	constricción
Konsum	consumption	consunción, tisis
kontagiös	contagious	contagioso, trasmisible
Kontakt	contact	contacto
Kontaktlinse	contact lens	lente de contacto
Kontraindikation	contraindication	contraindicación
Kontraktion	contraction	contracción
Kontraktur	contracture	contractura
kontralateral	contralateral	contralateral
kontrazeptiv	contraceptive	anticonceptivo
Kontrazeptivum	contraceptive	anticonceptivo
Kontrazeptivum, orales (Kombinationspräparat)	combined oral contraceptive	anticonceptivo oral combinado
Konvulsion	convulsion	convulsión
Koordinationsstörung	ataxia	ataxia
Kopf	head	cabeza
Kopf-	cephalic	cefálico
Kopfhaut	scalp	cuero cabelludo
Kopfschmerzen	headache	cefalea
Koplik-Flecken	Koplik's spots	manchas de Koplik
Kornährenverband	spica	espica
Kornea	cornea	córnea
Korneaplastik	corneal graft	injerto corneal
koronar	coronary	coronario
Koronararterie	coronary	coronario
koronare Herzkrankheit (KHK)	coronary heart disease (CHD)	enfermedad coronaria, cardiopatía isquémica
Koronarinsuffizienz, chronische	chronic coronary insufficiency (CCI)	insuficiencia coronaria crónico
Koronaropathie	coronary artery disease (CAD)	enfermadad arterial coronaria, cardiopatía isquémica
Körpergewicht	total body weight (TBW)	peso corporal total
körperlich	somatic	somático
Körpermassenindex	body mass index (BMI)	índice de masa corporal (IMC)
Korsakow-Psychose	Korsakoff's psychosis	psicosis de Korsakoff
Kortikosteroide	corticosteroid	corticosteroide
Koryza	coryza	coriza
kostal	costal	costal
Kot	faeces (Eng), feces (Am), stool	heces, deposición
kotig	faecal (Eng), fecal (Am)	fecal
Kotstein	faecalith (Eng), fecalith (Am)	fecalito
Krampf	convulsion, cramp, spasm	convulsión, calambre, espasmo
Krampfadern	varicose veins	varices

FRENCH	ITALIAN	GERMAN
conjonctive	congiuntiva	**Konjunktiva**
conjonctivite	congiuntivite	**Konjunktivitis**
conjonctivite aiguë contagieuse	congiuntivite batterica acuta contagiosa, congiuntivite catarrale	**Konjunktivitis, epidemische**
consolidation	solidificazione, addensamento	**Konsolidierung**
constriction	costrizione	**Konstriktion**
consommation	consunzione	**Konsum**
contagieux	contagioso	**kontagiös**
contact	contatto	**Kontakt**
verre de contact	lente a contatto	**Kontaktlinse**
contre-indication	controindicazione	**Kontraindikation**
contraction	contrazione	**Kontraktion**
contracture	contrattura	**Kontraktur**
controlatéral	controlaterale	**kontralateral**
contraceptif	anticoncezionale	**kontrazeptiv**
contraceptif	anticoncezionale	**Kontrazeptivum**
contraceptif oral combiné	contraccettivo orale estro-progestinico	**Kontrazeptivum, orales (Kombinationspräparat)**
convulsion	convulsione	**Konvulsion**
ataxie	atassia	**Koordinationsstörung**
tête	testa	**Kopf**
céphalique	cefalico	**Kopf-**
épicrâne	cuoio capelluto	**Kopfhaut**
mal de tête, céphalée	mal di testa	**Kopfschmerzen**
points de Koplik	segni di Koplik	**Koplik-Flecken**
spica	spiga	**Kornährenverband**
cornée	cornea	**Kornea**
greffe de la cornée	trapianto corneale	**Korneaplastik**
coronaire, coronarien	coronarico	**koronar**
coronaire	coronaria	**Koronararterie**
insuffisance coronarienne cardiaque	malattia cardiaca coronarica (MCC)	**koronare Herzkrankheit (KHK)**
insuffisance coronarienne chronique	insufficienza coronarica cronica	**Koronarinsuffizienz, chronische**
coronaropathie, cardiopathie ischémique, insuffisance coronarienne globale	malattia delle arterie coronarica (MAC)	**Koronaropathie**
poids corporel total	peso corporeo totale	**Körpergewicht**
somatique	somatico	**körperlich**
indice de masse corporelle (IMC)	indice di massa corporea (IMC)	**Körpermassenindex**
psychose de Korsakoff	psicosi di Korsakoff	**Korsakow-Psychose**
corticostéroïde	corticosteroide	**Kortikosteroide**
coryza	coriza	**Koryza**
costal	costale	**kostal**
fèces, selle	feci, feci	**Kot**
fécal	fecale	**kotig**
concrétion fécale	fecalito	**Kotstein**
convulsion, crampe, spasme	convulsione, crampo, spasmo	**Krampf**
varices	vene varicose	**Krampfadern**

GERMAN	ENGLISH	SPANISH
krampfartig	paroxysmal	paroxístico
krampfhaft	spastic	espástico
krampflösend	antispasmodic	antiespasmódico
Kraniosynostose	cranio-synostosis	craneosinostosis
Kranium	cranium	cráneo
Krankenhaus	hospital	hospital
Krankenschwester	nurse	enfermera
Krankhaftigkeit	morbidity	morbilidad
Krankheit	disease, illness	enfermedad
Krankheitserreger	pathogen	patógeno
Krätze	scabies	sarna
Kreatin	creatine	creatina
Kreatinin	creatinine	creatinina
Krebs	cancer, carcinoma	cáncer, carcinoma
kreisförmig	circinate	circinado
Kreislauf	circulation	circulación
Kreislauf-	cardiovascular	cardiovascular
Krepitation	crepitation	crepitación
Kretinismus	cretinism	cretinismo
Kreuzbein	sacrum	sacro
Kreuzbein-	sacral	sacral
Kreuzschmerzen	low back pain	lumbalgia
krikoid	cricoid	cricoideo
Krise	crisis	crisis
Kropf	goiter (Am), goitre (Eng)	bocio
Krupp	croup	garrotillo, crup, difteria laríngea
Kruste	scab	costra
Kryochirurgie	cryosurgery	criocirugía
Kryotherapie	cryotherapy	crioterapia
Krypte	crypt	cripta
kryptogenetisch	cryptogenic	criptogénico
Kryptomenorrhoe	cryptomenorrhea (Am), cryptomenorrhoea (Eng)	criptomenorrea
Kryptorchismus	undescended testes	testículos no descendidos
Kugelzellanämie	spherocytosis	esferocitosis
Kultur	culture	cultivo
Kunstfehler	malpractice	malpraxis
künstliche Befruchtung	artificial insemination (AI)	inseminación artificial
Kürettage	curettage, curetting	raspado, legrado, curetaje, material de legrado
Kürette	curette (Eng), curet (Am)	cureta, cucharilla de legrado
kürettieren	curette (Eng), curet (Am)	legrar
Kurzatmigkeit	shortness of breath	disnea
Kurzsichtiger	myope	miope
Kurzsichtigkeit	myopia	miopía
kutan	cutaneous	cutáneo
Kveim-Test	Kveim test	prueba de Kveim

FRENCH	ITALIAN	GERMAN
paroxysmal	parossistico	**krampfartig**
spastique	spastico	**krampfhaft**
antispasmodique	antispastico	**krampflösend**
craniosynostose	craniosinostosi	**Kraniosynostose**
boîte crânienne	cranio	**Kranium**
hôpital	ospedale	**Krankenhaus**
infirmière	infermiere	**Krankenschwester**
morbidité	morbilità	**Krankhaftigkeit**
maladie	malattia, affezione, infermità	**Krankheit**
pathogène	patogeno	**Krankheitserreger**
gale	scabbia	**Krätze**
créatine	creatina	**Kreatin**
créatinine	creatinina	**Kreatinin**
cancer, carcinome	cancro, carcinoma	**Krebs**
circinal	circinato	**kreisförmig**
circulation	circolazione	**Kreislauf**
cardiovasculaire	cardiovascolare	**Kreislauf-**
crépitation	crepitazione	**Krepitation**
crétinisme	cretinismo	**Kretinismus**
sacrum	sacro	**Kreuzbein**
sacré	sacrale	**Kreuzbein-**
douleurs lombaires basses	rachialgia lombosacrale	**Kreuzschmerzen**
cricoïde	cricoide	**krikoid**
crise	crisi	**Krise**
goitre	gozzo	**Kropf**
croup	ostruzione laringea	**Krupp**
croûte	crosta, escara	**Kruste**
cryochirurgie	criochirurgia	**Kryochirurgie**
cryothérapie	crioterapia	**Kryotherapie**
crypte	cripta	**Krypte**
cryptogène	criptogenico	**kryptogenetisch**
cryptoménorrhée	criptomenorrea	**Kryptomenorrhoe**
ectopie testiculaire	testicoli ritenuti	**Kryptorchismus**
sphérocytose	sferocitosi	**Kugelzellanämie**
culture	coltura	**Kultur**
faute professionnelle	pratica errata o disonesta	**Kunstfehler**
insémination artificielle (IA)	inseminazione artificiale	**künstliche Befruchtung**
curetage, curetages	curettage, raschiamento	**Kürettage**
curette	curette, cucchiaio chirurgico	**Kürette**
cureter	raschiare, scarificare	**kürettieren**
essoufflement	respiro affannoso	**Kurzatmigkeit**
myope	miope	**Kurzsichtiger**
myopie	miopia	**Kurzsichtigkeit**
cutané	cutaneo	**kutan**
test de Kveim	test di Kveim	**Kveim-Test**

GERMAN	ENGLISH	SPANISH
Kwashiorkor	kwashiorkor	kwashiorkor
Kypholordose	kypholordosis	cifolordosis
Kyphose	kyphosis	cifosis
Kyphoskoliose	kyphoscoliosis	cifoscoliosis

FRENCH	ITALIAN	GERMAN
kwashiorkor	kwashiorkor	**Kwashiorkor**
cypholordose	cifolordosi	**Kypholordose**
cyphose	cifosi	**Kyphose**
cyphoscoliose	cifoscoliosi	**Kyphoskoliose**

L

German	English	Spanish
Labia	labia	labios
labil	labile	lábil
Labilität	lability	labilidad
Labyrinth	labyrinth	laberinto
Labyrinthitis	labyrinthitis	laberintitis
Lackmus	litmus	tornasol
Lage	presentation	presentación
Lage-	postural	postural
Lageanomalie	malposition	malposición
Lähmung	palsy, paralysis, paresis	parálisis, paresia
Laktase	lactase	lactasa
Laktat	lactate	lactato
Laktation	lactation	lactación
Laktose	lactose	lactosa
Laktulose	lactulose	lactulosa
Lambliasis	giardiasis	giardiasis
Lamina	lamina	lámina
Laminektomie	laminectomy	laminectomía
Lancefield-Gruppen	Lancefield's groups	grupos de Lancefield
Langerhans-Inseln	islets of Langerhans, pancreatic islets	islotes de Langerhans, islotes pancreáticos
Lanugo	lanugo	lanugo
Laparoskopie	laparoscopy	laparoscopia
Laparotomie	laparotomy	laparotomía
Läppchen	lobule	lóbulo
Läppchenprobe	patch test	prueba del parche
Lappen	flap	colgajo, injerto
Lappen (Organ-)	lobe	lóbulo
Larve	maggot	antojo
laryngeal	laryngeal	laríngeo
Laryngitis	laryngitis	laringitis
Laryngologie	laryngology	laringología
Laryngoskop	laryngoscope	laringoscopio
Laryngospasmus	laryngospasm	laringospasmo
Laryngo-Tracheobronchitis	laryngotracheobronchitis	laringotraqueobronquitis
Larynx	larynx	laringe
Laser	laser	láser
Läsion	lesion	lesión
Lassafieber	Lassa fever	fiebre de Lassa
lateral	lateral	lateral
Lauge	alkali	álcali
Laus	louse	piojo
Läusebefall	pediculosis	pediculosis
Laut	tone	tono

FRENCH	ITALIAN	GERMAN
lèvres	labbra	**Labia**
labile	labile	**labil**
labilité	labilità	**Labilität**
labyrinthe	labirinto	**Labyrinth**
labyrinthite	labirintite	**Labyrinthitis**
tournesol	tornasole	**Lackmus**
présentation	presentazione	**Lage**
postural	posturale	**Lage-**
malposition	malposizione	**Lageanomalie**
paralysie, parésie	paralisi, paresi	**Lähmung**
lactase	lattasi	**Laktase**
lactate	lattato	**Laktat**
lactation	lattazione	**Laktation**
lactose	lattosio	**Laktose**
lactulose	lattulosio	**Laktulose**
giardiase	giardiasi	**Lambliasis**
lame	lamina	**Lamina**
laminectomie	laminectomia	**Laminektomie**
groupes de streptocoques suivant la classification de Lancefield	gruppi di Lancefield	**Lancefield-Gruppen**
îlots de Langerhans, îlots pancréatiques	isole di Langerhans, isolotti pancreatici	**Langerhans-Inseln**
lanugo	lanugine	**Lanugo**
coelioscopie	laparoscopia	**Laparoskopie**
laparotomie	laparotomia	**Laparotomie**
lobule	lobulo	**Läppchen**
tache, plaque, pièce	test epicutaneo	**Läppchenprobe**
lambeau	lembo, innesto	**Lappen**
lobe	lobo	**Lappen (Organ-)**
asticot	larva	**Larve**
laryngien	laringeo	**laryngeal**
laryngite	laringite	**Laryngitis**
laryngologie	laringologia	**Laryngologie**
laryngoscope	laringoscopio	**Laryngoskop**
laryngospasme	laringospasmo	**Laryngospasmus**
laryngotrachéobronchite	laringotracheobronchite	**Laryngo-Tracheobronchitis**
larynx	laringe	**Larynx**
laser	laser	**Laser**
lésion	lesione	**Läsion**
fièvre de Lassa	febbre di Lassa	**Lassafieber**
latéral	laterale	**lateral**
alcali	alcali	**Lauge**
pou	pidocchio	**Laus**
pédiculose	pediculosi	**Läusebefall**
tonus	tono	**Laut**

GERMAN	ENGLISH	SPANISH
Laxans	aperient, laxative	laxante
laxierend	aperient, laxative	laxante, laxativo
lebensfähig	viable	viable
Leber	liver	hígado
Leber-	hepatic	hepático
Leberfleck	liver spot	cloasma
Leberfunktionstest	liver function test (LFT)	prueba de función hepática
Leberpforte	portahepatitis	portohepatitis
leberschädigend	hepatotoxic	hepatotóxico
Legionärskrankheit	legionnaires' disease	enfermedad del legionario
Leib-Seele-	psychosomatic	psicosomático
Leiche	cadaver, corpse	cadáver
Leichenbeschauer	coroner	médico forense
Leiden	disease, mal	enfermedad, mal
Leimschnüffeln	glue sniffing	inhalación de pegamento
Leishman-Donovan-Körper	Leishman-Donovan body	cuerpo de Leishman-Donovan
Leishmaniose	leishmaniasis	leishmaniasis
Leiste	groin	ingle
Leisten-	inguinal	inguinal
Leitungsanästhesie	nerve block	bloqueo nervioso
Lende	loin	lomo
Lenden-	lumbar	lumbar
Lentigo	lentigo	lentigo
Lepra	leprosy	lepra
Leptospirose	leptospirosis	leptospirosis
lesbisch	lesbian	lesbiana
letal	lethal	letal
Lethargie	lethargy	letargo
letzte Menstruationsperiode	last menstrual period (LMP)	fecha última regla (FUR)
Leukämie	leukaemia (Eng), leukemia (Am)	leucemia
Leukopenie	leucopenia (Eng), leukopenia (Am)	leucopenia
Leukoplakie	leucoplakia (Eng), leukoplakia (Am)	leucoplasia
Leukorrhoe	leucorrhea (Eng), leukorrhea (Am)	leucorrea
Leukotomie	leucotomy (Eng), leukotomy (Am), lobotomy	leucotomía, lobotomía
Leukozyt	leucocyte (Eng), leukocyte (Am)	leucocito
Leukozytose	leucocytosis (Eng), leukocytosis (Am)	leucocitosis
Levator	levator	elevador
Lezithin	lecithin	lecitina
LH-luteinizing hormone releasing factor (LHRF)	LH-releasing factor (LHRF)	factor liberador de la hormona luteinizante
Libido	libido	líbido
Lichen	lichen	líquen
Lichenifikation	lichenification	liquenificación
lichtempfindlich	photosensitive	fotosensible
Lichtscheue	photophobia	fotofobia
Lid	palpebra	párpado

FRENCH	ITALIAN	GERMAN
laxatif	lassativo	**Laxans**
laxatif	lassativo	**laxierend**
viable	vitale, in grado di vivere	**lebensfähig**
foie	fegato	**Leber**
hépatique	epatico	**Leber-**
tache hépatique	cloasma	**Leberfleck**
test de la fonction hépatique (TFH)	test di funzionalità epatica (TFE)	**Leberfunktionstest**
porto-hépatite	portaepatite	**Leberpforte**
hépatotoxique	epatotossico	**leberschädigend**
maladie des légionnaires	malattia dei legionari	**Legionärskrankheit**
psychosomatique	psicosomatico	**Leib-Seele-**
cadavre	cadavere	**Leiche**
médecin légiste	medico legale	**Leichenbeschauer**
maladie, mal	malattia, affezione, infermità, male	**Leiden**
intoxication par inhalation de solvant	inalazione di toluene o collanti	**Leimschnüffeln**
Leishmania donovani	corpi di Leishman-Donovan	**Leishman-Donovan-Körper**
leishmaniose	leishmaniosi	**Leishmaniose**
aine	inguine	**Leiste**
inguinal	inguinale	**Leisten-**
anesthésie par blocage nerveux	blocco nervoso	**Leitungsanästhesie**
région lombaire	regione lombare	**Lende**
lombaire	lombare	**Lenden-**
lentigo	lentiggine	**Lentigo**
lèpre	lebbra	**Lepra**
leptospirose	leptospirosi	**Leptospirose**
lesbien	lesbismo	**lesbisch**
létal, léthal	letale	**letal**
léthargie	letargia	**Lethargie**
dernières règles	ultimo periodo mestruale	**letzte Menstruationsperiode**
leucémie	leucemia	**Leukämie**
leucopénie	leucopenia	**Leukopenie**
leucoplasie	leucoplachia	**Leukoplakie**
leucorrhée	leucorrea	**Leukorrhoe**
leucotomie, lobotomie	leucotomia, lobotomia	**Leukotomie**
leucocyte	leucocito	**Leukozyt**
leucocytose	leucocitosi	**Leukozytose**
releveur	muscolo elevatore	**Levator**
lécithine	lecitina	**Lezithin**
substance libératrice de l'hormone lutéotrope	releasing factor dell'ormone LH	**LH-luteinizing hormone releasing factor (LHRF)**
libido	desiderio sessuale	**Libido**
lichen	lichene	**Lichen**
lichénification	lichenificazione	**Lichenifikation**
photosensible	fotosensibile	**lichtempfindlich**
photophobie	fotofobia	**Lichtscheue**
paupière	palpebra	**Lid**

GERMAN	ENGLISH	SPANISH
Lidentzündung	blepharitis	blefaritis
Lidknorpel	tarsus	tarso
Lidkrampf	blepharospasm	blefarospasmo
liegend	recumbent	recumbente, de pie
Ligament	cord, ligament	cordón, cuerda, médula espinal, ligamento
Ligamentopexie	ventrosuspension	ventrosuspensión
ligamentum latum uteri	broad ligament	ligamento ancho
Ligatur	ligature	ligadura
Linctus	linctus	linctus
Linea	linea	línea
Linie	linea	línea
Liniment	liniment	linimento
linkshändig	left-handed	zurdo
Linse	lens	cristalino
Lipämie	lipaemia (Eng), lipemia (Am)	lipemia
Lipase	lipase	lipasa
Lipid	lipid	lípido
Lipidose	lipidosis	lipidosis
Lipochondrodystrophie	lipochondrodystrophy	lipocondrodistrofia
Lipodystrophie	lipodystrophy	lipodistrofia
Lipolyse	lipolysis	lipolisis
Lipom	lipoma	lipoma
Lipoprotein	lipoprotein	lipoproteína
Lipoprotein sehr geringer Dichte	very low density lipoprotein (VLDL)	lipoproteína de muy baja densidad (VLDL)
lipotroph	lipotrophic	lipotrófico
Lippe	lip	labio
Liquor	cerebrospinal fluid (CSF), liquor	liquido cefalorraquídeo (LCR), licor
Lithotomie	lithotomy	litotomía
Lithotripsie	lithotripsy	litotripsia
Lithotriptor	lithotriptor, lithotrite	litotriptor, litotritor
livide	livid	lívido
Lobektomie	lobectomy	lobectomía
Lobotomie	lobotomy	lobotomía
Lobulus	lobule	lóbulo
Lochien	lochia	loquios
Löffelnagel	koilonychia	coiloniquia
lokalisieren	localize	localizar
Lordose	lordosis	lordosis
löslich (teilweise)	partly soluble (p.sol)	semisoluble
Lösung	solution	solución
Lösungsmittel	solvent	disolvente
low density lipoprotein (LDL)	low density lipoprotein (LDL)	lipoproteína de baja densidad (LDL)
Lues	syphilis	sífilis
Luftröhre	trachea, windpipe	tráquea

blépharite	blefarite	**Lidentzündung**
tarse	tarso	**Lidknorpel**
blépharospasme	blefarospasmo	**Lidkrampf**
couché	supino, sdraiato	**liegend**
cordon, ligament	corda, cordone, notocorda, ligamento	**Ligament**
ventro-suspension	ventrosospensione, ventrofissazione	**Ligamentopexie**
ligaments larges	legamento largo	**ligamentum latum uteri**
ligature	legatura	**Ligatur**
linctus	sciroppo	**Linctus**
ligne	linea	**Linea**
ligne	linea	**Linie**
liniment	linimento	**Liniment**
gaucher	mancino	**linkshändig**
lentille	lente	**Linse**
lipémie	lipemia	**Lipämie**
lipase	lipasi	**Lipase**
lipide	lipide	**Lipid**
lipidose, dyslipoïdose	lipoidosi	**Lipidose**
maladie de Hurler, lipochondrodystrophie	lipocondrodistrofia	**Lipochondrodystrophie**
lipodystrophie	lipodistrofia	**Lipodystrophie**
lipolyse	lipolisi	**Lipolyse**
lipome	lipoma	**Lipom**
lipoprotéine	lipoprotcina	**Lipoprotein**
lipoprotéine de très faible densité	lipoproteina a bassissima densità	**Lipoprotein sehr geringer Dichte**
hormone lipotrope hypophysaire	lipotrofico	**lipotroph**
lèvre	labbro	**Lippe**
liquide céphalo-rachidien, liquide	liquido cerebrospinale (LCS), liquido	**Liquor**
lithotomie	litotomia	**Lithotomie**
lithotripsie, lithotritie	litotripsia	**Lithotripsie**
lithotriteur	litotritore	**Lithotriptor**
livide	livido	**livide**
lobectomie	lobectomia	**Lobektomie**
lobotomie	lobotomia	**Lobotomie**
lobule	lobulo	**Lobulus**
lochies	lochi puerperali	**Lochien**
koïlonychie	coilonichia	**Löffelnagel**
localiser	localizzare	**lokalisieren**
lordose	lordosi	**Lordose**
partiellement soluble	parzialmente solubile	**löslich (teilweise)**
solution	soluzione	**Lösung**
solvant	solvente	**Lösungsmittel**
lipoprotéine de basse densité (LBD)	lipoproteina a bassa densità (LBD)	**low density lipoprotein (LDL)**
syphilis	sifilide	**Lues**
trachée	trachea	**Luftröhre**

GERMAN	ENGLISH	SPANISH
Luftröhrenschnitt	tracheotomy	traqueotomía
Luftschlucken	aerophagia	aerofagia
Luftwege Atmung und Kreislauf (ABC-Regel)	airway breathing and circulation (ABC)	vías respiratorias y circulación
Lumbago	lumbago	lumbago
Lumbal-	lumbar	lumbar
Lumbalpunktion	lumbar puncture (LP)	punción lumbar (PL)
lumbosakral	lumbosacral	lumbosacro
Lumen	lumen	luz
Lumpektomie	lumpectomy	exéresis de tumores benignos de la mama
Lunge	lung	pulmón
Lungen-	pulmonary	pulmonar
Lungenembolie	pulmonary embolism (PE)	embolismo pulmonar
Lungenentzündung	pneumonia	neumonía
Lungenerkrankung, chronische obstruktive	chronic obstructive airway disease (COAD)	enfermedad obstructiva crónica de las vias respiratorias
Lungengefäßerkrankung	pulmonary vascular disease (PVD)	vasculopatia pulmonar
Lungenkapillardruck	pulmonary capillary pressure (PCP)	presión capilar pulmonar (PCP)
Lungenlappenresektion	lobectomy	lobectomía
Lungenresektion	pneumonectomy	neumonectomía
Lupus	lupus	lupus
Lupus erythematodes	lupus erythematosus	lupus eritematoso
Lupus erythematodes visceralis (SLE)	systemic lupus erythematosus (SLE)	lupus eritematoso sistémico (LES)
luteinisierendes Hormon	luteinizing hormone (LH)	hormona luteinizante (LH)
Luteinom	luteum	lúteo
Luteom	luteum	lúteo
Lyme-Arthritis	Lyme disease	enfermedad de Lyme
Lyme-Borreliose	Lyme disease	enfermedad de Lyme
Lymph-	lymphatic	linfático
Lymphadenektomie	lymphadenectomy	linfadenectomía
Lymphadenitis	lymphadenitis	linfadenitis
Lymphadenopathie	lymphadenopathy	linfadenopatía
Lymphangitis	lymphangitis	linfangitis
lymphatisch	lymphatic	linfático
Lymphe	lymph	linfa
Lymphknoten	lymph node	ganglio linfático
Lymphknotentuberkulose	scrofula	escrófula
Lymphoblast	lymphoblast	linfoblasto
Lymphödem	lymphedema (Am), lymphoedema (Eng)	linfedema
Lymphogranuloma inguinale	lymphogranuloma inguinale	linfogranuloma inguinal
Lymphokine	lymphokine	linfocinesis
Lymphom	lymphoma	linfoma
Lymphosarkom	lymphosarcoma	linfosarcoma
Lymphozyt	lymphocyte	linfocito

trachéotomie	tracheotomia	**Luftröhrenschnitt**
aérophagie	aerofagia	**Luftschlucken**
intubation, ventilation et circulation	ventilazione e respirazione nelle vie respiratorie	**Luftwege Atmung und Kreislauf (ABC-Regel)**
lumbago	lombaggine	**Lumbago**
lombaire	lombare	**Lumbal-**
ponction lombaire	puntura lombare, rachicentesi	**Lumbalpunktion**
lombo-sacré	lombosacrale	**lumbosakral**
lumière	lume	**Lumen**
exérèse locale d'une tumeur du sein	mastectomia parziale	**Lumpektomie**
poumon	polmoni	**Lunge**
pulmonaire	polmonare	**Lungen-**
embolie pulmonaire (EP)	embolia polmonare (EP)	**Lungenembolie**
pneumonie	polmonite	**Lungenentzündung**
bronchopneumopathie chronique obstructive, syndrome respiratoire obstructif chronique	malattia ostruttiva cronica delle vie respiratorie	**Lungenerkrankung, chronische obstruktive**
pneumopathie vasculaire	vasculopatia polmonare	**Lungengefäßerkrankung**
pression capillaire pulmonaire (PCP), pression artérielle bloquée moyenne	pressione polmonare di incuneamento	**Lungenkapillardruck**
lobectomie	lobectomia	**Lungenlappenresektion**
pneumonectomie	pneumonectomia	**Lungenresektion**
lupus	lupus	**Lupus**
lupus érythémateux	lupus eritematoso	**Lupus erythematodes**
lupus érythémateux systémique	lupus eritematoso sistemico (LES)	**Lupus erythematodes visceralis (SLE)**
hormone lutéinisante (HL)	ormone luteinizzante (LH)	**luteinisierendes Hormon**
corps jaune	luteo	**Luteinom**
corps jaune	luteo	**Luteom**
arthrite de Lyme, maladie de Lyme	malattia di Lyme	**Lyme-Arthritis**
arthrite de Lyme, maladie de Lyme	malattia di Lyme	**Lyme-Borreliose**
lymphatique	linfatico	**Lymph-**
lymphadénectomie	linfoadenectomia	**Lymphadenektomie**
lymphadénite	linfadenite	**Lymphadenitis**
lymphadénopathie	linfadenopatia	**Lymphadenopathie**
lymphangite	linfangite	**Lymphangitis**
lymphatique	linfatico	**lymphatisch**
lymphe	linfa	**Lymphe**
ganglion lymphatique	linfonodo	**Lymphknoten**
scrofule	scrofola, linfadenite tubercolare	**Lymphknotentuberkulose**
lymphoblaste	linfoblasto	**Lymphoblast**
lymphoedème	linfedema	**Lymphödem**
lymphogranulome vénérien	linfogranuloma inguinale	**Lymphogranuloma inguinale**
lymphokine	linfochina	**Lymphokine**
lymphome	linfoma	**Lymphom**
lymphosarcome	linfosarcoma	**Lymphosarkom**
lymphocyte	linfocito	**Lymphozyt**

GERMAN	ENGLISH	SPANISH
Lymphozytose	lymphocytosis	linfocitosis
Lysis	lysis	lisis
Lysosom	lysosome	lisosoma
Lysozym	lysozyme	lisozima

FRENCH	ITALIAN	GERMAN
lymphocytose	linfocitosi	**Lymphozytose**
lyse	lisi	**Lysis**
lysosome	lisosoma	**Lysosom**
lysozyme	lisozima	**Lysozym**

M

German	English	Spanish
Made	maggot	antojo
Magen	stomach	estómago
Magen-	gastric	gástrico
Magendarm-	gastrointestinal	gastrointestinal
Mageneingang	cardia	cardias
Magenresektion	gastrectomy	gastrectomía
magensaftresistente Tablette	enteric-coated tablet (ECT)	comprimido entérico
Magenschleimhautentzündung	gastritis	gastritis
Magenschmerz	gastrodynia	gastrodinia
Magenspiegel	gastroscope	gastroscopio
Magenverstimmung	indigestion	indigestión
Magersucht	anorexia	anorexia
magersüchtig	anorectic	anoréxico
Magersüchtige(r)	anorectic	anoréxico
makroskopisch	macroscopic	macroscópico
Makrozephalie	macrocephaly	macrocefalia
Makrozyt	macrocyte	macrocito
Makula	macula, macule	mácula
makulopapulär	maculopapular	maculopapular
Malabsorption	malabsorption	malabsorción
Malaria	malaria	paludismo
Malariamittel	antimalarial	antipalúdico
Malathion	malathion	malathion
Malazie	malacia	malacia
maligne	malignant	maligno
Malignität	malignancy	malignidad
Malleolus	malleolus	maléolo
Malleus	malleus	martillo
Malokklusion	malocclusion	maloclusión
Maltose	maltose	maltosa
Malum Potti	Pott's disease	enfermedad de Pott
Mamille	nipple	pezón
Mammaplastik	mammoplasty	mamoplastia
Mammographie	mammography	mamografía
Mandelentfernung	tonsillectomy	tonsilectomía
Mandelentzündung	tonsillitis	amigdalitis
Mandeln	tonsils	amígdalas
Mandibula	mandible	mandíbula
Mangel	defect	defecto
Manie	mania	manía
Manipulation	manipulation	manipulación
manisch-depressive Psychose	manic-depressive psychosis	psicosis maniacodepresiva
Manubrium	manubrium	manubrio
Marasmus	marasmus	marasmo

FRENCH	ITALIAN	GERMAN
asticot	larva	**Made**
estomac	stomaco	**Magen**
gastrique	gastrico	**Magen-**
gastro-intestinal	gastrointestinale	**Magendarm-**
cardia	cardias	**Mageneingang**
gastrectomie	gastrectomia	**Magenresektion**
dragée entérosoluble, comprimé à délitement entérique	compressa enterica rivestita (passano lo stomaco senza sciogliersi)	**magensaftresistente Tablette**
gastrite	gastrite	**Magenschleimhautentzündung**
gastrodynie	gastrodinia	**Magenschmerz**
gastroscope	gastroscopio	**Magenspiegel**
indigestion	indigestione	**Magenverstimmung**
anorexie	anoressia	**Magersucht**
anorexique	anoressico	**magersüchtig**
anorexique	anoressico	**Magersüchtige(r)**
macroscopique	macroscopico	**makroskopisch**
macrocéphalie	macrocefalia	**Makrozephalie**
macrocyte	macrocito	**Makrozyt**
macule	macula	**Makula**
maculopapuleux	maculopapulare	**makulopapulär**
malabsorption	malassorbimento	**Malabsorption**
paludisme	malaria	**Malaria**
antipaludique	antimalarico	**Malariamittel**
malathion	malathion	**Malathion**
malacie	malacia	**Malazie**
malin	maligno	**maligne**
malignité	neoplasia maligna	**Malignität**
malléole	malleolo	**Malleolus**
marteau	martello	**Malleus**
malocclusion	malocclusione	**Malokklusion**
maltose	maltosio	**Maltose**
mal de Pott	malattia di Pott	**Malum Potti**
mamelon	capezzolo	**Mamille**
mammoplastie	mammoplastica	**Mammaplastik**
mammographie	mammografia	**Mammographie**
amygdalectomie	tonsillectomia	**Mandelentfernung**
angine	tonsillite	**Mandelentzündung**
amygdales	tonsille	**Mandeln**
mandibule	mandibola	**Mandibula**
anomalie, défaut	difetto	**Mangel**
manie	mania	**Manie**
manipulation	manipolazione	**Manipulation**
psychose maniacodépressive	psicosi maniaco-depressiva	**manisch-depressive Psychose**
manubrium	manubrio	**Manubrium**
athrepsie	marasma	**Marasmus**

GERMAN	ENGLISH	SPANISH
Mark	medulla	médula
Markenname	proprietary name	nombre de patente
Marsupialisation	marsupialization	marsupialización
Masern	measles	sarampión
masernähnlich	morbilliform	morbiliforme
Masern Mumps und Röteln	measles mumps and rubella (MMR)	sarampión parotiditis y rubéola
Massage	massage	masaje
Mastektomie	mastectomy	mastectomía
Mastitis	mastitis	mastitis
Mastodynie	mastalgia	mastalgia
Mastoidektomie	mastoidectomy	mastoidectomía
mastoideus	mastoid	mastoideo
Mastoiditis	mastoiditis	mastoiditis
Masturbation	masturbation	masturbación
Matrix	matrix	matriz
Maxilla	maxilla	maxilar
maxillofazial	maxillofacial	maxilofacial
maximale exspiratorische Atemgeschwindigkeit	peak expiratory velocity (PEV)	velocidad espiratoria máxima (VEM)
maximale exspiratorische Atemstromstärke	peak expiratory flow rate (PEFR)	velocidad máxima del flujo espiratorio (VMFE)
Mazeration	maceration	maceración
McBurney-Punkt	McBurney's point	punto de McBurney
Meckel-Divertikel	Meckel's diverticulum	divertículo de Meckel
medial	medial	medial
Median-	median	mediana
Mediansyndrom	whiplash	latigazo
Mediastinitis	mediastinitis	mediastinitis
Mediastinum	mediastinum	mediastino
Medikament	medicament	medicamento
Medium	medium	medio
Medizin	medicine	medicina
medizinisch	medicated	medicado
Medulla	medulla	médula
Medulloblastom	medulloblastoma	meduloblastoma
Megacoloncongenitum	megacolon	megacolon
Megaloblast	megaloblast	megaloblasto
Meiose	meiosis	meiossis
Mekonium	meconium	meconio
Meläna	melaena (Eng), melena (Am)	melena
Melancholie	melancholia	melancolía
Melanin	melanin	melanina
Melanom	melanoma	melanoma
meldepflichtige Erkrankung	notifiable disease	enfermedad declarable
Membran	membrane	membrana
Menarche	menarche	menarquía
Mendelson-Syndrom	Mendelson's syndrome	síndrome de Mendelson

FRENCH	ITALIAN	GERMAN
moelle	midollo	Mark
nom de marque	marchio depositato	Markenname
marsupialisation	marsupializzazione	Marsupialisation
rougeole	morbillo	Masern
morbilliforme	morbilliforme	masernähnlich
oreillons rougeole et rubéole	parotide epidemica morbillo e rosolia	Masern Mumps und Röteln
massage	massaggio	Massage
mastectomie	mastectomia	Mastektomie
mastite	mastite	Mastitis
mastalgie, mammalgie	mastalgia	Mastodynie
mastoïdectomie	mastoidectomia	Mastoidektomie
mastoïde	mastoide, mastoideo	mastoideus
mastoïdite	mastoidite	Mastoiditis
masturbation	masturbazione	Masturbation
matrice	matrice	Matrix
maxillaire	mascella superiore	Maxilla
maxillofacial	maxillofacciale	maxillofazial
volume expiratoire maximum (VEM)	velocità espiratoria massima (VEM)	maximale exspiratorische Atemgeschwindigkeit
débit expiratoire de pointe	tasso di picco del flusso espiratorio	maximale exspiratorische Atemstromstärke
macération	macerazione	Mazeration
point de McBurney	punto di McBurney	McBurney-Punkt
diverticule de Meckel	diverticolo di Meckel	Meckel-Divertikel
interne	mediale	medial
médian	mediano	Median-
coup de fouet	colpo di frusta	Mediansyndrom
médiastinite	mediastinite	Mediastinitis
médiastin	mediastino	Mediastinum
médicament	medicamento	Medikament
milieu	mezzo	Medium
médecine	medicina	Medizin
médicamenté	medicato, medicamentoso	medizinisch
moelle	midollo	Medulla
médulloblastome	medulloblastoma	Medulloblastom
mégacôlon	megacolon	Megacoloncongenitum
mégaloblaste	megaloblasto	Megaloblast
méiose	meiosi	Meiose
méconium	meconio	Mekonium
méléna	melena	Meläna
mélancolie	melanconia	Melancholie
mélanine	melanina	Melanin
mélanome	melanoma	Melanom
maladie à déclaration obligatoire	malattia da denunciare alle autorità sanitarie	meldepflichtige Erkrankung
membrane	membrana	Membran
établissement de la menstruation	menarca	Menarche
syndrome de Mendelson	sindrome di Mendelson	Mendelson-Syndrom

GERMAN	ENGLISH	SPANISH
Meningen	meninges	meninges
Meningiom	meningioma	meningioma
Meningismus	meningism	meningismo
Meningitis	meningitis	meningitis
Meningoenzephalitis	meningoencephalitis	meningoencefalitis
Meningomyelozele	meningomyelocele	mielomeningocele
Meningozele	meningocele	meningocele
Meniskus	meniscus	menisco
Meniskusentfernung	meniscectomy	meniscectomía
Menopause	menopause	menopausia
Menorrhagie	menorrhagia	menorragia
Menstruation	menorrhea (Am), menorrhoea (Eng), menstruation	menorrea, menstruación
menstruell	menstrual	menstrual
mentoanterior	mentoanterior	mentoanterior
mentoposterior	mentoposterior	mentoposterior
Merkmal	character	carácter
Mesenterium	mesentery	mesenterio
Mesotheliom	mesothelioma	mesotelioma
metabolisch	metabolic	metabólico
Metabolismus	metabolism	metabolismo
Metabolit	metabolite	metabolito
metakarpophalangeal	metacarpophalangeal	metacarpofalángico
Metakarpus	metacarpus	metacarpo
Metastase	metastasis	metástasis
Metatarsalgie	metatarsalgia	metatarsalgia
metatarsophalangeal	metatarsophalangeal	metatarsofalángico
Metatarsus	metatarsus	metatarso
Methämoglobin	methaemoglobin (Eng), methemoglobin (Am)	metahemoglobina
Methämoglobinämie	methaemoglobinaemia (Eng), methemoglobinemia (Am)	metahemoglobinemia
Methylzellulose	methylcellulose	metilcelulosa
Metropathia haemorrhagica	metropathia haemorrhagica (Eng), metropathia hemorrhagica (Am)	metropatía hemorrágica
Metrorrhagie	metrorrhagia	metrorragia
mg/l	parts per million (ppm)	partes por millón (ppm)
Migräne	migraine	migraña
Mikrobiologie	microbiology	microbiología
Mikrochirurgie	microsurgery	microcirugía
Mikrofilarie	microfilaria	microfilaria
Mikroorganismus	microorganism	microorganismo
Mikroskop	microscope	microscopio
mikroskopisch	microscopic	microscópico
Mikrovilli	microvilli	microvellosidad
Mikrozephalie	microcephaly	microcefalia
Mikrozirkulation	microcirculation	microcirculación
Mikrozyt	microcyte	microcito

FRENCH	ITALIAN	GERMAN
méninges	meningi	**Meningen**
méningiome	meningioma	**Meningiom**
méningisme	meningismo	**Meningismus**
méningite	meningite	**Meningitis**
méningo-encéphalite	meningoencefalite	**Meningoenzephalitis**
méningomyélocèle	meningomielocele	**Meningomyelozele**
méningocèle	meningocele	**Meningozele**
ménisque	menisco	**Meniskus**
méniscectomie	meniscectomia	**Meniskusentfernung**
ménopause	menopausa	**Menopause**
ménorrhagie	menorragia	**Menorrhagie**
ménorrhée, menstruation	menorrea, mestruazione	**Menstruation**
menstruel	mestruale	**menstruell**
posture antéromentonnière	mentoanteriorc	**mentoanterior**
posture postmentonnière	mentoposteriore	**mentoposterior**
caractère	carattere	**Merkmal**
mésentère	mesentere	**Mesenterium**
mésothéliome	mesotelioma	**Mesotheliom**
métabolique	metabolico	**metabolisch**
métabolisme	metabolismo	**Metabolismus**
métabolite	metabolita	**Metabolit**
métacarpophalangien	metacarpofalangeo	**metakarpophalangeal**
métacarpe	metacarpo	**Metakarpus**
métastase	metastasi	**Metastase**
métatarsalgie	metatarsalgia	**Metatarsalgie**
métatarsophalangien	metatarsofalangeo	**metatarsophalangeal**
métatarse	metatarso	**Metatarsus**
méthémoglobine	metemoglobina	**Methämoglobin**
méthémoglobinémie	metemoglobinemia	**Methämoglobinämie**
méthylcellulose	metilcellulosa	**Methylzellulose**
métropathie hémorragique	metropatia emorragica	**Metropathia haemorrhagica**
métrorragie	metrorragia	**Metrorrhagie**
parties par million (ppm)	parti per milione (ppm)	**mg/l**
migraine	emicrania	**Migräne**
microbiologie	microbiologia	**Mikrobiologie**
microchirurgie	microchirurgia	**Mikrochirurgie**
microfilaire	microfilaria	**Mikrofilarie**
micro-organisme	microoganismo	**Mikroorganismus**
microscope	microscopio	**Mikroskop**
microscopique	microscopico	**mikroskopisch**
micropoils	microvilli	**Mikrovilli**
microcéphalie	microcefalia	**Mikrozephalie**
microcirculation	microcircolazione	**Mikrozirkulation**
microcyte	microcita	**Mikrozyt**

GERMAN	ENGLISH	SPANISH
Milch	milk	leche
Milchbildung	lactation	lactación
Milchsäure	lactic acid	ácido láctico
Milchschorf	cradle cap	costra láctea, dermatitis del cuero cabelludo
Milchzucker	lactose	lactosa
Milchzusammensetzung	formula	fórmula, receta
miliar	miliary	miliar
Miliaria	miliaria	miliaria
Milli-Äquivalent	milliequivalent (mEq)	miliequivalente (mEq)
Milz	spleen	bazo
Milzbrand	anthrax	carbunco
minderwertig	inferior	inferior
Mineralokortikoid	mineralocorticoid	mineralocorticoide
Miosis	miosis	miosis
Mißbildung	malformation	malformación
Mißbrauch	abuse	abuso
missed abortion	missed abortion	aborto diferido
Mitesser	pimple	grano
Mitochondrium	mitochondrion	mitocondria
Mitose	mitosis	mitosis
mitral	mitral	mitral
Mittelfuß	metatarsus	metatarso
Mittelhand	metacarpus	metacarpo
Mittelhirn	midbrain	mesencéfalo
Mittelmeeranämie	thalassaemia (Eng), thalassemia (Am)	talasemia
Mittelohrentzündung	otitis	otitis
Mittelschmerz	mittelschmerz	mittelschmerz
Mittelstrahlurin	midstream urine specimen (MUS)	muestra de orina de la parte media de la micción
mittleres Erythrozytenvolumen (MCV)	mean corpuscular volume (MCV)	volumen corpuscular medio (VCM)
molar	molar	molar
Mole	mole	nevo
Molekül	molecule	molécula
Molluscum	molluscum	molusco
Monatsblutung	menorrhea (Am), menorrhoea (Eng), menstruation	menorrea, menstruación
Mongolismus	Down's syndrome	síndrome de Down
Monoaminoxydase-Hemmer	monoamine oxidase inhibitor (MAOI)	inhibidor de la monoaminooxidasa (IMAO)
Monochromat	monochromat	monocromato
monochrom Farbenblinder	monochromat	monocromato
monoklonaler Antikörper	monoclonal antibody	anticuerpo monoclonal
mononukleär	mononuclear	mononuclear
Mononukleose	glandular fever, mononucleosis	fiebre glandular, mononucleosis
Mononukleose, infektiöse	infectious mononucleosis	mononucleosis infecciosa

FRENCH	ITALIAN	GERMAN
lait	latte	**Milch**
lactation	lattazione	**Milchbildung**
acide lactique	acido lattico	**Milchsäure**
casque séborrhéique	stecca, rima di frattura	**Milchschorf**
lactose	lattosio	**Milchzucker**
formule	formula	**Milchzusammensetzung**
miliaire	miliare	**miliar**
miliaire	miliaria, esantema miliare	**Miliaria**
milliéquivalent (mEq)	milliequivalente (mEq)	**Milli-Äquivalent**
rate	milza	**Milz**
anthrax	antrace, carbonchio	**Milzbrand**
inférieur	inferiore	**minderwertig**
minéralocorticoïde	mineralcorticoide	**Mineralokortikoid**
myosis	miosi	**Miosis**
malformation	malformazione	**Mißbildung**
abus	abuso	**Mißbrauch**
rétention foetale	aborto interno, aborto ritenuto	**missed abortion**
bouton	pustola, piccolo foruncolo	**Mitesser**
mitochondrie	mitocondrio	**Mitochondrium**
mitose	mitosi	**Mitose**
mitral	mitrale, mitralico	**mitral**
métatarse	metatarso	**Mittelfuß**
métacarpe	metacarpo	**Mittelhand**
mésencéphale	mesencefelo	**Mittelhirn**
thalassémie	talassemia	**Mittelmeeranämie**
otite	otite	**Mittelohrentzündung**
crise intermenstruelle	dolore intermestruale	**Mittelschmerz**
urine du milieu du jet	campione urinario del mitto intermedio (CUM)	**Mittelstrahlurin**
volume globulaire moyen (VGM)	volume corpuscolare medio (VCM)	**mittleres Erythrozytenvolumen (MCV)**
molaire	molare	**molar**
naevus	neo	**Mole**
molécule	molecula	**Molekül**
molluscum	mollusco	**Molluscum**
ménorrhée, menstruation	menorrea, mestruazione	**Monatsblutung**
trisomie 21	mongoloidismo, sindrome di Down	**Mongolismus**
inhibiteur de la monoamine-oxydase (IMAO)	inibitore monoaminoossidasi (IMAO)	**Monoaminoxydase-Hemmer**
monochromat	monocromatico	**Monochromat**
monochromat	monocromatico	**monochrom Farbenblinder**
anticorps monoclonal	anticorpo monoclonale	**monoklonaler Antikörper**
mononucléaire	mononucleare	**mononukleär**
fièvre glandulaire, mononucléose	mononucleosi infettiva, mononucleosi	**Mononukleose**
mononucléose infectieuse	mononucleosi infettiva	**Mononuklcose, infektiöse**

GERMAN	ENGLISH	SPANISH
Monoplegie	monoplegia	monoplegia
Morbidität	morbidity	morbilidad
morbilliform	morbilliform	morbiliforme
Morbus Boeck	sarcoidosis	sarcoidosis
Morbus haemolyticus neonatorum	haemolytic disease of the newborn (HDN) (Eng), hemolytic disease of the newborn (HDN) (Am)	enfermedad hemolítica del recién nacido
Morbus haemorrhagicus neonatorum	haemorrhagic disease of the newborn (Eng), hemorrhagic disease of the newborn (Am)	enfermedad hemorrágica neonatal
Morbus Hodgkin	Hodgkin's disease	enfermedad de Hodgkin
Morbus Ménière	Ménière's disease	enfermedad de Ménière
Morbus Paget	Paget's disease	enfermedad de Paget
Mord	homicide	homicidio
Morgagni-Stokes-Adams-Syndrom	Stokes-Adams syndrome	síndrome de Stokes-Adams
morgendliche Übelkeit der Schwangeren	morning sickness	náuseas matinales
moribund	moribund	moribundo
Moro-Reflex	Moro reflex	reflejo de Moro
Morphologie	morphology	morfología
Mortalität	mortality	mortalidad
Motoneuron	motor neurone	neurona motora
motorisch	motor	motor
motorischer Nerv	motor nerve	nervio motor
Mouches volantes	floaters	flotadores
mukoid	mucoid	mucoide
mukokutan	mucocutaneous	mucocutáneo
Mukopolysaccharidose	mucopolysaccharidosis	mucopolisacaridosis
mukopurulent	mucopurulent	mucopurulento
mukös	mucous (Eng), mucus (Am)	moco
Mukosa	mucosa	mucosa
Mukoviszidose	cystic fibrosis (CF)	fibrosis quística
Mukozele	mucocele (Am), mucocoele (Eng)	mucocele
Mull	gauze	gasa
Multigravida	multigravida	multípara
multilokulär	multilocular	multilocular
multiple Sklerose (MS)	multiple sclerosis (MS)	esclerosis múltiple
Mumps	mumps	paperas
Münchhausen-Syndrom	Münchhausen's syndrome	síndrome de Münchhausen
Mund	mouth, stoma	boca, estoma
Mundeckenschrunden	cheilosis	queilosis
Mundgeruch	halitosis	halitosis
Mundhöhlenentzündung	stomatitis	estomatitis
Mundrachenhöhle	oropharynx	orofaringe
Mund-zu-Mund-Wiederbelebung	kiss of life, mouth to mouth resuscitation	beso de vida, respiración boca a boca
mural	mural	mural
Musculi peronei	peroneus muscles	músculos peroneos

FRENCH	ITALIAN	GERMAN
monoplégie	monoplegia	**Monoplegie**
morbidité	morbilità	**Morbidität**
morbilliforme	morbilliforme	**morbilliform**
sarcoïdose	sarcoidosi	**Morbus Boeck**
hémolyse des nouveau-nés	ittero dei neonati, eritroblastosi fetale (da incompatibilità Rh)	**Morbus haemolyticus neonatorum**
hémorragies des nouveau-nés	malattia emorragica del neonato	**Morbus haemorrhagicus neonatorum**
maladie de Hodgkin	malattia di Hodgkin	**Morbus Hodgkin**
syndrome de Ménière	sindrome di Ménière	**Morbus Ménière**
maladie de Paget	malattia di Paget	**Morbus Paget**
homicide	omicidio	**Mord**
syndrome de Stokes-Adams	sindrome di Stokes-Adams	**Morgagni-Stokes-Adams-Syndrom**
nausées matinales	malessere mattutino	**morgendliche Übelkeit der Schwangeren**
moribond	moribondo	**moribund**
réflexe de Moro	riflesso di Moro	**Moro-Reflex**
morphologie	morfologia	**Morphologie**
mortalité	mortalità	**Mortalität**
neurone moteur	neurone motore	**Motoneuron**
moteur	motore	**motorisch**
nerf moteur	nervo motore	**motorischer Nerv**
flottants	corpuscoli vitreali sospesi visibili	**Mouches volantes**
mucoïde	mucoide	**mukoid**
mucocutané	mucocutaneo	**mukokutan**
mucopolysaccharidose	mucopolisaccaridosi	**Mukopolysaccharidose**
mucopurulent	mucopurulento	**mukopurulent**
muqueux	mucoso	**mukös**
muqueuse	mucosa	**Mukosa**
fibrose cystique	mucoviscidosi, malattia fibrocistica del pancreas	**Mukoviszidose**
mucocèle	mucocele	**Mukozele**
gaze	garza	**Mull**
multigeste	plurigravida	**Multigravida**
multiloculaire	multiloculare	**multilokulär**
sclérose en plaques	sclerosi multipla	**multiple Sklerose (MS)**
oreillons	parotite epidemica	**Mumps**
syndrome de Münchhausen	sindrome di Münchhausen	**Münchhausen-Syndrom**
bouche, stoma	bocca, stoma, orifizio	**Mund**
chéilose	cheilosi	**Mundeckenschrunden**
halitose	alitosi	**Mundgeruch**
stomatite	stomatite	**Mundhöhlenentzündung**
oropharynx	orofaringe	**Mundrachenhöhle**
bouche-à-bouche, réanimation au bouche-à-bouche	respirazione bocca a bocca, rianimazione bocca a bocca	**Mund-zu-Mund-Wiederbelebung**
pariétal	murale, parietale	**mural**
muscles péroniers	muscoli peronei	**Muscull peronei**

GERMAN	ENGLISH	SPANISH
Musculi trapezii	trapezius muscles	músculos trapecios
Musculus sternocleidomastoideus	sternocleidomastoid muscle	músculo esternocleidomastoideo
Muskel	muscle	músculo
Muskeldystrophie	muscular dystrophy	distrofia muscular
Muskelerkrankung	myopathy	miopatía
Muskelschmerz	myalgia	mialgia
Muskelschwäche	myasthenia	miastenia
muskulokutan	musculocutaneous	musculocutáneo
Mutagen	mutagen	mutágeno
Mutante	mutant	mutante
Mutation	mutation	mutación
Mutismus	mutism	mutismo
Muttermal	birthmark, mole, naevus (Eng), nevus (Am)	mancha de nacimiento, nevo
Muzin	mucin	mucina
Myalgie	myalgia	mialgia
myalgische Enzephalomyelitis	myalgic encephalomyelitis (ME)	encefalomielitis miálgica
Myasthenie	myasthenia	miastenia
myasthenische Krise	myasthenic crisis	crisis miasténica
Mydriasis	mydriasis	midriasis
Mydriatikum	mydriatic	midriático
mydriatisch	mydriatic	midriático
Myelin	myelin	mielina
Myelitis	myelitis	mielitis
Myelofibrose	myelofibrosis	mielofibrosis
Myelographie	myelography	mielografía
myeloisch	myeloid	mieloide
Myelom	myeloma	mieloma
Myelomatose	myelomatosis	mielomatosis
Myelopathie	myelopathy	mielopatía
Mykose	mycosis	micosis
Myofibrose	myofibrosis	miofibrosis
Myokard	myocardium	miocardio
Myokardinfarkt	myocardial infarction (MI)	infarto de miocardio (IM)
Myokarditis	myocarditis	miocarditis
Myom	myoma	mioma
Myomektomie	myomectomy	miomectomía
Myometrium	myometrium	miometrio
Myopathie	myopathy	miopatía
Myoper	myope	miope
Myopie	myopia	miopía
Myositis	myositis	miositis
Myxödem	myxedema (Am), myxoedema (Eng)	mixedema
Myxom	myxoma	mixoma
Myxovirus	myxovirus	mixovirus

FRENCH	ITALIAN	GERMAN
muscles trapèzes	muscoli trapezi	**Musculi trapezii**
muscle sternocléidomastoïdien	muscolo sternocleidomastoideo	**Musculus sternocleidomastoideus**
muscle	muscolo	**Muskel**
dystrophie musculaire	distrofia muscolare	**Muskeldystrophie**
myopathie	miopatia	**Muskelerkrankung**
myalgie	mialgia	**Muskelschmerz**
myasthénie	miastenia	**Muskelschwäche**
musculo-cutané	muscolocutaneo	**muskulokutan**
mutagène	mutageno	**Mutagen**
mutant	mutante	**Mutante**
mutation	mutazione	**Mutation**
mutisme	mutismo	**Mutismus**
naevus, envie	nevo congenito, neo, nevo	**Muttermal**
mucine	mucina	**Muzin**
myalgie	mialgia	**Myalgie**
encéphalomyélite myalgique	encefalomielite mialgica	**myalgische Enzephalomyelitis**
myasthénie	miastenia	**Myasthenie**
crise myasthénique	crisi miastenica	**myasthenische Krise**
mydriase	midriasi	**Mydriasis**
mydriatique	midriatico	**Mydriatikum**
mydriatique	midriatico	**mydriatisch**
myéline	mielina	**Myelin**
myélite	mielite	**Myelitis**
myélofibrose	mielofibrosi	**Myelofibrose**
myélographie	mielografia	**Myelographie**
myéloïde	mieloide	**myeloisch**
myélome	mieloma, plasmacitoma maligno	**Myelom**
myélomatose	mielomatosi	**Myelomatose**
myélopathie	mielopatia	**Myelopathie**
mycose	micosi	**Mykose**
myofibrose	miosite	**Myofibrose**
myocarde	miocardio	**Myokard**
infarctus du myocarde	infarto miocardico	**Myokardinfarkt**
myocardite	miocardite	**Myokarditis**
myome	leiomioma dell'utero, mioma	**Myom**
myomectomie	miomectomia	**Myomektomie**
myomètre	miometrio	**Myometrium**
myopathie	miopatia	**Myopathie**
myope	miope	**Myoper**
myopie	miopia	**Myopie**
myosite	miosite	**Myositis**
myxoedème	mixedema	**Myxödem**
myxome	mixoma	**Myxom**
myxovirus	myxovirus	**Myxovirus**

N

Nabel	navel, umbilicus	ombligo
Nabelbruch	exomphalos, umbilical hernia	exónfalo, hernia umbilical
Nabelschnur	umbilical cord	cordón umbilical
Naboth-Eier	nabothian follicles	folículos de Naboth
Nachbehandlung	aftercare	cuidados postoperatorios
Nachgeburt	afterbirth, placenta	secundinas, expulsión de la placenta y membranas, placenta
Nachlässigkeit	negligence	negligencia
Nachsorge	aftercare	cuidados postoperatorios
Nacht-	nocturnal	nocturno
Nachtblindheit	night blindness	ceguera nocturna
nächtlich	nocturnal	nocturno
Nachtschweiß	night sweat	sudoración nocturna
Nachwehen	afterpains	entuertos
Nacken	nape, neck	nuca, cuello
Nadel	needle	aguja
Naevus arachnoideus	spider naevus (Eng), spider nevus (Am)	araña vascular
Nagel	nail	uña
Nagelablösung	onycholysis	onicólisis
nähen	suture	suturar
nahrhaft	nutrient	nutriente
Nahrungsmittel	nutrient	nutriente
Nahrungsmittelallergie	food allergy	alergia alimentaria
Nahrungsmittelvergiftung	food poisoning	intoxicación alimentaria
Nahrung, ungesunde	junk food	comidas preparadas poco nutritivas
Naht	suture	sutura
Narbe	scar	cicatriz
Narkolepsie	narcolepsy	narcolepsia
Narkose	anaesthesia (Eng), anesthesia (Am), narcosis	anestesia, narcosis
Narkosemittel	anaesthetic (Eng), anesthetic (Am), narcotic	anestésico, narcótico
narkotisch	narcotic	narcótico
nasal	nasal	nasal
Nase	nose	nariz
Nasenbluten	epistaxis, nosebleed	epistaxis
Nasenloch	nostril	fosa nasale
Nasenmuschel	turbinate	turbinado
Nasenpolypen	adenoids	adenoides
Nasenrachenraum	nasopharynx	nasofaringe
nasogastrisch	nasogastric	nasogástrico
nasolakrimal	nasolacrimal	nasolacrimal
Nasopharynx	nasopharynx	nasofaringe
Nausea	nausea	náusea
Nävus	naevus (Eng), nevus (Am)	nevo

FRENCH	ITALIAN	GERMAN
nombril	ombelico	**Nabel**
exomphale, hernie ombilicale	ernia ombelicale, protrusione dell'ombelico	**Nabelbruch**
cordon ombilical	cordone ombelicale	**Nabelschnur**
oeufs de Naboth	follicoli di Naboth	**Naboth-Eier**
postcure	assistenza post-operatoria	**Nachbehandlung**
arrière-faix, placenta	secondine, membrane fetali e placenta, placenta	**Nachgeburt**
négligence	negligenza	**Nachlässigkeit**
postcure	assistenza post-operatoria	**Nachsorge**
nocturne	notturno	**Nacht-**
cécité nocturne	emeralopia	**Nachtblindheit**
nocturne	notturno	**nächtlich**
sueurs nocturnes	sudorazione notturna	**Nachtschweiß**
tranchées utérines	contrazioni uterine post partum	**Nachwehen**
nuque, cou	nuca, collo	**Nacken**
aiguille	ago	**Nadel**
naevi	angioma stellare	**Naevus arachnoideus**
ongle	unghia	**Nagel**
onycholyse	onicolisi	**Nagelablösung**
suturer	suturare, cucire	**nähen**
nourricier	nutriente	**nahrhaft**
nutriment	sostanza nutritiva	**Nahrungsmittel**
allergie alimentaire	allergia alimentare	**Nahrungsmittelallergie**
intoxication alimentaire	avvelenamento alimentare	**Nahrungsmittelvergiftung**
aliments non nutritifs	cibo contenente additivi chimici	**Nahrung, ungesunde**
suture	sutura	**Naht**
cicatrice	cicatrice	**Narbe**
narcolepsie	narcolessia	**Narkolepsie**
anesthésie, narcose	anestesia, narcosi	**Narkose**
anesthésique, narcotique	anestetico, narcotico	**Narkosemittel**
narcotique	narcotico	**narkotisch**
nasal	nasale	**nasal**
nez	naso	**Nase**
épistaxis, saignement de nez	epistassi	**Nasenbluten**
narine	narice	**Nasenloch**
cornet	turbinato	**Nasenmuschel**
végétations adénoïdes	adenoidi	**Nasenpolypen**
rhinopharynx	nasofaringe	**Nasenrachenraum**
nasogastrique	nasogastrico	**nasogastrisch**
nasolacrymal	nasolacrimale	**nasolakrimal**
rhinopharynx	nasofaringe	**Nasopharynx**
nausée	nausea	**Nausea**
naevus	nevo	**Nävus**

GERMAN	ENGLISH	SPANISH
Nebenhoden	epididymis	epidídimo
Nebenhodenentzündung	epididymitis	epididimitis
Nebenhöhle	sinus	seno
Nebennieren-	adrenal	adrenal
Nebennierenrindenhormon (ACH)	adrenal cortical hormone (ACH)	hormona corticosuprarrenal (HCS)
Nebenschilddrüse	parathyroid gland	glándula paratiroidea
Nebenwirkung	side effect	efecto secundario
Nekrose	necrosis	necrosis
Nematode	nematode	nematodo
Neonatalperiode	neonatal period	período neonatal
Neoplasie	neoplasia	neoplasia
Neoplasma	neoplasm	neoplasma
Nephralgie	nephralgia	nefralgia
Nephrektomie	nephrectomy	nefrectomía
Nephritis	nephritis	nefritis
nephrogen	nephrogenic	nefrógeno
Nephrolithotomie	lithonephrotomy	litonefrotomía
Nephrologie	nephrology	nefrología
Nephron	nephron	nefrona
Nephrose	nephrosis	nefrosis
Nephrostomie	nephrostomy	nefrostomía
nephrotisches Syndrom	nephrotic syndrome	síndrome nefrótico
nephrotoxisch	nephrotoxic	nefrotóxico
Nerv	nerve	nervio
Nervenendigung	nerve ending	terminación nerviosa
Nervenentzündung	neuritis	neuritis
Nervus hypoglossus	hypoglossal nerve	hipogloso
Nervus ischiadicus	sciatic nerve	nervio ciático
Nervus peroneus	peroneal nerve	nervio peroneo
Nesselfieber	hives, nettle rash	urticaria
Nesselsucht	urticaria	urticaria
Netz	omentum	epiplón
Netzhaut	retina	retina
Netzhaut, abgelöste	detached retina	desprendimiento de retina
Netzhautentzündung	retinitis	retinitis
neugeboren	neonate, newborn	neonato
Neugeborenenperiode	neonatal period	período neonatal
Neugeborenes	neonate, newborn	neonato
Neugeborenes, zyanotisches	blue baby	niño azul
neural	neural	nervioso
Neuralgie	neuralgia	neuralgia
Neurapraxie	neurapraxia	neuropraxia
Neurasthenie	neurasthenia	neurastenia
Neuritis	neuritis	neuritis
Neuroblastom	neuroblastoma	neuroblastoma
Neurochirurgie	neurosurgery	neurocirugía

FRENCH	ITALIAN	GERMAN
épididyme	epididimo	**Nebenhoden**
épididymite	epididimite	**Nebenhodenentzündung**
sinus	seno, fistula suppurante	**Nebenhöhle**
surrénale	surrenale	**Nebennieren-**
hormone cortico-surrénale	ormone corticosurrenale	**Nebennierenrindenhormon (ACH)**
glande parathyroïde	ghiandola paratiroide	**Nebenschilddrüse**
effet latéral	effetto collaterale	**Nebenwirkung**
nécrose	necrosi	**Nekrose**
nématode	nematode	**Nematode**
période néonatale	periodo neonatale	**Neonatalperiode**
néoplasie	neoplasia	**Neoplasie**
néoplasme	neoplasma	**Neoplasma**
néphralgie	nevralgia	**Nephralgie**
néphrectomie	nefrectomia	**Nephrektomie**
néphrite	nefrite	**Nephritis**
d'origine rénale	nefrogenico	**nephrogen**
lithonéphrotomie	litonefrotomia	**Nephrolithotomie**
néphrologie	nefrologia	**Nephrologie**
néphron	nefrone	**Nephron**
néphrose	nefrosi, nefropatia	**Nephrose**
néphrostomie	nefrostomia	**Nephrostomie**
syndrome néphrotique	sindrome nefrosica	**nephrotisches Syndrom**
néphrotoxique	nefrotossico	**nephrotoxisch**
nerf	nervo	**Nerv**
terminaison nerveuse	terminazione nervosa	**Nervenendigung**
névrite	neurite	**Nervenentzündung**
hypoglosse	ipoglosso	**Nervus hypoglossus**
nerf grand sciatique	nervo sciatico	**Nervus ischiadicus**
nerf péronier	nervo peroneo	**Nervus peroneus**
éruption, urticaire	orticaria	**Nesselfieber**
urticaire	orticaria	**Nesselsucht**
épiploon	omento	**Netz**
rétine	retina	**Netzhaut**
rétine décollée	distacco di retina	**Netzhaut, abgelöste**
rétinite	retinite	**Netzhautentzündung**
nouveau-né	neonato	**neugeboren**
période néonatale	periodo neonatale	**Neugeborenenperiode**
nouveau né	neonato	**Neugeborenes**
enfant bleu, enfant atteint de la maladie bleue	'blue baby' (cianosi da cardiopatia congenita)	**Neugeborenes, zyanotisches**
neural	neurale	**neural**
névralgie	nevralgia	**Neuralgie**
neurapraxie	neuroaprassia	**Neurapraxie**
neurasthénie	neuroastenia	**Neurasthenie**
névrite	neurite	**Neuritis**
neuroblastome	neuroblastoma	**Neuroblastom**
neurochirurgie	neurochirurgia	**Neurochirurgie**

GERMAN	ENGLISH	SPANISH
Neurofibromatose	neurofibromatosis	neurofibromatosis
neurogen	neurogenic	neurógeno
Neurolemm	neurolemma	neurolema
Neuroleptikum	antipsychotic, neuroleptic	antipsicótico, neuroléptico
neuroleptisch	antipsychotic, neuroleptic	antipsicótico, neuroléptico
Neurologie	neurology	neurología
neuromuskulär	neuromuscular	neuromuscular
Neuron	neuron	neurona
Neuropathie	neuropathy	neuropatia
Neuropharmakologie	neuropharmacology	neurofarmacología
Neuropsychiatrie	neuropsychiatry	neuropsiquiatría
Neurose	neurosis	neurosis
Neurosyphilis	neurosyphilis	neurosífilis
neurotrop	neurotropic	neurotrópico
Neutropenie	neutropenia	neutropenia
neutrophil	neutrophil	neutrófilo
Neutrophiler	neutrophil	neutrófilo
nichtinvasiv	non-invasive	no invasivo
nicht perforiert	imperforate	imperforado
nicht unfallbedingte Verletzung	non-accidental injury (NAI)	lesión no accidental
Nidus	nidus	nido
Niere	kidney	riñón
Nieren-	renal	renal
Nierenbeckenentzündung	pyelitis	pielitis
Nierendurchblutung	renal blood flow (RBF)	flujo sanguíneo renal (FSR)
Nierenentzündung	nephritis	nefritis
nierenschädigend	nephrotoxic	nefrotóxico
Niesen	sneeze	estornudo
niesen	sneeze	estornudar
Nikotin	nicotine	nicotina
Nisse	nit	liendre
noch nicht diagnostiziert	not yet diagnosed (NYD)	todavía no diagnosticado
Nodulus	nodule	nódulo
Noncompliance	noncompliance	incumplimiento
non-insulin dependent diabetes mellitus (NIDDM)	non-insulin dependent diabetes mellitus (NIDDM)	diabetes mellitus no insulinodependiente
Noradrenalin	noradrenaline, norepinephrine	noradrenalina, norepinefrina
Norepinephrin	norepinephrine	norepinefrina
Normoblast	normoblast	normoblasto
Normoglykämie	normoglycaemic (Eng), normoglycemic (Am)	normoglucémico
normoton	normotonic	normotónico
Normozyt	normocyte	normocito
Notfallstation	emergency treatment/trauma unit (ETU)	servicio de urgencias/traumatologia
Nüchternblutzucker (NBZ)	fasting blood sugar (FBS)	glucemia en ayunas
Nukleus	nucleus	núcleo
Nullipara	nullipara	nulípara

FRENCH	ITALIAN	GERMAN
neurofibromatose	neurofibromatosi	Neurofibromatose
neurogène	neurogenico	neurogen
neurilemme	neurilemma	Neurolemm
antipsychotique, neuroleptique	antipsicotico, neurolettico	Neuroleptikum
antipsychotique, neuroleptique	antipsicotico, neurolettico	neuroleptisch
neurologie	neurologia	Neurologie
neuromusculaire	neuromuscolare	neuromuskulär
neurone	neurone	Neuron
neuropathie	neuropatia	Neuropathie
neuropharmacologie	neurofarmacologia	Neuropharmakologie
neuropsychiatrie	neuropsichiatria	Neuropsychiatrie
névrose	nevrosi	Neurose
neurosyphilis	neurosifilide	Neurosyphilis
neurotrope	neurotropo	neurotrop
neutropénie	neutropenia	Neutropenie
neutrophile	neutrofilo	neutrophil
polynucléaire neutrophile	granulocito neutrofilo	Neutrophiler
non-invasif	non invasivo	nichtinvasiv
imperforé	imperforato	nicht perforiert
traumatisme non accidentel	lesione non accidentale	nicht unfallbedingte Verletzung
foyer morbide	nido	Nidus
rein	rene	Niere
rénal	renale	Nieren-
pyélite	pielite	Nierenbeckenentzündung
débit sanguin rénal	perfusione renale	Nierendurchblutung
néphrite	nefrite	Nierenentzündung
néphrotoxique	nefrotossico	nierenschädigend
éternuement	starnuto	Niesen
éternuer	starnutire	niesen
nicotine	nicotina	Nikotin
lente	lendine	Nisse
non encore diagnostiqué	non ancora diagnosticato	noch nicht diagnostiziert
nodule	nodulo	Nodulus
non observance	inadempienza a prescrizioni	Noncompliance
diabète sucré non insulinodépendant	diabete mellito non insulinodipendente	non-insulin dependent diabetes mellitus (NIDDM)
noradrénaline, norépinéphrine	noradrenalina, norepinefrina	Noradrenalin
norépinéphrine, noradrénaline	norepinefrina	Norepinephrin
normoblaste	normoblasto	Normoblast
normoglycémique	normoglicemico	Normoglykämie
normotonique	normotonico	normoton
normocyte	normocito	Normozyt
service des urgences/des traumatismes	pronto soccorso	Notfallstation
glycémie à jeun	glicemia a digiuno	Nüchternblutzucker (NBZ)
noyau	nucleo	Nukleus
nullipare	nullipara	Nullipara

GERMAN	ENGLISH	SPANISH
Nyktalgie	nyctalgia	nictalgia
Nykturie	nocturia, nycturia	nicturia
Nystagmus	nystagmus	nistagmo

FRENCH	ITALIAN	GERMAN
nyctalgie	nictalgia	**Nyktalgie**
nycturie	nicturia	**Nykturie**
nystagmus	nistagmo	**Nystagmus**

O

GERMAN	ENGLISH	SPANISH
Obduktion	dissection	disección
O-Bein	genu varum	genu varum
oben	superior	superior
Oberarmknochen	humerus	húmero
Oberbauch	epigastrium	epigastrio
Oberkieferknochen	maxilla	maxilar
Obesitas	obesity	obesidad
obstruktiv	obstructive	obstructivo
Obturator	obturator	obturador
Oculomotorius-	oculomotor	oculomotor
Ödem	edema (Am), oedema (Eng)	edema
Odonto-	odontic	dentario
odontoid	odontoid	odontoides
offen	patent	permeable
Öffnung	orifice	orificio
Ohnmacht	faint	vahído, síncope
ohnmächtig werden	faint	desmayar
Ohr	ear	oído
Ohr-	aural	aural
Ohrenfluß	otorrhea (Am), otorrhoea (Eng)	otorrea
Ohrenheilkunde	otology	otología
Ohrenschmalz	ear wax	cerumen
Ohrenschmerz	otalgia	otalgia
Ohrenspiegel	auriscope, otoscope	auriscopio, otoscopio
Ohrmuschel	pinna	pabellón de la oreja
Ohrspeicheldrüse	parotid gland	glándula parótida
Okklusion	occlusion	oclusión
okkult	occult	oculta
okkultes Blut	occult blood	sangre oculta
okkultes Blut (im Stuhl)	faecal occult blood (FOB) (Eng), fecal occult blood (FOB) (Am)	sangre oculta fecal
okular	ocular	ocular
okzipital	occipital	occipital
okzipitofrontal	occipitofrontal	occipitofrontal
Okziput	occiput	occipucio
Olekranon	olecranon (process)	olécranon
olfaktorisch	olfactory	olfatorio
Oligämie	oligaemia (Eng), oligemia (Am)	oligohemia
Oligomenorrhoe	oligomenorrhea (Am), oligomenorrhoea (Eng)	oligomenorrea
Oligurie	oliguria	oliguria
Omentum	omentum	epiplón
Onchozerkose	onchocerciasis, ringworm	oncocerciasis, tiña
Onkogen	oncogene	oncogén
Onkologie	oncology	oncología
Onychogryposis	onychogryphosis	onicogriposis

FRENCH	ITALIAN	GERMAN
dissection	dissezione	**Obduktion**
genu varum	ginocchio varo	**O-Bein**
supérieur	superiore	**oben**
humérus	omero	**Oberarmknochen**
épigastre	epigastrio	**Oberbauch**
maxillaire	mascella superiore	**Oberkieferknochen**
obésité	obesità	**Obesitas**
obstructif	ostruttivo	**obstruktiv**
obturateur	otturatorio	**Obturator**
oculomoteur	oculomotore	**Oculomotorius-**
oedème	edema	**Ödem**
dentaire	dentario	**Odonto-**
odontoïde	odontoide	**odontoid**
libre	aperto, esposto	**offen**
orifice	orifizio	**Öffnung**
syncope	svenimento	**Ohnmacht**
s'évanouir	svenire	**ohnmächtig werden**
oreille	orecchio	**Ohr**
aural	auricolare	**Ohr-**
otorrhée	otorrea	**Ohrenfluß**
otologie	otologia	**Ohrenheilkunde**
cérumen	cerume	**Ohrenschmalz**
otalgie	otite	**Ohrenschmerz**
auriscope, otoscope	otoscopio	**Ohrenspiegel**
pavillon de l'oreille	padiglione auricolare	**Ohrmuschel**
glande parotide	ghiandola parotide	**Ohrspeicheldrüse**
occlusion	occlusione	**Okklusion**
occulte	occulto	**okkult**
sang occulte	sangue occulto	**okkultes Blut**
sang occulte fécal	sangue occulto fecale	**okkultes Blut (im Stuhl)**
oculaire	oculare	**okular**
occipital	occipitale	**okzipital**
occipito-frontal	occipitofrontale	**okzipitofrontal**
occiput	occipite	**Okziput**
olécrane	olecrano	**Olekranon**
olfactif	olfattorio	**olfaktorisch**
hypovolémie	oligoemia	**Oligämie**
spanioménorrhée	oligomenorrea	**Oligomenorrhoe**
oligurie	oliguria	**Oligurie**
épiploon	omento	**Omentum**
onchocercose, dermatophytose	oncocerchiasi, tricofizia, tinea	**Onchozerkose**
oncogène	oncogene	**Onkogen**
oncologie	oncologia	**Onkologie**
onychogryphose	onicogrifosi	**Onychogryposis**

Onycholyse	onycholysis	onicólisis
Oophorektomie	oophorectomy	ooforectomía
Opazität	opacity	opacidad
Operation	operation	intervención quirúrgica
Operationsmikroskop	operating microscope	microscopio quirúrgico
Ophthalmie	ophthalmia	oftalmía
Ophthalmologie	ophthalmology	oftalmología
Ophthalmoplegie	ophthalmoplegia	oftalmoplejía
Ophthalmoskop	ophthalmoscope	oftalmoscopio
Optiker	optician	óptico
optimal	optimum	óptimo
optisch	optic	óptico
oral	oral	oral
Orangenhaut	peau d'orange	piel de naranja
Orbita	orbit	órbita
Orchidektomie	orchidectomy	orquidectomía
Orchidopexie	orchidopexy	orquidopexia
Orchidotomie	orchidotomy	orquidotomía
Orchipexie	orchiopexy	orquiopexia
Orchitis	orchitis	orquitis
organisch	organic	orgánico
Organismus	organism	organismo
Orgasmus	orgasm	orgasmo
Orientierung	orientation	orientación
Ornithose	psittacosis	psitacosis
orthopädisch	orthopaedic (Eng), orthopedic (Am)	ortopedia
Orthopnoe	orthopnea (Am), orthopnoea (Eng)	ortopnea
Orthoptik	orthoptics	ortóptica
Orthose	orthosis	ortosis
orthostatisch	orthostatic	ortostático
örtlich	topical	tópico
Öse	grommet	cánula ótica
Osgood-Schlatter-Krankheit	Osgood-Schlatter disease	enfermedad de Osgood-Schlatter
Os hyeoideum	hyoid	hioides
Os ilium	ilium	ilion
Osler-Knötchen	Osler's nodes	nódulos de Osler
Osmolalität	osmolality	osmolalidad
Osmolarität	osmolarity	osmolaridad
Osmose	osmosis	osmosis
osmotischer Druck	osmotic pressure	presión osmótica
ösophageal	esophageal (Am), oesophageal (Eng)	esofágico
Ösophagitis	esophagitis (Am), oesophagitis (Eng)	esofagitis
Ösophagus	esophagus (Am), oesophagus (Eng)	esófago
Os pubis	pubis	pubis
Ossikel	ossicle	huesecillos
Osteoarthritis	osteoarthritis (OA)	osteoartritis

FRENCH	ITALIAN	GERMAN
onycholyse	onicolisi	**Onycholyse**
ovariectomie	ovariectomia, ooforectomia	**Oophorektomie**
opacité	opacità	**Opazität**
opération	operazione	**Operation**
microscope opératoire	microscopio chirurgico	**Operationsmikroskop**
ophtalmie	oftalmia	**Ophthalmie**
ophtalmologie	oftalmologia	**Ophthalmologie**
ophtalmoplégie	oftalmoplegia	**Ophthalmoplegie**
ophtalmoscope	oftalmoscopio	**Ophthalmoskop**
opticien	ottico	**Optiker**
optimum	optimum	**optimal**
optique	ottico	**optisch**
oral	orale	**oral**
peau d'orange	buccia d'arancia	**Orangenhaut**
orbite	orbita	**Orbita**
orchidectomie	orchidectomia	**Orchidektomie**
orchidopexie	orchidopessia	**Orchidopexie**
orchodotomie	orchidectomia	**Orchidotomie**
orchidopexie	orchidopessia	**Orchipexie**
orchite	orchite	**Orchitis**
organique	organico	**organisch**
organisme	organismo	**Organismus**
orgasme	orgasmo	**Orgasmus**
orientation	orientamento	**Orientierung**
psittacose	psittacosi	**Ornithose**
orthopédique	ortopedia	**orthopädisch**
orthopnée	ortopnea	**Orthopnoe**
orthoptique	ortottica	**Orthoptik**
orthèse	raddrizzamento, correzione di una deformità	**Orthose**
orthostatique	ortostatico	**orthostatisch**
topique	topico, locale	**örtlich**
grommet	catetere per drenaggio auricolare	**Öse**
maladie d'Osgood-Schlatter	malattia di Osgood-Schlatter	**Osgood-Schlatter-Krankheit**
hyoïde	ioide	**Os hyeoideum**
ilion	ilio, osso dell'anca	**Os ilium**
nodules d'Osler	noduli di Osler	**Osler-Knötchen**
osmolalité	osmolalità	**Osmolalität**
osmolarité	osmolarità	**Osmolarität**
osmose	osmosi	**Osmose**
pression osmotique	pressione osmotica	**osmotischer Druck**
oesophagien	esofageo	**ösophageal**
oesophagite	esofagite	**Ösophagitis**
oesophage	esofago	**Ösophagus**
pubis	pube	**Os pubis**
osselet	ossicino	**Ossikel**
ostéo-arthrite	osteoartrosi (OA)	**Osteoarthritis**

GERMAN	ENGLISH	SPANISH
Osteoarthrose	osteoarthropathy	osteoartropatía
Osteoblast	osteoblast	osteoblasto
Osteochondritis	osteochondritis	osteocondritis
Osteochondrom	osteochondroma	osteocondroma
Osteochondrose	osteochondrosis	osteocondrosis
Osteodystrophie	osteodystrophy	osteodistrofia
osteogen	osteogenic	osteogénico
Osteoklast	osteoclast	osteoclasto
osteolytisch	osteolytic	osteolítico
Osteom	osteoma	osteoma
Osteomalazie	osteomalacia	osteomalacia
Osteomyelitis	osteomyelitis	osteomielitis
Osteopathie	osteopathy	osteopatía
Osteopetrose	osteopetrosis	osteopetrosis
Osteophyt	osteophyte	osteofito
Osteoplastik	bone graft	injerto óseo, osteoplastia
Osteoporose	osteoporosis	osteoporosis
Osteosarkom	osteosarcoma	osteosarcoma
Osteosklerose	osteosclerosis	osteosclerosis
Osteotomie	osteotomy, ostomy	osteotomía, ostomía
Osteozyt	osteocyte	osteocito
Ostitis	osteitis	osteítis
Östradiol	estradiol (Am), oestradiol (Eng)	estradiol
Östriol	estriol (Am), oestriol (Eng)	estriol
Östrogen	estrogen (Am), oestrogen (Eng)	estrógeno
Oszillation	oscillation	oscilación
Otalgie	otalgia	otalgia
Otitis	otitis	otitis
Otolaryngologie	otolaryngology	otolaringología
Otologie	otology	otología
Otorrhoe	otorrhea (Am), otorrhoea (Eng)	otorrea
Otosklerose	otosclerosis	otosclerosis
Otoskop	otoscope	otoscopio
ototoxisch	ototoxic	ototóxico
ovarial	ovarian	ovárico
Ovarium	ovary	ovario
Ovulation	ovulation	ovulación
Ovum	egg, ovum	huevo, óvulo
Oxydation	oxidation	oxidación
Oxygenierung	oxygenation	oxigenación
Oxytozin	oxytocin	oxitocina
Oxyuris	whipworm	trichuris trichiura

ostéo-arthropathie	osteoartropatia	**Osteoarthrose**
ostéoblaste	osteoblasto	**Osteoblast**
ostéochondrite	osteocondrite	**Osteochondritis**
ostéochondrome	osteocondroma	**Osteochondrom**
ostéochondrose	osteocondrosi	**Osteochondrose**
ostéodystrophie	osteodistrofia	**Osteodystrophie**
ostéogène	osteogenico	**osteogen**
ostéoclaste	osteoclasto	**Osteoklast**
ostéolytique	osteolitico	**osteolytisch**
ostéome	osteoma	**Osteom**
ostéomalacie	osteomalacia	**Osteomalazie**
ostéomyélite	osteomielite	**Osteomyelitis**
ostéopathie	osteopatia	**Osteopathie**
ostéopétrose	osteoporosi	**Osteopetrose**
ostéophyte	osteofito	**Osteophyt**
greffe osseuse	trapianto osseo	**Osteoplastik**
ostéoporose	osteoporosi	**Osteoporose**
ostéosarcome	sarcoma osteogenico	**Osteosarkom**
ostéosclérose	osteosclerosi	**Osteosklerose**
ostéotomie	osteotomia, otalgia	**Osteotomie**
ostéocyte	osteocito	**Osteozyt**
ostéite	osteite	**Ostitis**
oestradiol	estradiolo	**Östradiol**
oestriol	estriolo	**Östriol**
oestrogène	estrogeno	**Östrogen**
oscillation	oscillazione	**Oszillation**
otalgie	otite	**Otalgie**
otite	otite	**Otitis**
otolaryngologie	otolaringologia	**Otolaryngologie**
otologie	otologia	**Otologie**
otorrhée	otorrea	**Otorrhoe**
otospongiose	otosclerosi	**Otosklerose**
otoscope	otoscopio	**Otoskop**
ototoxique	ototossico	**ototoxisch**
ovarien	ovarico	**ovarial**
ovaire	ovaio	**Ovarium**
ovulation	ovulazione	**Ovulation**
oeuf, ovule, ovocyte de premier ordre	uovo, gamete femminile	**Ovum**
oxydation	ossidazione	**Oxydation**
oxygénation	ossigenazione	**Oxygenierung**
oxytocine	ossitocina	**Oxytozin**
flagellé	verme a frusta, tricocefalo	**Oxyuris**

P

GERMAN	ENGLISH	SPANISH
Pädiatrie	paediatrics (Eng), pediatrics (Am)	pediatría
palatal	palatine	palatino
palliativ	palliative	paliativo
Palliativum	palliative	paliativo
palmar	palmar	palmar
palpabel	palpable	palpable
Palpation	palpation	palpación
Palpebra	palpebra	párpado
Palpitation	palpitation	palpitación
Panaritium	whitlow	panadizo
Pandemie	pandemic	pandémico
pandemisch	pandemic	pandémico
Pankreas	pancreas	páncreas
Pankreatitis	pancreatitis	pancreatitis
Panzytopenie	pancytopenia	pancitopenia
Papanicolaou-Färbung (Pap)	Papanicolaou's stain test (Pap test)	prueba de tinción de Papanicolaou
Papel	papule	pápula
papillär	papillary	papilar
Papille	blind spot	mancha ciega
Papillenödem	papilledema (Am), papilloedema (Eng)	papiledema
Papillom	papilloma	papiloma
Paralyse	palsy, paralysis	parálisis
paralytisch	paralytic	paralítico
paramedizinisch	paramedical	paramédico
Paranoia	paranoia	paranoia
paranoide Schizophrenie	paranoid schizophrenia	esquizofrenia paranoica
Paraphimose	paraphimosis	parafimosis
Paraphrenie	paraphrenia	parafrenia
Paraplegie	paraplegia	paraplejía
Parasit	parasite	parásito
Parästhesie	paraesthesia (Eng), paresthesia (Am)	parestesia
parasuizidale Handlung	parasuicide	parasuicidio
parasympathisch	parasympathetic	parasimpático
Parathormon	parathormone	parathormona
Parathyreoidea	parathyroid gland	glándula paratiroidea
Parathyreoidektomie	parathyroidectomy	paratiroidectomía
Paratyphus	paratyphoid fever	fiebre paratifoidea
paravertebral	paravertebral	paravertebral
Parazentese	myringotomy	miringotomía
Parenchym	parenchyma	parénquima
parenteral	parenteral	parenteral
Parese	paresis	paresia
parietal	parietal	parietal
Parkinsonismus	parkinsonism	parkinsonismo
Paronychie	paronychia	paroniquia

FRENCH	ITALIAN	GERMAN
pédiatrie	pediatria	**Pädiatrie**
palatin	palatale, palatino	**palatal**
palliatif	palliativo	**palliativ**
palliatif	palliativo	**Palliativum**
palmaire	palmare	**palmar**
palpable	palpabile	**palpabel**
palpation	palpazione	**Palpation**
paupière	palpebra	**Palpebra**
palpitation	palpitazione	**Palpitation**
panaris	patereccio	**Panaritium**
pandémie	pandemia	**Pandemie**
pandémique	pandemico	**pandemisch**
pancréas	pancreas	**Pankreas**
pancréatite	pancreatite	**Pankreatitis**
pancytopénie	pancitopenia	**Panzytopenie**
test de Papanicolaou	test di Papanicolaou (Pap test)	**Papanicolaou-Färbung (Pap)**
papule	papula	**Papel**
papillaire	papillare	**papillär**
tache aveugle	punto cieco	**Papille**
oedème papillaire	papilledema	**Papillenödem**
papillome	papilloma	**Papillom**
paralysie	paralisi	**Paralyse**
paralytique	paralitico	**paralytisch**
paramédical	paramedico	**paramedizinisch**
paranoïa	paranoia	**Paranoia**
schizophrénie paranoïaque	schizofrenia paranoide	**paranoide Schizophrenie**
paraphimosis	parafimosi	**Paraphimose**
paraphrénie	parafrenia	**Paraphrenie**
paraplégie	paraplegia	**Paraplegie**
parasite	parassita	**Parasit**
paresthésie	parestesia	**Parästhesie**
parasuicide	suicidio figurato	**parasuizidale Handlung**
parasympathique	parasimpatico	**parasympathisch**
parathormone	paratormone	**Parathormon**
glande parathyroïde	ghiandola paratiroide	**Parathyreoidea**
parathyroïdectomie	paratiroidectomia	**Parathyreoidektomie**
fièvre paratyphoïde	febbre paratifoide	**Paratyphus**
paravertébral	paravertebrale	**paravertebral**
myringotomie	miringotomia	**Parazentese**
parenchyme	parenchima	**Parenchym**
parentéral	parenterale	**parenteral**
parésie	paresi	**Parese**
pariétal	parietale	**parietal**
parkinsonisme	parkinsonismo	**Parkinsonismus**
panaris superficiel	paronichia	**Paronychie**

GERMAN	ENGLISH	SPANISH
Parotis	parotid gland	glándula parótida
Parotitis	parotitis	parotiditis
paroxysmal	paroxysmal	paroxístico
Partialdruck	partial pressure	presión parcial
passiv	passive	pasivo
Paste	paste	pasta
Pasteurisierung	pasteurization	pasteurización
Pastille	lozenge	pastilla
Patella	patella	rótula
Pathogenese	pathogenesis	patogenia
Pathogenität	pathogenicity	patogenicidad
pathognomonisch	pathognomonic	patognomónico
Pathologie	pathology	patología
pathologische Fraktur	pathological fracture	fractura patológica
Paul-Bunnell-Reaktion	Paul-Bunnell test	prueba de Paul-Bunnell
Peak-Flowmeter	peak expiratory flow meter (PEFM)	medida de la velocidad máxima del flujo espiratorio
Pedikulose	pediculosis	pediculosis
Pediküre	chiropody	podología
Peitschenhiebsyndrom	whiplash	latigazo
Peitschenwurm	whipworm	trichuris trichiura
pektoral	pectoral	pectoral
Pellagra	pellagra	pelagra
Pelvimetrie	pelvimetry	pelvimetría
Pelvis	pelvis	pelvis
pemphigoid	pemphigoid	penfigoide
Pemphigus	pemphigus	pénfigo
Penis	penis, phallus	pene, falo
Pepsin	pepsin	pepsina
Peptide	peptide	péptido
peptisch	peptic	péptico
Perforation	perforation	perforación
perianal	perianal	perianal
Periarthritis humeroscapularis	frozen shoulder	hombro congelado/rígido
Perichondrium	perichondrium	pericondrio
Perikard	pericardium	pericardio
Perikarditis	pericarditis	pericarditis
perinatal	perinatal	perinatal
Perineum	perineum	perineo
Periodontitis	periodontal disease	enfermedad periodontal
perioperativ	perioperative	perioperatorio
perioral	perioral	perioral
Periost	periosteum	periostio
peripher	peripheral	periférico
Peristaltik	peristalsis	peristalsis
Peritonealdialyse	peritoneal dialysis	diálisis peritoneal
Peritoneum	peritoneum	peritoneo

FRENCH	ITALIAN	GERMAN
glande parotide	ghiandola parotide	**Parotis**
parotite	parotite	**Parotitis**
paroxysmal	parossistico	**paroxysmal**
pression partielle	pressione parziale	**Partialdruck**
passif	passivo	**passiv**
pâte	pasta, pasta gelificante	**Paste**
pasteurisation	pastorizzazione	**Pasteurisierung**
pastille	pastiglia	**Pastille**
rotule	patella, rotula	**Patella**
pathogenèse	patogenesi	**Pathogenese**
pouvoir pathogène	patogeneticità	**Pathogenität**
pathognomonique	patognomonico	**pathognomonisch**
pathologie	patologia	**Pathologie**
fracture spontanée	frattura patologica	**pathologische Fraktur**
réaction de Paul et Bunnell	test di Paul-Bunnell	**Paul-Bunnell-Reaktion**
appareil de mesure du débit expiratoire de pointe	misuratore del flusso espiratorio massimo	**Peak-Flowmeter**
pédiculose	pediculosi	**Pedikulose**
chiropodie	chiropodia	**Pediküre**
coup de fouet	colpo di frusta	**Peitschenhiebsyndrom**
flagellé	verme a frusta, tricocefalo	**Peitschenwurm**
pectoral	pettorale	**pektoral**
pellagre	pellagra	**Pellagra**
pelvimétrie	pelvimetria	**Pelvimetrie**
pelvis	pelvi	**Pelvis**
pemphigoïde	pemfigoide	**pemphigoid**
pemphigus	pemfigo	**Pemphigus**
pénis, phallus	pene, fallo	**Penis**
pepsine	pepsina	**Pepsin**
peptide	peptide	**Peptide**
peptique	peptico	**peptisch**
perforation	perforazione	**Perforation**
périanal	perianale	**perianal**
épaule ankylosée	'spalla congelata', periartrite scapoloomerale	**Periarthritis humeroscapularis**
périchondre	pericondrio	**Perichondrium**
péricarde	pericardio	**Perikard**
péricardite	pericardite	**Perikarditis**
périnatal	perinatale	**perinatal**
périnée	perineo	**Perineum**
paradontolyse	periodontopatia	**Periodontitis**
périopératoire	perioperatorio	**perioperativ**
périoral	periorale	**perioral**
périoste	periostio	**Periost**
périphérique	periferico	**peripher**
péristaltisme	peristalsi	**Peristaltik**
dialyse péritonéale	dialisi peritoneale	**Peritonealdialyse**
péritoine	peritoneo	**Peritoneum**

GERMAN	ENGLISH	SPANISH
Peritonitis	peritonitis	peritonitis
Peritonsillarabszeß	peritonsillar abscess, quinsy	absceso periamigdalino, angina
periumbilikal	periumbilical	periumbilical
Perkussion	percussion	percusión
perkutan	percutaneous	percutáneo
Perkutieren	tapping	paracentesis
permeabel	permeable	permeable
Pernio	chilblain	sabañón
perniziöse Anämie	pernicious anaemia (Eng), pernicious anemia (Am)	anemia perniciosa
peroral	peroral	peroral
Perseveration	perseveration	perseverancia
Persönlichkeit	personality	personalidad
Persönlichkeit, asoziale	antisocial personality	personalidad antisocial
Perthes-Krankheit	Perthes' disease	enfermedad de Perthes
Pertussis	pertussis	tos ferina
Perzeption	perception	percepción
pes equinovarus	talipes	talipes
Pessar	pessary	pesario
Pest	plague	peste, plaga
Petechie	petechia	petequia
Petit mal	petit mal	petit mal
Petrischale	Petri dish	disco de Petri
Peyer Plaques	Peyer's patches	placas de Peyer
Pfeiffersches Drüsenfieber	glandular fever, infectious mononucleosis, mononucleosis	fiebre glandular, mononucleosis infecciosa, mononucleosis
Pflaster	plaster	yeso
Pflege	fostering	adopción
pflegen	nurse	cuidar
Pflegerin	nurse	enfermera
Pflege Sterbender	terminal care	cuidados terminales
Pfortader	portal vein	vena porta
Pfortaderhochdruck	portal hypertension	hipertensión portal
Pfortaderkreislauf	portal circulation	circulación portal
Phagozyt	macrophage, phagocyte	macrófago, fagocito
Phagozytose	phagocytosis	fagocitosis
Phallus	phallus	falo
Phänotyp	phenotype	fenotipo
Phäochromozytom	phaeochromocytoma (Eng), pheochromocytoma (Am)	feocromocitoma
Pharmakogenetik	pharmacogenetics	farmacogenético
Pharmakokinetik	pharmacokinetics	farmacocinética
Pharmakologie	pharmacology	farmacología
Pharmazeut	pharmacist	farmacéutico
pharmazeutisch	pharmaceutical	farmacéutico
Pharyngitis	pharyngitis	faringitis

540

péritonite	peritonite	**Peritonitis**
abcès périamygdalien, phlegmon amygdalien ou périamygdalien	ascesso peritonsillare	**Peritonsillarabszeß**
périombilical	periombelicale	**periumbilikal**
percussion	percussione	**Perkussion**
percutané	percutaneo	**perkutan**
ponction	aspirazione di fluido	**Perkutieren**
perméable	permeabile	**permeabel**
engelure	gelone	**Pornio**
anémie pernicieuse	anemia perniciosa	**perniziöse Anämie**
peroral	perorale	**peroral**
persévération	perseverazione	**Perseveration**
personnalité	personalità	**Persönlichkeit**
personnalité psychopathique	personalità antisociale	**Persönlichkeit, asoziale**
coxa plana	malattia di Perthes	**Perthes-Krankheit**
pertussis	pertosse	**Pertussis**
perception	percezione	**Perzeption**
pied bot	piede talo	**pes equinovarus**
pessaire	pessario	**Pessar**
peste	peste	**Pest**
pétéchie	petecchia	**Petechie**
petit mal	piccolo male	**Petit mal**
boîte de Pétri	capsula di Petri	**Petrischale**
plaques de Peyer	placche di Peyer	**Peyer Plaques**
flèvre glandulaire, mononucléose infectieuse, mononucléose	mononucleosi infettiva, mononucleosi	**Pfeiffersches Drüsenfieber**
plâtre	gesso	**Pflaster**
prise en nourrice	affido	**Pflege**
soigner	assistere	**pflegen**
infirmière	infermiere	**Pflegerin**
soins pour malades en phase terminale	cura terminale	**Pflege Sterbender**
veine porte	vena porta	**Pfortader**
circulation porte	ipertensione portale	**Pfortaderhochdruck**
hypertension porte	circolazione portale	**Pfortaderkreislauf**
macrophage, phagocyte	macrofago, fagocito	**Phagozyt**
phagocytose	fagocitosi	**Phagozytose**
phallus	fallo	**Phallus**
phénotype	fenotipo	**Phänotyp**
phéochromocytome	feocromocitoma	**Phäochromozytom**
pharmacogénétique	farmacogenetica	**Pharmakogenetik**
pharmacocinétique	farmacocinetica	**Pharmakokinetik**
pharmacologie	farmacologia	**Pharmakologie**
pharmacien	farmacista	**Pharmazeut**
pharmaceutique	farmaceutico	**pharmazeutisch**
pharyngite	faringite	**Pharyngitis**

GERMAN	ENGLISH	SPANISH
Pharyngotomie	pharyngotomy	faringotomía
Pharynx	pharynx	faringe
Phenylketonurie (PKU)	phenylketonuria (PKU)	fenilcetonuria
Phimose	phimosis	fimosis
Phlebektomie	phlebectomy	flebectomía
Phlebitis	phlebitis	flebitis
Phlebographie	venography	venografía
Phlebolith	phlebolith	flebolito
Phlegma	phlegm	flema
Phobie	phobia	fobia
Phokomelie	phocomelia	focomelia
Photophobie	photophobia	fotofobia
Phototherapie	phototherapy	fototerapia
physiologisch	physiological	fisiológico
Pica	pica	pica
Pickel	pimple, pustule, spot	grano, pústula, mancha
Pigment	pigment	pigmento
Pigmentierung	pigmentation	pigmentación
Pille	pill	píldora
pilonidal	pilonidal	pilonidal
Pilz	fungus	hongo
Pilzinfektion	mycosis	micosis
Pinguekula	pinguecula	pinguécula
Pinta	pinta	mal de pinto
Pinzette	forceps	fórceps
Pityriasis	pityriasis	pitiriasis
plantar	plantar	plantar
Plaque	plaque	placa
Plasma	plasma	plasma
Plasmapherese	plasmapheresis	plasmaféresis
Plastik	graft	injerto
Plättchen-Aggregations-Test (PAT)	platelet aggregation test (PAT)	prueba de la agregación plaquetaria
Plattfuß	flat-foot	pie plano
Platzangst	agoraphobia	agorafobia
Plazebo	placebo	placebo
Plazenta	afterbirth, placenta	secundinas, expulsión de la placenta y membranas, placenta
Plazentaablösung	placental abruption	desprendimiento prematuro de la placenta
Plazentainsuffizienz	placental insufficiency	insuficiencia placentaria
Plethora	plethora	plétora
Pleura	pleura	pleura
Pleuralgie	pleurodynia	pleurodinia
Pleuritis	pleurisy (pleuritis)	pleuresia, pleuritis
Pleurodese	pleurodesis	pleurodesis
Plexus	plexus	plexo

FRENCH	ITALIAN	GERMAN
pharyngotomie	faringotomia	**Pharyngotomie**
pharynx	faringe	**Pharynx**
phénylcétonurie	fenilchetonuria	**Phenylketonurie (PKU)**
phimosis	fimosi	**Phimose**
phlébectomie	flebectomia	**Phlebektomie**
phlébite	flebite	**Phlebitis**
phlébographie	flebografia	**Phlebographie**
phlébolithe	flebolito	**Phlebolith**
phlegme	flemma	**Phlegma**
phobie	fobia	**Phobie**
phocomélie	focomelia	**Phokomelie**
photophobie	fotofobia	**Photophobie**
photothérapie	fototerapia	**Phototherapie**
physiologique	fisiologico	**physiologisch**
pica	picacismo	**Pica**
bouton, pustule	pustola, piccolo foruncolo, foruncolo	**Pickel**
pigment	pigmento	**Pigment**
pigmentation	pigmentazione	**Pigmentierung**
pilule	pillola	**Pille**
pilonidal	pilonidale	**pilonidal**
mycète	fungo	**Pilz**
mycose	micosi	**Pilzinfektion**
pinguécula	pinguecula	**Pinguekula**
pinta	pinta, spirochetosi discromica	**Pinta**
forceps	forcipe	**Pinzette**
pityriasis	pitiriasi	**Pityriasis**
plantaire	plantare	**plantar**
plaque	placca	**Plaque**
plasma	plasma	**Plasma**
plasmaphérèse	plasmaferesi	**Plasmapherese**
greffe	trapianto, innesto	**Plastik**
test d'agrégation plaquettaire (PAT)	test di aggregazione plastrinico	**Plättchen-Aggregations-Test (PAT)**
pied plat	piede piatto	**Plattfuß**
agoraphobie	agorafobia	**Platzangst**
placebo	placebo	**Plazebo**
arrière-faix, placenta	secondine, membrane fetali e placenta, placenta	**Plazenta**
rupture placentaire	distacco prematuro della placenta	**Plazentaablösung**
insuffisance placentaire	insufficienza placentare	**Plazentainsuffizienz**
pléthore	pletora	**Plethora**
plèvre	pleura	**Pleura**
pleurodynie	pleurodinia	**Pleuralgie**
pleurésie	pleurite	**Pleuritis**
pleurodèse	pleurodesi	**Pleurodese**
plexus	plesso	**Plexus**

GERMAN	ENGLISH	SPANISH
plötzlicher Säuglingstod	cot death, sudden infant death syndrome (SIDS)	muerte en la cuna, muerte súbita infantil, síndrome de muerte súbita infantil
Pneumaturie	pneumaturia	neumaturia
Pneumokoniose	pneumoconiosis	neumoconiosis
Pneumonektomie	pneumonectomy	neumonectomía
Pneumonie	pneumonia	neumonía
Pneumonitis	pneumonitis	neumonitis
Pneumoperitoneum	pneumoperitoneum	neumoperitoneo
Pneumothorax	pneumothorax	neumotórax
Pneumozephalus	pneumocephalus	neumocéfalo
Pneumozyt	pneumocyte	neumocito
Pocken	smallpox	viruela
Poliomyelitis	poliomyelitis	poliomielitis
Poliovirus	poliovirus	poliovirus
Polyarteritis	polyarteritis	poliarteritis
Polyarthralgie	polyarthralgia	poliartralgia
Polyarthritis	polyarthritis	poliartritis
Polyarthritis rheumatica (PCP)	rheumatoid arthritis (RA)	artritis reumatoide (AR)
Polydipsie	polydipsia	polidipsia
Polymyalgia rheumatica	polymyalgia rheumatica	polimialgia reumática
Polymyositis	polymyositis	polimiositis
Polyneuritis	polyneuritis	polineuritis
Polyp	polyp	pólipo
Polypektomie	polypectomy	polipectomía
Polypenentfernung	adenoidectomy	adenoidectomía
Polyposis	polyposis	poliposis
Polypragmasie	polypharmacy	polifarmacia
Polysaccharid	polysaccharide	polisacárido
Polyurie	polyuria	poliuria
polyzystisch	polycystic	poliquístico
Polyzythämie	polycythaemia (Eng), polycythemia (Am)	policitemia
Pompholyx	pompholyx	ponfólix
popliteal	popliteal	poplíteo
popliteus	popliteus	poplíteo
Pore	pore	poro
Porphyrie	porphyria	porfiria
Porphyrin	porphyrin	porfirinas
Porta hepatis	portahepatitis	portohepatitis
Portalkreislauf	portal circulation	circulación portal
portokaval	portacaval	portocava
postenzephalitisch	postencephalitic	postencefalítico
posteriore	posterior	posterior
posthepatisch	posthepatic	posthepático
postherpetisch	postherpetic	postherpético

FRENCH	ITALIAN	GERMAN
mort subite de nourrisson, syndrome de mort subite de nourrisson	sindrome da morte improvvisa del lattante, sindrome della morte neonatale improvvisa (SIDS)	plötzlicher Säuglingstod
pneumaturie	pneumaturia	Pneumaturie
pneumoconiose	pneumoconiosi	Pneumokoniose
pneumonectomie	pneumonectomia	Pneumonektomie
pneumonie	polmonite	Pneumonie
pneumonite	polmonite	Pneumonitis
pneumopéritoine	pneumoperitoneo	Pneumoperitoneum
pneumothorax	pneumotorace	Pneumothorax
pneumo-encéphale, pneumocéphale	pneumocefalo	Pneumozephalus
cellule alvéolaire	pneumocito	Pneumozyt
variole	vaiolo	Pocken
poliomyélite	poliomielite	Poliomyelitis
poliovirus	virus della poliomielite	Poliovirus
polyartérite	poliarterite	Polyarteritis
polyarthralgie	poliartralgia	Polyarthralgie
polyarthrite	poliartrite	Polyarthritis
polyarthrite rhumatoïde (PR), polyarthrite chronique évolutive (PCE)	artrite reumatoide (AR)	Polyarthritis rheumatica (PCP)
polydipsie	polidipsia	Polydipsie
polymyalgie rhumatismale	polimialgia reumatica	Polymyalgia rheumatica
polymyosite	polimiosite	Polymyositis
polynévrite	polineurite	Polyneuritis
polype	polipo	Polyp
polypectomie	polipectomia	Polypektomie
adénoïdectomie	adenoidectomia	Polypenentfernung
polypose	poliposi	Polyposis
polypharmacie	prescrizione multipla di farmaci, abuso di farmaci	Polypragmasie
polysaccharide	polisaccaride	Polysaccharid
polyurie	poliuria	Polyurie
polykystique	policistico	polyzystisch
polycythémie	policitemia	Polyzythämie
pompholyx	ponfolice (disidrosi vescicolare)	Pompholyx
poplité	popliteo	popliteal
poplité	popliteo	popliteus
pore	poro	Pore
porphyrie	porfiria	Porphyrie
porphyrine	porfirina	Porphyrin
porto-hépatite	portaepatite	Porta hepatis
hypertension porte	circolazione portale	Portalkreislauf
porto-cave	portocavale	portokaval
postencéphalitique	postencefalitico	postenzephalitisch
postérieur	posteriore	posteriore
posthépatique	postepatico	posthepatisch
postherpétique	posterpetico	postherpetisch

GERMAN	ENGLISH	SPANISH
Postkoital-	postcoital	postcoital
postmenopausal	postmenopausal	postmenopáusico
postmortal	post-mortem	postmortem
postnasal	postnasal	postnasal
postnatal	postnatal	postnatal
postoperativ	postoperative	postoperatorio
post partum	postpartum	postpartum
postprandial	postprandial	postprandial
Pott-Fraktur	Pott's fracture	fractura de Pott
pounds per square inch (psi)	pounds per square inch (psi)	libras por pulgada cuadrada (psi)
ppm	parts per million (ppm)	partes por millón (ppm)
Prädisposition	predisposition	predisposición
Präeklampsie	pre-eclampsia	preeclampsia
präkanzerös	precancerous	precanceroso
präkordial	precordial	precordial
Präkursor	precursor	precursor
Prämedikation	premedication	premedicación
prämenstruell	premenstrual	premenstrual
prämenstruelles Syndrom	premenstrual tension (PMT)	tensión premenstrual
pränatal	antenatal, prenatal	antenatal, prenatal
präoperativ	preoperative	preoperatorio
Präpubertäts-	prepubertal	prepubertal
Präputium	foreskin, prepuce	prepucio
prärenal	prerenal	prerrenal
Präservativ	condom	condón
Prellung	bruise	contusión, equímosis
Pressen	bearing down	postración
Primärkomplex	primary complex	complejo primario
Primärversorgung	primary care	asistencia primaria
Primigravida	primigravida	primigrávida
Primipara	primipara	primípara
prodromal	prodromal	prodrómico
pro-drug (Pharmakon-Vorform)	pro-drug	profármaco
Prognose	prognosis	pronóstico
progressive Paralyse	general paralysis of the insane	parálisis cerebral
Proktalgie	proctalgia	proctalgia
Proktitis	proctitis	proctitis
Proktokolektomie	proctocolectomy	proctocolectomia
Proktokolitis	proctocolitis	proctocolitis
Prolaps	procidentia, prolapse	procidencia, prolapso
proliferieren	proliferate	proliferar
Pronator	pronator	pronador
pronieren	pronate	pronar
Prophylaxe	prophylaxis	profilaxis
Prostaglandine	prostaglandin	prostaglandina
Prostata	prostate	próstata

FRENCH	ITALIAN	GERMAN
après rapport	postcoitale	**Postkoital-**
postménopausique	postmenopausale	**postmenopausal**
post mortem	post mortem	**postmortal**
rétronasal	retronasale	**postnasal**
postnatal	postnatale	**postnatal**
postopératoire	postoperatorio	**postoperativ**
postpartum	post partum	**post partum**
postprandial	postprandiale	**postprandial**
fracture de Pott	frattura di Pott	**Pott-Fraktur**
livres par pouce carré (psi)	libbre per pollici quadrati	**pounds per square inch (psi)**
parties par million (ppm)	parti per milione (ppm)	**ppm**
prédisposition	predisposizione	**Prädisposition**
éclampsisme	preeclampsia	**Präeklampsie**
précancéreux	precanceroso	**präkanzerös**
précordial	precordiale, epigastrico	**präkordial**
précurseur	precursore	**Präkursor**
prémédication	premedicazione, preanestesia	**Prämedikation**
prémenstruel	premestruale	**prämenstruell**
syndrome de tension prémenstruelle	tensione premenstruale	**prämenstruelles Syndrom**
anténatal, prénatal	prenatale	**pränatal**
préopératoire	preoperatorio	**präoperativ**
prépubertaire	prepubertale	**Präpubertäts-**
prépuce	prepuzio	**Präputium**
prérénal	prerenale	**prärenal**
préservatif	profilattico maschile	**Präservativ**
contusion	contusione	**Prellung**
efforts expulsifs	fase espulsiva del parto	**Pressen**
complexe primaire	complesso primario, complesso di Ghon	**Primärkomplex**
soins de santé primaires	primaria, neoplasia primitiva	**Primärversorgung**
primigeste	primigravida	**Primigravida**
primipare	primipara	**Primipara**
prodromique	prodromico	**prodromal**
précurseur de médicament	profarmaco (precursore inattivo)	**pro-drug (Pharmakon-Vorform)**
pronostic	prognosi	**Prognose**
paralysie générale des aliénés	paralisi progressiva luetica	**progressive Paralyse**
proctalgie	proctalgia	**Proktalgie**
rectite	proctite	**Proktitis**
proctocolectomie	proctocolectomia, rettocolectomia	**Proktokolektomie**
rectocolite	proctocolite	**Proktokolitis**
procidence, prolapsus	procidenza, prolasso	**Prolaps**
proliférer	proliferare	**proliferieren**
pronateur	pronatore	**Pronator**
mettre en pronation	pronare	**pronieren**
prophylaxie	profilassi	**Prophylaxe**
prostaglandine	prostaglandina	**Prostaglandine**
prostate	prostata	**Prostata**

GERMAN	ENGLISH	SPANISH
Prostataleiden, chronisches	prostatism	prostatismo
Prostatektomie	prostatectomy	prostatectomía
Protein	protein	proteína
Proteinurie	proteinuria	proteinuria
proteolytisches Enzym	proteolytic enzyme	enzima proteolítico
Prothese	prosthesis	prótesis
Protozoe	protozoa	protozoos
proximal	proximal	proximal
Pruritus	pruritus	prurito
Pseudopolypse	pseudopolyposis	pseudopoliposis
Psittakose	psittacosis	psitacosis
Psoas	psoas	psoas
Psoralen	psoralen	psoralen
Psoriasis	psoriasis	psoriasis
Psychiatrie	psychiatry	psiquiatría
psychiatrisch	psychiatric	psiquiátrico
psychisch	psychic	psíquico
Psychoanalyse	psychoanalysis	psicoanálisis
Psychodynamik	psychodynamics	psicodinámica
psychogen	psychogenic	psicógeno
Psychologie	psychology	psicología
psychomotorisch	psychomotor	psicomotor
Psychopath	psychopath	psicópata
Psychopathie	psychopathy	psicopatía
psychopathische Persönlichkeit	psychopathic personality	personalidad psicopática
Psychopathologie	psychopathology	psicopatología
Psychose	psychosis	psicosis
psychosomatisch	psychosomatic	psicosomático
Psychotherapie	psychotherapy	psicoterapia
psychotrop	psychotropic	psicotrópico
Pterygium	pterygium	pterigión
Ptose	ptosis	ptosis
Pubertät	puberty	pubertad
Pudendusblock	pudendal block	bloqueo del pudendo
puerperal	puerperal	puerperal
Puerperium	puerperium	puerperio
Puls	pulse	pulso
Pulsieren	pulsation	pulsación
pulsierend	pulsatile	pulsátil
Pulsloskrankheit	pulseless disease	enfermedad sin pulso
Pulsschlag	pulsation	pulsación
Pulsus alternans	pulsus alternans	pulso alternante
Pulsus paradoxus	pulsus paradoxus	pulso paradójico
Punktieren	tapping	paracentesis
pupillar	pupillary	pupilar
Pupille	pupil	pupila
Pupillen-	pupillary	pupilar

FRENCH	ITALIAN	GERMAN
prostatisme	prostatismo	**Prostataleiden, chronisches**
prostatectomie	prostatectomia	**Prostatektomie**
protéine	proteina	**Protein**
protéinurie	proteinuria	**Proteinurie**
enzyme protéolytique	enzima proteolitico, proteasi	**proteolytisches Enzym**
prothèse	protesi	**Prothese**
protozoaires	protozoi	**Protozoe**
proximal	prossimale	**proximal**
prurit	prurito	**Pruritus**
pseudopolypose	pseudopoliposi	**Pseudopolyhpse**
psittacose	psittacosi	**Psittakose**
psoas	psoas	**Psoas**
psoralène	psoralene	**Psoralen**
psoriasis	psoriasi	**Psoriasis**
psychiatrie	psichiatria	**Psychiatrie**
psychiatrique	psichiatrico	**psychiatrisch**
psychique	psichico	**psychisch**
psychanalyse	psicoanalisi	**Psychoanalyse**
psychodynamique	psicodinamica	**Psychodynamik**
psychogène	psicogenico	**psychogen**
psychologie	psicologia	**Psychologie**
psychomoteur	psicomotorio	**psychomotorisch**
psychopathe	psicopatico	**Psychopath**
psychopathie	psicopatia	**Psychopathie**
personnalité psychopathique	personalità psicopatica	**psychopathische Persönlichkeit**
psychopathologie	psicopatologia	**Psychopathologie**
psychose	psicosi	**Psychose**
psychosomatique	psicosomatico	**psychosomatisch**
psychothérapie	psicoterapia	**Psychotherapie**
psychotrope	psicotropo	**psychotrop**
ptérygion	pterigio, eponichio	**Pterygium**
ptose	ptosi	**Ptose**
puberté	pubertà	**Pubertät**
vulve	anestesia della regione pubica	**Pudendusblock**
puerpéral	puerperale	**puerperal**
puerpérium	puerperio	**Puerperium**
pouls	polso	**Puls**
pulsation	pulsazione	**Pulsieren**
pulsatile	pulsatile	**pulsierend**
syndrome de Takayashu	sindrome dell'arco aortico	**Pulsloskrankheit**
pulsation	pulsazione	**Pulsschlag**
pouls alternant	polso alternante	**Pulsus alternans**
pouls paradoxal	polso paradosso	**Pulsus paradoxus**
ponction	aspirazione di fluido	**Punktieren**
pupillaire	pupillare	**pupillar**
pupille	pupilla	**Pupille**
pupillaire	pupillare	**Pupillen-**

GERMAN	ENGLISH	SPANISH
pupillenerweiternd	mydriatic	midriático
Pupillenerweiterung	mydriasis	midriasis
Pupillenverengung	miosis	miosis
Purgativum	purgative	purga
purgierend	purgative	purgante
Purpura	purpura	púrpura
Purpura Schönlein-Henoch	Henoch-Schönlein purpura	púrpura de Schönlein-Henoch
purulent	purulent	purulento
Pustel	pustule	pústula
Pyämie	pyaemia (Eng), pyemia (Am)	piemia
Pyarthrose	pyarthrosis	piartrosis
Pyelitis	pyelitis	pielitis
Pyelographie	pyelography	pielografía
Pyelonephritis	pyelonephritis	pielonefritis
Pyloromyotomie	pyloromyotomy	piloromiotomía
Pyloroplastik	pyloroplasty	piloroplastia
Pylorospasmus	pylorospasm	pilorospasmo
Pylorus	pylorus	píloro
Pyodermie	pyoderma	pioderma
pyogen	pyogenic	piógeno
Pyometra	pyometra	piómetra
Pyonephrose	pyonephrosis	pionefrosis
Pyosalpinx	pyosalpinx	piosalpinx
pyramidal	pyramidal	piramidal
Pyurie	pyuria	piuria

FRENCH	ITALIAN	GERMAN
mydriatique	midriatico	pupillenerweiternd
mydriase	midriasi	Pupillenerweiterung
myosis	miosi	Pupillenverengung
purgatif	lassativo	Purgativum
purgatif	purgante	purgierend
purpura	porpora	Purpura
purpura rhumatoïde	porpora di Schönlein-Henoch	Purpura Schönlein-Henoch
purulent	purulento	purulent
pustule	pustola	Pustel
septicopyohémie	piemia	Pyämie
pyarthrose	pioartrosi, piartro	Pyarthrose
pyélite	pielite	Pyelitis
pyélographie	pielografia	Pyelographie
pyélonéphrite	pielonefrite	Pyelonephritis
pylorotomie	piloromiotomia, intervento di Ramstedt	Pyloromyotomie
pyloroplastie	piloroplastica	Pyloroplastik
pylorospasme	pilorospasmo	Pylorospasmus
pylore	piloro	Pylorus
pyodermie	piodermite, pioderma	Pyodermie
pyogène	piogenico	pyogen
pyométrie	piometra	Pyometra
pyonéphrose	pionefrosi	Pyonephrose
pyosalpinx	piosalpinge	Pyosalpinx
pyramidal	piramidale	pyramidal
pyurie	piuria	Pyurie

Q

German	English	Spanish
Q-Fieber	Q fever	fiebre Q
Quadrizeps	quadriceps	cuádriceps
qualitativ	qualitative	cualitativo
quantitativ	quantitative	cuantitativo
Quarantäne	quarantine	cuarentena
quartana (Malaria)	quartan	cuartana
Quecksilber	mercury	mercurio
Querschnitt	transection	transección
Querschnittslähmung	paraplegia	paraplejía
quetschen	bruise	magullar, contundir
Quetschung	bruise	contusión, equímosis
Quicksilberchlorid	sublimate	sublimado
Quincke-Ödem	angioneurotic edema (solidus) (Am), angioneurotic oedema (solidus) (Eng)	edema angioneurótico (sólido)

FRENCH	ITALIAN	GERMAN
fièvre Q	febbre Q	**Q-Fieber**
quadriceps	quadricipite	**Quadrizeps**
qualitatif	qualitativo	**qualitativ**
quantitatif	quantitativo	**quantitativ**
quarantaine	quarantena	**Quarantäne**
quarte	quartana	**quartana (Malaria)**
mercure	mercurio	**Quecksilber**
transsection	sezione trasversale	**Querschnitt**
paraplégie	paraplegia	**Querschnittslähmung**
contusionner	ammaccare	**quetschen**
contusion	contusione	**Quetschung**
sublimé	sublimato	**Quicksilberchlorid**
oedème angioneurotique	edema angioneurotico	**Quincke-Ödem**

R

GERMAN	ENGLISH	SPANISH
Rachen	fauces, pharynx	fauces, faringe
Rachitis	rickets	raquitismo
rachitischer Rosenkranz	rickety rosary	rosario raquítico
radikal	radical	radical
radioaktiv	radioactive	radiactivo
Radio-Allergo-Sorbent-Test (RAST)	radioallergosorbent test (RAST)	prueba radioalergosorbente (RAST)
Radioisotop	radioisotope	radioisótopo
Radiologie	radiology	radiología
Radiotherapie	radiotherapy	radioterapia
Radius	radius	radio
Ramsay-Hunt-Syndrom	Ramsay Hunt syndrome	síndrome de Ramsay-Hunt
Ramstedt-(Weber)-Operation	Ramstedt's operation	operación de Ramstedt
rapid eye movement (REM)	rapid eye movement (REM)	movimiento rápido de los ojos (REM)
Rasselgeräusch	rhonchus	roncus
Rasseln	crepitation	crepitación
rassisch	ethnic	étnico
Rauschgift	drug, narcotic	fármaco, narcótico
Raynaud-Krankheit	Raynaud's disease	enfermedad de Raynaud
Reagens	reagent	reactivo
Reagenzglas	test tube	tubo de ensayo
Reaktion	reaction	reacción
Reanimation	cardiopulmonary resuscitation (CPR), resuscitation	resucitación cardiopulmonar, resucitación
Rechtsmedizin	forensic medicine	medicina forense
rechtsmedizinisch	medicolegal	médicolegal
Reflex	reflex	reflejo
Reflex, bedingter	conditioned reflex	reflejo condicionado
Reflex, konditionierter	conditioned reflex	reflejo condicionado
Reflux	reflux	reflujo
refraktär	refractory	refractario
Refraktion	refraction	refracción
Regeneration	regeneration	regeneración
Regression	regression	regresión
Regurgitation bei Säuglingen	posseting	regurgitación láctea del neonato
Regurgitieren	regurgitation	regurgitación
Rehabilitation	rehabilitation	rehabilitación
Reibung	friction	fricción
Reihenuntersuchung	screening	criba, despistaje
Reinigungsmittel	detergent	detergente
Reiter-Syndrom	Reiter's syndrome	síndrome de Reiter
Reiz	impulse	impulso
reizbar	irritable	irritable
Reizbarkeit	excitability	excitabilidad

FRENCH	ITALIAN	GERMAN
fosse gutturale, pharynx	fauci, faringe	**Rachen**
rachitisme	rachitismo	**Rachitis**
chapelet costal	rosario rachitico	**rachitischer Rosenkranz**
radical	radicale	**radikal**
radioactif	radioattivo	**radioaktiv**
technique du RAST	test di radioallergoassorbimento (RAST)	**Radio-Allergo-Sorbent-Test (RAST)**
radio-isotope	radioisotopo	**Radioisotop**
radiologie	radiologia	**Radiologie**
radiothérapie	radioterapia	**Radiotherapie**
radius	radio	**Radius**
maladie de Ramsay Hunt	sindrome di Ramsay Hunt	**Ramsay-Hunt-Syndrom**
opération de Ramstedt	intervento di Ramstedt, piloromiotomia	**Ramstedt-(Weber)-Operation**
période des mouvements oculaires	fase REM del sonno, movimento oculare rapido	**rapid eye movement (REM)**
ronchus	ronco	**Rasselgeräusch**
crépitation	crepitazione	**Rasseln**
ethnique	etnico	**rassisch**
médicament, narcotique	farmaco, medicinale, droga, narcotico	**Rauschgift**
maladie de Raynaud	malattia di Raynaud	**Raynaud-Krankheit**
réactif	reagente	**Reagens**
tube à essai, éprouvette	provetta	**Reagenzglas**
réaction	reazione	**Reaktion**
réanimation cardiorespiratoire, ressuscitation	rianimazione cardiorespiratoria, rianimazione	**Reanimation**
médecine légale	medicina forense	**Rechtsmedizin**
médico-légal	medicolegale	**rechtsmedizinisch**
réflexe	riflesso	**Reflex**
réflexe conditionné	riflesso condizionato	**Reflex, bedingter**
réflexe conditionné	riflesso condizionato	**Reflex, konditionierter**
reflux	reflusso	**Reflux**
réfractaire	refrattario	**refraktär**
réfraction	rifrazione	**Refraktion**
régénération	rigenerazione	**Regeneration**
régression	regressione	**Regression**
régurgitation	rigurgito	**Regurgitation bei Säuglingen**
régurgitation	regurgito	**Regurgitieren**
réadaptation	riabilitazione	**Rehabilitation**
friction	attrito, frizione	**Reibung**
dépistage	selezione	**Reihenuntersuchung**
détergent	detergente	**Reinigungsmittel**
syndrome de Fiessinger-Leroy-Reiter	sindrome di Reiter	**Reiter-Syndrom**
impulsion	impulso	**Reiz**
irritable	irritabile	**reizbar**
excitabilité	eccitabilità	**Reizbarkeit**

GERMAN	ENGLISH	SPANISH
Reizdarm	irritable bowel syndrome	síndrome del intestino irritable
reizend	irritant	irritante
Reizung	excitation	excitación
Rektoskop	proctoscope	proctoscopio
Rektozele	rectocele	rectocele
Rektum	rectum	recto
Relaxans	relaxant	relajante
relaxierend	relaxant	relajante
Remission	remission	remisión
remittierend	remittent	remitente
REM-Schlaf	REM sleep	sueño REM
renal	renal	renal
renaler Blutfluß (RBF)	renal blood flow (RBF)	flujo sanguíneo renal (FSR)
Renin	renin	renina
Rentner	old age pensioner (OAP)	jubilado
Resektion	resection	resección
Resektionszystoskop	resectoscope	resectoscopio
Resektoskop	resectoscope	resectoscopio
Residual-	residual	residual
Resonanz	resonance	resonancia
Resorption	resorption	resorción
Respiration	respiration	respiración
Respirator	respirator	respirador
respiratorische Insuffizienz	respiratory failure	insuficiencia respiratoria
Respiratory-distress-Syndrom	respiratory distress syndrome (RDS)	síndrome de distress respiratorio
Retardmittel	slow release drug	medicamento de liberación lenta
Retention	retention	retención
retikulär	reticular	reticular
retikuloendotheliales System	reticuloendothelial system (RES)	sistema reticuloendotelial (SRE)
Retikulozyt	reticulocyte	reticulocito
Retikulozytose	reticulocytosis	reticulocitosis
Retina	retina	retina
Retinitis	retinitis	retinitis
Retinoblastom	retinoblastoma	retinoblastoma
Retinopathie	retinopathy	retinopatía
retraktionsfähig	retractile	retráctil
Retraktor	retractor	retractor
retrobulbär	retrobulbar	retrobulbar
retrograd	retrograde	retrógrado
retrolentale Fibroplasie	retrolental fibroplasia	fibroplasia retrolental
retroperitoneal	retroperitoneal	retroperitoneal
retropharyngeal	retropharyngeal	retrofaríngeo
retroplazentar	retroplacental	retroplacentario
retrosternal	retrosternal	retrosternal
Retroversion	retroversion	retroversión
retrozökal	retrocaecal (Eng), retrocecal (Am)	retrocecal

FRENCH	ITALIAN	GERMAN
syndrome de l'intestin irritable	sindrome dell'intestino irritable	Reizdarm
irritant	irritante	reizend
excitation	eccitazione	Reizung
rectoscope	proctoscopio	Rektoskop
rectocèle	rettocele	Rektozele
rectum	retto	Rektum
relaxant	rilassante	Relaxans
relaxant	rilassante	relaxierend
rémission	remissione	Remission
rémittent	remittente	remittierend
sommeil paradoxal	sonno REM, fase dei movimenti oculari rapidi	REM-Schlaf
rénal	renale	renal
débit sanguin rénal	perfusione renale	renaler Blutfluß (RBF)
rénine	renina	Renin
retraité(e)	anziano pensionato	Rentner
résection	resezione	Resektion
résectoscope	resettore endoscopico	Resektionszystoskop
résectoscope	resettore endoscopico	Resektoskop
résiduel	residuo	Residual-
résonance	risonanza	Resonanz
résorption	riassorbimento	Resorption
respiration	respirazione	Respiration
respirateur	respiratore	Respirator
insuffisance respiratoire	insufficienza respiratoria	respiratorische Insuffizienz
syndrome de membrane hyaline et de souffrance respiratoire	sindrome di sofferenza respiratoria	Respiratory-distress-Syndrom
médicament retard	farmaco a lenta dismissione	Retardmittel
rétention	ritenzione	Retention
réticulaire	reticolare	retikulär
système réticulo-endothélial	sistema reticoloendoteliale (RES)	retikuloendotheliales System
réticulocyte	reticolocito	Retikulozyt
réticulocytose	reticolocitosi	Retikulozytose
rétine	retina	Retina
rétinite	retinite	Retinitis
rétinoblastome	retinoblastoma	Retinoblastom
rétinopathie	retinopatia	Retinopathie
rétractile	retrattile	retraktionsfähig
rétracteur	divaricatore	Retraktor
rétrobulbaire	retrobulbare	retrobulbär
rétrograde	retrogrado	retrograd
fibroplasie rétrolentale	fibroplasia retrolenticolare	retrolentale Fibroplasie
rétropéritonéal	retroperitoneale	retroperitoneal
rétropharyngien	retrofaringeo	retropharyngeal
rétroplacentaire	retroplacentare	retroplazentar
rétrosternal	retrosternale	retrosternal
rétroversion	retroversione	Retroversion
rétrocaecal	retrociecale	retrozökal

GERMAN	ENGLISH	SPANISH
Revaskularisation	revascularization	revascularización
Reye-Syndrom	Reye's syndrome	síndrome de Reye
Rezept	prescription	receta
rezeptfrei	over the counter (OTC)	sin receta médica
Rezeptor	receptor	receptor
rezessiv	recessive	recesivo
Rezidiv	recurrence, relapse	periódico, recidiva
rezidivieren	relapse	recaer
Rhesusfaktor	Rhesus factor	factor Rhesus
rheumatisch	rheumatoid	reumatoide
rheumatisches Fieber	rheumatic fever	fiebre reumática
Rheumatismus	rheumatism	reumatismo
Rheumatoide Arthritis	rheumatoid arthritis (RA)	artritis reumatoide (AR)
Rheumatologie	rheumatology	reumatología
Rhinitis	rhinitis	rinitis
Rhinophym	rhinophyma	rinofima
Rhinoplastik	rhinoplasty	rinoplastia
Rhinorrhoe	rhinorrhea (Am), rhinorrhoea (Eng)	rinorrea
Rhinovirus	rhinovirus	rinovirus
Rh-negativ	rhesus negative (Rh−)	rhesus negativo (Rh−)
Rhonchus	rhonchus	roncus
Rh-positiv	rhesus positive (Rh+)	rhesus positivo (Rh+)
Rh-Unverträglichkeit	Rhesus incompatibility	incompatibilidad Rhesus
Rhythmusstörung	arrhythmia, dysrhythmia	arritmia, disritmia
Ribonukleinsäure (RNA)	ribonucleic acid (RNA)	ácido ribonucléico (ARN)
Riesenzellarteriitis	giant cell arteritis	arteritis de células gigantes
Rigor	rigor	rigor
Rinde	cortex	corteza
Rinderwahnsinn	bovine spongiform encephalitis (BSE)	encefalitis espongiforme bovina
ringförmig	annular	anular
Rippe	rib	costilla
Rippen-	costal	costal
Rippenfellentzündung	pleurisy (pleuritis)	pleuresia, pleuritis
Rippenknorpel-	costochondral	costocondral
Riß	rupture	ruptura
Rocky Mountain spotted fever	Rocky Mountain spotted fever	fiebre manchada de las Montañas Rocosas
Röhrchen	tubule	túbulo
Röntgen	radiography	radiografía
Röntgenaufnahme	radiograph	radiografía
Röntgenaufnahmen	X-rays	rayos X
röntgendicht	radio-opaque	radiopaco
Röntgenologie	radiology	radiología
Röntgenstrahlen	X-rays	rayos X
Rosacea	rosacea	rosácea

FRENCH	ITALIAN	GERMAN
revascularisation	rivascolarizzazione	**Revaskularisation**
syndrome de Reye	sindrome di Reye	**Reye-Syndrom**
ordonnance	prescrizione, ricetta	**Rezept**
spécialités pharmaceutiques grand public	(farmaco) ottenibile senza prescrizione medica	**rezeptfrei**
récepteur	recettore	**Rezeptor**
récessif	recessivo	**rezessiv**
répétition, réapparition, rechute	recidiva, ricaduta	**Rezidiv**
rechuter	recidivare	**rezidivieren**
facteur Rhésus	fattore Rh	**Rhesusfaktor**
rhumatoïde	reumatoide	**rheumatisch**
rhumatisme articulaire aigu	febbre reumatica	**rheumatisches Fieber**
rhumatisme	reumatismo	**Rheumatismus**
polyarthrite rhumatoïde (PR), polyarthrite chronique évolutive (PCE)	artrite reumatoide (AR)	**Rheumatoide Arthritis**
rhumatologie	reumatologia	**Rheumatologie**
rhinite	rinite	**Rhinitis**
rhinophyma	rinofima	**Rhinophym**
rhinoplastie	rinoplastica	**Rhinoplastik**
rhinorrhée	rinorrea	**Rhinorrhoe**
rhinovirus	rhinovirus	**Rhinovirus**
rhésus négatif (Rh−)	Rh negativo (Rh−)	**Rh-negativ**
ronchus	ronco	**Rhonchus**
rhésus positif (Rh+)	Rh positivo (Rh+)	**Rh-positiv**
incompatibilité Rhésus	incompatibilità Rh	**Rh-Unverträglichkeit**
arythmie, dysrythmie	aritmia, disritmia	**Rhythmusstörung**
acide ribonucléique (RNA)	acido ribonucleico (RNA)	**Ribonukleinsäure (RNA)**
artérite temporale	arterite a cellule giganti	**Riesenzellarteriitis**
rigor	rigor, ipertonia extrapiramidale	**Rigor**
cortex	corteccia	**Rinde**
encéphalite spongiforme bovine	encefalite spongiforme bovina	**Rinderwahnsinn**
annulaire	anulare	**ringförmig**
côte	costa	**Rippe**
costal	costale	**Rippen-**
pleurésie	pleurite	**Rippenfellentzündung**
costochondral	costocondrale	**Rippenknorpel**
hernie	rottura	**Riß**
fièvre pourprée des montagnes Rocheuses	febbre purpurica delle Montagne Rocciose	**Rocky Mountain spotted fever**
tube	tubulo	**Röhrchen**
radiographic	radiografia	**Röntgen**
radiographe	immagine radiologica	**Röntgenaufnahme**
rayons X	raggi X	**Röntgenaufnahmen**
radio-opaque	radioopaco	**röntgendicht**
radiologie	radiologia	**Röntgenologie**
rayons X	raggi X	**Röntgenstrahlen**
acné rosacée	rosacea, acne rosacea	**Rosacea**

GERMAN	ENGLISH	SPANISH
Roseole	roseola	roséola
Rotator	rotator	rotatorio
Rotavirus	rotavirus	rotavirus
Röteln	German measles, rubella	rubéola
rotes Blutkörperchen	erythrocyte	eritrocito
Rötung	rubor	rubor
RS-Virus	respiratory syncytial virus (RSV)	virus sincitial respiratorio (VSR)
Rubella	German measles, rubella	rubéola
Rubor	rubor	rubor
Rückbildung	involution, regression	involución, regresión
Rücken-	dorsal	dorsal
Rückenmarks-	spinal	espinal
Rückfall	relapse	recidiva
Rückfall erleiden	relapse	recaer
Rückgang	resolution	resolución
Rückgrat	spine, vertebral column	raquis, columna vertebral
rückläufig	retrograde	retrógrado
ruhend	recumbent	recumbente, de pie
Ruhr	dysentery	disentería
Rundwurm	roundworm	áscaris

FRENCH	ITALIAN	GERMAN
roséole	roseola	**Roseole**
rotateur	muscolo rotatore	**Rotator**
rotavirus	rotavirus	**Rotavirus**
rubéole	rosolia	**Röteln**
érythrocyte	eritrocito	**rotes Blutkörperchen**
rougeur	arrossamento infiammatorio	**Rötung**
virus respiratoire syncytial	virus respiratorio sinciziale (RSV)	**RS-Virus**
rubéole	rosolia	**Rubella**
rougeur	arrossamento infiammatorio	**Rubor**
involution, régression	involuzione, regressione	**Rückbildung**
dorsal	dorsale	**Rücken-**
spinal	spinale	**Rückenmarks-**
rechute	ricaduta, recidiva	**Rückfall**
rechuter	recidivare	**Rückfall erlciden**
résolution	risoluzione	**Rückgang**
colonne vertébrale	spina, colonna vertebrale	**Rückgrat**
rétrograde	retrogrado	**rückläufig**
couché	supino, sdraiato	**ruhend**
dysenterie	dissenteria	**Ruhr**
ascaris	ascaride, nematelminto	**Rundwurm**

S

Sack	sac	saco
sagittal	sagittal	sagital
sakral	sacral	sacral
Sakroiliitis	sacroiliitis	sacroileítis
sakrokokkygeal	sacrococcygeal	sacrococcígeo
Sakrum	sacrum	sacro
Salbe	ointment, paste, salve	ungüento, pasta
Salbentopf	gallipot	bote
salinisch	saline	salino
Salpingektomie	salpingectomy	salpingectomía
Salpingitis	pelvic inflammatory disease (PID), salpingitis	enfermedad inflamatoria de la pelvis, salpingitis
Samen	semen, sperm	semen, esperma
Samen-	seminal, spermatic	seminal, espermático
Samenerguß	ejaculation	eyaculación
saphenus	saphenous	safeno
Sarkoidose	sarcoidosis	sarcoidosis
Sarkom	sarcoma	sarcoma
sauer	acid	ácido
Sauerstoffentzug	deoxygenation	desoxigenación
Sauerstoffmangel	anoxia	anoxia
Sauerstoffsättigung	oxygenation	oxigenación
Saugglocke	vacuum extractor	extractor al vacío
Säugling	infant	lactante
Säuglings-Intensivstation	special care baby unit (SCBU)	unidad para cuidados especiales neonatales
Säure	acid	ácido
säurealkoholbeständig	acid-alcohol-fast	ácido-alcohol-resistente
säurebeständig	acid-fast	ácido-resistente
Säuregehalt	acidity	acidez
Scan	scan	exploración, barrido
Scaphoid	scaphoid	escafoides
Schädel	cranium, skull	cráneo
Schädel-	cephalic	cefálico
Schädelmessung	cephalometry	cefalometría
Schälen (Haut)	peeling	exfoliación
Schall	resonance	resonancia
Schambein	pubis	pubis
Schamlippenkommissur, hintere	fourchette	horquilla, frenillo pudendo
Schanker	chancre	chancro
scharf	acute	agudo
Schärfe	acuity	agudeza
Scharlach	scarlet fever	escarlatina
Scheide	vagina	vagina
Scheidewand	septum	septo, tabique
scheinkrank	malingering	simulación de síntomas

sac	sacco, sacca	**Sack**
sagittal	sagittale	**sagittal**
sacré	sacrale	**sakral**
sacro-ilite	sacroiliite	**Sakroiliitis**
sacrococcygien	sacrococcigeo	**sakrokokkygeal**
sacrum	sacro	**Sakrum**
pommade, pâte	unguento, pasta, pasta gelificante	**Salbe**
petit pot	ampolla o vasetto unguentario	**Salbentopf**
salin	salino	**salinisch**
salpingectomie	salpingectomia	**Salpingektomie**
pelvipéritonite, salpingite	malattia infiammatoria della pelvi (PID), salpingite	**Salpingitis**
sperme, sperme	seme, sperma	**Samen**
séminal, spermatique	seminale, spermatico	**Samen-**
éjaculation	eiaculazione	**Samenerguß**
saphène	safeno	**saphenus**
sarcoïdose	sarcoidosi	**Sarkoidose**
sarcome	sarcoma	**Sarkom**
acide	acido	**sauer**
désoxygénation	deossigenazione	**Sauerstoffentzug**
anoxie	anossia	**Sauerstoffmangel**
oxygénation	ossigenazione	**Sauerstoffsättigung**
ventouse obstétricale	ventosa ostetrica, ventosa cefalica	**Saugglocke**
enfant, nourrisson	infante	**Säugling**
pavillon de soins spéciaux aux nouveau-nés	unità di cure speciali pediatriche	**Säuglings-Intensivstation**
acide	acido	**Säure**
résistant à l'alcool et à l'acide	alcool-acido-resistente	**säurealkoholbeständig**
acido-résistant	acido resistente	**säurebeständig**
acidité	acidità	**Säuregehalt**
échogramme	ecografia, scintigrafia	**Scan**
scaphoïde	scafoide	**Scaphoid**
boîte crânienne, crâne	cranio	**Schädel**
céphalique	cefalico	**Schädel-**
céphalométrie	cefalometria	**Schädelmessung**
desquamation	desquamazione	**Schälen (Haut)**
résonance	risonanza	**Schall**
pubis	pube	**Schambein**
fourchette	forchetta	**Schamlippenkommissur, hintere**
chancre	cancroide, ulcera venerea	**Schanker**
aigu(ë)	acuto	**scharf**
acuité	acuità	**Schärfe**
scarlatine	scarlattina	**Scharlach**
vagin	vagina	**Scheide**
septum	setto	**Scheidewand**
simulation	simulazione di malattia	**scheinkrank**

GERMAN	ENGLISH	SPANISH
Scheinschwangerschaft	phantom pregnancy	embarazo fantasma
Scheitel	vertex	vértice
Schicht	stratum	estrato
Schick-Test	Schick test	prueba de Schick
Schiefhals (angeborener)	wry-neck	tortícolis
Schielen	squint, strabismus	estrabismo
Schienbein	shin bone, tibia	tibia
Schiene	caliper, splint	compás, calibrador, astilla
Schilddrüse	thyroid	tiroides
Schilddrüsenüberfunktion	hyperthyroidism	hipertiroidismo
Schistosomiasis	schistosomiasis	esquistosomiasis
schizoide Persönlichkeit	schizoid personality	personalidad esquizoide
Schizophrenie	schizophrenia	esquizofrenia
Schlaf	sleep	sueño
Schläfe	temple	sien
Schläfen-	temporal	temporal
schlaff	flaccid	fláccido
Schlaflosigkeit	insomnia	insomnio
Schlafmittel	hypnotic, soporific	hipnótico, soporífero
Schlafwandeln	somnambulism	sonambulismo
Schlag	stroke	ictus
Schlagader	artery	arteria
Schlaganfall	cerebrovascular accident (CVA), stroke	accidente vascular cerebral (ACV), ictus
Schlangenserum	antivenin	antídoto
Schlatter-Krankheit	Schlatter's disease	enfermedad de Schlatter
schleichend	insidious	insidioso
Schleimbeutelentzündung	bursitis	bursitis
Schleimhaut	mucosa	mucosa
schleimig	mucous (Eng), mucus (Am)	moco
schleimig-eitrig	mucopurulent	mucopurulento
schleimlösend	expectorant	expectorante
schleimlösendes Mittel	mucolytic	mucolítico
Schließmuskel	sphincter	esfínter
Schlitz	dehiscence	dehiscencia
Schluckauf	hiccup	hipo
Schluckbeschwerden	dysphagia	disfagia
schlucken	swallow	tragar
Schlund	fauces	fauces
Schlundtasche	pharyngeal pouch	bolsa faringea
Schlüsselbein	clavicle	clavícula
Schmarotzer	parasite	parásito
Schmerz	dolor, pain	dolor
Schmerz, ausstrahlender	referred pain	dolor referido
Schmerz, brennender	causalgia	causalgia

FRENCH	ITALIAN	GERMAN
fausse grossesse	pseudociesi	Scheinschwangerschaft
vertex	vertice	Scheitel
couche	strato	Schicht
réaction de Schick	test di Schick	Schick-Test
torticolis	torcicollo	Schiefhals (angeborener)
strabisme	strabismo	Schielen
tibia	tibia	Schienbein
armature orthopédique, attelle	compasso per pelvi-craniometria, stecca ortopedica	Schiene
thyroïde	tiroide	Schilddrüse
hyperthyroïdisme	ipertiroidismo	Schilddrüsenüberfunktion
schistosomiase	schistosomiasi	Schistosomiasis
personnalité schizoïde	personalità schizoide	schizoide Persönlichkeit
schizophrénie	schizofrenia	Schizophrenie
sommeil	sonno	Schlaf
tempe	tempia	Schläfe
temporal	temporale	Schläfen-
mou	flaccido	schlaff
insomnie	insonnia	Schlaflosigkeit
hypnotique, soporifique	ipnotico	Schlafmittel
somnambulisme	sonnambulismo	Schlafwandeln
apoplexie	ictus, colpo apoplettico, accidente cerebrovascolare	Schlag
artère	arteria	Schlagader
accident cérébrovasculaire, apoplexie	ictus, accidente cerebrovascolare (ACV), colpo apoplettico	Schlaganfall
sérum antivenimeux	antiveleno, contravveleno	Schlangenserum
maladie d'Osgood-Schlatter	malattia di Schlatter	Schlatter-Krankheit
insidieux	insidioso	schleichend
bursite	borsite	Schleimbeutelentzündung
muqueuse	mucosa	Schleimhaut
muqueux	mucoso	schleimig
mucopurulent	mucopurulento	schleimig-eitrig
expectorant	espettorante	schleimlösend
mucolytique	mucolitico	schleimlösendes Mittel
sphincter	sfintere	Schließmuskel
déhiscence	deiscenza	Schlitz
hoquet	singhiozzo	Schluckauf
dysphagie	disfagia	Schluckbeschwerden
avaler	inghiottire	schlucken
fosse gutturale	fauci	Schlund
poche ectobranchiale et entobranchiale	tasca faringea	Schlundtasche
clavicule	clavicola	Schlüsselbein
parasite	parassita	Schmarotzer
douleur	dolore	Schmerz
douleur irradiée	dolore riferito	Schmerz, ausstrahlender
causalgie	causalgia	Schmerz, brennender

Schmerz, fortgeleiteter	referred pain	dolor referido
schmerzhaft	sore	doloroso
schmerzlindernd	analgesic	analgésico
Schmerzlosigkeit	analgesia	analgesia
Schmerzmittel	analgesic	analgésico
schmerzunempfindlich	analgesic	analgésico
Schnarchen	snore	ronquido
schnarchen	snore	roncar
Schnecke	cochlea	cóclea
Schneidezahn	incisor	incisivo
schnellender Finger	trigger finger	dedo en gatillo
Schnüffeln	glue sniffing	inhalación de pegamento
Schnupfen	coryza	coriza
Schnur	cord	cordón, cuerda, médula espinal
Schock	shock	shock
Schokoladenzyste	chocolate cyst	quiste de chocolate
Schorf	slough, scab	esfacelo, costra
Schorfabtragung	desloughing	desesfacelación
Schrittmacher	pacemaker	marcapasos
Schröpfkopf	ventouse extraction	extracción con ventosa
Schulter	shoulder	hombro
Schulterblatt	scapula	omoplato
Schultergelenk-	glenoid	glenoide
Schultergürtel	shoulder girdle	cintura escapular
Schuppen	dandruff	caspa
Schuppenflechte	psoriasis	psoriasis
schuppig	squamous	escamoso
Schuppung	desquamation, peeling	desescamación, exfoliación
Schütteln	succussion	sucusión
Schützengrabenfuß	trench foot	pie de trinchera
Schutzimpfung	immunization	inmunización
Schwäche	debility, weakness	debilidad
schwammartig	cancellous	esponjoso, reticulado
Schwangerschaft	cyesis, gestation, pregnancy	ciesis, embarazo, gestación
Schwangerschaft, ektope	ectopic pregnancy	embarazo ectópico
Schwangerschaft, hysterische	phantom pregnancy	embarazo fantasma
Schwangerschaftsabbruch	termination of pregnancy (TOP)	interrupción del embarazo
Schwankung	oscillation	oscilación
Schwarzwasserfieber	blackwater fever	fiebre hemoglobinúrica
Schweiß	perspiration, sweat	sudor
Schweißabsonderung	diaphoresis, hidrosis	diaforesis, hidrosis
Schweißmangel	hypoidrosis	hipohidrosis
Schweißtest	sweat test	prueba del sudor
Schwere (der Erkrankung)	gravity	gravedad
schwerhörig	deaf	sordo
Schwerhörigkeit	deafness	sordera

FRENCH	ITALIAN	GERMAN
douleur irradiée	dolore riferito	Schmerz, fortgeleiteter
douloureux	dolente	schmerzhaft
analgésique	analgesico	schmerzlindernd
analgésie	analgesia	Schmerzlosigkeit
analgésique	analgesico	Schmerzmittel
analgésique	analgesico	schmerzunempfindlich
ronflement	russo	Schnarchen
ronfler	russare	schnarchen
limaçon osseux	coclea	Schnecke
incisive	incisore	Schneidezahn
index	dito a scatto	schnellender Finger
intoxication par inhalation de solvant	inalazione di toluene o collanti	Schnüffeln
coryza	coriza	Schnupfen
cordon	corda, cordone, notocorda	Schnur
choc	shock	Schock
kyste chocolat	cisti cioccolato (c. emosiderinica dell'endometriosi)	Schokoladenzyste
escarre, croûte	crosta, escara	Schorf
curetage	rimozione di escara da una ferita	Schorfabtragung
stimulateur cardiaque	pacemaker	Schrittmacher
extraction par ventouse	estrazione con ventosa ostetrica	Schröpfkopf
épaule	spalla	Schulter
omoplate	scapola	Schulterblatt
glénoïde	glenoide	Schultergelenk-
ceinture scapulaire	cingolo scapolare	Schultergürtel
pellicules	forfora	Schuppen
psoriasis	psoriasi	Schuppenflechte
squameux	squamoso	schuppig
desquamation	desquamazione	Schuppung
succussion	succussione, scuotimento	Schütteln
pied gelé	piede da trincea	Schützengrabenfuß
immunisation	immunizzazione	Schutzimpfung
débilité, faiblesse	debilità, debolezza	Schwäche
spongieux	spugnoso, trabecolare	schwammartig
grossesse, gestation	gravidanza, gestazione	Schwangerschaft
grossesse ectopique	gravidanza ectopica	Schwangerschaft, ektope
fausse grossesse	pseudociesi	Schwangerschaft, hysterische
interruption de grossesse (IG)	interruzione di gravidanza (IG)	Schwangerschaftsabbruch
oscillation	oscillazione	Schwankung
hématurie	febbre emoglobinurica da Plasmodium falciparum	Schwarzwasserfieber
perspiration, sueur	perspirazione, sudore	Schweiß
diaphorèse, transpiration	diaforesi, idrosi, sudorazione	Schweißabsonderung
hypohidrose	ipoidrosi	Schweißmangel
test de sueur	test del sudore, prova del sudore	Schweißtest
gravité	gravità	Schwere (der Erkrankung)
sourd	sordo	schwerhörig
surdité	sordità	Schwerhörigkeit

GERMAN	ENGLISH	SPANISH
Schwester	nurse	enfermera
Schwiele	callosity, weal	callosidad, verdugón
Schwindel	dizziness, vertigo	desvanecimiento, mareo, vértigo
Schwinden	wasting away	consunción
schwindlig	giddy	mareado
Schwindsucht	tabes	tabes
Schwirren	thrill	frémito
schwitzen	sweat	sudar
Screening	screening	criba, despistaje
Seborrhoe	seborrhea (Am), seborrhoea (Eng)	seborrea
Sectio	caesarean section (Eng), cesarean section (Am)	cesárea
Sedativum	sedative	sedante
sedierend	sedative	sedante
Sedierung	sedation	sedación
seelisch	mental, psychic	mental, psíquico
Segment	segment	segmento
Seh-	optic, visual	óptico, visual
Sehne	tendon	tendón
Sehnenentzündung	tendinitis (Am), tendonitis (Eng)	tendinitis
Sehnenscheidenentzündung	tenosynovitis	tenosinovitis
Sehschärfe	visual acuity	agudeza visual
Sehschwäche	amblyopia	ambliopía
seitlich	lateral	lateral
Sekretion	secretion	secreción
Sekretionsmangel	hyposecretion	hiposecreción
Sekretionsschwäche	hyposecretion	hiposecreción
Sekretolytikum	expectorant	expectorante
sekretorisch	secretory	secretorio
Sektion	autopsy	autopsia
Selbstbefriedigung	masturbation	masturbación
Selbstmord	suicide	suicidio
Selbstschädigung	self-harm	autolesión
Selbstuntersuchung der Brust	breast self-examination (BSE)	autoexamen de la mama
Selbstvergiftung	self-poisoning	autointoxicación
semilunar	semilunar	semilunar
Seminom	seminoma	seminoma
semiotisch	semeiotic	semiótica
semipermeabel	semipermeable	semipermeable
Seneszenz	senescence	senescencia
senil	senile	senil
sensitiv	sensitive	sensible
Sensitivierung	sensitization	sensibilización
sensorisch	sensory	sensorio
Sepsis	sepsis	sepsis

FRENCH	ITALIAN	GERMAN
infirmière	infermiere	Schwester
callosité, marque	callosità, pomfo	Schwiele
étourdissement, vertige	stordimento, capogiro, vertigine	Schwindel
dépérissement	cachessia	Schwinden
pris de vertige	stordito, affetto da vertigini o capogiro	schwindlig
tabès	tabe dorsale	Schwindsucht
murmure respiratoire	fremito	Schwirren
suer	sudare	schwitzen
dépistage	selezione	Screening
séborrhée	seborrea	Seborrhoe
césarienne	taglio cesareo	Sectio
sédatif	sedativo	Sedativum
sédatif	sedativo	sedierend
sédation	sedazione	Sedierung
mental, psychique	mentale, psichico	seelisch
segment	segmento	Segment
optique, visuel	ottico, visivo	Seh-
tendon	tendine	Sehne
tendinite	tendinite	Sehnenentzündung
ténosynovite	tenosinovite	Sehnenscheidenentzündung
acuité visuelle	acutezza visiva	Sehschärfe
amblyopie	ambliopia	Sehschwäche
latéral	laterale	seitlich
sécrétion	secrezione	Sekretion
hyposécrétion	iposecrezione	Sekretionsmangel
hyposécrétion	iposecrezione	Sekretionsschwäche
expectorant	espettorante	Sekretolytikum
secréteur	secretorio	sekretorisch
autopsie	autopsia	Sektion
masturbation	masturbazione	Selbstbefriedigung
suicide	suicidio	Selbstmord
automutilation	autolesionismo	Selbstschädigung
auto-examen des seins	autopalpazione mammaria	Selbstuntersuchung der Brust
intoxication volontaire	autoavvelenamento	Selbstvergiftung
semi-lunaire	semilunare	semilunar
séminome	seminoma	Seminom
sémiologique	semiotico	semiotisch
semi-perméable	semipermeabile	semipermeabel
sénescence	senescenza	Seneszenz
sénile	senile	senil
sensible	sensibile	sensitiv
sensibilisation	sensibilizzazione	Sensitivierung
sensitif	sensoriale	sensorisch
septicémie	sepsi	Sepsis

Septikämie	septicaemia (Eng), septicemia (Am)	septicemia
Septum	septum	septo, tabique
Sequester	sequestrum	secuestro
Serologie	serology	serología
seropositiv	seropositive	seropositivo
serös	serous	seroso
Serosa	serosa	serosa
Serum	serum	suero
Serum-	serous	seroso
seßhaft	sedentary	sedentario
Seuche	plague	peste, plaga
sexueller Mißbrauch	sexual abuse	abuso sexual
Shirodkar-Operation	Shirodkar's operation	operación de Shirodkar
Shunt	shunt	derivación
Sichelzellanämie	sickle-cell anaemia (Eng), sickle-cell anemia (Am)	anemia drepanocítica
(sich) erinnern	recall	recordar
sich übergeben	vomit	vomitar
Siebbein	ethmoid	etmoides
sigmoid	sigmoid	sigmoideo
Sigmoidoskop	sigmoidoscope	sigmoidoscopio
Sigmoidostomie	sigmoidostomy	sigmoidostomía
Silikose	silicosis	silicosis
Sims-Lage	Sims' position	posición de Sim
Sims-Spekulum	Sims' speculum	espéculo de Sim
Sinn	sense	sentido
Sinnes-	sensory	sensorio
Sinneswahrnehmung	sensation	sensación
Sinne u Nerven betr	sensorineural	sensorineural
Sinus	sinus	seno
Sinusitis	sinusitis	sinusitis
Sinusknoten	sinoatrial node	nodo sinoauricular
Sitzbein	ischium	isquión
sitzend	sedentary	sedentario
Sjögren-Syndrom	Sjögren-Larsson syndrome	síndrome de Sjögren
Skabies	scabies	sarna
Skalpell	scalpel	escalpelo
Skapula	scapula	omoplato
Skelett	skeleton	esqueleto
Skelettmuskulatur betr	musculoskeletal	musculoesquelético
Sklera	sclera	esclerótica
Sklera-	sclerotic	esclerótico
Skleritis	scleritis	escleritis
Sklerödem	scleredema (Am), scleredoema (Eng)	escleredema
Sklerodermie	scleroderma	escleroderma

FRENCH	ITALIAN	GERMAN
septicémie	setticemia	**Septikämie**
septum	setto	**Septum**
séquestre	sequestro	**Sequester**
sérologie	sierologia	**Serologie**
séropositif	siero-positivo	**seropositiv**
séreux	sieroso	**serös**
séreuse	sierosa, membrana sierosa	**Serosa**
sérum	siero	**Serum**
séreux	sieroso	**Serum-**
sédentaire	sedentario	**seßhaft**
peste	peste	**Seuche**
sévices sexuels	violenza sessuale, violenza carnale	**sexueller Mißbrauch**
opération de Shirodkar	intervento di Shirodkar	**Shirodkar-Operation**
dérivation	derivazione	**Shunt**
drépanocytose	anemia drepanocitica	**Sichelzellanämie**
évoquer	ricordare	**(sich) erinnern**
vomir	vomitare	**sich übergeben**
ethmoïde	etmoide	**Siebbein**
sigmoïde	sigmoide	**sigmoid**
sigmoïdoscope	sigmoidoscopio	**Sigmoidoskop**
sigmoïdostomie	sigmoidostomia	**Sigmoidostomie**
silicose	silicosi	**Silikose**
position de Sim	posizione di Sim	**Sims-Lage**
spéculum de Sim	speculum di Sim	**Sims-Spekulum**
sens	sensi	**Sinn**
sensitif	sensoriale	**Sinnes-**
sensation	sensazione, sensibilità	**Sinneswahrnehmung**
de perception	neurosensoriale	**Sinne u Nerven betr**
sinus	seno, fistula suppurante	**Sinus**
sinusite	sinusite	**Sinusitis**
noeud sinusal de Keith et Flack	nodo sinoatriale	**Sinusknoten**
ischion	ischio	**Sitzbein**
sédentaire	sedentario	**sitzend**
syndrome de Sjögren	sindrome di Sjögren-Larsson (eritrodermia ittiosiforme con oligofrenia spastica)	**Sjögren-Syndrom**
gale	scabbia	**Skabies**
scalpel	bisturi	**Skalpell**
omoplate	scapola	**Skapula**
squelette	scheletro	**Skelett**
musculo-squelettique	muscoloscheletrico	**Skelettmuskulatur betr**
sclérotique	sclera, sclerotica	**Sklera**
sclérotique	sclerotico	**Sklera-**
sclérite	sclerite	**Skleritis**
scléroderme	scleredema	**Sklerödem**
scléroderme	sclerodermia	**Sklerodermie**

GERMAN	ENGLISH	SPANISH
Sklerose	sclerosis	esclerosis
Sklerotherapie	sclerotherapy	escleroterapia
sklerotisch	sclerotic	esclerótico
Skoliose	scoliosis	escoliosis
Skorbut	scurvy	escorbuto
Skotom	scotoma	escotoma
Skrofula	scrofula	escrófula
Skrotum	scrotum	escroto
Sodbrennen	heartburn, pyrosis	ardor de estómago, pirosis
Solarplexus	solar plexus	plexo solar
somatisch	somatic	somático
Somnambulismus	somnambulism	sonambulismo
Sonnenstich	sunstroke	insolación
Sonographie	ultrasonography	ultrasonografía, ecografía
Soor	thrush	muguet
sozialmedizinisch	medicosocial, sociomedical	médicosocial
Spaltung	fission	fisión
Spann	instep	empeine
Spannungskopfschmerz	tension headache	cefalea por tensión
Spasmolytikum	antispasmodic	antiespasmódico
spasmolytisch	antispasmodic	antiespasmódico
Spasmus	spasm	espasmo
spastisch	spastic	espástico
spastische Dysmenorrhoe	spasmodic dysmenorrhoea	dismenorrea espasmódica
Spatel	spatula	espátula
Speichel	saliva, spittle	saliva, salivazo
Speicheldrüse	salivary gland	glándula salivar
Speiseröhre	esophagus (Am), gullet, oesophagus (Eng)	esófago, gaznate
Spekulum	speculum	espéculo
Spender	donor	donante
Sperma	sperm	esperma
Sperma-	spermatic	espermático
Spermatozele	spermatocele	espermatocele
Spermien-	seminal	seminal
Spermizid	spermicide	espermicida
speziell	specific	específico
Spezies	species	especie
spezifisch	specific	específico
Sphärozytose	spherocytosis	esferocitosis
Sphenoid	sphenoid	esfenoides
Sphinkter	sphincter	esfínter
Spider naevus	spider naevus (Eng), spider nevus (Am)	araña vascular
Spiegel	speculum	espéculo
Spikulum	spicule	espícula
Spina bifida	spina bifida	espina bífida

FRENCH	ITALIAN	GERMAN
sclérose	sclerosi	**Sklerose**
sclérothérapie	scleroterapia	**Sklerotherapie**
sclérotique	sclerotico	**sklerotisch**
scoliose	scoliosi	**Skoliose**
scorbut	scorbuto	**Skorbut**
scotome	scotoma	**Skotom**
scrofule	scrofola, linfadenite tubercolare	**Skrofula**
scrotum	scroto	**Skrotum**
aigreurs, pyrosis	pirosi	**Sodbrennen**
plexus solaire	plesso solare, plesso celiaco	**Solarplexus**
somatique	somatico	**somatisch**
somnambulisme	sonnambulismo	**Somnambulismus**
insolation	colpo di sole	**Sonnenstich**
échographie	ultrasonografia, ecografia	**Sonographie**
aphte	stomatite de Candida albicans, mughetto	**Soor**
médico-social, sociomédical	medicosociale, sociosanitario	**sozialmedizinisch**
fission	fissione	**Spaltung**
tarse	dorso del piede	**Spann**
céphalée due à la tension	cefalea muscolotensiva	**Spannungskopfschmerz**
antispasmodique	antispastico	**Spasmolytikum**
antispasmodique	antispastico	**spasmolytisch**
spasme	spasmo	**Spasmus**
spastique	spastico	**spastisch**
dysménorrhée spasmodique	dismenorrea spastica	**spastische Dysmenorrhoe**
spatule	spatola	**Spatel**
salive, crachat	saliva	**Speichel**
glande salivaire	ghiandola salivare	**Speicheldrüse**
oesophage	esofago (gola)	**Speiseröhre**
spéculum	speculum	**Spekulum**
donneur	donatore	**Spender**
sperme	sperma	**Sperma**
spermatique	spermatico	**Sperma-**
spermatocèle	spermatocele	**Spermatozele**
séminal, spermatique	seminale	**Spermien-**
spermicide	spermicida	**Spermizid**
spécifique	specifico	**speziell**
espèce	specie	**Spezies**
spécifique	specifico	**spezifisch**
sphérocytose	sferocitosi	**Sphärozytose**
sphénoïde	sfenoide	**Sphenoid**
sphincter	sfintere	**Sphinkter**
naevi	angioma stellare	**Spider naevus**
spéculum	speculum	**Spiegel**
spicule	spicola, picco	**Spikulum**
spina bifida	spina bifida	**Spina bifida**

GERMAN	ENGLISH	SPANISH
spinal	spinal	espinal
Spirochäte	spirochaete (Eng), spirochete (Am)	espiroqueta
Spirograph	spirograph	espirografía
Spirometer	spirometer	espirómetro
spitz	acute	agudo
Spitze	apex	ápex
Splenektomie	splenectomy	esplenectomía
Splenomegalie	splenomegaly	esplenomegalia
Splitterbruch	comminuted fracture	fractura conminuta
Spondylitis	spondylitis	espondilitis
Spondylolisthesis	spondylolisthesis	espondilolistesis
spongiös	cancellous	esponjoso, reticulado
sporadisch	sporadic	esporádico
Sporn	spica	espica
Sprachtherapie	speech therapy	logopedia
Spreizer	retractor	retractor
Spritze	injection, syringe	inyección, jeringuilla
spritzen	inject	inyectar
Sprue	sprue, thrush	esprue, muguet
Spülung	douche, irrigation, lavage	ducha, irrigación, lavado
Spulwurm	roundworm, ascaris	áscaris
Sputum	sputum	esputo
squamös	squamous	escamoso
Stachel	sting	picadura
Stapedektomie	stapedectomy	estapedectomía
Stapes	stapes	estribo
stärkehaltig	amyloid	amiloideo
Stärkungsmittel	tonic	tónico
Starre	rigor	rigor
Stase	stasis	estasis
Status	status	status
Staublunge	pneumoconiosis	neumoconiosis
Stauung	congestion, engorgement	congestión, estancamiento
Stauungsherz	congestive cardiac failure (CCF), congestive heart failure (CHF)	insuficiencia cardíaca congestiva (ICC),
Steatorrhoe	steatorrhea (Am), steatorrhoea (Eng)	esteatorrea
Stechen	stitch	punto de sutura
stechen	puncture	pinchar
Steigbügel	stapes	estribo
Stein	calculus, stone	cálculo
Steinkohlenteer	coal tar	alquitrán, brea
Stein-Leventhal-Syndrom	Stein-Leventhal syndrome	síndrome de Stein-Leventhal
Steinmann Knochennagel	Steinmann's pin	clavo de Steinmann
Steiß	breech	nalgas
Steißbein	coccyx	cóccix

FRENCH	ITALIAN	GERMAN
spinal	spinale	spinal
spirochète	spirocheta	Spirochäte
spirographe	spirografo	Spirograph
spiromètre	spirometro	Spirometer
aigu(ë)	acuto	spitz
apex	apice	Spitze
splénectomie	splenectomia	Splenektomie
splénomégalie	splenomegalia	Splenomegalie
fracture esquilleuse	frattura comminuta	Splitterbruch
spondylite	spondilite	Spondylitis
spondylolisthésis	spondilolistesi	Spondylolisthesis
spongieux	spugnoso, trabecolare	spongiös
sporadique	sporadico	sporadisch
spica	spiga	Sporn
orthophonie	terapia del linguaggio	Sprachtherapie
rétracteur	divaricatore	Spreizer
injection, seringue	iniezione, siringa	Spritze
injecter	iniettare	spritzen
sprue, aphte	sprue, stomatite de Candida albicans, mughetto	Sprue
douche, irrigation, lavage	lavanda vaginale, irrigazione, lavaggio	Spülung
ascaris	ascaride, nematelminto	Spulwurm
salive	sputo, escreato	Sputum
squameux	squamoso	squamös
piqûre	dolore acuto, puntura	Stachel
stapédectomie	stapedectomia	Stapedektomie
étrier	staffa	Stapes
amyloïde	amiloide	stärkehaltig
tonique	tonico	Stärkungsmittel
rigor	rigor, ipertonia extrapiramidale	Starre
stase	stasi, ristagno	Stase
statut	stato	Status
pneumoconiose	pneumoconiosi	Staublunge
congestion, engorgement	congestione	Stauung
insuffisance cardiaque globale	insufficienza cardiaca congestizia, scompenso cardiaco congestizio	Stauungsherz
stéatorrhée	steatorrea, seborrea	Steatorrhoe
point de suture	punto	Stechen
ponctionner	pungere	stechen
étrier	staffa	Steigbügel
calcul, caillou	calcolo	Stein
coaltar	catrame	Steinkohlenteer
syndrome de Stein-Leventhal	sindrome di Stein-Leventhal	Stein-Leventhal-Syndrom
broche de Steinmann	chiodo per estensione di Steinmann	Steinmann Knochennagel
siège	natica	Steiß
coccyx	coccige	Steißbein

GERMAN	ENGLISH	SPANISH
Steißlage	breech-birth presentation	presentación de nalgas
Stenose	stenosis	estenosis
Sterbehilfe	euthanasia	eutanasia
sterbend	moribund	moribundo
Sterblichkeit	mortality	mortalidad
steril	sterile	estéril
Sterilisation	sterilization	esterilización
Sterilisationsapparat	autoclave	autoclave
Sterilisierung	sterilization	esterilización
Sternalpunktion	sternal puncture	punción esternal
sternokostal	sternocostal	esternocostal
Sternum	sternum	esternón
Steroid	steroid	esteroide
Stethoskop	stethoscope	estetoscopio
Stevens-Johnson-Syndrom	Stevens-Johnson syndrome	síndrome de Stevens-Johnson
Stich	sting, puncture	picadura, punción
Stiel	peduncle	pedúnculo
Stigmata	stigmata	estigmas
Stillen	lactation	lactación
stillen	nurse	cuidar
Still-Krankheit	Still's disease	enfermedad de Still
Stimmband	vocal cord	cuerda vocal
Stimmbandresektion	cordotomy	cordotomía
Stimmritze	glottis	glotis
Stimulans	stimulant	estimulante
stimulierend	stimulant	estimulante
Stirn	forehead	frente
Stirn-	frontal	frontal
Stoffwechsel	metabolism	metabolismo
Stoffwechsel-	metabolic	metabólico
Stoffwechselprodukt	metabolite	metabolito
Stoma	stoma	estoma
Stomatitis	stomatitis	estomatitis
Storchenbiß	birthmark	mancha de nacimiento
Störung	defect	defecto
stoßen	bruise	magullar, contundir
Stottern	stammer	tartamudeo
Strabismus	strabismus	estrabismo
strahlenempfindlich	radiosensitive	radiosensible
Strahlentherapie	radiotherapy	radioterapia
Strang	cord	cordón, cuerda, médula espinal
Strangulation	strangulation	estrangulación
Stratum	stratum	estrato
Streck-	extension	extensión
Streckmuskel	extensor	extensor
Streifen	striae	estrias
Streß	stress	stress, estrés

FRENCH	ITALIAN	GERMAN
présentation, naissance par le siège	presentazione podalica	**Steißlage**
sténose	stenosi	**Stenose**
euthanasie	eutanasia	**Sterbehilfe**
moribond	moribondo	**sterbend**
mortalité	mortalità	**Sterblichkeit**
stérile	sterile	**steril**
stérilisation	sterilizzazione	**Sterilisation**
autoclave	autoclave	**Sterilisationsapparat**
stérilisation	sterilizzazione	**Sterilisierung**
ponction sternale	puntura sternale	**Sternalpunktion**
sternocostal	sternocostale	**sternokostal**
sternum	sterno	**Sternum**
stéroïde	steroide	**Steroid**
stéthoscope	stetoscopio	**Stethoskop**
syndrome de Stevens-Johnson	sindrome di Stevens-Johnson	**Stevens-Johnson-Syndrom**
piqûre, ponction	dolore acuto, puntura	**Stich**
pédoncule	peduncolo	**Stiel**
stigmate	stigmate	**Stigmata**
lactation	lattazione	**Stillen**
soigner	assistere	**stillen**
maladie de Still	malattia di Still	**Still-Krankheit**
corde vocale	corda vocale	**Stimmband**
cordotomie	cordotomia	**Stimmbandresektion**
glotte	glottide	**Stimmritze**
stimulant	stimolante	**Stimulans**
stimulant	stimolante	**stimulierend**
front	fronte	**Stirn**
frontal	frontale	**Stirn-**
métabolisme	metabolismo	**Stoffwechsel**
métabolique	metabolico	**Stoffwechsel-**
métabolite	metabolita	**Stoffwechselprodukt**
stoma	stoma, orifizio	**Stoma**
stomatite	stomatite	**Stomatitis**
naevus, envie	nevo congenito	**Storchenbiß**
anomalie, défaut	difetto	**Störung**
contusionner	ammaccare	**stoßen**
bégaiement	balbuzie	**Stottern**
strabisme	strabismo	**Strabismus**
radiosensible	radiosensibile	**strahlenempfindlich**
radiothérapie	radioterapia	**Strahlentherapie**
cordon	corda, cordone, notocorda	**Strang**
strangulation	strangolamento	**Strangulation**
couche	strato	**Stratum**
extension	estensione	**Streck-**
extenseur	estensore	**Streckmuskel**
stries	stria	**Streifen**
stress	stress	**Streß**

GERMAN	ENGLISH	SPANISH
Striae	striae	estrias
Stridor	stridor	estridor
Striemen	weal	verdugón
Striktur	stricture	estrictura
Struma	goiter (Am), goitre (Eng)	bocio
Stuhl	stool	deposición
Stuhlgang	evacuation, motion, stool	evacuación, movimiento, deposición
Stummheit	mutism	mutismo
Stupor	stupor	estupor
Styloid-	styloid	estiloides
subakut	subacute	subagudo
Subarachnoidalblutung	subarachnoid haemorrhage (Eng), subarachnoid hemorrhage (Am)	hemorragia subaracnoidea
Subarachnoidalraum	subarachnoid space	espacio subaracnoideo
subdiaphragmatisch	subphrenic	subfrénico
subdural	subdural	subdural
Subfertilität	subfertility	subfertilidad
subjektiv	subjective	subjetivo
Subklavia-	subclavian	subclavia
subklinisch	subclinical	subclínico
subkonjunktival	subconjunctival	subconjuntival
subkostal	subcostal	subcostal
subkutan	hypodermic, subcutaneous (SC, SQ)	hipodérmico, subcutáneo (SC)
Sublimat	sublimate	sublimado
sublingual	sublingual	sublingual
Subluxation	subluxation	subluxación
submandibulär	submandibular	submandibular
Submukosa	submucosa	submucosa
Subnormalität	subnormality	subnormalidad
subokzipital	suboccipital	suboccipital
Substanznahme	generic	genérico
Sucht	addiction	adicción, toxicomanía
Sudden-infant-death-Syndrom (SIDS)	sudden infant death syndrome (SIDS)	síndrome de muerte súbita infantil
Suggestion	suggestion	sugestión
Suizid	suicide	suicidio
Sulcus	sulcus	surco
Sulfonamid	sulfonamide (Am), sulphonamide (Eng)	sulfonamida
Sulfonylharnstoff	sulfonylurea (Am), sulphonylurea (Eng)	sulfonilurea
Supination	supination	supinar
Supinator	supinator	supinador
supiniert	supine	supino
Suppositorium	suppository	supositorio
Suppuration	suppuration	supuración
supraklavikulär	supraclavicular	supraclavicular

FRENCH	ITALIAN	GERMAN
stries	stria	**Striae**
stridor	stridore	**Stridor**
marque	pomfo	**Striemen**
rétrécissement	stenosi, restringimento	**Striktur**
goitre	gozzo	**Struma**
selle	feci	**Stuhl**
évacuation, mouvement, selle	evacuazione, movimento, feci	**Stuhlgang**
mutisme	mutismo	**Stummheit**
stupeur	stupore	**Stupor**
styloïde	stiloide, stiloideo	**Styloid-**
subaigu	subacuto	**subakut**
hémorragie sous-arachnoïdienne	emorragia subaracnoidea	**Subarachnoidalblutung**
espace sous-arachnoïdien	spazio subaracnoideo	**Subarachnoidalraum**
sous-phrénique	subfrenico, sottodiaframmatico	**subdiaphragmatisch**
sous-dural	subdurale, sottodurale	**subdural**
sous-fertilité	subfertilità	**Subfertilität**
subjectif	soggettivo	**subjektiv**
sous-clavier	succlavio, sottoclavicolare	**Subklavia-**
sous-clinique	subclinico	**subklinisch**
sous-conjonctival	sottocongiuntivale	**subkonjunktival**
sous-costal	sottocostale	**subkostal**
hypodermique, sous-cutané (SC)	ipodermico, sottocutaneo	**subkutan**
sublimé	sublimato	**Sublimat**
sublingual	sublinguale	**sublingual**
subluxation	sublussazione	**Subluxation**
submandibulaire	sottomandibolare	**submandibulär**
tissu sous-muqueux	sottomucosa	**Submukosa**
subnormalité	subnormalità	**Subnormalität**
sous-occipital	suboccipitale	**subokzipital**
dénomination commune d'un médicament	medico generico	**Substanznahme**
accoutumance	tossicomania	**Sucht**
syndrome de mort subite de nourrisson	sindrome della morte neonatale improvvisa (SIDS)	**Sudden-infant-death-Syndrom (SIDS)**
suggestion	suggestione	**Suggestion**
suicide	suicidio	**Suizid**
sillon, gouttière, scissure	solco	**Sulcus**
sulfamide	sulfonammide	**Sulfonamid**
sulfonylurée	sulfonilurea	**Sulfonylharnstoff**
supination	supinazione	**Supination**
supinateur	supinatore	**Supinator**
en supination	supino	**supiniert**
suppositoire	supposta	**Suppositorium**
suppuration	suppurazione	**Suppuration**
supraclaviculaire	sopraclavicolare	**supraklavikulär**

GERMAN	ENGLISH	SPANISH
suprakondylär	supracondylar	supracondilar
suprapubisch	suprapubic	suprapúbico
suprasternal	suprasternal	supraesternal
Surfactant-Faktor	surfactant	tensoactivo
Symbiose	symbiosis	simbiosis
Sympathektomie	sympathectomy	simpatectomía
sympathisches Nervensystem	sympathetic nervous system	sistema nervioso simpático
Sympathomimetikum	sympathomimetic	simpaticomimético
sympathomimetisch	sympathomimetic	simpaticomimético
Symphyse	symphysis	sínfisis
Symptom	sign, symptom	signo, síntoma
Synapse	synapse	sinapsis
Syndrom	syndrome	síndrome
Syndrom der blinden Schlinge	blind loop syndrome	síndrome del asa ciega
Synechie	synechia	sinequia
Synergie	synergy	sinergia
Synkope	syncope	síncope
Synovia	synovial membrane	membrana sinovial
Synovialflüssigkeit	synovial fluid	líquido sinovial
Syphilis	syphilis	sífilis
Syringomyelie	syringomyelia	siringomielia
systemischer Lupus erythematodes	systemic lupus erythematosus (SLE)	lupus eritematoso sistémico (LES)
Systole	systole	sístole
Systolikum	systolic murmur	soplo sistólico

FRENCH	ITALIAN	GERMAN
supracondylaire	sopracondiloideo, epicondiloideo	suprakondylär
suprapubien	soprapubico	suprapubisch
suprasternal	soprasternale	suprasternal
surfactant	tensioattivo, surfattante	Surfactant-Faktor
symbiose	simbiosi	Symbiose
sympathectomie	simpatectomia, simpaticectomia	Sympathektomie
système nerveux sympathique	sistema nervoso simpatico	sympathisches Nervensystem
sympathomimétique	simpaticomimetico	Sympathomimetikum
sympathomimétique	simpaticomimetico	sympathomimetisch
symphyse	sinfisi	Symphyse
signe, symptôme	segno, sintomo	Symptom
synapse	sinapsi, giunzione	Synapse
syndrome	sindrome	Syndrom
syndrome de l'anse borgne	sindrome dell'ansa cieca	Syndrom der blinden Schlinge
synéchie	sinechia, aderenza	Synechie
synergie	sinergia	Synergie
syncope	sincope	Synkope
membrane synoviale	membrana sinoviale	Synovia
fluide synovial	liquido sinoviale	Synovialflüssigkeit
syphilis	sifilide	Syphilis
syringomyélie	siringomielia	Syringomyelie
lupus érythémateux systémique	lupus eritematoso sistemico (LES)	systemischer Lupus erythematodes
systole	sistole	Systole
murmure systolique	soffio sistolico	Systolikum

T

Tablette	tablet	comprimido
Tachykardie	tachycardia	taquicardia
Tachypnoe	tachypnea (Am), tachypnoea (Eng)	taquipnea
Tagesdosis, empfohlene	recommended daily allowance (RDA)	dosis diaria recomendada
Tagesklinik	day hospital	hospital de día
taktil	tactile	táctil
Talg	sebum	sebo
Talg-	sebaceous	sebáceo
talgig	sebaceous	sebáceo
Talkum	talc	talco
Talus	ankle, talus	tobillo, astrágalo
Tamponade	tamponade	taponamiento
Tänia	Taenia, tapeworm	tenia, tenia solitaria
Tarsalgie	tarsalgia	tarsalgia
Tarsorrhaphie	tarsorrhaphy	tarsorrafia
Tasche	pouch	bolsa
tastbar	palpable, tactile	palpable, táctil
Tätigkeit	action	acción
taub	deaf	sordo
Taubheit	deafness	sordera
Tay-Sachs-Krankheit	Tay-Sachs disease	enfermedad de Tay-Sachs
Teerzyste	chocolate cyst	quiste de chocolate
teilnahmslos	passive	pasivo
Teleangiektasie	telangiectasis	telangiectasia
Temperament	temperament	temperamento
temporal	temporal	temporal
Tendinitis	tendinitis (Am), tendonitis (Eng)	tendinitis
Tendosynovitis	tenosynovitis	tenosinovitis
Tendovaginitis	tenosynovitis	tenosinovitis
Tenesmus	tenesmus	tenesmo
Tennisellenbogen	tennis elbow	codo del tenista
Tenotomie	tenotomy	tenotomía
Teratogen	teratogen	teratógeno
Teratom	teratoma	teratoma
termingemäß klein	small-for-dates (SFD)	útero pequeño para la edad gestacional
tertiär	tertiary	terciario
Test	test	prueba
testen	test	probar
Tetanie	tetany	tetania
Tetanus	tetanus	tétanos
Tetraplegie	quadriplegia, tetraplegia	cuadriplejía, tetraplejía
Thalamus	thalamus	tálamo

FRENCH	ITALIAN	GERMAN
comprimé	pasticca, compressa	**Tablette**
tachycardie	tachicardia	**Tachykardie**
tachypnée	tachipnea	**Tachypnoe**
taux quotidien recommandé	dose giornaliera raccomandata	**Tagesdosis, empfohlene**
hôpital de jour	ospedale diurno	**Tagesklinik**
tactile	tattile	**taktil**
sébum	sebo	**Talg**
sébacé	sebaceo	**Talg-**
sébacé	sebaceo	**talgig**
talc	talco	**Talkum**
cheville, astragale	caviglia, astragalo, talo	**Talus**
tamponnement	tamponamento	**Tamponade**
ténia	Tenia, cestode	**Tänia**
tarsalgie	tarsalgia	**Tarsalgie**
tarsorraphie	tarsorrafia	**Tarsorrhaphie**
poche	tasca	**Tasche**
palpable, tactile	palpabile, tattile	**tastbar**
action	azione	**Tätigkeit**
sourd	sordo	**taub**
surdité	sordità	**Taubheit**
maladie de Tay-Sachs	malattia di Tay-Sachs	**Tay-Sachs-Krankheit**
kyste chocolat	cisti cioccolato (c. emosiderinica dell'endometriosi)	**Teerzyste**
passif	passivo	**teilnahmslos**
télangiectasie	telangectasia	**Teleangiektasie**
tempérament	temperamento	**Temperament**
temporal	temporale	**temporal**
tendinite	tendinite	**Tendinitis**
ténosynovite	tenosinovite	**Tendosynovitis**
ténosynovite	tenosinovite	**Tendovaginitis**
ténesme	tenesmo	**Tenesmus**
'tennis elbow'	epicondilite radio-omerale, gomito del tennista	**Tennisellenbogen**
ténotomie	tenotomia	**Tenotomie**
tératogène	teratogeno	**Teratogen**
tératome	teratoma	**Teratom**
présentant un retard de croissance	basso peso alla nascita	**termingemäß klein**
tertiaire	terziario	**tertiär**
test	test, prova	**Test**
tester	valutare	**testen**
tétanie	tetania	**Tetanie**
tétanos	tetano	**Tetanus**
quadriplégie, tétraplégie	tetraplegia	**Tetraplegie**
thalamus	talamo	**Thalamus**

GERMAN	ENGLISH	SPANISH
Thalassämie	thalassaemia (Eng), thalassemia (Am)	talasemia
Thenar-	thenar	tenar
Therapeutik	therapeutics	terapéutica
Therapie	therapy	terapéutica
-therapie	therapeutics	terapéutica
thermal	thermal	termal
Thermometer	thermometer	termómetro
thorakal	thoracic	torácico
Thorakoplastik	thoracoplasty	toracoplastia
Thorakotomie	thoracotomy	toracotomía
Thorax	thorax	tórax
Thrombektomie	thrombectomy	trombectomía
thromboembolisch	thromboembolic	tromboembólico
thrombolytisch	thrombolytic	trombolítico
Thrombopenie	thrombocytopenia	trombocitopenia
Thrombophlebitis	thrombophlebitis	tromboflebitis
Thrombose	thrombosis	trombosis
Thrombozyt	platelet, thrombocyte	plaqueta, trombocito
Thrombozythämie	thrombocythaemia (Eng), thrombocythemia (Am)	trombocitemia
Thrombozytose	thrombocytosis	trombocitosis
Thrombus	thrombus	trombo
Thymus	thymus	timo
thyreoglossus	thyroglossal	tirogloso
Thyreoidea	thyroid	tiroides
Thyreoidektomie	thyroidectomy	tiroidectomía
Thyreoiditis	thyroiditis	tiroiditis
Thyreotoxikose	thyrotoxicosis	tirotoxicosis
thyreotoxische Krise	thyrotoxic crisis	crisis tirotóxica
Thyreotropin	thyroid stimulating hormone (TSH)	hormona estimulante del tiroides (TSH)
Tibia	tibia	tibia
tibiofibular	tibiofibular	tibioperoneo
Tic	tic	tic
Tic douloureux	tic douloureux	tic doloroso
tiefer gelegen	inferior	inferior
Tierkrankheit	zoonosis	zoonosis
Tietze Syndrom	costochondritis	costocondritis
Tinea	ringworm, tinea	tiña
Tinnitus	tinnitus	tinnitus
Titer	titer (Am), titre (Eng)	titulo
Titration	titration	titulación
Tod	death	muerte
Todesfall	death	muerte
Todesursache	cause of death (COD)	causa de la muerte
tödlich	lethal	letal
Toleranz	tolerance	tolerancia

FRENCH	ITALIAN	GERMAN
thalassémie	talassemia	**Thalassämie**
thénar	pertinente al palmo della mano	**Thenar-**
thérapeutique	terapia	**Therapeutik**
thérapie	terapia	**Therapie**
thérapeutique	terapia	**-therapie**
thermique	termale	**thermal**
thermomètre	termometro	**Thermometer**
thoracique	toracico	**thorakal**
thoracoplastie	toracoplastica	**Thorakoplastik**
thoracotomie	toracotomia	**Thorakotomie**
thorax	torace	**Thorax**
thrombectomie	trombectomia	**Thrombektomie**
thrombo-embolique	tromboembolico	**thromboembolisch**
thrombolytique	trombolitico	**thrombolytisch**
thrombopénie	trombocitopenia	**Thrombopenie**
thrombophlébite	tromboflebite	**Thrombophlebitis**
thrombose	trombosi	**Thrombose**
plaquette, thrombocyte	piastrina, trombocito	**Thrombozyt**
thrombocytémie	trombocitemia	**Thrombozythämie**
thrombocytose	trombocitosi	**Thrombozytose**
thrombus	trombo	**Thrombus**
thymus	timo	**Thymus**
thyroglossien	tireoglosso	**thyreoglossus**
thyroïde	tiroide	**Thyreoidea**
thyroïdectomie	tiroidectomia	**Thyreoidektomie**
thyroïdite	tiroidite	**Thyreoiditis**
thyrotoxicose	tireotossicosi, ipertiroidismo	**Thyreotoxikose**
crise thyrotoxique	crisi tireotossica	**thyreotoxische Krise**
thyrotrophine, thyréostimuline	ormone tireotropo (TSH)	**Thyreotropin**
tibia	tibia	**Tibia**
tibiofibulaire	tibiofibulare	**tibiofibular**
tic	tic	**Tic**
tic douloureux	tic doloroso, nevralgia del trigemino	**Tic douloureux**
inférieur	inferiore	**tiefer gelegen**
zoonose	zoonosi	**Tierkrankheit**
costochondrite	costocondrite	**Tietze Syndrom**
dermatophytose, teigne	tricofizia, tinea, tigna	**Tinea**
tintement	tinnito	**Tinnitus**
titre	titolo	**Titer**
titrage	titolazione	**Titration**
mort	morte	**Tod**
mort	morte	**Todesfall**
cause du décès	causa di morte	**Todesursache**
létal, léthal	letale	**tödlich**
tolérance	tolleranza	**Toleranz**

GERMAN	ENGLISH	SPANISH
Tollwut	rabies	rabia
Ton	sound, tone	sonido, tono
Tonikum	tonic	tónico
Tonometer	tonometer	tonómetro
Tonsillektomie	tonsillectomy	tonsilectomía
Tonsillen	tonsils	amígdalas
Tonsillitis	tonsillitis	amigdalitis
Tophus	tophus	tofo
topisch	topical	tópico
Torsion	torsion	torsión
Tortikollis	wry-neck	tortícolis
tot	dead	muerto
totale Eisenbindungskapazität (TEBK)	total iron binding capacity (TIBC)	capacidad total de unión con el hierro
Totalkapazität (TK)	total lung capacity (TLC)	capacidad pulmonar total (CPT)
tot bei Einlieferung	dead on arrival (DOA)	muerto al llegar
Toter	corpse	cadáver
totgeboren	stillborn	mortinato, nacido muerto
Totschlag	homicide	homicidio
Tourniquet	tourniquet	torniquete
Toxämie	toxaemia (Eng), toxemia (Am)	toxemia
Toxikämie	toxaemia (Eng), toxemia (Am)	toxemia
Toxin	toxin	toxina
toxisch	toxic	tóxico
toxisches Schocksyndrom (TSS)	toxic shock syndrome	síndrome de shock tóxico
Toxizität	toxicity	toxicidad
Toxoid	toxoid	toxoide
Toxoplasmose	toxoplasmosis	toxoplasmosis
Tracer	tracer	trazador
Trachea	trachea, windpipe	tráquea
Tracheitis	tracheitis	traqueitis
Tracheoösophageal-	tracheoesophageal (Am), tracheo-oesophageal (Eng)	traqueoesofágico
Tracheostomie	tracheostomy	traqueostomía
Tracheotomie	tracheotomy	traqueotomía
Trachom	trachoma, trachoma inclusion conjunctivitis (TRIC)	tracoma, conjuntivitis de inclusion por tracomas
Trägerstoff	carrier	portador
Trägheitsmoment	inertia	inercia
Traktion	traction	tracción
Tränen	tears	lágrimas
Tränen-	lacrimal	lagrimal
Tränengangs-	lacrimal	lagrimal
Tranquilizer	tranquilizer	tranquilizante
transabdominal	transabdominal	transabdominal
transamniotisch	transamniotic	transamniótico
Transfusion	transfusion	transfusión

FRENCH	ITALIAN	GERMAN
rage	rabbia	Tollwut
son, tonus	suono, tono	Ton
tonique	tonico	Tonikum
tonomètre	tonometro	Tonometer
amygdalectomie	tonsillectomia	Tonsillektomie
amygdales	tonsille	Tonsillen
angine	tonsillite	Tonsillitis
tophus	tofo, concrezione tofacea	Tophus
topique	topico, locale	topisch
torsion	torsione	Torsion
torticolis	torcicollo	Tortikollis
mort	morto	tot
capacité totale de fixation du fer	capacità totale di legame del ferro (TIBC)	totale Eisenbindungskapazität (TEBK)
capacité pulmonaire totale	capacità polmonare totale	Totalkapazität (TK)
mort à l'arrivée	deceduto all'arrivo in ospedale	tot bei Einlieferung
cadavre	cadavere	Toter
mort-né	nato morto	totgeboren
homicide	omicidio	Totschlag
tourniquet	laccio emostatico	Tourniquet
toxémie	tossiemia	Toxämie
toxémie	tossiemia	Toxikämie
toxine	tossina	Toxin
toxique	tossico	toxisch
syndrome de choc toxique staphylococcique	sindrome da shock tossico	toxisches Schocksyndrom (TSS)
toxicité	tossicità	Toxizität
toxoïde	tossoide	Toxoid
toxoplasmose	toxoplasmosi	Toxoplasmose
traceur	tracciante	Tracer
trachée	trachea	Trachea
trachéite	tracheite	Tracheitis
trachéo-oesophagien	tracheoesofageo	Tracheoösophageal-
trachéostomie	tracheostomia	Tracheostomie
trachéotomie	tracheotomia	Tracheotomie
trachome, conjonctivite à inclusions trachomateuses	tracoma, congiuntivite tracomatosa	Trachom
porteur	portatore	Trägerstoff
inertie	inerzia	Trägheitsmoment
traction	trazione, attrazione	Traktion
larmes	lacrime	Tränen
lacrymal	lacrimale	Tränen-
lacrymal	lacrimale	Tränengangs-
tranquillisant	tranquillante	Tranquilizer
transabdominal	transaddominale	transabdominal
transamniotique	transamniotico	transamniotisch
transfusion	trasfusione	Transfusion

GERMAN	ENGLISH	SPANISH
transitorische ischämische Attacke (TIA)	transient ischaemic attack (TIA) (Eng), transient ishemic attack (TIA) (Am)	ataque isquémico transitorio (AIT)
transkutan	transcutaneous	transcutáneo
Translokation	translocation	translocación
transmural	transmural	transmural
Transplantat	graft, transplant	injerto, trasplante
Transplantation	graft, transplant	injerto, trasplante
transplantieren	graft, transplant	injertar, trasplantar
Transsudat	transudate	trasudado
transthorakal	transthoracic	transtorácico
transurethral	transurethral	transuretral
Traubenzucker	glucose	glucosa
Trauma	trauma	trauma
Trematode	fluke	trematodo
Tremor	tremor	temblor
Tremor, feinschlägiger	fine tremor	temblor fino
Trendelenburg-Zeichen	Trendelenburg sign	signo de Trendelenburg
Trennung	dissociation	disociación
Trepan	trephine	trépano
trepanieren	trephine	trepanar
Triage	triage	triage
Trichotillomanie	trichotillomania	tricotilomanía
Trigeminus-	trigeminal	trigémino
Trikuspidal	tricuspid	tricúspide
Trimester	trimester	trimestre
Tripper	gonorrhea (Am), gonorrhoea (Eng)	gonorrea
Trisomie	trisomy	trisomía
Trizeps	triceps	tríceps
Trochanter	trochanter	trocánter
Trommelfell	eardrum, tympanum	tímpano
Trommelfell-	tympanic	timpánico
Trommelschlegelfinger	clubbing	dedos en palillo de tambor, dedos hipocráticos
Tropenkrankheit	tropical disease	enfermedad tropical
tröpfeln	drip	infundir
tropfen	drip	infundir
Tropfinfusion	drip	gota a gota intravenoso
trophisches Ulkus	trophic ulcer	úlcera trófica
Trypanosomiasis	trypanosomiasis	tripanosomiasis
Tsetsefliege	tsetse	mosca tsetsé
Tube	Fallopian tube	trompa de Falopio
Tuben-	tubal	tubárico
Tuberkel	tubercle	tubérculo
tuberkuloid	tuberculoid	tuberculoide
Tuberkulose	tuberculosis (TB)	tuberculosis (TB)
tuberöse Sklerose	tuberous sclerosis	esclerosis tuberosa
Tuberositas	tuberosity	tuberosidad
Tubulus	tubule	túbulo

accès ischémique transitoire cérébral	attacco ischemico transitorio	**transitorische ischämische Attacke (TIA)**
transcutané	percutaneo	**transkutan**
translocation	traslocazione	**Translokation**
transmural	transmurale	**transmural**
greffe, transplantation	trapianto, innesto	**Transplantat**
greffe, transplantation	trapianto, innesto	**Transplantation**
greffer, transplanter	trapiantare	**transplantieren**
transsudat	trasudato	**Transsudat**
transthoracique	transtoracico	**transthorakal**
transurétral	transuretrale	**transurethral**
glucose	glucosio	**Traubenzucker**
traumatisme	trauma	**Trauma**
douve	trematode, Digeneum	**Trematode**
tremblement	tremore	**Tremor**
tremblement fin	tremore fino	**Tremor, feinschlägiger**
signe de Trendelenburg	segno di Trendelenburg	**Trendelenburg-Zeichen**
dissociation	dissociazione	**Trennung**
tréphine	trapano	**Trepan**
trépaner	trapanare	**trepanieren**
triage	selezione e distribuzione dei malati	**Triage**
trichotillomanie	tricotillomania	**Trichotillomanie**
trigéminal	trigemino	**Trigeminus-**
tricuspide	tricuspide	**Trikuspidal**
trimestre	trimestre	**Trimester**
gonorrhée	gonorrea	**Tripper**
trisomie	trisomia	**Trisomie**
triceps	tricipite	**Trizeps**
trochanter	trocantere	**Trochanter**
tympan	timpano	**Trommelfell**
tympanique	timpanico, risonante	**Trommelfell-**
hippocratisme digital	dita a clava, ippocratismo	**Trommelschlegelfinger**
maladie tropicale	malattia tropicale	**Tropenkrankheit**
perfuser	gocciolare, far gocciolare	**tröpfeln**
perfuser	gocciolare, far gocciolare	**tropfen**
perfusion	fleboclisi	**Tropfinfusion**
ulcère trophique	ulcera trofica	**trophisches Ulkus**
trypanosomiase	tripanosomiasi	**Trypanosomiasis**
mouche tsé-tsé	tse-tse	**Tsetsefliege**
trompe de Fallope	tuba di Falloppio	**Tube**
tubaire	tubarico	**Tuben-**
tubercule	tubercolo	**Tuberkel**
tuberculoïde	tubercoloide	**tuberkuloid**
tuberculose (TB)	tubercolosi (TBC)	**Tuberkulose**
sclérose tubéreuse du cerveau	sclerosi tuberosa	**tuberöse Sklerose**
tubérosité	tuberosità	**Tuberositas**
tube	tubulo	**Tubulus**

GERMAN	ENGLISH	SPANISH
Tubulsnekrose	tubular necrosis	necrosis tubular
Tumeszenz	tumescence	tumescencia
Tumor	growth, neoplasm, tumor (Am), tumour (Eng)	crecimiento, neoplasma, tumor
Tupfer	swab	torunda
Turner-Syndrom	Turner's syndrome	síndrome de Turner
Tympanon	tympanum	tímpano
Tympanoplastik	tympanoplasty	timpanoplastia
Typ	type	tipo
Typhus	typhoid fever, typhus	fiebre tifoidea, tifus

FRENCH	ITALIAN	GERMAN
nécrose tubulaire	necrosi tubulare	**Tubulusnekrose**
tumescence	tumefazione	**Tumeszenz**
croissance, néoplasme, tumeur	crescita, neoplasma, tumore, tumefazione	**Tumor**
tampon	tampone	**Tupfer**
syndrome de Turner	sindrome di Turner, disgenesia gonadica	**Turner-Syndrom**
tympan	timpano	**Tympanon**
tympanoplastie	timpanoplastica	**Tympanoplastik**
type	tipo	**Typ**
fièvre typhoïde, typhus	febbre tifoide, tifo addominale, ileotifo, tifo	**Typhus**

U

GERMAN	ENGLISH	SPANISH
Übel	mal	mal
übel	queasy	nauseabundo
Übelkeit	nausea	náusea
Überaktivität	hyperactivity	hiperactividad
Überbein	ganglion	ganglio
Überdehnung	hyperextension	hiperextensión
Überdruckbeatmung	positive pressure ventilation	ventilación con presión positiva
Überempfindlichkeit	hypersensitive	hipersensibilidad
überlegen	superior	superior
Überreife	postmaturity	postmaduro
Überstreckung	hyperextension	hiperextensión
übertragen	graft	injertar
Überträger	vector	vector
Ulcus rodens	rodent ulcer	úlcera corrosiva
Ulkus	ulcer	úlcera
Ulna	ulna	cúbito
Ultraschallmethode	ultrasonography	ultrasonografía, ecografía
ultraviolett	ultraviolet (UV)	ultravioleta (UV)
ulzerierend	ulcerative	ulcerativo
Umgebung	environment	ambiente
Umkehrung	inversion	inversión
Umschlag	dressing	cura, vendaje
Umstülpung	eversion	eversión
Umwelt	environment	ambiente
unabsichtlich	involuntary	involuntario
unbekannten Ursprungs	cryptogenic	criptogénico
undurchsichtig	opaque	opaco
unempfindlich	insensible	insensible
unfruchtbar	sterile	estéril
unmittelbar nach Krankheitsausbruch	immediately after onset (IAO)	inmediatamente después del comienzo
unreduzierbar	irreducible	irreductible
unschädlich	innocent, innocuous	inocente, inocuo
unschuldig	innocent	inocente
Untätigkeit	inertia	inercia
Unterarm	forearm	antebrazo
Unterarmvene	cubital vein	vena cubital
unterbewußt	subconscious	subconsciente
Unterdrückung	repression, suppression	represión, supresión
unterempfindlich	hyposensitive	hiposensibilidad
Unterernährung	malnutrition	desnutrición
Unterfunktion	hypofunction	hipofunción
Unterkiefer	mandible	mandíbula
unterschwellig	subliminal	subliminal
untersuchen	test	probar

FRENCH	ITALIAN	GERMAN
mal	male, malattia	**Übel**
indigeste, délicat	nauseabondo, nauseato, a disagio	**übel**
nausée	nausea	**Übelkeit**
hyperactivité	iperattività	**Überaktivität**
ganglion	ganglio	**Überbein**
hyperextension	iperestensione	**Überdehnung**
ventilation à pression positive	ventilazione a pressione positiva	**Überdruckbeatmung**
hypersensibilité	ipersensitività, ipersensibilità	**Überempfindlichkeit**
supérieur	superiore	**überlegen**
postmature	postmaturo, ipermaturo	**Überreife**
hyperextension	iperestensione	**Überstreckung**
greffer	trapiantare	**übertragen**
vecteur	vettore	**Überträger**
ulcus rodens	ulcus rodens, basalioma	**Ulcus rodens**
ulcère	ulcera	**Ulkus**
cubitus	ulna	**Ulna**
échographie	ultrasonografia, ecografia	**Ultraschallmethode**
ultraviolet (UV)	ultravioletto (UV)	**ultraviolett**
ulcératif	ulcerativo, ulceroso	**ulzerierend**
milieu	ambiente	**Umgebung**
inversion	inversione	**Umkehrung**
pansement	medicazione	**Umschlag**
éversion	eversione, estrofia	**Umstülpung**
milieu	ambiente	**Umwelt**
involontaire	involontario	**unabsichtlich**
cryptogène	criptogenico	**unbekannten Ursprungs**
opaque	opaco	**undurchsichtig**
insensible	insensibile	**unempfindlich**
stérile	sterile	**unfruchtbar**
immédiatement après le début	immediatamente dopo l'attacco	**unmittelbar nach Krankheitsausbruch**
irréductible	irriducibile	**unreduzierbar**
innocent, inoffensif	innocente, innocuo	**unschädlich**
innocent	innocente	**unschuldig**
inertie	inerzia	**Untätigkeit**
avant-bras	avambraccio	**Unterarm**
veine de l'avant-bras	vena cubitale	**Unterarmvene**
subconscient	subconscio	**unterbewußt**
répression, suppression	repressione, soppressione	**Unterdrückung**
hyposensibilité	iposensitività, iposensibilità	**unterempfindlich**
malnutrition	malnutrizione	**Unterernährung**
hypofonction	ipofunzione	**Unterfunktion**
mandibule	mandibola	**Unterkiefer**
subliminal	subliminale	**unterschwellig**
tester	valutare	**untersuchen**

GERMAN	ENGLISH	SPANISH
Untersuchung	test	prueba
Unterziehtuch	drawsheet	alezo, faja
Unverträglichkeit	incompatibility, intolerance	incompatibilidad, intolerancia
unwillkürlich	involuntary	involuntario
unwohl	queasy	nauseabundo
Unwohlsein	malaise	destemplanza, malestar
Urämie	uraemia (Eng), uremia (Am)	uremia
Urat	urate	urato
Urea	urea	urea
Ureter	ureter	uréter
Ureterkolik	ureterocolic	ureterocólico
Urethra	urethra	uretra
Urethralsyndrom	urethral syndrome	síndrome uretral
Urethritis	urethritis	uretritis
Urethritis, nicht durch Gonokokken bedingte	non-gonococcal urethritis	uretritis no gonocócica
Urethritis, unspezifische	non-specific urethritis (NSU)	uretritis inespecífica
Urethrozele	urethrocele	uretrocele
Urikämie	uricaemia (Eng), uricemia (Am)	uricemia
Urikosurie	uricosuria	uricosúrico
Urin	urine	orina
Urinanalyse	urinalysis	urinálisis
Urinuntersuchung	urinalysis	urinálisis
urogenital	genitourinary (GU)	genitourinario
Urographie	urography	urografía
Urologie	urology	urología
Ursprung	origin	origen
Urtikaria	urticaria	urticaria
uterosakral	uterosacral	uterosacro
uterovesikal	uterovesical	uterovesical
Uterus	uterus, womb	útero, matriz
Uterusblutung, dysfunktionale	dysfunctional uterine bleeding (DUB)	hemorragia uterina funcional
Uveitis	uveitis	uveitis
Uvula	uvula	úvula
Uvulitis	uvulitis	uvulitis

FRENCH	ITALIAN	GERMAN
test	test, prova	**Untersuchung**
alèse	traversa	**Unterziehtuch**
incompatibilité, intolérance	incompatibilità, intolleranza	**Unverträglichkeit**
involontaire	involontario	**unwillkürlich**
indigeste, délicat	nauseabondo, nauseato, a disagio	**unwohl**
malaise	indisposizione, malessere	**Unwohlsein**
urémie	uremia	**Urämie**
urate	urato	**Urat**
urée	urea, carbammide	**Urea**
uretère	uretere	**Ureter**
urétérocolique	ureterocolico	**Ureterkolik**
urètre	uretra	**Urethra**
syndrome urétral	sindrome uretrale	**Urethralsyndrom**
urétrite	uretrite	**Urethritis**
urétrite non gonococcique	uretrite non gonococcica	**Urethritis, nicht durch Gonokokken bedingte**
urétrite aspécifique	uretrite aspecifica	**Urethritis, unspezifische**
urétrocèle	uretrocele	**Urethrozele**
uricémie	uricemia	**Urikämie**
uricosurique	uricuria	**Urikosurie**
urine	urina	**Urin**
analyse d'urine	esame dell'urina	**Urinanalyse**
analyse d'urine	esame dell'urina	**Urinuntersuchung**
génito-urinaire (GT)	genito-urinario	**urogenital**
urographie	urografia	**Urographie**
urologie	urologia	**Urologie**
origine	origine	**Ursprung**
urticaire	orticaria	**Urtikaria**
utéro-sacré	uterosacrale	**uterosakral**
utéro-vésical	uterovescicale	**uterovesikal**
utérus	utero	**Uterus**
ménométrorragies fonctionnelles	sanguinamento uterino funzionale	**Uterusblutung, dysfunktionale**
uréite	uveite	**Uveitis**
uvule	ugola	**Uvula**
uvulite	stafilite	**Uvulitis**

V

GERMAN	ENGLISH	SPANISH
vagal	vagal	vagal
Vagina	vagina	vagina
Vaginismus	vaginismus	vaginismo
Vaginitis	vaginitis	vaginitis
Vagotomie	vagotomy	vagotomía
Vagus-	vagal	vagal
Vakuumextraktor	vacuum extractor	extractor al vacío
Vakzination	vaccination	vacunación
Vakzine	vaccine	vacuna
valgus	valgus	valgus
Valvotomie	valvotomy	valvotomía
Vanillylmandelsäure	vanyl mandelic acid (VMA)	ácido vanilmandélico (AVM)
Variola	smallpox	viruela
Varizellen	chickenpox, varicella	varicela
Varizen	varicose veins	varices
varus	varus	varus
Vasektomie	vasectomy	vasectomía
vaskulär	vascular	vascular
Vaskulitis	vasculitis	vasculitis
Vasodilatator	vasodilator	vasodilatador
vasodilatatorisch	vasodilator	vasodilatador
Vasokonstriktor	vasoconstrictor	vasoconstrictor
vasokonstriktorisch	vasoconstrictor	vasoconstrictor
vasomotorische Nerven	vasomotor nerves	nervios vasomotores
Vasopressor	vasopressor	vasopresor
vasopressorisch	pressor, vasopressor	presor, vasopresor
Vasoresektion	vasectomy	vasectomía
Vasospasmus	vasospasm	vasospasmo
vasovagale Synkope	vasovagal attack	ataque vasovagal
Veitstanz	chorea	corea
Vektor	vector	vector
Vena cava	vena cava	vena cava
Venae sectio	phlebotomy, venesection	flebotomía, venisección
Vena femoralis	femoral vein	vena femoral
Vena jugularis	jugular vein	vena yugular
Vena radialis	radial vein	vena radial
Vene	vein	vena
Venenentzündung	phlebitis	flebitis
Venenpunktion	venepuncture, venipuncture	venopuntura, venipuntura
Venenthrombose, tiefe	deep vein thrombosis (DVT)	trombosis venosa profunda
venerisch	venereal	venéreo
Venerologie	venereology	venereología
Ventil	valve	válvula
Ventilator	ventilator	ventilador
ventral	ventral	ventral

FRENCH	ITALIAN	GERMAN
vague	vagale	vagal
vagin	vagina	Vagina
vaginisme	vaginismo	Vaginismus
vaginite	vaginite	Vaginitis
vagotomie	vagotomia	Vagotomie
vague	vagale	Vagus-
ventouse obstétricale	ventosa ostetrica, ventosa cefalica	Vakuumextraktor
vaccination	vaccinazione	Vakzination
vaccin	vaccino	Vakzine
valgus	valgo	valgus
valvulotomie	valvulotomia	Valvotomie
acide vanillyl-mandélique	acido vanilmandelico	Vanillylmandelsäure
variole	vaiolo	Variola
varicelle	varicella	Varizellen
varices	vene varicose	Varizen
varus	varo	varus
vasectomie	vasectomia	Vasektomie
vasculaire	vascolare	vaskulär
vasculite	vasculite	Vaskulitis
vasodilatateur	vasodilatatore	Vasodilatator
vasodilatateur	vasodilatatore	vasodilatatorisch
vasoconstricteur	vasocostrittore	Vasokonstriktor
vasoconstricteur	vasocostrittore	vasokonstriktorisch
nerfs vasomoteurs	nervi vasomotori	vasomotorische Nerven
vasopresseur	vasopressore	Vasopressor
pressif, vasopresseur	pressorio, vasopressore	vasopressorisch
vasectomie	vasectomia	Vasoresektion
spasme d'un vaisseau	vasospasmo, angiospasmo	Vasospasmus
malaise vasovagal	crisi vagale	vasovagale Synkope
chorée	corea	Veitstanz
vecteur	vettore	Vektor
veine cave	vena cava	Vena cava
phlébotomie	flebotomia	Venae sectio
veine fémorale	vena femorale	Vena femoralis
veine jugulaire	vena giugulare	Vena jugularis
veine radiale	vena radiale	Vena radialis
veine	vena	Vene
phlébite	flebite	Venenentzündung
ponction d'une veine	puntura di vena	Venenpunktion
thrombose veineuse profonde (TVP)	trombosi venosa profonda (TVP)	Venenthrombose, tiefe
vénérien	venereo	venerisch
vénéréologie	venereologia	Venerologie
valve	valvola	Ventil
appareil de ventilation artificielle	ventilatore	Ventilator
ventral	ventrale	ventral

GERMAN	ENGLISH	SPANISH
Ventrikel	ventricle	ventrículo
Ventrofixation	ventrosuspension	ventrosuspensión
Venula	venule	vénula
veranlagt	prone	prono, inclinado
Verband	bandage, dressing	vendaje, cura
Verbandmaterial	wound dressing	curas para heridas
Verbindung	compound	compuesto
Verbrauch	consumption	consunción, tisis
verbrennen	burn	quemar
Verbrennung	burn	quemadura
Verbrühung	scald	escaldadura
verdampfen	evaporate	evaporar
Verdauung	digestion	digestión
Verdauungsapparat	digestive system	aparato digestivo
Verdauungsstörung	dyspepsia, indigestion	dispepsia, indigestión
Verdrängung	repression, suppression	represión, supresión
Verdünnung	attenuation	atenuación
verdunsten	evaporate	evaporar
Verengung	isthmus	istmo
Vererbung	heredity	herencia
Verfall	degeneration	degeneración
Verfettung	fatty degeneration	degeneración grasa
vergiften	poison	envenenar
vergrößert	swollen	hinchado
Verhalten	behavior (Am), behaviour (Eng)	comportamiento
Verhärtung	induration	induración
Verhornung	keratinization	queratinización
Verhütungs-	contraceptive	anticonceptivo
Verhütungsmittel	contraceptive	anticonceptivo
Verkalkung	calcification	calcificación
Verkapselung	encapsulation	encapsulación
Verkehrsunfall	road traffic accident (RTA)	accidente de circulacion
verkrusten	scab	formar una costra
Verletzung	injury, lesion, wound	lesión, herida
Verletzung, penetrierende	penetrating wound	herida penetrante
Vernebler	nebulizer	nebulizador
Verrenkung	dislocation	dislocación
Verruca	verruca	verruga
verschattet (radiolog)	opaque	opaco
Verschlechterung	deterioration	deterioro
Verschlimmerung	exacerbation	exacerbación
Verschluß	occlusion	oclusión
Verschreibung	prescription	receta
Versio	version	versión
Verstand	brain	cerebro
verstauchen	sprain	torcer
Verstauchung	sprain	esguince

ventricule	ventricolo	**Ventrikel**
ventro-suspension	ventrosospensione, ventrofissazione	**Ventrofixation**
veinule	venula	**Venula**
en pronation	prono	**veranlagt**
bandage, pansement	benda, medicazione	**Verband**
pansements	medicazione di ferita	**Verbandmaterial**
composé	composto	**Verbindung**
consommation	consunzione	**Verbrauch**
brûler	bruciare	**verbrennen**
brûlure	ustione, scottatura	**Verbrennung**
échaudure	scottatura	**Verbrühung**
évaporer	evaporare	**verdampfen**
digestion	digestione	**Verdauung**
système digestif	sistema digestivo	**Verdauungsapparat**
dyspepsie, indigestion	dispepsia, indigestione	**Verdauungsstörung**
répression, uppression	repressione, soppressione	**Verdrängung**
atténuation	attenuazione	**Verdünnung**
évaporer	evaporare	**verdunsten**
isthme	istmo	**Verengung**
hérédité	eredità	**Vererbung**
dégénération	degenerazione	**Verfall**
dégénérescence graisseuse	degenerazione grassa	**Verfettung**
empoisonner	avvelenare	**vergiften**
enflé	gonfio, tumefatto	**vergrößert**
comportement	comportamento	**Verhalten**
induration	indurimento	**Verhärtung**
kératinisation	cheratinizzazione	**Verhornung**
contraceptif	anticoncezionale	**Verhütungs-**
contraceptif	anticoncezionale	**Verhütungsmittel**
calcification	calcificazione	**Verkalkung**
capsulage	incapsulamento	**Verkapselung**
accident de la route	incidente stradale	**Verkehrsunfall**
former une croûte	ricoprirsi di croste	**verkrusten**
blessure, lésion, plaie	lesione, ferita	**Verletzung**
plaie par pénétration	ferita penetrante	**Verletzung, penetrierende**
nébuliseur	nebulizzatore, atomizzatore	**Vernebler**
dislocation	dislocazione	**Verrenkung**
verrue	verruca	**Verruca**
opaque	opaco	**verschattet (radiolog)**
détérioration	deterioramento	**Verschlechterung**
exacerbation	esacerbazione	**Verschlimmerung**
occlusion	occlusione	**Verschluß**
ordonnance	prescrizione, ricetta	**Verschreibung**
version	versione	**Versio**
cerveau	cervello	**Verstand**
se fouler	distorcere	**verstauchen**
foulure	distorsione	**Verstauchung**

GERMAN	ENGLISH	SPANISH
Versteifung	ankylosis	anquilosis
Verstopfung	constipation	estreñimiento
verstreut	disseminated	diseminado
Verstümmelung	mutilation	mutilación
vertebrobasiläre Insuffizienz	vertebrobasilar insufficiency (VBI)	insuficiencia vertebrobasilar
Vertex	vertex	vértice
Vertigo	vertigo	vértigo
Verträglichkeit	compatibility	compatibilidad
Verwachsung	synechia	sinequia
Verwesung	putrefaction	putrefacción
Verwirrung	confusion	confusión
Verzögerung	retardation	retraso
verzweigtes Geschwür	dendritic ulcer	úlcera dendrítica
vesikoureteral	vesicoureteric	vesicoureteral
vesikovaginal	vesicovaginal	vesicovaginal
Vesikula	vesicle	vesícula
Vestibulum	vestibule	vestíbulo
Vibrationssyndrom	vibration syndrome	síndrome de vibración
Vibrieren	thrill	frémito
Virämie	viraemia (Er,g), viremia (Am)	viremia
Virilismus	virilism	virilismo
Virologie	virology	virología
Virulenz	virulence	virulencia
Virus	virus	virus
Virushepatitis	viral hepatitis	hepatitis vírica
visuell	visual	visual
Viszera	viscera	visceras
viszeral	splanchnic	esplácnico
Vitalfunktionserhaltung	basic life support	soporte de vida básico
Vitalkapazität	vital capacity	capacidad vital
Vitamin	vitamin	vitamina
Vitiligo	vitiligo	vitíligo
Volkmann-Kontraktur	Volkmann's ischaemic contracture (Eng), Volkmann's ischemic contracture (Am)	contractura isquémica de Volkmann
Volvulus	volvulus	vólvulo
von Recklinghausen, Morbus	von Recklinghausen's disease	enfermedad de von Recklinghausen
Vorbeugung	prophylaxis	profilaxis
Vorder-	anterior	anterior
vor der Entbindung	ante-partum	ante partum, preparto
vor Empfängnis	preconceptual	preconceptual
Vorfall	procidentia, prolapse, proptosis	procidencia, prolapso, proptosis
vorgeburtlich	prenatal	prenatal
Vorhaut	foreskin, prepuce	prepucio
vorherrschend	dominant	dominante
Vorhof	atrium, vestibule	aurícula, vestíbulo
Vorhofflattern	atrial flutter	aleteo auricular

FRENCH	ITALIAN	GERMAN
ankylose	anchilosi	**Versteifung**
constipation	stipsi	**Verstopfung**
disséminé	disseminato	**verstreut**
mutilation	mutilazione	**Verstümmelung**
insuffisance vertébro-basilaire	insufficienza vertebrobasilare	**vertebrobasiläre Insuffizienz**
vertex	vertice	**Vertex**
vertige	vertigine	**Vertigo**
compatibilité	compatibilità	**Verträglichkeit**
synéchie	sinechia, aderenza	**Verwachsung**
putréfaction	putrefazione	**Verwesung**
confusion	confusione	**Verwirrung**
retard	ritardo mentale, psicomotorio	**Verzögerung**
ulcère dendritique	ulcera dendritica	**verzweigtes Geschwür**
vésico-urétérique	vescicoureterale	**vesikoureteral**
vésico-vaginal	vescicovaginale	**vesikovaginal**
vésicule	vescicola	**Vesikula**
vestibule	vestibolo	**Vestibulum**
syndrome de vibrations	sindrome vibratoria	**Vibrationssyndrom**
murmure respiratoire	fremito	**Vibrieren**
virémie	viremia	**Virämie**
virilisme	virilismo	**Virilismus**
virologie	virologia	**Virologie**
virulence	virulenza	**Virulenz**
virus	virus	**Virus**
hépatite virale	epatite virale	**Virushepatitis**
visuel	visivo	**visuell**
viscères	visceri	**Viszera**
splanchnique	splancnico	**viszeral**
équipement de survie	mantenimento delle funzioni vitali	**Vitalfunktionserhaltung**
capacité vitale	capacità vitale	**Vitalkapazität**
vitamine	vitamina	**Vitamin**
vitiligo	vitiligine	**Vitiligo**
contracture ischémique de Volkmann	paralisi ischemica di Volkmann	**Volkmann-Kontraktur**
volvulus	volvolo	**Volvulus**
maladie de von Recklinghausen	malattia di von Recklinghausen, neurofibromatosi	**von Recklinghausen, Morbus**
prophylaxie	profilassi	**Vorbeugung**
antérieur	anteriore	**Vorder-**
ante partum	preparto	**vor der Entbindung**
préconceptuel	precedente il concepimento	**vor Empfängnis**
procidence, prolapsus, proptose	procidenza, prolasso, proptosi	**Vorfall**
prénatal	prenatale	**vorgeburtlich**
prépuce	prepuzio	**Vorhaut**
dominant	dominante	**vorherrschend**
oreillette, vestibule	atrio, vestibolo	**Vorhof**
flutter auriculaire	flutter atriale	**Vorhofflattern**

GERMAN	ENGLISH	SPANISH
Vorhofflimmern	atrial fibrillation	fibrilación auricular
Vorhofseptumdefekt	atrial septal defect (ASD)	defecto del septum auricular
Vormilch	colostrum	calostro
Vorschlag	suggestion	sugestión
Vorstellung	idea	idea
Vorstufe	precursor	precursor
Vorzeichen	precursor	precursor
vorzeitig	premature	prematuro
Vulva	vulva	vulva
Vulvitis	vulvitis	vulvitis
vulvovaginal	vulvovaginal	vulvovaginal

FRENCH	ITALIAN	GERMAN
fibrillation auriculaire	fibrillazione atriale	**Vorhofflimmern**
communication auriculaire	difetto atriosettale	**Vorhofseptumdefekt**
colostrum	colostro	**Vormilch**
suggestion	suggestione	**Vorschlag**
idée	idea	**Vorstellung**
précurseur	precursore	**Vorstufe**
précurseur	precursore	**Vorzeichen**
prématuré	preamaturo	**vorzeitig**
vulve	vulva	**Vulva**
vulvite	vulvite	**Vulvitis**
vulvo-vaginal	vulvovaginale	**vulvovaginal**

W

German	English	Spanish
Wachstum	growth	crecimiento
Wachstumshormon	growth hormone (GH)	hormona del crecimiento (HC)
Wade	calf	pantorrilla
Wadenbein	fibula	peroné
Wahn	delusion	idea delusiva, delirio
Wahnvorstellung	delusion	idea delusiva, delirio
Wahrnehmung	cognition, perception	cognición, percepción
wandständig	parietal	parietal
Wange	cheek	mejilla
Wärme-	thermal	termal
Warteliste	waiting list	lista de espera
Warze	verruca, wart	verruga
Wasserbruch	hydrocele	hidrocele
wasserhaltig	aqueous	acuoso
Wasserlassen	micturition	micción
Wassermann-Reaktion	Wassermann reaction	reacción de Wassermann
wässrig	aqueous	acuoso
Weber-Ramstedt-Operation	Ramstedt's operation	operación de Ramstedt
Wechseljahre	climacteric, menopause	climatérico, menopausia
Wechselwirkung	interaction	interacción
Wehen	labor (Am), labour (Eng)	parto
weiblich	female	hembra
Weil Krankheit	Weil's disease	enfermedad de Weil
Weisheitszahn	wisdom tooth	muela del juicio
Weitsichtigkeit	hypermetropia	hipermetropía
Wendung	version	versión
Wendung auf den Kopf, äußere	external cephalic version (ECV)	versión cefálica externa
Widal-Reaktion	Widal reaction	reacción de Widal
Wiederbelebung	resuscitation	resucitación
Willebrand-Krankheit	von Willebrand's disease	enfermedad de von Willebrand
Wilms-Tumor	Wilms' tumor (Am), Wilms' tumour (Eng)	tumor de Wilms
Wilson-Krankheit	Wilson's disease	enfermedad de Wilson
Wimper	lash	pestaña
Wimpern	cilia	cilios
Wimpern-	ciliary	ciliar
Wind	flatus, gas, wind	flato, gas, flatulencia, ventosidad
Windeldermatitis	diaper rash (Am), napkin rash (Eng)	exantema del pañal
Windpocken	chickenpox, varicella	varicela
Wirbel	vertebra	vértebra
Wirbelbogenresektion	laminectomy	laminectomía
Wirbelsäule	spine, vertebral column	raquis, columna vertebral

croissance	crescita	**Wachstum**
hormone de croissance (HGH), somatotrophine (STH)	ormone della crescita (GH)	**Wachstumshormon**
mollet	polpaccio	**Wade**
fibula	fibula	**Wadenbein**
hallucination	allucinazione, fissazione	**Wahn**
hallucination	allucinazione, fissazione	**Wahnvorstellung**
cognition, perception	cognizione, percezione	**Wahrnehmung**
pariétal	parietale	**wandständig**
joue	guancia	**Wange**
thermique	termale	**Wärme-**
liste d'attente	lista d'attesa	**Warteliste**
verrue	verruca volgare	**Warze**
hydrocèle	idrocele	**Wasserbruch**
aqueux	acquoso	**wasserhaltig**
micturition	minzione	**Wasserlassen**
réaction de Wassermann	reazione di Wassermann	**Wassermann-Reaktion**
aqueux	acquoso	**wässrig**
opération de Ramstedt	intervento di Ramstedt, piloromiotomia	**Weber-Ramstedt-Operation**
climatérique, ménopause	climaterio, menopausa	**Wechseljahre**
interaction	interazione	**Wechselwirkung**
travail	travaglio di parto	**Wehen**
femelle	femmina	**weiblich**
maladie de Weil	malattia di Weil	**Weil Krankheit**
dent de sagesse	dente del giudizio	**Weisheitszahn**
hypermétropie	ipermetropia	**Weitsichtigkeit**
version	versione	**Wendung**
version céphalique externe	versione cefalica esterna	**Wendung auf den Kopf, äußere**
réaction de Widal	reazione di Widal	**Widal-Reaktion**
ressuscitation	rianimazione	**Wiederbelebung**
maladie de von Willebrand	malattia di von Willebrand	**Willebrand-Krankheit**
tumeur de Wilms	tumore di Wilms	**Wilms-Tumor**
maladie de Wilson	malattia di Wilson	**Wilson-Krankheit**
mèche, lanière	ciglio	**Wimper**
cils	ciglia	**Wimpern**
ciliaire	ciliare	**Wimpern-**
flatuosité, gaz	flatulenza, gas intestinale, gas, ventosità	**Wind**
érythème fessier du nourrisson, érythème papulo-érosif	eruzione cutanea da pannolino	**Windeldermatitis**
varicelle	varicella	**Windpocken**
vertèbre	vertebra	**Wirbel**
laminectomie	laminectomia	**Wirbelbogenresektion**
colonne vertébrale	spina, colonna vertebrale	**Wirbelsäule**

GERMAN	ENGLISH	SPANISH
Wirbelsäulen-	spinal	espinal
wirksam	active	activo
Wirt	host	huésped
Wittmaack-Ekbom-Syndrom	restless legs syndrome	síndrome de piernas inquietas
Wochenbett	puerperium	puerperio
Wochenfluß	lochia	loquios
wund	sore	doloroso
Wunde	wound	herida
Wundhaken	retractor	retractor
Wundrose	erysipelas	erisipela
Wundstarrkrampf	tetanus	tétanos
Wundtoilette	debridement	desbridamiento
Würgen	retching	arcadas
Wurm	worm	lombriz
Wurzel-	radical	radical
Wurzelhautentzündung	periodontal disease	enfermedad periodontal

X

GERMAN	ENGLISH	SPANISH
Xanthämie	xanthaemia (Eng), xanthemia (Am)	xantemia
Xanthelasma	xanthelasma	xantelasma
Xanthom	xanthoma	xantoma
X-Bein	genu valgum, knock-knee	genu valgum
Xerodermie	xeroderma	xeroderma
Xerophthalmie	xerophthalmia	xeroftalmia

FRENCH	ITALIAN	GERMAN
spinal	spinale	**Wirbelsäulen-**
actif	attivo	**wirksam**
hôte	ospite	**Wirt**
syndrome d'impatience musculaire	sindrome delle gambe irrequiete, sindrome di Ekbom	**Wittmaack-Ekbom-Syndrom**
puerpérium	puerperio	**Wochenbett**
lochies	lochi puerperali	**Wochenfluß**
douloureux	dolente	**wund**
plaie	ferita	**Wunde**
rétracteur	divaricatore	**Wundhaken**
érysipèle	erisipela	**Wundrose**
tétanos	tetano	**Wundstarrkrampf**
débridement	sbrigliamento	**Wundtoilette**
haut-le-coeur	conati di vomito	**Würgen**
ver	verme	**Wurm**
radical	radicale	**Wurzel-**
paradontolyse	periodontopatia	**Wurzelhautentzündung**
xanthémie, caroténémie	xantemia	**Xanthämie**
xanthélasma	xantelasma	**Xanthelasma**
xanthome	xantoma, malattia di Rayer	**Xanthom**
genu valgum, genou cagneux	ginocchio valgo	**X-Bein**
xérodermie	xerodermia	**Xerodermie**
xérophtalmie	xeroftalmia	**Xerophthalmie**

Z

zäh	viscid	viscoso
Zahn	tooth	diente
Zahn-	odontic	dentario
Zahnarzt	dentist	dentista
Zahnbelag	plaque	placa
Zähne	teeth	dientes
Zahnfleisch	gingiva	encía
Zahnfleischentzündung	gingivitis	gingivitis
Zahnheilkunde	dentistry	odontologia
zahnlos	edentulous	desdentado
Zahntechnik	dentistry	odontologia
Zahnung	dentition	dentición
Zange	forceps	fórceps
Zäpfchen	suppository, uvula	supositorio, úvula
Zecke	tick	garrapata
Zehe	toe	dedo del pie
Zehenglieder	phalanges	falanges
Zeichen	sign	signo
Zelle	cell	célula
Zellmembran	cell membrane	membrana celular
zellschädigend	cytotoxic	citotóxico
Zellulitis	cellulitis	celulitis
zentraler Venendruck (ZVD)	central venous pressure (CVP)	presión venosa central (PVC)
Zentralnervensystem (ZNS)	central nervous system (CNS)	sistema nervioso central (SNC)
zentrifugal	centrifugal	centrífugo
Zentrifuge	centrifuge	centrífugo
zentrifugieren	centrifuge	centrifugar
zentripetal	centripetal	centrípeto
zerebral	cerebral	cerebral
Zerebralparese	cerebral palsy	parálisis cerebral
zerebrospinal	cerebrospinal	cerebroespinal
zerebrovaskulär	cerebrovascular	cerebrovascular
zerrissen	lacerated	lacerado
Zerstäuber	nebulizer	nebulizador
Zerumen	ear wax	cerumen
zervikal	cervical	cervical
zervikale intraepitheliale Neoplasie (CIN)	cervical intraepithelial neoplasia (CIN)	neoplasia intraepitelial cervical
Zervix	cervix	cuello uterino
Ziegenpeter	mumps	paperas
ziliar	ciliary	ciliar
Zilien	cilia	cilios
Zirbeldrüse	epiphysis	epífisis
Zirkulation	circulation	circulación
zirkumoral	circumoral	circumoral, peroral

visqueux	viscido	zäh
dent	dente	Zahn
dentaire	dentario	Zahn-
dentiste	dentista	Zahnarzt
plaque	placca	Zahnbelag
dents	denti	Zähne
gencive	gengiva	Zahnfleisch
gingivite	gengivite	Zahnfleischentzündung
médecine dentaire, dentisterie	odontoiatria	Zahnheilkunde
édenté	edentulo	zahnlos
médecine dentaire, dentisterie	odontoiatria	Zahntechnik
dentition	dentizione	Zahnung
forceps	forcipe	Zange
suppositoire, uvule	supposta, ugola	Zäpfchen
tique	zecca	Zecke
orteil	dito del piede	Zehe
phalanges	falangi	Zehenglieder
signe	segno	Zeichen
cellule	cellula	Zelle
membrane cellulaire	membrana cellulare	Zellmembran
cytotoxique	citotossico	zellschädigend
cellulite	cellulite	Zellulitis
tension veineuse centrale	pressione venosa centrale	zentraler Venendruck (ZVD)
système nerveux central (CNS)	sistema nervoso centrale	Zentralnervensystem (ZNS)
centrifuge	centrifugo	zentrifugal
centrifugeur	centrifuga	Zentrifuge
centrifuger	centrifugare	zentrifugieren
centripète	centripeto	zentripetal
cérébral	cerebrale	zerebral
infirmité motrice cérébrale	paralisi cerebrale	Zerebralparese
cérébrospinal	cerebrospinale	zerebrospinal
cérébrovasculaire	cerebrovascolare	zerebrovaskulär
lacéré	lacerato	zerrissen
nébuliseur	nebulizzatore, atomizzatore	Zerstäuber
cérumen	cerume	Zerumen
cervical	cervicale	zervikal
néoplasie intra-épithéliale cervicale	neoplasia intraepiteliale della cervice uterina (CIN)	zervikale intraepitheliale Neoplasie (CIN)
cou	cervice	Zervix
oreillons	parotite epidemica	Ziegenpeter
ciliaire	ciliare	ziliar
cils	ciglia	Zilien
épiphyse	epifisi	Zirbeldrüse
circulation	circolazione	Zirkulation
péribuccal	circumorale	zirkumoral

GERMAN	ENGLISH	SPANISH
Zirkumzision	circumcision	circuncisión
Zirrhose	cirrhosis	cirrosis
Zökostomie	caecostomy (Eng), cecostomy (Am)	cecostomía
Zökum	caecum (Eng), cecum (Am)	ciego
Zöliakie	gluten-induced enteropathy	enteropatía provocada por glúten
Zoonose	zoonosis	zoonosis
Zotte	villus	vellosidad
Zuckerkrankheit	diabetes mellitus (DM)	diabetes mellitus
Zuckung	convulsion	convulsión
zuführend	afferent	aferente
Zug	traction, trait	tracción, rasgo
Zunahme	growth	crecimiento
Zunge	glossa, tongue	lengua
Zungenbändchendurchtrennung	frenotomy	frenotomía
Zungenschmerz	glossodynia	glosodinia
zupfen	tease	separar con aguja
zurechnungsfähig	compos mentis	compos mentis, de espíritu sano
Zusammensetzung	compound	compuesto
zusammenwachsen	coalesce	coalescer
zusammenziehen	adduct	aducir
Zustand	status	status
Zwang	compulsion	compulsión, apremio
Zwangsneurose	obsessional neurosis	neurosis obsesiva
zweiklappig	bivalve	bivalvo
zweiseitig	bilateral	bilateral
Zwerchfell	diaphragm, midriff	diafragma
Zwerchfell-	phrenic	frénico
Zwergwuchs	dwarfism	enanismo
Zwilling	twin	mellizo
Zwillinge, eineiige	identical twins	gemelos idénticos
Zwischenblutung	metrorrhagia	metrorragia
Zwischenwirbel-	intervertebral	intervertebral
Zwitter	hermaphrodite	hermafrodita
Zwölffingerdarm	duodenum	duodeno
Zwölffingerdarmentzündung	duodenitis	duodenitis
Zwölffingerdarmgeschwür	duodenal ulcer	úlcera duodenal
Zyanose	cyanosis	cianosis
Zygoma	zygoma	cigoma
Zygote	zygote	cigoto
Zyklus	cycle	ciclo
Zyste	cyst	quiste
Zystektomie	cystectomy	quistectomía
Zystenentfernung	cystectomy	quistectomía
Zystitis	cystitis	cistitis
Zystometrie	cystometry	cistometría
Zystopexie	cystopexy	cistopexia

FRENCH	ITALIAN	GERMAN
circoncision	circoncisione	**Zirkumzision**
cirrhose	cirrosi	**Zirrhose**
caecostomie	ciecostomia	**Zökostomie**
caecum	intestino cieco	**Zökum**
maladie coeliaque	enteropatia da glutine	**Zöliakie**
zoonose	zoonosi	**Zoonose**
villosité	villo	**Zotte**
diabète sucré	diabete mellito	**Zuckerkrankheit**
convulsion	convulsione	**Zuckung**
afférent	afferente	**zuführend**
traction, trait	trazione, attrazione, tratto, carattere ereditario	**Zug**
croissance	crescita	**Zunahme**
langue	lingua	**Zunge**
frénotomie	frenulotomia	**Zungenbändchendurçhtrennung**
glossodynie	glossodinia	**Zungenschmerz**
défilocher	dissociare i tessuti	**zupfen**
compos mentis	mentalmente sano	**zurechnungsfähig**
composé	composto	**Zusammensetzung**
se combiner	aggregarsi	**zusammenwachsen**
produire l'adduction	addurre	**zusammenziehen**
statut	stato	**Zustand**
compulsion	compulsione	**Zwang**
névrose obsessionnelle	nevrosi ossessiva	**Zwangsneurose**
bivalve	bivalve	**zweiklappig**
bilatéral	bilaterale	**zweiseitig**
diaphragme	diaframma, parte bassa del torace	**Zwerchfell**
psychique	frenico (diaframmatico mentale)	**Zwerchfell-**
nanisme	nanismo	**Zwergwuchs**
jumeau	gemello	**Zwilling**
jumeaux univitellins	gemelli omozigoti	**Zwillinge, eineiige**
métrorragie	metrorragia	**Zwischenblutung**
intervertébral	intervertebrale	**Zwischenwirbel-**
hermaphrodite	ermafrodito	**Zwitter**
duodénum	duodeno	**Zwölffingerdarm**
duodénite	duodenite	**Zwölffingerdarmentzündung**
ulcère duodénal	ulcera duodenale	**Zwölffingerdarmgeschwür**
cyanose	cianosi	**Zyanose**
zygoma	zigomo, osso zigomatico	**Zygoma**
zygote	zigote	**Zygote**
cycle	ciclo	**Zyklus**
kyste	cisti	**Zyste**
cystectomie	cistectomia	**Zystektomie**
cystectomie	cistectomia	**Zystenentfernung**
cystite	cistite	**Zystitis**
cystométrie	cistometria	**Zystometrie**
cystopexie	cistopessia	**Zystopexie**

GERMAN	ENGLISH	SPANISH
Zystoskop	cystoscope	citoscopio
Zystoskopie	cystoscopy	citoscopía
Zystozele	cystocele	cistocele
Zytologie	cytology	citología
Zytomegalie-Virus (CMV)	cytomegalovirus (CMV)	citomegalovirus
zytotoxisch	cytotoxic	citotóxico

FRENCH	ITALIAN	GERMAN
cystoscope	cistoscopio	**Zystoskop**
cystoscopie	cistoscopia	**Zystoskopie**
cystocèle	cistocele	**Zystozele**
cytologie	citologia	**Zytologie**
cytomégalovirus	citomegalovirus	**Zytomegalie-Virus (CMV)**
cytotoxique	citotossico	**zytotoxisch**

ABRÉVIATIONS ALLEMANDES
DEUTSCHE ABKÜRZUNGEN
ABBREVIAZIONI TEDESCHE
ABREVIATURAS ALEMANAS

ABC-Regel	Luftwege Atmung und Kreislauf
ACH	Nebennierenrindenhormon
ACTH	adrenokortikotropes Hormon
AIDS	erworbenes Immundefektsyndrom
BCG	Bacillus Calmette-Guérin
BKS	Blutkörperchen-Senkungsgeschwindigkeit
BSE	Bovine Spongiforme Enzephalitis
BSG	Blutkörperchen-Senkungsgeschwindigkeit
CIN	zervikale intraepitheliale Neoplasie
CMV	Zytomegalie-Virus
CRP	C-reaktives Protein
CT	Computertomographie
DIC	disseminierte intravasale Gerinnung
DNS	Desoxyribonukleinsäure
EBV	Epstein-Barr-Virus
EEG	Elektroenzephalogramm
EKG	Elektrokardiogramm
ELISA	enzyme-linked immunosorbent assay
ERCP	endoskopische retrograde Cholangiopankreatographie
FSH	follikelstimulierendes Hormon
FT	freies Thyroxin
FTi	freier Thyroxinindex
GFR	glomeruläre Filtrationsrate
gGt	Gammaglutamyltransferase
HBsAG	Australia-Antigen
HCG	Choriongonadotropin
HCS	human chorionic somatomammotropin
HDL-Cholesterol	high density lipoprotein-cholesterol
HIV	human immunodeficiency virus
HKT	Hämatokrit
HLA	human lymphocytic antigen
HSV	Herpes simplex-Virus
HTLV	human T-cell leukemia virus
IHK	ischämische Herzkrankheit
IUP	Intrauterinpessar
KHK	koronare Herzkrankheit
LDL	low density lipoprotein
LHRF	LH-luteinizing hormone releasing factor
MCV	mittleres Erythrozytenvolumen
MS	multiple Sklerose
NBZ	Nüchternblutzucker
NIDDM	non-insulin dependent diabetes mellitus
NMR	Kernspintomographie
Pap	Papanicolaou (-Färbung, -Abstrich)
PAT	Plättchen-Aggregations-Test
PCP	Polyarthritis rheumatica
PKU	Phenylketonurie
psi	pounds per square inch
RAST	Radio-Allergo-Sorbent-Test

RBF	renaler Blutfluß
REM	rapid eye movement
RNA	Ribonukleinsäure
SIDS	Sudden-infant-death-Syndrom
SLE	systemischer Lupus erythematodes
TEBK	totale Eisenbindungskapazität
TIA	transitorische ischämische Attacke
TK	Totalkapazität
TSS	toxisches Schocksyndrom
ZNS	Zentralnervensystem
ZVD	zentraler Venendruck

ITALIAN
English
German
Spanish
French
ITALIAN

A

abdurre	abduct	abduzieren
abduttore	abductor	Abduktor
abduzione	abduction	Abduktion
aberrante	aberrant	aberrans, abartig
aberrazione	aberration	Aberration, Abweichung
abilità	ability	Fähigkeit
abitudine	habit	Gewohnheit
ablazione	ablation	Ablatio, Absetzung
abortire	abort	fehlgebären
aborto	abortion, miscarriage	Abort, Fehlgeburt
aborto interno	missed abortion	verhaltener Abort, missed abortion
aborto procurato	induced abortion	Abtreibung, künstlicher Abort
aborto ritenuto	missed abortion	verhaltener Abort, missed abortion
aborto terapeutico	therapeutic abortion	indizierter Abort
abrasione	abrasion	Abschabung, Ausschabung
abreazione	abreaction	Abreaktion
abuso	abuse	Abusus, Mißbrauch
abuso di droga	drug abuse	Arzneimittelmißbrauch, Drogenmißbrauch
abuso di farmaci	drug abuse, polypharmacy	Arzneimittelmißbrauch, Drogenmißbrauch, Polypragmasie
acalasia	achalasia	Achalasie
acalasia esofagea	cardiospasm	Kardiospasmus
accidente cerebrovascolare (ACV)	cerebrovascular accident (CVA), stroke	Schlaganfall, Apoplex, Schlag
accomodazione	accommodation	Akkommodation
acetabolo	acetabulum	Azetabulum, Hüftgelenkspfanne
acidità	acidity	Säuregehalt
acido (n)	acid (n)	Säure (n)
acido (a)	acid (a)	sauer (a)
acido deossiribonucleico	deoxyribonucleic acid (DNA)	Desoxyribonukleinsäure (DNS)
acido folico	folic acid	Folsäure
acido grasso	fatty acid	Fettsäure
acido grasso essenziale	essential fatty acid	essentielle Fettsäure
acido lattico	lactic acid	Milchsäure
acido omovanillico	homovanillic acid (HVA)	Homovanillinsäure
acido resistente	acid-fast	säurebeständig
acido ribonucleico (RNA)	ribonucleic acid (RNA)	Ribonukleinsäure (RNA)
acidosi	acidosis	Azidose
acido urico	uric acid	Harnsäure
acido vanilmandelico	vanyl mandelic acid (VMA)	Vanillylmandelsäure
acinetico	akinetic	akinetisch
acne	acne	Akne
acne rosacea	rosacea	Rosacea
acondroplasia	achondroplasia	Achondroplasie
acquedotto	aqueduct	Aquädukt

SPANISH	FRENCH	ITALIAN
abducir	produire l'abduction	**abdurre**
abductor	abducteur	**abduttore**
abducción	abduction	**abduzione**
aberrante, desviado	aberrant	**aberrante**
aberración	aberration	**aberrazione**
habilidad, capacidad	capacité, aptitude, compétence	**abilità**
hábito	habitude	**abitudine**
ablación, excisión	ablation	**ablazione**
abortar	avorter	**abortire**
aborto	avortement, fausse couche	**aborto**
aborto diferido	rétention foetale	**aborto interno**
aborto inducido	avortement provoqué	**aborto procurato**
aborto diferido	rétention foetale	**aborto ritenuto**
aborto terapéutico	avortement thérapeutique	**aborto terapeutico**
abrasión	abrasion	**abrasione**
abreacción, catarsis	abréaction	**abreazione**
abuso	abus	**abuso**
abuso de drogas	toxicomanie	**abuso di droga**
abuso de drogas, polifarmacia	toxicomanie, polypharmacie	**abuso di farmaci**
acalasia	achalasie	**acalasia**
cardiospasmo	cardiospasme	**acalasia esofagea**
accidente vascular cerebral (ACV), ictus	accident cérébrovasculaire, apoplexie	**accidente cerebrovascolare (ACV)**
acomodación	accommodation	**accomodazione**
acetábulo	acétabule	**acetabolo**
acidez	acidité	**acidità**
ácido (n)	acide (n)	**acido** (n)
ácido (a)	acide (a)	**acido** (a)
ácido desoxirribonucléico (ADN)	acide désoxyribonucléique (ADN)	**acido deossiribonucleico**
ácido fólico	acide folique	**acido folico**
ácido graso	acide gras	**acido grasso**
ácido graso esenciale	acide gras essentiel	**acido grasso essenziale**
ácido láctico	acide lactique	**acido lattico**
ácido homovaníllico	acide homovanillique	**acido omovanillico**
ácido-resistente	acido-résistant	**acido resistente**
ácido ribonucléico (ARN)	acide ribonucléique (RNA)	**acido ribonucleico (RNA)**
acidosis	acidose	**acidosi**
ácido úrico	acide urique	**acido urico**
ácido vanilmandélico (AVM)	acide vanillyl-mandélique	**acido vanilmandelico**
acinético	acinétique	**acinetico**
acné	acné	**acne**
rosácea	acné rosacée	**acne rosacea**
acondroplasia	achondroplasic	**acondroplasia**
acueducto	aqueduc	**acquedotto**

ITALIAN	ENGLISH	GERMAN
acquiescenza alle prescrizioni	patient compliance	Compliance
acquoso	aqueous	wässrig, wasserhaltig
acromatopsia	color blindness (Am), colour blindness (Eng)	Farbenblindheit
acromegalia	acromegaly	Akromegalie
acromioclavicolare	acromioclavicular	akromioklavikular
acromion	acromion	Akromion
actinomicosi	actinomycosis	Aktinomykose
acuità	acuity	Schärfe
acustico	acoustic, auditory	akustisch, Gehör-, Hör-
acutezza visiva	visual acuity	Sehschärfe
acuto	acute	spitz, scharf
addensamento	consolidation	Konsolidierung, Festigung
addome	abdomen, belly	Abdomen, Bauch
addominale	abdominal	abdominal
addomino-perineale	abdomino-perineal	abdominoperineal
addurre	adduct	adduzieren, zusammenziehen
adduttore	adductor	Adduktor
adduzione	adduction	Adduktion
adenocarcinoma	adenocarcinoma	Adenokarzinom
adenoidectomia	adenoidectomy	Adenoidektomie, Polypenentfernung
adenoidi	adenoids	Adenoide, Nasenpolypen
adenoma	adenoma	Adenom
adenomioma	adenomyoma	Adenomyom
adenotonsillectomia	adenotonsillectomy	Adenotonsillektomie
adenovirus	adenovirus	Adenovirus
aderenza	synechia	Synechie, Verwachsung
adesione	adhesion	Adhäsion, Anhaften
adipe	fat	Fett
adiposo	adipose	adipös, fettleibig
a disagio	queasy	unwohl, übel
adiuvante	adjuvant	Adjuvans
adolescenza	adolescence	Adoleszenz, Jugendalter
adozione	adoption	Adoption
adrenalina	adrenaline, epinephrine	Adrenalin
adrenergico	adrenergic	adrenerg
adsorbimento	adsorption	Adsorption
aerobio	aerobe	Aerobier
aerofagia	aerophagia	Aerophagie, Luftschlucken
aerosol	aerosol	Aerosol
afasia	aphasia	Aphasie
afebbrile	afebrile	fieberfrei
afferente	afferent	afferent, zuführend
affettivo	affective	affektiv
affetto da vertigini o capogiro	giddy	schwindlig
affezione	disease	Krankheit, Leiden
affido	fostering	Pflege

SPANISH	FRENCH	ITALIAN
cumplimiento del paciente	observance du patient	**acquiescenza alle prescrizioni**
acuoso	aqueux	**acquoso**
daltonismo, ceguera de colores	daltonisme	**acromatopsia**
acromegalia	acromégalie	**acromegalia**
acromioclavicular	acromio-claviculaire	**acromioclavicolare**
acromion	acromion	**acromion**
actinomicosis	actinomycose	**actinomicosi**
agudeza	acuité	**acuità**
acústico, auditorio	acoustique, auditif	**acustico**
agudeza visual	acuité visuelle	**acutezza visiva**
agudo	aigu(ë)	**acuto**
consolidación	consolidation	**addensamento**
abdomen, vientre	abdomen, ventre	**addome**
abdominal	abdominal	**addominale**
abdominoperineal	abdomino-périnéal	**addomino-perineale**
aducir	produire l'adduction	**addurre**
aductor	adducteur	**adduttore**
aducción	adduction	**adduzione**
adenocarcinoma	adénocarcinome	**adenocarcinoma**
adenoidectomía	adénoïdectomie	**adenoidectomia**
adenoides	végétations adénoïdes	**adenoidi**
adenoma	adénome	**adenoma**
adenomioma	adénomyome	**adenomioma**
amigdaloadenoidectomía	adéno-amygdalectomie	**adenotonsillectomia**
adenovirus	adénovirus	**adenovirus**
sinequia	synéchie	**aderenza**
adherencia	adhésion	**adesione**
grasa	graisse	**adipe**
adiposo, graso	adipeux	**adiposo**
nauseabundo	indigeste, délicat	**a disagio**
coadyuvante	adjuvant	**adiuvante**
adolescencia	adolescence	**adolescenza**
adopción	adoption	**adozione**
adrenalina, epinefrina	adrénaline, épinéphrine	**adrenalina**
adrenérgico	adrénergique	**adrenergico**
adsorción	adsorption	**adsorbimento**
aerobio, aeróbico	aérobie	**aerobio**
aerofagia	aérophagie	**aerofagia**
aerosol	aérosol	**aerosol**
afasia	aphasie	**afasia**
apirético, afebril	afébrile	**afebbrile**
aferente	afférent	**afferente**
afectivo	affectif	**affettivo**
mareado	pris de vertige	**affetto da vertigini o capogiro**
enfermedad	maladie	**affezione**
adopción	prise en nourrice	**affido**

ITALIAN	ENGLISH	GERMAN
afte	aphthae	Aphthe
agenesia	agenesis	Agenesie
agente chelante	chelating agent	Chelatbildner
agglutinazione	agglutination	Agglutination
agglutinine	agglutinin	Agglutinin
aggregarsi	coalesce	zusammenwachsen
aggressività	aggression	Aggression
agnazia	agnathia	Agnathie
agnosia	agnosia	Agnosie
ago	needle	Nadel, Kanüle
agonista	agonist	Agonist
agopuntura	acupuncture	Akupunktur
agorafobia	agoraphobia	Agoraphobie, Platzangst
agranulocitosi	agranulocytosis	Agranulozytose
albumina	albumin	Albumin
albuminuria	albuminuria	Albuminurie
alcali	alkali	Alkali, Lauge, Base
alcalino	alkaline	alkalisch, basisch
alcalosi	alkalosis	Alkalose
alcolismo	alcoholism	Alkoholismus, Alkoholvergiftung
alcool	alcohol	Alkohol
alcool-acido-resistente	acid-alcohol-fast	säurealkoholbeständig
alcool-resistente	alcohol-fast	alkoholresistent
alfafetoproteina	alpha-fetoprotein (AFP)	Alpha-Fetoprotein
alimentazione	alimentation	Ernährung
alimento ricco di fibre	roughage	Ballaststoff
alitosi	halitosis	Foetor ex ore, Mundgeruch
allergene	allergen	Allergen
allergia	allergy	Allergie
allergia alimentare	food allergy	Nahrungsmittelallergie
allopurinolo	allopurinol	Allopurinol
alluce	hallux	Hallux, Großzeh
allucinazione	delusion, hallucination	Wahn, Wahnvorstellung, Halluzination
alopecia	alopecia	Alopezie, Haarausfall
alveolite	alveolitis	Alveolitis
alveolo	alveolus	Alveole
amaurosi	amaurosis	Amaurose
ambiente	environment	Umgebung, Umwelt
ambliopia	amblyopia	Amblyopie, Sehschwäche
ambulatoriale	ambulatory	ambulant
ambulatorio	ambulant	ambulant
ameba	ameba (Am), amoeba (Eng)	Amöbe
amebiasi	amebiasis (Am), amoebiasis (Eng)	Amöbenkrankheit, Amöbiasis
ameboma	ameboma (Am), amoeboma (Eng)	Amöbengranulom
amenorrea	amenorrhea (Am), amenorrhoea (Eng)	Amenorrhoe
amilasi	diastasis	Diastase

aftas	aphtes	afte
agenesia	agénésie	agenesia
quelantes	agent chélateur	agente chelante
aglutinación	agglutination	agglutinazione
aglutinina	agglutinine	agglutinine
coalescer	se combiner	aggregarsi
agresión	agression	aggressività
agnatia	agnathie	agnazia
agnosia	agnosie	agnosia
aguja	aiguille	ago
agonista	agoniste	agonista
acupuntura	acupuncture	agopuntura
agorafobia	agoraphobie	agorafobia
agranulocitosis	agranulocytose	agranulocitosi
albúmina	albumine	albumina
albuminuria	albuminurie	albuminuria
álcali	alcali	alcali
alcalino	alcalin	alcalino
alcalosis	alcalose	alcalosi
alcoholismo	alcoolisme	alcolismo
alcohol	alcool	alcool
ácido-alcohol-resistente	résistant à l'alcool et à l'acide	alcool-acido-resistente
resistente al alcohol	résistant à l'alcool	alcool-resistente
alfafetoproteína (AFP)	alpha-foetoprotéine	alfafetoproteina
alimentación	alimentation	alimentazione
fibra alimentaria	ballant intestinal	alimento ricco di fibre
halitosis	halitose	alitosi
alérgeno	allergène	allergene
alergia	allergie	allergia
alergia alimentaria	allergie alimentaire	allergia alimentare
alopurinol	allopurinol	allopurinolo
dedo gordo del pie	hallux	alluce
idea delusiva, delirio, alucinación	hallucination	allucinazione
alopecia, calvicie	alopécie	alopecia
alveolitis	alvéolite	alveolite
alvéolo	alvéole	alveolo
amaurosis, ceguera	amaurose	amaurosi
ambiente	milieu	ambiente
ambliopía	amblyopie	ambliopia
ambulatorio	ambulatoire	ambulatoriale
ambulante	ambulant	ambulatorio
ameba	amibe	ameba
amebiasis	amibiase	amebiasi
ameboma	amibome	ameboma
amenorrea	aménorrhée	amenorrea
diastasis	diastasis	amilasi

amiloide *(n)*	amyloid *(n)*	Amyloid *(n)*
amiloide *(a)*	amyloid *(a)*	amyloid *(a)*, stärkehaltig *(a)*
amiloidosi	amyloidosis	Amyloidose
aminoacido	amino acid	Aminosäure
aminoacido essenziale	essential amino acid	essentielle Aminosäure
ammaccare	bruise	stoßen, quetschen
amnesia	amnesia	Amnesie
amniocentesi	amniocentesis	Amniozentese
amnios	amnion	Amnion
amnioscopia	amnioscopy	Amnioskopie
amniotomia	amniotomy	Amnionpunktur
amorfo	amorphous	amorph
ampolla	ampoule (Eng), ampule (Am), ampulla	Ampulle
ampolla o vasetto unguentario	gallipot	Salbentopf
amputato	amputee	Amputierter
amputazione	amputation	Amputation
anabolismo	anabolism	Anabolismus, Aufbaustoffwechsel
anaerobio	anaerobe (Eng), anerobe (Am)	Anaerobier
anafilassi	anaphylaxis	Anaphylaxie
analettico *(n)*	analeptic *(n)*	Analeptikum *(n)*
analettico *(a)*	analeptic *(a)*	analeptisch *(a)*
analgesia	analgesia	Analgesie, Schmerzlosigkeit
analgesico *(n)*	analgesic *(n)*	Analgetikum *(n)*, Schmerzmittel *(n)*
analgesico *(a)*	analgesic *(a)*	analgetisch *(a)*, schmerzlindernd *(a)*, schmerzunempfindlich *(a)*
analisi	analysis	Analyse
anaplasia	anaplasia	Anaplasie
anartria	anarthria	Anarthrie
anastomosi	anastomosis	Anastomose
anatomia	anatomy	Anatomie
anca	hip	Hüfte
anchilosi	ankylosis	Ankylose, Versteifung
andatura	gait	Gang
androgeni	androgens	Androgene
anemia	anaemia (Eng), anemia (Am)	Anämie
anemia drepanocitica	sickle-cell anaemia (Eng), sickle-cell anemia (Am)	Sichelzellanämie
anemia perniciosa	pernicious anaemia (Eng), pernicious anemia (Am)	perniziöse Anämie
anencefalia	anencephaly	Anenzephalie
anestesia	anaesthesia (Eng), anesthesia (Am)	Anästhesie, Betäubung, Narkose
anestesia della regione pubica	pudendal block	Pudendusblock
anestetico *(n)*	anaesthetic (Eng) *(n)*, anesthetic (Am) *(n)*	Anästhetikum *(n)*, Betäubungsmittel *(n)*, Narkosemittel *(n)*
anestetico *(a)*	anaesthetic (Eng) *(a)*, anesthetic (Am) *(a)*	anästhetisch *(a)*, betäubend *(a)*, gefühllos *(a)*
aneurisma	aneurysm	Aneurysma

amiloide *(n)*	amyloïde *(n)*	**amiloide** *(n)*
amiloideo *(a)*	amyloïde *(a)*	**amiloide** *(a)*
amiloidosis	amylose	**amiloidosi**
aminoácido	acide aminé	**aminoacido**
aminoácido esencial	acide aminé essentiel	**aminoacido essenziale**
magullar, contundir	contusionner	**ammaccare**
amnesia	amnésie	**amnesia**
amniocentesis	amniocentèse	**amniocentesi**
amnios	amnion	**amnios**
amnioscopia	amnioscopie	**amnioscopia**
amniotomía	amniotomie	**amniotomia**
amorfo	amorphe	**amorfo**
ampolla, víal	ampoule	**ampolla**
bote	petit pot	**ampolla o vasetto unguentario**
amputado	amputé	**amputato**
amputación	amputation	**amputazione**
anabolismo	anabolisme	**anabolismo**
anaerobio	anaérobie	**anaerobio**
anafilaxis	anaphylaxie	**anafilassi**
analéptico, estimulante *(n)*	analeptique *(n)*	**analettico** *(n)*
analéptico, estimulante *(a)*	analeptique *(a)*	**analettico** *(a)*
analgesia	analgésie	**analgesia**
analgésico *(n)*	analgésique *(n)*	**analgesico** *(n)*
analgésico *(a)*	analgésique *(a)*	**analgesico** *(n)*
análisis	analyse	**analisi**
anaplasia	anaplasie	**anaplasia**
anartria	anarthrie	**anartria**
anastómosis	anastomose	**anastomosi**
anatomía	anatomie	**anatomia**
cadera	hanche	**anca**
anquilosis	ankylose	**anchilosi**
marcha	démarche	**andatura**
andrógenos	androgènes	**androgeni**
anemia	anémie	**anemia**
anemia drepanocítica	drépanocytose	**anemia drepanocitica**
anemia perniciosa	anémie pernicieuse	**anemia perniciosa**
anencefalia	anencéphalie	**anencefalia**
anestesia	anesthésie	**anestesia**
bloqueo del pudendo	vulve	**anestesia della regione pubica**
anestésico *(n)*	anesthésique *(n)*	**anestetico** *(n)*
anestésico *(a)*	anesthésique *(a)*	**anestetico** *(a)*
aneurisma	anévrisme	**aneurisma**

angina	angina	Angina
angioma stellare	spider naevus (Eng), spider nevus (Am)	Spider naevus, Naevus arachnoideus
angioplastica	angioplasty	Angioplastie
angiospasmo	vasospasm	Vasospasmus
angiotensina	angiotensin	Angiotensin
anisocitosi	anisocytosis	Anisozytose
annessi	adnexa	Adnexe
ano	anus	Anus, After
anogenitale	anogenital	anogenital
anomala motilità respiratoria della cassa toracica in conseguenza di fratture	flail chest	Flatterbrust
anomalia	anomaly	Anomalie, Fehlbildung
anoressia	anorexia	Anorexie, Magersucht
anoressico (n)	anorectic (n)	Anorektiker(in) (n), Magersüchtige(r) (n), Apettitzügler (n)
anoressico (a)	anorectic (a)	anorektisch (a), magersüchtig (a)
anorettale	anorectal	anorektal
anormale	abnormal	abnormal
anosmia	anosmia	Anosmie
anossia	anoxia	Anoxie, Sauerstoffmangel
anovulare	anovular	anovulatorisch
ansietà	anxiety	Angst
ansiolitico (n)	anxiolytic (n)	Anxiolytikum (n)
ansiolitico (a)	anxiolytic (a)	anxiolytisch (a)
antagonismo	antagonism	Antagonismus
antagonista	antagonist	Antagonist
antagonista H2	H2 antagonist	H2-Antagonist
anteriore	anterior	anterior, Vorder-
anterogrado	anterograde	anterograd
antiacido	antacid	Antazidum
anti-aritmico	anti-arrhythmic	antiarrhythmisch
antibatterico	antibacterial	antibakteriell
antibechico (n)	antitussive (n)	Antitussivum (n), Hustenmittel (n)
antibechico (a)	antitussive (a)	antitussiv (a)
antibiotici	antibiotics	Antibiotika
anticoagulante	anticoagulant	Antikoagulans, Gerinnungshemmer
anticolinergico	anticholinergic	anticholinerg
anticomiziale (n)	anti-epileptic (n)	Antiepileptikum (n), Antikonvulsivum (n)
anticomiziale (a)	anti-epileptic (a)	antiepileptisch (a), antikonvulsiv (a)
anticoncezionale (n)	contraceptive (n)	Kontrazeptivum (n), Verhütungsmittel (n)
anticoncezionale (a)	contraceptive (a)	kontrazeptiv (a), Verhütungs- (a)
anticonvulsivante (n)	anticonvulsant (n)	Antiepileptikum (n), Antikonvulsivum (n)
anticonvulsivante (a)	anticonvulsant (a)	antiepileptisch (a), antikonvulsiv (a)
anticorpi (Ac)	antibodies (Ab)	Antikörper

SPANISH	FRENCH	ITALIAN
angina	angor	**angina**
araña vascular	naevi	**angioma stellare**
angioplastia	angioplastie	**angioplastica**
vasospasmo	spasme d'un vaisseau	**angiospasmo**
angiotensina	angiotensine	**angiotensina**
anisocitosis	anisocytose	**anisocitosi**
anejos, anexos	annexes	**annessi**
ano	anus	**ano**
anogenital	anogénital	**anogenitale**
volet torácico	volet thoracique	**anomala motilità respiratoria della cassa toracica in conseguenza di fratture**
anomalía	anomalie	**anomalia**
anorexia	anorexie	**anoressia**
anoréxico (n)	anorexique (n)	**anoressico (n)**
anoréxico (a)	anorexique (a)	**anoressico (a)**
anorrectal	anorectal	**anorettale**
anormal	anormal	**anormale**
anosmia	anosmie	**anosmia**
anoxia	anoxie	**anossia**
anovular	anovulaire	**anovulare**
ansiedad	anxiété	**ansietà**
ansiolítico (n)	anxiolytique (n)	**ansiolitico (n)**
ansiolítico (a)	anxiolytique (a)	**ansiolitico (a)**
antagonismo	antagonisme	**antagonismo**
antagonista	antagoniste	**antagonista**
antagonista H2	antagoniste H2	**antagonista H2**
anterior	antérieur	**anteriore**
anterógrado	antérograde	**anterogrado**
antiácido	antiacide	**antiacido**
antiarrítmico	antiarythmique	**anti-aritmico**
antibacteriano	antibactérien	**antibatterico**
antitusígeno (n)	antitussif (n)	**antibechico (n)**
antitusígeno (a)	antitussif (a)	**antibechico (a)**
antibióticos	antibiotiques	**antibiotici**
anticoagulante	anticoagulant	**anticoagulante**
anticolinérgico	anticholinergique	**anticolinergico**
antiepiléptico (n)	antiépileptique (n)	**anticomiziale (n)**
antiepiléptico (a)	antiépileptique (a)	**anticomiziale (a)**
anticonceptivo (n)	contraceptif (n)	**anticoncezionale (n)**
anticonceptivo (a)	contraceptif (a)	**anticoncezionale (a)**
anticonvulsivo (n)	anticonvulsant (n)	**anticonvulsivante (n)**
anticonvulsivo (a)	anticonvulsant (a)	**anticonvulsivante (a)**
anticuerpos	anticorps	**anticorpi (Ac)**

anticorpo immuno-fluorescente anti-treponema	fluorescent treponemal antibody (FTA)	Fluoreszenz-Treponemen-Antikörper
anticorpo monoclonale	monoclonal antibody	monoklonaler Antikörper
anti-D	anti-D	Anti-D-Immununglobulin
antidepressivo	antidepressant	Antidepressivum
antidoto	antidote	Antidot
anti-emetico (n)	antiemetic (n)	Antiemetikum (n)
anti-emetico (a)	antiemetic (a)	antiemetisch (a)
antigene	antigen	Antigen
antigene Australia	Australian antigen	Australia-Antigen (HBsAG)
antigene di istocompatibilità	histocompatibility antigen	Histokompatibilitäts-Antigen
antigene eritrocitico umano	human erythrocyte antigen (HEA)	menschliches Erythrozyten-Antigen
antigene linfocitario umano	human lymphocytic antigen (HLA)	human lymphocytic antigen (HLA)
antigene triplo	triple antigen	Dreifachantigen
anti-infiammatorio	anti-inflammatory	entzündungshemmend
anti-ipertensivo (n)	antihypertensive (n)	Antihypertonikum (n), Antihypertensivum (n)
anti-ipertensivo (a)	antihypertensive (a)	blutdrucksenkend (a), antihypertensiv (a)
anti-istaminico	antihistamine	Antihistamine
antimalarico (n)	antimalarial (n)	Antimalariamittel (n), Malariamittel (n)
antimalarico (a)	antimalarial (a)	Antimalaria- (a)
antimetabolita	antimetabolite	Antimetabolit
antimicotico (n)	antimycotic (n)	Antimykotikum (n)
antimicotico (a)	antimycotic (a)	antimykotisch (a)
antimicrobico	antimicrobial	antimikrobiell
anti-piretico (n)	antipyretic (n)	Antipyretikum (n), Fiebermittel (n)
anti-piretico (a)	antipyretic (a)	antipyretisch (a), fiebersenkend (a)
antipruriginoso (n)	antipruritic (n)	Antipruriginosum (n)
antipruriginoso (a)	antipruritic (a)	antipruriginös (a), juckreizlindernd (a)
antipsicotico (n)	antipsychotic (n)	Antipsychotikum (n), Neuroleptikum (n)
antipsicotico (a)	antipsychotic (a)	antipsychotisch (a), neuroleptisch (a)
antisepsi	antisepsis	Antisepsis
antisettico (n)	antiseptic (n)	Antiseptikum (n)
antisettico (a)	antiseptic (a)	antiseptisch (a)
anti-siero	antiserum	Antiserum, Immunserum
antisociale	antisocial	dissozial
antispastico (n)	antispasmodic (n)	Spasmolytikum (n)
antispastico (a)	antispasmodic (a)	spasmolytisch (a), krampflösend (a)
antitossina	antitoxin	Antitoxin, Gegengift
antiveleno	antivenin	Schlangenserum
antiversione	anteversion	Anteversion
antrace	anthrax, carbuncle	Anthrax, Milzbrand, Karbunkel
antro	antrum	Antrum
antropoide	anthropoid	anthropoid
antropologia	anthropology	Anthropologie

SPANISH	FRENCH	ITALIAN
anticuerpo anti-treponema fluorescente	test d'immunofluorescence absorbée pour le diagnostic sérologique de la syphilis	anticorpo immuno-fluorescente anti-treponema
anticuerpo monoclonal	anticorps monoclonal	anticorpo monoclonale
anti-D	anti-D	anti-D
antidepresivo	antidépresseur	antidepressivo
antídoto	antidote	antidoto
antiemético (n)	antiémétique (n)	anti-emetico (n)
antiemético (a)	antiémétique (a)	anti-emetico (a)
antígeno	antigène	antigene
antígeno Australia	antigène australien	antigene Australia
antígeno de histocompatibilidad	antigène d'histocompatibilité	antigene di istocompatibilità
antígeno eritrocitario humano	antigène humain des erythrocytes	antigene eritrocitico umano
antígeno linfocitario humano (HLA)	antigène lymphocytaire humain	antigene linfocitario umano
antígeno triple	triple antigène	antigene triplo
antiinflamatorio	anti-inflammatoire	anti-infiammatorio
hipotensor (n)	antihypertenseur (n)	anti-ipertensivo (n)
hipotensor (a)	antihypertensif (a)	anti-ipertensivo (a)
antihistamínico	antihistamine	anti-istaminico
antipalúdico (n)	antipaludique (n)	antimalarico (n)
antipalúdico (a)	antipaludique (a)	antimalarico (a)
antimetabolito	antimétabolite	antimetabolita
antimicótico (n)	antimycotique (n)	antimicotico (n)
antimicótico (a)	antimycotique (a)	antimicotico (a)
antimicrobiano	antimicrobien	antimicrobico
antipirético (n)	antipyrétique (n)	anti-piretico (n)
antipirético (a)	antipyrétique (a)	anti-piretico (a)
antipruriginoso (n)	antiprurigineux (n)	antipruriginoso (n)
antipruriginoso (a)	antiprurigineux (a)	antipruriginoso (a)
antipsicótico (n)	antipsychotique (n)	antipsicotico (n)
antipsicótico (a)	antipsychotique (a)	antipsicotico (a)
antisepsia	antisepsie	antisepsi
antiséptico (n)	antiseptique (n)	antisettico (n)
antiséptico (a)	antiseptique (a)	antisettico (a)
antisuero	anti-serum	anti-siero
antisocial	antisocial	antisociale
antiespasmódico (n)	antispasmodique (n)	antispastico (n)
antiespasmódico (a)	antispasmodique (a)	antispastico (a)
antitoxina	antitoxine	antitossina
antídoto	sérum antivenimeux	antiveleno
anteversión	antéversion	antiversione
carbunco, ántrax	anthrax, charbon	antrace
antro	antre	antro
antropoide	anthropoïde	antropoide
antropología	anthropologie	antropologia

629

antrostomia	antrostomy	Antrumeröffnung
anulare	annular	ringförmig
anuria	anuria	Anurie, Harnverhaltung
anziano pensionato	old age pensioner (OAP)	Rentner
aorta	aorta	Aorta, Hauptschlagader
apatia	apathy	Apathie
aperto	patent	offen, durchgängig
apice	apex	Apex, Spitze
apiressia	apyrexia	Apyrexie
apnea	apnea (Am), apnoea (Eng)	Apnoe, Atemstillstand
appendice	appendix	Appendix, Blinddarm
appendicectomia	appendectomy, appendicectomy	Appendektomie, Blinddarmoperation
appendicite	appendicitis	Appendizitis, Blinddarmentzündung
applicatore	applicator	Applikator
apposizione	apposition	Apposition
aprassia	apraxia	Apraxie
aracnoidea	arachnoid	arachnoid
arbovirus	arbovirus	ARBO-Virus
arcata sopracciliare	brow	Augenbraue
area di Broca	Broca's area	Broca-Sprachzentrum
area di pressione	pressure area	Druckfläche
areola	areola	Areola, Brustwarzenhof
aritmia	arrhythmia	Arrhythmie, Rhythmusstörung
arrossamento infiammatorio	rubor	Rubor, Rötung
artefatto	artefact (Eng), artifact (Am)	Artefakt
arteria	artery	Arterie, Schlagader
arteria femorale	femoral artery	Arteria femoralis
arteria radiale	radial artery	Arteria radialis
arteriola	arteriole	Arteriole
arteriopatia	arteriopathy	Arteriopathie, Arterienerkrankung
arteriosclerosi	arteriosclerosis	Arteriosklerose, Arterienverkalkung
arterite	arteritis	Arteriitis
arterite a cellule giganti	giant cell arteritis	Riesenzellarteriitis
arterovenosa	arteriovenous	arteriovenös
articolare	articular	Gelenk-
articolazione	articulation, joint	Artikulation, Gelenk
articolazione interfalangea	knuckle	Knöchel
arto	leg	Bein
artralgia	arthralgia	Arthralgie, Gelenkschmerz
artrite	arthritis	Arthritis, Gelenkentzündung
artrite reumatoide (AR)	rheumatoid arthritis (RA)	Polyarthritis rheumatica (PCP), Rheumatoide Arthritis
artrodesi	arthrodesis	Arthrodese
artrografia	arthrography	Arthrographie
artropatia	arthropathy	Arthropathie, Gelenkleiden
artropatia di Charcot	Charcot's joint	Charcot-Gelenk
artropatia psoriasica	psoriatic arthritis	Arthritis psoriatica

antrostomía	antrostomie	**antrostomia**
anular	annulaire	**anulare**
anuria	anurie	**anuria**
jubilado	retraité(e)	**anziano pensionato**
aorta	aorte	**aorta**
apatía	apathie	**apatia**
permeable	libre	**aperto**
ápex	apex	**apice**
apirexia	apyrexie	**apiressia**
apnea	apnée	**apnea**
apéndice	appendice	**appendice**
apendicectomía	appendicectomie	**appendicectomia**
apendicitis	appendicite	**appendicite**
aplicador	applicateur	**applicatore**
aposición	apposition	**apposizione**
apraxia	apraxie	**aprassia**
aracnoideo	arachnoïde	**aracnoidea**
arbovirus	arbovirus	**arbovirus**
ceja	front, sourcil	**arcata sopracciliare**
área de Broca	centre moteur de Broca	**area di Broca**
zona de decúbito	zone particulièrement sensible	**area di pressione**
areola	aréole	**areola**
arritmia	arythmie	**aritmia**
rubor	rougeur	**arrossamento infiammatorio**
artefacto	artefact	**artefatto**
arteria	artère	**arteria**
arteria femoral	artère fémorale	**arteria femorale**
arteria radial	artère radiale	**arteria radiale**
arteriola	artériole	**arteriola**
arteriopatía	artériopathie	**arteriopatia**
arteriosclerosis	artériosclérose	**arteriosclerosi**
arteritis	artérite	**arterite**
arteritis de células gigantes	artérite temporale	**arterite a cellule giganti**
arteriovenoso	artérioveineux	**arterovenosa**
articular	articulaire	**articolare**
articulación	articulation	**articolazione**
nudillo	jointure	**articolazione interfalangea**
pierna	jambe	**arto**
artralgia	arthralgie	**artralgia**
artritis	arthrite	**artrite**
artritis reumatoide (AR)	polyarthrite rhumatoïde (PR), polyarthrite chronique évolutive (PCE)	**artrite reumatoide (AR)**
artrodesis	arthrodèse	**artrodesi**
artrografía	arthrographie	**artrografia**
artropatía	arthropathie	**artropatia**
articulación de Charcot	arthropathie neurogène	**artropatia di Charcot**
artritis psoriásica	rhumatisme psoriasique	**artropatia psoriasica**

ITALIAN	ENGLISH	GERMAN
artroplastica	arthroplasty	Arthroplastik, Gelenkplastik
artroscopia	arthroscopy	Arthroskopie, Gelenkendoskopie
asbesto	asbestos	Asbest
asbestosi	asbestosis	Asbestose
ascaride	ascaris, roundworm	Rundwurm, Spulwurm
ascella	axilla	Axilla, Achsel(höhle)
ascesso	abscess	Abszeß
ascesso freddo	cold abscess	kalter Abszeß
ascesso peritonsillare	peritonsillar abscess, quinsy	Peritonsillarabszeß
ascite	ascites	Aszites
asepsi	asepsis	Asepsis
asfissia	asphyxia	Asphyxie
asimmetria	asymmetry	Asymmetrie
asintomatico	asymptomatic	asymptomatisch
asma	asthma	Asthma
asma bronchiale	bronchial asthma	Asthma bronchiale
aspergillosi	aspergillosis	Aspergillose
aspirazione	aspiration	Aspiration
aspirazione di fluido	tapping	Abzapfen, Punktieren, Perkutieren
asportazione di disco intervertebrale	discectomy (Eng), diskectomy (Am)	Diskektomie
asse	axis	Achse
assestamento difettoso	maladjustment	Fehlanpassung
assimilazione	assimilation	Assimilation
assistenza post-operatoria	aftercare	Nachbehandlung, Nachsorge
assistere	nurse	stillen, pflegen
associazione	association	Assoziation
assone	axon	Axon
assorbimento	absorption	Absorption
assuefazione	habituation	Habituation, Gewöhnung
astenia	fatigue	Ermüdung
astereognosia	astereognosis	Astereognosie
astigmatismo	astigmatism	Astigmatismus
astinenza	withdrawal	Entzug
astragalo	talus	Talus
astringente	astringent	adstringierend
atassia	ataxia	Ataxie, Koordinationsstörung
atelettasia	atelectasis	Atelektase
aterogenico	atherogenic	atherogen
ateroma	atheroma	Atherom, Grützbeutel
aterosclerosi	atherosclerosis	Atherosklerose
atetosi	athetosis	Athetose
atipico	atypical	atypisch, heterolog
atomizzatore	nebulizer	Zerstäuber, Vernebler
atomo	atom	Atom
atonico	atonic	atonisch

SPANISH	FRENCH	ITALIAN
artroplastia	arthroplastie	artroplastica
artroscopia	arthroscopie	artroscopia
asbesto	asbeste	asbesto
asbestosis	asbestose	asbestosi
áscaris	ascaris	ascaride
axila	aisselle	ascella
absceso	abcès	ascesso
absceso frío	abcès froid	ascesso freddo
absceso periamigdalino, angina	abcès périamygdalien, phlegmon amygdalien ou périamygdalien	ascesso peritonsillare
ascitis	ascite	ascite
asepsia	asepsie	asepsi
asfixia	asphyxie	asfissia
asimetría	asymétrie	asimmetria
asintomático	asymptomatique	asintomatico
asma	asthme	asma
asma bronquial	asthme bronchique	asma bronchiale
aspergilosis	aspergillose	aspergillosi
aspiración	aspiration	aspirazione
paracentesis	ponction	aspirazione di fluido
disquectomía	discectomie	asportazione di disco intervertebrale
eje	axe	asse
inadaptación	inadaptation	assestamento difettoso
asimilación	assimilation	assimilazione
cuidados postoperatorios	postcure	assistenza post-operatoria
cuidar	soigner	assistere
asociación	association	associazione
axón	axone	assone
absorción	absorption	assorbimento
habituación	accoutumance	assuefazione
fatiga, cansancio	fatigue	astenia
astereognosia	astéréognosie	astereognosia
astigmatismo	astigmatisme	astigmatismo
supresión, abstinencia	retrait, sevrage, suppression	astinenza
astrágalo	astragale	astragalo
astringente	astringent	astringente
ataxia	ataxie	atassia
atelectasia	atélectasie	atelettasia
aterogénico	athérogène	aterogenico
ateroma	athérome	ateroma
aterosclerosis	athérosclérose	aterosclerosi
atetosis	athétose	atetosi
atípico	atypique	atipico
nebulizador	nébuliseur	atomizzatore
átomo	atome	atomo
atono	atonique	atonico

633

ITALIAN	ENGLISH	GERMAN
atresia	atresia	Atresie
atrio	atrium	Atrium, Vorhof
atrioventricolare	atrioventricular (AV)	atrioventrikulär
atrofia	atrophy	Atrophie
atropina	atropine	Atropin
attaccare	affect	befallen
attacco	attack, seizure	Anfall, Attacke
attacco ischemico transitorio	transient ischaemic attack (TIA) (Eng), transient ishemic attack (TIA) (Am)	transitorische ischämische Attacke (TIA)
attenuazione	attenuation	Verdünnung, Abschwächung
attivo	active	aktiv, wirksam
attrazione	traction	Traktion, Zug
attrito	friction	Friktion, Reibung
audiogramma	audiogram	Audiogramm, Hörkurve
audiologia	audiology	Audiologie
auditivo	auditory	Gehör-, Hör-
aura	aura	Aura
auricolare	aural	Gehör-, Ohr-, Aura-
auscultazione	auscultation	Auskultation, Abhören
autismo	autism	Autismus
autistico	autistic	autistisch
autoanticorpo	autoantibody	Autoantikörper
autoantigene	autoantigen	Autoantigen
autoavvelenamento	self-poisoning	Selbstvergiftung
autoclave	autoclave	Autoklav, Sterilisationsapparat
autoimmunizzazione	autoimmunity	Autoimmunität
autoinnesto	autograft	Autoplastik
autolesionismo	self-harm	Selbstschädigung
autolisi	autolysis	Autolyse
autologo	autologous	autolog
autonomo	autonomic	autonom
autopalpazione mammaria	breast self-examination (BSE)	Selbstuntersuchung der Brust
autopsia	autopsy	Autopsie, Sektion
avambraccio	forearm	Unterarm
avascolare	avascular	gefäßlos
avulsione	avulsion	Abriß, Ausreißen
avvelenamento alimentare	food poisoning	Nahrungsmittelvergiftung
avvelenare	poison	vergiften
azione	action	Tätigkeit
azotemia	blood urea	Blutharnstoff
azygos	azygous	azygos

SPANISH	FRENCH	ITALIAN
atresia	atrésie	**atresia**
aurícula	oreillette	**atrio**
atrioventricular, aurículo-ventricular (AV)	atrio-ventriculaire	**atrioventricolare**
atrofia	atrophie	**atrofia**
atropina	atropine	**atropina**
afectar	affecter	**attaccare**
ataque, acceso	attaque, accès	**attacco**
ataque isquémico transitorio (AIT)	accès ischémique transitoire cérébral	**attacco ischemico transitorio**
atenuación	atténuation	**attenuazione**
activo	actif	**attivo**
tracción	traction	**attrazione**
fricción	friction	**attrito**
audiograma	audiogramme	**audiogramma**
audiología	audiologie	**audiologia**
auditorio	auditif	**auditivo**
aura	aura	**aura**
aural	aural	**auricolare**
auscultación	auscultation	**auscultazione**
autismo	autisme	**autismo**
persona autística	autiste	**autistico**
autoanticuerpo	auto-anticorps	**autoanticorpo**
autoantígeno	auto-antigène	**autoantigene**
autointoxicación	intoxication volontaire	**autoavvelenamento**
autoclave	autoclave	**autoclave**
autoinmunización	auto-immunisation	**autoimmunizzazione**
autoinjerto	autogreffe	**autoinnesto**
autolesión	automutilation	**autolesionismo**
autólisis	autolyse	**autolisi**
autólogo	autologue	**autologo**
autónomo	autonome	**autonomo**
autoexamen de la mama	auto-examen des seins	**autopalpazione mammaria**
autopsia	autopsie	**autopsia**
antebrazo	avant-bras	**avambraccio**
avascular	avasculaire	**avascolare**
avulsión	avulsion	**avulsione**
intoxicación alimentaria	intoxication alimentaire	**avvelenamento alimentare**
envenenar	empoisonner	**avvelenare**
acción	action	**azione**
urea sérica	urée du sang	**azotemia**
ácigos	azygos	**azygos**

B

ITALIAN	ENGLISH	GERMAN
bacillo	bacillus	Bazillus
bacillo di Calmette e Guérin	bacille Calmette-Guérin (BCG)	Bacillus Calmette-Guérin (BCG)
bagno	bath	Bad
balanite	balanitis	Balanitis
balanopostite	balanoposthitis	Balanoposthitis
balbuzie	stammer	Stottern
ballottamento	ballottement	Ballottement
banca del sangue	blood bank	Blutbank
barriera ematoencefalica	blood-brain barrier (BBB)	Blut-Hirn-Schranke
basalioma	rodent ulcer	Ulcus rodens
basso peso alla nascita	low birth weight (LBW), small-for-dates (SFD)	niedriges Geburtsgewicht, termingemäß klein
bastoncello retiníco (per anestetizzare la dentina)	Harrington rod	Harrington Stab
batteri	bacteria	Bakterien
battericida	bactericide	Bakterizid
batteriemia	bacteraemia (Eng), bacteremia (Am)	Bakteriämie
batteriologia	bacteriology	Bakteriologie
batteriostasi	bacteriostasis	Bakteriostase
batteriuria	bacteriuria	Bakteriurie
battito cardiaco	heartbeat	Herzschlag
battito cardiaco fetale	fetal heart rate (FHR)	fetale Herzfrequenz
'belle indifference'	'belle indifference'	belle indifference
benda	bandage	Verband
benigno	benign	benigne, gutartig
beri-beri	beri-beri	Beriberi
beta-bloccante	beta blocker	Betablocker
bicipite	biceps	Bizeps
bicorne	bicornuate	bicornis
bicuspide	bicuspid	bicuspidal
bifido	bifid	bifidus
biforcazione	bifurcation	Bifurkation
bilaterale	bilateral	zweiseitig
bile	bile	Galle
biliare	biliary, bilious	biliär, biliös
bilirubina	bilirubin	Bilirubin
biliuria	biliuria	Bilirubinurie
bimanuale	bimanual	bimanuell, beidhändig
biologico	biological	biologisch
biopsia	biopsy	Biopsie
biopsia dei villi coriali	chorionic villus biopsy	Chorionzottenbiopsie
biopsia digiunale	jejunal biopsy	Jejunumbiopsie
bioritmo	biorhythm	Biorhythmus
bipolare	bipolar	bipolar
bisessuale	bisexual	bisexuell

636

SPANISH	FRENCH	ITALIAN
bacilo	bacille	bacillo
bacilo de Calmette-Guérin (BCG)	bacille de Calmette-Guérin (BCG)	bacillo di Calmette e Guérin
baño	bain	bagno
balanitis	balanite	balanite
balanopostitis	balanoposthite	balanopostite
tartamudeo	bégaiement	balbuzie
peloteo	ballottement	ballottamento
banco de sangre	banque de sang	banca del sangue
barrera hematoencefálica (BHE)	barrière hémato-encéphalique	barriera ematoencefalica
úlcera corrosiva	ulcus rodens	basalioma
bajo peso al nacer, útero pequeño para la edad gestacional	hypotrophie, présentant un retard de croissance	basso peso alla nascita
varilla de Harrington	tige de Harrington	bastoncello retinico (per anestetizzare la dentina)
bacteria	bactérie	batteri
bactericida	bactéricide	battericida
bacteriemia	bactériémie	batteriemia
bacteriología	bactériologie	batteriologia
bacteriostasis	bactériostase	batteriostasi
bacteriuria	bactériurie	batteriuria
patido cardíaco	pulsation (de coeur)	battito cardiaco
frecuencia cardíaca fetal (FCF)	fréquence cardiaque foetale	battito cardiaco fetale
la belle indifférence	indifférence	'belle indifference'
vendaje	bandage	benda
benigno	bénin (bénigne)	benigno
beri-beri	béribéri	beri-beri
beta-bloqueador	bêtabloquant	beta-bloccante
bíceps	biceps	bicipite
bicornio	bicorne	bicorne
bicúspide	bicuspide	bicuspide
bífido	bifide	bifido
bifurcación	bifurcation	biforcazione
bilateral	bilatéral	bilaterale
bilis	bile	bile
biliar, bilioso	biliaire, bilieux	biliare
bilirrubina	bilirubine	bilirubina
biliuria	biliurie	biliuria
bimanual	bimanuel	bimanuale
biológico	biologique	biologico
biopsia	biopsie	biopsia
biopsia de las vellosidades coriónicas	biopsie du villus chorionique	biopsia dei villi coriali
biopsia del yeyuno	biopsie jéjunale	biopsia digiunale
biorritmo	biorythme	bioritmo
bipolar	bipolaire	bipolare
bisexual	bisexuel	bisessuale

ITALIAN	ENGLISH	GERMAN
bisturi	scalpel	Skalpell
bivalve	bivalve	zweiklappig
blefarite	blepharitis	Blepharitis, Lidentzündung
blefarospasmo	blepharospasm	Blepharospasmus, Lidkrampf
blocco nervoso	nerve block	Leitungsanästhesie
'blue baby' (cianosi da cardiopatia congenita)	blue baby	zyanotisches Neugeborenes
bocca	mouth	Mund
bolla	blister, bulla	Blase, Hautblase, Brandblase, Bulla
bolo	bolus	Bolus
bolo isterico	globus hystericus	Globus hystericus, Globusgefühl
borreliosi	borreliosis	Borreliose
borsa	bursa	Bursa
borsite	bursitis	Bursitis, Schleimbeutelentzündung
borsite dell'alluce	bunion	entzündeter Fußballen
botulismo	botulism	Botulismus
braccio	arm, limb	Arm, Glied, Extremität
brachiale	brachial	Arm-
bradicardia	bradycardia	Bradykardie
branchiale	branchial	branchial-
bronchi	bronchi	Bronchien
bronchiettasia	bronchiectasis	Bronchiektase
bronchiolite	bronchiolitis	Bronchiolitis
bronchiolo	bronchiole	Bronchiolus, Bronchiole
bronchite	bronchitis	Bronchitis
bronco	bronchus	Bronchus
broncocostrittore	bronchoconstrictor	Bronchokonstriktor
broncodilatatore	bronchodilator	Bronchodilatator
broncopolmonare	bronchopulmonary	bronchopulmonal
broncopolmonite	bronchopneumonia	Bronchopneumonie
broncoscopio	bronchoscope	Bronchoskop
broncospasmo	bronchospasm	Bronchospasmus
brucellosi	brucellosis	Brucellose
bruciare	burn	brennen, verbrennen
buccale	buccal	bukkal
buccia d'arancia	peau d'orange	Orangenhaut
bulbare	bulbar	bulbär
bulimia	bulimia	Bulimie

SPANISH	FRENCH	ITALIAN
escalpelo	scalpel	bisturi
bivalvo	bivalve	bivalve
blefaritis	blépharite	blefarite
blefarospasmo	blépharospasme	blefarospasmo
bloqueo nervioso	anesthésie par blocage nerveux	blocco nervoso
niño azul	enfant bleu, enfant atteint de la maladie bleue	'blue baby' (cianosi da cardiopatia congenita)
boca	bouche	bocca
vesícula, ampolla, flictena, bulla	ampoule, bulle	bolla
bolo	bol	bolo
globo histérico	boule hystérique	bolo isterico
borreliosis	borréliose	borreliosi
bolsa	bourse	borsa
bursitis	bursite	borsite
juanete	hallux valgus	borsite dell'alluce
botulismo	botulisme	botulismo
brazo, extremidad	bras, membre	braccio
braquial	brachial	brachiale
bradicardia	bradycardie	bradicardia
branquial	branchial	branchiale
bronquios	bronches	bronchi
bronquiectasia	bronchectasie	bronchiettasia
bronquiolitis	bronchiolite	bronchiolite
bronquiolo	bronchiole	bronchiolo
bronquitis	bronchite	bronchite
bronquio	bronche	bronco
broncoconstrictor	bronchoconstricteur	broncocostrittore
broncodilatador	bronchodilatateur	broncodilatatore
broncopulmonar	bronchopulmonaire	broncopolmonare
bronconeumonia	bronchopneumonie	broncopolmonite
broncoscopio	bronchoscope	broncoscopio
broncospasmo	bronchospasme	broncospasmo
brucelosis	brucellose	brucellosi
quemar	brûler	bruciare
bucal	buccal	buccale
piel de naranja	peau d'orange	buccia d'arancia
bulbar	bulbaire	bulbare
bulimia	boulimie	bulimia

C

ITALIAN	ENGLISH	GERMAN
cachessia	cachexia, wasting away	Kachexie, Schwinden
cadavere	cadaver, corpse	Kadaver, Leiche, Toter
caffeina	caffeine	Koffein
calazion	chalazion	Chalazion, Hagelkorn
calcificazione	calcification	Kalzifikation, Verkalkung
calcio	calcium	Kalzium
calcoli biliari	gallstones	Gallensteine
calcolo	calculus, stone	Stein
callista	chiropodist	Fußpfleger
callo	callus, corn	Kallus, Klavus, Hühnerauge
callosità	callosity	Schwiele, Hornhaut
calore	calor	Fieber, Hitze
caloria	calorie	Kalorie
campione urinario del mitto intermedio (CUM)	midstream urine specimen (MUS)	Mittelstrahlurin
campo visivo	field of vision	Gesichtsfeld
canale	canal	Kanal, Gang
canale semicircolare	semicircular canal	Bogengang
cancro	cancer	Karzinom, Krebs
cancroide	chancre	Schanker
candidiasi	candidiasis	Candidiasis
canino	canine	Hunde-
cannula	cannula	Kanüle
capacità	ability	Fähigkeit
capacità di legame del ferro	iron binding capacity (IBC)	Eisenbindungskapazität
capacità di legame dell'antigene	antigen binding capacity (ABC)	Antigen-Bindungskapazität
capacità polmonare totale	total lung capacity (TLC)	Totalkapazität (TK)
capacità totale di legame del ferro (TIBC)	total iron binding capacity (TIBC)	totale Eisenbindungskapazität (TEBK)
capacità vitale	vital capacity	Vitalkapazität
capello	hair	Haar
capezzolo	nipple	Brustwarze, Mamille
capillare	capillary	Kapillare
capogiro	dizziness	Schwindel
capsula	capsule	Kapsel
capsula di Petri	Petri dish	Petrischale
capsulite	capsulitis	Kapselentzündung
carattere	character	Charakter, Merkmal
carattere ereditario	trait	Zug, Charakterzug, Eigenschaft
carbammide	urea	Urea, Harnstoff
carboidrato	carbohydrate (CHO)	Kohlenhydrat, Kohlenwasserstoff
carbonchio	anthrax, carbuncle	Anthrax, Milzbrand, Karbunkel
carbone vegetale	charcoal	Holzkohle
carbossiemoglobina	carboxyhaemoglobin (Eng), carboxyhemoglobin (Am)	Carboxyhämoglobin

SPANISH	FRENCH	ITALIAN
caquexia, consunción	cachexie, dépérissement	cachessia
cadáver	cadavre	cadavere
cafeína	caféine	caffeina
chalacio, orzuelo	chalazion	calazion
calcificación	calcification	calcificazione
calcio	calcium	calcio
cálculos biliares	calculs biliaires	calcoli biliari
cálculo	calcul, caillou	calcolo
callista, podólogo	pédicure	callista
callo, papiloma	cal, cor	callo
callosidad	callosité	callosità
calor	chaleur	calore
caloría	calorie	caloria
muestra de orina de la parte media de la micción	urine du milieu du jet	campione urinario del mitto intermedio (CUM)
campo de visión	champ de vision	campo visivo
canal	canal	canale
conducto semicircular	canal semi-circulaire	canale semicircolare
cáncer	cancer	cancro
chancro	chancre	cancroide
candidiasis	candidose	candidiasi
canino	canin	canino
cánula	canule	cannula
habilidad, capacidad	capacité, aptitude, compétence	capacità
capacidad de unión con el hierro	pouvoir sidéropexique, capacité de fixation du fer	capacità di legame del ferro
capacidad de unión con antígenos	capacité de liaison d'un antigène, capacité de fixation d'un antigène	capacità di legame dell'antigene
capacidad pulmonar total (CPT)	capacité pulmonaire totale	capacità polmonare totale
capacidad total de unión con el hierro	capacité totale de fixation du fer	capacità totale di legame del ferro (TIBC)
capacidad vital	capacité vitale	capacità vitale
pelo	poil	capello
pezón	mamelon	capezzolo
capilar	capillaire	capillare
desvanecimiento, mareo	étourdissement	capogiro
cápsula	capsule	capsula
disco de Petri	boîte de Pétri	capsula di Petri
capsulitis	capsulite	capsulite
carácter	caractère	carattere
rasgo	trait	carattere ereditario
urea	urée	carbammide
hidrato de carbono	glucide	carboidrato
carbunco, ántrax	anthrax, charbon	carbonchio
carbón vegetal	charbon	carbone vegetale
carboxihemoglobina	carboxyhémoglobine	carbossiemoglobina

ITALIAN	ENGLISH	GERMAN
carcinogenesi	carcinogenesis	Karzinogenese
carcinogeno	carcinogen	Karzinogen
carcinoma	carcinoma	Karzinom, Krebs
carcinoma a piccole cellule	oat cell cancer	kleinzelliges Bronchialkarzinom
carcinomatosi	carcinomatosis	Karzinose, Karzinomatose
cardiaco	cardiac	Herz-
cardias	cardia	Kardia, Mageneingang
cardiogeno	cardiogenic	kardiogen
cardiologia	cardiology	Kardiologie
cardiomegalia	cardiomegaly	Kardiomegalie
cardiomiopatia	cardiomyopathy	Kardiomyopathie
cardiopatia ischemica	ischaemic heart disease (IHD) (Eng), ischemic heart disease (IHD) (Am)	ischämische Herzkrankheit (IHK)
cardiopolmonare	cardiopulmonary	kardiopulmonal, Herz-Lungen-
cardiorespiratorio	cardiorespiratory	kardiorespiratorisch
cardiotocografia	cardiotocograph	Kardiotokograph
cardiotoracico	cardiothoracic	kardiothorakal
cardiotossico	cardiotoxic	kardiotoxisch, herzschädigend
cardiovascolare	cardiovascular	kardiovaskulär, Kreislauf-
cardioversione	cardioversion	Kardioversion
carena tracheale	carina	Carina
carie	caries	Karies
cariotipo	karyotype	Karyotyp
carminativo (n)	carminative (n)	Karminativum (n)
carminativo (a)	carminative (a)	karminativ (a), entblähend (a)
carotene	carotene	Karotin
carotide	carotid	Karotis-
carpometacarpale	carpometacarpal	karpometakarpal
carpopedalico	carpopedal	karpopedal
cartilagine	cartilage	Knorpel
cartilagine costale	haemoptysis (Eng), hemoptysis (Am)	Hämoptoe, Bluthusten
caruncola	caruncle	Karunkel
castrazione	castration	Kastration
catabolismo	catabolism	Katabolismus, Abbaustoffwechsel
catalizzatore	catalyst	Katalysator
cataratta	cataract	Katarakt, grauer Star
catarro	catarrh	Katarrh
catarsi	abreaction	Abreaktion
catatonico	catatonic	kataton
catetere	catheter	Katheter
catetere per drenaggio auricolare	grommet	Öse
cateterizzazione	catheterization	Katheterisierung
catgut	catgut	Catgut
catrame	coal tar	Steinkohlenteer
causa di morte	cause of death (COD)	Todesursache
causalgia	causalgia	Kausalgie, brennender Schmerz
caustico (n)	caustic (n)	Ätzmittel (n), Kaustikum (n)

SPANISH	FRENCH	ITALIAN
carcinogénesis	carcinogenèse	carcinogenesi
carcinogénico	carcinogène	carcinogeno
carcinoma	carcinome	carcinoma
carcinoma de células de avena	épithélioma à petites cellules	carcinoma a piccole cellule
carcinomatosis	carcinomatose	carcinomatosi
cardíaco	cardiaque	cardiaco
cardias	cardia	cardias
cardiógenico	cardiogène	cardiogeno
cardiología	cardiologie	cardiologia
cardiomegalia	cardiomégalie	cardiomegalia
cardiomiopatía, miocardiopatía	cardiomyopathie	cardiomiopatia
cardiopatía isquémica	cardiopathie ischémique	cardiopatia ischemica
cardiopulmonar	cardiopulmonaire	cardiopolmonare
cardiorespiratorio	cardiorespiratoire	cardiorespiratorio
tococardiógrafo	cardiotocographe	cardiotocografia
cardiotorácico	cardiothoracique	cardiotoracico
cardiotóxico	cardiotoxique	cardiotossico
cardiovascular	cardiovasculaire	cardiovascolare
cardioversión	cardioversion	cardioversione
carina	carène	carena tracheale
caries	carie	carie
cariotipo	karyotype	cariotipo
carminativo (n)	carminatif (n)	carminativo (n)
carminativo (a)	carminatif (a)	carminativo (a)
carotenos	carotène	carotene
carótida	carotide	carotide
carpometacarpiano	carpo-métarcarpien	carpometacarpale
carpopedal	carpo-pédal	carpopedalico
cartílago	cartilage	cartilagine
hemoptisis	hémoptysie	cartilagine costale
carúncula	caroncule	caruncola
castración	castration	castrazione
catabolismo	catabolisme	catabolismo
catalizador	catalyseur	catalizzatore
catarata	cataracte	cataratta
catarro	catarrhe	catarro
abreacción, catarsis	abréaction	catarsi
catatónico	catatonique	catatonico
catéter	cathéter	catetere
cánula ótica	grommet	catetere per drenaggio auricolare
cateterismo	cathétérisme	cateterizzazione
catgut	catgut	catgut
alquitrán, brea	coaltar	catrame
causa de la muerte	cause du décès	causa di morte
causalgia	causalgie	causalgia
cáustico (n)	caustique (n)	caustico (n)

ITALIAN	ENGLISH	GERMAN
caustico (a)	caustic (a)	ätzend (a), brennend (a)
cauterizzare	cauterize	kauterisieren, ätzen, brennen
cavernoso	cavernous	kavernös
caviglia	ankle	Knöchel, Talus
cavità	cavity	Höhle
cavità amniotica	amniotic cavity	Amnionhöhle
cecità	blindness	Blindheit
cecità ai colori	color blindness (Am), colour blindness (Eng)	Farbenblindheit
cecità fluviale	river blindness	Flußblindheit
cefalea muscolotensiva	tension headache	Spannungskopfschmerz
cefalico	cephalic	Kopf-, Schädel-
cefaloematoma	cephalhaematoma (Eng), cephalhematoma (Am)	Kephalhämatom
cefalometria	cephalometry	Kephalometrie, Schädelmessung
celiaco	celiac (Am), coeliac (Eng)	abdominal
cellula	cell	Zelle
cellulite	cellulitis	Zellulitis
centigrado	centigrade	Celsiusgrad
centrifuga	centrifuge	Zentrifuge
centrifugare	centrifuge	zentrifugieren
centrifugo	centrifugal	zentrifugal
centripeto	centripetal	zentripetal
cerebrale	cerebral	zerebral, Gehirn-
cerebrospinale	cerebrospinal	zerebrospinal
cerebrovascolare	cerebrovascular	zerebrovaskulär
cerume	ear wax	Zerumen, Ohrenschmalz
cerume nell orecchio	glue ear	glue ear
cervelletto	cerebellum	Cerebellum, Kleinhirn
cervello	brain, cerebrum	Gehirn, Verstand, Großhirn
cervicale	cervical	zervikal
cervice	cervix	Zervix, Gebärmutterhals
cestode	tapeworm	Bandwurm, Tänia
che ha avuto figli	parous	geboren habend
cheilosi	cheilosis	Mundeckenschrunden
cheloide	keloid	Keloid
chemioprofilassi	chemoprophylaxis	Chemoprophylaxe
chemiotassi	chemotaxis	Chemotaxis
chemioterapia	chemotherapy	Chemotherapie
chemorecettore	chemoreceptor	Chemorezeptor
chemosi	chemosis	Chemosis
cheratina	keratin	Keratin
cheratinizzazione	keratinization	Keratinisation, Verhornung
cheratite	keratitis	Keratitis, Hornhautentzündung
cheratocele	keratocele	Keratozele
cheratocongiuntivite	keratoconjunctivitis	Keratokonjunktivitis
cheratomalacia	keratomalacia	Keratomalazie

644

SPANISH	FRENCH	ITALIAN
cáustico (a)	caustique (a)	caustico (a)
cauterizar	cautériser	cauterizzare
cavernoso	caverneux	cavernoso
tobillo	cheville	caviglia
cavidad	cavité	cavità
cavidad amniótica	cavité amniotique	cavità amniotica
ceguera	cécité	cecità
daltonismo, ceguera de colores	daltonisme	cecità ai colori
oncocerciasis ocular	cécité des rivières	cecità fluviale
cefalea por tensión	céphalée due à la tension	cefalea muscolotensiva
cefálico	céphalique	cefalico
hematoma cefálico	céphalhématome	cefaloematoma
cefalometría	céphalométrie	cefalometria
celíaco	coeliaque	celiaco
célula	cellule	cellula
celulitis	cellulite	cellulite
centígrado	centigrade	centigrado
centrífugo	centrifugeur	centrifuga
centrifugar	centrifuger	centrifugare
centrífugo	centrifuge	centrifugo
centrípeto	centripète	centripeto
cerebral	cérébral	cerebrale
cerebroespinal	cérébrospinal	cerebrospinale
cerebrovascular	cérébrovasculaire	cerebrovascolare
cerumen	cérumen	cerume
otitis media exudativa crónica, tapon de oído	otite moyenne adhésive	cerume nell orecchio
cerebelo	cervelet	cervelletto
cerebro	cerveau	cervello
cervical	cervical	cervicale
cuello uterino	cou	cervice
tenia solitaria	ténia	cestode
parir	poreux	che ha avuto figli
queilosis	chéilose	cheilosi
queloide	chéloïde	cheloide
quimioprofilaxis	chimioprophylaxie	chemioprofilassi
quimiotaxis	chimiotaxie	chemiotassi
quimioterapia	chimiothérapie	chemioterapia
quimiorreceptor	chimiorécepteur	chemorecettore
quemosis	chémosis	chemosi
queratina	kératine	cheratina
queratinización	kératinisation	cheratinizzazione
queratitis	kératite	cheratite
queratocele	kératocèle	cheratocele
queratoconjuntivitis	kératoconjonctivite	cheratocongiuntivite
queratomalacia	kératomalacie	cheratomalacia

cheratomo	keratome	Keratotom
cheratosi	keratosis	Keratose
chetoacidosi	ketoacidosis	Ketoazidose
chetogenesi	ketogenesis	Ketogenese
chetoni	ketone	Keton, Ketonkörper
chetonuria	ketonuria	Ketonurie
chetosi	ketosis	Ketose
chiasma	chiasma	Chiasma
chilo	chyle	Chylus
chinasi	kinase	Kinase
chiodo per estensione di Steinmann	Steinmann's pin	Steinmann Knochennagel
chiropodia	chiropody	Pediküre, Fußpflege
chiropratica	chiropractic	Chiropraktik
chiropratico	chiropractor	Chiropraktiker
chirurgia	surgery	Chirurgie
chirurgo	surgeon	Chirurg
cianosi	cyanosis	Zyanose
cibo contenente additivi chimici	junk food	ungesunde Nahrung
cicatrice	scar	Narbe
cicatrizzazione	healing	Heilung
ciclo	cycle	Zyklus
ciecostomia	caecostomy (Eng), cecostomy (Am)	Zökostomie
cifolordosi	kypholordosis	Kypholordose
cifoscoliosi	kyphoscoliosis	Kyphoskoliose
cifosi	kyphosis	Kyphose
ciglia	cilia	Zilien, Wimpern
ciglio	lash	Wimper
ciliare	ciliary	ziliar, Wimpern-
cilindrasse	axon	Axon
cingolo pelvico	pelvic girdle	Beckengürtel
cingolo scapolare	shoulder girdle	Schultergürtel
cintura	girdle	Gürtel
circinato	circinate	kreisförmig
circolazione	circulation	Kreislauf, Zirkulation, Durchblutung
circolazione collaterale	collateral circulation	Kollateralkreislauf
circolazione fetale	fetal circulation	fetaler Kreislauf
circolazione portale	portal circulation	Portalkreislauf, Pfortaderkreislauf
circolazione sistemica	systemic circulation	Großer Kreislauf
circoncisione	circumcision	Zirkumzision, Beschneidung
circumorale	circumoral	zirkumoral
cirrosi	cirrhosis	Zirrhose
cistectomia	cystectomy	Zystektomie, Zystenentfernung
cisti	cyst	Zyste
cisti cioccolato (c. emosiderinica dell'endometriosi)	chocolate cyst	Schokoladenzyste, Teerzyste
cistifellea	gall bladder	Gallenblase
cisti idatidea	hydatid	Hydatide

SPANISH	FRENCH	ITALIAN
queratoma	kératome	**cheratomo**
queratosis	kératose	**cheratosi**
cetoacidosis	céto-acidose	**chetoacidosi**
cetogénesis	cétogenèse	**chetogenesi**
acetona	cétone	**chetoni**
cetonuria	cétonurie	**chetonuria**
cetosis	cétose	**chetosi**
quiasma	chiasma	**chiasma**
quilo	chyle	**chilo**
cinasa	kinase	**chinasi**
clavo de Steinmann	broche de Steinmann	**chiodo per estensione di Steinmann**
podología	chiropodie	**chiropodia**
quiropráctica	chiropractique	**chiropratica**
quiropractor	chiropracteur	**chiropratico**
cirugía	chirurgie	**chirurgia**
cirujano	chirurgien	**chirurgo**
cianosis	cyanose	**cianosi**
comidas preparadas poco nutritivas	aliments non nutritifs	**cibo contenente additivi chimici**
cicatriz	cicatrice	**cicatrice**
curación	curatif	**cicatrizzazione**
ciclo	cycle	**ciclo**
cecostomía	caecostomie	**ciecostomia**
cifolordosis	cypholordose	**cifolordosi**
cifoscoliosis	cyphoscoliose	**cifoscoliosi**
cifosis	cyphose	**cifosi**
cilios	cils	**ciglia**
pestaña	mèche, lanière	**ciglio**
ciliar	ciliaire	**ciliare**
axón	axone	**cilindrasse**
cintura pélvica	ceinture pelvienne	**cingolo pelvico**
cintura escapular	ceinture scapulaire	**cingolo scapolare**
cintura	ceinture	**cintura**
circinado	circinal	**circinato**
circulación	circulation	**circolazione**
circulación colateral	circulation collatérale	**circolazione collaterale**
circulación fetal	circulation foetale	**circolazione fetale**
circulación portal	hypertension porte	**circolazione portale**
circulación sistémica	circulation systémique	**circolazione sistemica**
circuncisión	circoncision	**circoncisione**
circumoral, peroral	péribuccal	**circumorale**
cirrosis	cirrhose	**cirrosi**
quistectomía	cystectomie	**cistectomia**
quiste	kyste	**cisti**
quiste de chocolate	kyste chocolat	**cisti cioccolato (c. emosiderinica dell'endometriosi)**
vesícula biliar	vésicule biliaire	**cistifellea**
quiste hidatídico	kyste hydatique	**cisti idatidea**

cistite	cystitis	Zystitis, Blasenentzündung
cistocele	cystocele	Zystozele
cistometria	cystometry	Zystometrie, Blasendruckmessung
cistopessia	cystopexy	Zystopexie
cistoscopia	cystoscopy	Zystoskopie, Blasenspiegelung
cistoscopio	cystoscope	Zystoskop, Blasenspiegel
citologia	cytology	Zytologie
citomegalovirus	cytomegalovirus (CMV)	Zytomegalie-Virus (CMV)
citotossico	cytotoxic	zytotoxisch, zellschädigend
claudicazione	claudication	Hinken, Claudicatio
claustrofobia	claustrophobia	Klaustrophobie
clavicola	clavicle	Schlüsselbein
climaterio	climacteric	Klimakterium, Wechseljahre
clinico	clinical	klinisch
clisma opaco	barium enema	Bariumeinlauf
clistere	enema	Klistier, Einlauf
clitoride	clitoris	Klitoris
cloasma	chloasma, liver spot	Chloasma, Hyperpigmentierung, Leberfleck
clone	clone	Klonus
clono	clonus	Klonus
coagulare	clot	gerinnen, koagulieren
coagulazione del sangue	blood coagulation	Blutgerinnung
coagulazione ematica	blood clotting	Blutgerinnung
coagulazione intravascolare disseminata (CID)	disseminated intravascular coagulation (DIC)	disseminierte intravasale Gerinnung (DIC)
coagulo	clot	Blutgerinnsel, Koagel
coartazione	coarctation	Coarctatio
coccige	coccyx	Steißbein
coclea	cochlea	Cochlea, Schnecke
cognizione	cognition	Erkennungsvermögen, Wahrnehmung
coilonichia	koilonychia	Koilonychie, Löffelnagel
coito	coitus, intercourse, pareunia, sexual intercourse	Koitus, Geschlechtsverkehr
colangiografia	cholangiography	Cholangiographie
colangio-pancreatografia retrograda endoscopica (ERCP)	endoscopic retrograde cholangiopancreatography (ERCP)	endoskopische retrograde Cholangiopankreatographie (ERCP)
colangite	cholangitis	Cholangitis
colecistectomia	cholecystectomy	Cholezystektomie
colecistite	cholecystitis	Cholezystitis
colecistografia	cholecystography	Cholezystographie
colectomia	colectomy	Kolektomie, Kolonresektion
coledocografia	choledochography	Choledochographie
coledocolitiasi	choledocholithiasis	Choledocholithiasis
colelitiasi	cholelithiasis	Cholelithiasis, Gallensteinleiden
colera	cholera	Cholera
colestasi	cholestasis	Cholestase, Gallenstauung
colesteatoma	cholesteatoma	Cholesteatom

cistitis	cystite	cistite
cistocele	cystocèle	cistocele
cistometría	cystométrie	cistometria
cistopexia	cystopexie	cistopessia
citoscopía	cystoscopie	cistoscopia
citoscopio	cystoscope	cistoscopio
citología	cytologie	citologia
citomegalovirus	cytomégalovirus	citomegalovirus
citotóxico	cytotoxique	citotossico
claudicación	claudication	claudicazione
claustrofobia	claustrophobie	claustrofobia
clavícula	clavicule	clavicola
climatérico	climatérique	climaterio
clínico	clinique	clinico
enema de bario	lavement au baryte	clisma opaco
enema	lavement	clistere
clítoris	clitoris	clitoride
cloasma	chloasma, tache hépatique	cloasma
clono	clone	clone
clono, clonus	clonus	clono
coagular	coaguler	coagulare
coagulación de la sangre	coagulation sanguine	coagulazione del sangue
coagulación de la sangre	coagulation du sang	coagulazione ematica
coagulación intravascular diseminada (CID)	coagulation intravasculaire disséminée (CID)	coagulazione intravascolare disseminata (CID)
coágulo	caillot	coagulo
coartación	coarctation	coartazione
cóccix	coccyx	coccige
cóclea	limaçon osseux	coclea
cognición	cognition	cognizione
coiloniquia	koïlonychie	coilonichia
coito, pareunia	coït, rapports, rapports sexuels	coito
colangiografía	cholangiographie	colangiografia
colangiopancreatografía endoscópica retrógrada	cholangio-pancréatographie rétrograde endoscopique (CPRE)	colangio-pancreatografia retrograda endoscopica (ERCP)
colangitis	cholangite	colangite
colecistectomía	cholécystectomie	colecistectomia
colecistitis	cholécystite	colecistite
colecistografía	cholécystographie	colecistografia
colectomía	colectomie	colectomia
coledocografía	cholédochographie	coledocografia
coledocolitiasis	cholédocholithiase	coledocolitiasi
colelitiasis	cholélithiase	colelitiasi
cólera	choléra	colera
colestasis	cholestase	colestasi
colesteatoma	cholestéatome	colesteatoma

ITALIAN	ENGLISH	GERMAN
colesterolo	cholesterol (chol)	Cholesterin
colesterolo legato a lipoproteina ad alta densità	high density lipoprotein cholesterol (HDLC)	high density lipoprotein-cholesterol (HDL-Cholesterol)
colica	colic	Kolik
colica addominale	gripe	Kolik, Bauchschmerzen
coliforme	coliform	coliform
colinergico	cholinergic	cholinergisch
colite	colitis	Kolitis
collageno	collagen	Kollagen
collassarsi	collapse	kollabieren
collasso	collapse	Kollaps
collasso da colpo di calore	heat exhaustion	Hitzschlag
collo	neck	Nacken, Hals
colloide	colloid	Kolloid
coloboma	coloboma	Kolobom
colon	colon	Kolon
colon ascendente	ascending colon	Colon ascendens
colon discendente	descending colon	Colon descendens
colonizzare	colonize	kolonisieren
colonna vertebrale	axis, vertebral column	Achse, Wirbelsäule, Rückgrat
colonne di eritrociti	rouleaux	Geldrollenagglutination
colonscopia	colonoscopy	Koloskopie
colon trasverso	transverse colon	Colon transversum
colorazione di Gram	Gram stain	Gramfärbung
colorettale	colorectal	kolorektal
colostomia	colostomy	Kolostomie
colostro	colostrum	Kolostrum, Vormilch
colpo apoplettico	stroke	Schlag, Schlaganfall
colpo di calore	heatstroke	Hitzschlag
colpo di frusta	whiplash	Peitschenhiebsyndrom, Mediansyndrom
colpo di sole	sunstroke	Sonnenstich
colporrafia	colporrhaphy	Kolporrhaphie
colposcopio	colposcope	Kolposkop
coltura	culture	Bakterienkultur, Kultur
coma	coma	Koma
comatoso	comatose	komatös
commessura	commissure	Kommissur
commozione	concussion	Erschütterung, Commotio
compasso per pelvi-craniometria	caliper	Schiene
compatibilità	compatibility	Kompatibilität, Verträglichkeit
compenso	compensation	Kompensation, Entschädigung
complemento	complement	Komplement
complesso AIDS-correlato	AIDS-related complex	AIDS-related complex
complesso di Ghon	primary complex	Primärkomplex
complesso primario	primary complex	Primärkomplex
comportamento	behavior (Am), behaviour (Eng)	Verhalten
composto	compound	Verbindung, Zusammensetzung

colesterol	cholestérol	colesterolo
colesterol unido a las lipoproteínas de alta densidad (HDLC)	cholestérol composé de lipoprotéines de haut	colesterolo legato a lipoproteina ad alta densità
cólico	colique	colica
cólico intestinal	colique	colica addominale
coliforme	coliforme	coliforme
colinérgico	cholinergique	colinergico
colitis	colite	colite
colágeno	collagène	collageno
colapsar	s'affaisser	collassarsi
colapso	affaissement	collasso
agotamiento por calor	échauffement	collasso da colpo di calore
cuello	cou	collo
coloide	colloïde	colloide
coloboma	colobome, coloboma	coloboma
colon	côlon	colon
colon ascendente	côlon ascendant	colon ascendente
colon descendente	côlon descendant	colon discendente
colonizar	coloniser	colonizzare
eje, columna vertebral	axe, colonne vertébrale	colonna vertebrale
rollos	rouleaux	colonne di eritrociti
colonoscopia	coloscopie	colonscopia
cólon transverso	côlon transversal	colon trasverso
tinción de Gram	coloration de Gram	colorazione di Gram
colorrectal	colorectal	colorettale
colostomía	colostomie	colostomia
calostro	colostrum	colostro
ictus	apoplexie	colpo apoplettico
insolación	coup de chaleur	colpo di calore
latigazo	coup de fouet	colpo di frusta
insolación	insolation	colpo di sole
colporrafia	colporraphie	colporrafia
colposcopio	colposcope	colposcopio
cultivo	culture	coltura
coma	coma	coma
comatoso	comateux	comatoso
comisura	commissure	commessura
concusión, contusión violenta	commotion	commozione
compás, calibrador	armature orthopédique	compasso per pelvi-craniometria
compatibilidad	compatibilité	compatibilità
compensación	compensation	compenso
complemento	complément	complemento
complejo relacionado con SIDA	para-SIDA	complesso AIDS-correlato
complejo primario	complexe primaire	complesso di Ghon
complejo primario	complexe primaire	complesso primario
comportamiento	comportement	comportamento
compuesto	composé	composto

ITALIAN	ENGLISH	GERMAN
compressa	tablet	Tablette
compressa enterica rivestita (passano lo stomaco senza sciogliersi)	enteric-coated tablet (ECT)	magensaftresistente Tablette
compressione	compression	Kompression
compressione digitale	digital compression	Fingerdruck
compresso	impacted	impaktiert
compulsione	compulsion	Zwang
conati di vomito	retching	Würgen, Brechreiz
concepimento	conception	Empfängnis
concrezione tofacea	tophus	Tophus, Gichtknoten
condrite	chondritis	Chondritis
condroma	chondroma	Chondrom
condromalacia	chondromalacia	Chondromalazie
confusione	confusion	Verwirrung
congelamento	frostbite	Erfrierung
congenito	congenital	angeboren
congestione	congestion, engorgement	Stauung, Anschoppung
congiuntiva	conjunctiva	Konjunktiva, Bindehaut
congiuntivite	conjunctivitis	Konjunktivitis, Bindehautentzündung
congiuntivite batterica acuta contagiosa	pinkeye	epidemische Konjunktivitis
congiuntivite catarrale	pinkeye	epidemische Konjunktivitis
congiuntivite tracomatosa	trachoma inclusion conjunctivitis (TRIC)	Trachom, Einschluß(körperchen)konjunktivitis
coniugata	conjugate	Beckendurchmesser
coniugato	conjugate	konjugiert
conscio	conscious	bewußt, bei Bewußtsein
consulenza eugenetica	counselling	Beratung
consunzione	consumption	Konsum, Verbrauch
contagioso	contagious	kontagiös, ansteckend
contatto	contact	Kontakt, Berührung
conteggio dei globuli bianchi (CGB, WBC)	white blood cell count (WBC)	weißes Blutbild
conteggio dei globuli rossi (CGR)	red blood cell count (RBC)	rotes Blutbild
contraccettivo orale estro-progestinico	combined oral contraceptive	orales Kontrazeptivum (Kombinationspräparat)
contraccolpo	contrecoup	contre coup
contrattura	contracture	Kontraktur
contravveleno	antivenin	Schlangenserum
contrazione	contraction	Kontraktion
contrazioni uterine post partum	afterpains	Nachwehen
controindicazione	contraindication	Kontraindikation, Gegenanzeige
controlaterale	contralateral	kontralateral
controllo delle nascite	family planning	Familienplanung
contusione	bruise	Quetschung, Prellung
convulsione	fit, seizure, convulsion	Anfall, Krampf, Zuckung, Konvulsion
corda	cord	Strang, Schnur, Ligament

SPANISH	FRENCH	ITALIAN
comprimido	comprimé	compressa
comprimido entérico	dragée entérosoluble, comprimé à délitement entérique	compressa enterica rivestita (passano lo stomaco senza sciogliersi)
compresión	compression	compressione
compresión digital	compression digitale	compressione digitale
impactado	enclavé	compresso
compulsión, apremio	compulsion	compulsione
arcadas	haut-le-coeur	conati di vomito
concepción	conception	concepimento
tofo	tophus	concrezione tofacea
condritis	chondrite	condrite
condroma	chondrome	condroma
condromalacia	chondromalacie	condromalacia
confusión	confusion	confusione
congelación, sabañón	gelure	congelamento
congénito	congénital	congenito
congestión, estancamiento	congestion, engorgement	congestione
conjuntiva	conjonctive	congiuntiva
conjuntivitis	conjonctivite	congiuntivite
conjuntivitis	conjonctivite aiguë contagieuse	congiuntivite batterica acuta contagiosa
conjuntivitis	conjonctivite aiguë contagieuse	congiuntivite catarrale
conjuntivitis de inclusion por tracomas	conjonctivite à inclusions trachomateuses	congiuntivite tracomatosa
conjugado	diamètre conjugué	coniugata
conjugado	conjugué	coniugato
consciente	conscient	conscio
asesoramiento, consejo, consulta psicológica	consultation	consulenza eugenetica
consunción, tisis	consommation	consunzione
contagioso, trasmisible	contagieux	contagioso
contacto	contact	contatto
recuento de leucocitos	nombre de globules blancs (NGB)	conteggio dei globuli bianchi (CGB, WBC)
recuento de glóbulos rojos	numération érythrocytaire	conteggio dei globuli rossi (CGR)
anticonceptivo oral combinado	contraceptif oral combiné	contraccettivo orale estro-progestinico
contragolpe	contrecoup	contraccolpo
contractura	contracture	contrattura
antídoto	sérum antivenimeux	contravveleno
contracción	contraction	contrazione
entuertos	tranchées utérines	contrazioni uterine post partum
contraindicación	contre-indication	controindicazione
contralateral	controlatéral	controlaterale
planificación familiar	contrôle des naissances	controllo delle nascite
contusión, equímosis	contusion	contusione
ataque, acceso, convulsión	attaque, accès, convulsion	convulsione
cordón, cuerda, médula espinal	cordon	corda

ITALIAN	ENGLISH	GERMAN
corda vocale	vocal cord	Stimmband
cordone	cord	Strang, Schnur, Ligament
cordone ombelicale	umbilical cord	Nabelschnur
cordotomia	cordotomy	Stimmbandresektion
corea	chorea	Chorea, Veitstanz
corea di Huntington	Huntington's chorea	Chorea Huntington
corion	chorion	Chorion
coriza	coryza	Koryza, Schnupfen
cornea	cornea	Kornea, Hornhaut (des Auges)
coroide	choroid	Choroidea, Aderhaut
coroidite	choroiditis	Choroiditis
coronaria	coronary	Koronararterie
coronarico	coronary	koronar
corpi di Leishman-Donovan	Leishman-Donovan body	Leishman-Donovan-Körper
corpo	corpus	Corpus
corpo vitreo	vitreous body	Glaskörper
corpuscoli vitreali sospesi visibili	floaters	Mouches volantes
corpuscolo	corpuscle	Corpusculum
correzione di una deformità	orthosis	Orthose
corteccia	cortex	Cortex, Rinde
corticosteroide	corticosteroid	Kortikosteroide
costa	rib	Rippe
costale	costal	kostal, Rippen-
costocondrale	costochondral	Rippenknorpel-
costocondrite	costochondritis	Tietze Syndrom
costrizione	constriction	Konstriktion, Einengung
crampo	cramp	Krampf
cranio	cranium, skull	Schädel, Kranium
craniosinostosi	cranio-synostosis	Kraniosynostose
craurosi vulvare	kraurosis vulvae	Craurosis vulvae
creatina	creatine	Kreatin
creatinina	creatinine	Kreatinin
crepitazione	crepitation	Krepitation, Rasseln
crescita	growth	Wachstum, Zunahme, Geschwulst, Tumor
cretinismo	cretinism	Kretinismus
cricoide	cricoid	krikoid
criochirurgia	cryosurgery	Kryochirurgie
crioterapia	cryotherapy	Kryotherapie
cripta	crypt	Krypte
criptogenico	cryptogenic	kryptogenetisch, unbekannten Ursprungs
criptomenorrea	cryptomenorrhea (Am), cryptomenorrhoea (Eng)	Kryptomenorrhoe
crisi	crisis	Krise
crisi miastenica	myasthenic crisis	myasthenische Krise
crisi tireotossica	thyrotoxic crisis	thyreotoxische Krise
crisi vagale	vasovagal attack	vasovagale Synkope

SPANISH	FRENCH	ITALIAN
cuerda vocal	corde vocale	corda vocale
cordón, cuerda, médula espinal	cordon	cordone
cordón umbilical	cordon ombilical	cordone ombelicale
cordotomía	cordotomie	cordotomia
corea	chorée	corea
corea de Huntington	chorée de Huntington	corea di Huntington
corion	chorion	corion
coriza	coryza	coriza
córnea	cornée	cornea
coroides	choroïde	coroide
coroiditis	choroïdite	coroidite
coronario	coronaire	coronaria
coronario	coronaire, coronarien	coronarico
cuerpo de Leishman-Donovan	Leishmania donovani	corpi di Leishman-Donovan
cuerpo	corps	corpo
vítreo	vitré	corpo vitreo
flotadores	flottants	corpuscoli vitreali sospesi visibili
corpúsculo	corpuscule	corpuscolo
ortosis	orthèse	correzione di una deformità
corteza	cortex	corteccia
corticosteroide	corticostéroïde	corticosteroide
costilla	côte	costa
costal	costal	costale
costocondral	costochondral	costocondrale
costocondritis	costochondrite	costocondrite
constricción	constriction	costrizione
calambre, espasmo	crampe	crampo
cráneo	boîte crânienne, crâne	cranio
craneosinostosis	craniosynostose	craniosinostosi
craurosis vulvar	kraurosis de la vulve	craurosi vulvare
creatina	créatine	creatina
creatinina	créatinine	creatinina
crepitación	crépitation	crepitazione
crecimiento	croissance	crescita
cretinismo	crétinisme	cretinismo
cricoideo	cricoïde	cricoide
criocirugía	cryochirurgie	criochirurgia
crioterapia	cryothérapie	crioterapia
cripta	crypte	cripta
criptogénico	cryptogène	criptogenico
criptomenorrea	cryptoménorrhée	criptomenorrea
crisis	crise	crisi
crisis miasténica	crise myasthénique	crisi miastenica
crisis tirotóxica	crise thyrotoxique	crisi tireotossica
ataque vasovagal	malaise vasovagal	crisi vagale

ITALIAN	ENGLISH	GERMAN
crollare	collapse	kollabieren
cromatografia	chromatography	Chromatographie
cromosoma	chromosome	Chromosom
cronico	chronic	chronisch
crosta	slough, scab	Schorf, Kruste
crusca	bran	Kleie
cucchiaio chirurgico	curette (Eng), curet (Am)	Kürette
cucire	suture	nähen
cuoio capelluto	scalp	Kopfhaut
cuore	heart	Herz
cuore polmonare	cor pulmonale	Cor pulmonale
cura terminale	terminal care	Pflege Sterbender
curettage	curettage, curetting	Kürettage, Ausschabung
curette	curette (Eng), curet (Am)	Kürette
cutaneo	cutaneous	kutan, Haut-
cuticola	cuticle	Cuticula, Häutchen

SPANISH	FRENCH	ITALIAN
colapsar	s'affaisser	crollare
cromatografía	chromatographie	cromatografia
cromosoma	chromosome	cromosoma
crónico	chronique	cronico
esfacelo, costra	escarre, croûte	crosta
salvado	son	crusca
cureta, cucharilla de legrado	curette	cucchiaio chirurgico
suturar	suturer	cucire
cuero cabelludo	épicrâne	cuoio capelluto
corazón	coeur	cuore
cor pulmonale	coeur pulmonaire	cuore polmonare
cuidados terminales	soins pour malades en phase terminale	cura terminale
raspado, legrado, curetaje, material de legrado	curetage, curetages	curettage
cureta, cucharilla de legrado	curette	curette
cutáneo	cutané	cutaneo
cutícula	cuticule	cuticola

D

Italian	English	German
dacriocistite	dacryocystitis	Dakryozystitis
data del concepimento	date of conception (DOC)	Empfängnisdatum
data di nascita	date of birth (DOB)	Geburtsdatum
data presunta delle doglie	expected date of confinement (EDC)	errechneter Geburtstermin
data prevista per il parto	expected date of delivery (EDD)	errechneter Geburtstermin
debilità	debility	Schwäche
debolezza	weakness	Schwäche
deceduto all'arrivo in ospedale	dead on arrival (DOA)	tot bei Einlieferung
decerebrato	decerebrate	dezerebriert
decidua	decidua	Dezidua
decompensazione	decompensation	Dekompensation, Insuffizienz
decompressione	decompression	Dekompression, Drucksenkung
decondizionamento	aversion therapy	Aversionstherapie
decongestionante	decongestant	Dekongestionsmittel
defecazione	defaecation (Eng), defecation (Am)	Defäkation, Darmentleerung
defibrillatore	defibrillator	Defibrillator
defibrillazione	defibrillation	Defibrillierung
degenerazione	degeneration	Degeneration, Verfall
degenerazione del cilindrasse	axonotmesis	Axonotmesis
degenerazione grassa	fatty degeneration	fettige Degeneration, Verfettung
deidratazione	dehydration	Dehydration, Flüssigkeitsmangel
deiscenza	dehiscence	Dehiszenz, Schlitz
delirio	delirium	Delirium, Fieberwahn
del piede	pedal	Fuß-
deltoide	deltoid	Deltoides, Deltamuskel
demarcazione	demarcation	Demarkation
demenza	dementia	Demenz
demenza presenile	presenile dementia	präsenile Demenz
demielinizzazione	demyelination	Demyelinisierung, Entmarkung
demografia	demography	Demographie
denervazione	denervation	Denervierung
dengue	dengue	Denguefieber
dentario	odontic	Odonto-, Zahn-
dente	tooth	Zahn
dente del giudizio	wisdom tooth	Weisheitszahn
denti	teeth	Zähne, Gebiß
dentiera	denture	Gebiß
dentista	dentist	Zahnarzt
dentizione	dentition	Dentition, Zahnung
deodorante (n)	deodorant (n)	Deodorant (n)
deodorante (a)	deodorant (a)	desodorierend (a)
deossigenazione	deoxygenation	Desoxydation, Sauerstoffentzug
depressione	depression	Depression
depressione agitata	agitated depression	agitierte Depression

SPANISH	FRENCH	ITALIAN
dacriocistitis	dacryocystite	dacriocistite
fecha de concepción	date du rapport fécondant	data del concepimento
fecha de nacimiento	date de naissance	data di nascita
fecha esperada del parto	date présumée de l'accouchement	data presunta delle doglie
fecha probable del parto (FPP)	date présumée de l'accouchement	data prevista per il parto
debilidad	débilité	debilità
debilidad	faiblesse	debolezza
muerto al llegar	mort à l'arrivée	deceduto all'arrivo in ospedale
descerebrado	décérébré	decerebrato
decidua	caduque	decidua
descompensación	décompensation	decompensazione
descompresión	décompression	decompressione
tratamiento por aversión	cure de dégoût	decondizionamento
descongestivo	décongestionnant	decongestionante
defecación	défécation	defecazione
desfibrilador	défibrillateur	defibrillatore
desfibrilación	défibrillation	defibrillazione
degeneración	dégénération	degenerazione
axonotmesis	axonotmésis	degenerazione del cilindrasse
degeneración grasa	dégénérescence graisseuse	degenerazione grassa
deshidratación	déshydratation	deidratazione
dehiscencia	déhiscence	deiscenza
delirio	délire	delirio
pedal	pédieux	del piede
deltoides	deltoïde	deltoide
demarcación	démarcation	demarcazione
demencia	démence	demenza
demencia presenil	démence présénile	demenza presenile
desmielinización	démyélinisation	demielinizzazione
demografía	démographie	demografia
denervación	énervation	denervazione
dengue	dengue	dengue
dentario	dentaire	dentario
diente	dent	dente
muela del juicio	dent de sagesse	dente del giudizio
dientes	dents	denti
dentadura	dentier	dentiera
dentista	dentiste	dentista
dentición	dentition	dentizione
desodorante (n)	déodorant (n)	deodorante (n)
desodorante (a)	déodorant (a)	deodorante (a)
desoxigenación	désoxygénation	deossigenazione
depresión	dépression	depressione
depresión agitada	dépression anxieuse	depressione agitata

659

ITALIAN	ENGLISH	GERMAN
depressioni puntiformi	pitting	Dellenbildung
derealizzazione	derealization	Derealisation
derivazione	shunt	Shunt
derma	dermis	Haut
dermatite	dermatitis	Dermatitis
dermatite seborroica	seborrheic dermatitis (Am), seborrhoeic dermatitis (Eng)	seborrhoisches Ekzem
dermatologia	dermatology	Dermatologie
dermatologo	dermatologist	Dermatologe
dermatomiosite	dermatomyositis	Dermatomyositis
dermatomo	dermatome	Dermatom, Hautmesser
dermatosi	dermatosis	Dermatose, Hauterkrankung
dermoide	dermoid	Dermoid, Dermoidzyste
desensibilizzazione	desensitization	Desensibilisierung
desiderio sessuale	libido	Libido
desquamazione	desquamation peeling	Desquamation, Schuppung Schälen (Haut), Schuppung
destrocardia	dextrocardia	Dextrokardie
detergente	detergent	Reinigungsmittel
deterioramento	deterioration	Verschlechterung
diabete	diabetes	Diabetes
diabete insipido	diabetes insipidus	Diabetes insipidus
diabete mellito	diabetes mellitus (DM)	Diabetes mellitus, Zuckerkrankheit
diabete mellito insulinodipendente	insulin dependent diabetes mellitus (IDDM)	insulinabhängiger Diabetes mellitus
diabete mellito non insulinodipendente	non-insulin dependent diabetes mellitus (NIDDM)	Diabetes mellitus Typ II, non-insulin dependent diabetes mellitus (NIDDM)
diafisi	diaphysis	Diaphyse, Knochenschaft
diaforesi	diaphoresis	Diaphorese, Schweißabsonderung
diaframma	diaphragm, midriff	Diaphragma, Zwerchfell
diagnosi	diagnosis	Diagnose
diagnosi differenziale	differential diagnosis	Differentialdiagnose
diagnostico	diagnostic	diagnostisch
dialisato	dialysate	Dialysat
dialisi	dialysis	Dialyse
dialisi peritoneale	peritoneal dialysis	Peritonealdialyse
dializzatore	dialyser (Eng), dialyzer (Am)	Dialysator
diarrea	diarrhea (Am), diarrhoea (Eng)	Diarrhoe, Durchfall
diarrea e vomito	diarrhea and vomiting (D & V) (Am), diarrhoea and vomiting (D & V) (Eng)	Brechdurchfall
diastasi	diastasis	Diastase
diastole	diastole	Diastole
diatermia	diathermy	Diathermie
dieta	diet, regimen	Ernährung, Diät
dieta chetogenica	ketogenic diet	ketogene Ernährung
dietetica	dietetics	Diätlehre, Ernährungskunde
dietista	dietitian	Diätspezialist

SPANISH	FRENCH	ITALIAN
cavitación	formation de godet	depressioni puntiformi
desrealización	déréalisation	derealizzazione
derivación	dérivation	derivazione
dermis	derme	derma
dermatitis	dermatite	dermatite
dermatitis seborréica	eczéma	dermatite seborroica
dermatología	dermatologie	dermatologia
dermatólogo	dermatologue	dermatologo
dermatomiositis	dermatomyosite	dermatomiosite
dermátomo	dermatome	dermatomo
dermatosis	dermatose	dermatosi
dermoide	dermoïde	dermoide
desensibilización	désensibilisation	desensibilizzazione
líbido	libido	desiderio sessuale
desescamación exfoliación	desquamation	desquamazione
dextrocardia	dextrocardie	destrocardia
detergente	détergent	detergente
deterioro	détérioration	deterioramento
diabetes	diabète	diabete
diabetes insípida	diabète insipide	diabete insipido
diabetes mellitus	diabète sucré	diabete mellito
diabetes mellitus insulinodependiente	diabète sucré insulinodépendant	diabete mellito insulinodipendente
diabetes mellitus no insulinodependiente	diabète sucré non insulinodépendant	diabete mellito non insulinodipendente
diáfisis	diaphyse	diafisi
diaforesis	diaphorèse	diaforesi
diafragma	diaphragme	diaframma
diagnóstico	diagnostic	diagnosi
diagnóstico diferencial	diagnostic différentiel	diagnosi differenziale
diagnóstico	diagnostique	diagnostico
dializado	dialysat	dialisato
diálisis	dialyse	dialisi
diálisis peritoneal	dialyse péritonéale	dialisi peritoneale
dializador	dialyseur	dializzatore
diarrea	diarrhée	diarrea
diarrea y vómitos	diarrhées et vomissements	diarrea e vomito
diastasis	diastasis	diastasi
diástole	diastole	diastole
diatermia	diathermie	diatermia
régimen	régime	dieta
dieta cetógena	régime cétogène	dieta chetogenica
dietética	diététique	dietetica
dietista	diététicien	dietista

ITALIAN	ENGLISH	GERMAN
dietologo	dietitian	Diätspezialist
difetto	defect	Defekt, Mangel, Störung
difetto atriosettale	atrial septal defect (ASD)	Vorhofseptumdefekt
difterite	diphtheria	Diphtherie
Digeneum	fluke	Trematode
digestione	digestion	Verdauung
digitale	digitalis	Digitalis, Fingerhut
digitalizzazione	digitalization	Digitalisierung
digiuno	jejunum	Jejunum
dilatazione	dilatation (Eng), dilation (Am)	Dilatation, Erweiterung
dilatazione e raschiamento	dilatation and curettage (D & C) (Eng), dilation and curettage (D & C) (Am)	Dilatation und Kürettage
diplegia	diplegia	Diplegie, doppelseitige Lähmung
diplopia	diplopia, double vision	Diplopie, Doppelsehen
disarticolazione	disarticulation	Exartikulation
disartria	dysarthria	Dysarthrie
discariosi	dyskaryosis	Kernanomalie, Dysplasie
discectomia	discectomy (Eng), diskectomy (Am)	Diskektomie
discinesia	dyskinesia	Dyskinesie
discrasia	dyscrasia	Dyskrasie
discreto	discrete	diskret
disfagia	dysphagia	Dysphagie, Schluckbeschwerden
disfasia	dysphasia	Dysphasie
disfunzione	dysfunction	Dysfunktion, Funktionsstörung
disgenesia gonadica	Turner's syndrome	Turner-Syndrom
disinfestazione	disinfestation	Entwesung, Entlausung
disinfettante	disinfectant	Desinfektionsmittel
disinfettare	disinfect	desinfizieren
disinfezione	disinfection	Desinfektion
dislessia	dyslexia	Dyslexie
dislocazione	dislocation	Dislokation, Verrenkung
dismenorrea	dysmenorrhea (Am), dysmenorrhoea (Eng)	Dysmenorrhoe
dismenorrea spastica	spasmodic dysmenorrhoea	spastische Dysmenorrhoe
disobliterazione	rebore	Desobliteration
disorientamento	disorientation	Desorientiertheit
dispareunia	dyspareunia	Dyspareunie
dispepsia	dyspepsia	Dyspepsie, Verdauungsstörung
displasia	dysplasia	Dysplasie, Fehlbildung
dispnea	dyspnea (Am), dyspnoea (Eng)	Dyspnoe, Atemnot
dispositivo anticoncezionale intrauterino (IUD)	intrauterine contraceptive device (IUD, IUCD)	Intrauterinpessar (IUP)
disprassia	dyspraxia	Dyspraxie
disritmia	dysrhythmia	Dysrhythmie, Rhythmusstörung
disseminato	disseminated	disseminiert, verstreut
dissenteria	dysentery	Dysenterie, Ruhr
dissezione	dissection	Sektion, Obduktion
dissociare i tessuti	tease	zupfen

SPANISH	FRENCH	ITALIAN
dietista	diététicien	dietologo
defecto	anomalie, défaut	difetto
defecto del septum auricular	communication auriculaire	difetto atriosettale
difteria	diphtérie	difterite
trematodo	douve	Digeneum
digestión	digestion	digestione
digital	digitale	digitale
digitalización	digitalisation	digitalizzazione
yeyuno	jéjunum	digiuno
dilatación	dilatation	dilatazione
dilatación y raspado/legrado	dilatation et curetage	dilatazione e raschiamento
diplejía, parálisis bilateral	diplégie	diplegia
diplopia, visión doble	diplopie, double vision	diplopia
desarticulación	désarticulation	disarticolazione
disartria	dysarthrie	disartria
discariosis	dyskaryose	discariosi
disquectomía	discectomie	discectomia
discinesia	dyskinésie	discinesia
discrasia	dyscrasie	discrasia
discreto	discret	discreto
disfagia	dysphagie	disfagia
disfasia	dysphasie	disfasia
disfunción	dysfonctionnement	disfunzione
síndrome de Turner	syndrome de Turner	disgenesia gonadica
desinfestación	désinfestation	disinfestazione
desinfectante	désinfectant	disinfettante
desinfectar	désinfecter	disinfettare
desinfección	désinfection	disinfezione
dislexia	dyslexie	dislessia
dislocación	dislocation	dislocazione
dismenorrea	dysménorrhée	dismenorrea
dismenorrea espasmódica	dysménorrhée spasmodique	dismenorrea spastica
desobliteración, repermeabilización	désobstruction	disobliterazione
desorientación	désorientation	disorientamento
dispareunia	dyspareunie	dispareunia
dispepsia	dyspepsie	dispepsia
displasia	dysplasie	displasia
disnea	dyspnée	dispnea
dispositivo intrauterino anticonceptivo (DIU)	dispositif intra-utérin (DIU), stérilet	dispositivo anticoncezionale intrauterino (IUD)
dispraxia	dyspraxie	disprassia
disritmia	dysrythmie	disritmia
diseminado	disséminé	disseminato
disentería	dysenterie	dissenteria
disección	dissection	dissezione
separar con aguja	défilocher	dissociare i tessuti

ITALIAN	ENGLISH	GERMAN
dissociazione	dissociation	Dissoziation, Trennung
distacco di retina	detached retina	abgelöste Netzhaut
distacco epifisario	slipped epiphysis	Epiphyseolyse
distacco prematuro della placenta	placental abruption	Plazentaablösung
distale	distal	distal
distorcere	sprain	verstauchen
distorsione	sprain	Verstauchung
distrofia	dystrophy	Dystrophie
distrofia muscolare	muscular dystrophy	Muskeldystrophie
disturbo funzionale	functional disorder	funktionelle Störung
disuria	dysuria	Dysurie
dita a clava	clubbing	Trommelschlegelfinger
dito	finger	Finger
dito a scatto	trigger finger	schnellender Finger
dito del piede	toe	Zehe
diuresi	diuresis	Diurese
diuretico (n)	diuretic (n)	Diuretikum (n)
diuretico (a)	diuretic (a)	diuretisch (a)
divaricatore	retractor	Wundhaken, Spreizer, Retraktor
diverticolite	diverticulitis	Divertikulitis
diverticolo	diverticulum	Divertikel
diverticolo di Meckel	Meckel's diverticulum	Meckel-Divertikel
diverticolosi	diverticulosis	Divertikulose
dolente	sore	wund, schmerzhaft
dolore	dolor, pain	Schmerz
dolore acuto	sting	Stachel, Stich
dolore intermestruale	mittelschmerz	Mittelschmerz
dolore riferito	referred pain	ausstrahlender Schmerz, fortgeleiteter Schmerz
dominante	dominant	dominant, vorherrschend
donatore	donor	Spender
dopammina	dopamine	Dopamin
dorsale	dorsal	dorsal, Rücken-
dorsiflessione	dorsiflexion	Dorsalflexion
dorso del piede	instep	Fußrücken, Spann
dosaggio immunologico	immunoassay	Immunoassay
dose giornaliera raccomandata	recommended daily allowance (RDA)	empfohlene Tagesdosis
dotto	duct	Ductus, Gang
dotto arterioso	ductus arteriosus	Ductus arteriosus
dottore	doctor	Arzt
drenaggio	drain	Drain
drenare	drain	drainieren
droga	drug	Arzneimittel, Rauschgift
duodenite	duodenitis	Duodenitis, Zwölffingerdarmentzündung
duodeno	duodenum	Duodenum, Zwölffingerdarm

SPANISH	FRENCH	ITALIAN
disociación	dissociation	dissociazione
desprendimiento de retina	rétine décollée	distacco di retina
epífisis desplazada	épiphysiolyse	distacco epifisario
desprendimiento prematuro de la placenta	rupture placentaire	distacco prematuro della placenta
distal	distal	distale
torcer	se fouler	distorcere
esguince	foulure	distorsione
distrofia	dystrophie	distrofia
distrofia muscular	dystrophie musculaire	distrofia muscolare
trastorno funcional	fonctionnel	disturbo funzionale
disuria	dysurie	disuria
dedos en palillo de tambor, dedos hipocráticos	hippocratisme digital	dita a clava
dedo de la mano	doigt	dito
dedo en gatillo	index	dito a scatto
dedo del pie	orteil	dito del piede
diuresis	diurèse	diuresi
diurético (n)	diurétique (n)	diuretico (n)
diurético (a)	diurétique (a)	diuretico (a)
retractor	rétracteur	divaricatore
diverticulitis	diverticulite	diverticolite
divertículo	diverticulum	diverticolo
divertículo de Meckel	diverticule de Meckel	diverticolo di Meckel
diverticulosis	diverticulose	diverticolosi
doloroso	douloureux	dolente
dolor	douleur	dolore
picadura	piqûre	dolore acuto
mittelschmerz	crise intermenstruelle	dolore intermestruale
dolor referido	douleur irradiée	dolore riferito
dominante	dominant	dominante
donante	donneur	donatore
dopamina	dopamine	dopammina
dorsal	dorsal	dorsale
dorsiflexión	dorsiflexion	dorsiflessione
empeine	tarse	dorso del piede
inmunoensayo	dosage immunologique, immunodosage	dosaggio immunologico
dosis diaria recomendada	taux quotidien recommandé	dose giornaliera raccomandata
conducto	conduit	dotto
ductus arteriosus	canal artériel	dotto arterioso
médico	médecin	dottore
drenaje	drain	drenaggio
drenar	drainer	drenare
fármaco	médicament	droga
duodenitis	duodénite	duodenite
duodeno	duodénum	duodeno

E

ebefrenia	hebephrenia	Hebephrenie
ecchimosi	ecchymosis	Ekchymose
eccitabilità	excitability	Reizbarkeit, Erregbarkeit
eccitazione	excitation	Reizung, Erregung
echovirus	echovirus	ECHO-Virus
eclampsia	eclampsia	Eklampsie
ecocardiografia	echocardiography	Echokardiographie
ecoencefalografia	echoencephalography	Echoenzephalographie
ecografia	scan, ultrasonography	Scan, Sonographie, Ultraschallmethode
ecolalia	echolalia	Echolalie
ectoderma	ectoderm	Ektoderm
ectoparassita	ectoparasite	Ektoparasit
ectopico	ectopic	ektop
ectropion	ectropion	Ektropion
eczema	eczema	Ekzem
edema	edema (Am), oedema (Eng)	Ödem, Flüssigkeitsansammlung
edema angioneurotico	angioneurotic edema (solidus) (Am), angioneurotic oedema (solidus) (Eng)	Quincke-Ödem
edentulo	edentulous	zahnlos
efedrina	ephedrine	Ephedrin
efferente	efferent	efferent
effetto collaterale	side effect	Nebenwirkung
effusione	effusion	Erguß
eiaculazione	ejaculation	Ejakulation, Samenerguß
elastina	elastin	Elastin
elefantiasi	elephantiasis	Elephantiasis
elettrocardiogramma (ECG)	electrocardiogram (ECG)	Elektrokardiogramm (EKG)
elettrodo	electrode	Elektrode
elettroencefalogramma (EEG)	electroencephalogram (EEG)	Elektroenzephalogramm (EEG)
elettrolisi	electrolysis	Elektrolyse
elettrolito	electrolyte	Elektrolyt
elettromiografia	electromyography	Elektromyographie
elettroshock	electroconvulsive therapy (ECT)	Elektroschocktherapie
eliminazione	elimination	Elimination, Ausscheidung
elisir	elixir	Elixier
ellissocitosi	elliptocytosis	Elliptozytose
emaciazione	emaciation	Auszehrung
emangioma	haemangioma (Eng), hemangioma (Am)	Hämangiom
emartrosi	haemarthrosis (Eng), hemarthrosis (Am)	Hämarthros
ematemesi	haematemesis (Eng), hematemesis (Am)	Hämatemesis, Bluterbrechen
ematocolpo	haematocolpos (Eng), hematocolpos (Am)	Hämatokolpos

SPANISH	FRENCH	ITALIAN
hebefrenia	hébéphrénie	ebefrenia
equímosis	ecchymose	ecchimosi
excitabilidad	excitabilité	eccitabilità
excitación	excitation	eccitazione
virus ECHO	échovirus	echovirus
eclampsia	éclampsie	eclampsia
ecocardiografía	échocardiographie	ecocardiografia
ecoencefalografía	écho-encéphalographie	ecoencefalografia
exploración, barrido, ultrasonografía, ecografía	échogramme, échographie	ecografia
ecolalia	écholalie	ecolalia
ectodermo	ectoderme	ectoderma
ectoparásito	ectoparasite	ectoparassita
ectópico	ectopique	ectopico
ectropión	ectropion	ectropion
eccema	eczéma	eczema
edema	oedème	edema
edema angioneurótico (sólido)	oedème angioneurotique	edema angioneurotico
desdentado	édenté	edentulo
efedrina	éphédrine	efedrina
eferente	efférent	efferente
efecto secundario	effet latéral	effetto collaterale
derrame	effusion	effusione
eyaculación	éjaculation	eiaculazione
elastina	élastine	elastina
elefantiasis	éléphantiasis	elefantiasi
electrocardiograma (ECG)	électrocardiogramme (ECG)	elettrocardiogramma (ECG)
electrodo	électrode	elettrodo
electroencefalograma (EEG)	électroencéphalogramme (EEG)	elettroencefalogramma (EEG)
electrólisis	électrolyse	elettrolisi
electrólito	électrolyte	elettrolito
electromiografía	électromyographie	elettromiografia
electrochoqueterapia (ECT)	électrochoc	elettroshock
eliminación	élimination	eliminazione
elixir	élixir	elisir
eliptocitosis	elliptocytose	ellissocitosi
emaciación	émaciation	emaciazione
hemangioma	hémangiome	emangioma
hemartrosis	hémarthrose	emartrosi
hematemesis	hématémèse	ematemesi
hematocolpos	hématocolpos	ematocolpo

ITALIAN	ENGLISH	GERMAN
ematologia	haematology (Eng), hematology (Am)	Hämatologie
ematoma	haematoma (Eng), hematoma (Am)	Hämatom, Bluterguß
ematopoiesi	haemopoiesis (Eng), hemopoiesis (Am)	Hämatopoese
ematrocrito	haematocrit (Eng), hematocrit (Am)	Hämatokrit (HKT)
ematuria	haematuria (Eng), hematuria (Am)	Hämaturie, Blut im Urin
embolia	embolism	Embolie
embolia polmonare (EP)	pulmonary embolism (PE)	Lungenembolie
embolico	embolic	embolisch
embolo	embolus	Embolus
embriologia	embryology	Embryologie
embrione	embryo	Embryo
embriopatia	embryopathy	Embryopathie
emeralopia	night blindness	Nachtblindheit
emesi	emesis	Erbrechen
emetico (n)	emetic (n)	Emetikum (n), Brechmittel (n)
emetico (a)	emetic (a)	emetisch (a)
emicolectomia	hemicolectomy	Hemikolektomie
emicrania	migraine	Migräne
eminenza ipotenar	hypothenar eminence	Antithenar
emiparesi	hemiparesis	Hemiparese, unvollständige Halbseitenlähmung
emiplegia	hemiplegia	Hemiplegie, Halbseitenlähmung
emocitometria	blood count	Blutbild
emocoltura	blood culture	Blutkultur
emocromatosi	haemochromatosis (Eng), hemochromatosis (Am)	Hämochromatose, Bronzediabetes
emodialisi	haemodialysis (Eng), hemodialysis (Am)	Hämodialyse
emofilia	haemophilia (Eng), hemophilia (Am)	Hämophilie, Bluterkrankheit
emoglobina (E)	haemoglobin (Hb) (Hg) (Eng), hemoglobin (Hb) (Hg) (Am)	Hämoglobin
emoglobinopatia	haemoglobinopathy (Eng), hemoglobinopathy (Am)	Hämoglobinopathie
emoglobinuria	haemoglobinuria (Eng) hemoglobinuria (Am)	Hämoglobinurie
emoliente (n)	emollient (n)	Emollientium (n)
emoliente (a)	emollient (a)	erweichend (a)
emolisi	haemolysis (Eng), hemolysis (Am)	Hämolyse
emopericardio	haemopericardium (Eng), hemopericardium (Am)	Hämatoperikard
emoperitoneo	haemoperitoneum (Eng), hemoperitoneum (Am)	Hämatoperitoneum
emopneumotorace	haemopneumothorax (Eng), hemopneumothorax (Am)	Hämatopneumothorax
emorragia	haemorrhage (Eng), hemorrhage (Am)	Hämorrhagie, Blutung

668

SPANISH	FRENCH	ITALIAN
hematología	hématologie	ematologia
hematoma	hématome	ematoma
hemopoyesis	hémopoïèse	ematopoiesi
hematócrito	hématocrite	ematrocrito
hematuria	hématurie	ematuria
embolia	embolisme	embolia
embolismo pulmonar	embolie pulmonaire (EP)	embolia polmonare (EP)
embólico	embolique	embolico
émbolo	embole	embolo
embriología	embryologie	embriologia
embrión	embryon	embrione
embriopatía	embryopathie	embriopatia
ceguera nocturna	cécité nocturne	emeralopia
emesis	vomissement	emesi
emético (n)	émétique (n)	emetico (n)
emético (a)	émétique (a)	emetico (a)
hemocolectomía	hémicolectomie	emicolectomia
migraña	migraine	emicrania
eminencia hipotenar	éminence hypothénar	eminenza ipotenar
hemiparesia	hémiparésie	emiparesi
hemiplejía	hémiplégie	emiplegia
recuento sanguíneo	dénombrement des hématies	emocitometria
hemocultivo	hémoculture	emocoltura
hemocromatosis	hémochromatose	emocromatosi
hemodiálisis	hémodialyse	emodialisi
hemofilia	hémophilie	emofilia
hemoglobina (Hb)	hémoglobine (Hb) (Hg)	emoglobina (E)
hemoglobinopatía	hémoglobinopathie	emoglobinopatia
hemoglobinuria	hémoglobinurie	emoglobinuria
emoliente (n)	émollient (n)	emoliente (n)
emoliente (a)	émollient (a)	emoliente (a)
hemólisis	hémolyse	emolisi
hemopericardio	hémopéricarde	emopericardio
hemoperitoneo	hémopéritoine	emoperitoneo
hemoneumotórax	hémopneumothorax	emopneumotorace
hemorragia	hémorragie	emorragia

ITALIAN	ENGLISH	GERMAN
emorragia subaracnoidea	subarachnoid haemorrhage (Eng), subarachnoid hemorrhage (Am)	Subarachnoidalblutung
emorroide	haemorrhoid (Eng), hemorrhoid (Am)	Hämorrhoide
emorroidectomia	haemorrhoidectomy (Eng), hemorrhoidectomy (Am)	Hämorrhoidektomie, Hämorrhoidenoperation
emorroidi	piles	Hämorrhoiden
emostasi	haemostasis (Eng), hemostasis (Am)	Hämostase, Blutgerinnung
emotivo	emotional	emotional
emotorace	haemothorax (Eng), hemothorax (Am)	Hämatothorax
emozione	emotion, affect	Emotion, Gefühl, Affekt, Erregung
empiema	empyema	Empyem
empirico	empirical	empirisch
emulsione	emulsion	Emulsion
encefalina	encephalin (Eng), enkephalin (Am)	Enzephalin
encefalite	encephalitis	Enzephalitis
encefalite spongiforme bovina	bovine spongiform encephalitis (BSE)	Rinderwahnsinn, Bovine Spongiforme Enzephalitis (BSE)
encefalomielite	encephalomyelitis	Enzephalomyelitis
encefalomielite mialgica	myalgic encephalomyelitis (ME)	myalgische Enzephalomyelitis
encefalopatia	encephalopathy	Enzephalopathie
encopresi	encopresis	Enkopresis, Einkoten
endemia	endemic	Endemie
endemico	endemic	endemisch
endoarterectomia	endarterectomy	Endarteriektomie
endoarterite	endarteritis	Endarteriitis
endocardite	endocarditis	Endokarditis
endocardite batterica subacuta	subacute bacterial endocarditis (SBE)	Endocarditis lenta
endocervicale	endocervical	endozervikal
endocrino	endocrine	endokrin
endocrinologia	endocrinology	Endokrinologie
endogeno	endogenous	endogen
endometrio	endometrium	Endometrium
endometriosi	endometriosis	Endometriose
endometrite	endometritis	Endometritis
endonevrio	endoneurium	Endoneurium
endoparassita	endoparasite	Endoparasit
endorfina	endorphin	Endorphin
endoscopia	endoscopy	Endoskopie
endoscopio	endoscope	Endoskop
endotelio	endothelium	Endothel
endotossina	endotoxin	Endotoxin
endotracheale	endotracheal	endotracheal
endovenoso (EV)	intravenous (IV)	intravenös, endovenös
enfisema	emphysema	Emphysem
enoftalmo	enophthalmos	Enophtalmus
enterale	enteral	enteral
enterico	enteric	enterisch

SPANISH	FRENCH	ITALIAN
hemorragia subaracnoidea	hémorragie sous-arachnoïdienne	emorragia subaracnoidea
hemorroide	hémorroïde	emorroide
hemorroidectomía	hémorroïdectomie	emorroidectomia
hemorroides	hémorroïdes	emorroidi
hemostasis	hémostase	emostasi
emocional	émotionnel	emotivo
hemotórax	hémothorax	emotorace
emoción, afecto	émotion, affect	emozione
empiema	empyème	empiema
empírico	empirique	empirico
emulsión	émulsion	emulsione
encefalina	encéphaline	encefalina
encefalitis	encéphalite	encefalite
encefalitis espongiforme bovina	encéphalite spongiforme bovine	encefalite spongiforme bovina
encefalomielitis	encéphalomyélite	encefalomielite
encefalomielitis miálgica	encéphalomyélite myalgique	encefalomielite mialgica
encefalopatía	encéphalopathie	encefalopatia
encopresis	encoprésie	encopresi
endémico	endémie	endemia
endémico	endémique	endemico
endarterectomía	endartériectomie	endoarterectomia
endarteritis	endartérite	endoarterite
endocarditis	endocardite	endocardite
endocarditis bacteriana subaguda	endocardite lente	endocardite batterica subacuta
endocervical	endocervical	endocervicale
endocrino	endocrine	endocrino
endocrinología	endocrinologie	endocrinologia
endógeno	endogène	endogeno
endometrio	endomètre	endometrio
endometriosis	endométriose	endometriosi
endometritis	endométrite	endometrite
endoneuro	endonèvre	endonevrio
endoparásito	endoparasite	endoparassita
endorfina	endorphine	endorfina
endoscopia	endoscopie	endoscopia
endoscopio	endoscope	endoscopio
endotelio	endothélium	endotelio
endotoxina	endotoxine	endotossina
endotraqueal	endotrachéique	endotracheale
intravenoso (IV)	intraveineux (IV)	endovenoso (EV)
enfisema	emphysème	enfisema
enoftalmos	énophtalmie	enoftalmo
enteral	entéral	enterale
entérico	entérique	enterico

enterite	enteritis	Enteritis
enteroanastomosi	enteroanastomosis	Enteroanastomose
enterocele	enterocele	Enterozele
enterocolite	enterocolitis	Enterokolitis
enterocolite necrotizzante	necrotizing enterocolitis (NEC)	nekrotisierende Enterokolitis
enteropatia da glutine	gluten-induced enteropathy	Zöliakie
enterostomia	enterostomy	Enterostomie
enterovirus	enterovirus	Enterovirus
entropion	entropion	Entropion
enucleazione	enucleation	Enukleation, Ausschälung
enuresi	enuresis	Enuresis, Bettnässen
enuresi notturna	bedwetting	Bettnässen
enzima	enzyme	Enzym
enzima proteolitico	proteolytic enzyme	proteolytisches Enzym
enzimologia	enzymology	Enzymologie
eosinofilia	eosinophilia	Eosinophilie
eosinofilo (n)	eosinophil (n)	Eosinophiler (n)
eosinofilo (a)	eosinophil (a)	eosinophil (a)
epatico	hepatic	hepatisch, Leber-
epatite	hepatitis	Hepatitis
epatite virale	viral hepatitis	Virushepatitis
epatocellulare	hepatocellular	hepatozellulär
epatoma	hepatoma	Hepatom
epatomegalia	hepatomegaly	Hepatomegalie
epatosplenomegalia	hepatosplenomegaly	Hepatosplenomegalie
epatotossico	hepatotoxic	leberschädigend
ependimoma	ependymoma	Ependymom
epicanto	epicanthus	Epikanthus
epicardio	epicardium	Epikard
epicondilite radio-omerale	tennis elbow	Tennisellenbogen
epicondiloideo	supracondylar	suprakondylär
epidemia	epidemic	Epidemie
epidemico	epidemic	epidemisch
epidemiologia	epidemiology	Epidemiologie
epidermide	epidermis	Epidermis
epididimite	epididymitis	Epididymitis, Nebenhodenentzündung
epididimo	epididymis	Epididymis, Nebenhoden
epididimo-orchite	epididymo-orchitis	Epididymoorchitis
epidurale	epidural	epidural
epifisi	epiphysis	Epiphyse, Zirbeldrüse
epigastrico	precordial	präkordial
epigastrio	epigastrium	Epigastrium, Oberbauch
epiglottide	epiglottis	Epiglottis
epiglottite	epiglottitis	Epiglottitis
epilessia	epilepsy	Epilepsie
epilettico	epileptic	epileptisch
epilettiforme	epileptiform	epileptiform

SPANISH	FRENCH	ITALIAN
enteritis	entérite	enterite
enteroanastómosis	entéro-anastomose	enteroanastomosi
enterocele	entérocèle, hernie intestinale	enterocele
enterocolitis	entérocolite	enterocolite
enterocolitis necrotizante	entérocolite nécrosante	enterocolite necrotizzante
enteropatía provocada por glúten	maladie coeliaque	enteropatia da glutine
enterostomía	entérostomie	enterostomia
enterovirus	entérovirus	enterovirus
entropión	entropion	entropion
enucleación	énucléation	enucleazione
enuresis	énurèse	enuresi
enuresis nocturna	incontinence nocturne	enuresi notturna
enzima	enzyme	enzima
enzima proteolítico	enzyme protéolytique	enzima proteolitico
enzimología	enzymologie	enzimologia
eosinofilia	éosinophilie	eosinofilia
eosinófilo (n)	éosinophile (n)	eosinofilo (n)
eosinófilo (a)	éosinophile (a)	eosinofilo (a)
hepático	hépatique	epatico
hepatitis	hépatite	epatite
hepatitis vírica	hépatite virale	epatite virale
hepatocelular	hépatocellulaire	epatocellulare
hepatoma	hépatome	epatoma
hepatomegalia	hépatomégalie	epatomegalia
hepatosplenomegalia	hépatosplénomégalie	epatosplenomegalia
hepatotóxico	hépatotoxique	epatotossico
ependimoma	épendymome	ependimoma
epicanto	épicanthus	epicanto
epicardio	épicarde	epicardio
codo del tenista	tennis elbow'	epicondilite radio-omerale
supracondilar	supracondylaire	epicondiloideo
epidemia	épidémie	epidemia
epidémico	épidémique	epidemico
epidemiología	épidémiologie	epidemiologia
epidermis	épiderme	epidermide
epididimitis	épididymite	epididimite
epidídimo	épididyme	epididimo
epididimoorquitis	orchi-épididymite	epididimo-orchite
epidural	épidural	epidurale
epífisis	épiphyse	epifisi
precordial	précordial	epigastrico
epigastrio	épigastre	epigastrio
epiglotis	épiglotte	epiglottide
epiglotitis	épiglottite	epiglottite
epilepsia	épilepsie	epilessia
epiléptico	épileptique	epilettico
epileptiforme	épileptiforme	epilettiforme

epilettogeno	epileptogenic	epileptogen
episclera	episclera	Episklera
episclerite	episcleritis	Episkleritis
episiotomia	episiotomy	Episiotomie, Dammschnitt
epistassi	epistaxis, nosebleed	Epistaxis, Nasenbluten
epitelio	epithelium	Epithel
epitelioma	epithelioma	Epitheliom
eponichio	pterygium	Pterygium
eredità	heredity	Erblichkeit, Vererbung
ereditario	hereditary	hereditär, erblich
erettile	erectile	erektil
erezione	erection	Erektion
ergoterapia	occupational therapy	Beschäftigungstherapie
erisipela	erysipelas	Erysipel, Wundrose
eritema	erythema	Erythem
eritema vasomotorio	flush	Flush
eritroblasto	erythroblast	Erythroblast
eritroblastosi fetale (da incompatibilità Rh)	haemolytic disease of the newborn (HDN) (Eng), hemolytic disease of the newborn (HDN) (Am)	Morbus haemolyticus neonatorum
eritrocito	erythrocyte, red blood cell (RBC)	Erythrozyt, rotes Blutkörperchen
eritrodermia	erythroderma	Erythrodermie
eritropoiesi	erythropoiesis	Erythropoese
eritropoietina	erythropoietin	Erythropoetin, erythropoetischer Faktor
ermafrodito	hermaphrodite	Hermaphrodit, Zwitter
ernia	hernia	Hernie, Bruch
ernia discale	slipped disc	Bandscheibenvorfall
ernia ombelicale	exomphalos, umbilical hernia	Exomphalos, Nabelbruch
ernia strozzata	strangulated hernia	inkarzerierte Hernie
erniorrafia	herniorraphy	Bruchoperation
erniotomia	herniotomy	Herniotomie
eruttazione	belching	Aufstoßen
eruzione	eruption	Ausbruch, Ausschlag
eruzione cutanea	rash	Ausschlag, Hautausschlag
eruzione cutanea da pannolino	diaper rash (Am), napkin rash (Eng)	Windeldermatitis
esacerbazione	exacerbation	Verschlimmerung
esame dell'urina	urinalysis	Urinanalyse, Urinuntersuchung
esame emocromocitometrico	complete blood count (CBC)	großes Blutbild
esantema miliare	miliaria	Miliaria
escara	eschar, slough, scab	Brandschorf, Schorf, Kruste
escissione	excision	Exzision
escoriazione	excoriation	Exkoriation, Abschürfung
escreato	sputum	Sputum, Auswurf
escrezione	excretion	Exkretion, Ausscheidung
esfoliazione	exfoliation	Exfoliation
esibizionismo	exhibitionism	Exhibitionismus

SPANISH	FRENCH	ITALIAN
epileptógeno	épileptogène	epilettogeno
episclera	épisclérotique	episclera
episcleritis	épisclérite	episclerite
episiotomía	épisiotomie	episiotomia
epistaxis	épistaxis, saignement de nez	epistassi
epitelio	épithélium	epitelio
epitelioma	épithélioma	epitelioma
pterigión	ptérygion	eponichio
herencia	hérédité	eredità
hereditario	héréditaire	ereditario
eréctil	érectile	erettile
erección	érection	erezione
terapéutica ocupacional	ergothérapie	ergoterapia
erisipela	érysipèle	erisipela
eritema	érythème	eritema
rubor	rougeur	eritema vasomotorio
eritroblasto	érythroblaste	eritroblasto
enfermedad hemolítica del recién nacido	hémolyse des nouveau-nés	eritroblastosi fetale (da incompatibilità Rh)
eritrocito, glóbulo rojo	érythrocyte, globule rouge	eritrocito
eritrodermia	érythroderme	eritrodermia
eritropoyesis	érythropoïèse	eritropoiesi
eritropoyetina	érythropoïétine	eritropoietina
hermafrodita	hermaphrodite	ermafrodito
hernia	hernie	ernia
hernia de disco	hernie discale	ernia discale
exónfalo, hernia umbilical	exomphale, hernie ombilicale	ernia ombelicale
hernia estrangulada	hernie étranglée	ernia strozzata
herniorrafia	herniorrhaphie	erniorrafia
herniotomía	herniotomie	erniotomia
eructo	éructation	eruttazione
erupción	éruption	eruzione
exantema	rash	eruzione cutanea
exantema del pañal	érythème fessier du nourrisson, érythème papulo-érosif	eruzione cutanea da pannolino
exacerbación	exacerbation	esacerbazione
urinálisis	analyse d'urine	esame dell'urina
hemograma completo	numération globulaire	esame emocromocitometrico
miliaria	miliaire	esantema miliare
escara, costra, esfacelo	escarre, croûte	escara
excisión	excision	escissione
excoriación	excoriation	escoriazione
esputo	salive	escreato
excreción	excrétion	escrezione
exfoliación	exfoliation	esfoliazione
exhibicionismo	exhibitionnisme	esibizionismo

ITALIAN	ENGLISH	GERMAN
esocrino	exocrine	exokrin
esofageo	esophageal (Am), oesophageal (Eng)	ösophageal
esofagite	esophagitis (Am), oesophagitis (Eng)	Ösophagitis
esofago	esophagus (Am), oesophagus (Eng)	Ösophagus, Speiseröhre
esofago (gola)	gullet	Speiseröhre
esoftalmo	exophthalmos	Exophthalmus
esogeno	exogenous	exogen
esostosi	exostosis	Exostose
esotossina	exotoxin	Exotoxin
espettorante (n)	expectorant (n)	Expektorans (n), Sekretolytikum (n)
espettorante (a)	expectorant (a)	schleimlösend (a)
espirazione	expiration	Exspiration, Ausatmen
esplorazione	exploration	Exploration
esposto	patent	offen, durchgängig
espressione	expression	Expressio
essenza	essence	Essenz
essudato	exudate	Exsudat
estensione	extension	Extension, Streck-
estensore	extensor	Extensor, Streckmuskel
estradiolo	estradiol (Am), oestradiol (Eng)	Östradiol
estrazione	extraction	Extraktion
estrazione con ventosa ostetrica	ventouse extraction	Schröpfkopf
estrinseco	extrinsic	exogen
estriolo	estriol (Am), oestriol (Eng)	Östriol
estrofia	eversion	Auswärtskehrung, Umstülpung
estrogeno	estrogen (Am), oestrogen (Eng)	Östrogen
eterogenico	heterogenous	heterogen
eterosessuale	heterosexual	heterosexuell
etmoide	ethmoid	Ethmoid, Siebbein
etnico	ethnic	ethnisch, rassisch
euforia	euphoria	Euphorie
eutanasia	euthanasia	Euthanasie, Sterbehilfe
evacuazione	evacuation	Ausleerung, Stuhlgang
evaporare	evaporate	verdampfen, verdunsten
eversione	eversion	Auswärtskehrung, Umstülpung
extraarticolare	extra-articular	extraartikulär
extracellulare	extracellular	extrazellulär
extradurale	extradural	extradural
extramurale	extramural	extramural
extrasistole	extrasystole	Extrasystole
extrauterino	extrauterine	extrauterin
eziologia	aetiology	Ätiologie

SPANISH	FRENCH	ITALIAN
exocrino	exocrine	esocrino
esofágico	oesophagien	esofageo
esofagitis	oesophagite	esofagite
esófago	oesophage	esofago
gaznate	oesophage	esofago (gola)
exoftalmía	exophthalmie	esoftalmo
exógeno	exogène	esogeno
exostosis	exostose	esostosi
exotoxina	exotoxine	esotossina
expectorante (n)	expectorant (n)	espettorante (n)
expectorante (a)	expectorant (a)	espettorante (a)
espiración	expiration	espirazione
exploración	exploration	esplorazione
permeable	libre	esposto
expresión	expression	espressione
esencia	essence	essenza
exudado	exsudat	essudato
extensión	extension	estensione
extensor	extenseur	estensore
estradiol	oestradiol	estradiolo
extracción	extraction	estrazione
extracción con ventosa	extraction par ventouse	estrazione con ventosa ostetrica
extrínseco	extrinsèque	estrinseco
estriol	oestriol	estriolo
eversión	éversion	estrofia
estrógeno	oestrogène	estrogeno
heterogéneo	hétérogène	eterogenico
heterosexual	hétérosexuel	eterosessuale
etmoides	ethmoïde	etmoide
étnico	ethnique	etnico
euforia	euphorie	euforia
eutanasia	euthanasie	eutanasia
evacuación	évacuation	evacuazione
evaporar	évaporer	evaporare
eversión	éversion	eversione
extraarticular	extra-articulaire	extraarticolare
extracelular	extracellulaire	extracellulare
extradural	extradural	extradurale
extramural	extramural	extramurale
extrasístole	extrasystole	extrasistole
extrauterino	extra-utérin	extrauterino
etiología	étiologie	eziologia

F

ITALIAN	ENGLISH	GERMAN
faccetta	facet	Facette
facciale	facial	Gesichts-
facies	facies	Facies, Gesicht
facoltativo	facultative	fakultativ
fagocito	phagocyte	Phagozyt
fagocitosi	phagocytosis	Phagozytose
falangi	phalanges	Fingerglieder, Zehenglieder
falciforme	falciform	falciformis
fallo	phallus	Phallus, Penis
fame	hunger	Hunger
familiare	familial	familiär
far gocciolare	drip	tröpfeln, tropfen
faringe	pharynx	Pharynx, Rachen
faringite	pharyngitis	Pharyngitis
faringotomia	pharyngotomy	Pharyngotomie
farmaceutico	pharmaceutical	pharmazeutisch, Apotheker-
farmaci antiparkinsoniani	antiparkinson(ism) drugs	Antiparkinsonmittel
farmacista	pharmacist	Apotheker, Pharmazeut
farmaco	drug	Arzneimittel, Rauschgift
farmaco a lenta dismissione	slow release drug	Retardmittel
farmaco antinfiammatorio non steroideo (FANS)	non-steroidal anti-inflammatory drug (NSAID)	nichtsteroidales Antiphlogistikum
farmacocinetica	pharmacokinetics	Pharmakokinetik
farmacogenetica	pharmacogenetics	Pharmakogenetik
farmacologia	pharmacology	Pharmakologie
(farmaco) ottenibile senza prescrizione medica	over the counter (OTC)	rezeptfrei
farmaco sottoposto a controllo	controlled drug	Betäubungsmittel (gemäß BTM)
fascia	fascia	Faszie
fascicolazione	fasciculation	Faszikulation
fase dei movimenti oculari rapidi	REM sleep	REM-Schlaf
fase espulsiva del parto	bearing down	Pressen
fase REM del sonno	rapid eye movement (REM)	rapid eye movement (REM)
fattore Rh	Rhesus factor	Rhesusfaktor
fauci	fauces	Rachen, Schlund
favo	carbuncle	Karbunkel
febbre	fever	Fieber
febbre da fieno	hay fever	Heuschnupfen
febbre di Lassa	Lassa fever	Lassafieber
febbre emoglobinurica da Plasmodium falciparum	blackwater fever	Schwarzwasserfieber
febbre gialla	yellow fever	Gelbfieber
febbre paratifoide	paratyphoid fever	Paratyphus
febbre purpurica delle Montagne Rocciose	Rocky Mountain spotted fever	Rocky Mountain spotted fever

SPANISH	FRENCH	ITALIAN
faceta	facette	faccetta
facial	facial	facciale
facies	faciès	facies
facultativo	facultatif	facoltativo
fagocito	phagocyte	fagocito
fagocitosis	phagocytose	fagocitosi
falanges	phalanges	falangi
falciforme	falciforme	falciforme
falo	phallus	fallo
hambre	faim	fame
familiar	familial	familiare
infundir	perfuser	far gocciolare
faringe	pharynx	faringe
faringitis	pharyngite	faringite
faringotomía	pharyngotomie	faringotomia
farmacéutico	pharmaceutique	farmaceutico
farmacos antiparkinsonianos	médicaments contre la maladie de Parkinson	farmaci antiparkinsoniani
farmacéutico	pharmacien	farmacista
fármaco	médicament	farmaco
medicamento de liberación lenta	médicament retard	farmaco a lenta dismissione
fármaco antiinflamatorio no esteroide (AINE)	anti-inflammatoire non stéroïdien	farmaco antinfiammatorio non steroideo (FANS)
farmacocinética	pharmacocinétique	farmacocinetica
farmacogenético	pharmacogénétique	farmacogenetica
farmacología	pharmacologie	farmacologia
sin receta médica	spécialités pharmaceutiques grand public	(farmaco) ottenibile senza prescrizione medica
fármaco controlado	médicament contrôlé	farmaco sottoposto a controllo
fascia, aponeurosis	fascia	fascia
fasciculación	fasciculation	fascicolazione
sueño REM	sommeil paradoxal	fase dei movimenti oculari rapidi
postración	efforts expulsifs	fase espulsiva del parto
movimiento rápido de los ojos (REM)	période des mouvements oculaires	fase REM del sonno
factor Rhesus	facteur Rhésus	fattore Rh
fauces	fosse gutturale	fauci
ántrax	charbon	favo
fiebre	fièvre	febbre
fiebre del heno	rhume des foins	febbre da fieno
fiebre de Lassa	fièvre de Lassa	febbre di Lassa
fiebre hemoglobinúrica	hématurie	febbre emoglobinurica da Plasmodium falciparum
fiebre amarilla	fièvre jaune	febbre gialla
fiebre paratifoidea	fièvre paratyphoïde	febbre paratifoide
fiebre manchada de las Montañas Rocosas	fièvre pourprée des montagnes Rocheuses	febbre purpurica delle Montagne Rocciose

ITALIAN	ENGLISH	GERMAN
febbre Q	Q fever	Q-Fieber
febbre reumatica	rheumatic fever	rheumatisches Fieber
febbre tifoide	typhoid fever	Typhus
febbrile	febrile	Fieber-, fieberhaft
fecale	faecal (Eng), fecal (Am)	fäkal, kotig
fecalito	faecalith (Eng), fecalith (Am)	Kotstein
feci	faeces (Eng), feces (Am), stool	Fäzes, Kot, Stuhl, Stuhlgang
fecondazione artificiale tramite donatore	artificial insemination by donor (AID)	heterologe Insemination
fegato	liver	Leber
femmina	female	weiblich
femore	femur	Femur
fenestrazione	fenestration	Fensterung
fenilchetonuria	phenylketonuria (PKU)	Phenylketonurie (PKU)
fenotipo	phenotype	Phänotyp
feocromocitoma	phaeochromocytoma (Eng), pheochromocytoma (Am)	Phäochromozytom
ferita	wound	Wunde, Verletzung
ferita penetrante	penetrating wound	penetrierende Verletzung
ferroso	ferrous (Eng), ferrus (Am)	Eisen-
fertilizzazione	fertilization	Befruchtung
fertilizzazione in vitro	in vitro fertilization (IVF)	In-vitro-Fertilisation
feto	fetus	Fetus
fetoscopia	fetoscopy	Fetoskopie
fiala	ampoule (Eng), ampule (Am), ampulla	Ampulle
fibra	fiber (Am), fibre (Eng)	Faser
fibra dietetica	dietary fiber (Am), dietary fibre (Eng)	Ballaststoff
fibrilla	fibril	Fibrille, Fäserchen
fibrillazione	fibrillation	Fibrillieren
fibrillazione atriale	atrial fibrillation	Vorhofflimmern
fibrina	fibrin	Fibrin
fibrinogeno	fibrinogen	Fibrinogen
fibroadenoma	fibroadenoma	Fibroadenom
fibroblasto	fibroblast	Fibroblast
fibrocistico	fibrocystic	fibrozystisch
fibroma	fibroma	Fibrom
fibromioma	fibromyoma	Fibromyom
fibroplasia retrolenticolare	retrolental fibroplasia	retrolentale Fibroplasie
fibrosarcoma	fibrosarcoma	Fibrosarkom
fibrosi	fibrosis	Fibrose
fibrosite	fibrositis	Fibrositis, Bindegewebsentzündung
fibula	fibula	Fibula, Wadenbein
filariasi	filariasis	Filariasis, Fadenwurmbefall
filtrato	filtrate	Filtrat
filtrazione	filtration	Filtrieren, Filtration
fimbria	fimbria	Fimbrie
fimosi	phimosis	Phimose
fisiologico	physiological	physiologisch

fiebre Q	fièvre Q	febbre Q
fiebre reumática	rhumatisme articulaire aigu	febbre reumatica
fiebre tifoidea	fièvre typhoïde	febbre tifoide
febril	fébrile	febbrile
fecal	fécal	fecale
fecalito	concrétion fécale	fecalito
heces, deposición	fèces, selle	feci
inseminación artificial por donante (AID)	insémination hétérologue	fecondazione artificiale tramite donatore
hígado	foie	fegato
hembra	femelle	femmina
fémur	fémur	femore
fenestración	fenestration	fenestrazione
fenilcetonuria	phénylcétonurie	fenilchetonuria
fenotipo	phénotype	fenotipo
feocromocitoma	phéochromocytome	feocromocitoma
herida	plaie	ferita
herida penetrante	plaie par pénétration	ferita penetrante
ferroso	ferreux	ferroso
fertilización	fertilisation	fertilizzazione
fertilización in vitro (FIV)	fertilisation in vitro	fertilizzazione in vitro
feto	foetus	feto
fetoscopia	fétoscopie	fetoscopia
ampolla, víal	ampoule	fiala
fibra	fibre	fibra
fibra dietética	fibre alimentaire	fibra dietetica
fibrilla	fibrille	fibrilla
fibrilación	fibrillation	fibrillazione
fibrilación auricular	fibrillation auriculaire	fibrillazione atriale
fibrina	fibrine	fibrina
fibrinógeno	fibrinogène	fibrinogeno
fibroadenoma	fibroadénome	fibroadenoma
fibroblasto	fibroblaste	fibroblasto
fibrocístico	fibrokystique	fibrocistico
fibroma	fibrome	fibroma
fibromioma	fibromyome	fibromioma
fibroplasia retrolental	fibroplasie rétrolentale	fibroplasia retrolenticolare
fibrosarcoma	fibrosarcome	fibrosarcoma
fibrosis	fibrose	fibrosi
fibrositis	fibrosite	fibrosite
peroné	fibula	fibula
filariasis	filariose	filariasi
filtrado	filtrat	filtrato
filtración	filtration	filtrazione
fimbria, franja	fimbria	fimbria
fimosis	phimosis	fimosi
fisiológico	physiologique	fisiologico

ITALIAN	ENGLISH	GERMAN
fissazione	delusion, fixation	Wahn, Wahnvorstellung, Fixation, Fixierung
fissione	fission	Spaltung
fistola	fistula	Fistel
fistula suppurante	sinus	Sinus, Nebenhöhle
flaccido	flaccid	schlaff
flatulenza	flatulence, flatus, wind	Flatulenz, Blähung, Flatus, Wind
flebectomia	phlebectomy	Phlebektomie
flebite	phlebitis	Phlebitis, Venenentzündung
fleboclisi	drip	Tropfinfusion
flebografia	venography	Phlebographie
flebolito	phlebolith	Phlebolith
flebotomia	phlebotomy, venesection	Venae sectio
flemma	phlegm	Phlegma
flessione	flexion	Flexion, Beugung
flessore	flexor	Flexor, Beugemuskel
flessura	flexure	Flexur
flettere	flex	beugen, flektieren
flittena	bleb	Bläschen
flora	flora	Flora
florido	florid	floride
fluido amniotico	amniotic fluid .	Amnionflüssigkeit, Fruchtwasser
fluoresceina	fluorescein	Fluorescin
fluoruro	fluoride	Fluorid
flutter atriale	atrial flutter	Vorhofflattern
fluttuazione	fluctuation	Fluktuation
fobia	phobia	Phobie
focomelia	phocomelia	Phokomelie
folgorazione	fulguration	Fulguration
follicoli di Naboth	nabothian follicles	Naboth-Eier
follicolite	folliculitis	Follikulitis
follicolo	follicle	Follikel
follicolo di Graaf	Graafian follicle	Graaf-Follikel
fondo	fundus	Fundus, Augenhintergrund
fontanella	fontanelle	Fontanelle
foramen	foramen	Foramen
forchetta	fourchette	hintere Schamlippenkommissur
forcipe	forceps	Zange, Pinzette, Klemme
forfora	dandruff	Schuppen
formula	formula	Formel, Milchzusammensetzung
formula leucocitaria	differential blood count	Differentialblutbild
formulario	formulary	Formelnbuch
fornice	fornix	Fornix
foruncolo	boil, furuncle, spot	Furunkel, Eiterbeule, Flecken, Pickel
fotofobia	photophobia	Photophobie, Lichtscheue
fotosensibile	photosensitive	lichtempfindlich
fototerapia	phototherapy	Phototherapie

idea delusiva, delirio, fijación	hallucination, fixation	**fissazione**
fisión	fission	**fissione**
fístula	fistule	**fistola**
seno	sinus	**fistula suppurante**
fláccido	mou	**flaccido**
flatulencia, flato, ventosidad	flatulence, flatuosité, gaz	**flatulenza**
flebectomía	phlébectomie	**flebectomia**
flebitis	phlébite	**flebite**
gota a gota intravenoso	perfusion	**fleboclisi**
venografía	phlébographie	**flebografia**
flebolito	phlébolithe	**flebolito**
flebotomía, venisección	phlébotomie	**flebotomia**
flema	phlegme	**flemma**
flexión	flexion	**flessione**
flexor	fléchisseur	**flessore**
flexura	angle	**flessura**
flexionar	fléchir	**flettere**
vesícula, bulla, ampolla	phlyctène	**flittena**
flora	flore	**flora**
florido, bien desarrollado	coloré	**florido**
líquido amniótico	liquide amniotique	**fluido amniotico**
fluoresceína	fluorescéine	**fluoresceina**
flúor	fluorure	**fluoruro**
aleteo auricular	flutter auriculaire	**flutter atriale**
fluctuación	variation	**fluttuazione**
fobia	phobie	**fobia**
focomelia	phocomélie	**focomelia**
fulguración	fulguration	**folgorazione**
folículos de Naboth	oeufs de Naboth	**follicoli di Naboth**
foliculitis	folliculite	**follicolite**
folículo	follicule	**follicolo**
folículo de De Graaf	follicule de De Graaf	**follicolo di Graaf**
fundus	fond	**fondo**
fontanela	fontanelle	**fontanella**
foramen	orifice	**foramen**
horquilla, frenillo pudendo	fourchette	**forchetta**
fórceps	forceps	**forcipe**
caspa	pellicules	**forfora**
fórmula, receta	formule	**formula**
fórmula leucocitaria	formule leucocytaire	**formula leucocitaria**
formulario	formulaire	**formulario**
fórnix, bóveda	fornix	**fornice**
forúnculo, mancha	furoncle, bouton	**foruncolo**
fotofobia	photophobie	**fotofobia**
fotosensible	photosensible	**fotosensibile**
fototerapia	photothérapie	**fototerapia**

fovea	fovea, pitting	Fovea, Dellenbildung
framboesia	yaws	Frambösie
fratello germano	sibling	Geschwister
frattura	fracture	Fraktur, Knochenbruch
frattura a legno verde	greenstick fracture	Grünholzfraktur
frattura comminuta	comminuted fracture	Splitterbruch
frattura con infossamento dei frammenti	depressed fracture	Impressionsfraktur
frattura di Colles	Colles' fracture	distale Radiusfraktur
frattura di Pott	Pott's fracture	Pott-Fraktur
frattura patologica	pathological fracture	pathologische Fraktur
fratturare	fracture	frakturieren, brechen
freddo	cold	kalt
fremito	thrill	Vibrieren, Schwirren
frenico (diaframmatico mentale)	phrenic	diaphragmatisch, Zwerchfell-
freno	frenum	Frenulum
frenulotomia	frenotomy	Frenotomie, Zungenbändchendurchtrennung
friabile	friable	bröckelig, brüchig
frigidità	frigidity	Frigidität, Kälte
frizione	friction	Friktion, Reibung
frontale	frontal	Stirn-, frontal
fronte	forehead	Stirn
fuga	fugue	Fugue
fuga delle idee	flight of ideas	Ideenflucht
fulminante	fulminant	fulminant
fundoplicazione	fundoplication	Fundoplikatio(n)
fungo	fungus	Pilz
funzionare	function	funktionieren
funzione	function	Funktion

SPANISH	FRENCH	ITALIAN
fóvea, cavitación	fovea, formation de godet	fovea
yaws, pian	pian	framboesia
hermano no gemelo	frère ou soeur	fratello germano
fractura	fracture	frattura
fractura en tallo verde	fracture incomplète	frattura a legno verde
fractura conminuta	fracture esquilleuse	frattura comminuta
fractura con hundimiento	enfoncement localisé	frattura con infossamento dei frammenti
fractura de Colles	fracture de Pouteau-Colles	frattura di Colles
fractura de Pott	fracture de Pott	frattura di Pott
fractura patológica	fracture spontanée	frattura patologica
fracturar	fracturer	fratturare
frío	froid	freddo
frémito	murmure respiratoire	fremito
frénico	psychique	frenico (diaframmatico mentale)
frenillo	frein	freno
frenotomía	frénotomie	frenulotomia
friable	friable	friabile
frigidez	frigidité	frigidità
fricción	friction	frizione
frontal	frontal	frontale
frente	front	fronte
fuga	fugue	fuga
fuga de ideas	fuite des idées	fuga delle idee
fulminante	fulminant	fulminante
fundoplicatura	fundoplication	fundoplicazione
hongo	mycète	fungo
funcionar	fonctionner	funzionare
función	fonction	funzione

G

Italian	English	German
galattagogo	galactagogue	Galaktagogum
galattorrea	galactorrhea (Am), galactorrhoea (Eng)	Galaktorrhoe
galattosemia	galactosaemia (Eng), galactosemia (Am)	Galaktosämie
galattosio	galactose	Galaktose
gamba	leg	Bein
gamete	gamete	Gamete
gamete femminile	ovum	Ovum, Ei
gammaglobulina	gammaglobulin	Gammaglobulin
gammaglobulina umana	human gamma globulin (HGG)	Human-Gammaglobulin
gangli basali	basal ganglia	Basalganglien
ganglio	ganglion	Ganglion, Überbein
gangrena	gangrene	Gangrän
gargarismi	gargle	Gurgelmittel
gargarizzare	gargle	gurgeln
garza	gauze	Gaze, Mull
gas	gas	Gas, Wind
gas intestinale	flatus	Flatus, Wind
gastrectomia	gastrectomy	Magenresektion
gastrico	gastric	gastrisch, Magen-
gastrina	gastrin	Gastrin
gastrite	gastritis	Gastritis, Magenschleimhautentzündung
gastrocnemio	gastrocnemius	gastrocnemius
gastrocolico	gastrocolic	gastrokolisch
gastrodigiunostomia	gastrojejunostomy	Gastrojejunostomie
gastrodinia	gastrodynia	Magenschmerz
gastroenterite	gastroenteritis	Gastroenteritis
gastroenterologia	gastroenterology	Gastroenterologie
gastroenteropatia	gastroenteropathy	Gastroenteropathie
gastroenterostomia	gastroenterostomy	Gastroenterostomie
gastroesofageo	gastroesophageal (Am), gastro-oesophageal (Eng)	gastroösophageal
gastrointestinale	gastrointestinal	gastrointestinal, Magendarm-
gastroschisi	gastroschisis	Gastroschisis
gastroscopio	gastroscope	Gastroskop, Magenspiegel
gastrostomia	gastrostomy	Gastrostomie
gelatina	gelatine (Eng), gelatin (Am)	Gelatine, Gallerte
gelone	chilblain	Frostbeule, Pernio
gemelli omozigoti	identical twins	eineiige Zwillinge
gemello	twin	Zwilling
gene	gene	Gen
genere	genus	Genus, Gattung

galactogogo	galactagogue	galattagogo
galactorrea	galactorrhée	galattorrea
galactosemia	galactosémie	galattosemia
galactosa	galactose	galattosio
pierna	jambe	gamba
gameto	gamète	gamete
óvulo	ovule, ovocyte de premier ordre, oeuf	gamete femminile
gammaglobulina	gamma-globuline	gammaglobulina
gammaglobulina humana	gamma-globuline humaine (GGH), globuline humaine	gammaglobulina umana
ganglios basales	noyau lenticulaire, noyau caudé, avant-mur et noyau amygdalien	gangli basali
ganglio	ganglion	ganglio
gangrena	gangrène	gangrena
gárgara, colutorio	gargarisme	gargarismi
gargajear	se gargariser	gargarizzare
gasa	gaze	garza
gas	gaz	gas
flato	flatuosité	gas intestinale
gastrectomía	gastrectomie	gastrectomia
gástrico	gastrique	gastrico
gastrina	gastrine	gastrina
gastritis	gastrite	gastrite
gastrocnemio, gemelos	gastrocnémien	gastrocnemio
gastrocólico	gastrocolique	gastrocolico
gastroyeyunostomía	gastrojéjunostomie	gastrodigiunostomia
gastrodinia	gastrodynie	gastrodinia
gastroenteritis	gastro-entérite	gastroenterite
gastroenterología	gastro-entérologie	gastroenterologia
gastroenteropatía	gastro-entéropathie	gastroenteropatia
gastroenterostomía	gastro-entérostomie	gastroenterostomia
gastroesofágico	gastro-oesophagien	gastroesofageo
gastrointestinal	gastro-intestinal	gastrointestinale
gastrosquisis	gastroschisis	gastroschisi
gastroscopio	gastroscope	gastroscopio
gastrotomía	gastrostomie	gastrostomia
gelatina	gélatine	gelatina
sabañón	engelure	gelone
gemelos idénticos	jumeaux univitellins	gemelli omozigoti
mellizo	jumeau	gemello
gen	gène	gene
género	genre	genere

ITALIAN	ENGLISH	GERMAN
generico	generic	generisch
genetica	genetics	Genetik
genetico	genetic	genetisch
gengiva	gingiva	Gingiva, Zahnfleisch
gengivite	gingivitis	Gingivitis, Zahnfleischentzündung
genitale	genital	genital, Geschlechts-
genito-urinario	genitourinary (GU)	urogenital
genoma	genome	Genom
genotipo	genotype	Genotyp
geriatra	geriatrician	Geriater
geriatria	geriatrics	Geriatrie
geriatrico	geriatric	geriatrisch
germe	germ	Erreger, Keim, Bazillus
gesso	gypsum, plaster	Gips, Pflaster
gesso di Parigi (calcio solfato diidrato)	plaster of Paris	Gips
gestazione	gestation	Gestation, Schwangerschaft
ghiandola	gland	Glandula, Drüse
ghiandola apocrina	apocrine gland	apokrine Drüse
ghiandola parotide	parotid gland	Parotis, Ohrspeicheldrüse
ghiandola paratiroide	parathyroid gland	Nebenschilddrüse, Parathyreoidea
ghiandola pineale	pineal body	Epiphyse
ghiandola pituitaria	pituitary gland	Hypophyse
ghiandola salivare	salivary gland	Speicheldrüse
ghiandole di Bartolini	Bartholin's glands	Bartholini-Drüsen
giardiasi	giardiasis	Lambliasis
ginecologia	gynaecology (Eng), gynecology (Am)	Gynäkologie, Frauenheilkunde
ginecomastia	gynaecomastia (Eng), gynecomastia (Am)	Gynäkomastie
ginocchio	knee	Knie
ginocchio valgo	genu valgum, knock-knee	Genu valgum, X-Bein
ginocchio varo	genu varum	Genu varum, O-Bein
giunzione	synapse	Synapse
glaucoma	glaucoma	Glaukom, grüner Star
glenoide	glenoid	Schultergelenk-
gleno-omerale	glenohumeral	glenohumeral
glicemia	blood sugar	Blutzucker
glicemia a digiuno	fasting blood sugar (FBS)	Nüchternblutzucker (NBZ)
glicocorticoide	glucocorticoid	Glukokortikoid
glicogenesi	glycogenesis	Glykogenese
glicolisi	glycolysis	Glykolyse, Glukoseabbau
glicosuria	glycosuria	Glykosurie, Glukoseausscheidung im Urin
glioma	glioma	Gliom
globulo rosso (RBC)	red blood cell (RBC)	Erythrozyt
glomerulite	glomerulitis	Glomerulitis
glomerulo	glomerulus	Glomerulus

SPANISH	FRENCH	ITALIAN
genérico	générique	generico
genética	génétique	genetica
genético	génétique	genetico
encía	gencive	gengiva
gingivitis	gingivite	gengivite
genital	génital	genitale
genitourinario	génito-urinaire (GT)	genito-urinario
genoma	génome	genoma
genotipo	génotype	genotipo
geriatra	gériatre	geriatra
geriatría	gériatrie	geriatria
geriátrico	gériatrique	geriatrico
gérmen	germe	germe
yeso	gypse, plâtre	gesso
escayola	sulfate de calcium hydraté, plâtre	gesso di Parigi (calcio solfato diidrato)
gestación	gestation	gestazione
glándula	glande	ghiandola
glándula apocrina	glande apocrine	ghiandola apocrina
glándula parótida	glande parotide	ghiandola parotide
glándula paratiroidea	glande parathyroïde	ghiandola paratiroide
cuerpo pineal	glande pinéale	ghiandola pineale
hipófisis	hypophyse	ghiandola pituitaria
glándula salivar	glande salivaire	ghiandola salivare
glándulas de Bartolino	glandes de Bartholin	ghiandole di Bartolini
giardiasis	giardiase	giardiasi
ginecología	gynécologie	ginecologia
ginecomastia	gynécomastie	ginecomastia
rodilla	genou	ginocchio
genu valgum	genu valgum, genou cagneux	ginocchio valgo
genu varum	genu varum	ginocchio varo
sinapsis	synapse	giunzione
glaucoma	glaucome	glaucoma
glenoide	glénoïde	glenoide
glenohumeral	gléno-huméral	gleno-omerale
glucemia	glycémie	glicemia
glucemia en ayunas	glycémie à jeun	glicemia a digiuno
glucocorticoide	glucocorticoïde	glicocorticoide
glucogénesis	glycogenèse	glicogenesi
glucolisis	glycolyse	glicolisi
glucosuria	glycosurie	glicosuria
glioma	gliome	glioma
eritrocito, glóbulo rojo	globule rouge	globulo rosso (RBC)
glomerulitis	glomérulite	glomerulite
glomérulo	glomérule	glomerulo

ITALIAN	ENGLISH	GERMAN
glomerulonefrite	glomerulonephritis	Glomerulonephritis
glomerulosclerosi	glomerulosclerosis	Glomerulosklerose
glossite	glossitis	Glossitis
glossodinia	glossodynia	Glossodynie, Zungenschmerz
glossofaringeo	glossopharyngeal	glossopharyngeal
glottide	glottis	Glottis, Stimmritze
glucagone	glucagon	Glukagon
glucogenesi	glucogenesis	Glukogenese
gluconeogenesi	gluconeogenesis	Glukoneogenese
glucosio	glucose	Glukose, Traubenzucker
gluteo	gluteal	gluteal
glutine	gluten	Gluten
gocciolare	drip	tröpfeln, tropfen
gomito del tennista	tennis elbow	Tennisellenbogen
gomma	gumma	Gumma
gonade	gonad	Gonade
gonadotropina	gonadotrophin (Eng), gonadotropin (Am)	Gonadotropin
gonadotropina corionica umana (GCU)	human chorionic gonadotrophin (HCG) (Eng), human chorionic gonadotropin (HCG) (Am)	Choriongonadotropin (HCG)
gonfio	swollen	geschwollen, vergrößert
gonorrea	gonorrhea (Am), gonorrhoea (Eng)	Gonorrhoe, Tripper
gotta	gout	Gicht
gozzo	goiter (Am), goitre (Eng)	Struma, Kropf
grande male	grand mal	Grand mal
granulazione	granulation	Granulation
granulocita	granulocyte	Granulozyt
granulocito neutrofilo	neutrophil	Neutrophiler
granuloma	granuloma	Granulom, Granulationsgeschwulst
grasso	fat	fett, fetthaltig
gravidanza	cyesis, pregnancy	Schwangerschaft, Gravidität
gravidanza a termine	full-term	ausgetragen
gravidanza ectopica	ectopic pregnancy	ektope Schwangerschaft
gravità	gravity	Schwere (der Erkrankung)
gravitazionale	gravitational	Gravitations-
gruppi di Lancefield	Lancefield's groups	Lancefield-Gruppen
gruppo sanguigno	blood group	Blutgruppe
guancia	cheek	Wange, Backe
guarigione	healing	Heilung

H

handicappato	handicap	Behinderung
herpes	cold sore, herpes	Herpes, Bläschenausschlag
herpes zoster	shingles, zoster	Herpes zoster, Gürtelrose

SPANISH	FRENCH	ITALIAN
glomerulonefritis	glomérulonéphrite	glomerulonefrite
glomerulosclerosis	glomérulosclérose	glomerulosclerosi
glositis	glossite	glossite
glosodinia	glossodynie	glossodinia
glosofaríngeo	glossopharyngien	glossofaringeo
glotis	glotte	glottide
glucagón	glucagon	glucagone
glucogénesis	glucogenèse	glucogenesi
gluconeogénesis	gluconéogenèse	gluconeogenesi
glucosa	glucose	glucosio
glúteo	fessier	gluteo
gluten	gluten	glutine
infundir	perfuser	gocciolare
codo del tenista	'tennis elbow'	gomito del tennista
goma	gomme	gomma
gónada	gonade	gonade
gonadotropina	gonadotrophine	gonadotropina
gonadotropina coriónica humana (GCH)	gonadotrophine chorionique humaine (GCH)	gonadotropina corionica umana (GCU)
hinchado	enflé	gonfio
gonorrea	gonorrhée	gonorrea
gota	goutte	gotta
bocio	goitre	gozzo
gran mal	grand mal	grande male
granulación	granulation	granulazione
granulocito	granulocyte	granulocita
neutrófilo	polynucléaire neutrophile	granulocito neutrofilo
granuloma	granulome	granuloma
graso	gras, obèse	grasso
ciesis, embarazo	grossesse	gravidanza
embarazo a término	à terme	gravidanza a termine
embarazo ectópico	grossesse ectopique	gravidanza ectopica
gravedad	gravité	gravità
gestacional	gravitationnel	gravitazionale
grupos de Lancefield	groupes de streptocoques suivant la classification de Lancefield	gruppi di Lancefield
grupo sanguíneo	groupe sanguin	gruppo sanguigno
mejilla	joue	guancia
curación	curatif	guarigione
disminución, minusvalía	handicapé	handicappato
herpes labial, herpes	herpès	herpes
herpes zóster, zóster	zona	herpes zoster

I

ialinite	hyalitis	Hyalitis
ialoideo	hyaloid	Glaskörper-
iatrogeno	iatrogenic	iatrogen
ictus	cerebrovascular accident (CVA), stroke	Schlaganfall, Apoplex, Schlag
idatiforme	hydatidiform mole	Blasenmole
idea	idea	Gedanke, Vorstellung
identificazione	empathy	Empathie, Einfühlungsvermögen
idiopatico	idiopathic	idiopathisch, essentiell
idiosincrasia	idiosyncrasy	Idiosynkrasie
idramnios	hydramnios	Hydramnion
idratare	hydrate	hydrieren, hydratisieren
idrato	hydrate	Hydrat
idrocefalo	hydrocephalus	Hydrozephalus
idrocele	hydrocele	Hydrozele, Wasserbruch
idrolisi	hydrolysis	Hydrolyse
idronefrosi	hydronephrosis	Hydronephrose
idrope fetale	hydrops fetalis	Hydrops fetalis
idrosalpinge	hydrosalpinx	Hydrosalpinx
idrosi	hidrosis	Hidrosis, Schweißabsonderung
ifema	hyphaema (Eng), hyphema (Am)	Hyphaema
igiene	hygiene	Hygiene
igroma	hygroma	Hygrom
ileectomia	ileectomy	Ileumresektion
ileite	ileitis	Ileitis
ileite regionale	regional ileitis	Ileitis regionalis
ileo	ileum, ileus	Ileum, Ileus, Darmverschluß
ileocecale	ileocaecal (Eng), ileocecal (Am)	ileozäkal
ileostomia	ileostomy	Ileostomie
ileotifo	typhoid fever	Typhus
iliaco	iliac	ileo-
ilio	ilium	Os ilium
illusione	illusion	Illusion
ilo	hilum	Hilus
imene	hymen	Hymen
imenectomia	hymenectomy	Hymenektomie
immagine radiologica	radiograph	Röntgenaufnahme
immedesimazione	empathy	Empathie, Einfühlungsvermögen
immediatamente dopo l'attacco	immediately after onset (IAO)	unmittelbar nach Krankheitsausbruch
immune	immune	immun
immunità	immunity	Immunität
immunizzazione	immunization	Immunisierung, Schutzimpfung
immunodeficienza	immunodeficiency	Immundefekt
immunofluorescenza	immunofluorescence	Immunfluoreszenz
immunoglobulina (Ig)	immunoglobulin (Ig)	Immunglobulin

SPANISH	FRENCH	ITALIAN
hialitis	hyalite	ialinite
hialoide	hyaloïde	ialoideo
yatrógeno	iatrogène	iatrogeno
accidente vascular cerebral (ACV), ictus	accident cérébrovasculaire, apoplexie	ictus
mola hidatidiforme	hydatidiforme	idatiforme
idea	idée	idea
empatía	empathie	identificazione
idiopático	idiopathique	idiopatico
idiosincrasia	idiosyncrasie	idiosincrasia
hidramnios	hydramnios	idramnios
hidratar	hydrater	idratare
hidrato	hydrate	idrato
hidrocéfalo	hydrocéphale	idrocefalo
hidrocele	hydrocèle	idrocele
hidrólisis	hydrolyse	idrolisi
hidronefrosis	hydronéphrose	idronefrosi
hydrops fetal	anasarque foeto-placentaire	idrope fetale
hidrosálpinx	hydrosalpinx	idrosalpinge
hidrosis	transpiration	idrosi
hipema	hyphéma	ifema
higiene	hygiène	igiene
higroma	hygroma	igroma
ileoctomía	iléoctomie	ileectomia
ileítis	iléite	ileite
ileítis regional	iléite régionale	ileite regionale
ileón, íleo	iléon, iléus	ileo
ileocecal	iléocaecal	ileocecale
ileostomía	iléostomie	ileostomia
fiebre tifoidea	fièvre typhoïde	ileotifo
ilíaco	iliaque	iliaco
ilion	ilion	ilio
ilusión	illusion	illusione
hilio	hile	ilo
himen	hymen	imene
himenectomía	hyménectomie	imenectomia
radiografía	radiographe	immagine radiologica
empatía	empathie	immedesimazione
inmediatamente después del comienzo	immédiatement après le début	immediatamente dopo l'attacco
inmune	immun	immune
inmunidad	immunité	immunità
inmunización	immunisation	immunizzazione
inmunodeficiencia	immunodéficience	immunodeficienza
inmunofluorescencia	immunofluorescence	immunofluorescenza
inmunoglobulina (Ig)	immunoglobuline (Ig)	immunoglobulina (Ig)

ITALIAN	ENGLISH	GERMAN
immunologia	immunology	Immunologie
immunoreazione	immune reaction	Immunreaktion
immunosoppressione	immunosuppression	Immunsuppression
impatto	impacted	impaktiert
imperforato	imperforate	nicht perforiert
impetigine	impetigo	Impetigo
impiantare	implant	implantieren
impianto	implantation	Implantation
impianto chirurgico sottocutaneo di farmaci	implant	Implantat
impotenza	impotence	Impotenz
improvvisa perdita della postura ad insorgenza periodica	drop attack	Drop attack
impulso	impulse	Impuls, Reiz
inadempienza a prescrizioni	noncompliance	Noncompliance
inalare	inhale	inhalieren, einatmen
inalazione	inhalation	Inhalation, Einatmen
inalazione di toluene o collanti	glue sniffing	Schnüffeln, Leimschnüffeln
incapacità ad agire	burnout syndrome	Helfer-Syndrom
incapsulamento	encapsulation	Verkapselung
incarcerato	incarcerated	inkarzeriert, eingeklemmt
incesto	incest	Inzest
incidente stradale	road traffic accident (RTA)	Verkehrsunfall
incidenza	incidence	Inzidenz
incipiente	incipient	beginnend
incisione	incision	Inzision, Einschnitt
incisore	incisor	Schneidezahn
incompatibilità	incompatibility	Inkompatibilität, Unverträglichkeit
incompatibilità Rh	Rhesus incompatibility	Rh-Unverträglichkeit
incompetenza	incompetence	Insuffizienz
inconscio	unconscious	bewußtlos
incontinenza	incontinence	Inkontinenz
incoordinazione	incoordination	Inkoordination
incoscio	id	Es
incubatore	incubator	Inkubator, Brutkasten
incubazione	incubation	Inkubation
incudine	incus	Incus, Amboß
incuneato	impacted	impaktiert
indagine morfologica con risonanza magnetica	magnetic resonance imaging (MRI)	Kernspintomographie (NMR)
indentificazione	identification	Identifizierung
indicatore	indicator	Indikator
indice del metabolismo basale (MB)	basal metabolic rate (BMR)	Grundumsatz
indice di Apgar	Apgar score	Apgar-Index
indice di massa corporea (IMC)	body mass index (BMI)	Körpermassenindex
indice di tiroxina libera	free thyroxine index (FTI)	freier Thyroxinindex (FTi)
indigeno	indigenous	eingeboren, einheimisch
indigestione	indigestion	Verdauungsstörung, Magenverstimmung

SPANISH	FRENCH	ITALIAN
inmunología	immunologie	**immunologia**
reacción inmunológica	réaction immunitaire	**immunoreazione**
inmunosupresión	immunosuppression	**immunosoppressione**
impactado	enclavé	**impatto**
imperforado	imperforé	**imperforato**
impétigo	impétigo	**impetigine**
implantar	implanter	**impiantare**
implantación	implantation	**impianto**
implante	implant	**impianto chirurgico sottocutaneo di farmaci**
impotencia	impotence	**impotenza**
ataque isquémico transitorio (AIT), caida	chute brusque par dérobement des jambes	**improvvisa perdita della postura ad insorgenza periodica**
impulso	impulsion	**impulso**
incumplimiento	non observance	**inadempienza a prescrizioni**
inhalar	inhaler	**inalare**
inhalación	inhalation	**inalazione**
inhalación de pegamento	intoxication par inhalation de solvant	**inalazione di toluene o collanti**
surmenage, neurastenia	syndrome de 'surmenage'	**incapacità ad agire**
encapsulación	capsulage	**incapsulamento**
incarcerado	incarcéré	**incarcerato**
incesto	inceste	**incesto**
accidente de circulacion	accident de la route	**incidente stradale**
incidencia	fréquence	**incidenza**
incipiente	débutant	**incipiente**
incisión	incision	**incisione**
incisivo	incisive	**incisore**
incompatibilidad	incompatibilité	**incompatibilità**
incompatibilidad Rhesus	incompatibilité Rhésus	**incompatibilità Rh**
incompetencia	incompétence	**incompetenza**
inconsciente, sin sentido	sans connaissance	**inconscio**
incontinencia	incontinence	**incontinenza**
incoordinación	incoordination	**incoordinazione**
id	ça	**incoscio**
incubadora	incubateur	**incubatore**
incubación	incubation	**incubazione**
incus, yunque	enclume	**incudine**
impactado	enclavé	**incuneato**
formación de imágenes por resonancia magnética	imagerie par résonance magnétique	**indagine morfologica con risonanza magnetica**
identificación	identification	**indentificazione**
indicador	indicateur	**indicatore**
tasa de metabolismo basal (MB)	taux du métabolisme basal	**indice del metabolismo basale (MB)**
índice de Apgar	indice d'Apgar	**indice di Apgar**
índice de masa corporal (IMC)	indice de masse corporelle (IMC)	**indice di massa corporea (IMC)**
indice de tiroxina libre	index de thyroxine libre	**indice di tiroxina libera**
indígena	indigène	**indigeno**
indigestión	indigestion	**indigestione**

indisposizione	malaise	Unwohlsein
indurimento	induration	Induration, Verhärtung
induzione	induction	Induktion, Einleitung
inerente	inherent	eigen, angeboren
inerzia	inertia	Trägheitsmoment, Untätigkeit
infante	infant	Kleinkind, Säugling
infantile	infantile	infantil, kindlich
infarto	infarction	Infarzierung
infarto miocardico	myocardial infarction (MI)	Myokardinfarkt, Herzinfarkt
inferiore	inferior	tiefer gelegen, minderwertig
infermiere	nurse	Krankenschwester, Schwester, Pflegerin
infermità	disease	Krankheit, Leiden
infertilità	infertility	Infertilität
infestazione	infestation	Befall
infettivo	infective	infektiös, ansteckend
infezione	infection	Infektion
infezione da Flavivirus ('febbre rompiossa')	dengue	Denguefieber
infezione delle vie urinarie (IVU)	urinary tract infection (UTI)	Harnwegsinfekt
infezione del tratto respiratorio inferiore (LRTI)	lower respiratory tract infection (LRTI)	Atemwegsinfekt (untere)
infezione del tratto respiratorio superiore (URTI)	upper respiratory tract infection (URTI)	Atemwegsinfekt
infezione opportunista	opportunistic infection	opportunistische Infektion
infiammazione	inflammation	Entzündung
infiltrazione	infiltration	Infiltration
influenza	influenza	Influenza, Grippe
influenzare	affect	befallen
infusione	infusion	Infusion
ingessatura	cast	Abdruck, Gipsverband
ingestione	ingestion	Einnahme, Aufnahme
inghiottire	swallow	schlucken
in grado di vivere	viable	lebensfähig
inguinale	inguinal	inguinal, Leisten-
inguine	groin	Leiste
inibitore monoaminoossidasi (IMAO)	monoamine oxidase inhibitor (MAOI)	Monoaminoxydase-Hemmer
inibizione	inhibition	Inhibierung, Hemmung
iniettare	inject	injizieren, spritzen
iniezione	injection	Injektion, Spritze
innato	innate	kongenital, angeboren
innervazione	innervation	Innervation
innesto	flap, graft	Lappen, Hautlappen, Transplantat, Transplantation, Plastik
innocente	innocent	unschuldig, unschädlich
innocuo	innocuous	unschädlich, harmlos
inoculazione	inoculation	Impfung
inorganico	inorganic	anorganisch

SPANISH	FRENCH	ITALIAN
destemplanza, malestar	malaise	**indisposizione**
induración	induration	**indurimento**
inducción	induction	**induzione**
inherente	inhérent	**inerente**
inercia	inertie	**inerzia**
lactante	enfant, nourrisson	**infante**
infantil	infantile	**infantile**
infarto	infarcissement	**infarto**
infarto de miocardio (IM)	infarctus du myocarde	**infarto miocardico**
inferior	inférieur	**inferiore**
enfermera	infirmière	**infermiere**
enfermedad	maladie	**infermità**
infertilidad	infertilité	**infertilità**
infestación	infestation	**infestazione**
infeccioso	infectieux	**infettivo**
infección	infection	**infezione**
dengue	dengue	**infezione da Flavivirus ('febbre rompiossa')**
infección de las vías urinarias (IVU)	infection des voies urinaires	**infezione delle vie urinarie (IVU)**
infección de las vías respiratorias bajas	infection du poumon profond	**infezione del tratto respiratorio inferiore (LRTI)**
infección de las vías respiratorias altas	infection des voies respiratoires supérieures	**infezione del tratto respiratorio superiore (URTI)**
infección oportunista	infection opportuniste	**infezione opportunista**
inflamación	inflammation	**infiammazione**
infiltración	infiltration	**infiltrazione**
influenza	grippe	**influenza**
afectar	affecter	**influenzare**
infusión	infusion	**infusione**
enyesado, vendaje de yeso	plâtre	**ingessatura**
ingestión	ingestion	**ingestione**
tragar	avaler	**inghiottire**
viable	viable	**in grado di vivere**
inguinal	inguinal	**inguinale**
ingle	aine	**inguine**
inhibidor de la monoaminooxidasa (IMAO)	inhibiteur de la monoamine-oxydase (IMAO)	**inibitore monoaminoossidasi (IMAO)**
inhibición	inhibition	**inibizione**
inyectar	injecter	**iniettare**
inyección	injection	**iniezione**
innato	endogène	**innato**
inervación	innervation	**innervazione**
colgajo, injerto	lambeau, greffe	**innesto**
inocente	innocent	**innocente**
inocuo	inoffensif	**innocuo**
inoculación	inoculation	**inoculazione**
inorgánico	inorganique	**inorganico**

inotropo	inotropic	inotrop
inseminazione	insemination	Befruchtung
inseminazione artificiale	artificial insemination (AI)	künstliche Befruchtung
insensibile	insensible	bewußtlos, unempfindlich
inserzione	insertion	Insertion
insidioso	insidious	heimtückisch, schleichend
in situ	in situ	in situ
insonnia '	insomnia	Schlaflosigkeit
inspessito	inspissated	kondensiert, eingedickt
inspirazione	inspiration	Inspiration, Einatmung
insufficienza cardiaca congestizia	congestive cardiac failure (CCF)	Stauungsherz, Herzinsuffizienz mit Stauungszeichen
insufficienza cardiaca coronarica	coronary heart failure (CHF)	Herzinfarkt
insufficienza coronarica cronica	chronic coronary insufficiency (CCI)	chronische Koronarinsuffizienz
insufficienza placentare	placental insufficiency	Plazentainsuffizienz
insufficienza respiratoria	respiratory failure	respiratorische Insuffizienz
insufficienza vertebrobasilare	vertebrobasilar insufficiency (VBI), basilar-vertebral insufficiency	vertebrobasiläre Insuffizienz, Basilarvertebralinsuffizienz
insufflazione	insufflation	Insufflation
insulina	insulin	Insulin
intelletto	intellect	Intellekt
intelligenza	intelligence	Intelligenz
interarticolare	interarticular	interartikulär
interazione	interaction	Wechselwirkung
intercorrente	intercurrent	interkurrent
intercostale	intercostal	interkostal
interleuchina	interleukin	Interleukin
intermestruale	intermenstrual	intermenstruel
intermittente	intermittent	intermittierend
interno	internal	intern, innerlich
interosseo	interosseous	interossär
interruzione di gravidanza (IG)	termination of pregnancy (TOP)	Schwangerschaftsabbruch
interspinoso	interspinous	interspinal
interstiziale	interstitial	interstitiell
intertrigine	intertrigo	Intertrigo
intertrocanterico	intertrochanteric	intertrochantär
intervento di Ramstedt	pyloromyotomy, Ramstedt's operation	Pyloromyotomie, Weber-Ramstedt-Operation, Ramstedt-(Weber)-Operation
intervento di Shirodkar	Shirodkar's operation	Shirodkar-Operation
intervertebrale	intervertebral	intervertebral, Zwischenwirbel-
intestinale	enteral	enteral
intestino	bowel, gut, intestine	Darm
intestino cieco	caecum (Eng), cecum (Am)	Zökum
intima	intima	Intima
intolleranza	intolerance	Intoleranz, Unverträglichkeit
intossicazione da piombo	plumbism	Bleivergiftung
intra-addominale	intra-abdominal	intraabdominal

SPANISH	FRENCH	ITALIAN
inotrópico	inotrope	inotropo
inseminación	insémination	inseminazione
inseminación artificial	insémination artificielle (IA)	inseminazione artificiale
insensible	insensible	insensibile
inserción	insertion	inserzione
insidioso	insidieux	insidioso
in situ	in situ	in situ
insomnio	insomnie	insonnia
espesado	épaissir	inspessito
inspiración	inspiration	inspirazione
insuficiencia cardíaca congestiva (ICC)	insuffisance cardiaque globale	insufficienza cardiaca congestizia
insuficiencia coronaria	insuffisance coronarienne cardiaque	insufficienza cardiaca coronarica
insuficiencia coronaria crónico	insuffisance coronarienne chronique	insufficienza coronarica cronica
insuficiencia placentaria	insuffisance placentaire	insufficienza placentare
insuficiencia respiratoria	insuffisance respiratoire	insufficienza respiratoria
insuficiencia vértebrobasilar	insuffisance vertébro-basilaire, insuffisance basilaire vertébrale	insufficienza vertebrobasilare
insuflación	insufflation	insufflazione
insulina	insuline	insulina
intelecto	intellect	intelletto
inteligencia	intelligence	intelligenza
interarticular	interarticulaire	interarticolare
interacción	interaction	interazione
intercurrente	intercurrent	intercorrente
intercostal	intercostal	intercostale
interleucina	interleukine	interleuchina
intermenstrual	intermenstruel	intermestruale
intermitente	intermittent	intermittente
interno	interne	interno
interóseo	interosseux	interosseo
interrupción del embarazo	interruption de grossesse (IG)	interruzione di gravidanza (IG)
interespinoso	interépineux	interspinoso
intersticial	interstitiel	interstiziale
intertrigo	intertrigo	intertrigine
intertrocantéreo	intertrochantérien	intertrocanterico
piloromiotomía, operación de Ramstedt	pylorotomie, opération de Ramstedt	intervento di Ramstedt
operación de Shirodkar	opération de Shirodkar	intervento di Shirodkar
intervertebral	intervertébral	intervertebrale
enteral	entéral	intestinale
intestino	intestin	intestino
ciego	caecum	intestino cieco
íntima	intima	intima
intolerancia	intolérance	intolleranza
plumbismo, saturnismo	saturnisme	intossicazione da piombo
intraabdominal	intra-abdominal	intra-addominale

ITALIAN	ENGLISH	GERMAN
intra-arterioso	intra-arterial	intraarteriell
intracapsulare	intracapsular	intrakapsulär
intracellulare	intracellular	intrazellulär
intradermico	intradermal	intradermal, intrakutan
intramurale	intramural	intramural
intramuscolare (IM)	intramuscular (IM)	intramuskulär
intranasale	intranasal	intranasal
intraoculare	intraocular	intraokulär
intraorale	intraoral	intraoral
intraparto	intrapartum	intra partum
intraperitoneale	intraperitoneal	intraperitoneal
intratecale	intrathecal	intrathekal
intrauterino	intrauterine	intrauterin
intravaginale	intravaginal	intravaginal
intrinseco	intrinsic	intrinsisch, endogen
introito	introitus	Introitus
introspezione	introspection	Introspektion
introversione	introversion	Introversion
introverso	introvert	Introvertierter
intubazione	intubation	Intubation
intussuscezione	intussusception	Intussuszeption
invaginazione	invagination	Invagination
invasione	invasion	Invasion
invecchiamento	ageing	Altern
inversione	inversion	Inversion, Umkehrung
in vitro	in vitro	in vitro
in vivo	in vivo	in vivo
involontario	involuntary	unabsichtlich, unwillkürlich
involuzione	involution	Involution, Rückbildung
iodio	iodine	Jod
ioide	hyoid	Os hyeoideum
ione	ion	Ion
iperacidità	hyperacidity	Hyperazidität
iperalgesia	hyperalgesia	Hyperalgesie
iperattività	hyperactivity	Überaktivität
iperbilirubinemia	hyperbilirubinaemia (Eng), hyperbilirubinemia (Am)	Hyperbilirubinämie
ipercalcemia	hypercalcaemia (Eng), hypercalcemia (Am)	Hyperkalzämie
ipercalciuria	hypercalciuria	Hyperkalziurie
ipercapnia	hypercapnia	Hyperkapnie
ipercolesterolemia	hypercholesterolaemia (Eng), hypercholesterolemia (Am)	Hypercholesterinämie
iperemesi	hyperemesis	Hyperemesis
iperemia	hyperaemia (Eng), hyperemia (Am)	Hyperämie
iperestensione	hyperextension	Überdehnung, Überstreckung
iperestesia	hyperaesthesia (Eng), hyperesthesia (Am)	Hyperästhesie

SPANISH	FRENCH	ITALIAN
intraarterial	intra-artériel	intra-arterioso
intracapsular	intracapsulaire	intracapsulare
intracelular	intracellulaire	intracellulare
intradérmico	intradermique	intradermico
intramural	intramural	intramurale
intramuscular (im)	intramusculaire (IM)	intramuscolare (IM)
intranasal	intranasal	intranasale
intraocular	intra-oculaire	intraoculare
intraoral	intra-oral	intraorale
intra partum	intrapartum	intraparto
intraperitoneal	intrapéritonéal	intraperitoneale
intratecal	intrathécal	intratecale
intrauterino	intra-utérin	intrauterino
intravaginal	intravaginal	intravaginale
intrínseco	intrinsèque	intrinseco
introito	orifice	introito
introspección	introspection	introspezione
introversión	introversion	introversione
introvertido	introverti	introverso
intubación	intubation	intubazione
intususcepción	intussusception	intussuscezione
invaginación	invagination	invaginazione
invasión	invasion	invasione
envejecimiento	vieillissement	invecchiamento
inversión	inversion	inversione
in vitro	in vitro	in vitro
in vivo	in vivo	in vivo
involuntario	involontaire	involontario
involución	involution	involuzione
yodo	iode	iodio
hioides	hyoïde	ioide
ión	ion	ione
hiperacidez	hyperacidité	iperacidità
hiperalgesia	hyperalgie, hyperalgésie	iperalgesia
hiperactividad	hyperactivité	iperattività
hiperbilirrubinemia	hyperbilirubinémie	iperbilirubinemia
hipercalcemia	hypercalcémie	ipercalcemia
hipercalciuria	hypercalciurie	ipercalciuria
hipercapnia	hypercapnie	ipercapnia
hipercolesterolemia	hypercholestérolémie	ipercolesterolemia
hiperemesis	hyperémèse	iperemesi
hiperemia	hyperémie	iperemia
hiperextensión	hyperextension	iperestensione
hiperestesia	hyperesthésie	iperestesia

ITALIAN	ENGLISH	GERMAN
iperflessione	hyperflexion	Hyperflexion
iperglicemia	hyperglycaemia (Eng), hyperglycemia (Am)	Hyperglykämie
iperidrosi	hyperidrosis	Hyperhidrosis
iperkaliemia	hyperkalaemia (Eng), hyperkalemia (Am)	Hyperkaliämie
iperlipemia	hyperlipaemia (Eng), hyperlipemia (Am)	Hyperlipämie
iperlipoproteinemia	hyperlipoproteinaemia (Eng), hyperlipoproteinemia (Am)	Hyperlipoproteinämie
ipermaturo	postmaturity	Überreife
ipermetropia	hypermetropia	Hypermetropie, Weitsichtigkeit
ipernefroma	hypernephroma	Hypernephrom
iperparatiroidismo	hyperparathyroidism	Hyperparathyreoidismus
iperpiressia	hyperpyrexia	Hyperpyrexie
iperplasia	hyperplasia	Hyperplasie
iperpnea	hyperpnea (Am), hyperpnoea (Eng)	Hyperpnoe
iperpotassiemia	hyperkalaemia (Eng), hyperkalemia (Am)	Hyperkaliämie
ipersensibilità	hypersensitive	Hypersensibilität, Überempfindlichkeit
ipersensitività	hypersensitive	Hypersensibilität, Überempfindlichkeit
ipertelorismo	hypertelorism	Hypertelorismus
ipertensione	hypertension	Hypertonie
ipertensione portale	portal hypertension	Pfortaderhochdruck
ipertermia	hyperthermia	Hyperthermie
ipertiroidismo	hyperthyroidism, thyrotoxicosis	Hyperthyreoidismus, Schilddrüsenüberfunktion, Thyreotoxikose
ipertonia	hypertonia	Hypertension, Hypertonus
ipertonia extrapiramidale	rigor	Rigor, Starre
ipertonico	hypertonic	hyperton
ipertrofia	hypertrophy	Hypertrophie
iperventilazione	hyperventilation	Hyperventilation
ipervolemia	hypervolaemia (Eng), hypervolemia (Am)	Hypervolämie
ipnosi	hypnosis	Hypnose
ipnoterapia	hypnotherapy	Hypnotherapie
ipnotico (n)	hypnotic (n), soporific (n)	Schlafmittel (n), Hypnotikum (n)
ipnotico (a)	hypnotic (a), soporific (a)	hypnotisch (a), einschläfernd (a)
ipocalcemia	hypocalcaemia (Eng), hypocalcemia (Am)	Hypokalzämie
ipocapnia	hypocapnia	Hypokapnie
ipocondria	hypochondria	Hypochondrie
ipocondrio	hypochondrium	Hypochondrium
ipocromico	hypochromic	hypochrom, farbarm
ipodermico	hypodermic	subkutan
ipoestesia	hypoaesthesia (Eng), hypoesthesia (Am)	Hypästhesie
ipofaringe	hypopharynx	Hypopharynx

702

hiperflexión	hyperflexion	**iperflessione**
hiperglucemia	hyperglycémic	**iperglicemia**
hiperhidrosis	hyperhidrose	**iperidrosi**
hipercaliemia	hyperkaliémie	**iperkaliemia**
hiperlipemia	hyperlipémie	**iperlipemia**
hiperlipoproteinemia	hyperlipoprotéinémie	**iperlipoproteinemia**
postmaduro	postmature	**ipermaturo**
hipermetropía	hypermétropie	**ipermetropia**
hipernefroma	hypernéphrome	**ipernefroma**
hiperparatiroidismo	hyperparathyroïdisme	**iperparatiroidismo**
hiperpirexia	hyperpyrexie	**iperpiressia**
hiperplasia	hyperplasie	**iperplasia**
hiperpnea	hyperpnoïa	**iperpnea**
hipercaliemia	hyperkaliémie	**iperpotassiemia**
hipersensibilidad	hypersensibilité	**ipersensibilità**
hipersensibilidad	hypersensibilité	**ipersensitività**
hipertelorismo	hypertélorisme	**ipertelorismo**
hipertensión	hypertension	**ipertensione**
hipertensión portal	circulation porte	**ipertensione portale**
hipertermia	hyperthermie	**ipertermia**
hipertiroidismo, tirotoxicosis	hyperthyroïdisme, thyrotoxicose	**ipertiroidismo**
hipertonía	hypertonie	**ipertonia**
rigor	rigor	**ipertonia extrapiramidale**
hipertónico	hypertonique	**ipertonico**
hipertrofia	hypertrophie	**ipertrofia**
hiperventilación	hyperventilation	**iperventilazione**
hipervolemia	hypervolémie	**ipervolemia**
hipnosis	hypnose	**ipnosi**
hipnoterapia	hypnothérapie	**ipnoterapia**
hipnótico (n), soporífero (n)	hypnotique (n), soporifique (n)	**ipnotico (n)**
hipnótico (a), soporífero (a)	hypnotique (n), soporifique (a)	**ipnotico (a)**
hipocalcemia	hypocalcémie	**ipocalcemia**
hipocapnia	hypocapnie	**ipocapnia**
hipocondría	hypocondrie	**ipocondria**
hipocondrio	hypocondre	**ipocondrio**
hipocrómico	hypochromique	**ipocromico**
hipodérmico	hypodermique	**ipodermico**
hipoestesia	hypoesthésie, hypesthésie	**ipoestesia**
hipofaringe	hypopharynx	**ipofaringe**

ITALIAN	ENGLISH	GERMAN
ipofisi	pituitary gland	Hypophyse
ipofunzione	hypofunction	Unterfunktion
ipogastrio	hypogastrium	Hypogastrium
ipoglicemia	hypoglycaemia (Eng), hypoglycemia (Am)	Hypoglykämie
ipoglosso	hypoglossal nerve	Nervus hypoglossus
ipoidrosi	hypoidrosis	Hypohidrosis, Schweißmangel
ipokalemia	hypokalaemia (Eng), hypokalemia (Am)	Hypokaliämie
ipomania	hypomania	Hypomanie
ipoparatiroidismo	hypoparathyroidism	Hypoparathyreoidismus
ipopion	hypopyon	Hypopyon
ipopituitarismo	hypopituitarism	Hypopituitarismus
ipoplasia	hypoplasia	Hypoplasie
ipopnea	hypopnea (Am), hypopnoea (Eng)	flache Atmung
ipoproteinemia	hypoproteinaemia (Eng), hypoproteinemia (Am)	Hypoproteinämie
iposecrezione	hyposecretion	Sekretionsmangel, Sekretionsschwäche
iposensibilità	hyposensitive	hyposensibel, unterempfindlich
iposensitività	hyposensitive	hyposensibel, unterempfindlich
ipospadia	hypospadias	Hypospadie
ipossia	hypoxia	Hypoxie
ipossiemia	hypoxaemia (Eng), hypoxemia (Am)	Hypoxämie
ipostasi	hypostasis	Hypostase
ipotalamo	hypothalamus	Hypothalamus
ipotensione	hypotension	Hypotonie
ipotermia	hypothermia	Hypothermie
ipotiroidismo	hypothyroidism	Hypothyreose
ipotonia	hypotonia	Hypotonie
ipotonico	hypotonic	hypoton
ipoventilazione	hypoventilation	Hypoventilation
ipovolemia	hypovolaemia (Eng), hypovolemia (Am)	Hypovolämie
ippocratismo	clubbing	Trommelschlegelfinger
ipsilaterale	ipsilateral	ipsilateral
iride	iris	Iris
irite	iritis	Iritis
irradiazione	irradiation	Bestrahlung
irriducibile	irreducible	unreduzierbar
irrigazione	irrigation	Spülung
irritabile	irritable	reizbar, erregbar
irritante	irritant	reizend
irsutismo	hirsuties, hirsutism	Hirsutismus
ischemia	ischaemia (Eng), ischemia (Am)	Ischämie
ischio	ischium	Ischium, Sitzbein
ischiorettale	ischiorectal	ischiorektal
isoimmunizzazione	isoimmunization	Isoimmunisierung

hipófisis	hypophyse	**ipofisi**
hipofunción	hypofonction	**ipofunzione**
hipogastrio	hypogastre	**ipogastrio**
hipoglucemia	hypoglycémie	**ipoglicemia**
hipogloso	hypoglosse	**ipoglosso**
hipohidrosis	hypohidrose	**ipoidrosi**
hipocaliemia	hypokalémie	**ipokalemia**
hipomanía	hypomanie	**ipomania**
hipoparatiroidismo	hypoparathyroïdisme	**ipoparatiroidismo**
hipopión	hypopyon	**ipopion**
hipopituitarismo	hypopituitarisme	**ipopituitarismo**
hipoplasia	hypoplasie	**ipoplasia**
hipopnea	hypopnée	**ipopnea**
hipoproteinemia	hypoprotéinémie	**ipoproteinemia**
hiposecreción	hyposécrétion	**iposecrezione**
hiposensibilidad	hyposensibilité	**iposensibilità**
hiposensibilidad	hyposensibilité	**iposensitività**
hipospadias	hypospadias	**ipospadia**
hipoxia	hypoxie	**ipossia**
hipoxemia	hypoxémie	**ipossiemia**
hipostasis	hypostase	**ipostasi**
hipotálamo	hypothalamus	**ipotalamo**
hipotensión	hypotension	**ipotensione**
hipotermia	hypothermie	**ipotermia**
hipotiroidismo	hypothyroïdisme	**ipotiroidismo**
hipotonía	hypotonie	**ipotonia**
hipotónico	hypotonique	**ipotonico**
hipoventilación	hypoventilation	**ipoventilazione**
hipovolemia	hypovolémie	**ipovolemia**
dedos en palillo de tambor, dedos hipocráticos	hippocratisme digital	**ippocratismo**
ipsilateral	ipsilatéral	**ipsilaterale**
iris	iris	**iride**
iritis	iritis	**irite**
irradiación	irradiation	**irradiazione**
irreductible	irréductible	**irriducibile**
irrigación	irrigation	**irrigazione**
irritable	irritable	**irritabile**
irritante	irritant	**irritante**
hirsutismo	hirsutisme	**irsutismo**
isquemia	ischémie	**ischemia**
isquión	ischion	**ischio**
isquiorrectal	ischio-rectal	**ischiorettale**
isoinmunización	iso-immunisation	**isoimmunizzazione**

ITALIAN	ENGLISH	GERMAN
isolamento	barrier nursing, isolation	Isolierung (auf Isolierstation)
isole di Langerhans	islets of Langerhans	Langerhans-Inseln
isolotti pancreatici	pancreatic islets	Langerhans-Inseln
isometrico	isometric	isometrisch
isotonico	isotonic	isotonisch
isterectomia	hysterectomy	Hysterektomie
isteria	hysteria	Hysterie
isterosalpingectomia	hysterosalpingectomy	Hysterosalpingektomie
isterosalpingografia	hysterosalpingography	Hysterosalpingographie
isterotomia	hysterotomy	Hysterotomie
istillazione	instillation	Einträufelung, Einflößung
istinto	instinct	Instinkt
istiocito	histiocyte	Histiozyt
istiocitoma	histiocytoma	Histiozytom
istituzionalizzazione	institutionalization	Institutionalisierung
istmo	isthmus	Isthmus, Verengung
istolisi	histolysis	Histolyse
istologia	histology	Histologie
ittero	icterus, jaundice	Ikterus, Gelbsucht
ittero dei neonati	haemolytic disease of the newborn (HDN) (Eng), hemolytic disease of the newborn (HDN) (Am)	Morbus haemolyticus neonatorum
ittero nucleare	kernicterus	Kernikterus
ittiosi	ichthyosis	Ichthyosis

K

kala-azar	kala-azar	Kala-Azar
kwashiorkor	kwashiorkor	Kwashiorkor

SPANISH	FRENCH	ITALIAN
enfermería por aislamiento, aislamiento	nursage de protection, isolement	isolamento
islotes de Langerhans	îlots de Langerhans, îlots pancréatiques	isole di Langerhans
islotes pancreáticos	îlots pancréatiques, îlots de Langerhans	isolotti pancreatici
isométrico	isométrique	isometrico
isotónico	isotonique	isotonico
histerectomía	hystérectomie	isterectomia
histeria	hystérie	isteria
histerosalpingectomía	hystérosalpingectomie	isterosalpingectomia
histerosalpingografía	hystérosalpingographie	isterosalpingografia
histerotomía	hystérotomie	isterotomia
instilación	instillation	istillazione
instinto	instinct	istinto
histiocito	histiocyte	istiocito
histiocitoma	histiocytome	istiocitoma
institucionalización	institutionalisation	istituzionalizzazione
istmo	isthme	istmo
histólisis	histolyse	istolisi
histología	histologie	istologia
ictericia	ictère, jaunisse	ittero
enfermedad hemolítica del recién nacido	hémolyse des nouveau-nés	ittero dei neonati
ictericia nuclear	ictère cérébral	ittero nucleare
ictiosis	ichthyose	ittiosi
kala-azar	kala-azar	kala-azar
kwashiorkor	kwashiorkor	kwashiorkor

L

Italian	English	German
labbra	labia	Labia
labbro	lip	Lippe
labbro leporino	harelip	Hasenscharte
labialis	cold sore	Herpes
labile	labile	labil
labilità	lability	Labilität
labirintite	labyrinthitis	Labyrinthitis
labirinto	labyrinth	Labyrinth
laccio emostatico	tourniquet	Tourniquet
lacerato	lacerated	eingerissen, zerrissen
lacrimale	lacrimal	Tränen-, Tränengangs-
lacrime	tears	Tränen
lamina	lamina	Lamina
laminectomia	laminectomy	Laminektomie, Wirbelbogenresektion
lanugine	lanugo	Lanugo
laparoscopia	laparoscopy	Laparoskopie, Bauchspiegelung
laparotomia	laparotomy	Laparotomie
laringe	larynx	Larynx, Kehlkopf
laringeo	laryngeal	laryngeal, Kehlkopf-
laringite	laryngitis	Laryngitis
laringologia	laryngology	Laryngologie
laringoscopio	laryngoscope	Laryngoskop, Kehlkopfspiegel
laringospasmo	laryngospasm	Laryngospasmus
laringotracheobronchite	laryngotracheobronchitis	Laryngo-Tracheobronchitis
larva	maggot	Larve, Made
laser	laser	Laser
lassativo (n)	aperient (n), laxative (n), purgative (n)	Abführmittel (n), Laxans (n), Purgativum (n)
lassativo (a)	aperient (a), laxative (a)	abführend (a), laxierend (a)
laterale	lateral	lateral, seitlich
lattasi	lactase	Laktase
lattato	lactate	Laktat
lattazione	lactation	Laktation, Milchbildung, Stillen
latte	milk	Milch
lattosio	lactose	Laktose, Milchzucker
lattulosio	lactulose	Laktulose
lavaggio	lavage	Spülung
lavanda vaginale	douche	Dusche, Spülung
lebbra	leprosy	Lepra, Aussatz
lecitina	lecithin	Lezithin
legame	bonding	Bindung
legamento largo	broad ligament	ligamentum latum uteri
legare	ligate	abbinden
legato al sesso	sex-linked	geschlechtsgebunden
legatura	ligature	Ligatur, Gefäßunterbindung

SPANISH	FRENCH	ITALIAN
labios	lèvres	labbra
labio	lèvre	labbro
labio leporino	bec-de-lièvre	labbro leporino
herpes labial	herpès	labialis
lábil	labile	labile
labilidad	labilité	labilità
laberintitis	labyrinthite	labirintite
laberinto	labyrinthe	labirinto
torniquete	tourniquet	laccio emostatico
lacerado	lacéré	lacerato
lagrimal	lacrymal	lacrimale
lágrimas	larmes	lacrime
lámina	lame	lamina
laminectomía	laminectomie	laminectomia
lanugo	lanugo	lanugine
laparoscopia	coelioscopie	laparoscopia
laparotomía	laparotomie	laparotomia
laringe	larynx	laringe
laríngeo	laryngien	laringeo
laringitis	laryngite	laringite
laringología	laryngologie	laringologia
laringoscopio	laryngoscope	laringoscopio
laringospasmo	laryngospasme	laringospasmo
laringotraqueobronquitis	laryngotrachéobronchite	laringotracheobronchite
antojo	asticot	larva
láser	laser	laser
laxante (n), purga (n)	laxatif (n), purgatif (n)	lassativo (n)
laxante (a), laxativo (a)	laxatif (a)	lassativo (a)
lateral	latéral	laterale
lactasa	lactase	lattasi
lactato	lactate	lattato
lactación	lactation	lattazione
leche	lait	latte
lactosa	lactose	lattosio
lactulosa	lactulose	lattulosio
lavado	lavage	lavaggio
ducha	douche	lavanda vaginale
lepra	lèpre	lebbra
lecitina	lécithine	lecitina
vinculación	attachement	legame
ligamento ancho	ligaments larges	legamento largo
ligar	ligaturer	legare
vinculado al sexo	lié au sexe	legato al sesso
ligadura	ligature	legatura

ITALIAN	ENGLISH	GERMAN
leiomioma dell'utero	myoma	Myom
leishmaniosi	leishmaniasis	Leishmaniose
lembo	flap	Lappen, Hautlappen
lendine	nit	Nisse
lente	lens	Linse
lente a contatto	contact lens	Kontaktlinse
lentiggine	lentigo	Lentigo
leptospirosi	leptospirosis	Leptospirose
lesbismo	lesbian	lesbisch
lesione	injury, lesion	Verletzung, Läsion
lesione non accidentale	non-accidental injury (NAI)	nicht unfallbedingte Verletzung
letale	lethal	letal, tödlich
letargia	lethargy	Lethargie
leucemia	leukaemia (Eng), leukemia (Am)	Leukämie
leucocito	leucocyte (Eng), leukocyte (Am)	Leukozyt
leucocitosi	leucocytosis (Eng), leukocytosis (Am)	Leukozytose
leucopenia	leucopenia (Eng), leukopenia (Am)	Leukopenie
leucoplachia	leucoplakia (Eng), leukoplakia (Am)	Leukoplakie
leucorrea	leucorrhea (Eng), leukorrhea (Am)	Leukorrhoe
leucotomia	leucotomy (Eng), leukotomy (Am)	Leukotomie
levatrice	midwife	Hebamme
libbre per pollici quadrati	pounds per square inch (psi)	pounds per square inch (psi)
lichene	lichen	Lichen
lichenificazione	lichenification	Lichenifikation
lievito	yeast	Hefe, Hefepilz
ligamento	ligament	Ligament, Band
linea	linea	Linea, Linie
linfa	lymph	Lymphe
linfadenite	lymphadenitis	Lymphadenitis
linfadenite tubercolare	scrofula	Skrofula, Lymphknotentuberkulose
linfadenopatia	lymphadenopathy	Lymphadenopathie
linfangite	lymphangitis	Lymphangitis
linfatico	lymphatic	lymphatisch, Lymph-
linfedema	lymphedema (Am), lymphoedema (Eng)	Lymphödem
linfoadenectomia	lymphadenectomy	Lymphadenektomie
linfoblasto	lymphoblast	Lymphoblast
linfochina	lymphokine	Lymphokine
linfocito	lymphocyte	Lymphozyt
linfocitosi	lymphocytosis	Lymphozytose
linfogranuloma inguinale	lymphogranuloma inguinale	Lymphogranuloma inguinale
linfoma	lymphoma	Lymphom
linfonodo	lymph node	Lymphknoten
linfosarcoma	lymphosarcoma	Lymphosarkom
lingua	glossa, tongue	Zunge
linimento	liniment	Liniment, Einreibemittel
lipasi	lipase	Lipase

SPANISH	FRENCH	ITALIAN
mioma	myome	leiomioma dell'utero
leishmaniasis	leishmaniose	leishmaniosi
colgajo, injerto	lambeau	lembo
liendre	lente	lendine
cristalino	lentille	lente
lente de contacto	verre de contact	lente a contatto
lentigo	lentigo	lentiggine
leptospirosis	leptospirose	leptospirosi
lesbiana	lesbien	lesbismo
lesión	blessure, lésion	lesione
lesión no accidental	traumatisme non accidentel	lesione non accidentale
letal	létal, léthal	letale
letargo	léthargie	letargia
leucemia	leucémie	leucemia
leucocito	leucocyte	leucocito
leucocitosis	leucocytose	leucocitosi
leucopenia	leucopénie	leucopenia
leucoplasia	leucoplasie	leucoplachia
leucorrea	leucorrhée	leucorrea
leucotomía	leucotomie	leucotomia
comadrona	sage-femme	levatrice
libras por pulgada cuadrada (psi)	livres par pouce carré (psi)	libbre per pollici quadrati
líquen	lichen	lichene
liquenificación	lichénification	lichenificazione
levadura	levure	lievito
ligamento	ligament	ligamento
línea	ligne	linea
linfa	lymphe	linfa
linfadenitis	lymphadénite	linfadenite
escrófula	scrofule	linfadenite tubercolare
linfadenopatía	lymphadénopathie	linfadenopatia
linfangitis	lymphangite	linfangite
linfático	lymphatique	linfatico
linfedema	lymphoedème	linfedema
linfadenectomía	lymphadénectomie	linfoadenectomia
linfoblasto	lymphoblaste	linfoblasto
linfocinesis	lymphokine	linfochina
linfocito	lymphocyte	linfocito
linfocitosis	lymphocytose	linfocitosi
linfogranuloma inguinal	lymphogranulome vénérien	linfogranuloma inguinale
linfoma	lymphome	linfoma
ganglio linfático	ganglion lymphatique	linfonodo
linfosarcoma	lymphosarcome	linfosarcoma
lengua	langue	lingua
linimento	liniment	linimento
lipasa	lipase	lipasi

ITALIAN	ENGLISH	GERMAN
lipemia	lipaemia (Eng), lipemia (Am)	Lipämie
lipide	lipid	Lipid
lipocondrodistrofia	lipochondrodystrophy	Lipochondrodystrophie
lipodistrofia	lipodystrophy	Lipodystrophie
lipoidosi	lipidosis	Lipidose
lipolisi	lipolysis	Lipolyse
lipoma	lipoma	Lipom
lipoproteina	lipoprotein	Lipoprotein
lipoproteina a bassa densità (LBD)	low density lipoprotein (LDL)	low density lipoprotein (LDL)
lipoproteina a bassissima densità	very low density lipoprotein (VLDL)	Lipoprotein sehr geringer Dichte
lipoproteina ad alta densità (LAD)	high density lipoprotein (HDL)	high density lipoprotein (HDL)
lipotrofico	lipotrophic	lipotroph
liquido	liquor	Liquor, Flüssigkeit
liquido cerebrospinale (LCS)	cerebrospinal fluid (CSF)	Liquor
liquido sinoviale	synovial fluid	Synovialflüssigkeit
lisi	lysis	Lysis
lisosoma	lysosome	Lysosom
lisozima	lysozyme	Lysozym
lista d'attesa	waiting list	Warteliste
litonefrotomia	lithonephrotomy	Nephrolithotomie
litotomia	lithotomy	Lithotomie
litotripsia	lithotripsy	Lithotripsie
litotritore	lithotriptor, lithotrite	Lithotriptor
livido	livid	livide, bleich
lobectomia	lobectomy	Lobektomie, Lungenlappenresektion
lobo	lobe	Lappen (Organ-)
lobotomia	lobotomy	Lobotomie, Leukotomie
lobulo	lobule	Lobulus, Läppchen
locale	topical	topisch, örtlich
localizzare	localize	lokalisieren
lochi puerperali	lochia	Lochien, Wochenfluß
locomotore	locomotor	fortbewegend, Bewegungs-
loculato	loculated	gekammert
lombaggine	lumbago	Lumbago, Hexenschuß
lombare	lumbar	Lumbal-, Lenden-
lombosacrale	lumbosacral	lumbosakral
lordosi	lordosis	Lordose
lucido	lucid	glänzend, bei Bewußtsein
lume	lumen	Lumen, Durchmesser
lupus	lupus	Lupus
lupus eritematoso	lupus erythematosus	Lupus erythematodes
lupus eritematoso sistemico (LES)	systemic lupus erythematosus (SLE)	systemischer Lupus erythematodes, Lupus erythematodes visceralis (SLE)
luteo	luteum	Luteom, Luteinom

SPANISH	FRENCH	ITALIAN
lipemia	lipémie	lipemia
lípido	lipide	lipide
lipocondrodistrofia	maladie de Hurler, lipochondrodystrophie	lipocondrodistrofia
lipodistrofia	lipodystrophie	lipodistrofia
lipidosis	lipidose, dyslipoïdose	lipoidosi
lipolisis	lipolyse	lipolisi
lipoma	lipome	lipoma
lipoproteína	lipoprotéine	lipoproteina
lipoproteína de baja densidad (LDL)	lipoprotéine de basse densité (LBD)	lipoproteina a bassa densità (LBD)
lipoproteína de muy baja densidad (VLDL)	lipoprotéine de très faible densité	lipoproteina a bassissima densità
lipoproteína de alta densidad (HDL)	lipoprotéine de haute densité (LHD)	lipoproteina ad alta densità (LAD)
lipotrófico	hormone lipotrope hypophysaire	lipotrofico
licor	liquide	liquido
líquido cefalorraquídeo (LCR)	liquide céphalo-rachidien	liquido cerebrospinale (LCS)
líquido sinovial	fluide synovial	liquido sinoviale
lisis	lyse	lisi
lisosoma	lysosome	lisosoma
lisozima	lysozyme	lisozima
lista de espera	liste d'attente	lista d'attesa
litonefrotomía	lithonéphrotomie	litonefrotomia
litotomía	lithotomie	litotomia
litotripsia	lithotripsie, lithotritie	litotripsia
litotriptor, litotritor	lithotriteur	litotritore
lívido	livide	livido
lobectomía	lobectomie	lobectomia
lóbulo	lobe	lobo
lobotomía	lobotomie	lobotomia
lóbulo	lobule	lobulo
tópico	topique	locale
localizar	localiser	localizzare
loquios	lochies	lochi puerperali
locomotor	locomoteur	locomotore
loculado	loculé	loculato
lumbago	lumbago	lombaggine
lumbar	lombaire	lombare
lumbosacro	lombo-sacré	lombosacrale
lordosis	lordose	lordosi
lúcido	lucide	lucido
luz	lumière	lume
lupus	lupus	lupus
lupus eritematoso	lupus érythémateux	lupus eritematoso
lupus eritematoso sistémico (LES)	lupus érythémateux systémique	lupus eritematoso sistemico (LES)
lúteo	corps jaune	luteo

M

Italian	English	German
macchina cuore-polmone	heart-lung machine	Herzlungenmaschine
macerazione	maceration	Mazeration
macrocefalia	macrocephaly	Makrozephalie
macrocito	macrocyte	Makrozyt
macrofago	macrophage	Phagozyt
macroscopico	macroscopic	makroskopisch
macula	macula, macule	Makula, Fleck
maculopapulare	maculopapular	makulopapulär
malacia	malacia	Malazie, Erweichung
malare	malar	Backe betr, Backen-
malaria	malaria	Malaria
malassorbimento	malabsorption	Malabsorption
malathion	malathion	Malathion
malattia	disease, illness, mal	Krankheit, Leiden, Übel
malattia a trasmissione sessuale (STD)	sexually transmitted disease (STD)	Geschlechtskrankheit
malattia autoimmune	autoimmune disease	Autoimmunerkrankung
malattia cardiaca	heart disease	Herzerkrankung, Herzleiden
malattia cardiaca coronarica (MCC)	coronary heart disease (CHD)	koronare Herzkrankheit (KHK)
malattia da denunciare alle autorità sanitarie	notifiable disease	meldepflichtige Erkrankung
malattia dei legionari	legionnaires' disease	Legionärskrankheit
malattia delle arterie coronarica (MAC)	coronary artery disease (CAD)	Koronaropathie
malattia delle membrane ialine	hyaline membrane disease	Hyalinmembrankrankheit
malattia di Bornholm	Bornholm disease	Bornholm-Krankheit
malattia di Crohn	Crohn's disease	Morbus Crohn
malattia di Friedreich	Friedreich's ataxia	Friedreich Ataxie
malattia di Hirschsprung	Hirschsprung's disease	Hirschsprung-Krankheit
malattia di Hodgkin	Hodgkin's disease	Morbus Hodgkin
malattia di Lyme	Lyme disease	Lyme-Arthritis, Lyme-Borreliose
malattia di Osgood-Schlatter	Osgood-Schlatter disease	Osgood-Schlatter-Krankheit
malattia di Paget	Paget's disease	Morbus Paget
malattia di Perthes	Perthes' disease	Perthes-Krankheit
malattia di Peyronie	Peyronie's disease	Induratio penis plastica
malattia di Pott	Pott's disease	Malum Potti
malattia di Rayer	xanthoma	Xanthom
malattia di Raynaud	Raynaud's disease	Raynaud-Krankheit
malattia di Schlatter	Schlatter's disease	Schlatter-Krankheit
malattia di Still	Still's disease	Still-Krankheit
malattia di Tay-Sachs	Tay-Sachs disease	Tay-Sachs-Krankheit
malattia di von Recklinghausen	von Recklinghausen's disease	Morbus von Recklinghausen
malattia di von Willebrand	von Willebrand's disease	Willebrand-Krankheit
malattia di Weil	Weil's disease	Weil Krankheit
malattia di Wilson	Wilson's disease	Wilson-Krankheit

máquina de circulación extracorpórea	poumon d'acier	macchina cuore-polmone
maceración	macération	macerazione
macrocefalia	macrocéphalie	macrocefalia
macrocito	macrocyte	macrocito
macrófago	macrophage	macrofago
macroscópico	macroscopique	macroscopico
mácula	macule	macula
maculopapular	maculopapuleux	maculopapulare
malacia	malacie	malacia
malar	malaire	malare
paludismo	paludisme	malaria
malabsorción	malabsorption	malassorbimento
malathion	malathion	malathion
enfermedad, mal	maladie, mal	malattia
enfermedad de transmisión sexual (ETS)	maladie sexuellement transmissible (MST)	malattia a trasmissione sessuale (STD)
enfermedad autoinmune	maladie auto-immune	malattia autoimmune
cardiopatía	insuffisance cardiaque	malattia cardiaca
enfermedad coronaria, cardiopatía isquémica	insuffisance coronarienne cardiaque	malattia cardiaca coronarica (MCC)
enfermedad declarable	maladie à déclaration obligatoire	malattia da denunciare alle autorità sanitarie
enfermedad del legionario	maladie des légionnaires	malattia dei legionari
enfermadad arterial coronaria, cardiopatía isquémica	coronaropathie, cardiopathie ischémique, insuffisance coronarienne globale	malattia delle arterie coronarica (MAC)
enfermedad de la membrana hialina	maladie des membranes hyalines	malattia delle membrane ialine
enfermedad de Bornholm	maladie de Bornholm	malattia di Bornholm
enfermedad de Crohn	mal de Crohn	malattia di Crohn
ataxia de Friedreich	maladie de Friedreich	malattia di Friedreich
enfermedad de Hirschsprung	maladie de Hirschsprung	malattia di Hirschsprung
enfermedad de Hodgkin	maladie de Hodgkin	malattia di Hodgkin
enfermedad de Lyme	arthrite de Lyme, maladie de Lyme	malattia di Lyme
enfermedad de Osgood-Schlatter	maladie d'Osgood-Schlatter	malattia di Osgood-Schlatter
enfermedad de Paget	maladie de Paget	malattia di Paget
enfermedad de Perthes	coxa plana	malattia di Perthes
enfermedad de Peyronie	maladie de La Peyronie	malattia di Peyronie
enfermedad de Pott	mal de Pott	malattia di Pott
xantoma	xanthome	malattia di Rayer
enfermedad de Raynaud	maladie de Raynaud	malattia di Raynaud
enfermedad de Schlatter	maladie d'Osgood-Schlatter	malattia di Schlatter
enfermedad de Still	maladie de Still	malattia di Still
enfermedad de Tay-Sachs	maladie de Tay-Sachs	malattia di Tay-Sachs
enfermedad de von Recklinghausen	maladie de von Recklinghausen	malattia di von Recklinghausen
enfermedad de von Willebrand	maladie de von Willebrand	malattia di von Willebrand
enfermedad de Weil	maladie de Weil	malattia di Weil
enfermedad de Wilson	maladie de Wilson	malattia di Wilson

malattia emorragica del neonato	haemorrhagic disease of the newborn (Eng), hemorrhagic disease of the newborn (Am)	Morbus haemorrhagicus neonatorum
malattia fibrocistica del pancreas	cystic fibrosis (CF)	Mukoviszidose
malattia industriale	industrial disease	Berufskrankheit
malattia infettiva	infectious disease	Infektionskrankheit
malattia infiammatoria della pelvi (PID)	pelvic inflammatory disease (PID)	Salpingitis
malattia ostruttiva cronica delle vie respiratorie	chronic obstructive airway disease (COAD)	chronische obstruktive Lungenerkrankung
malattia professionale	occupational disease	Berufskrankheit
malattia respiratoria acuta febbrile	acute febrile respiratory disease/illness (AFRD/I)	Atemwegsinfekt (akut fieberhaft)
malattia tropicale	tropical disease	Tropenkrankheit
malattia venerea (MV)	venereal disease (VD)	Geschlechtskrankheit
mal di montagna	altitude sickness	Höhenkrankheit
mal di testa	headache	Kopfschmerzen
male	mal	Übel, Leiden
malessere	malaise	Unwohlsein
malessere mattutino	morning sickness	morgendliche Übelkeit der Schwangeren
malformazione	malformation	Mißbildung
maligno	malignant	maligne, bösartig
malleolo	malleolus	Malleolus, Knöchel
malnutrizione	malnutrition	Unterernährung, Fehlernährung
malocclusione	malocclusion	Malokklusion
malposizione	malposition	Lageanomalie
maltosio	maltose	Maltose
maltrattamento a bambini	child abuse	Kindesmißhandlung
mammella	breast	Brust
mammografia	mammography	Mammographie
mammoplastica	mammoplasty	Mammaplastik
mancino	left-handed	linkshändig
mandibola	mandible	Mandibula, Unterkiefer
mania	mania	Manie
manipolazione	manipulation	Manipulation, Handhabung
mano	hand	Hand
mantenimento delle funzioni vitali	basic life support	Vitalfunktionserhaltung
manubrio	manubrium	Manubrium
marasma	marasmus	Marasmus
marasma infantile	failure to thrive (FTT)	Gedeihstörung
marchio depositato	proprietary name	Markenname
marsupializzazione	marsupialization	Marsupialisation
martello	malleus	Malleus, Hammer
mascella superiore	maxilla	Maxilla, Oberkieferknochen
massaggio	massage	Massage
mastalgia	mastalgia	Mastodynie
mastectomia	mastectomy	Mastektomie, Brustamputation

SPANISH	FRENCH	ITALIAN
enfermedad hemorrágica neonatal	hémorragies des nouveau-nés	malattia emorragica del neonato
fibrosis quística	fibrose cystique	malattia fibrocistica del pancreas
enfermedad industrial	maladie professionnelle	malattia industriale
enfermedad infecciosa	maladie infectieuse	malattia infettiva
enfermedad inflamatoria de la pelvis	pelvipéritonite	malattia infiammatoria della pelvi (PID)
enfermedad obstructiva crónica de las vias respiratorias	bronchopneumopathie chronique obstructive, syndrome respiratoire	malattia ostruttiva cronica delle vie respiratorie
enfermedad profesional	maladie professionnelle	malattia professionale
enfermedad respiratoria febril aguda	affection/maladie respiratoire fébrile aiguë	malattia respiratoria acuta febbrile
enfermedad tropical	maladie tropicale	malattia tropicale
enfermedad venérea	maladie vénérienne (MV)	malattia venerea (MV)
mal de altura	mal d'altitude, mal des montagnes	mal di montagna
cefalea	mal de tète, céphalée	mal di testa
mal	mal	male
destemplanza, malestar	malaise	malessere
náuseas matinales	nausées matinales	malessere mattutino
malformación	malformation	malformazione
maligno	malin	maligno
maléolo	malléole	malleolo
desnutrición	malnutrition	malnutrizione
maloclusión	malocclusion	malocclusione
malposición	malposition	malposizione
maltosa	maltose	maltosio
abuso de menores	sévices infligés aux enfants, martyre d'enfants	maltrattamento a bambini
mama, pecho	sein	mammella
mamografía	mammographie	mammografia
mamoplastia	mammoplastie	mammoplastica
zurdo	gaucher	mancino
mandíbula	mandibule	mandibola
manía	manie	mania
manipulación	manipulation	manipolazione
mano	main	mano
soporte de vida básico	équipement de survie	mantenimento delle funzioni vitali
manubrio	manubrium	manubrio
marasmo	athrepsie	marasma
desmedro, marasmo	absence de développement pondéro-statural normal	marasma infantile
nombre de patente	nom de marque	marchio depositato
marsupialización	marsupialisation	marsupializzazione
martillo	marteau	martello
maxilar	maxillaire	mascella superiore
masaje	massage	massaggio
mastalgia	mastalgie, mammalgie	mastalgia
mastectomía	mastectomie	mastectomia

ITALIAN	ENGLISH	GERMAN
mastectomia parziale	lumpectomy	Lumpektomie
masticazione	mastication	Kauen, Kauvermögen
mastite	mastitis	Mastitis, Brustdrüsenentzündung
mastoide	mastoid	mastoideus
mastoidectomia	mastoidectomy	Mastoidektomie
mastoideo	mastoid	mastoideus
mastoidite	mastoiditis	Mastoiditis
masturbazione	masturbation	Masturbation, Selbstbefriedigung
matrice	matrix	Matrix
maxillofacciale	maxillofacial	maxillofazial
meconio	meconium	Mekonium
mediale	medial	medial
mediano	median	Median-
mediastinite	mediastinitis	Mediastinitis
mediastino	mediastinum	Mediastinum
medicamento	medicament	Medikament, Arzneimittel
medicamentoso	medicated	medizinisch
medicato	medicated	medizinisch
medicazione	dressing	Verband, Umschlag
medicazione di ferita	wound dressing	Verbandmaterial
medicina	medicine	Medizin, Arznei
medicina alternativa	alternative medicine	Alternativmedizin
medicina complementare	complementary medicine	komplementäre Medizin
medicina del lavoro	occupational health	Gewerbehygiene
medicina forense	forensic medicine	Gerichtsmedizin, Rechtsmedizin
medicinale	drug	Arzneimittel, Rauschgift
medico	doctor, physician	Arzt
medico generico	generic	Substanznahme, Generic
medico legale	coroner	Leichenbeschauer
medicolegale	medicolegal	rechtsmedizinisch
medicosociale	medicosocial	sozialmedizinisch
medulloblastoma	medulloblastoma	Medulloblastom
megacolon	megacolon	Megacoloncongenitum, Hirschsprung-Krankheit
megaloblasto	megaloblast	Megaloblast
meiosi	meiosis	Meiose
melanconia	melancholia	Melancholie
melanina	melanin	Melanin
melanoma	melanoma	Melanom
melena	melaena (Eng), melena (Am)	Meläna, Blutstuhl
membrana	membrane	Membran
membrana cellulare	cell membrane	Zellmembran
membrana sierosa	serosa	Serosa
membrana sinoviale	synovial membrane	Synovia
membrane fetali e placenta	afterbirth	Plazenta, Nachgeburt

SPANISH	FRENCH	ITALIAN
exéresis de tumores benignos de la mama	exérèse locale d'une tumeur du sein	mastectomia parziale
masticación	mastication	masticazione
mastitis	mastite	mastite
mastoideo	mastoïde	mastoide
mastoidectomía	mastoïdectomie	mastoidectomia
mastoideo	mastoïde	mastoideo
mastoiditis	mastoïdite	mastoidite
masturbación	masturbation	masturbazione
matriz	matrice	matrice
maxilofacial	maxillofacial	maxillofacciale
meconio	méconium	meconio
medial	interne	mediale
mediana	médian	mediano
mediastinitis	médiastinite	mediastinite
mediastino	médiastin	mediastino
medicamento	médicament	medicamento
medicado	médicamenté	medicamentoso
medicado	médicamenté	medicato
cura, vendaje	pansement	medicazione
curas para heridas	pansements	medicazione di ferita
medicina	médecine	medicina
medicina alternativa	médecine complémentaire	medicina alternativa
medicina complementaria	traitement complémentaire	medicina complementare
higiene profesional	hygiène du travail	medicina del lavoro
medicina forense	médecine légale	medicina forense
fármaco	médicament	medicinale
médico, facultativo	médecin	medico
genérico	dénomination commune d'un médicament	medico generico
médico forense	médecin légiste	medico legale
médicolegal	médico-légal	medicolegale
médicosocial	médico-social	medicosociale
meduloblastoma	médulloblastome	medulloblastoma
megacolon	mégacôlon	megacolon
megaloblasto	mégaloblaste	megaloblasto
meiossis	méiose	meiosi
melancolía	mélancolie	melanconia
melanina	mélanine	melanina
melanoma	mélanome	melanoma
melena	méléna	melena
membrana	membrane	membrana
membrana celular	membrane cellulaire	membrana cellulare
serosa	séreuse	membrana sierosa
membrana sinovial	membrane synoviale	membrana sinoviale
secundinas, expulsión de la placenta y membranas	arrière faix	membrane fetali e placenta

membro	leg	Bein
memoria	memory, recall	Gedächtnis, Erinnerungsvermögen, Errinerung
menarca	menarche	Menarche
meningi	meninges	Meningen, Hirnhäute
meningioma	meningioma	Meningiom
meningismo	meningism	Meningismus
meningite	meningitis	Meningitis, Gehirnhautentzündung
meningocele	meningocele	Meningozele
meningoencefalite	meningoencephalitis	Meningoenzephalitis
meningomielocele	meningomyelocele	Meningomyelozele
meniscectomia	meniscectomy	Meniskusentfernung
menisco	meniscus	Meniskus
menopausa	menopause	Menopause, Wechseljahre
menorragia	menorrhagia	Menorrhagie
menorrea	menorrhea (Am), menorrhoea (Eng)	Monatsblutung, Menstruation
mentale	mental	geistig, seelisch
mentalmente sano	compos mentis	zurechnungsfähig
mento	chin, mentum	Kinn
mentoanteriore	mentoanterior	mentoanterior
mentoposteriore	mentoposterior	mentoposterior
mercurio	mercury	Quecksilber
mesencefelo	midbrain	Mittelhirn
mesentere	mesentery	Mesenterium
mesotelioma	mesothelioma	Mesotheliom
mestruale	menstrual	menstruell
mestruazione	menstruation	Menstruation, Monatsblutung
metabolico	metabolic	metabolisch, Stoffwechsel-
metabolismo	metabolism	Metabolismus, Stoffwechsel
metabolita	metabolite	Metabolit, Stoffwechselprodukt
metacarpo	metacarpus	Metakarpus, Mittelhand
metacarpofalangeo	metacarpophalangeal	metakarpophalangeal
metastasi	metastasis	Metastase
metatarsalgia	metatarsalgia	Metatarsalgie
metatarso	metatarsus	Metatarsus, Mittelfuß
metatarsofalangeo	metatarsophalangeal	metatarsophalangeal
metemoglobina	methaemoglobin (Eng), methemoglobin (Am)	Methämoglobin
metemoglobinemia	methaemoglobinaemia (Eng), methemoglobinemia (Am)	Methämoglobinämie
metilcellulosa	methylcellulose	Methylzellulose
metropatia emorragica	metropathia haemorrhagica (Eng), metropathia hemorrhagica (Am)	Metropathia haemorrhagica
metrorragia	metrorrhagia	Metrorrhagie, Zwischenblutung
mezzo	medium	Medium
mialgia	myalgia	Myalgie, Muskelschmerz
mialgia epidemica	Bornholm disease	Bornholm-Krankheit
miastenia	myasthenia	Myasthenie, Muskelschwäche

SPANISH	FRENCH	ITALIAN
pierna	jambe	membro
memoria, recuerdo	mémoire, évocation	memoria
menarquía	établissement de la menstruation	menarca
meninges	méninges	meningi
meningioma	méningiome	meningioma
meningismo	méningisme	meningismo
meningitis	méningite	meningite
meningocele	méningocèle	meningocele
meningoencefalitis	méningo-encéphalite	meningoencefalite
mielomeningocele	méningomyélocèle	meningomielocele
meniscectomía	méniscectomie	meniscectomia
menisco	ménisque	menisco
menopausia	ménopause	menopausa
menorragia	ménorrhagie	menorragia
menorrea	ménorrhée	menorrea
mental	mental	mentale
compos mentis, de espíritu sano	compos mentis	mentalmente sano
barbilla, mentón	menton	mento
mentoanterior	posture antéromentonnière	mentoanteriore
mentoposterior	posture postmentonnière	mentoposteriore
mercurio	mercure	mercurio
mesencéfalo	mésencéphale	mesencefelo
mesenterio	mésentère	mesentere
mesotelioma	mésothéliome	mesotelioma
menstrual	menstruel	mestruale
menstruación	menstruation	mestruazione
metabólico	métabolique	metabolico
metabolismo	métabolisme	metabolismo
metabolito	métabolite	metabolita
metacarpo	métacarpe	metacarpo
metacarpofalángico	métacarpophalangien	metacarpofalangeo
metástasis	métastase	metastasi
metatarsalgia	métatarsalgie	metatarsalgia
metatarso	métatarse	metatarso
metatarsofalángico	métatarsophalangien	metatarsofalangeo
metahemoglobina	méthémoglobine	metemoglobina
metahemoglobinemia	méthémoglobinémie	metemoglobinemia
metilcelulosa	méthylcellulose	metilcellulosa
metropatía hemorrágica	métropathie hémorragique	metropatia emorragica
metrorragia	métrorragie	metrorragia
medio	milieu	mezzo
mialgia	myalgie	mialgia
enfermedad de Bornholm	maladie de Bornholm	mialgia epidemica
miastenia	myasthénie	miastenia

micosi	mycosis	Mykose, Pilzinfektion
microbiologia	microbiology	Mikrobiologie
microcefalia	microcephaly	Mikrozephalie
microchirurgia	microsurgery	Mikrochirurgie
microcircolazione	microcirculation	Mikrozirkulation
microcita	microcyte	Mikrozyt
microcitoma	oat cell cancer	kleinzelliges Bronchialkarzinom
microfilaria	microfilaria	Mikrofilarie
microoganismo	microorganism	Mikroorganismus
microscopico	microscopic	mikroskopisch
microscopio	microscope	Mikroskop
microscopio chirurgico	operating microscope	Operationsmikroskop
microvilli	microvilli	Mikrovilli
midollo	medulla	Medulla, Mark
midollo osseo	bone marrow	Knochenmark
midriasi	mydriasis	Mydriasis, Pupillenerweiterung
midriatico (n)	mydriatic (n)	Mydriatikum (n)
midriatico (a)	mydriatic (a)	mydriatisch (a), pupillenerweiternd (a)
mielina	myelin	Myelin
mielite	myelitis	Myelitis
mielofibrosi	myelofibrosis	Myelofibrose
mielografia	myelography	Myelographie
mieloide	myeloid	myeloisch
mieloma	myeloma	Myelom
mielomatosi	myelomatosis	Myelomatose
mielopatia	myelopathy	Myelopathie
miglioramento	amelioration	Besserung
miliare	miliary	miliar
miliaria	miliaria	Miliaria
milliequivalente (mEq)	milliequivalent (mEq)	Milli-Äquivalent
milza	spleen	Milz
minaccia d'aborto	threatened abortion	drohender Abort
mineralcorticoide	mineralocorticoid	Mineralokortikoid
minorato	handicap	Behinderung
minzione	micturition	Wasserlassen, Blasenentleerung
miocardio	myocardium	Myokard, Herzmuskel
miocardite	myocarditis	Myokarditis, Herzmuskelentzündung
mioma	myoma	Myom
miomectomia	myomectomy	Myomektomie
miometrio	myometrium	Myometrium
miopatia	myopathy	Myopathie, Muskelerkrankung
miope	myope	Myoper, Kurzsichtiger
miopia	myopia	Myopie, Kurzsichtigkeit
miosi	miosis	Miosis, Pupillenverengung
miosite	myofibrosis, myositis	Myofibrose, Myositis
miringotomia	myringotomy	Parazentese
misuratore del flusso espiratorio massimo	peak expiratory flow meter (PEFM)	Peak-Flowmeter

SPANISH	FRENCH	ITALIAN
micosis	mycose	micosi
microbiología	microbiologie	microbiologia
microcefalia	microcéphalie	microcefalia
microcirugía	microchirurgie	microchirurgia
microcirculación	microcirculation	microcircolazione
microcito	microcyte	microcita
carcinoma de células de avena	épithélioma à petites cellules	microcitoma
microfilaria	microfilaire	microfilaria
microorganismo	micro-organisme	microoganismo
microscópico	microscopique	microscopico
microscopio	microscope	microscopio
microscopio quirúrgico	microscope opératoire	microscopio chirurgico
microvellosidad	micropoils	microvilli
médula	moelle	midollo
médula ósea	moelle osseuse	midollo osseo
midriasis	mydriase	midriasi
midriático (n)	mydriatique (n)	midriatico (n)
midriático (a)	mydriatique (a)	midriatico (a)
mielina	myéline	mielina
mielitis	myélite	mielite
mielofibrosis	myélofibrose	mielofibrosi
mielografía	myélographie	mielografia
mieloide	myéloïde	mieloide
mieloma	myélome	mieloma
mielomatosis	myélomatose	mielomatosi
mielopatía	myélopathie	mielopatia
mejoría	amélioration	miglioramento
miliar	miliaire	miliare
miliaria	miliaire	miliaria
miliequivalente (mEq)	milliéquivalent (mEq)	milliequivalente (mEq)
bazo	rate	milza
amenaza de aborto	risque d'avortement	minaccia d'aborto
mineralocorticoide	minéralocorticoïde	mineralcorticoide
disminución, minusvalía	handicapé	minorato
micción	micturition	minzione
miocardio	myocarde	miocardio
miocarditis	myocardite	miocardite
mioma	myome	mioma
miomectomía	myomectomie	miomectomia
miometrio	myomètre	miometrio
miopatía	myopathie	miopatia
miope	myope	miope
miopía	myopie	miopia
miosis	myosis	miosi
miofibrosis, miositis	myofibrose, myosite	miosite
miringotomía	myringotomie	miringotomia
medida de la velocidad máxima del flujo espiratorio	appareil de mesure du débit expiratoire de pointe	misuratore del flusso espiratorio massimo

ITALIAN	ENGLISH	GERMAN
mitocondrio	mitochondrion	Mitochondrium
mitosi	mitosis	Mitose
mitrale	mitral	mitral
mitralico	mitral	mitral
mixedema	myxedema (Am), myxoedema (Eng)	Myxödem
mixoma	myxoma	Myxom
mobile	motile	bewegungsfähig, beweglich
molare	molar	molar
molecula	molecule	Molekül
mollusco	molluscum	Molluscum
mongoloidismo	Down's syndrome	Down-Syndrom, Mongolismus
monocromatico	monochromat	Monochromat, monochrom Farbenblinder
monoculare	uniocular	einäugig
mononucleare	mononuclear	mononukleär
mononucleosi	mononucleosis	Mononukleose, Pfeiffersches Drüsenfieber
mononucleosi infettiva	glandular fever, infectious mononucleosis	Mononukleose, Pfeiffersches Drüsenfieber, infektiöse Mononukleose
monoplegia	monoplegia	Monoplegie
morbilità	morbidity	Morbidität, Krankhaftigkeit
morbilliforme	morbilliform	morbilliform, masernähnlich
morbillo	measles	Masern
morbo di Addison	Addison's disease	Addison Krankheit
morbo di Alzheimer	Alzheimer's disease	Alzheimer Krankheit
morbo di Graves	Graves' disease	Basedow-Krankheit
morfologia	morphology	Morphologie
moribondo	moribund	moribund, sterbend
mortalità	mortality	Mortalität, Sterblichkeit
morte	death	Tod, Todesfall
morto	dead	tot
motore	motor	motorisch
movimento	motion	Bewegung, Stuhlgang
movimento oculare rapido	rapid eye movement (REM)	rapid eye movement (REM)
mucina	mucin	Muzin
mucocele	mucocele (Am), mucocoele (Eng)	Mukozele
mucocutaneo	mucocutaneous	mukokutan
mucoide	mucoid	mukoid
mucolitico	mucolytic	schleimlösendes Mittel
mucopolisaccaridosi	mucopolysaccharidosis	Mukopolysaccharidose
mucopurulento	mucopurulent	mukopurulent, schleimig-eitrig
mucosa	mucosa	Mukosa, Schleimhaut
mucoso	mucous (Eng), mucus (Am)	mukös, schleimig
mucoviscidosi	cystic fibrosis (CF)	Mukoviszidose
mughetto	thrush	Soor, Sprue
multiloculare	multilocular	multilokulär
murale	mural	mural

SPANISH	FRENCH	ITALIAN
mitocondria	mitochondrie	**mitocondrio**
mitosis	mitose	**mitosi**
mitral	mitral	**mitrale**
mitral	mitral	**mitralico**
mixedema	myxoedème	**mixedema**
mixoma	myxome	**mixoma**
móvil	mobile	**mobile**
molar	molaire	**molare**
molécula	molécule	**molecula**
molusco	molluscum	**mollusco**
síndrome de Down	trisomie 21	**mongoloidismo**
monocromato	monochromat	**monocromatico**
uniocular	unioculé	**monoculare**
mononuclear	mononucléaire	**mononucleare**
mononucleosis	mononucléose	**mononucleosi**
fiebre glandular, mononucleosis infecciosa	fièvre glandulaire, mononucléose infectieuse	**mononucleosi infettiva**
monoplegia	monoplégie	**monoplegia**
morbilidad	morbidité	**morbilità**
morbiliforme	morbilliforme	**morbilliforme**
sarampión	rougeole	**morbillo**
enfermedad de Addison	maladie d'Addison	**morbo di Addison**
enfermedad de Alzheimer	maladie d'Alzheimer	**morbo di Alzheimer**
enfermedad de Graves	goitre exophtalmique	**morbo di Graves**
morfología	morphologie	**morfologia**
moribundo	moribond	**moribondo**
mortalidad	mortalité	**mortalità**
muerte	mort	**morte**
muerto	mort	**morto**
motor	moteur	**motore**
movimiento	mouvement	**movimento**
movimiento rápido de los ojos (REM)	période des mouvements oculaires	**movimento oculare rapido**
mucina	mucine	**mucina**
mucocele	mucocèle	**mucocele**
mucocutáneo	mucocutané	**mucocutaneo**
mucoide	mucoïde	**mucoide**
mucolítico	mucolytique	**mucolitico**
mucopolisacaridosis	mucopolysaccharidose	**mucopolisaccaridosi**
mucopurulento	mucopurulent	**mucopurulento**
mucosa	muqueuse	**mucosa**
moco	muqueux	**mucoso**
fibrosis quística	fibrose cystique	**mucoviscidosi**
muguet	aphte	**mughetto**
multilocular	multiloculaire	**multiloculare**
mural	pariétal	**murale**

ITALIAN	ENGLISH	GERMAN
muscoli glutei	gluteus muscles	Glutealmuskulatur, Gesäßmuskulatur
muscoli peronei	peroneus muscles	Musculi peronei
muscoli trapezi	trapezius muscles	Musculi trapezii
muscolo	muscle	Muskel
muscolocutaneo	musculocutaneous	muskulokutan
muscolo elevatore	levator	Levator
muscolo rotatore	rotator	Rotator
muscoloscheletrico	musculoskeletal	Skelettmuskulatur betr
muscolo sternocleidomastoideo	sternocleidomastoid muscle	Musculus sternocleidomastoideus
mutageno	mutagen	Mutagen
mutante	mutant	Mutante
mutazione	mutation	Mutation
mutilazione	mutilation	Verstümmelung
mutismo	mutism	Mutismus, Stummheit
myxovirus	myxovirus	Myxovirus

SPANISH	FRENCH	ITALIAN
músculos glúteos	muscles fessiers	muscoli glutei
músculos peroneos	muscles péroniers	muscoli peronei
músculos trapecios	muscles trapèzes	muscoli trapezi
músculo	muscle	muscolo
musculocutáneo	musculo-cutané	muscolocutaneo
elevador	releveur	muscolo elevatore
rotatorio	rotateur	muscolo rotatore
muscoloesquelético	musculo-squelettique	muscoloscheletrico
músculo esternocleidomastoideo	muscle sternocléidomastoïdien	muscolo sternocleidomastoideo
mutágeno	mutagène	mutageno
mutante	mutant	mutante
mutación	mutation	mutazione
mutilación	mutilation	mutilazione
mutismo	mutisme	mutismo
mixovirus	myxovirus	myxovirus

N

nanismo	dwarfism	Zwergwuchs
narcolessia	narcolepsy	Narkolepsie
narcosi	narcosis	Narkose, Anästhesie
narcotico (n)	narcotic (n)	Narkosemittel (n), Betäubungsmittel (n), Rauschgift (n)
narcotico (a)	narcotic (a)	narkotisch (a)
narice	nostril	Nasenloch
nasale	nasal	nasal
nascita	birth	Geburt
naso	nose	Nase
nasofaringe	nasopharynx	Nasopharynx, Nasenrachenraum
nasogastrico	nasogastric	nasogastrisch
nasolacrimale	nasolacrimal	nasolakrimal
natica	breech, buttock	Steiß, Gesäß, Gesäßbacke
nato morto	stillborn	totgeboren
nausea	nausea	Nausea, Übelkeit, Brechreiz
nauseabondo	queasy	unwohl, übel
nauseato	queasy	unwohl, übel
nebulizzatore	nebulizer	Zerstäuber, Vernebler
nebulizzatore per farmaci	spinhaler	Drehinhaliergerät
necrosi	necrosis	Nekrose
necrosi tubulare	tubular necrosis	Tubulusnekrose
nefrectomia	nephrectomy	Nephrektomie
nefrite	nephritis	Nephritis, Nierenentzündung
nefrogenico	nephrogenic	nephrogen
nefrologia	nephrology	Nephrologie
nefrone	nephron	Nephron
nefropatia	nephrosis	Nephrose
nefrosi	nephrosis	Nephrose
nefrostomia	nephrostomy	Nephrostomie
nefrotossico	nephrotoxic	nephrotoxisch, nierenschädigend
negligenza	negligence	Nachlässigkeit
nematelminto	roundworm	Rundwurm, Spulwurm
nematode	nematode	Nematode, Fadenwurm
neo	mole	Mole, Muttermal
neonato (n)	neonate (n), newborn (n)	Neugeborenes (n)
neonato (a)	neonate (a), newborn (a)	neugeboren (a)
neoplasia	neoplasia	Neoplasie
neoplasia intraepiteliale della cervice uterina (CIN)	cervical intraepithelial neoplasia (CIN)	zervikale intraepitheliale Neoplasie (CIN)
neoplasia maligna	malignancy	Malignität, Bösartigkeit
neoplasia primitiva	primary care	Primärversorgung
neoplasma	neoplasm	Neoplasma, Tumor
nervi vasomotori	vasomotor nerves	vasomotorische Nerven
nervo	nerve	Nerv

SPANISH	FRENCH	ITALIAN
enanismo	nanisme	nanismo
narcolepsia	narcolepsie	narcolessia
narcosis	narcose	narcosi
narcótico (n)	narcotique (n)	narcotico (n)
narcótico (a)	narcotique (a)	narcotico (a)
fosa nasale	narine	narice
nasal	nasal	nasale
nacimiento, parto	naissance	nascita
nariz	nez	naso
nasofaringe	rhinopharynx	nasofaringe
nasogástrico	nasogastrique	nasogastrico
nasolacrimal	nasolacrymal	nasolacrimale
nalgas, nalga	siège, fesse	natica
mortinato, nacido muerto	mort-né	nato morto
náusea	nausée	nausea
nauseabundo	indigeste, délicat	nauseabondo
nauseabundo	indigeste, délicat	nauseato
nebulizador	nébuliseur	nebulizzatore
inhalador spinhaler	turbo-inhalateur	nebulizzatore per farmaci
necrosis	nécrose	necrosi
necrosis tubular	nécrose tubulaire	necrosi tubulare
nefrectomía	néphrectomie	nefrectomia
nefritis	néphrite	nefrite
nefrógeno	d'origine rénale	nefrogenico
nefrología	néphrologie	nefrologia
nefrona	néphron	nefrone
nefrosis	néphrose	nefropatia
nefrosis	néphrose	nefrosi
nefrostomía	néphrostomie	nefrostomia
nefrotóxico	néphrotoxique	nefrotossico
negligencia	négligence	negligenza
áscaris	ascaris	nematelminto
nematodo	nématode	nematode
nevo	naevus	neo
neonato (n)	nouveau-né (n)	neonato (n)
neonato (a)	nouveau-né (a)	neonato (a)
neoplasia	néoplasie	neoplasia
neoplasia intraepitelial cervical	néoplasie intra-épithéliale cervicale	neoplasia intraepiteliale della cervice uterina (CIN)
malignidad	malignité	neoplasia maligna
asistencia primaria	soins de santé primaires	neoplasia primitiva
neoplasma	néoplasme	neoplasma
nervios vasomotores	nerfs vasomoteurs	nervi vasomotori
nervio	nerf	nervo

ITALIAN	ENGLISH	GERMAN
nervo craniale	cranial nerve	Hirnnerv
nervo motore	motor nerve	motorischer Nerv
nervo peroneo	peroneal nerve	Nervus peroneus
nervo sciatico	sciatic nerve	Ischiasnerv, Nervus ischiadicus
neurale	neural	neural
neurilemma	neurolemma	Neurolemm
neurite	neuritis	Neuritis, Nervenentzündung
neuroaprassia	neurapraxia	Neurapraxie
neuroastenia	neurasthenia	Neurasthenie
neuroblastoma	neuroblastoma	Neuroblastom
neurochirurgia	neurosurgery	Neurochirurgie
neurofarmacologia	neuropharmacology	Neuropharmakologie
neurofibromatosi	neurofibromatosis, von Recklinghausen's disease	Neurofibromatose, Morbus von Recklinghausen
neurogenico	neurogenic	neurogen
neurolettico (n)	neuroleptic (n)	Neuroleptikum (n)
neurolettico (a)	neuroleptic (a)	neuroleptisch (a)
neurologia	neurology	Neurologie
neuromuscolare	neuromuscular	neuromuskulär
neurone	neuron	Neuron
neurone motore	motor neurone	Motoneuron
neuropatia	neuropathy	Neuropathie
neuropsichiatria	neuropsychiatry	Neuropsychiatrie
neurosensoriale	sensorineural	Sinne u Nerven betr
neurosifilide	neurosyphilis	Neurosyphilis
neurotropo	neurotropic	neurotrop
neutrofilo	neutrophil	neutrophil
neutropenia	neutropenia	Neutropenie
nevo	naevus (Eng), nevus (Am)	Nävus, Muttermal
nevo congenito	birthmark	Muttermal, Storchenbiß
nevralgia	nephralgia, neuralgia	Nephralgie, Neuralgie
nevralgia del trigemino	tic douloureux	Tic douloureux
nevrosi	neurosis	Neurose
nevrosi ossessiva	obsessional neurosis	Zwangsneurose
nicotina	nicotine	Nikotin
nictalgia	nyctalgia	Nyktalgie
nicturia	nocturia, nycturia	Nykturie
nido	nidus	Nidus
nistagmo	nystagmus	Nystagmus
nodo	node	Knoten
nodo sinoatriale	sinoatrial node	Sinusknoten
noduli di Osler	Osler's nodes	Osler-Knötchen
nodulo	nodule	Nodulus, Knötchen
non ancora diagnosticato	not yet diagnosed (NYD)	noch nicht diagnostiziert
non invasivo	non-invasive	nichtinvasiv
noradrenalina	noradrenaline	Noradrenalin
norepinefrina	norepinephrine	Norepinephrin, Noradrenalin

SPANISH	FRENCH	ITALIAN
nervio craneal	nerf crânien	**nervo craniale**
nervio motor	nerf moteur	**nervo motore**
nervio peroneo	nerf péronier	**nervo peroneo**
nervio ciático	nerf grand sciatique	**nervo sciatico**
nervioso	neural	**neurale**
neurolema	neurilemme	**neurilemma**
neuritis	névrite	**neurite**
neuropraxia	neurapraxie	**neuroaprassia**
neurastenia	neurasthénie	**neuroastenia**
neuroblastoma	neuroblastome	**neuroblastoma**
neurocirugía	neurochirurgie	**neurochirurgia**
neurofarmacología	neuropharmacologie	**neurofarmacologia**
neurofibromatosis, enfermedad de von Recklinghausen	neurofibromatose, maladie de von Recklinghausen	**neurofibromatosi**
neurógeno	neurogène	**neurogenico**
neuroléptico (n)	neuroleptique (n)	**neurolettico (n)**
neuroléptico (a)	neuroleptique (a)	**neurolettico (a)**
neurología	neurologie	**neurologia**
neuromuscular	neuromusculaire	**neuromuscolare**
neurona	neurone	**neurone**
neurona motora	neurone moteur	**neurone motore**
neuropatia	neuropathie	**neuropatia**
neuropsiquiatría	neuropsychiatrie	**neuropsichiatria**
sensorineural	de perception	**neurosensoriale**
neurosífilis	neurosyphilis	**neurosifilide**
neurotrópico	neurotrope	**neurotropo**
neutrófilo	neutrophile	**neutrofilo**
neutropenia	neutropénie	**neutropenia**
nevo	naevus	**nevo**
mancha de nacimiento	naevus, envie	**nevo congenito**
nefralgia, neuralgia	néphralgie, névralgie	**nevralgia**
tic doloroso	tic douloureux	**nevralgia del trigemino**
neurosis	névrose	**nevrosi**
neurosis obsesiva	névrose obsessionnelle	**nevrosi ossessiva**
nicotina	nicotine	**nicotina**
nictalgia	nyctalgie	**nictalgia**
nicturia	nycturie	**nicturia**
nido	foyer morbide	**nido**
nistagmo	nystagmus	**nistagmo**
nodo	noeud	**nodo**
nodo sinoauricular	noeud sinusal de Keith et Flack	**nodo sinoatriale**
nódulos de Osler	nodules d'Osler	**noduli di Osler**
nódulo	nodule	**nodulo**
todavía no diagnosticado	non encore diagnostiqué	**non ancora diagnosticato**
no invasivo	non invasif	**non invasivo**
noradrenalina	noradrénaline	**noradrenalina**
norepinefrina	norépinéphrine, noradrénaline	**norepinefrina**

ITALIAN	ENGLISH	GERMAN
normoblasto	normoblast	Normoblast
normocito	normocyte	Normozyt
normoglicemico	normoglycaemic (Eng), normoglycemic (Am)	Normoglykämie
normotonico	normotonic	normoton
notocorda	cord	Strang, Schnur, Ligament
notturno	nocturnal	nächtlich, Nacht-
nuca	nape	Nacken
nucleo	nucleus	Nukleus, Kern
nullipara	nullipara	Nullipara
numero di gravidanze pregresse	parity	Gebärfähigkeit, Ähnlichkeit
nutriente	nutrient	nahrhaft
nutrizione	nutrition	Ernährung
nutrizione parenterale totale	total parenteral nutrition (TPN)	parenterale Ernährung

SPANISH	FRENCH	ITALIAN
normoblasto	normoblaste	normoblasto
normocito	normocyte	normocito
normoglucémico	normoglycémique	normoglicemico
normotónico	normotonique	normotonico
cordón, cuerda, médula espinal	cordon	notocorda
nocturno	nocturne	notturno
nuca	nuque	nuca
núcleo	noyau	nucleo
nulípara	nullipare	nullipara
paridad	parité	numero di gravidanze pregresse
nutriente	nourricier	nutriente
nutrición	nutrition	nutrizione
nutrición parenteral total	alimentation parentérale totale	nutrizione parenterale totale

O

obesità	obesity	Adipositas, Obesitas
occhio	eye	Auge
occipitale	occipital	okzipital
occipite	occiput	Okziput, Hinterkopf
occipitoanteriore	occipitoanterior	vordere Hinterhauptslage
occipitoanteriore sinistro (OAS)	left occipito-anterior (LOA)	linke vordere Hinterhauptslage
occipitofrontale	occipitofrontal	okzipitofrontal
occipitoposteriore	occipitoposterior	hintere Hinterhauptslage
occlusione	occlusion	Okklusion, Verschluß
occlusione intestinale acuta	ileus	Ileus, Darmverschluß
occulto	occult	okkult
oculare	ocular	okular
oculogiro	oculogyric	Bewegung der Augen betr
oculomotore	oculomotor	Oculomotorius-
odontoiatria	dentistry	Zahnheilkunde, Zahntechnik
odontoide	odontoid	odontoid
oftalmia	ophthalmia	Ophthalmie
oftalmico	ophthalmic	Augen-
oftalmologia	ophthalmology	Ophthalmologie, Augenheilkunde
oftalmoplegia	ophthalmoplegia	Ophthalmoplegie, Augenmuskellähmung
oftalmoscopio	ophthalmoscope	Ophthalmoskop, Augenspiegel
olecrano	olecranon (process)	Olekranon, Ellenbozen
olfattorio	olfactory	olfaktorisch
oligoemia	oligaemia (Eng), oligemia (Am)	Oligämie, Blutmangel
oligomenorrea	oligomenorrhea (Am), oligomenorrhoea (Eng)	Oligomenorrhoe
oliguria	oliguria	Oligurie
ombelico	navel, umbilicus	Nabel
omento	omentum	Omentum, Netz
omeopatia	homeopathy (Am), homoeopathy (Eng)	Homöopathie
omeostasi	homeostasis	Homöostase
omero	humerus	Humerus, Oberarmknochen
omicidio	homicide	Totschlag, Mord
omogeneo	homogeneous (Eng), homogenous (Am)	homogen
omolaterale	ipsilateral	ipsilateral
omologo	homologous	homolog
omonimo	homonymous	homonym
omosessuale (n)	homosexual (n)	Homosexueller (n)
omosessuale (a)	homosexual (a)	homosexuell (a)
omozigote	homozygous	homozygot
oncocerchiasi	onchocerciasis, river blindness	Onchozerkose, Flußblindheit
oncogene	oncogene	Onkogen
oncologia	oncology	Onkologie

SPANISH	FRENCH	ITALIAN
obesidad	obésité	obesità
ojo	oeil	occhio
occipital	occipital	occipitale
occipucio	occiput	occipite
occipitoanterior	occipito-antérieur	occipitoanteriore
occipito anterior izquierdo	occipito-antérieur gauche	occipitoanteriore sinistro (OAS)
occipitofrontal	occipito-frontal	occipitofrontale
occipitoposterior	occipito-postérieur	occipitoposteriore
oclusión	occlusion	occlusione
íleo	iléus	occlusione intestinale acuta
oculta	occulte	occulto
ocular	oculaire	oculare
oculógiro	oculogyre	oculogiro
oculomotor	oculomoteur	oculomotore
odontologia	médecine dentaire, dentisterie	odontoiatria
odontoides	odontoïde	odontoide
oftalmía	ophtalmie	oftalmia
oftálmico	ophtalmique	oftalmico
oftalmología	ophtalmologie	oftalmologia
oftalmoplejía	ophtalmoplégie	oftalmoplegia
oftalmoscopio	ophtalmoscope	oftalmoscopio
olécranon	olécrane	olecrano
olfatorio	olfactif	olfattorio
oligohemia	hypovolémie	oligoemia
oligomenorrea	spanioménorrhée	oligomenorrea
oliguria	oligurie	oliguria
ombligo	nombril	ombelico
epiplón	épiploon	omento
homeopatía	homéopathie	omeopatia
homeostasis	homéostasie	omeostasi
húmero	humérus	omero
homicidio	homicide	omicidio
homogéneo	homogène	omogeneo
ipsilateral	ipsilatéral	omolaterale
homólogo	homologue	omologo
homónimo	homonyme	omonimo
homosexual (n)	homosexuel (n)	omosessuale (n)
homosexual (a)	homosexuel (a)	omosessuale (a)
homocigoto	homozygote	omozigote
oncocerciasis, oncocerciasis ocular	onchocercose, cécité des rivières	oncocerchiasi
oncogén	oncogène	oncogene
oncología	oncologie	oncologia

ITALIAN	ENGLISH	GERMAN
onicogrifosi	onychogryphosis	Onychogryposis
onicolisi	onycholysis	Onycholyse, Nagelablösung
ooforectomia	oophorectomy	Oophorektomie
opacità	opacity	Opazität
opaco	opaque	undurchsichtig, verschattet (radiolog)
operazione	operation	Operation, Einwirkung, Eingriff
operazione di Billroth	Billroth's operation	Billroth-Magenresektion
operazione di Caldwell-Luc	Caldwell-Luc operation	Caldwell-Luc-Operation
optimum	optimum	optimal
orale	oral	oral
orbita	orbit	Orbita, Augenhöhle
orchidectomia	orchidectomy, orchidotomy	Orchidektomie, Orchidotomie
orchidopessia	orchidopexy, orchiopexy	Orchidopexie, Orchipexie
orchite	orchitis	Orchitis
orecchio	ear	Ohr
orecchio naso e gola	ear nose and throat (ENT)	Hals- Nasen- Ohren-
organico	organic	organisch
organi genitali	genitalia	Genitalien
organismo	organism	Organismus, Keim
orgasmo	orgasm	Orgasmus
orientamento	orientation	Orientierung
orifizio	orifice, stoma	Öffnung, Stoma, Mund
origine	origin	Ursprung
ormone	hormone	Hormon
ormone corticosurrenale	adrenal cortical hormone (ACH)	Nebennierenrindenhormon (ACH)
ormone corticotropo (ACTH)	adrenocorticotrophic hormone (ACTH)	adrenokortikotropes Hormon (ACTH)
ormone della crescita (GH)	growth hormone (GH)	Wachstumshormon
ormone follicolostimolante (FSH)	follicle stimulating hormone (FSH)	follikelstimulierendes Hormon (FSH)
ormone luteinizzante (LH)	luteinizing hormone (LH)	luteinisierendes Hormon
ormone tireotropo (TSH)	thyroid stimulating hormone (TSH)	Thyreotropin
orofaringe	oropharynx	Mundrachenhöhle
orticaria	hives, nettle rash, urticaria	Ausschlag, Nesselfieber, Urtikaria, Nesselsucht
ortodonzia	orthodontics	Kieferorthopädie
ortopedia	orthopaedic (Eng), orthopedic (Am)	orthopädisch
ortopnea	orthopnea (Am), orthopnoea (Eng)	Orthopnoe
ortostatico	orthostatic	orthostatisch
ortottica	orthoptics	Orthoptik
orzaiolo	stye	Hordeolum, Gerstenkorn
oscillazione	oscillation	Oszillation, Schwankung
osmolalità	osmolality	Osmolalität
osmolarità	osmolarity	Osmolarität
osmosi	osmosis	Osmose
ospedale	hospital	Krankenhaus, Hospital
ospedale diurno	day hospital	Tagesklinik

736

SPANISH	FRENCH	ITALIAN
onicogriposis	onychogryphose	onicogrifosi
onicólisis	onycholyse	onicolisi
ooforectomía	ovariectomie	ooforectomia
opacidad	opacité	opacità
opaco	opaque	opaco
intervención quirúrgica	opération	operazione
operación de Billroth	opération de Billroth	operazione di Billroth
operación de Caldwell-Luc	opération de Caldwell-Luc	operazione di Caldwell-Luc
óptimo	optimum	optimum
oral	oral	orale
órbita	orbite	orbita
orquidectomía, orquidotomía	orchidectomie, orchodotomie	orchidectomia
orquidopexia, orquiopexia	orchidopexie	orchidopessia
orquitis	orchite	orchite
oído	oreille	orecchio
otorrinolaringología (ORL)	oto-rhino-laryngologie (ORL)	orecchio naso e gola
orgánico	organique	organico
genitales	organes génitaux	organi genitali
organismo	organisme	organismo
orgasmo	orgasme	orgasmo
orientación	orientation	orientamento
orificio, estoma	orifice, stoma	orifizio
origen	origine	origine
hormona	hormone	ormone
hormona corticosuprarrenal (HCS)	hormone cortico-surrénale	ormone corticosurrenale
hormona adrenocorticotropa (ACTH)	hormone adrénocorticotrope (ACTH)	ormone corticotropo (ACTH)
hormona del crecimiento (HC)	hormone de croissance (HGH), somatotrophine (STH)	ormone della crescita (GH)
hormona estimulante del folículo (FSH)	hormone folliculo-stimulante, gonadotrophine A	ormone follicolostimolante (FSH)
hormona luteinizante (LH)	hormone lutéinisante (HL)	ormone luteinizzante (LH)
hormona estimulante del tiroides (TSH)	thyrotrophine, thyréostimuline	ormone tireotropo (TSH)
orofaringe	oropharynx	orofaringe
urticaria	éruption, urticaire	orticaria
ortodoncia	orthodontie	ortodonzia
ortopedia	orthopédique	ortopedia
ortopnea	orthopnée	ortopnea
ortostático	orthostatique	ortostatico
ortóptica	orthoptique	ortottica
orzuelo	orgelet	orzaiolo
oscilación	oscillation	oscillazione
osmolalidad	osmolalité	osmolalità
osmolaridad	osmolarité	osmolarità
osmosis	osmose	osmosi
hospital	hôpital	ospedale
hospital de día	hôpital de jour	ospedale diurno

ITALIAN	ENGLISH	GERMAN
ospite	host	Wirt
osseo	osseous	knöchern, Knochen-
ossicino	ossicle	Gehörknöchelchen, Ossikel
ossidazione	oxidation	Oxydation
ossigenazione	oxygenation	Sauerstoffsättigung, Oxygenierung
ossigenoterapia iperbarica	hyperbaric oxygen treatment	hyperbare Sauerstoffbehandlung
ossitocina	oxytocin	Oxytozin
ossiuro	threadworm	Fadenwurm
osso	bone	Knochen, Gräte
osso dell'anca	ilium	Os ilium
osso iliaco	hip bone	Hüftknochen
osso mandibolare	jaw-bone	Kieferknochen
osso zigomatico	zygoma	Zygoma, Jochbein
osteite	osteitis	Ostitis, Knochenentzündung
osteoartropatia	osteoarthropathy	Osteoarthrose
osteoartrosi (OA)	osteoarthritis (OA)	Osteoarthritis
osteoblasto	osteoblast	Osteoblast
osteocito	osteocyte	Osteozyt
osteoclasto	osteoclast	Osteoklast
osteocondrite	osteochondritis	Osteochondritis
osteocondroma	osteochondroma	Osteochondrom
osteocondrosi	osteochondrosis	Osteochondrose
osteodistrofia	osteodystrophy	Osteodystrophie
osteofito	osteophyte	Osteophyt
osteogenico	osteogenic	osteogen
osteolitico	osteolytic	osteolytisch
osteoma	osteoma	Osteom
osteomalacia	osteomalacia	Osteomalazie
osteomielite	osteomyelitis	Osteomyelitis, Knochenmarksentzündung
osteopatia	osteopathy	Osteopathie
osteoporosi	osteopetrosis, osteoporosis	Osteopetrose, Osteoporose
osteosclerosi	osteosclerosis	Osteosklerose, Eburnifikation
osteotomia	osteotomy	Osteotomie
ostetricia	obstetrics	Geburtshilfe
ostruttivo	obstructive	obstruktiv
ostruzione laringea	croup	Krupp
otalgia	ostomy	Osteotomie
otite	otalgia, otitis	Otalgie, Ohrenschmerz, Otitis, Mittelohrentzündung
otolaringologia	otolaryngology	Otolaryngologie
otologia	otology	Otologie, Ohrenheilkunde
otorinolaringoiatria	ear nose and throat (ENT)	Hals- Nasen- Ohren-
otorrea	otorrhea (Am), otorrhoea (Eng)	Otorrhoe, Ohrenfluß
otosclerosi	otosclerosis	Otosklerose
otoscopio	auriscope, otoscope	Ohrenspiegel, Otoskop
ototossico	ototoxic	ototoxisch
ottico (n)	optician (n)	Optiker (n)

SPANISH	FRENCH	ITALIAN
huésped	hôte	ospite
óseo	osseux	osseo
huesecillos	osselet	ossicino
oxidación	oxydation	ossidazione
oxigenación	oxygénation	ossigenazione
tratamiento con oxígeno hiperbárico	oxygénothérapie hyperbase	ossigenoterapia iperbarica
oxitocina	oxytocine	ossitocina
enterobius vermincularis, oxiuros	ascaride	ossiuro
hueso	os	osso
ilion	ilion	osso dell'anca
hueso coxal o ilíaco	os coxal	osso iliaco
mandíbula	mâchoire	osso mandibolare
cigoma	zygoma	osso zigomatico
osteítis	ostéite	osteite
osteoartropatía	ostéo-arthropathie	osteoartropatia
osteoartritis	ostéo-arthrite	osteoartrosi (OA)
osteoblasto	ostéoblaste	osteoblasto
osteocito	ostéocyte	osteocito
osteoclasto	ostéoclaste	osteoclasto
osteocondritis	ostéochondrite	osteocondrite
osteocondroma	ostéochondrome	osteocondroma
osteocondrosis	ostéochondrose	osteocondrosi
osteodistrofia	ostéodystrophie	osteodistrofia
osteofito	ostéophyte	osteofito
osteogénico	ostéogène	osteogenico
osteolítico	ostéolytique	osteolitico
osteoma	ostéome	osteoma
osteomalacia	ostéomalacie	osteomalacia
osteomielitis	ostéomyélite	osteomielite
osteopatía	ostéopathie	osteopatia
osteopetrosis, osteoporosis	ostéopétrose, ostéoporose	osteoporosi
osteosclerosis	ostéosclérose	osteosclerosi
osteotomía	ostéotomie	osteotomia
obstetricia	obstétrique	ostetricia
obstructivo	obstructif	ostruttivo
garrotillo, crup, difteria laríngea	croup	ostruzione laringea
ostomía	ostéotomie	otalgia
otalgia, otitis	otalgie, otite	otite
otolaringología	otolaryngologie	otolaringologia
otología	otologie	otologia
otorrinolaringología (ORL)	oto-rhino-laryngologie (ORL)	otorinolaringoiatria
otorrea	otorrhée	otorrea
otosclerosis	otospongiose	otosclerosi
auriscopio, otoscopio	auriscope, otoscope	otoscopio
ototóxico	ototoxique	ototossico
óptico (n)	opticien (n)	ottico (n)

ITALIAN	ENGLISH	GERMAN
ottico *(a)*	optic *(a)*	optisch *(a)*, Seh- *(a)*
otturatorio	obturator	Obturator, Gaumenverschlußplatte
ovaio	ovary	Ovarium, Eierstock
ovarico	ovarian	ovarial, Eierstock-
ovariectomia	oophorectomy	Oophorektomie
ovulazione	ovulation	Ovulation, Eisprung

SPANISH	FRENCH	ITALIAN
óptico *(a)*	optique *(a)*	**ottico** *(a)*
obturador	obturateur	**otturatorio**
ovario	ovaire	**ovaio**
ovárico	ovarien	**ovarico**
ooforectomía	ovariectomie	**ovariectomia**
ovulación	ovulation	**ovulazione**

P

Italian	English	German
pacemaker	pacemaker	Schrittmacher
padiglione auricolare	pinna	Ohrmuschel
palatale	palatine	palatal
palatino	palatine	palatal
palato	palate	Gaumen
palato molle	soft palate	weicher Gaumen
palatoschisi	cleft palate	Gaumenspalte
palliativo (n)	palliative (n)	Palliativum (n)
palliativo (a)	palliative (a)	palliativ (a)
pallore	pallor	Blässe
palmare	palmar	palmar
palmo	palm	Handinnenfläche
palpabile	palpable	palpabel, tastbar
palpazione	palpation	Palpation
palpebra	palpebra	Palpebra, Lid
palpitazione	palpitation	Palpitation, Herzklopfen
pancitopenia	pancytopenia	Panzytopenie
pancreas	pancreas	Pankreas, Bauchspeicheldrüse
pancreatite	pancreatitis	Pankreatitis, Bauchspeicheldrüsenentzündung
pandemia	pandemic	Pandemie
pandemico	pandemic	pandemisch
papillare	papillary	papillär
papilledema	papilledema (Am), papilloedema (Eng)	Papillenödem
papilloma	papilloma	Papillom
papula	papule	Papel, Knötchen
parafimosi	paraphimosis	Paraphimose
parafrenia	paraphrenia	Paraphrenie
paralisi	palsy, paralysis	Paralyse, Lähmung
paralisi cerebrale	cerebral palsy	Zerebralparese
paralisi di Bell	Bell's palsy	Bell-Fazialisparese
paralisi ischemica di Volkmann	Volkmann's ischaemic contracture (Eng), Volkmann's ischemic contracture (Am)	Volkmann-Kontraktur
paralisi progressiva luetica	general paralysis of the insane	progressive Paralyse
paralitico	paralytic	paralytisch, gelähmt
paramedico	paramedical	paramedizinisch
paranoia	paranoia	Paranoia
paraplegia	paraplegia	Paraplegie, Querschnittslähmung
parasimpatico	parasympathetic	parasympathisch
parassita	parasite	Parasit, Schmarotzer
paratiroidectomia	parathyroidectomy	Parathyreoidektomie
paratormone	parathormone	Parathormon
paravertebrale	paravertebral	paravertebral
parenchima	parenchyma	Parenchym

marcapasos	stimulateur cardiaque	pacemaker
pabellón de la oreja	pavillon de l'oreille	padiglione auricolare
palatino	palatin	palatale
palatino	palatin	palatino
paladar	palais	palato
paladar blando	voile du palais	palato molle
paladar hendido	fente palatine	palatoschisi
paliativo (n)	palliatif (n)	palliativo (n)
paliativo (a)	palliatif (a)	palliativo (a)
palidez	pâleur	pallore
palmar	palmaire	palmare
palma	paume	palmo
palpable	palpable	palpabile
palpación	palpation	palpazione
párpado	paupière	palpebra
palpitación	palpitation	palpitazione
pancitopenia	pancytopénie	pancitopenia
páncreas	pancréas	pancreas
pancreatitis	pancréatite	pancreatite
pandémico	pandémie	pandemia
pandémico	pandémique	pandemico
papilar	papillaire	papillare
papiledema	oedème papillaire	papilledema
papiloma	papillome	papilloma
pápula	papule	papula
parafimosis	paraphimosis	parafimosi
parafrenia	paraphrénie	parafrenia
parálisis	paralysie	paralisi
parálisis cerebral	infirmité motrice cérébrale	paralisi cerebrale
parálisis de Bell	paralysie de Bell	paralisi di Bell
contractura isquémica de Volkmann	contracture ischémique de Volkmann	paralisi ischemica di Volkmann
parálisis cerebral	paralysie générale des aliénés	paralisi progressiva luetica
paralítico	paralytique	paralitico
paramédico	paramédical	paramedico
paranoia	paranoïa	paranoia
paraplejía	paraplégie	paraplegia
parasimpático	parasympathique	parasimpatico
parásito	parasite	parassita
paratiroidectomía	parathyroïdectomie	paratiroidectomia
parathormona	parathormone	paratormone
paravertebral	paravertébral	paravertebrale
parénquima	parenchyme	parenchima

parenterale	parenteral	parenteral
paresi	paresis	Parese, Lähmung
parestesia	paraesthesia (Eng), paresthesia (Am)	Parästhesie
parietale	mural, parietal	mural, parietal, wandständig
parità	parity	Gebärfähigkeit, Ähnlichkeit
parkinsonismo	parkinsonism	Parkinsonismus
paronichia	paronychia	Paronychie
parossistico	paroxysmal	paroxysmal, krampfartig
parotide epidemica morbillo e rosolia	measles mumps and rubella (MMR)	Masern Mumps und Röteln
parotite	parotitis	Parotitis
parotite epidemica	mumps	Mumps, Ziegenpeter
parte bassa del torace	midriff	Zwerchfell, Diaphragma
parti per milione (ppm)	parts per million (ppm)	ppm, mg/l
parto	delivery, parturition	Entbindung, Geburt, Gebären
partoriente	parturient	gebärend
parzialmente solubile	partly soluble (p.sol)	teilweise löslich
passivo	passive	passiv, teilnahmslos
pasta	paste	Paste, Salbe
pasta gelificante	paste	Paste, Salbe
pasticca	tablet	Tablette
pastiglia	lozenge	Pastille
pastorizzazione	pasteurization	Pasteurisierung
patella	patella	Patella, Kniescheibe
patereccio	whitlow	Panaritium
patogenesi	pathogenesis	Pathogenese
patogeneticità	pathogenicity	Pathogenität
patogeno	pathogen	Krankheitserreger, Erreger
patognomonico	pathognomonic	pathognomonisch
patologia	pathology	Pathologie
pavimento pelvico	pelvic floor	Beckenboden
paziente immunocompromesso	immunocompromised patient	immungestörter Patient
paziente immunosoppresso	immunosuppressed patient	immunsupprimierter Patient
pazzia	insanity	Geisteskrankheit
pediatria	paediatrics (Eng), pediatrics (Am)	Pädiatrie, Kinderheilkunde
pediculosi	pediculosis	Pedikulose, Läusebefall
peduncolo	peduncle	Stiel
pellagra	pellagra	Pellagra
pelle	skin	Haut
pelo	hair	Haar
pelvi	pelvis	Pelvis, Becken
pelvimetria	pelvimetry	Pelvimetrie
pemfigo	pemphigus	Pemphigus
pemfigoide	pemphigoid	pemphigoid
pendulo	pendulous	hängend, gestielt
pene	penis	Penis
pepsina	pepsin	Pepsin

SPANISH	FRENCH	ITALIAN
parenteral	parentéral	**parenterale**
paresia	parésie	**paresi**
parestesia	paresthésie	**parestesia**
mural, parietal	pariétal	**parietale**
paridad	parité	**parità**
parkinsonismo	parkinsonisme	**parkinsonismo**
paroniquia	panaris superficiel	**paronichia**
paroxístico	paroxysmal	**parossistico**
sarampión parotiditis y rubéola	oreillons rougeole et rubéole	**parotide epidemica morbillo e rosolia**
parotiditis	parotite	**parotite**
paperas	oreillons	**parotite epidemica**
diafragma	diaphragme	**parte bassa del torace**
partes por millón (ppm)	parties par million (ppm)	**parti per milione (ppm)**
parto, parturición	livraison, accouchement, parturition	**parto**
parturienta	parturient	**partoriente**
semisoluble	partiellement soluble	**parzialmente solubile**
pasivo	passif	**passivo**
pasta	pâte	**pasta**
pasta	pâte	**pasta gelificante**
comprimido	comprimé	**pasticca**
pastilla	pastille	**pastiglia**
pasteurización	pasteurisation	**pastorizzazione**
rótula	rotule	**patella**
panadizo	panaris	**patereccio**
patogenia	pathogenèse	**patogenesi**
patogenicidad	pouvoir pathogène	**patogeneticità**
patógeno	pathogène	**patogeno**
patognomónico	pathognomonique	**patognomonico**
patología	pathologie	**patologia**
suelo de la pelvis	plancher pelvien	**pavimento pelvico**
paciente inmunocomprometido	malade à déficit immunitaire	**paziente immunocompromesso**
paciente inmunosuprimido	malade à suppression immunitaire	**paziente immunosoppresso**
locura, demencia	aliénation	**pazzia**
pediatría	pédiatrie	**pediatria**
pediculosis	pédiculose	**pediculosi**
pedúnculo	pédoncule	**peduncolo**
pelagra	pellagre	**pellagra**
piel	peau	**pelle**
pelo	poil	**pelo**
pelvis	pelvis	**pelvi**
pelvimetría	pelvimétrie	**pelvimetria**
pénfigo	pemphigus	**pemfigo**
penfigoide	pemphigoïde	**pemfigoide**
péndulo	pendant	**pendulo**
pene	pénis	**pene**
pepsina	pepsine	**pepsina**

ITALIAN	ENGLISH	GERMAN
peptico	peptic	peptisch
peptide	peptide	Peptide
percezione	perception	Perzeption, Wahrnehmung
percussione	percussion	Perkussion
percutaneo	percutaneous, transcutaneous	perkutan, transkutan
perdita di peso	weight loss	Gewichtsverlust
perdita ematica che precede il parto o la mestruazione	'show'	Geburtsbeginn (Anzeichen)
perforazione	perforation	Perforation
perfusione	perfusion	Durchblutung
perfusione renale	renal blood flow (RBF)	Nierendurchblutung, renaler Blutfluß (RBF)
perianale	perianal	perianal
periartrite scapoloomerale	frozen shoulder	Frozen shoulder, Periarthritis humeroscapularis
pericardio	pericardium	Perikard, Herzbeutel
pericardite	pericarditis	Perikarditis
pericondrio	perichondrium	Perichondrium, Knorpelhaut
periferico	peripheral	peripher
perinatale	perinatal	perinatal
perineo	perineum	Perineum, Damm
periodo neonatale	neonatal period	Neonatalperiode, Neugeborenenperiode
periodontopatia	periodontal disease	Periodontitis, Wurzelhautentzündung
periombelicale	periumbilical	periumbilikal
perioperatorio	perioperative	perioperativ
periorale	perioral	perioral
periostio	periosteum	Periost, Knochenhaut
peristalsi	peristalsis	Peristaltik
peritoneo	peritoneum	Peritoneum, Bauchfell
peritonite	peritonitis	Peritonitis
permeabile	permeable	permeabel, durchlässig
perorale	peroral	peroral
perseverazione	perseveration	Perseveration
personalità	personality	Persönlichkeit
personalità antisociale	antisocial personality	asoziale Persönlichkeit
personalità psicopatica	psychopathic personality	psychopathische Persönlichkeit
personalità schizoide	schizoid personality	schizoide Persönlichkeit
perspirazione	perspiration	Schweiß
pertinente al palmo della mano	thenar	Thenar-
pertosse	pertussis, whooping cough	Pertussis, Keuchhusten
peso atomico	atomic weight (at wt)	Atomgewicht
peso corporeo totale	total body weight (TBW)	Körpergewicht
pessario	pessary	Pessar
peste	plague	Pest, Seuche
petecchia	petechia	Petechie
pettorale	pectoral	pektoral, Brust-
piaga da decubito	bedsore	Dekubitus, Durchliegen

SPANISH	FRENCH	ITALIAN
péptico	peptique	peptico
péptido	peptide	peptide
percepción	perception	percezione
percusión	percussion	percussione
percutáneo, transcutáneo	percutané, transcutané	percutaneo
pérdida de peso	perte de poids	perdita di peso
'señal sanguinolenta menstrual'	eaux de l'amnios	perdita ematica che precede il parto o la mestruazione
perforación	perforation	perforazione
perfusión	perfusion	perfusione
flujo sanguíneo renal (FSR)	débit sanguin rénal	perfusione renale
perianal	périanal	perianale
hombro congelado/rígido	épaule ankylosée	periartrite scapoloomerale
pericardio	péricarde	pericardio
pericarditis	péricardite	pericardite
pericondrio	périchondre	pericondrio
periférico	périphérique	periferico
perinatal	périnatal	perinatale
perineo	périnée	perineo
período neonatal	période néonatale	periodo neonatale
enfermedad periodontal	paradontolyse	periodontopatia
periumbilical	périombilical	periombelicale
perioperatorio	périopératoire	perioperatorio
perioral	périoral	periorale
periostio	périoste	periostio
peristalsis	péristaltisme	peristalsi
peritoneo	péritoine	peritoneo
peritonitis	péritonite	peritonite
permeable	perméable	permeabile
peroral	peroral	perorale
perseverancia	persévération	perseverazione
personalidad	personnalité	personalità
personalidad antisocial	personnalité psychopathique	personalità antisociale
personalidad psicopática	personnalité psychopathique	personalità psicopatica
personalidad esquizoide	personnalité schizoïde	personalità schizoide
sudor	perspiration	perspirazione
tenar	thénar	pertinente al palmo della mano
tos ferina	pertussis, coqueluche	pertosse
peso atómico	poids atomique	peso atomico
peso corporal total	poids corporel total	peso corporeo totale
pesario	pessaire	pessario
peste, plaga	peste	peste
petequia	pétéchie	petecchia
pectoral	pectoral	pettorale
úlcera por decúbito	escarre de décubitus	piaga da decubito

ITALIAN	ENGLISH	GERMAN
pian	yaws	Frambösie
piartro	pyarthrosis	Pyarthrose, eitrige Gelenkentzündung
piastrina	platelet	Thrombozyt, Blutplättchen
picacismo	pica	Pica
picco	spicule	Spikulum
piccolo foruncolo	pimple	Pickel, Mitesser
piccolo male	petit mal	Petit mal
pidocchio	louse	Laus
piede	foot	Fuß
piede da trincea	trench foot	Schützengrabenfuß
piede di atleta	athlete's foot	Fußpilz
piede piatto	flat-foot	Plattfuß
piede talo	talipes	Klumpfuß, pes equinovarus
piede torto	club-foot	Klumpfuß
piegatura	plication	Faltenbildung
pielite	pyelitis	Pyelitis, Nierenbeckenentzündung
pielografia	pyelography	Pyelographie
pielografia endovenosa (PE)	intravenous pyelogram (IVP)	i.v. − Pyelogramm
pielonefrite	pyelonephritis	Pyelonephritis
piemia	pyaemia (Eng), pyemia (Am)	Pyämie
pigmentazione	pigmentation	Pigmentierung, Färbung
pigmento	pigment	Pigment, Farbstoff
pillola	pill	Pille
pilonidale	pilonidal	pilonidal
piloro	pylorus	Pylorus
piloromiotomia	pyloromyotomy, Ramstedt's operation	Pyloromyotomie, Weber-Ramstedt-Operation, Ramstedt-(Weber)-Operation
piloroplastica	pyloroplasty	Pyloroplastik
pilorospasmo	pylorospasm	Pylorospasmus
pinguecula	pinguecula	Pinguekula
pinta	pinta	Pinta
pioartrosi	pyarthrosis	Pyarthrose, eitrige Gelenkentzündung
pioderma	pyoderma	Pyodermie
piodermite	pyoderma	Pyodermie
piogenico	pyogenic	pyogen
piombo derivazione	lead	Ableitung
piometra	pyometra	Pyometra
pionefrosi	pyonephrosis	Pyonephrose
piosalpinge	pyosalpinx	Pyosalpinx
piramidale	pyramidal	pyramidal
piressia	pyrexia	Fieber
piressia di origine sconosciuta (POS)	pyrexia of unknown origin (PUO, FUO)	Fieber unklarer Genese
pirosi	heartburn, pyrosis	Sodbrennen
pitiriasi	pityriasis	Pityriasis
piuria	pyuria	Pyurie
placca	plaque	Plaque, Zahnbelag

SPANISH	FRENCH	ITALIAN
yaws, pian	pian	**pian**
piartrosis	pyarthrose	**piartro**
plaqueta	plaquette	**piastrina**
pica	pica	**picacismo**
espícula	spicule	**picco**
grano	bouton	**piccolo foruncolo**
petit mal	petit mal	**piccolo male**
piojo	pou	**pidocchio**
pie	pied	**piede**
pie de trinchera	pied gelé	**piede da trincea**
pie de atleta	pied d'athlète	**piede di atleta**
pie plano	pied plat	**piede piatto**
talipes	pied bot	**piede talo**
pie zambo	pied bot	**piede torto**
plicatura	plicature	**plegatura**
pielitis	pyélite	**pielite**
pielografía	pyélographie	**pielografia**
pielograma intravenoso	urographie intraveineuse (UIV)	**pielografia endovenosa (PE)**
pielonefritis	pyélonéphrite	**pielonefrite**
piemia	septicopyohémie	**piemia**
pigmentación	pigmentation	**pigmentazione**
pigmento	pigment	**pigmento**
píldora	pilule	**pillola**
pilonidal	pilonidal	**pilonidale**
píloro	pylore	**piloro**
piloromiotomía, operación de Ramstedt	pylorotomie, opération de Ramstedt	**piloromiotomia**
piloroplastia	pyloroplastie	**piloroplastica**
pilorospasmo	pylorospasme	**pilorospasmo**
pinguécula	pinguécula	**pinguecula**
mal de pinto	pinta	**pinta**
piartrosis	pyarthrose	**pioartrosi**
pioderma	pyodermie	**pioderma**
pioderma	pyodermie	**piodermite**
piógeno	pyogène	**piogenico**
plomo	plomb	**piombo derivazione**
piómetra	pyométrie	**piometra**
pionefrosis	pyonéphrose	**pionefrosi**
piosalpinx	pyosalpinx	**piosalpinge**
piramidal	pyramidal	**piramidale**
pirexia, fiebre	pyrexie	**piressia**
fiebre de origen desconocido	fièvre d'origine inconnue	**piressia di origine sconosciuta (POS)**
ardor de estómago, pirosis	aigreurs, pyrosis	**pirosi**
pitiriasis	pityriasis	**pitiriasi**
piuria	pyurie	**piuria**
placa	plaque	**placca**

ITALIAN	ENGLISH	GERMAN
placche di Peyer	Peyer's patches	Peyer Plaques
placebo	placebo	Plazebo
placenta	placenta	Plazenta, Nachgeburt
plantare	plantar	plantar
plasma	plasma	Plasma
plasmacitoma maligno	myeloma	Myelom
plasmaferesi	plasmapheresis	Plasmapherese
plesso	plexus	Plexus
plesso celiaco	solar plexus	Solarplexus
plesso solare	solar plexus	Solarplexus
pletora	plethora	Plethora
pleura	pleura	Pleura
pleurite	pleurisy (pleuritis)	Pleuritis, Rippenfellentzündung
pleurodesi	pleurodesis	Pleurodese
pleurodinia	pleurodynia	Pleuralgie
plicazione	plication	Faltenbildung
plurigravida	multigravida	Multigravida
pneumaturia	pneumaturia	Pneumaturie
pneumocefalo	pneumocephalus	Pneumozephalus
pneumocito	pneumocyte	Pneumozyt
pneumoconiosi	pneumoconiosis	Pneumokoniose, Staublunge
pneumonectomia	pneumonectomy	Pneumonektomie, Lungenresektion
pneumoperitoneo	pneumoperitoneum	Pneumoperitoneum
pneumotorace	pneumothorax	Pneumothorax
poliarterite	polyarteritis	Polyarteritis
poliartralgia	polyarthralgia	Polyarthralgie
poliartrite	polyarthritis	Polyarthritis
policistico	polycystic	polyzystisch
policitemia	polycythaemia (Eng), polycythemia (Am)	Polyzythämie
polidipsia	polydipsia	Polydipsie
polimialgia reumatica	polymyalgia rheumatica	Polymyalgia rheumatica
polimiosite	polymyositis	Polymyositis
polineurite	polyneuritis	Polyneuritis
poliomielite	poliomyelitis	Poliomyelitis, Kinderlähmung
polipectomia	polypectomy	Polypektomie
polipo	polyp	Polyp
poliposi	polyposis	Polyposis
polisaccaride	polysaccharide	Polysaccharid
poliuria	polyuria	Polyurie
pollice	thumb	Daumen
polmonare	pulmonary	Lungen-
polmoni	lung	Lunge
polmonite	pneumonia, pneumonitis	Pneumonie, Lungenentzündung, Pneumonitis
polpaccio	calf	Wade
polso	pulse, wrist	Puls, Handgelenk, Karpus
polso alternante	pulsus alternans	Pulsus alternans

SPANISH	FRENCH	ITALIAN
placas de Peyer	plaques de Peyer	placche di Peyer
placebo	placebo	placebo
placenta	placenta	placenta
plantar	plantaire	plantare
plasma	plasma	plasma
mieloma	myélome	plasmacitoma maligno
plasmaféresis	plasmaphérèse	plasmaferesi
plexo	plexus	plesso
plexo solar	plexus solaire	plesso celiaco
plexo solar	plexus solaire	plesso solare
plétora	pléthore	pletora
pleura	plèvre	pleura
pleuresia, pleuritis	pleurésie	pleurite
pleurodesis	pleurodèse	pleurodesi
pleurodinia	pleurodynie	pleurodinia
plicatura	plicature	plicazione
multípara	multigeste	plurigravida
neumaturia	pneumaturie	pneumaturia
neumocéfalo	pneumo-encéphale, pneumocéphale	pneumocefalo
neumocito	cellule alvéolaire	pneumocito
neumoconiosis	pneumoconiose	pneumoconiosi
neumonectomía	pneumonectomie	pneumonectomia
neumoperitoneo	pneumopéritoine	pneumoperitoneo
neumotórax	pneumothorax	pneumotorace
poliarteritis	polyartérite	poliarterite
poliartralgia	polyarthralgie	poliartralgia
poliartritis	polyarthrite	poliartrite
poliquístico	polykystique	policistico
policitemia	polycythémie	policitemia
polidipsia	polydipsie	polidipsia
polimialgia reumática	polymyalgie rhumatismale	polimialgia reumatica
polimiositis	polymyosite	polimiosite
polineuritis	polynévrite	polineurite
poliomielitis	poliomyélite	poliomielite
polipectomía	polypectomie	polipectomia
pólipo	polype	polipo
poliposis	polypose	poliposi
polisacárido	polysaccharide	polisaccaride
poliuria	polyurie	poliuria
pulgar	pouce	pollice
pulmonar	pulmonaire	polmonare
pulmón	poumon	polmoni
neumonía, neumonitis	pneumonie, pneumonite	polmonite
pantorrilla	mollet	polpaccio
pulso, muñeca	pouls, poignet	polso
pulso alternante	pouls alternant	polso alternante

polso paradosso	pulsus paradoxus	Pulsus paradoxus
pomfo	weal	Schwiele, Striemen
pomo di Adamo	Adam's apple	Adamsapfel
ponfolice (disidrosi vescicolare)	pompholyx	Pompholyx
popliteo	popliteal, popliteus	popliteal, popliteus
porfiria	porphyria	Porphyrie
porfirina	porphyrin	Porphyrin
poro	pore	Pore
porpora	purpura	Purpura
porpora di Schönlein-Henoch	Henoch-Schönlein purpura	Purpura Schönlein-Henoch
porta	porta	Eingang
portaepatite	portahepatitis	Porta hepatis, Leberpforte
portatore	carrier	Ausscheider, Trägerstoff
portocavale	portacaval	portokaval
posizione di Sim	Sims' position	Sims-Lage
postcoitale	postcoital	Postkoital-
postencefalitico	postencephalitic	postenzephalitisch
postepatico	posthepatic	posthepatisch
posteriore	posterior	posteriore, hintere, Gesäß-
posterpetico	postherpetic	postherpetisch
postmaturo	postmaturity	Überreife
postmenopausale	postmenopausal	postmenopausal
post mortem	post-mortem	postmortal
postnatale	postnatal	postnatal
postoperatorio	postoperative	postoperativ
post partum	postpartum	post partum
postprandiale	postprandial	postprandial
posturale	postural	Lage-
pratica errata o disonesta	malpractice	Kunstfehler
preamaturo	premature	frühreif, vorzeitig
preanestesia	premedication	Prämedikation
precanceroso	precancerous	präkanzerös
precedente il concepimento	preconceptual	vor Empfängnis
precordiale	precordial	präkordial
precursore	precursor	Vorzeichen, Vorstufe, Präkursor
predisposizione	predisposition	Prädisposition, Anfälligkeit
preeclampsia	pre-eclampsia	Präeklampsie, Eklampsiebereitschaft
premedicazione	premedication	Prämedikation
premestruale	premenstrual	prämenstruell
prenatale	antenatal, prenatal	pränatal, vorgeburtlich
preoperatorio	preoperative	präoperativ
preparto	ante-partum	ante partum, vor der Entbindung
prepubertale	prepubertal	Präpubertäts-
prepuzio	foreskin, prepuce	Präputium, Vorhaut
prerenale	prerenal	prärenal
prescrizione	prescription	Rezept, Verschreibung
prescrizione dietetica	regimen	Diät

SPANISH	FRENCH	ITALIAN
pulso paradójico	pouls paradoxal	polso paradosso
verdugón	marque	pomfo
huez de Adán	pomme d'Adam	pomo di Adamo
ponfólix	pompholyx	ponfolice (disidrosi vescicolare)
poplíteo	poplité	popliteo
porfiria	porphyrie	porfiria
porfirinas	porphyrine	porfirina
poro	pore	poro
púrpura	purpura	porpora
púrpura de Schönlein-Henoch	purpura rhumatoïde	porpora di Schönlein-Henoch
porta	porte	porta
portohepatitis	porto-hépatite	portaepatite
portador	porteur	portatore
portocava	porto-cave	portocavale
posición de Sim	position de Sim	posizione di Sim
postcoital	après rapport	postcoitale
postencefalítico	postencéphalitique	postencefalitico
posthepático	posthépatique	postepatico
posterior	postérieur	posteriore
postherpético	postherpétique	posterpetico
postmaduro	postmature	postmaturo
postmenopáusico	postménopausique	postmenopausale
postmortem	post mortem	post mortem
postnatal	postnatal	postnatale
postoperatorio	postopératoire	postoperatorio
postpartum	postpartum	post partum
postprandial	postprandial	postprandiale
postural	postural	posturale
malpraxis	faute professionnelle	pratica errata o disonesta
prematuro	prématuré	preamaturo
premedicación	prémédication	preanestesia
precanceroso	précancéreux	precanceroso
preconceptual	préconceptuel	precedente il concepimento
precordial	précordial	precordiale
precursor	précurseur	precursore
predisposición	prédisposition	predisposizione
preeclampsia	éclampsisme	preeclampsia
premedicación	prémédication	premedicazione
premenstrual	prémenstruel	premestruale
antenatal, prenatal	anténatal, prénatal	prenatale
preoperatorio	préopératoire	preoperatorio
ante partum, preparto	ante partum	preparto
prepubertal	prépubertaire	prepubertale
prepucio	prépuce	prepuzio
prerrenal	prérénal	prerenale
receta	ordonnance	prescrizione
régimen	régime	prescrizione dietetica

ITALIAN	ENGLISH	GERMAN
prescrizione multipla di farmaci	polypharmacy	Polypragmasie
presentazione	presentation	Lage, Kindslage
presentazione fetale anomala	malpresentation	anomale Kindslage
presentazione podalica	breech-birth presentation	Steißlage
pressione arteriosa	blood pressure (BP)	Blutdruck
pressione continua positiva delle vie aeree	continuous positive airway pressure (CPAP)	kontinuierlich positiver Atemwegsdruck
pressione intracranica	intracranial pressure (ICP)	Hirndruck, intrakranieller Druck
pressione osmotica	osmotic pressure	osmotischer Druck
pressione parziale	partial pressure	Partialdruck
pressione polmonare di incuneamento	pulmonary capillary pressure (PCP)	Lungenkapillardruck
pressione venosa centrale	central venous pressure (CVP)	zentraler Venendruck (ZVD)
pressorio	pressor	blutdruckerhöhend, vasopressorisch
primaria	primary care	Primärversorgung
primigravida	primigravida	Primigravida
primipara	primipara	Primipara, Erstgebärende
procidenza	procidentia	Prolaps, Vorfall
proctalgia	proctalgia	Proktalgie
proctite	proctitis	Proktitis
proctocolectomia	proctocolectomy	Proktokolektomie
proctocolite	proctocolitis	Proktokolitis
proctoscopio	proctoscope	Rektoskop
prodromico	prodromal	prodromal
profarmaco (precursore inattivo)	pro-drug	pro-drug (Pharmakon-Vorform)
profilassi	prophylaxis	Prophylaxe, Vorbeugung
profilattico maschile	condom	Kondom, Präservativ
prognosi	prognosis	Prognose
prolasso	prolapse	Prolaps, Vorfall
proliferare	proliferate	proliferieren
pronare	pronate	pronieren
pronatore	pronator	Pronator
prono	prone	veranlagt, empfänglich
pronto soccorso	emergency treatment/trauma unit (ETU), first aid	Notfallstation, Erste Hilfe
proptosi	proptosis	Vorfall, Exophthalmus
prossimale	proximal	proximal
prostaglandina	prostaglandin	Prostaglandine
prostata	prostate	Prostata
prostatectomia	prostatectomy	Prostatektomie
prostatismo	prostatism	chronisches Prostataleiden
proteasi	proteolytic enzyme	proteolytisches Enzym
proteina	protein	Protein
proteina che lega il ferro	iron binding protein (IBP)	eisenbindendes Protein
proteina C reattiva	C-reactive protein (CRP)	C-reaktives Protein (CRP)
proteina di Bence-Jones	Bence-Jones protein (BJ)	Bence-Jones-Proteine
proteinuria	proteinuria	Proteinurie

SPANISH	FRENCH	ITALIAN
polifarmacia	polypharmacie	**prescrizione multipla di farmaci**
presentación	présentation	**presentazione**
malpresentación	présentation vicieuse	**presentazione fetale anomala**
presentación de nalgas	présentation, naissance par le siège	**presentazione podalica**
presión arterial (PA)	tension artérielle (TA)	**pressione arteriosa**
presión continua positiva de las vías respiratorias	ventilation spontanée en pression positive continue	**pressione continua positiva delle vie aeree**
presión intracraneal (PIC)	pression intracrânienne	**pressione intracranica**
presión osmótica	pression osmotique	**pressione osmotica**
presión parcial	pression partielle	**pressione parziale**
presión capilar pulmonar (PCP)	pression capillaire pulmonaire (PCP), pression artérielle bloquée moyenne	**pressione polmonare di incuneamento**
presión venosa central (PVC)	tension veineuse centrale	**pressione venosa centrale**
presor	pressif	**pressorio**
asistencia primaria	soins de santé primaires	**primaria**
primigrávida	primigeste	**primigravida**
primípara	primipare	**primipara**
procidencia	procidence	**procidenza**
proctalgia	proctalgie	**proctalgia**
proctitis	rectite	**proctite**
proctocolectomia	proctocolectomie	**proctocolectomia**
proctocolitis	rectocolite	**proctocolite**
proctoscopio	rectoscope	**proctoscopio**
prodrómico	prodromique	**prodromico**
profármaco	précurseur de médicament	**profarmaco (precursore inattivo)**
profilaxis	prophylaxie	**profilassi**
condón	préservatif	**profilattico maschile**
pronóstico	pronostic	**prognosi**
prolapso	prolapsus	**prolasso**
proliferar	proliférer	**proliferare**
pronar	mettre en pronation	**pronare**
pronador	pronateur	**pronatore**
prono, inclinado	en pronation	**prono**
servicio de urgencias/traumatologia, primeros auxilios	service des urgences/des traumatismes, secourisme, premiers soins	**pronto soccorso**
proptosis	proptose	**proptosi**
proximal	proximal	**prossimale**
prostaglandina	prostaglandine	**prostaglandina**
próstata	prostate	**prostata**
prostatectomía	prostatectomie	**prostatectomia**
prostatismo	prostatisme	**prostatismo**
enzima proteolítico	enzyme protéolytique	**proteasi**
proteína	protéine	**proteina**
proteína de unión con el hierro	sidérophyline	**proteina che lega il ferro**
proteína C-reactiva	test de protéine C-réactive	**proteina C reattiva**
proteína de Bence-Jones	protéine de Bence Jones (BJ)	**proteina di Bence-Jones**
proteinuria	protéinurie	**proteinuria**

protesi	prosthesis	Prothese
protozoi	protozoa	Protozoe
protrusione dell'ombelico	exomphalos	Exomphalos, Nabelbruch
prova	test	Test, Untersuchung
prova del sudore	sweat test	Schweißtest
provetta	test tube	Reagenzglas
prurito	itch, pruritus	Jucken, Pruritus
pseudociesi	phantom pregnancy	Scheinschwangerschaft, hysterische Schwangerschaft
pseudopoliposi	pseudopolyposis	Pseudopolype
psichiatria	psychiatry	Psychiatrie
psichiatrico	psychiatric	psychiatrisch
psichico	psychic	psychisch, seelisch
psicoanalisi	psychoanalysis	Psychoanalyse
psicodinamica	psychodynamics	Psychodynamik
psicogenico	psychogenic	psychogen
psicogeriatrico	psychogeriatric	gerontopsychiatrisch
psicologia	psychology	Psychologie
psicomotorio (n)	retardation (n)	Verzögerung (n), Hemmung (n)
psicomotorio (a)	psychomotor (a)	psychomotorisch (a)
psicopatia	psychopathy	Psychopathie
psicopatico	psychopath	Psychopath
psicopatologia	psychopathology	Psychopathologie
psicosi	psychosis	Psychose
psicosi di Korsakoff	Korsakoff's psychosis	Korsakow-Psychose
psicosi maniaco-depressiva	manic-depressive psychosis	manisch-depressive Psychose
psicosomatico	psychosomatic	psychosomatisch, Leib-Seele-
psicoterapia	psychotherapy	Psychotherapie
psicotropo	psychotropic	psychotrop
psittacosi	psittacosis	Psittakose, Ornithose
psoas	psoas	Psoas
psoralene	psoralen	Psoralen
psoriasi	psoriasis	Psoriasis, Schuppenflechte
psoriasi artropatica	psoriatic arthritis	Arthritis psoriatica
pterigio	pterygium	Pterygium
ptosi	ptosis	Ptose
pube	pubis	Os pubis, Schambein
pubertà	puberty	Pubertät
puerperale	puerperal	puerperal, Kindbett-
puerperio	puerperium	Wochenbett, Puerperium
pulce	flea	Floh
pulsatile	pulsatile	pulsierend
pulsazione	pulsation	Pulsieren, Pulsschlag
pungere	puncture	stechen, injizieren
punto	stitch	Stechen
punto cieco	blind spot	blinder Fleck, Papille
punto cutaneo sensibile alla pressione	pressure point	Druckpunkt, Dekubitus

SPANISH	FRENCH	ITALIAN
prótesis	prothèse	protesi
protozoos	protozoaires	protozoi
exónfalo, hernia umbilical	exomphale	protrusione dell'ombelico
prueba	test	prova
prueba del sudor	test de sueur	prova del sudore
tubo de ensayo	tube à essai, éprouvette	provetta
picor, prurito	démangeaison, prurit	prurito
embarazo fantasma	fausse grossesse	pseudociesi
pseudopoliposis	pseudopolypose	pseudopoliposi
psiquiatría	psychiatrie	psichiatria
psiquiátrico	psychiatrique	psichiatrico
psíquico	psychique	psichico
psicoanálisis	psychanalyse	psicoanalisi
psicodinámica	psychodynamique	psicodinamica
psicógeno	psychogène	psicogenico
psicogeriátrico	psychogériatrique	psicogeriatrico
psicología	psychologie	psicologia
retraso (n)	retard (n)	psicomotorio (n)
psicomotor (a)	psychomoteur (a)	psicomotorio (a)
psicopatía	psychopathie	psicopatia
psicópata	psychopathe	psicopatico
psicopatología	psychopathologie	psicopatologia
psicosis	psychose	psicosi
psicosis de Korsakoff	psychose de Korsakoff	psicosi di Korsakoff
psicosis maniacodepresiva	psychose maniacodépressive	psicosi maniaco-depressiva
psicosomático	psychosomatique	psicosomatico
psicoterapia	psychothérapie	psicoterapia
psicotrópico	psychotrope	psicotropo
psitacosis	psittacose	psittacosi
psoas	psoas	psoas
psoralen	psoralène	psoralène
psoriasis	psoriasis	psoriasi
artritis psoriásica	rhumatisme psoriasique	psoriasi artropatica
pterigión	ptérygion	pterigio
ptosis	ptose	ptosi
pubis	pubis	pube
pubertad	puberté	pubertà
puerperal	puerpéral	puerperale
puerperio	puerpérium	puerperio
pulga	puce	pulce
pulsátil	pulsatile	pulsatile
pulsación	pulsation	pulsazione
pinchar	ponctionner	pungere
punto de sutura	point de suture	punto
mancha ciega	tache aveugle	punto cieco
punto de presión	point particulièrement sensible	punto cutaneo sensibile alla pressione

ITALIAN	ENGLISH	GERMAN
punto di McBurney	McBurney's point	McBurney-Punkt
puntura	sting, puncture	Stachel, Stich, Injektion
puntura di vena	venepuncture, venipuncture	Venenpunktion
puntura lombare	lumbar puncture (LP)	Lumbalpunktion
puntura sternale	sternal puncture	Sternalpunktion
pupilla	pupil	Pupille
pupillare	pupillary	pupillar, Pupillen-
purgante	purgative	purgierend, abführend
purulento	purulent	purulent, eitrig
pus	pus	Eiter
pustola	pimple, pustule	Pickel, Mitesser, Pustel
putrefazione	putrefaction	Verwesung, Fäulnis

Q

ITALIAN	ENGLISH	GERMAN
quadricipite	quadriceps	Quadrizeps
qualitativo	qualitative	qualitativ
quantitativo	quantitative	quantitativ
quarantena	quarantine	Quarantäne
quartana	quartan	quartana (Malaria)

SPANISH	FRENCH	ITALIAN
punto de McBurney	point de McBurney	punto di McBurney
picadura, punción	piqûre, ponction	puntura
venopuntura, venipuntura	ponction d'une veine	puntura di vena
punción lumbar (PL)	ponction lombaire	puntura lombare
punción esternal	ponction sternale	puntura sternale
pupila	pupille	pupilla
pupilar	pupillaire	pupillare
purgante	purgatif	purgante
purulento	purulent	purulento
pus	pus	pus
grano, pústula	bouton, pustule	pustola
putrefacción	putréfaction	putrefazione

cuádriceps	quadriceps	quadricipite
cualitativo	qualitatif	qualitativo
cuantitativo	quantitatif	quantitativo
cuarentena	quarantaine	quarantena
cuartana	quarte	quartana

R

ITALIAN	ENGLISH	GERMAN
rabbia	rabies	Tollwut
rachialgia lombosacrale	low back pain	Kreuzschmerzen
rachicentesi	lumbar puncture (LP)	Lumbalpunktion
rachitismo	rickets	Rachitis
raddrizzamento	orthosis	Orthose
radicale	radical	radikal, Wurzel-
radio	radius	Radius, Halbmesser
radioattivo	radioactive	radioaktiv
radiografia	radiography	Röntgen
radioisotopo	radioisotope	Radioisotop
radiologia	radiology	Radiologie, Röntgenologie
radioopaco	radio-opaque	röntgendicht
radiosensibile	radiosensitive	strahlenempfindlich
radioterapia	radiotherapy	Strahlentherapie, Radiotherapie
raffreddore	cold	Kälte, Erkältung
raffreddore da fieno	hay fever	Heuschnupfen
raggi X	X-rays	Röntgenstrahlen, Röntgenaufnahmen
raschiamento	curettage, curetting	Kürettage, Ausschabung
raschiare	curette (Eng), curet (Am)	kürettieren
reagente	reagent	Reagens
reazione	reaction	Reaktion
reazione anafilattica	anaphylactic reaction	anaphylaktische Reaktion
reazione dannosa (indesiderata) da farmaci	adverse drug reaction (ADR)	unerwünschte Arzneimittelreaktion
reazione di Wassermann	Wassermann reaction	Wassermann-Reaktion
reazione di Widal	Widal reaction	Widal-Reaktion
reazione immune	immune reaction	Immunreaktion
reazioni collaterali extrapiramidali da farmaci	extrapyramidal side effects	extrapyramidale Nebenwirkungen
recessivo	recessive	rezessiv
recettore	receptor	Rezeptor
recidiva	recurrence, relapse	Rezidiv, Rückfall
recidivare	relapse	rezidivieren, Rückfall erleiden
reflusso	reflux	Reflux
refrattario	refractory	refraktär
regime	diet	Ernährung, Diät
regione lombare	loin	Lende
regressione	regression	Regression, Rückbildung
regurgito	regurgitation	Regurgitieren
releasing factor dell'ormone LH	LH-releasing factor (LHRF)	LH-luteinizing hormone releasing factor (LHRF)
remissione	remission	Remission
remittente	remittent	remittierend, abfallend
renale	renal	renal, Nieren-
rene	kidney	Niere

rabia	rage	**rabbia**
lumbalgia	douleurs lombaires basses	**rachialgia lombosacrale**
punción lumbar (PL)	ponction lombaire	**rachicentesi**
raquitismo	rachitisme	**rachitismo**
ortosis	orthèse	**raddrizzamento**
radical	radical	**radicale**
radio	radius	**radio**
radiactivo	radioactif	**radioattivo**
radiografía	radiographie	**radiografia**
radioisótopo	radio-isotope	**radioisotopo**
radiología	radiologie	**radiologia**
radiopaco	radio-opaque	**radioopaco**
radiosensible	radiosensible	**radiosensibile**
radioterapia	radiothérapie	**radioterapia**
resfriado	rhume	**raffreddore**
fiebre del heno	rhume des foins	**raffreddore da fieno**
rayos X	rayons X	**raggi X**
raspado, legrado, curetaje, material de legrado	curetage, curetages	**raschiamento**
legrar	cureter	**raschiare**
reactivo	réactif	**reagente**
reacción	réaction	**reazione**
reacción anafiláctica	réaction anaphylactique	**reazione anafilattica**
reacción adversa a un medicamento	réaction médicamenteuse indésirable	**reazione dannosa (indesiderata) da farmaci**
reacción de Wassermann	réaction de Wassermann	**reazione di Wassermann**
reacción de Widal	réaction de Widal	**reazione di Widal**
reacción inmunológica	réaction immunitaire	**reazione immune**
efectos secundarios extrapiramidales	effets latéraux extrapyramidaux	**reazioni collaterali extrapiramidali da farmaci**
recesivo	récessif	**recessivo**
receptor	récepteur	**recettore**
periódico, recidiva	répétition, réapparition, rechute	**recidiva**
recaer	rechuter	**recidivare**
reflujo	reflux	**reflusso**
refractario	réfractaire	**refrattario**
régimen	régime	**regime**
lomo	région lombaire	**regione lombare**
regresión	régression	**regressione**
regurgitación	régurgitation	**regurgito**
factor liberador de la hormona luteinizante	substance libératrice de l'hormone lutéotrope	**releasing factor dell'ormone LH**
remisión	rémission	**remissione**
remitente	rémittent	**remittente**
renal	rénal	**renale**
riñón	rein	**rene**

renina	renin	Renin
reparto coronarico	coronary care unit (CCU)	Infarktpflegestation
reparto di terapia intensiva neonatale	neonatal intensive care unit (NICU) (Am)	Frühgeborenen-Intensivstation
repressione	repression	Unterdrückung, Verdrängung
resettore endoscopico	resectoscope	Resektoskop, Resektionszystoskop
resezione	resection	Resektion
residuo	residual	Residual-
respiratore	respirator	Respirator, Beatmungsgerät
respirazione	respiration	Respiration, Atmung
respirazione anaerobica	anaerobic respiration (Eng), anerobic respiration (Am)	anaerobe Respiration
respirazione bocca a bocca	kiss of life	Mund-zu-Mund-Wiederbelebung
respiro	breath	Atem, Atemzug
respiro affannoso	shortness of breath	Kurzatmigkeit
respiro di Cheyne-Stokes	Cheyne-Stokes respiration	Cheyne-Stokes-Atmung
restringimento	stricture	Striktur
reticolare	reticular	retikulär
reticolocito	reticulocyte	Retikulozyt
reticolocitosi	reticulocytosis	Retikulozytose
retina	retina	Retina, Netzhaut
retinite	retinitis	Retinitis, Netzhautentzündung
retinoblastoma	retinoblastoma	Retinoblastom
retinopatia	retinopathy	Retinopathie
retrattile	retractile	retraktionsfähig
retrobulbare	retrobulbar	retrobulbär
retrociecale	retrocaecal (Eng), retrocecal (Am)	retrozökal
retrofaringeo	retropharyngeal	retropharyngeal
retrogrado	retrograde	retrograd, rückläufig
retronasale	postnasal	postnasal
retroperitoneale	retroperitoneal	retroperitoneal
retroplacentare	retroplacental	retroplazentar
retrosternale	retrosternal	retrosternal
retroversione	retroversion	Retroversion
retto	rectum	Rektum
rettocele	rectocele	Rektozele
rettocolectomia	proctocolectomy	Proktokolektomie
reumatismo	rheumatism	Rheumatismus
reumatoide	rheumatoid	rheumatisch
reumatologia	rheumatology	Rheumatologie
rhinovirus	rhinovirus	Rhinovirus
Rh negativo (Rh−)	rhesus negative (Rh−)	Rh-negativ
Rh positivo (Rh+)	rhesus positive (Rh+)	Rh-positiv
riabilitazione	rehabilitation	Rehabilitation
rianimazione	resuscitation	Reanimation, Wiederbelebung
rianimazione bocca a bocca	mouth to mouth resuscitation	Mund-zu-Mund-Wiederbelebung
rianimazione cardiorespiratoria	cardiopulmonary resuscitation (CPR)	Herz-Lungen-Wiederbelebung, Reanimation

SPANISH	FRENCH	ITALIAN
renina	rénine	renina
unidad de cuidados coronarios (UCC)	unité de soins intensifs coronaires	reparto coronarico
unidad de cuidados intensivos para recién nacidos	service de soins intensifs néonatals	reparto di terapia intensiva neonatale
represión	répression	repressione
resectoscopio	résectoscope	resettore endoscopico
resección	résection	resezione
residual	résiduel	residuo
respirador	respirateur	respiratore
respiración	respiration	respirazione
respiración anaerobia	respiration anaérobie	respirazione anaerobica
beso de vida	bouche-à-bouche	respirazione bocca a bocca
aliento	haleine, souffle	respiro
disnea	essoufflement	respiro affannoso
respiración de Cheyne-Stokes	dyspnée de Cheyne-Stokes	respiro di Cheyne-Stokes
estrictura	rétrécissement	restringimento
reticular	réticulaire	reticolare
reticulocito	réticulocyte	reticolocito
reticulocitosis	réticulocytose	reticolocitosi
retina	rétine	retina
retinitis	rétinite	retinite
retinoblastoma	rétinoblastome	retinoblastoma
retinopatía	rétinopathie	retinopatia
retráctil	rétractile	retrattile
retrobulbar	rétrobulbaire	retrobulbare
retrocecal	rétrocaecal	retrociecale
retrofaríngeo	rétropharyngien	retrofaringeo
retrógrado	rétrograde	retrogrado
postnasal	rétronasal	retronasale
retroperitoneal	rétropéritonéal	retroperitoneale
retroplacentario	rétroplacentaire	retroplacentare
retrosternal	rétrosternal	retrosternale
retroversión	rétroversion	retroversione
recto	rectum	retto
rectocele	rectocèle	rettocele
proctocolectomia	proctocolectomie	rettocolectomia
reumatismo	rhumatisme	reumatismo
reumatoide	rhumatoïde	reumatoide
reumatología	rhumatologie	reumatologia
rinovirus	rhinovirus	rhinovirus
rhesus negativo (Rh−)	rhésus négatif (Rh−)	Rh negativo (Rh−)
rhesus positivo (Rh+)	rhésus positif (Rh+)	Rh positivo (Rh+)
rehabilitación	réadaptation	riabilitazione
resucitación	ressuscitation	rianimazione
respiración boca a boca	réanimation au bouche-à-bouche	rianimazione bocca a bocca
resucitación cardiopulmonar	réanimation cardiorespiratoire	rianimazione cardiorespiratoria

ITALIAN	ENGLISH	GERMAN
riassorbimento	resorption	Resorption
ricaduta	relapse	Rückfall, Rezidiv
ricetta	prescription	Rezept, Verschreibung
ricevente	recipient	Empfänger
ricoprirsi di croste	scab	verkrusten
ricordare	recall	(sich) erinnern
ricovero	hospice	Hospiz
riduzione	disimpaction	Fragmentlösung
riflesso	reflex	Reflex
riflesso condizionato	conditioned reflex	bedingter Reflex, konditionierter Reflex
riflesso di Babinski	Babinski's reflex	Babinski-Reflex
riflesso di Moro	Moro reflex	Moro-Reflex
rifrazione	refraction	Refraktion, Brechung
rigenerazione	regeneration	Regeneration
rigetto	rejection	Abstoßung
rigor	rigor	Rigor, Starre
rigurgito	posseting	Regurgitation bei Säuglingen
rilassante (n)	relaxant (n)	Relaxans (n)
rilassante (a)	relaxant (a)	entspannend (a), relaxierend (a)
rima di frattura	cradle cap	Milchschorf
rimozione di escara da una ferita	desloughing	Schorfabtragung
rinite	rhinitis	Rhinitis
rinofima	rhinophyma	Rhinophym
rinoplastica	rhinoplasty	Rhinoplastik
rinorrea	rhinorrhea (Am), rhinorrhoea (Eng)	Rhinorrhoe
riproduttivo	generative	fertil, Fortpflanzungs-
risoluzione	resolution	Auflösung, Rückgang
risonante	tympanic	Trommelfell-
risonanza	resonance	Resonanz, Schall
ristagno	stasis	Stase
ritardo mentale	retardation	Verzögerung, Hemmung
ritenzione	retention	Retention
ritiro	withdrawal	Entzug
rivascolarizzazione	revascularization	Revaskularisation
ronco	rhonchus	Rhonchus, Rasselgeräusch
rosacea	rosacea	Rosacea
rosario rachitico	rickety rosary	rachitischer Rosenkranz
roseola	roseola	Roseole
rosolia	German measles, rubella	Rubella, Röteln
rotavirus	rotavirus	Rotavirus
rottura	rupture	Riß, Bruch
rotula	patella	Patella, Kniescheibe
rullio	murmur	Herzgeräusch, Geräusch
russare	snore	schnarchen
russo	snore	Schnarchen

SPANISH	FRENCH	ITALIAN
resorción	résorption	riassorbimento
recidiva	rechute	ricaduta
receta	ordonnance	ricetta
recipiente	receveur	ricevente
formar una costra	former une croûte	ricoprirsi di croste
recordar	évoquer	ricordare
hospicio	hospice, asile	ricovero
desimpactación	désimpaction	riduzione
reflejo	réflexe	riflesso
reflejo condicionado	réflexe conditionné	riflesso condizionato
reflejo de Babinski	réflexe de Babinski	riflesso di Babinski
reflejo de Moro	réflexe de Moro	riflesso di Moro
refracción	réfraction	rifrazione
regeneración	régénération	rigenerazione
rechazo	rejet	rigetto
rigor	rigor	rigor
regurgitación láctea del neonato	régurgitation	rigurgito
relajante (n)	relaxant (n)	rilassante (n)
relajante (a)	relaxant (a)	rilassante (a)
costra láctea, dermatitis del cuero cabelludo	casque séborrhéique	rima di frattura
desesfacelación	curetage	rimozione di escara da una ferita
rinitis	rhinite	rinite
rinofima	rhinophyma	rinofima
rinoplastia	rhinoplastie	rinoplastica
rinorrea	rhinorrhée	rinorrea
generador	génératif	riproduttivo
resolución	résolution	risoluzione
timpánico	tympanique	risonante
resonancia	résonance	risonanza
estasis	stase	ristagno
retraso	retard	ritardo mentale
retención	rétention	ritenzione
supresión, abstinencia	retrait, sevrage, suppression	ritiro
revascularización	revascularisation	rivascolarizzazione
roncus	ronchus	ronco
rosácea	acné rosacée	rosacea
rosario raquítico	chapelet costal	rosario rachitico
roséola	roséole	roseola
rubéola	rubéole	rosolia
rotavirus	rotavirus	rotavirus
ruptura	hernie	rottura
rótula	rotule	rotula
soplo	murmure	rullio
roncar	ronfler	russare
ronquido	ronflement	russo

ITALIAN	ENGLISH	GERMAN

S

sacca	sac	Sack, Beutel
sacco	sac	Sack, Beutel
sacrale	sacral	sakral, Kreuzbein-
sacro	sacrum	Sakrum, Kreuzbein
sacrococcigeo	sacrococcygeal	sakrokokkygeal
sacroiliaco	sacroiliac	Iliosakral-
sacroiliite	sacroiliitis	Sakroiliitis
safeno	saphenous	saphenus
sagittale	sagittal	sagittal
salino	saline	salinisch
saliva	saliva, spittle	Speichel
salpingectomia	salpingectomy	Salpingektomie
salpingite	salpingitis	Salpingitis, Eileiterentzündung
salute	health	Gesundheit
sangue	blood	Blut
sangue occulto	occult blood	okkultes Blut
sangue occulto fecale	faecal occult blood (FOB) (Eng), fecal occult blood (FOB) (Am)	okkultes Blut (im Stuhl)
sanguinamento uterino funzionale	dysfunctional uterine bleeding (DUB)	dysfunktionale Uterusblutung
sanguinare	bleed	bluten
sanità	sanity	geistige Gesundheit
sarcoideo	sarcoid	fleischähnlich
sarcoidosi	sarcoidosis	Sarkoidose, Morbus Boeck
sarcoma	sarcoma	Sarkom
sarcoma di Kaposi	Kaposi's sarcoma	Kaposi-Sarkom
sarcoma osteogenico	osteosarcoma	Osteosarkom, Knochensarkom
sbadiglio	yawn	Gähnen
sbrigliamento	debridement	Debridement, Wundtoilette
scabbia	scabies	Skabies, Krätze
scafoide	scaphoid	Scaphoid
scapola	scapula	Skapula, Schulterblatt
scarificare	curette (Eng), curet (Am)	kürettieren
scarlattina	scarlet fever	Scharlach
scheletro	skeleton	Skelett
schistosomiasi	schistosomiasis	Schistosomiasis, Bilharziose
schizofrenia	schizophrenia	Schizophrenie
schizofrenia paranoide	paranoid schizophrenia	paranoide Schizophrenie
sciatica	sciatica	Ischias
sciatico	sciatic	ischiadicus
scintigrafia	scan	Scan
sciroppo	linctus	Linctus
sclera	sclera	Sklera
scleredema	scleredema (Am), scleredoema (Eng)	Sklerödem
sclerite	scleritis	Skleritis
sclerodermia	scleroderma	Sklerodermie

SPANISH	FRENCH	ITALIAN
saco	sac	sacca
saco	sac	sacco
sacral	sacré	sacrale
sacro	sacrum	sacro
sacrococcígeo	sacrococcygien	sacrococcigeo
sacroílíaco	sacro-iliaque	sacroiliaco
sacroileítis	sacro-ilite	sacroilíte
safeno	saphène	safeno
sagital	sagittal	sagittale
salino	salin	salino
saliva, salivazo	salive, crachat	saliva
salpingectomía	salpingectomie	salpingectomia
salpingitis	salpingite	salpingite
salud	santé	salute
sangre	sang	sangue
sangre oculta	sang occulte	sangue occulto
sangre oculta fecal	sang occulte fécal	sangue occulto fecale
hemorragia uterina funcional	ménométrorragies fonctionnelles	sanguinamento uterino funzionale
sangrar	saigner	sanguinare
cordura	santé mentale	sanità
sarcoideo	sarcoïde	sarcoideo
sarcoidosis	sarcoïdose	sarcoidosi
sarcoma	sarcome	sarcoma
sarcoma de Kaposi	sarcome de Kaposi	sarcoma di Kaposi
osteosarcoma	ostéosarcome	sarcoma osteogenico
bostezo	bâillement	sbadiglio
desbridamiento	débridement	sbrigliamento
sarna	gale	scabbia
escafoides	scaphoïde	scafoide
omoplato	omoplate	scapola
legrar	cureter	scarificare
escarlatina	scarlatine	scarlattina
esqueleto	squelette	scheletro
esquistosomiasis	schistosomiase	schistosomiasi
esquizofrenia	schizophrénie	schizofrenia
esquizofrenia paranoica	schizophrénie paranoïaque	schizofrenia paranoide
ciática	sciatique	sciatica
ciático	sciatique	sciatico
exploración, barrido	échogramme	scintigrafia
linctus	linctus	sciroppo
esclerótica	sclérotique	sclera
escleredema	scléroderme	scleredema
escleritis	sclérite	sclerite
escleroderma	scléroderme	sclerodermia

ITALIAN	ENGLISH	GERMAN
sclerosi	sclerosis	Sklerose
sclerosi multipla	multiple sclerosis (MS)	multiple Sklerose (MS)
sclerosi tuberosa	tuberous sclerosis	tuberöse Sklerose
scleroterapia	sclerotherapy	Sklerotherapie
sclerotica	sclera	Sklera
sclerotico	sclerotic	sklerotisch, Sklera-
scoliosi	scoliosis	Skoliose
scompenso cardiaco	heart failure	Herzinsuffizienz, Herzversagen
scompenso cardiaco congestizio	congestive heart failure (CHF)	Stauungsherz, Herzinsuffizienz mit Stauungszeichen
scorbuto	scurvy	Skorbut
scotoma	scotoma	Skotom, Gesichtsfeldausfall
scottatura	scald, burn	Verbrühung, Brandwunde, Verbrennung
scrofola	scrofula	Skrofula, Lymphknotentuberkulose
scroto	scrotum	Skrotum, Hodensack
scuotimento	succussion	Erschütterung, Schütteln
sdraiato	recumbent	liegend, ruhend
sebaceo	sebaceous	Talg-, talgig
sebo	sebum	Talg
seborrea	seborrhea (Am), seborrhoea (Eng), steatorrhea (Am), steatorrhoea (Eng)	Seborrhoe, Steatorrhoe, Fettstuhl
secondine	afterbirth	Plazenta, Nachgeburt
secretorio	secretory	sekretorisch
secrezione	secretion	Sekretion
sedativo (n)	sedative (n)	Sedativum (n), Beruhigungsmittel (n)
sedativo (a)	sedative (a)	sedierend (a), beruhigend (a)
sedazione	sedation	Sedierung
sedentario	sedentary	sitzend, seßhaft
segmento	segment	Segment
segni di Koplik	Koplik's spots	Koplik-Flecken
segno	sign	Zeichen, Symptom
segno di Chvostek	Chvostek's sign	Chvostek-Zeichen
segno di Kernig	Kernig's sign	Kernig Zeichen
segno di Trendelenburg	Trendelenburg sign	Trendelenburg-Zeichen
selezione	screening	Screening, Reihenuntersuchung
selezione e distribuzione dei malati	triage	Triage
seme	semen	Samen
semilunare	semilunar	semilunar, halbmondförmig
seminale	seminal	Samen-, Spermien-
seminoma	seminoma	Seminom
semiotico	semeiotic	semiotisch
semipermeabile	semipermeable	semipermeabel
senescenza	ageing, senescence	Altern, Seneszenz
senile	senile	senil, Alters-
seno	sinus	Sinus, Nebenhöhle
sensazione	sensation	Sinneswahrnehmung, Gefühl

SPANISH	FRENCH	ITALIAN
esclerosis	sclérose	sclerosi
esclerosis múltiple	sclérose en plaques	sclerosi multipla
esclerosis tuberosa	sclérose tubéreuse du cerveau	sclerosi tuberosa
escleroterapia	sclérothérapie	scleroterapia
esclerótica	sclérotique	sclerotica
esclerótico	sclérotique	sclerotico
escoliosis	scoliose	scoliosi
insuficiencia cardíaca	cardiopathie, maladie du coeur	scompenso cardiaco
insuficiencia cardíaca congestiva (ICC)	insuffisance cardiaque globale	scompenso cardiaco congestizio
escorbuto	scorbut	scorbuto
escotoma	scotome	scotoma
escaldadura, quemadura	échaudure, brûlure	scottatura
escrófula	scrofule	scrofola
escroto	scrotum	scroto
sucusión	succussion	scuotimento
recumbente, de pie	couché	sdraiato
sebáceo	sébacé	sebaceo
sebo	sébum	sebo
seborrea, esteatorrea	séborrhée, stéatorrhée	seborrea
secundinas, expulsión de la placenta y membranas	arrière-faix	secondine
secretorio	secréteur	secretorio
secreción	sécrétion	secrezione
sedante (n)	sédatif (n)	sedativo (n)
sedante (a)	sédatif (a)	sedativo (a)
sedación	sédation	sedazione
sedentario	sédentaire	sedentario
segmento	segment	segmento
manchas de Koplik	points de Koplik	segni di Koplik
signo	signe	segno
signo de Chvostek	signe de Chvostek	segno di Chvostek
signo de Kernig	signe de Kernig	segno di Kernig
signo de Trendelenburg	signe de Trendelenburg	segno di Trendelenburg
criba, despistaje	dépistage	selezione
triage	triage	selezione e distribuzione dei malati
semen	sperme	seme
semilunar	semi-lunaire	semilunare
seminal	séminal, spermatique	seminale
seminoma	séminome	seminoma
semiótica	sémiologique	semiotico
semipermeable	semi-perméable	semipermeabile
envejecimiento, senescencia	vieillissement, sénescence	senescenza
senil	sénile	senile
seno	sinus	seno
sensación	sensation	sensazione

ITALIAN	ENGLISH	GERMAN
sensi	sense	Sinn
sensibile	sensitive	sensitiv, empfindlich
sensibilità	sensation, sensitivity	Sinneswahrnehmung, Gefühl, Empfindlichkeit, Feingefühl
sensibilizzazione	sensitization	Sensitivierung, Allergisierung
sensoriale	sensory	sensorisch, Sinnes-
sepsi	sepsis	Sepsis
sequela	sequela	Folgeerscheinung, Folgezustand
sequestro	sequestrum	Sequester
sete	thirst	Durst
setticemia	septicaemia (Eng), septicemia (Am)	Septikämie
setto	septum	Septum, Scheidewand
sezione trasversale	transection	Querschnitt
sfenoide	sphenoid	Sphenoid, Keilbein
sferocitosi	spherocytosis	Sphärozytose, Kugelzellanämie
sfigmomanometro	sphygmomanometer	Blutdruckmeßgerät
sfintere	sphincter	Sphinkter, Schließmuskel
shock	shock	Schock
sibilo	wheeze	Giemen
siero	serum	Serum, Blutserum
sierologia	serology	Serologie
siero-positivo	seropositive	seropositiv
sierosa	serosa	Serosa
sieroso	serous	serös, Serum-
sifilide	syphilis	Syphilis, Lues
sigmoide	sigmoid	sigmoid
sigmoidoscopio	sigmoidoscope	Sigmoidoskop
sigmoidostomia	sigmoidostomy	Sigmoidostomie
silicosi	silicosis	Silikose
simbiosi	symbiosis	Symbiose
simpatectomia	sympathectomy	Sympathektomie
simpaticectomia	sympathectomy	Sympathektomie
simpaticomimetico (n)	sympathomimetic (n)	Sympathomimetikum (n)
simpaticomimetico (a)	sympathomimetic (a)	sympathomimetisch (a)
simulazione di malattia	malingering	scheinkrank
sinapsi	synapse	Synapse
sincope	syncope	Synkope
sindrome	syndrome	Syndrom
sindrome cerebrale cronica	chronic brain syndrome (CBS)	chronisches Gehirnsyndrom
sindrome da alcolismo materno	fetal alcohol syndrome	fetales Alkoholsyndrom
sindrome da alcool	alcohol syndrome	Alkoholsyndrom
sindrome da carcinoide	carcinoid syndrome	Karzinoid-Syndrom
sindrome da immunodeficienza acquisita (AIDS)	acquired immune deficiency syndrome (AIDS)	erworbenes Immundefektsyndrom (AIDS)
sindrome da morte improvvisa del lattante	cot death	plötzlicher Säuglingstod
sindrome da shock tossico	toxic shock syndrome	toxisches Schocksyndrom (TSS)

SPANISH	FRENCH	ITALIAN
sentido	sens	sensi
sensible	sensible	sensibile
sensación, sensibilidad	sensation, sensibilité	sensibilità
sensibilización	sensibilisation	sensibilizzazione
sensorio	sensitif	sensoriale
sepsis	septicémie	sepsi
secuela	séquelle	sequela
secuestro	séquestre	sequestro
sed	soif	sete
septicemia	septicémie	setticemia
septo, tabique	septum	setto
transección	transsection	sezione trasversale
esfenoides	sphénoïde	sfenoide
esferocitosis	sphérocytose	sferocitosi
esfigmomanómetro	sphygmomanomètre	sfigmomanometro
esfínter	sphincter	sfintere
shock	choc	shock
jadeo	wheezing	sibilo
suero	sérum	siero
serología	sérologie	sierologia
seropositivo	séropositif	siero-positivo
serosa	séreuse	sierosa
seroso	séreux	sieroso
sífilis	syphilis	sifilide
sigmoideo	sigmoïde	sigmoide
sigmoidoscopio	sigmoïdoscope	sigmoidoscopio
sigmoidostomía	sigmoïdostomie	sigmoidostomia
silicosis	silicose	silicosi
simbiosis	symbiose	simbiosi
simpatectomía	sympathectomie	simpatectomia
simpatectomía	sympathectomie	simpaticectomia
simpaticomimético (n)	sympathomimétique (n)	simpaticomimetico (n)
simpaticomimético (a)	sympathomimétique (a)	simpaticomimetico (a)
simulación de síntomas	simulation	simulazione di malattia
sinapsis	synapse	sinapsi
síncope	syncope	sincope
síndrome	syndrome	sindrome
síndrome cerebral crónico	syndrome chronique du cerveau	sindrome cerebrale cronica
síndrome alcohólico fetal	syndrome d'alcoolisme foetal	sindrome da alcolismo materno
síndrome alcohólico	syndrome d'alcoolisme	sindrome da alcool
síndrome carcinoide	syndrome carcinoïde	sindrome da carcinoide
síndrome de inmunodeficiencia adquirida (SIDA)	syndrome d'immuno-déficience acquise (SIDA)	sindrome da immunodeficienza acquisita (AIDS)
muerte en la cuna, muerte súbita infantil	mort subite de nourrisson	sindrome da morte improvvisa del lattante
síndrome de shock tóxico	syndrome de choc toxique staphylococcique	sindrome da shock tossico

771

ITALIAN	ENGLISH	GERMAN
sindrome del bambino maltrattato	battered baby syndrome	Kindesmißhandlung (Folgen)
sindrome del gastroresecato	dumping syndrome	Dumping-Syndrom
sindrome della morte neonatale improvvisa (SIDS)	sudden infant death syndrome (SIDS)	plötzlicher Säuglingstod, Sudden-infant-death-Syndrom (SIDS)
sindrome dell'ansa cieca	blind loop syndrome	Syndrom der blinden Schlinge
sindrome dell'arco aortico	pulseless disease	Pulsloskrankheit
sindrome dell'articolazione temporomandibolare	temporomandibular joint syndrome	Costen-Syndrom
sindrome delle gambe irrequiete	restless legs syndrome	Wittmaack-Ekbom-Syndrom
sindrome dell'intestino irritable	irritable bowel syndrome	Reizdarm
sindrome del tunnel carpale	carpal tunnel syndrome	Karpaltunnelsyndrom
sindrome di Arnold Chiari	Arnold-Chiari malformation	Arnold-Chiari-Mißbildung
sindrome di Behçet	Behçet syndrome	Behçet-Syndrom
sindrome di Cushing	Cushing's syndrome	Cushing-Syndrom
sindrome di Down	Down's syndrome	Down-Syndrom, Mongolismus
sindrome di Ekbom	restless legs syndrome	Wittmaack-Ekbom-Syndrom
sindrome di esaurimento professionale	burnout syndrome	Helfer-Syndrom
sindrome di Horner	Horner's syndrome	Horner-Syndrom
sindrome di Klinefelter	Klinefelter's syndrome	Klinefelter-Syndrom
sindrome di Mendelson	Mendelson's syndrome	Mendelson-Syndrom
sindrome di Münchhausen	Münchhausen's syndrome	Münchhausen-Syndrom
sindrome di Ménière	Ménière's disease	Morbus Ménière
sindrome di Ramsay Hunt	Ramsay Hunt syndrome	Ramsay-Hunt-Syndrom
sindrome di Reiter	Reiter's syndrome	Reiter-Syndrom
sindrome di Reye	Reye's syndrome	Reye-Syndrom
sindrome di Sjögren-Larsson (eritrodermia ittiosiforme con oligofrenia spastica)	Sjögren-Larsson syndrome	Sjögren-Syndrom
sindrome di sofferenza respiratoria	respiratory distress syndrome (RDS)	Respiratory-distress-Syndrom, Atemnotsyndrom
sindrome di Stein-Leventhal	Stein-Leventhal syndrome	Stein-Leventhal-Syndrom
sindrome di Stevens-Johnson	Stevens-Johnson syndrome	Stevens-Johnson-Syndrom
sindrome di Stokes-Adams	Stokes-Adams syndrome	Morgagni-Stokes-Adams-Syndrom
sindrome di Turner	Turner's syndrome	Turner-Syndrom
sindrome emolitico-uremica	haemolytic uraemic syndrome (HUS) (Eng), hemolytic uremic syndrome (HUS) (Am)	hämolytisch-urämisches Syndrom
sindrome ipercinetica	hyperkinetic syndrome	hyperkinetisches Syndrom
sindrome nefrosica	nephrotic syndrome	nephrotisches Syndrom
sindrome uretrale	urethral syndrome	Urethralsyndrom
sindrome vibratoria	vibration syndrome	Vibrationssyndrom
sinechia	synechia	Synechie, Verwachsung
sinergia	synergy	Synergie
sinfisi	symphysis	Symphyse
singhiozzo	hiccup	Schluckauf
sintomo	symptom	Symptom
sinusite	sinusitis	Sinusitis

SPANISH	FRENCH	ITALIAN
síndrome del niño apaleado	syndrome des enfants maltraités	sindrome del bambino maltrattato
síndrome de dumping, síndrome del vaciamiento en gastrectomizados	syndrome de chasse	sindrome del gastroresecato
síndrome de muerte súbita infantil	syndrome de mort subite de nourrisson	sindrome della morte neonatale improvvisa (SIDS)
síndrome del asa ciega	syndrome de l'anse borgne	sindrome dell'ansa cieca
enfermedad sin pulso	syndrome de Takayashu	sindrome dell'arco aortico
síndrome de la articulación temporomandibular	syndrome de Costen	sindrome dell'articolazione temporomandibolare
síndrome de piernas inquietas	syndrome d'impatience musculaire	sindrome delle gambe irrequiete
síndrome del intestino irritable	syndrome de l'intestin irritable	sindrome dell'intestino irritabile
síndrome del túnel carpiano	syndrome du canal carpien	sindrome del tunnel carpale
malformación de Arnold-Chiari	malformation d'Arnold Chiari	sindrome di Arnold Chiari
síndrome de Behçet	syndrome de Behçet	sindrome di Behçet
síndrome de Cushing	syndrome de Cushing	sindrome di Cushing
síndrome de Down	trisomie 21	sindrome di Down
síndrome de piernas inquietas	syndrome d'impatience musculaire	sindrome di Ekbom
surmenage, neurastenia	syndrome de 'surmenage'	sindrome di esaurimento professionale
síndrome de Horner	syndrome de Bernard-Horner, syndrome oculaire sympathique	sindrome di Horner
síndrome de Klinefelter	syndrome de Klinefelter	sindrome di Klinefelter
síndrome de Mendelson	syndrome de Mendelson	sindrome di Mendelson
síndrome de Münchhausen	syndrome de Münchhausen	sindrome di Münchhausen
enfermedad de Ménière	syndrome de Ménière	sindrome di Ménière
síndrome de Ramsay-Hunt	maladie de Ramsay Hunt	sindrome di Ramsay Hunt
síndrome de Reiter	syndrome de Fiessinger-Leroy-Reiter	sindrome di Reiter
síndrome de Reye	syndrome de Reye	sindrome di Reye
síndrome de Sjögren	syndrome de Sjögren	sindrome di Sjögren-Larsson (eritrodermia ittiosiforme con oligofrenia spastica)
síndrome de distress respiratorio	syndrome de membrane hyaline et de souffrance respiratoire	sindrome di sofferenza respiratoria
síndrome de Stein-Leventhal	syndrome de Stein-Leventhal	sindrome di Stein-Leventhal
síndrome de Stevens-Johnson	syndrome de Stevens-Johnson	sindrome di Stevens-Johnson
síndrome de Stokes-Adams	syndrome de Stokes-Adams	sindrome di Stokes-Adams
síndrome de Turner	syndrome de Turner	sindrome di Turner
síndrome hemolítico urémico	hémolyse urémique des nouveau-nés	sindrome emolitico-uremica
síndrome hipercinético	syndrome hyperkinétique	sindrome ipercinetica
síndrome nefrótico	syndrome néphrotique	sindrome nefrosica
síndrome uretral	syndrome urétral	sindrome uretrale
síndrome de vibración	syndrome de vibrations	sindrome vibratoria
sinequia	synéchie	sinechia
sinergia	synergie	sinergia
sínfisis	symphyse	sinfisi
hipo	hoquet	singhiozzo
síntoma	symptôme	sintomo
sinusitis	sinusite	sinusite

ITALIAN	ENGLISH	GERMAN
siringa	syringe	Spritze
siringomielia	syringomyelia	Syringomyelie
sistema digestivo	digestive system	Verdauungsapparat
sistema nervoso centrale	central nervous system (CNS)	Zentralnervensystem (ZNS)
sistema nervoso simpatico	sympathetic nervous system	sympathisches Nervensystem
sistema respiratorio	respiratory system	Atmungsapparat, Atmungsorgane
sistema reticoloendoteliale (RES)	reticuloendothelial system (RES)	retikuloendotheliales System
sistema riproduttivo	reproductive system	Fortpflanzungsapparat
sistole	systole	Systole
smalto	enamel	Emaille
sociosanitario	sociomedical	sozialmedizinisch
soffio	murmur	Herzgeräusch, Geräusch
soffio sistolico	systolic murmur	systolisches Geräusch, Systolikum
soffocamento	suffocation	Ersticken, Erstickung
soggettivo	subjective	subjektiv
solco	sulcus	Sulcus, Furche
solfato di calcio	gypsum	Gips
solidificazione	consolidation	Konsolidierung, Festigung
soluzione	solution	Lösung, Auflösung
soluzione di Brompton	Brompton's mixture	Brompton-Lösung (Alkohol, Morphin, Kokain)
soluzione di Hartmann	Hartmann's solution	Hartmann-Lösung
soluzione fisiologica	saline	Kochsalzlösung
solvente	solvent	Lösungsmittel
somatico	somatic	somatisch, körperlich
somatomammotropina corionica umana	human chorionic somatomammotrophin (HCS) (Eng), human chorionic somatomammotropin (HCS, HPL) (Am)	human chorionic somatomammotropin (HCS)
sonnambulismo	somnambulism	Somnambulismus, Schlafwandeln
sonno	sleep	Schlaf
sonno REM	REM sleep	REM-Schlaf
soppressione	suppression	Unterdrückung, Verdrängung
sopracciglio	brow	Augenbraue
sopraclavicolare	supraclavicular	supraklavikulär
sopracondiloideo	supracondylar	suprakondylär
soprapubico	suprapubic	suprapubisch
soprasternale	suprasternal	suprasternal
sordità	deafness	Taubheit, Schwerhörigkeit
sordo	deaf	taub, schwerhörig
sospensione	withdrawal	Entzug
sostanza nutritiva	nutrient	Nahrungsmittel
sottoclavicolare	subclavian	Subklavia-
sottocongiuntivale	subconjunctival	subkonjunktival
sottocostale	subcostal	subkostal
sottocutaneo	subcutaneous (SC, SQ)	subkutan
sottodiaframmatico	subphrenic	subdiaphragmatisch
sottodurale	subdural	subdural

SPANISH	FRENCH	ITALIAN
jeringuilla	seringue	siringa
siringomielia	syringomyélie	siringomielia
aparato digestivo	système digestif	sistema digestivo
sistema nervioso central (SNC)	système nerveux central (CNS)	sistema nervoso centrale
sistema nervioso simpático	système nerveux sympathique	sistema nervoso simpatico
aparato respiratorio	système respiratoire	sistema respiratorio
sistema reticuloendotelial (SRE)	système réticulo-endothélial	sistema reticoloendoteliale (RES)
aparato reproductor	système reproducteur	sistema riproduttivo
sístole	systole	sistole
esmalte	émail	smalto
médico-social	sociomédical	sociosanitario
soplo	murmure	soffio
soplo sistólico	murmure systolique	soffio sistolico
asfixia	suffocation	soffocamento
subjetivo	subjectif	soggettivo
surco	sillon, gouttière, scissure	solco
yeso	gypse	solfato di calcio
consolidación	consolidation	solidificazione
solución	solution	soluzione
mezcla de Brompton	liquide de Brompton	soluzione di Brompton
solución de Hartmann	liquide de Hartmann	soluzione di Hartmann
solución salina	solution physiologique	soluzione fisiologica
disolvente	solvant	solvente
somático	somatique	somatico
somatomamotropina corionica humana	somatomammotropine chorionique humaine (HCS), somatoprolactine chorionique humain	somatomammotropina corionica umana
sonambulismo	somnambulisme	sonnambulismo
sueño	sommeil	sonno
sueño REM	sommeil paradoxal	sonno REM
supresión	suppression	soppressione
ceja	front, sourcil	sopracciglio
supraclavicular	supraclaviculaire	sopraclavicolare
supracondilar	supracondylaire	sopracondiloideo
suprapúbico	suprapubien	soprapubico
supraesternal	suprasternal	soprasternale
sordera	surdité	sordità
sordo	sourd	sordo
supresión, abstinencia	retrait, sevrage, suppression	sospensione
nutriente	nutriment	sostanza nutritiva
subclavia	sous-clavier	sottoclavicolare
subconjuntival	sous-conjonctival	sottocongiuntivale
subcostal	sous-costal	sottocostale
subcutáneo (SC)	sous-cutané (SC)	sottocutaneo
subfrénico	sous-phrénique	sottodiaframmatico
subdural	sous-dural	sottodurale

ITALIAN	ENGLISH	GERMAN
sottomandibolare	submandibular	submandibulär
sottomucosa	submucosa	Submukosa
spalla	shoulder	Schulter
'spalla congelata'	frozen shoulder	Frozen shoulder, Periarthritis humeroscapularis
spasmo	spasm	Spasmus, Krampf
spasmo cardiale	cardiospasm	Kardiospasmus
spastico	spastic	spastisch, krampfhaft
spatola	spatula	Spatel
spazio subaracnoideo	subarachnoid space	Subarachnoidalraum
specie	species	Spezies, Art
specifico	specific	spezifisch, speziell
speculum	speculum	Spekulum, Spiegel
speculum di Sim	Sims' speculum	Sims-Spekulum
sperma	sperm	Sperma, Samen
spermatico	spermatic	Sperma-, Samen-
spermatocele	spermatocele	Spermatozele
spermicida	spermicide	Spermizid
spicola	spicule	Spikulum
spiga	spica	Kornährenverband, Sporn
spina	spine	Wirbelsäule, Rückgrat
spina bifida	spina bifida	Spina bifida
spinale	spinal	spinal, Rückenmarks-, Wirbelsäulen-
spirocheta	spirochaete (Eng), spirochete (Am)	Spirochäte
spirochetosi discromica	pinta	Pinta
spirografo	spirograph	Spirograph
spirometro	spirometer	Spirometer
splancnico	splanchnic	viszeral, Eingeweide-
splenectomia	splenectomy	Splenektomie
splenomegalia	splenomegaly	Splenomegalie
spondilite	spondylitis	Spondylitis
spondilolistesi	spondylolisthesis	Spondylolisthesis
sporadico	sporadic	sporadisch
sprue	sprue	Sprue
spugnoso	cancellous	spongiös, schwammartig
sputo	sputum	Sputum, Auswurf
squamoso	squamous	squamös, schuppig
squilibrio	imbalance	Gleichgewichtsstörung
staffa	stapes	Stapes, Steigbügel
stafilite	uvulitis	Uvulitis
stanchezza	fatigue	Ermüdung
stapedectomia	stapedectomy	Stapedektomie
starnutire	sneeze	niesen
starnuto	sneeze	Niesen
stasi	stasis	Stase
stato	status	Status, Zustand
steatorrea	steatorrhea (Am), steatorrhoea (Eng)	Steatorrhoe, Fettstuhl

SPANISH	FRENCH	ITALIAN
submandibular	submandibulaire	sottomandibolare
submucosa	tissu sous-muqueux	sottomucosa
hombro	épaule	spalla
hombro congelado/rígido	épaule ankylosée	'spalla congelata'
espasmo	spasme	spasmo
cardiospasmo	cardiospasme	spasmo cardiale
espástico	spastique	spastico
espátula	spatule	spatola
espacio subaracnoideo	espace sous-arachnoïdien	spazio subaracnoideo
especie	espèce	specie
específico	spécifique	specifico
espéculo	spéculum	speculum
espéculo de Sim	spéculum de Sim	speculum di Sim
esperma	sperme	sperma
espermático	spermatique	spermatico
espermatocele	spermatocèle	spermatocele
espermicida	spermicide	spermicida
espícula	spicule	spicola
espica	spica	spiga
raquis	colonne vertébrale	spina
espina bífida	spina bifida	spina bifida
espinal	spinal	spinale
espiroqueta	spirochète	spirocheta
mal de pinto	pinta	spirochetosi discromica
espirografía	spirographe	spirografo
espirómetro	spiromètre	spirometro
esplácnico	splanchnique	splancnico
esplenectomía	splénectomie	splenectomia
esplenomegalia	splénomégalie	splenomegalia
espondilitis	spondylite	spondilite
espondilolistesis	spondylolisthésis	spondilolistesi
esporádico	sporadique	sporadico
esprue	sprue	sprue
esponjoso, reticulado	spongieux	spugnoso
esputo	salive	sputo
escamoso	squameux	squamoso
desequilibrio	déséquilibre	squilibrio
estribo	étrier	staffa
uvulitis	uvulite	stafilite
fatiga, cansancio	fatigue	stanchezza
estapedectomía	stapédectomie	stapedectomia
estornudar	éternuer	starnutire
estornudo	éternuement	starnuto
estasis	stase	stasi
status	statut	stato
esteatorrea	stéatorrhée	steatorrea

ITALIAN	ENGLISH	GERMAN
stecca	cradle cap	Milchschorf
stecca ortopedica	splint	Schiene
steccatura	cast	Abdruck, Gipsverband
stenosi	stenosis, stricture	Stenose, Striktur
sterile	sterile	steril, keimfrei, unfruchtbar
sterilizzazione	sterilization	Sterilisation, Sterilisierung
sterno	sternum	Sternum, Brustbein
sternocostale	sternocostal	sternokostal
steroide	steroid	Steroid
stetoscopio	stethoscope	Stethoskop
stigmate	stigmata	Stigmata, Kennzeichen
stilbestrolo	stilbestrol (Am), stilboestrol (Eng)	Diäthylstilboestrol
stiloide	styloid	Styloid-
stiloideo	styloid	Styloid-
stimolante (n)	stimulant (n)	Stimulans (n)
stimolante (a)	stimulant (a)	stimulierend (a)
stipsi	constipation	Verstopfung
stoma	stoma	Stoma, Mund
stomaco	stomach	Magen
stomatite	stomatitis	Stomatitis, Mundhöhlenentzündung
stomatite de Candida albicans	thrush	Soor, Sprue
stordimento	dizziness	Schwindel
stordito	giddy	schwindlig
strabismo	squint, strabismus	Schielen, Strabismus
strangolamento	strangulation	Strangulation, Einklemmung
stranguria	strangury	Harnzwang
strato	stratum	Stratum, Schicht
stravaso	extravasation	Extravasat
stress	stress	Belastung, Streß
stria	striae	Striae, Streifen
stridore	stridor	Stridor
striscio	smear	Belag, Abstrich
strongiloide	hookworm	Hakenwurm
stupore	stupor	Stupor, Benommenheit
subacuto	subacute	subakut
subclinico	subclinical	subklinisch
subconscio	subconscious	unterbewußt
subdurale	subdural	subdural
subfertilità	subfertility	Subfertilität
subfrenico	subphrenic	subdiaphragmatisch
sublimato	sublimate	Sublimat, Quicksilberchlorid
subliminale	subliminal	unterschwellig
sublinguale	sublingual	sublingual
sublussazione	subluxation	Subluxation
subnormalità	subnormality	Subnormalität
suboccipitale	suboccipital	subokzipital

SPANISH	FRENCH	ITALIAN
costra láctea, dermatitis del cuero cabelludo	casque séborrhéique	stecca
astilla	attelle	stecca ortopedica
enyesado, vendaje de yeso	plâtre	steccatura
estenosis, estrictura	sténose, rétrécissement	stenosi
estéril	stérile	sterile
esterilización	stérilisation	sterilizzazione
esternón	sternum	sterno
esternocostal	sternocostal	sternocostale
esteroide	stéroïde	steroide
estetoscopio	stéthoscope	stetoscopio
estigmas	stigmate	stigmate
estilbestrol	stilboestrol	stilbestrolo
estiloides	styloïde	stiloide
estiloides	styloïde	stiloideo
estimulante (n)	stimulant (n)	stimolante (n)
estimulante (a)	stimulant (a)	stimolante (a)
estreñimiento	constipation	stipsi
estoma	stoma	stoma
estómago	estomac	stomaco
estomatitis	stomatite	stomatite
muguet	aphte	stomatite de Candida albicans
desvanecimiento, mareo	étourdissement	stordimento
mareado	pris de vertige	stordito
estrabismo	strabisme	strabismo
estrangulación	strangulation	strangolamento
estranguria	strangurie	stranguria
estrato	couche	strato
extravasación	extravasation	stravaso
stress, estrés	stress	stress
estrias	stries	stria
estridor	stridor	stridore
frotis	frottis	striscio
anquilostoma duodenal	ankylostome	strongiloide
estupor	stupeur	stupore
subagudo	subaigu	subacuto
subclínico	sous-clinique	subclinico
subconsciente	subconscient	subconscio
subdural	sous-dural	subdurale
subfertilidad	sous-fertilité	subfertilità
subfrénico	sous-phrénique	subfrenico
sublimado	sublimé	sublimato
subliminal	subliminal	subliminale
sublingual	sublingual	sublinguale
subluxación	subluxation	sublussazione
subnormalidad	subnormalité	subnormalità
suboccipital	sous-occipital	suboccipitale

ITALIAN	ENGLISH	GERMAN
succlavio	subclavian	Subklavia-
succussione	succussion	Erschütterung, Schütteln
sudare	sweat	schwitzen
sudorazione	hidrosis	Hidrosis, Schweißabsonderung
sudorazione notturna	night sweat	Nachtschweiß
sudore	sweat	Schweiß
suggestione	suggestion	Vorschlag, Suggestion
suicidio	suicide	Suizid, Selbstmord
suicidio figurato	parasuicide	parasuizidale Handlung
sulfonammide	sulfonamide (Am), sulphonamide (Eng)	Sulfonamid
sulfonilurea	sulfonylurea (Am), sulphonylurea (Eng)	Sulfonylharnstoff
suono	sound	Ton, Klang
superiore	superior	oben, überlegen
supinatore	supinator	Supinator
supinazione	supination	Supination
supino	recumbent, supine	liegend, ruhend, supiniert
supposta	suppository	Suppositorium, Zäpfchen
suppurazione	suppuration	Suppuration, Eiterung
surfattante	surfactant	Surfactant-Faktor
surrenale	adrenal	Nebennieren-
suscettibilità	susceptibility	Anfälligkeit, Empfindlichkeit
sutura	suture	Naht
suturare	suture	nähen
svenimento	faint	Ohnmacht
svenire	faint	ohnmächtig werden

SPANISH	FRENCH	ITALIAN
subclavia	sous-clavier	succlavio
sucusión	succussion	succussione
sudar	suer	sudare
hidrosis	transpiration	sudorazione
sudoración nocturna	sueurs nocturnes	sudorazione notturna
sudor	sueur	sudore
sugestión	suggestion	suggestione
suicidio	suicide	suicidio
parasuicidio	parasuicide	suicidio figurato
sulfonamida	sulfamide	sulfonammide
sulfonilurea	sulfonylurée	sulfonilurea
sonido	son	suono
superior	supérieur	superiore
supinador	supinateur	supinatore
supinar	supination	supinazione
recumbente, de pie, supino	couché, en supination	supino
supositorio	suppositoire	supposta
supuración	suppuration	suppurazione
tensoactivo	surfactant	surfattante
adrenal	surrénale	surrenale
susceptibilidad	susceptibilité	suscettibilità
sutura	suture	sutura
suturar	suturer	suturare
vahído, síncope	syncope	svenimento
desmayar	s'évanouir	svenire

T

tabe dorsale	tabes	Auszehrung, Schwindsucht
tachicardia	tachycardia	Tachykardie
tachipnea	tachypnea (Am), tachypnoea (Eng)	Tachypnoe
taglio cesareo	caesarean section (Eng), cesarean section (Am)	Kaiserschnitt, Sectio
talamo	thalamus	Thalamus
talassemia	thalassaemia (Eng), thalassemia (Am)	Thalassämie, Mittelmeeranämie
talco	talc	Talkum
tallone	heel	Ferse
talo	talus	Talus
tamponamento	tamponade	Tamponade
tampone	swab	Tupfer, Abstrichtupfer
tarsalgia	tarsalgia	Tarsalgie
tarso	tarsus	Fußwurzel, Lidknorpel
tarsorrafia	tarsorrhaphy	Tarsorrhaphie
tasca	pouch	Beutel, Tasche
tasca faringea	pharyngeal pouch	Schlundtasche
tasso di picco del flusso espiratorio	peak expiratory flow rate (PEFR)	maximale exspiratorische Atemstromstärke
tattile	tactile	taktil, tastbar
tecnica asettica	aseptic technique	aseptische Technik
tecnica ultrasonografica Doppler	Doppler ultrasound technique	Doppler-Sonographie
telangectasia	telangiectasis	Teleangiektasie
temperamento	temperament	Temperament, Gemütsart
tempia	temple	Schläfe
tempo di sanguinamento	'bleeding time'	Blutungszeit
temporale	temporal	temporal, Schläfen-
tendine	tendon	Sehne
tendine del ginocchio	hamstring	Kniesehne
tendine di Achille	Achilles tendon	Achillessehne
tendinite	tendinitis (Am), tendonitis (Eng)	Tendinitis, Sehnenentzündung
tenesmo	tenesmus	Tenesmus
Tenia	Taenia	Bandwurm, Tänia
tenosinovite	tenosynovitis	Tendovaginitis, Tendosynovitis, Sehnenscheidenentzündung
tenotomia	tenotomy	Tenotomie
tensioattivo	surfactant	Surfactant-Faktor
tensione	strain	Anstrengung, Belastung
tensione premenstruale	premenstrual tension (PMT)	prämenstruelles Syndrom
terapia	therapeutics, therapy	Therapeutik, -therapie, Therapie, Behandlung
terapia del linguaggio	speech therapy	Sprachtherapie
terapia elettroconvulsiva	electroconvulsive therapy (ECT)	Elektroschocktherapie
terapia sostitutiva ormonale	hormone replacement therapy (HRT)	Hormonsubstitutionstherapie

SPANISH	FRENCH	ITALIAN
tabes	tabès	tabe dorsale
taquicardia	tachycardie	tachicardia
taquipnea	tachypnée	tachipnea
cesárea	césarienne	taglio cesareo
tálamo	thalamus	talamo
talasemia	thalassémie	talassemia
talco	talc	talco
talón	talon	tallone
astrágalo	astragale	talo
taponamiento	tamponnement	tamponamento
torunda	tampon	tampone
tarsalgia	tarsalgie	tarsalgia
tarso	tarse	tarso
tarsorrafia	tarsorraphie	tarsorrafia
bolsa	poche	tasca
bolsa faringea	poche ectobranchiale et entobranchiale	tasca faringea
velocidad máxima del flujo espiratorio (VMFE)	débit expiratoire de pointe	tasso di picco del flusso espiratorio
táctil	tactile	tattile
técnica aséptica	technique aseptique	tecnica asettica
técnica de ultrasonidos Doppler	échographie de Doppler	tecnica ultrasonografica Doppler
telangiectasia	télangiectasie	telangectasia
temperamento	tempérament	temperamento
sien	tempe	tempia
tiempo de sangría	temps de saignement	tempo di sanguinamento
temporal	temporal	temporale
tendón	tendon	tendine
tendón del hueso poplíteo	tendon du jarret	tendine del ginocchio
tendón de Aquiles	tendon d'Achille	tendine di Achille
tendinitis	tendinite	tendinite
tenesmo	ténesme	tenesmo
tenia	ténia	Tenia
tenosinovitis	ténosynovite	tenosinovite
tenotomía	ténotomie	tenotomia
tensoactivo	surfactant	tensioattivo
cepa	entorse	tensione
tensión premenstrual	syndrome de tension prémenstruelle	tensione premenstruale
terapéutica	thérapeutique, thérapie	terapia
logopedia	orthophonie	terapia del linguaggio
electrochoqueterapia (ECT)	électrochoc	terapia elettroconvulsiva
terapéutica de reposición de hormonas	traitement hormonal substitutif, hormonothérapie supplétive	terapia sostitutiva ormonale

ITALIAN	ENGLISH	GERMAN
teratogeno	teratogen	Teratogen
teratoma	teratoma	Teratom
termale	thermal	thermal, Wärme-
terminazione nervosa	nerve ending	Nervenendigung
termine	expiration	Exspiration, Ausatmen
termometro	thermometer	Thermometer
terziario	tertiary	tertiär, dritten Grades
tessuto	tissue	Gewebe
test	test	Test, Untersuchung
testa	head	Kopf
test alla tubercolina	Heaf test	Heaf-Test
test audiometrici	hearing test	Hörtest
test calorico	caloric test	kalorische Prüfung
test del sudore	sweat test	Schweißtest
test di aggregazione piastrinico	platelet aggregation test (PAT)	Plättchen-Aggregations-Test (PAT)
test di funzionalità epatica (TFE)	liver function test (LFT)	Leberfunktionstest
test di funzionalità respiratoria	respiratory function test	Atemfunktionstest
test di Guthrie per la fenilchetonuria	Guthrie test	Guthrie-Test
test di immunoassorbimento enzimatico	enzyme-linked immunosorbent assay (ELISA)	enzyme-linked immunosorbent assay (ELISA)
test di Kveim	Kveim test	Kveim-Test
test di Papanicolaou (Pap test)	Papanicolaou's stain test (Pap test)	Papanicolaou-Färbung (Pap)
test di Paul-Bunnell	Paul-Bunnell test	Paul-Bunnell-Reaktion
test di radioallergoassorbimento (RAST)	radioallergosorbent test (RAST)	Radio-Allergo-Sorbent-Test (RAST)
test di Schick	Schick test	Schick-Test
test di tolleranza al glucosio (TTG)	glucose tolerance test (GTT)	Glukose-Toleranztest
test di tolleranza all' insulina	insulin tolerance test (ITT)	Insulintoleranztest
test epicutaneo	patch test	Läppchenprobe, Einreibeprobe
testicoli ritenuti	undescended testes	Kryptorchismus
testicolo	orchis, testis	Hoden
test insulinico di tolleranza al glucosio	glucose insulin tolerance test (GITT)	Glukose-Insulin-Toleranztest
tetania	tetany	Tetanie
tetano	lock jaw, tetanus	Kiefersperre, Tetanus, Wundstarrkrampf
tetralogia di Fallot	Fallot's tetralogy, tetralogy of Fallot	Fallot-Tetralogie
tetraplegia	quadriplegia, tetraplegia	Tetraplegie
tibia	shin bone, tibia	Schienbein, Tibia
tibiofibulare	tibiofibular	tibiofibular
tic	tic	Tic
tic doloroso	tic douloureux	Tic douloureux
tifo	typhus	Typhus, Fleckfieber
tifo addominale	typhoid fever	Typhus
tigna	tinea	Tinea
timo	thymus	Thymus
timpanico	tympanic	Trommelfell-
timpano	eardrum, tympanum	Trommelfell, Tympanon

SPANISH	FRENCH	ENGLISH	ITALIAN

SPANISH	FRENCH	ITALIAN
teratógeno	tératogène	teratogeno
teratoma	tératome	teratoma
termal	thermique	termale
terminación nerviosa	terminaison nerveuse	terminazione nervosa
espiración	expiration	termine
termómetro	thermomètre	termometro
terciario	tertiaire	terziario
tejido	tissu	tessuto
prueba	test	test
cabeza	tête	testa
prueba de Heaf	cuti-réaction de Heaf	test alla tubercolina
prueba auditiva	test auditif	test audiometrici
prueba calórica	essai calorique	test calorico
prueba del sudor	test de sueur	test del sudore
prueba de la agregación plaquetaria	test d'agrégation plaquettaire (PAT)	test di aggregazione piastrinico
prueba de función hepática	test de la fonction hépatique (TFH)	test di funzionalità epatica (TFE)
prueba de función respiratoria	test de la fonction respiratoire	test di funzionalità respiratoria
prueba de Guthrie	test de Guthrie	test di Guthrie per la fenilchetonuria
análisis enzimático por inmunoabsorción	dosage par la méthode (ELISA)	test di immunoassorbimento enzimatico
prueba de Kveim	test de Kveim	test di Kveim
prueba de tinción de Papanicolaou	test de Papanicolaou	test di Papanicolaou (Pap test)
prueba de Paul-Bunnell	réaction de Paul et Bunnell	test di Paul-Bunnell
prueba radioalergosorbente (RAST)	technique du RAST	test di radioallergoassorbimento (RAST)
prueba de Schick	réaction de Schick	test di Schick
prueba de tolerancia a la glucosa	épreuve d'hyperglycémie provoquée	test di tolleranza al glucosio (TTG)
prueba de la tolerancia a la insulina	épreuve de tolérance à l'insuline	test di tolleranza all' insulina
prueba del parche	tache, plaque, pièce	test epicutaneo
testículos no descendidos	ectopie testiculaire	testicoli ritenuti
testículo	testicule	testicolo
prueba de resistencia a la insulina	épreuve de tolérance au glucose et à l'insuline	test insulinico di tolleranza al glucosio
tetania	tétanie	tetania
trismo, tétanos	tétanos	tetano
tetralogía de Fallot	trilogie de Fallot, tétralogie de Fallot	tetralogia di Fallot
cuadriplejía, tetraplejía	quadriplégie, tétraplégie	tetraplegia
tibia	tibia	tibia
tibioperoneo	tibiofibulaire	tibiofibulare
tic	tic	tic
tic doloroso	tic douloureux	tic doloroso
tifus	typhus	tifo
fiebre tifoidea	fièvre typhoïde	tifo addominale
tiña	teigne	tigna
timo	thymus	timo
timpánico	tympanique	timpanico
tímpano	tympan	timpano

ITALIAN	ENGLISH	GERMAN
timpanoplastica	tympanoplasty	Tympanoplastik
tinea	ringworm	Tinea, Fadenpilzerkrankung, Onchozerkose
tinnito	tinnitus	Tinnitus
tipo	type	Typ, Art
tireoglosso	thyroglossal	thyreoglossus
tireotossicosi	thyrotoxicosis	Thyreotoxikose
tiroide	thyroid	Thyreoidea, Schilddrüse
tiroidectomia	thyroidectomy	Thyreoidektomie
tiroidite	thyroiditis	Thyreoiditis
tiroidite di Hashimoto	Hashimoto's disease	Hashimoto-Struma
tiroxina libera (FT)	free thyroxine (FT)	freies Thyroxin (FT)
titolazione	titration	Titration
titolo	titer (Am), titre (Eng)	Titer
tofo	tophus	Tophus, Gichtknoten
tolleranza	tolerance	Toleranz
tomografia assiale computerizzata (TAC)	computerized axial tomography (CAT)	axiale Computertomographie
tomografia computerizzata	computerized tomography	Computertomographie (CT)
tonico	tonic	Tonikum, Stärkungsmittel
tono	tone	Ton, Laut
tonometro	tonometer	Tonometer
tonsille	tonsils	Tonsillen, Mandeln
tonsillectomia	tonsillectomy	Tonsillektomie, Mandelentfernung
tonsillite	tonsillitis	Tonsillitis, Mandelentzündung
topico	topical	topisch, örtlich
torace	thorax	Thorax, Brustkorb
torace carenato	pigeon chest	Hühnerbrust
toracico	thoracic	thorakal, Brust-
toracoplastica	thoracoplasty	Thorakoplastik
toracotomia	thoracotomy	Thorakotomie
torcicollo	wry-neck	Tortikollis, (angeborener) Schiefhals
tornasole	litmus	Lackmus
torsione	torsion	Torsion
tosse	cough	Husten
tossicità	toxicity	Toxizität
tossico	toxic	toxisch, giftig
tossicomania	addiction	Sucht, Gewöhnung
tossiemia	toxaemia (Eng), toxemia (Am)	Toxämie, Toxikämie, Blutvergiftung
tossina	toxin	Toxin
tossire	cough	husten
tossoide	toxoid	Toxoid
toxoplasmosi	toxoplasmosis	Toxoplasmose
trabecolare	cancellous	spongiös, schwammartig
tracciante	tracer	Tracer
trachea	trachea, windpipe	Trachea, Luftröhre
tracheite	tracheitis	Tracheitis

SPANISH	FRENCH	ITALIAN
timpanoplastia	tympanoplastie	timpanoplastica
tiña	dermatophytose	tinea
tinnitus	tintement	tinnito
tipo	type	tipo
tirogloso	thyroglossien	tireoglosso
tirotoxicosis	thyrotoxicose	tireotossicosi
tiroides	thyroïde	tiroide
tiroidectomía	thyroïdectomie	tiroidectomia
tiroiditis	thyroïdite	tiroidite
enfermedad de Hashimoto	maladie d'Hashimoto	tiroidite di Hashimoto
tiroxina libre	thyroxine libre (TL)	tiroxina libera (FT)
titulación	titrage	titolazione
titulo	titre	titolo
tofo	tophus	tofo
tolerancia	tolérance	tolleranza
tomografía axial computerizada (TAC)	tacographie	tomografia assiale computerizzata (TAC)
tomografía computerizada	tomographie avec ordinateur, scanographie	tomografia computerizzata
tónico	tonique	tonico
tono	tonus	tono
tonómetro	tonomètre	tonometro
amígdalas	amygdales	tonsille
tonsilectomía	amygdalectomie	tonsillectomia
amigdalitis	angine	tonsillite
tópico	topique	topico
tórax	thorax	torace
tórax de pichón	thorax en carène	torace carenato
torácico	thoracique	toracico
toracoplastia	thoracoplastie	toracoplastica
toracotomía	thoracotomie	toracotomia
tortícolis	torticolis	torcicollo
tornasol	tournesol	tornasole
torsión	torsion	torsione
tos	toux	tosse
toxicidad	toxicité	tossicità
tóxico	toxique	tossico
adicción, toxicomanía	accoutumance	tossicomania
toxemia	toxémie	tossiemia
toxina	toxine	tossina
toser	tousser	tossire
toxoide	toxoïde	tossoide
toxoplasmosis	toxoplasmose	toxoplasmosi
esponjoso, reticulado	spongieux	trabecolare
trazador	traceur	tracciante
tráquea	trachée	trachea
traqueitis	trachéite	tracheite

ITALIAN	ENGLISH	GERMAN
tracheoesofageo	tracheoesophageal (Am), tracheo-oesophageal (Eng)	Tracheoösophageal-
tracheostomia	tracheostomy	Tracheostomie
tracheotomia	tracheotomy	Tracheotomie, Luftröhrenschnitt
tracoma	trachoma	Trachom, ägyptische Augenkrankheit
tranquillante	tranquilizer	Tranquilizer, Beruhigungsmittel
transaddominale	transabdominal	transabdominal
transaminasi	gamma glutamyl transferase (GGT)	Gammaglutamyltransferase (gGT)
transamniotico	transamniotic	transamniotisch
transferasi glutammica	gamma glutamyl transferase (GGT)	Gammaglutamyltransferase (gGT)
translucido	translucent	durchscheinend, durchsichtig
transmurale	transmural	transmural
transtoracico	transthoracic	transthorakal
transuretrale	transurethral	transurethral
trapanare	trephine	trepanieren
trapano	trephine	Trepan
trapiantare	graft, transplant	transplantieren, übertragen
trapianto	graft, transplant	Transplantat, Transplantation, Plastik
trapianto corneale	corneal graft	Korneaplastik
trapianto osseo	bone graft	Osteoplastik, Knochentransplantation
trasfusione	transfusion	Transfusion, Bluttransfusion
traslocazione	translocation	Translokation
trasudato	transudate	Transsudat
tratto	trait	Zug, Charakterzug, Eigenschaft
trauma	trauma	Trauma
travaglio di parto	labor (Am), labour (Eng)	Wehen
traversa	drawsheet	Unterziehtuch
trazione	traction	Traktion, Zug
trematode	fluke	Trematode
tremore	tremor	Tremor
tremore fino	fine tremor	feinschlägiger Tremor
tricipite	triceps	Trizeps
tricocefalo	whipworm	Oxyuris, Peitschenwurm
tricofizia	ringworm	Tinea, Fadenpilzerkrankung, Onchozerkose
tricotillomania	trichotillomania	Trichotillomanie
tricuspide	tricuspid	Trikuspidal
trigemino	trigeminal	Trigeminus-
trimestre	trimester	Trimester
tripanosomiasi	trypanosomiasis	Trypanosomiasis
triplo vaccino	triple vaccine	Dreifachimpfstoff
trisma	lock jaw	Kiefersperre
trisomia	trisomy	Trisomie
trocantere	trochanter	Trochanter
trombectomia	thrombectomy	Thrombektomie
trombo	thrombus	Thrombus
trombocitemia	thrombocythaemia (Eng), thrombocythemia (Am)	Thrombozythämie

SPANISH	FRENCH	ITALIAN
traqueoesofágico	trachéo-oesophagien	tracheoesofageo
traqueostomía	trachéostomie	tracheostomia
traqueotomía	trachéotomie	tracheotomia
tracoma	trachome	tracoma
tranquilizante	tranquillisant	tranquillante
transabdominal	transabdominal	transaddominale
gamma glutamil transferasa (GGT)	gamma-glutamyl-transférase (GGT)	transaminasi
transamniótico	transamniotique	transamniotico
gamma glutamil transferasa (GGT)	gamma-glutamyl-transférase (GGT)	transferasi glutammica
translúcido	translucide	translucido
transmural	transmural	transmurale
transtorácico	transthoracique	transtoracico
transuretral	transurétral	transuretrale
trepanar	trépaner	trapanare
trépano	tréphine	trapano
injertar, trasplantar	greffer, transplanter	trapiantare
injerto, transplante	greffe, transplantation	trapianto
injerto corneal	greffe de la cornée	trapianto corneale
injerto óseo, osteoplastia	greffe osseuse	trapianto osseo
transfusión	transfusion	trasfusione
translocación	translocation	traslocazione
trasudado	transsudat	trasudato
rasgo	trait	tratto
trauma	traumatisme	trauma
parto	travail	travaglio di parto
alezo, faja	alèse	traversa
tracción	traction	trazione
trematodo	douve	trematode
temblor	tremblement	tremore
temblor fino	tremblement fin	tremore fino
tríceps	triceps	tricipite
trichuris trichiura	flagellé	tricocefalo
tiña	dermatophytose	tricofizia
tricotilomanía	trichotillomanie	tricotillomania
tricúspide	tricuspide	tricuspide
trigémino	trigéminal	trigemino
trimestre	trimestre	trimestre
tripanosomiasis	trypanosomiase	tripanosomiasi
vacuna triple	triple vaccin	triplo vaccino
trismo	tétanos	trisma
trisomía	trisomie	trisomia
trocánter	trochanter	trocantere
trombectomía	thrombectomie	trombectomia
trombo	thrombus	trombo
trombocitemia	thrombocytémie	trombocitemia

ITALIAN	ENGLISH	GERMAN
trombocito	thrombocyte	Thrombozyt, Blutplättchen
trombocitopenia	thrombocytopenia	Thrombopenie
trombocitosi	thrombocytosis	Thrombozytose
tromboembolico	thromboembolic	thromboembolisch
tromboflebite	thrombophlebitis	Thrombophlebitis
trombolitico	thrombolytic	thrombolytisch
trombosi	thrombosis	Thrombose
trombosi venosa profonda (TVP)	deep vein thrombosis (DVT)	tiefe Venenthrombose
tse-tse	tsetse	Tsetsefliege
tuba d'Eustachio	Eustachian tube	Eustachische Röhre
tuba di Falloppio	Fallopian tube	Tube, Eileiter
tubarico	tubal	Tuben-, Eileiter-
tubercolo	tubercle	Tuberkel
tubercoloide	tuberculoid	tuberkuloid
tubercolosi (TBC)	tuberculosis (TB)	Tuberkulose
tuberosità	tuberosity	Tuberositas
tubulo	tubule	Tubulus, Röhrchen
tumefatto	swollen	geschwollen, vergrößert
tumefazione	tumescence, tumor (Am), tumour (Eng)	Tumeszenz, diffuse Anschwellung, Tumor
tumore	tumor (Am), tumour (Eng)	Tumor
tumore da parto	caput succedaneum	Geburtsgeschwulst
tumore di Ewing	Ewing's tumour	Ewing-Sarkom
tumore di Wilms	Wilms' tumor (Am), Wilms' tumour (Eng)	Wilms-Tumor
turbinato	turbinate	Nasenmuschel
turgido	turgid	geschwollen

SPANISH	FRENCH	ITALIAN
trombocito	thrombocyte	**trombocito**
trombocitopenia	thrombopénie	**trombocitopenia**
trombocitosis	thrombocytose	**trombocitosi**
tromboembólico	thrombo-embolique	**tromboembolico**
tromboflebitis	thrombophlébite	**tromboflebite**
trombolítico	thrombolytique	**trombolitico**
trombosis	thrombose	**trombosi**
trombosis venosa profunda	thrombose veineuse profonde (TVP)	**trombosi venosa profonda (TVP)**
mosca tsetsé	mouche tsé-tsé	**tse-tse**
trompa de Eustaquio	trompe d'Eustache	**tuba d'Eustachio**
trompa de Falopio	trompe de Fallope	**tuba di Falloppio**
tubárico	tubaire	**tubarico**
tubérculo	tubercule	**tubercolo**
tuberculoide	tuberculoïde	**tubercoloide**
tuberculosis (TB)	tuberculose (TB)	**tubercolosi (TBC)**
tuberosidad	tubérosité	**tuberosità**
túbulo	tube	**tubulo**
hinchado	enflé	**tumefatto**
tumescencia, tumor	tumescence, tumeur	**tumefazione**
tumor	tumeur	**tumore**
caput succedaneum	caput succedaneum	**tumore da parto**
sarcoma de Ewing	tumeur d'Ewing	**tumore di Ewing**
tumor de Wilms	tumeur de Wilms	**tumore di Wilms**
turbinado	cornet	**turbinato**
túrgido	enflé	**turgido**

U

Italian	English	German
udito	hearing	Gehör, Hören
ugola	uvula	Uvula, Zäpfchen
ulcera	ulcer	Ulkus, Geschwür
ulcera da decubito	pressure sore	Druckgeschwür, Dekubitus
ulcera dendritica	dendritic ulcer	verzweigtes Geschwür
ulcera duodenale	duodenal ulcer	Duodenalulkus, Zwölffingerdarmgeschwür
ulcerativo	ulcerative	ulzerierend, geschwürig
ulcera trofica	trophic ulcer	trophisches Ulkus
ulcera venerea	chancre	Schanker
ulceroso	ulcerative	ulzerierend, geschwürig
ulcus rodens	rodent ulcer	Ulcus rodens
ulna	ulna	Ulna, Elle
ultimo periodo mestruale	last menstrual period (LMP)	letzte Menstruationsperiode
ultrasonografia	ultrasonography	Sonographie, Ultraschallmethode
ultravioletto (UV)	ultraviolet (UV)	ultraviolett
unghia	nail	Nagel
unguento	ointment, salve	Salbe
unilaterale	unilateral	einseitig
unione difettosa	malunion	Fehlstellung (Frakturenden)
unità di cura intensiva	intensive care unit (ICU)	Intensivstation
unità di cure speciali pediatriche	special care baby unit (SCBU)	Säuglings-Intensivstation
unità di terapia intensiva	intensive therapy unit (ITU)	Intensivstation
unità pediatrica di cure speciali	special care unit (SCU)	Intensivstation
uovo	egg, ovum	Ei, Ovum
urato	urate	Urat
urea	urea	Urea, Harnstoff
uremia	uraemia (Eng), uremia (Am)	Urämie, Harnvergiftung
uretere	ureter	Ureter, Harnleiter
ureterocolico	ureterocolic	Ureterkolik
uretra	urethra	Urethra, Harnröhre
uretrite	urethritis	Urethritis
uretrite aspecifica	non-specific urethritis (NSU)	unspezifische Urethritis
uretrite non gonococcica	non-gonococcal urethritis (NGU)	nicht durch Gonokokken bedingte Urethritis
uretrocele	urethrocele	Urethrozele
uricaemia	uricaemia (Eng), uricemia (Am)	Urikämie
uricuria	uricosuria	Urikosurie
urina	urine	Urin, Harn
urografia	urography	Urographie
urologia	urology	Urologie
ustione	burn	Verbrennung, Brandwunde
utero	uterus, womb	Uterus, Gebärmutter

SPANISH	FRENCH	ITALIAN
oído	audition	udito
úvula	uvule	ugola
úlcera	ulcère	ulcera
úlcera de decúbito	plaie de décubitus	ulcera da decubito
úlcera dendrítica	ulcère dendritique	ulcera dendritica
úlcera duodenal	ulcère duodénal	ulcera duodenale
ulcerativo	ulcératif	ulcerativo
úlcera trófica	ulcère trophique	ulcera trofica
chancro	chancre	ulcera venerea
ulcerativo	ulcératif	ulceroso
úlcera corrosiva	ulcus rodens	ulcus rodens
cúbito	cubitus	ulna
fecha última regla (FUR)	dernières règles	ultimo periodo mestruale
ultrasonografía, ecografía	échographie	ultrasonografia
ultravioleta (UV)	ultraviolet (UV)	ultravioletto (UV)
uña	ongle	unghia
ungüento	pommade	unguento
unilateral	unilatéral	unilaterale
unión defectuosa	cal vicieux	unione difettosa
unidad de cuidados intensivos (UCI)	unité de soins intensifs	unità di cura intensiva
unidad para cuidados especiales neonatales	pavillon de soins spéciaux aux nouveau-nés	unità di cure speciali pediatriche
unidad de cuidados intensivos (UCI)	service de réanimation	unità di terapia intensiva
unidad de cuidados especiales	unité de soins spéciaux	unità pediatrica di cure speciali
huevo, óvulo	oeuf, ovule, ovocyte de premier ordre	uovo
urato	urate	urato
urea	urée	urea
uremia	urémie	uremia
uréter	uretère	uretere
ureterocólico	urétérocolique	ureterocolico
uretra	urètre	uretra
uretritis	urétrite	uretrite
uretritis inespecífica	urétrite aspécifique	uretrite aspecifica
uretritis no gonocócica	urétrite non gonococcique	uretrite non gonococcica
uretrocele	urétrocèle	uretrocele
uricemia	uricémie	uricaemia
uricosúrico	uricosurique	uricuria
orina	urine	urina
urografía	urographie	urografia
urología	urologie	urologia
quemadura	brûlure	ustione
útero, matriz	utérus	utero

ITALIAN	ENGLISH	GERMAN
uterosacrale	uterosacral	uterosakral
uterovescicale	uterovesical	uterovesikal
uveite	uveitis	Uveitis

SPANISH	FRENCH	ITALIAN
uterosacro	utéro-sacré	uterosacrale
uterovesical	utéro-vésical	uterovescicale
uveitis	uréite	uveite

V

Italian	English	German
vaccinazione	vaccination	Impfung, Vakzination
vaccino	vaccine	Vakzine, Impfstoff
vagale	vagal	vagal, Vagus-
vagina	vagina	Vagina, Scheide
vaginismo	vaginismus	Vaginismus
vaginite	vaginitis	Vaginitis
vagotomia	vagotomy	Vagotomie
vaiolo	smallpox	Variola, Pocken
valgo	valgus	valgus
valutare	test	testen, untersuchen
valvola	valve	Klappe, Ventil
valvulotomia	valvotomy	Valvotomie
varicella	chickenpox, varicella	Varizellen, Windpocken
varo	varus	varus
vascolare	vascular	vaskulär, Gefäß-
vasculite	vasculitis	Vaskulitis
vasculopatia polmonare	pulmonary vascular disease (PVD)	Lungengefäßerkrankung
vasectomia	vasectomy	Vasektomie, Vasoresektion
vaso	vessel	Gefäß, Ader
vasocostrittore (n)	vasoconstrictor (n)	Vasokonstriktor (n)
vasocostrittore (a)	vasoconstrictor (a)	vasokonstriktorisch (a)
vasodilatatore (n)	vasodilator (n)	Vasodilatator (n)
vasodilatatore (a)	vasodilator (a)	vasodilatatorisch (a)
vasopressore (n)	vasopressor (n)	Vasopressor (n)
vasopressore (a)	vasopressor (a)	vasopressorisch (a)
vasospasmo	vasospasm	Vasospasmus
veleno	poison	Gift
velocità di eritrosedimentazione (VES)	blood sedimentation rate (BSR), erythrocyte sedimentation rate (ESR), sedimentation rate (SR)	Blutkörperchen-Senkungsgeschwindigkeit (BSG, BKS)
velocità espiratoria massima (VEM)	peak expiratory velocity (PEV)	maximale exspiratorische Atemgeschwindigkeit
vena	vein	Vene
vena cava	vena cava	Vena cava
vena cubitale	cubital vein	Unterarmvene
vena femorale	femoral vein	Vena femoralis
vena giugulare	jugular vein	Vena jugularis
vena porta	portal vein	Pfortader
vena radiale	radial vein	Vena radialis
venereo	venereal	venerisch
venereologia	venereology	Venerologie
vene varicose	varicose veins	Varizen, Krampfadern
ventilatore	ventilator	Ventilator
ventilazione a pressione positiva	positive pressure ventilation	Überdruckbeatmung
ventilazione e respirazione nelle vie respiratorie	airway breathing and circulation (ABC)	Luftwege Atmung und Kreislauf (ABC-Regel)

796

SPANISH	FRENCH	ITALIAN
vacunación	vaccination	vaccinazione
vacuna	vaccin	vaccino
vagal	vague	vagale
vagina	vagin	vagina
vaginismo	vaginisme	vaginismo
vaginitis	vaginite	vaginite
vagotomía	vagotomie	vagotomia
viruela	variole	vaiolo
valgus	valgus	valgo
probar	tester	valutare
válvula	valve	valvola
valvotomía	valvulotomie	valvulotomia
varicela	varicelle	varicella
varus	varus	varo
vascular	vasculaire	vascolare
vasculitis	vasculite	vasculite
vasculopatia pulmonar	pneumopathie vasculaire	vasculopatia polmonare
vasectomía	vasectomie	vasectomia
vaso	vaisseau	vaso
vasoconstrictor (n)	vasoconstricteur (n)	vasocostrittore (n)
vasoconstrictor (a)	vasoconstricteur (a)	vasocostrittore (a)
vasodilatador (n)	vasodilatateur (n)	vasodilatatore (n)
vasodilatador (a)	vasodilatateur (a)	vasodilatatore (a)
vasopresor (n)	vasopresseur (n)	vasopressore (n)
vasopresor (a)	vasopresseur (a)	vasopressore (a)
vasospasmo	spasme d'un vaisseau	vasospasmo
veneno	poison	veleno
velocidad de sedimentación globular (VSG)	vitesse de sédimentation sanguine, vitesse de sédimentation globulaire, vitesse de sédimentation (VS)	velocità di eritrosedimentazione (VES)
velocidad espiratoria máxima (VEM)	volume expiratoire maximum (VEM)	velocità espiratoria massima (VEM)
vena	veine	vena
vena cava	veine cave	vena cava
vena cubital	veine de l'avant bras	vena cubitale
vena femoral	veine fémorale	vena femorale
vena yugular	veine jugulaire	vena giugulare
vena porta	veine porte	vena porta
vena radial	veine radiale	vena radiale
venéreo	vénérien	venereo
venereología	vénéréologie	venereologia
varices	varices	vene varicose
ventilador	appareil de ventilation artificielle	ventilatore
ventilación con presión positiva	ventilation à pression positive	ventilazione a pressione positiva
vías respiratorias y circulación	intubation, ventilation et circulation	ventilazione e respirazione nelle vie respiratorie

ITALIAN	ENGLISH	GERMAN
ventosa cefalica	vacuum extractor	Vakuumextraktor, Saugglocke
ventosa ostetrica	vacuum extractor	Vakuumextraktor, Saugglocke
ventosità	wind	Blähung, Wind
ventrale	ventral	ventral, Bauch-
ventre	belly	Bauch
ventricolo	ventricle	Ventrikel, Kammer
ventrofissazione	ventrofixation, ventrosuspension	Hysteropexie, Ventrofixation, Ligamentopexie
ventrosospensione	ventrosuspension	Ventrofixation, Ligamentopexie
venula	venule	Venula
verme	worm	Wurm
verme a frusta	whipworm	Oxyuris, Peitschenwurm
verruca	verruca	Warze, Verruca
verruca volgare	wart	Warze
versione	version	Versio, Wendung
versione cefalica esterna	external cephalic version (ECV)	äußere Wendung auf den Kopf
vertebra	vertebra	Wirbel
vertice	vertex	Vertex, Scheitel
vertigine	vertigo	Schwindel, Vertigo
vertigini	dizziness	Schwindel
vescica	bladder	Blase, Harnblase
vescica ileale (protesi mediante segmento ileale)	ileal conduit	Ileumconduit
vescichetta	bleb	Bläschen
vescicola	blister, vesicle	Blase, Hautblase, Brandblase, Vesikula, Bläschen
vescicoureterale	vesicoureteric	vesikoureteral
vescicovaginale	vesicovaginal	vesikovaginal
vestibolo	vestibule	Vestibulum, Vorhof
vettore	vector	Überträger, Vektor
villi coriali	chorionic villi	Chorionzotten
villo	villus	Zotte
violenza carnale	sexual abuse	sexueller Mißbrauch
violenza sessuale	sexual abuse	sexueller Mißbrauch
viremia	viraemia (Eng), viremia (Am)	Virämie
virilismo	virilism	Virilismus
virologia	virology	Virologie
virulenza	virulence	Virulenz
virus	virus	Virus
virus coxsackie	Coxsackie virus	Coxsackie-Virus
virus della famiglia dell'herpes	herpes-like virus (HLV)	Herpes-ähnlicher Virus
virus della leucemia a cellule T	human T-cell leukaemia virus (HTLV) (Eng), human T-cell leukemia virus (HTLV) (Am)	human T-cell leukemia virus (HTLV)
virus della poliomielite	poliovirus	Poliovirus
virus dell'immunodeficienza umana (HIV)	human immunodeficiency virus (HIV)	human immunodeficiency virus (HIV), AIDS-Virus
virus di Epstein Barr	Epstein-Barr virus (EBV)	Epstein-Barr-Virus (EBV)
virus herpes simplex	herpes simplex virus (HSV)	Herpes simplex-Virus (HSV)

SPANISH	FRENCH	ITALIAN
extractor al vacío	ventouse obstétricale	ventosa cefalica
extractor al vacío	ventouse obstétricale	ventosa ostetrica
flatulencia, ventosidad	gaz	ventosità
ventral	ventral	ventrale
vientre	ventre	ventre
ventrículo	ventricule	ventricolo
ventrofijación, ventrosuspensión	hystéropexie abdominale, ventro-suspension	ventrofissazione
ventrosuspensión	ventro-suspension	ventrosospensione
vénula	veinule	venula
lombriz	ver	verme
trichuris trichiura	flagellé	verme a frusta
verruga	verrue	verruca
verruga	verrue	verruca volgare
versión	version	versione
versión cefálica externa	version céphalique externe	versione cefalica esterna
vértebra	vertèbre	vertebra
vértice	vertex	vertice
vértigo	vertige	vertigine
desvanecimiento, mareo	étourdissement	vertigini
vejiga	vessie	vescica
conducto ileal	conduit iléal	vescica ileale (protesi mediante segmento ileale)
vesícula, bulla, ampolla	phlyctène	vescichetta
vesícula, ampolla, flictena	ampoule, vésicule	vescicola
vesicoureteral	vésico-urétérique	vescicoureterale
vesicovaginal	vésico-vaginal	vescicovaginale
vestíbulo	vestibule	vestibolo
vector	vecteur	vettore
vellosidades coriónicas	villosités du chorion	villi coriali
vellosidad	villosité	villo
abuso sexual	sévices sexuels	violenza carnale
abuso sexual	sévices sexuels	violenza sessuale
viremia	virémie	viremia
virilismo	virilisme	virilismo
virología	virologie	virologia
virulencia	virulence	virulenza
virus	virus	virus
virus Coxsackie	virus Coxsackie	virus coxsackie
virus semejante al del herpes (HLV)	virus de type herpétique (HLV)	virus della famiglia dell'herpes
leucemia por virus humano de las células T	leucémie humaine à lymphocytes T	virus della leucemia a cellule T
poliovirus	poliovirus	virus della poliomielite
virus de la inmunodeficiencia humana (VIH)	virus de l'immunodéficience humaine	virus dell'immunodeficienza umana (HIV)
virus de Epstein-Barr	virus d'Epstein-Barr	virus di Epstein Barr
virus del herpes simple (VHS)	virus de l'herpès simplex (HSV)	virus herpes simplex

ITALIAN	ENGLISH	GERMAN
virus respiratorio sinciziale (RSV)	respiratory syncytial virus (RSV)	RS-Virus
visceri	viscera	Eingeweide, Viszera
viscido	viscid	zäh, klebrig
visione binoculare	binocular vision	binokulares Sehen, beidäugiges Sehen
visivo	visual	visuell, Seh-
vitale	viable	lebensfähig
vitamina	vitamin	Vitamin
vitiligine	vitiligo	Vitiligo
volume cellulare (VC)	packed cell volume (PCV)	Hämatokrit (HKT)
volume corpuscolare medio (VCM)	mean corpuscular volume (MCV)	mittleres Erythrozytenvolumen (MCV)
volume di filtrazione glomerulare (VFG)	glomerular filtration rate (GFR)	glomeruläre Filtrationsrate (GFR)
volume espiratorio forzato	forced expiratory volume (FEV)	forciertes Exspirationsvolumen, Atemstoßwert
volume sanguigno	blood volume (BV)	Blutvolumen
volvolo	volvulus	Volvulus
vomitare	vomit	sich übergeben, erbrechen
vomito	emesis	Erbrechen
vomito ciclico	cyclical vomiting	zyklisches Erbrechen
vulva	vulva	Vulva
vulvite	vulvitis	Vulvitis
vulvovaginale	vulvovaginal	vulvovaginal

X

ITALIAN	ENGLISH	GERMAN
xantelasma	xanthelasma	Xanthelasma
xantemia	xanthaemia (Eng), xanthemia (Am)	Xanthämie
xantoma	xanthoma	Xanthom
xerodermia	xeroderma	Xerodermie
xeroftalmia	xerophthalmia	Xerophthalmie

Z

ITALIAN	ENGLISH	GERMAN
zecca	tick	Zecke
zigomo	zygoma	Zygoma, Jochbein
zigote	zygote	Zygote
zoonosi	zoonosis	Zoonose, Tierkrankheit

SPANISH	FRENCH	ITALIAN
virus sincitial respiratorio (VSR)	virus respiratoire syncytial	**virus respiratorio sinciziale (RSV)**
visceras	viscères	**visceri**
viscoso	visqueux	**viscido**
visión binocular	vision binoculaire	**visione binoculare**
visual	visuel	**visivo**
viable	viable	**vitale**
vitamina	vitamine	**vitamina**
vitíligo	vitiligo	**vitiligine**
volumen de células agregadas	hématocrite	**volume cellulare (VC)**
volumen corpuscular medio (VCM)	volume globulaire moyen (VGM)	**volume corpuscolare medio (VCM)**
tasa de filtración glomerular (FG)	taux de filtration glomérulaire	**volume di filtrazione glomerulare (VFG)**
volumen espiratorio forzado (VEF)	volume expiratoire maximum (VEM)	**volume espiratorio forzato**
volumen hemático	masse sanguine	**volume sanguigno**
vólvulo	volvulus	**volvolo**
vomitar	vomir	**vomitare**
emesis	vomissement	**vomito**
vómito cíclico	vomissement cyclique	**vomito ciclico**
vulva	vulve	**vulva**
vulvitis	vulvite	**vulvite**
vulvovaginal	vulvo-vaginal	**vulvovaginale**
xantelasma	xanthélasma	**xantelasma**
xantemia	xanthémie, caroténémie	**xantemia**
xantoma	xanthome	**xantoma**
xeroderma	xérodermie	**xerodermia**
xeroftalmia	xérophtalmie	**xeroftalmia**
garrapata	tique	**zecca**
cigoma	zygoma	**zigomo**
cigoto	zygote	**zigote**
zoonosis	zoonose	**zoonosi**

ITALIAN ABBREVIATIONS

ABRÉVIATIONS ITALIENNES
ITALIENISCHE ABKÜRZUNGEN
ABBREVIAZIONI ITALIANE
ABREVIATURAS ITALIANAS

Ac	anticorpi
ACTH	ormone corticotropo
ACV	accidente cerebrovascolare
AIDS	sindrome da immunodeficienza acquisita
AR	artrite reumatoide
CGB	conteggio dei globuli bianchi
CGR	conteggio dei globuli rossi
CID	coagulazione intravascolare disseminata
CIN	neoplasia intraepiteliale della cervice uterina
CUM	campione urinario del mitto intermedio
E	emoglobina
ECG	elettrocardiogramma
EEG	elettroencefalogramma
EP	embolia polmonare
ERCP	colangio-pancreatografia retrograda endoscopica
EV	endovenoso
FANS	farmaco antinfiammatorio non steroideo
FSH	ormone follicolostimolante
FT	tiroxina libera
GCU	gonadotropina corionica umana
GH	ormone della crescita
HIV	virus dell'immunodeficienza umana
Ig	immunoglobulina
IG	interruzione di gravidanza
IM	intramuscolare
IMAO	inibitore monoaminoossidasi
IMC	indice di massa corporea
IUD	dispositivo anticoncezionale intrauterino
IVU	infezione delle vie urinarie
LAD	lipoproteina ad alta densità
LBD	lipoproteina a bassa densità
LCS	liquido cerebrospinale
LES	lupus eritematoso sistemico
LH	ormone luteinizzante
LRTI	infezione del tratto respiratorio inferiore
MAC	malattia delle arterie coronarica
MCC	malattia cardiaca coronarica
mEq	milliequivalente
MV	malattia venerea
OA	osteoartrosi
OAS	occipitoanteriore sinistro
PE	pielografia endovenosa
PID	malattia infiammatoria della pelvi
POS	piressia di origine sconosciuta
ppm	parti per milione
RAST	test di radioallergoassorbimento
RBC	eritrocito
RES	sistema reticoloendoteliale
Rh−	Rh negativo

Rh+	Rh positivo
RNA	acido ribonucleico
RSV	virus respiratorio sinciziale
SIDS	sindrome della morte neonatale improvvisa
STD	malattia a trasmissione sessuale
TAC	tomografia assiale computerizzata
TBC	tubercolosi
TFE	test di funzionalità epatica
TIBC	capacità totale di legame del ferro
TSH	ormone tireotropo
TTG	test di tolleranza al glucosio
TVP	trombosi venosa profonda
URTI	infezione del tratto respiratorio superiore
UV	ultravioletto
VC	volume cellulare
VCM	volume corpuscolare medio
VEM	velocità espiratoria massima
VES	velocità di eritrosedimentazione
VFG	volume di filtrazione glomerulare
WBC	conteggio dei globuli bianchi

SPANISH
English
French
Italian
German
SPANISH

SPANISH	ENGLISH	FRENCH
A		
abdomen	abdomen	abdomen
abdominal	abdominal	abdominal
abdominoperineal	abdomino-perineal	abdomino-périnéal
abducción	abduction	abduction
abducir	abduct	produire l'abduction
abductor	abductor	abducteur
aberración	aberration	aberration
aberrante	aberrant	aberrant
ablación	ablation	ablation
abortar	abort	avorter
aborto	abortion, miscarriage	avortement, fausse couche
aborto diferido	missed abortion	rétention foetale
aborto inducido	induced abortion	avortement provoqué
aborto terapéutico	therapeutic abortion	avortement thérapeutique
abrasión	abrasion	abrasion
abreacción	abreaction	abréaction
absceso	abscess	abcès
absceso frío	cold abscess	abcès froid
absceso periamigdalino	peritonsillar abscess, quinsy	abcès périamygdalien, phlegmon amygdalien ou périamygdalien
absorción	absorption	absorption
abstinencia	withdrawal	retrait, sevrage, suppression
abuso	abuse	abus
abuso de drogas	drug abuse	toxicomanie
abuso de menores	child abuse	sévices infligés aux enfants, martyre d'enfants
abuso sexual	sexual abuse	sévices sexuels
acalasia	achalasia	achalasie
acceso	fit, seizure	attaque, accès
accidente de circulacion	road traffic accident (RTA)	accident de la route
accidente vascular cerebral (ACV)	cerebrovascular accident (CVA)	accident cérébrovasculaire
acción	action	action
acetábulo	acetabulum	acétabule
acetona	ketone	cétone
acidez	acidity	acidité
ácido (n)	acid (n)	acide (n)
ácido (a)	acid (a)	acide (a)
ácido-alcohol-resistente	acid-alcohol-fast	résistant à l'alcool et à l'acide
ácido desoxirribonucléico (ADN)	deoxyribonucleic acid (DNA)	acide désoxyribonucléique (ADN)
ácido fólico	folic acid	acide folique
ácido graso	fatty acid	acide gras
ácido graso esencial	essential fatty acid	acide gras essentiel
ácido homovanílico	homovanillic acid (HVA)	acide homovanillique
ácido láctico	lactic acid	acide lactique

ITALIAN	GERMAN	SPANISH
addome	Abdomen	abdomen
addominale	abdominal	abdominal
addomino-perineale	abdominoperineal	abdominoperineal
abduzione	Abduktion	abducción
abdurre	abduzieren	abducir
abduttore	Abduktor	abductor
aberrazione	Aberration, Abweichung	aberración
aberrante	aberrans, abartig	aberrante
ablazione	Ablatio, Absetzung	ablación
abortire	fehlgebären	abortar
aborto	Abort, Fehlgeburt	aborto
aborto interno, aborto ritenuto	verhaltener Abort, missed abortion	aborto diferido
aborto procurato	Abtreibung, künstlicher Abort	aborto inducido
aborto terapeutico	indizierter Abort	aborto terapéutico
abrasione	Abschabung, Ausschabung	abrasión
abreazione, catarsi	Abreaktion	abreacción
ascesso	Abszeß	absceso
ascesso freddo	kalter Abszeß	absceso frío
ascesso peritonsillare	Peritonsillarabszeß	absceso periamigdalino
assorbimento	Absorption	absorción
ritiro, astinenza, sospensione	Entzug	abstinencia
abuso	Abusus, Mißbrauch	abuso
abuso di droga, abuso di farmaci	Arzneimittelmißbrauch, Drogenmißbrauch	abuso de drogas
maltrattamento a bambini	Kindesmißhandlung	abuso de menores
violenza sessuale, violenza carnale	sexueller Mißbrauch	abuso sexual
acalasia	Achalasie	acalasia
convulsione, attacco	Anfall	acceso
incidente stradale	Verkehrsunfall	accidente de circulacion
ictus, accidente cerebrovascolare (ACV)	Schlaganfall, Apoplex	accidente vascular cerebral (ACV)
azione	Tätigkeit	acción
acetabolo	Azetabulum, Hüftgelenkspfanne	acetábulo
chetoni	Keton, Ketonkörper	acetona
acidità	Säuregehalt	acidez
acido (n)	Säure (n)	ácido (n)
acido (a)	sauer (a)	ácido (a)
alcool-acido-resistente	säurealkoholbeständig	ácido-alcohol-resistente
acido deossiribonucleico	Desoxyribonukleinsäure (DNS)	ácido desoxirribonucléico (ADN)
acido folico	Folsäure	ácido fólico
acido grasso	Fettsäure	ácido graso
acido grasso essenziale	essentielle Fettsäure	ácido graso esencial
acido omovanillico	Homovanillinsäure	ácido homovanílico
acido lattico	Milchsäure	ácido láctico

SPANISH	ENGLISH	FRENCH
ácido-resistente	acid-fast	acido-résistant
ácido ribonucléico (ARN)	ribonucleic acid (RNA)	acide ribonucléique (RNA)
acidosis	acidosis	acidose
ácido úrico	uric acid	acide urique
ácido vanilmandélico (AVM)	vanyl mandelic acid (VMA)	acide vanillyl-mandélique
ácigos	azygous	azygos
acinético	akinetic	acinétique
acné	acne	acné
acomodación	accommodation	accommodation
acondroplasia	achondroplasia	achondroplasie
acromegalia	acromegaly	acromégalie
acromioclavicular	acromioclavicular	acromio-claviculaire
acromion	acromion	acromion
actinomicosis	actinomycosis	actinomycose
activo	active	actif
acueducto	aqueduct	aqueduc
acuoso	aqueous	aqueux
acupuntura	acupuncture	acupuncture
acústico	acoustic	acoustique
adenocarcinoma	adenocarcinoma	adénocarcinome
adenoidectomía	adenoidectomy	adénoïdectomie
adenoides	adenoids	végétations adénoïdes
adenoma	adenoma	adénome
adenomioma	adenomyoma	adénomyome
adenovirus	adenovirus	adénovirus
adherencia	adhesion	adhésion
adicción	addiction	accoutumance
adiposo	adipose	adipeux
adolescencia	adolescence	adolescence
adopción	adoption, fostering	adoption, prise en nourrice
adrenal	adrenal	surrénale
adrenalina	adrenaline	adrénaline
adrenérgico	adrenergic	adrénergique
adsorción	adsorption	adsorption
aducción	adduction	adduction
aducir	adduct	produire l'adduction
aductor	adductor	adducteur
aeróbico	aerobe	aérobie
aerobio	aerobe	aérobie
aerofagia	aerophagia	aérophagie
aerosol	aerosol	aérosol
afasia	aphasia	aphasie
afebril	afebrile	afébrile
afectar	affect	affecter
afectivo	affective	affectif
afecto	affect	affect
aferente	afferent	afférent

808

ITALIAN	GERMAN	SPANISH
acido resistente	säurebeständig	ácido-resistente
acido ribonucleico (RNA)	Ribonukleinsäure (RNA)	ácido ribonucléico (ARN)
acidosi	Azidose	acidosis
acido urico	Harnsäure	ácido úrico
acido vanilmandelico	Vanillylmandelsäure	ácido vanilmandélico (AVM)
azygos	azygos	ácigos
acinetico	akinetisch	acinético
acne	Akne	acné
accomodazione	Akkommodation	acomodación
acondroplasia	Achondroplasie	acondroplasia
acromegalia	Akromegalie	acromegalia
acromioclavicolare	akromioklavikular	acromioclavicular
acromion	Akromion	acromion
actinomicosi	Aktinomykose	actinomicosis
attivo	aktiv, wirksam	activo
acquedotto	Aquädukt	acueducto
acquoso	wässrig, wasserhaltig	acuoso
agopuntura	Akupunktur	acupuntura
acustico	akustisch, Gehör-	acústico
adenocarcinoma	Adenokarzinom	adenocarcinoma
adenoidectomia	Adenoidektomie, Polypenentfernung	adenoidectomía
adenoidi	Adenoide, Nasenpolypen	adenoides
adenoma	Adenom	adenoma
adenomioma	Adenomyom	adenomioma
adenovirus	Adenovirus	adenovirus
adesione	Adhäsion, Anhaften	adherencia
tossicomania	Sucht, Gewöhnung	adicción
adiposo	adipös, fettleibig	adiposo
adolescenza	Adoleszenz, Jugendalter	adolescencia
adozione, affido	Adoption, Pflege	adopción
surrenale	Nebennieren-	adrenal
adrenalina	Adrenalin	adrenalina
adrenergico	adrenerg	adrenérgico
adsorbimento	Adsorption	adsorción
adduzione	Adduktion	aducción
addurre	adduzieren, zusammenziehen	aducir
adduttore	Adduktor	aductor
aerobio	Aerobier	aeróbico
aerobio	Aerobier	aerobio
aerofagia	Aerophagie, Luftschlucken	aerofagia
aerosol	Aerosol	aerosol
afasia	Aphasie	afasia
afebbrile	fieberfrei	afebril
attaccare, influenzare	befallen	afectar
affettivo	affektiv	afectivo
emozione	Affekt, Erregung	afecto
afferente	afferent, zuführend	aferente

SPANISH	ENGLISH	FRENCH
aftas	aphthae	aphtes
agenesia	agenesis	agénésie
aglutinación	agglutination	agglutination
aglutinina	agglutinin	agglutinine
agnatia	agnathia	agnathie
agnosia	agnosia	agnosie
agonista	agonist	agoniste
agorafobia	agoraphobia	agoraphobie
agotamiento por calor	heat exhaustion	échauffement
agranulocitosis	agranulocytosis	agranulocytose
agresión	aggression	agression
agudeza	acuity	acuité
agudeza visual	visual acuity	acuité visuelle
agudo	acute	aigu(ë)
aguja	needle	aiguille
aislamiento	isolation	isolement
albúmina	albumin	albumine
albuminuria	albuminuria	albuminurie
álcali	alkali	alcali
alcalino	alkaline	alcalin
alcalosis	alkalosis	alcalose
alcohol	alcohol	alcool
alcoholismo	alcoholism	alcoolisme
alérgeno	allergen	allergène
alergia	allergy	allergie
alergia alimentaria	food allergy	allergie alimentaire
aleteo auricular	atrial flutter	flutter auriculaire
alezo	drawsheet	alèse
alfafetoproteína (AFP)	alpha-fetoprotein (AFP)	alpha-foetoprotéine
aliento	breath	haleine, souffle
alimentación	alimentation	alimentation
alopecia	alopecia	alopécie
alopurinol	allopurinol	allopurinol
alquitrán	coal tar	coaltar
alucinación	hallucination	hallucination
alveolitis	alveolitis	alvéolite
alvéolo	alveolus	alvéole
amaurosis	amaurosis	amaurose
ambiente	environment	milieu
ambliopía	amblyopia	amblyopie
ambulante	ambulant	ambulant
ambulatorio	ambulatory	ambulatoire
ameba	ameba (Am), amoeba (Eng)	amibe
amebiasis	amebiasis (Am), amoebiasis (Eng)	amibiase
ameboma	ameboma (Am), amoeboma (Eng)	amibome

ITALIAN	GERMAN	SPANISH
afte	Aphthe	aftas
agenesia	Agenesie	agenesia
agglutinazione	Agglutination	aglutinación
agglutinine	Agglutinin	aglutinina
agnazia	Agnathie	agnatia
agnosia	Agnosie	agnosia
agonista	Agonist	agonista
agorafobia	Agoraphobie, Platzangst	agorafobia
collasso da colpo di calore	Hitzschlag	agotamiento por calor
agranulocitosi	Agranulozytose	agranulocitosis
aggressività	Aggression	agresión
acuità	Schärfe	agudeza
acutezza visiva	Sehschärfe	agudeza visual
acuto	spitz, scharf	agudo
ago	Nadel, Kanüle	aguja
isolamento	Isolierung	aislamiento
albumina	Albumin	albúmina
albuminuria	Albuminurie	albuminuria
alcali	Alkali, Lauge, Base	álcali
alcalino	alkalisch, basisch	alcalino
alcalosi	Alkalose	alcalosis
alcool	Alkohol	alcohol
alcolismo	Alkoholismus, Alkoholvergiftung	alcoholismo
allergene	Allergen	alérgeno
allergia	Allergie	alergia
allergia alimentare	Nahrungsmittelallergie	alergia alimentaria
flutter atriale	Vorhofflattern	aleteo auricular
traversa	Unterziehtuch	alezo
alfafetoproteina	Alpha-Fetoprotein	alfafetoproteína (AFP)
respiro	Atem, Atemzug	aliento
alimentazione	Ernährung	alimentación
alopecia	Alopezie, Haarausfall	alopecia
allopurinolo	Allopurinol	alopurinol
catrame	Steinkohlenteer	alquitrán
allucinazione	Halluzination	alucinación
alveolite	Alveolitis	alveolitis
alveolo	Alveole	alvéolo
amaurosi	Amaurose	amaurosis
ambiente	Umgebung, Umwelt	ambiente
ambliopia	Amblyopie, Sehschwäche	ambliopía
ambulatorio	ambulant	ambulante
ambulatoriale	ambulant	ambulatorio
ameba	Amöbe	ameba
amebiasi	Amöbenkrankheit, Amöbiasis	amebiasis
ameboma	Amöbengranulom	ameboma

SPANISH	ENGLISH	FRENCH
amenaza de aborto	threatened abortion	risque d'avortement
amenorrea	amenorrhea (Am), amenorrhoea (Eng)	aménorrhée
amígdalas	tonsils	amygdales
amigdalitis	tonsillitis	angine
amigdaloadenoidectomía	adenotonsillectomy	adéno-amygdalectomie
amiloide	amyloid	amyloïde
amiloideo	amyloid	amyloïde
amiloidosis	amyloidosis	amylose
aminoácido	amino acid	acide aminé
aminoácido esenciale	essential amino acid	acide aminé essentiel
amnesia	amnesia	amnésie
amniocentesis	amniocentesis	amniocentèse
amnios	amnion	amnion
amnioscopia	amnioscopy	amnioscopie
amniotomía	amniotomy	amniotomie
amorfo	amorphous	amorphe
ampolla	ampoule (Eng), ampule (Am), ampulla, bleb, blister	ampoule, phlyctène
amputación	amputation	amputation
amputado	amputee	amputé
anabolismo	anabolism	anabolisme
anaerobio	anaerobe (Eng), anerobe (Am)	anaérobie
anafilaxis	anaphylaxis	anaphylaxie
analéptico (n)	analeptic (n)	analeptique (n)
analéptico (a)	analeptic (a)	analeptique (a)
analgesia	analgesia	analgésie
analgésico (n)	analgesic (n)	analgésique (n)
analgésico (a)	analgesic (a)	analgésique (a)
análisis	analysis	analyse
análisis enzimático por inmunoabsorción	enzyme-linked immunosorbent assay (ELISA)	dosage par la méthode (ELISA)
anaplasia	anaplasia	anaplasie
anartria	anarthria	anarthrie
anastómosis	anastomosis	anastomose
anatomía	anatomy	anatomie
andrógenos	androgens	androgènes
anejos	adnexa	annexes
anemia	anaemia (Eng), anemia (Am)	anémie
anemia drepanocítica	sickle-cell anaemia (Eng), sickle-cell anemia (Am)	drépanocytose
anemia perniciosa	pernicious anaemia (Eng), pernicious anemia (Am)	anémie pernicieuse
anencefalia	anencephaly	anencéphalie
anestesia	anaesthesia (Eng), anesthesia (Am)	anesthésie
anestésico (n)	anaesthetic (Eng) (n), anesthetic (Am) (n)	anesthésique (n)

minaccia d'aborto	drohender Abort	amenaza de aborto
amenorrea	Amenorrhoe	amenorrea
tonsille	Tonsillen, Mandeln	amígdalas
tonsillite	Tonsillitis, Mandelentzündung	amigdalitis
adenotonsillectomia	Adenotonsillektomie	amigdaloadenoidectomía
amiloide	Amyloid	amiloide
amiloide	amyloid, stärkehaltig	amiloideo
amiloidosi	Amyloidose	amiloidosis
aminoacido	Aminosäure	aminoácido
aminoacido essenziale	essentielle Aminosäure	aminoácido esencial
amnesia	Amnesie	amnesia
amniocentesi	Amniozentese	amniocentesis
amnios	Amnion	amnios
amnioscopia	Amnioskopie	amnioscopia
amniotomia	Amnionpunktur	amniotomía
amorfo	amorph	amorfo
ampolla, fiala, vescichetta, flittena, vescicola, bolla	Ampulle, Bläschen Blase, Hautblase, Brandblase	ampolla
amputazione	Amputation	amputación
amputato	Amputierter	amputado
anabolismo	Anabolismus, Aufbaustoffwechsel	anabolismo
anaerobio	Anaerobier	anaerobio
anafilassi	Anaphylaxie	anafilaxis
analettico (n)	Analeptikum (n)	analéptico (n)
analettico (a)	analeptisch (a)	analéptico (a)
analgesia	Analgesie, Schmerzlosigkeit	analgesia
analgesico (n)	Analgetikum (n), Schmerzmittel (n)	analgésico (n)
analgesico (a)	analgetisch (a), schmerzlindernd (a), schmerzunempfindlich (a)	analgésico (a)
analisi	Analyse	análisis
test di immunoassorbimento enzimatico	enzyme-linked immunosorbent assay (ELISA)	análisis enzimático por inmunoabsorción
anaplasia	Anaplasie	anaplasia
anartria	Anarthrie	anartria
anastomosi	Anastomose	anastómosis
anatomia	Anatomie	anatomía
androgeni	Androgene	andrógenos
annessi	Adnexe	anejos
anemia	Anämie	anemia
anemia drepanocitica	Sichelzellanämie	anemia drepanocítica
anemia perniciosa	perniziöse Anämie	anemia perniciosa
anencefalia	Anenzephalie	anencefalia
anestesia	Anästhesie, Betäubung, Narkose	anestesia
anestetico (n)	Anästhetikum (n), Betäubungsmittel (n), Narkosemittel (n)	anestésico (n)

SPANISH	ENGLISH	FRENCH
anestésico *(a)*	anaesthetic (Eng) *(a)*, anesthetic (Am) *(a)*	anesthésique *(a)*
aneurisma	aneurysm	anévrisme
anexos	adnexa	annexes
angina	angina quinsy	angor, phlegmon amygdalien ou périamygdalien
angioplastia	angioplasty	angioplastie
angiotensina	angiotensin	angiotensine
anisocitosis	anisocytosis	anisocytose
ano	anus	anus
anogenital	anogenital	anogénital
anomalía	anomaly	anomalie
anorexia	anorexia	anorexie
anoréxico *(n)*	anorectic *(n)*	anorexique *(n)*
anoréxico *(a)*	anorectic *(a)*	anorexique *(a)*
anormal	abnormal	anormal
anorrectal	anorectal	anorectal
anosmia	anosmia	anosmie
anovular	anovular	anovulaire
anoxia	anoxia	anoxie
anquilosis	ankylosis	ankylose
anquilostoma duodenal	hookworm	ankylostome
ansiedad	anxiety	anxiété
ansiolítico *(n)*	anxiolytic *(n)*	anxiolytique *(n)*
ansiolítico *(a)*	anxiolytic *(a)*	anxiolytique *(a)*
antagonismo	antagonism	antagonisme
antagonista	antagonist	antagoniste
antagonista H2	H2 antagonist	antagoniste H2
antebrazo	forearm	avant-bras
antenatal	antenatal	anténatal
ante partum	ante-partum	ante partum
anterior	anterior	antérieur
anterógrado	anterograde	antérograde
anteversión	anteversion	antéversion
antiácido	antacid	antiacide
antiarrítmico	anti-arrhythmic	antiarythmique
antibacteriano	antibacterial	antibactérien
antibióticos	antibiotics	antibiotiques
anticoagulante	anticoagulant	anticoagulant
anticolinérgico	anticholinergic	anticholinergique
anticonceptivo *(n)*	contraceptive *(n)*	contraceptif *(n)*
anticonceptivo *(a)*	contraceptive *(a)*	contraceptif *(a)*
anticonceptivo oral combinado	combined oral contraceptive	contraceptif oral combiné
anticonvulsivo *(n)*	anticonvulsant *(n)*	anticonvulsant *(n)*

ITALIAN	GERMAN	SPANISH
anestetico *(a)*	anästhetisch *(a)*, betäubend *(a)*, gefühllos *(a)*	anestésico *(a)*
aneurisma	Aneurysma	aneurisma
annessi	Adnexe	anexos
angina, ascesso peritonsillare	Angina, Peritonsillarabszeß	angina
angioplastica	Angioplastie	angioplastia
angiotensina	Angiotensin	angiotensina
anisocitosi	Anisozytose	anisocitosis
ano	Anus, After	ano
anogenitale	anogenital	anogenital
anomalia	Anomalie, Fehlbildung	anomalía
anoressia	Anorexie, Magersucht	anorexia
anoressico *(n)*	Anorektiker(in) *(n)*, Magersüchtige(r) *(n)*, Apettitzügler *(n)*	anoréxico *(n)*
anoressico *(a)*	anorektisch *(a)*, magersüchtig *(a)*	anoréxico *(a)*
anormale	abnormal	anormal
anorettale	anorektal	anorrectal
anosmia	Anosmie	anosmia
anovulare	anovulatorisch	anovular
anossia	Anoxie, Sauerstoffmangel	anoxia
anchilosi	Ankylose, Versteifung	anquilosis
strongiloide	Hakenwurm	anquilostoma duodenal
ansietà	Angst	ansiedad
ansiolitico *(n)*	Anxiolytikum *(n)*	ansiolítico *(n)*
ansiolitico *(a)*	anxiolytisch *(a)*	ansiolítico *(a)*
antagonismo	Antagonismus	antagonismo
antagonista	Antagonist	antagonista
antagonista H2	H2-Antagonist	antagonista H2
avambraccio	Unterarm	antebrazo
prenatale	pränatal	antenatal
preparto	ante partum, vor der Entbindung	ante partum
anteriore	anterior, Vorder-	anterior
anterogrado	anterograd	anterógrado
antiversione	Anteversion	anteversión
antiacido	Antazidum	antiácido
anti-aritmico	antiarrhythmisch	antiarrítmico
antibatterico	antibakteriell	antibacteriano
antibiotici	Antibiotika	antibióticos
anticoagulante	Antikoagulans, Gerinnungshemmer	anticoagulante
anticolinergico	anticholinerg	anticolinérgico
anticoncezionale *(n)*	Kontrazeptivum *(n)*, Verhütungsmittel *(n)*	anticonceptivo *(n)*
anticoncezionale *(a)*	kontrazeptiv *(a)*, Verhütungs- *(a)*	anticonceptivo *(a)*
contraccettivo orale estro-progestinico	orales Kontrazeptivum (Kombinationspräparat)	anticonceptivo oral combinado
anticonvulsivante *(n)*	Antiepileptikum *(n)*, Antikonvulsivum *(n)*	anticonvulsivo *(n)*

SPANISH	ENGLISH	FRENCH
anticonvulsivo *(a)*	anticonvulsant *(a)*	anticonvulsant *(a)*
anticuerpo anti-treponema fluorescente	fluorescent treponemal antibody (FTA)	test d'immunofluorescence absorbée pour le diagnostic sérologique de la syphilis
anticuerpo monoclonal	monoclonal antibody	anticorps monoclonal
anticuerpos	antibodies (Ab)	anticorps
anti-D	anti-D	anti-D
antidepresivo	antidepressant	antidépresseur
antídoto	antidote, antivenin	antidote, sérum antivenimeux
antiemético *(n)*	antiemetic *(n)*	antiémétique *(n)*
antiemético *(a)*	antiemetic *(a)*	antiémétique *(a)*
antiepiléptico *(n)*	anti-epileptic *(n)*	antiépileptique *(n)*
antiepiléptico *(a)*	anti-epileptic *(a)*	antiépileptique *(a)*
antiespasmódico *(n)*	antispasmodic *(n)*	antispasmodique *(n)*
antiespasmódico *(a)*	antispasmodic *(a)*	antispasmodique *(a)*
antígeno	antigen	antigène
antígeno Australia	Australian antigen	antigène australien
antígeno de histocompatibilidad	histocompatibility antigen	antigène d'histocompatibilité
antígeno eritrocitario humano	human erythrocyte antigen (HEA)	antigène humain des erythrocytes
antígeno linfocitario humano (HLA)	human lymphocytic antigen (HLA)	antigène lymphocytaire humain
antígeno triple	triple antigen	triple antigène
antihistamínico	antihistamine	antihistamine
antiinflamatorio	anti-inflammatory	anti-inflammatoire
antimetabolito	antimetabolite	antimétabolite
antimicótico *(n)*	antimycotic *(n)*	antimycotique *(n)*
antimicótico *(a)*	antimycotic *(a)*	antimycotique *(a)*
antimicrobiano	antimicrobial	antimicrobien
antipalúdico *(n)*	antimalarial *(n)*	antipaludique *(n)*
antipalúdico *(a)*	antimalarial *(a)*	antipaludique *(a)*
antipirético *(n)*	antipyretic *(n)*	antipyrétique *(n)*
antipirético *(a)*	antipyretic *(a)*	antipyrétique *(a)*
antipruriginoso *(n)*	antipruritic *(n)*	antiprurigineux *(n)*
antipruriginoso *(a)*	antipruritic *(a)*	antiprurigineux *(a)*
antipsicótico *(n)*	antipsychotic *(n)*	antipsychotique *(n)*
antipsicótico *(a)*	antipsychotic *(a)*	antipsychotique *(a)*
antisepsia	antisepsis	antisepsie
antiséptico *(n)*	antiseptic *(n)*	antiseptique *(n)*
antiséptico *(a)*	antiseptic *(a)*	antiseptique *(a)*
antisocial	antisocial	antisocial
antisuero	antiserum	anti-serum
antitoxina	antitoxin	antitoxine
antitusígeno *(n)*	antitussive *(n)*	antitussif *(n)*
antitusígeno *(a)*	antitussive *(a)*	antitussif *(a)*
antojo	maggot	asticot
ántrax	carbuncle	charbon
antro	antrum	antre

anticonvulsivante *(a)*	antiepileptisch *(a)*, antikonvulsiv *(a)*	**anticonvulsivo** *(a)*
anticorpo immuno-fluorescente anti-treponema	Fluoreszenz-Treponemen-Antikörper	**anticuerpo anti-treponema fluorescente**
anticorpo monoclonale	monoklonaler Antikörper	**anticuerpo monoclonal**
anticorpi (Ac)	Antikörper	**anticuerpos**
anti-D	Anti-D-Immununglobulin	**anti-D**
antidepressivo	Antidepressivum	**antidepresivo**
antidoto, antiveleno, contravveleno	Antidot, Schlangenserum	**antídoto**
anti-emetico *(n)*	Antiemetikum *(n)*	**antiemético** *(n)*
anti-emetico *(a)*	antiemetisch *(a)*	**antiemético** *(a)*
anticomiziale *(n)*	Antiepileptikum *(n)*, Antikonvulsivum *(n)*	**antiepiléptico** *(n)*
anticomiziale *(a)*	antiepileptisch *(a)*, antikonvulsiv *(a)*	**antiepiléptico** *(a)*
antispastico *(n)*	Spasmolytikum *(n)*	**antiespasmódico** *(n)*
antispastico *(a)*	spasmolytisch *(a)*, krampflösend *(a)*	**antiespasmódico** *(a)*
antigene	Antigen	**antígeno**
antigene Australia	Australia-Antigen (HBsAG)	**antígeno Australia**
antigene di istocompatibilità	Histokompatibilitäts-Antigen	**antígeno de histocompatibilidad**
antigene eritrocitico umano	menschliches Erythrozyten-Antigen	**antígeno eritrocitario humano**
antigene linfocitario umano	human lymphocytic antigen (HLA)	**antígeno linfocitario humano (HLA)**
antigene triplo	Dreifachantigen	**antígeno triple**
anti istaminico	Antihistamine	**antihistamínico**
anti-infiammatorio	entzündungshemmend	**antiinflamatorio**
antimetabolita	Antimetabolit	**antimetabolito**
antimicotico *(n)*	Antimykotikum *(n)*	**antimicótico** *(n)*
antimicotico *(a)*	antimykotisch *(a)*	**antimicótico** *(a)*
antimicrobico	antimikrobiell	**antimicrobiano**
antimalarico *(n)*	Antimalariamittel *(n)*, Malariamittel *(n)*	**antipalúdico** *(n)*
antimalarico *(a)*	Antimalaria- *(a)*	**antipalúdico** *(a)*
anti-piretico *(n)*	Antipyretikum *(n)*, Fiebermittel *(n)*	**antipirético** *(n)*
anti-piretico *(a)*	antipyretisch *(a)*, fiebersenkend *(a)*	**antipirético** *(a)*
antipruriginoso *(n)*	Antipruriginosum *(n)*	**antipruriginoso** *(n)*
antipruriginoso *(a)*	antipruriginös *(a)*, juckreizlindernd *(a)*	**antipruriginoso** *(a)*
antipsicotico *(n)*	Antipsychotikum *(n)*, Neuroleptikum *(n)*	**antipsicótico** *(n)*
antipsicotico *(a)*	antipsychotisch *(a)*, neuroleptisch *(a)*	**antipsicótico** *(a)*
antisepsi	Antisepsis	**antisepsia**
antisettico *(n)*	Antiseptikum *(n)*	**antiséptico** *(n)*
antisettico *(a)*	antiseptisch *(a)*	**antiséptico** *(a)*
antisociale	dissozial	**antisocial**
anti-siero	Antiserum, Immunserum	**antisuero**
antitossina	Antitoxin, Gegengift	**antitoxina**
antibechico *(n)*	Antitussivum *(n)*, Hustenmittel *(n)*	**antitusígeno** *(n)*
antibechico *(a)*	antitussiv *(a)*	**antitusígeno** *(a)*
larva	Larve, Made	**antojo**
carbonchio, antrace, favo	Karbunkel	**ántrax**
antro	Antrum	**antro**

SPANISH	ENGLISH	FRENCH
antropoide	anthropoid	anthropoïde
antropología	anthropology	anthropologie
antrostomía	antrostomy	antrostomie
anular	annular	annulaire
anuria	anuria	anurie
aorta	aorta	aorte
aparato digestivo	digestive system	système digestif
aparato reproductor	reproductive system	système reproducteur
aparato respiratorio	respiratory system	système respiratoire
apatía	apathy	apathie
apéndice	appendix	appendice
apendicectomía	appendectomy, appendicectomy	appendicectomie
apendicitis	appendicitis	appendicite
ápex	apex	apex
apirético	afebrile	afébrile
apirexia	apyrexia	apyrexie
aplicador	applicator	applicateur
apnea	apnea (Am), apnoea (Eng)	apnée
aponeurosis	fascia	fascia
aposición	apposition	apposition
apraxia	apraxia	apraxie
apremio	compulsion	compulsion
aracnoideo	arachnoid	arachnoïde
araña vascular	spider naevus (Eng), spider nevus (Am)	naevi
arbovirus	arbovirus	arbovirus
arcadas	retching	haut-le-coeur
ardor de estómago	heartburn	aigreurs
área de Broca	Broca's area	centre moteur de Broca
areola	areola	aréole
arritmia	arrhythmia	arythmie
artefacto	artefact (Eng), artifact (Am)	artefact
arteria	artery	artère
arteria femoral	femoral artery	artère fémorale
arteria radial	radial artery	artère radiale
arteriola	arteriole	artériole
arteriopatía	arteriopathy	artériopathie
arteriosclerosis	arteriosclerosis	artériosclérose
arteriovenoso	arteriovenous	artérioveineux
arteritis	arteritis	artérite
arteritis de células gigantes	giant cell arteritis	artérite temporale
articulación	articulation, joint	articulation
articulación de Charcot	Charcot's joint	arthropathie neurogène
articular	articular	articulaire
artralgia	arthralgia	arthralgie
artritis	arthritis	arthrite

ITALIAN	GERMAN	SPANISH
antropoide	anthropoid	antropoide
antropologia	Anthropologie	antropología
antrostomia	Antrumeröffnung	antrostomía
anulare	ringförmig	anular
anuria	Anurie, Harnverhaltung	anuria
aorta	Aorta, Hauptschlagader	aorta
sistema digestivo	Verdauungsapparat	aparato digestivo
sistema riproduttivo	Fortpflanzungsapparat	aparato reproductor
sistema respiratorio	Atmungsapparat, Atmungsorgane	aparato respiratorio
apatia	Apathie	apatía
appendice	Appendix, Blinddarm	apéndice
appendicectomia	Appendektomie, Blinddarmoperation	apendicectomía
appendicite	Appendizitis, Blinddarmentzündung	apendicitis
apice	Apex, Spitze	ápex
afebbrile	fieberfrei	apirético
apiressia	Apyrexie	apirexia
applicatore	Applikator	aplicador
apnea	Apnoe, Atemstillstand	apnea
fascia	Faszie	aponeurosis
apposizione	Apposition	aposición
aprassia	Apraxie	apraxia
compulsione	Zwang	apremio
aracnoidea	arachnoid	aracnoideo
angioma stellare	Spider naevus, Naevus arachnoideus	araña vascular
arbovirus	ARBO-Virus	arbovirus
conati di vomito	Würgen, Brechreiz	arcadas
pirosi	Sodbrennen	ardor de estómago
area di Broca	Broca-Sprachzentrum	área de Broca
areola	Areola, Brustwarzenhof	areola
aritmia	Arrhythmie, Rhythmusstörung	arritmia
artefatto	Artefakt	artefacto
arteria	Arterie, Schlagader	arteria
arteria femorale	Arteria femoralis	arteria femoral
arteria radiale	Arteria radialis	arteria radial
arteriola	Arteriole	arteriola
arteriopatia	Arteriopathie, Arterienerkrankung	arteriopatía
arteriosclerosi	Arteriosklerose, Arterienverkalkung	arteriosclerosis
arterovenosa	arteriovenös	arteriovenoso
arterite	Arteriitis	arteritis
arterite a cellule giganti	Riesenzellarteriitis	arteritis de células gigantes
articolazione	Artikulation, Gelenk	articulación
artropatia di Charcot	Charcot-Gelenk	articulación de Charcot
articolare	Gelenk-	articular
artralgia	Arthralgie, Gelenkschmerz	artralgia
artrite	Arthritis, Gelenkentzündung	artritis

SPANISH	ENGLISH	FRENCH
artritis psoriásica	psoriatic arthritis	rhumatisme psoriasique
artritis reumatoide (AR)	rheumatoid arthritis (RA)	polyarthrite rhumatoïde (PR), polyarthrite chronique évolutive (PCE)
artrodesis	arthrodesis	arthrodèse
artrografía	arthrography	arthrographie
artropatía	arthropathy	arthropathie
artroplastia	arthroplasty	arthroplastie
artroscopia	arthroscopy	arthroscopie
asbesto	asbestos	asbeste
asbestosis	asbestosis	asbestose
áscaris	ascaris, roundworm	ascaris
ascitis	ascites	ascite
asepsia	asepsis	asepsie
asesoramiento	counselling	consultation
asfixia	asphyxia, suffocation	asphyxie, suffocation
asimetría	asymmetry	asymétrie
asimilación	assimilation	assimilation
asintomático	asymptomatic	asymptomatique
asistencia primaria	primary care	soins de santé primaires
asma	asthma	asthme
asma bronquial	bronchial asthma	asthme bronchique
asociación	association	association
aspergilosis	aspergillosis	aspergillose
aspiración	aspiration	aspiration
astereognosia	astereognosis	astéréognosie
astigmatismo	astigmatism	astigmatisme
astilla	splint	attelle
astrágalo	talus	astragale
astringente	astringent	astringent
ataque	attack, fit, seizure	attaque, accès
ataque isquémico transitorio (AIT)	transient ischaemic attack (TIA) (Eng), transient ishemic attack (TIA) (Am), drop attack	accès ischémique transitoire cérébral, chute brusque par dérobement des jambes
ataque vasovagal	vasovagal attack	malaise vasovagal
ataxia	ataxia	ataxie
ataxia de Friedreich	Friedreich's ataxia	maladie de Friedreich
atelectasia	atelectasis	atélectasie
atenuación	attenuation	atténuation
aterogénico	atherogenic	athérogène
ateroma	atheroma	athérome
aterosclerosis	atherosclerosis	athérosclérose
atetosis	athetosis	athétose
atípico	atypical	atypique
átomo	atom	atome
atono	atonic	atonique

ITALIAN	GERMAN	SPANISH
artropatia psoriasica, psoriasi artropatica	Arthritis psoriatica	artritis psoriásica
artrite reumatoide (AR)	Polyarthritis rheumatica (PCP), Rheumatoide Arthritis	artritis reumatoide (AR)
artrodesi	Arthrodese	artrodesis
artrografia	Arthrographie	artrografía
artropatia	Arthropathie, Gelenkleiden	artropatía
artroplastica	Arthroplastik, Gelenkplastik	artroplastia
artroscopia	Arthroskopie, Gelenkendoskopie	artroscopia
asbesto	Asbest	asbesto
asbestosi	Asbestose	asbestosis
ascaride, nematelminto	Rundwurm, Spulwurm	áscaris
ascite	Aszites	ascitis
asepsi	Asepsis	asepsia
consulenza eugenetica	Beratung	asesoramiento
asfissia, soffocamento	Asphyxie, Ersticken, Erstickung	asfixia
asimmetria	Asymmetrie	asimetría
assimilazione	Assimilation	asimilación
asintomatico	asymptomatisch	asintomático
primaria, neoplasia primitiva	Primärversorgung	asistencia primaria
asma	Asthma	asma
asma bronchiale	Asthma bronchiale	asma bronquial
associazione	Assoziation	asociación
aspergillosi	Aspergillose	aspergilosis
aspirazione	Aspiration	aspiración
astereognosia	Astereognosie	astereognosia
astigmatismo	Astigmatismus	astigmatismo
stecca ortopedica	Schiene	astilla
astragalo, talo	Talus	astrágalo
astringente	adstringierend	astringente
attacco, convulsione	Attacke, Anfall	ataque
attacco ischemico transitorio, improvvisa perdita della postura ad insorgenza periodica	transitorische ischämische Attacke (TIA), Drop attack	ataque isquémico transitorio (AIT)
crisi vagale	vasovagale Synkope	ataque vasovagal
atassia	Ataxie, Koordinationsstörung	ataxia
malattia di Friedreich	Friedreich Ataxie	ataxia de Friedreich
atelettasia	Atelektase	atelectasia
attenuazione	Verdünnung, Abschwächung	atenuación
aterogenico	atherogen	aterogénico
ateroma	Atherom, Grützbeutel	ateroma
aterosclerosi	Atherosklerose	aterosclerosis
atetosi	Athetose	atetosis
atipico	atypisch, heterolog	atípico
atomo	Atom	átomo
atonico	atonisch	atono

SPANISH	ENGLISH	FRENCH
atresia	atresia	atrésie
atrioventricular	atrioventricular (AV)	atrio-ventriculaire
atrofia	atrophy	atrophie
atropina	atropine	atropine
audiograma	audiogram	audiogramme
audiología	audiology	audiologie
auditorio	auditory	auditif
aura	aura	aura
aural	aural	aural
aurícula	atrium	oreillette
aurículo-ventricular (AV)	atrioventricular (AV)	atrio-ventriculaire
auriscopio	auriscope	auriscope
auscultación	auscultation	auscultation
autismo	autism	autisme
autoanticuerpo	autoantibody	auto-anticorps
autoantígeno	autoantigen	auto-antigène
autoclave	autoclave	autoclave
autoexamen de la mama	breast self-examination (BSE)	auto-examen des seins
autoinjerto	autograft	autogreffe
autoinmunización	autoimmunity	auto-immunisation
autointoxicación	self-poisoning	intoxication volontaire
autolesión	self-harm	automutilation
autólisis	autolysis	autolyse
autólogo	autologous	autologue
autónomo	autonomic	autonome
autopsia	autopsy	autopsie
avascular	avascular	avasculaire
avulsión	avulsion	avulsion
axila	axilla	aisselle
axón	axon	axone
axonotmesis	axonotmesis	axonotmésis

ITALIAN	GERMAN	SPANISH
atresia	Atresie	atresia
atrioventricolare	atrioventrikulär	atrioventricular
atrofia	Atrophie	atrofia
atropina	Atropin	atropina
audiogramma	Audiogramm, Hörkurve	audiograma
audiologia	Audiologie	audiología
acustico, auditivo	Gehör-, Hör-	auditorio
aura	Aura	aura
auricolare	Gehör-, Ohr-, Aura-	aural
atrio	Atrium, Vorhof	aurícula
atrioventricolare	atrioventrikulär	aurículo-ventricular (AV)
otoscopio	Ohrenspiegel	auriscopio
auscultazione	Auskultation, Abhören	auscultación
autismo	Autismus	autismo
autoanticorpo	Autoantikörper	autoanticuerpo
autoantigene	Autoantigen	autoantígeno
autoclave	Autoklav, Sterilisationsapparat	autoclave
autopalpazione mammaria	Selbstuntersuchung der Brust	autoexamen de la mama
autoinnesto	Autoplastik	autoinjerto
autoimmunizzazione	Autoimmunität	autoinmunización
autoavvelenamento	Selbstvergiftung	autointoxicación
autolesionismo	Selbstschädigung	autolesión
autolisi	Autolyse	autólisis
autologo	autolog	autólogo
autonomo	autonom	autónomo
autopsia	Autopsie, Sektion	autopsia
avascolare	gefäßlos	avascular
avulsione	Abriß, Ausreißen	avulsión
ascella	Axilla, Achsel(höhle)	axila
cilindrasse, assone	Axon	axón
degenerazione del cilindrasse con possibile rigenerazione	Axonotmesis	axonotmesis

B

SPANISH	ENGLISH	FRENCH
bacilo	bacillus	bacille
bacilo de Calmette-Guérin (BCG)	bacille Calmette-Guérin (BCG)	bacille de Calmette-Guérin (BCG)
bacteria	bacteria	bactérie
bactericida	bactericide	bactéricide
bacteriemia	bacteraemia (Eng), bacteremia (Am)	bactériémie
bacteriología	bacteriology	bactériologie
bacteriostasis	bacteriostasis	bactériostase
bacteriuria	bacteriuria	bactériurie
bajo peso al nacer	low birth weight (LBW)	hypotrophie
balanitis	balanitis	balanite
balanopostitis	balanoposthitis	balanoposthite
banco de sangre	blood bank	banque de sang
baño	bath	bain
barbilla	chin	menton
barrera hematoencefálica (BHE)	blood-brain barrier (BBB)	barrière hémato-encéphalique
barrido	scan	échogramme
bazo	spleen	rate
benigno	benign	bénin (bénigne)
beri-beri	beri-beri	béribéri
beso de vida	kiss of life	bouche-à-bouche
beta-bloqueador	beta blocker	bêtabloquant
bíceps	biceps	biceps
bicornio	bicornuate	bicorne
bicúspide	bicuspid	bicuspide
bien desarrollado	florid	coloré
bífido	bifid	bifide
bifurcación	bifurcation	bifurcation
bilateral	bilateral	bilatéral
biliar	biliary	biliaire
bilioso	bilious	bilieux
bilirrubina	bilirubin	bilirubine
bilis	bile	bile
biliuria	biliuria	biliurie
bimanual	bimanual	bimanuel
biológico	biological	biologique
biopsia	biopsy	biopsie
biopsia de las vellosidades coriónicas	chorionic villus biopsy	biopsie du villus chorionique
biopsia del yeyuno	jejunal biopsy	biopsie jéjunale
biorritmo	biorhythm	biorythme
bipolar	bipolar	bipolaire
bisexual	bisexual	bisexuel
bivalvo	bivalve	bivalve
blefaritis	blepharitis	blépharite
blefarospasmo	blepharospasm	blépharospasme

ITALIAN	GERMAN	SPANISH
bacillo	Bazillus	bacilo
bacillo di Calmette e Guérin	Bacillus Calmette-Guérin (BCG)	bacilo de Calmette-Guérin (BCG)
batteri	Bakterien	bacteria
battericida	Bakterizid	bactericida
batteriemia	Bakteriämie	bacteriemia
batteriologia	Bakteriologie	bacteriología
batteriostasi	Bakteriostase	bacteriostasis
batteriuria	Bakteriurie	bacteriuria
basso peso alla nascita	niedriges Geburtsgewicht	bajo peso al nacer
balanite	Balanitis	balanitis
balanopostite	Balanoposthitis	balanopostitis
banca del sangue	Blutbank	banco de sangre
bagno	Bad	baño
mento	Kinn	barbilla
barriera ematoencefalica	Blut-Hirn-Schranke	barrera hematoencefálica (BHE)
ecografia, scintigrafia	Scan	barrido
milza	Milz	bazo
benigno	benigne, gutartig	benigno
beri beri	Beriberi	beri-beri
respirazione bocca a bocca	Mund-zu-Mund-Wiederbelebung	beso de vida
beta-bloccante	Betablocker	beta-bloqueador
bicipite	Bizeps	bíceps
bicorne	bicornis	bicornio
bicuspide	bicuspidal	bicúspide
florido	floride	bien desarrollado
bifido	bifidus	bífido
biforcazione	Bifurkation	bifurcación
bilaterale	zweiseitig	bilateral
biliare	biliär	biliar
biliare	biliös	bilioso
bilirubina	Bilirubin	bilirrubina
bile	Galle	bilis
biliuria	Bilirubinurie	biliuria
bimanuale	bimanuell, beidhändig	bimanual
biologico	biologisch	biológico
biopsia	Biopsie	biopsia
biopsia dei villi coriali	Chorionzottenbiopsie	biopsia de las vellosidades coriónicas
biopsia digiunale	Jejunumbiopsie	biopsia del yeyuno
bioritmo	Biorhythmus	biorritmo
bipolare	bipolar	bipolar
bisessuale	bisexuell	bisexual
bivalve	zweiklappig	bivalvo
blefarite	Blepharitis, Lidentzündung	blefaritis
blefarospasmo	Blepharospasmus, Lidkrampf	blefarospasmo

SPANISH	ENGLISH	FRENCH
bloqueo del pudendo	pudendal block	vulve
bloqueo nervioso	nerve block	anesthésie par blocage nerveux
boca	mouth	bouche
bocio	goiter (Am), goitre (Eng)	goitre
bolo	bolus	bol
bolsa	bursa, pouch	bourse, poche
bolsa faringea	pharyngeal pouch	poche ectobranchiale et entobranchiale
borreliosis	borreliosis	borréliose
bostezo	yawn	bâillement
bote	gallipot	petit pot
botulismo	botulism	botulisme
bóveda	fornix	fornix
bradicardia	bradycardia	bradycardie
branquial	branchial	branchial
braquial	brachial	brachial
brazo	arm	bras
brea	coal tar	coaltar
broncoconstrictor	bronchoconstrictor	bronchoconstricteur
broncodilatador	bronchodilator	bronchodilatateur
bronconeumonia	bronchopneumonia	bronchopneumonie
broncopulmonar	bronchopulmonary	bronchopulmonaire
broncoscopio	bronchoscope	bronchoscope
broncospasmo	bronchospasm	bronchospasme
bronquiectasia	bronchiectasis	bronchectasie
bronquio	bronchus	bronche
bronquiolitis	bronchiolitis	bronchiolite
bronquiolo	bronchiole	bronchiole
bronquios	bronchi	bronches
bronquitis	bronchitis	bronchite
brucelosis	brucellosis	brucellose
bucal	buccal	buccal
bulbar	bulbar	bulbaire
bulimia	bulimia	boulimie
bulla	bleb, bulla	phlyctène, bulle
bursitis	bursitis	bursite

ITALIAN	GERMAN	SPANISH
anestesia della regione pubica	Pudendusblock	bloqueo del pudendo
blocco nervoso	Leitungsanästhesie	bloqueo nervioso
bocca	Mund	boca
gozzo	Struma, Kropf	bocio
bolo	Bolus	bolo
borsa, tasca	Bursa, Beutel, Tasche	bolsa
tasca faringea	Schlundtasche	bolsa faringea
borreliosi	Borreliose	borreliosis
sbadiglio	Gähnen	bostezo
ampolla o vasetto unguentario	Salbentopf	bote
botulismo	Botulismus	botulismo
fornice	Fornix	bóveda
bradicardia	Bradykardie	bradicardia
branchiale	branchial-	branquial
brachiale	Arm-	braquial
braccio	Arm	brazo
catrame	Steinkohlenteer	brea
broncocostrittore	Bronchokonstriktor	broncoconstrictor
broncodilatatore	Bronchodilatator	broncodilatador
broncopolmonite	Bronchopneumonie	bronconeumonia
broncopolmonare	bronchopulmonal	broncopulmonar
broncoscopio	Bronchoskop	broncoscopio
broncospasmo	Bronchospasmus	broncospasmo
bronchiettasia	Bronchiektase	bronquiectasia
bronco	Bronchus	bronquio
bronchiolite	Bronchiolitis	bronquiolitis
bronchiolo	Bronchiolus, Bronchiole	bronquiolo
bronchi	Bronchien	bronquios
bronchite	Bronchitis	bronquitis
brucellosi	Brucellose	brucelosis
buccale	bukkal	bucal
bulbare	bulbär	bulbar
bulimia	Bulimie	bulimia
vescichetta, flittena, bolla	Bläschen, Bulla, Blase	bulla
borsite	Bursitis, Schleimbeutelentzündung	bursitis

C

SPANISH	ENGLISH	FRENCH
cabeza	head	tête
cadáver	cadaver, corpse	cadavre
cadera	hip	hanche
cafeína	caffeine	caféine
caida	drop attack	chutes brusques par dérobement des jambes
calambre	cramp	crampe
calcificación	calcification	calcification
calcio	calcium	calcium
cálculo	calculus, stone	calcul, caillou
cálculos biliares	gallstones	calculs biliaires
calibrador	caliper	armature orthopédique
callista	chiropodist	pédicure
callo	callus, corn	cal, cor
callosidad	callosity	callosité
calor	calor	chaleur
caloría	calorie	calorie
calostro	colostrum	colostrum
calvicie	alopecia	alopécie
campo de visión	field of vision	champ de vision
canal	canal	canal
cáncer	cancer	cancer
candidiasis	candidiasis	candidose
canino	canine	canin
cansancio	fatigue	fatigue
cánula	cannula	canule
cánula ótica	grommet	grommet
capacidad	ability	capacité, aptitude, compétence
capacidad de unión con antígenos	antigen binding capacity (ABC)	capacité de liaison d'un antigène, capacité de fixation d'un antigène
capacidad de unión con el hierro	iron binding capacity (IBC)	pouvoir sidéropexique, capacité de fixation du fer
capacidad pulmonar total (CPT)	total lung capacity (TLC)	capacité pulmonaire totale
capacidad total de unión con el hierro	total iron binding capacity (TIBC)	capacité totale de fixation du fer
capacidad vital	vital capacity	capacité vitale
capilar	capillary	capillaire
cápsula	capsule	capsule
capsulitis	capsulitis	capsulite
caput succedaneum	caput succedaneum	caput succedaneum
caquexia	cachexia	cachexie
carácter	character	caractère
carbón vegetal	charcoal	charbon
carboxihemoglobina	carboxyhaemoglobin (Eng), carboxyhemoglobin (Am)	carboxyhémoglobine
carbunco	anthrax	anthrax
carcinogénesis	carcinogenesis	carcinogenèse

ITALIAN	GERMAN	SPANISH
testa	Kopf	cabeza
cadavere	Kadaver, Leiche, Toter	cadáver
anca	Hüfte	cadera
caffeina	Koffein	cafeína
improvvisa perdita della postura ad insorgenza periodica	Drop attack	caida
crampo	Krampf	calambre
calcificazione	Kalzifikation, Verkalkung	calcificación
calcio	Kalzium	calcio
calcolo	Stein	cálculo
calcoli biliari	Gallensteine	cálculos biliares
compasso per pelvi-craniometria	Schiene	calibrador
callista	Fußpfleger	callista
callo	Kallus, Klavus, Hühnerauge	callo
callosità	Schwiele, Hornhaut	callosidad
calore	Fieber, Hitze	calor
caloria	Kalorie	caloría
colostro	Kolostrum, Vormilch	calostro
alopecia	Alopezie, Haarausfall	calvicie
campo visivo	Gesichtsfeld	campo de visión
canale	Kanal, Gang	canal
cancro	Karzinom, Krebs	cáncer
candidiasi	Candidiasis	candidiasis
canino	Hunde-	canino
stanchezza, astenia	Ermüdung	cansancio
cannula	Kanüle	cánula
catetere per drenaggio auricolare	Öse	cánula ótica
abilità, capacità	Fähigkeit	capacidad
capacità di legame dell'antigene	Antigen-Bindungskapazität	capacidad de unión con antígenos
capacità di legame del ferro	Eisenbindungskapazität	capacidad de unión con el hierro
capacità polmonare totale	Totalkapazität (TK)	capacidad pulmonar total (CPT)
capacità totale di legame del ferro (TIBC)	totale Eisenbindungskapazität (TEBK)	capacidad total de unión con el hierro
capacità vitale	Vitalkapazität	capacidad vital
capillare	Kapillare	capilar
capsula	Kapsel	cápsula
capsulite	Kapselentzündung	capsulitis
tumore da parto	Geburtsgeschwulst	caput succedaneum
cachessia	Kachexie	caquexia
carattere	Charakter, Merkmal	carácter
carbone vegetale	Holzkohle	carbón vegetal
carbossiemoglobina	Carboxyhämoglobin	carboxihemoglobina
antrace, carbonchio	Anthrax, Milzbrand	carbunco
carcinogenesi	Karzinogenese	carcinogénesis

SPANISH	ENGLISH	FRENCH
carcinogénico	carcinogen	carcinogène
carcinoma	carcinoma	carcinome
carcinoma de células de avena	oat cell cancer	épithélioma à petites cellules
carcinomatosis	carcinomatosis	carcinomatose
cardíaco	cardiac	cardiaque
cardias	cardia	cardia
cardiógenico	cardiogenic	cardiogène
cardiología	cardiology	cardiologie
cardiomegalia	cardiomegaly	cardiomégalie
cardiomiopatía	cardiomyopathy	cardiomyopathie
cardiopatía	heart disease	insuffisance cardiaque
cardiopatía isquémica	coronary artery disease (CAD), coronary heart disease (CHD), ischaemic heart disease (IHD) (Eng), ischemic heart disease (IHD) (Am)	coronaropathie, cardiopathie ischémique, insuffisance coronarienne globale, insuffisance coronarienne cardiaque
cardiopulmonar	cardiopulmonary	cardiopulmonaire
cardiorespiratorio	cardiorespiratory	cardiorespiratoire
cardiospasmo	cardiospasm	cardiospasme
cardiotorácico	cardiothoracic	cardiothoracique
cardiotóxico	cardiotoxic	cardiotoxique
cardiovascular	cardiovascular	cardiovasculaire
cardioversión	cardioversion	cardioversion
caries	caries	carie
carina	carina	carène
cariotipo	karyotype	karyotype
carminativo (n)	carminative (n)	carminatif (n)
carminativo (a)	carminative (a)	carminatif (a)
carotenos	carotene	carotène
carótida	carotid	carotide
carpometacarpiano	carpometacarpal	carpo-métarcarpien
carpopedal	carpopedal	carpo-pédal
cartílago	cartilage	cartilage
carúncula	caruncle	caroncule
caspa	dandruff	pellicules
castración	castration	castration
catabolismo	catabolism	catabolisme
catalizador	catalyst	catalyseur
catarata	cataract	cataracte
catarro	catarrh	catarrhe
catarsis	abreaction	abréaction
catatónico	catatonic	catatonique
catéter	catheter	cathéter
cateterismo	catheterization	cathétérisme
catgut	catgut	catgut
causa de la muerte	cause of death (COD)	cause du décès
causalgia	causalgia	causalgie

ITALIAN	GERMAN	SPANISH
carcinogeno	Karzinogen	carcinogénico
carcinoma	Karzinom, Krebs	carcinoma
microcitoma, carcinoma a piccole cellule	kleinzelliges Bronchialkarzinom	carcinoma de células de avena
carcinomatosi	Karzinose, Karzinomatose	carcinomatosis
cardiaco	Herz-	cardíaco
cardias	Kardia, Mageneingang	cardias
cardiogeno	kardiogen	cardiógenico
cardiologia	Kardiologie	cardiología
cardiomegalia	Kardiomegalie	cardiomegalia
cardiomiopatia	Kardiomyopathie	cardiomiopatía
malattia cardiaca	Herzerkrankung, Herzleiden	cardiopatía
malattia delle arterie coronarica (MAC), malattia cardiaca coronarica (MCC), cardiopatia ischemica	Koronaropathie, koronare Herzkrankheit (KHK), ischämische Herzkrankheit (IHK)	cardiopatía isquémica
cardiopolmonare	kardiopulmonal, Herz-Lungen-	cardiopulmonar
cardiorespiratorio	kardiorespiratorisch	cardiorespiratorio
spasmo cardiale, acalasia esofagea	Kardiospasmus	cardiospasmo
cardiotoracico	kardiothorakal	cardiotorácico
cardiotossico	kardiotoxisch, herzschädigend	cardiotóxico
cardiovascolare	kardiovaskulär, Kreislauf-	cardiovascular
cardioversione	Kardioversion	cardioversión
carie	Karies	caries
carena tracheale	Carina	carina
cariotipo	Karyotyp	cariotipo
carminativo (n)	Karminativum (n)	carminativo (n)
carminativo (a)	karminativ (a), entblähend (a)	carminativo (a)
carotene	Karotin	carotenos
carotide	Karotis-	carótida
carpometacarpale	karpometakarpal	carpometacarpiano
carpopedalico	karpopedal	carpopedal
cartilagine	Knorpel	cartílago
caruncola	Karunkel	carúncula
forfora	Schuppen	caspa
castrazione	Kastration	castración
catabolismo	Katabolismus, Abbaustoffwechsel	catabolismo
catalizzatore	Katalysator	catalizador
cataratta	Katarakt, grauer Star	catarata
catarro	Katarrh	catarro
abreazione, catarsi	Abreaktion	catarsis
catatonico	kataton	catatónico
catetere	Katheter	catéter
cateterizzazione	Katheterisierung	cateterismo
catgut	Catgut	catgut
causa di morte	Todesursache	causa de la muerte
causalgia	Kausalgie, brennender Schmerz	causalgia

SPANISH	ENGLISH	FRENCH
cáustico *(n)*	caustic *(n)*	caustique *(n)*
cáustico *(a)*	caustic *(a)*	caustique *(a)*
cauterizar	cauterize	cautériser
cavernoso	cavernous	caverneux
cavidad	cavity	cavité
cavidad amniótica	amniotic cavity	cavité amniotique
cavitación	pitting	formation de godet
cecostomía	caecostomy (Eng), cecostomy (Am)	caecostomie
cefalea	headache	mal de tête, céphalée
cefalea por tensión	tension headache	céphalée due à la tension
cefálico	cephalic	céphalique
cefalometría	cephalometry	céphalométrie
ceguera	amaurosis, blindness	amaurose, cécité
ceguera de colores	color blindness (Am), colour blindness (Eng)	daltonisme
ceguera nocturna	night blindness	cécité nocturne
ceja	brow	front, sourcil
celíaco	celiac (Am), coeliac (Eng)	coeliaque
célula	cell	cellule
celulitis	cellulitis	cellulite
centígrado	centigrade	centigrade
centrifugar	centrifuge	centrifuger
centrífugo *(n)*	centrifuge *(n)*	centrifugeur *(n)*
centrífugo *(a)*	centrifugal *(a)*	centrifuge *(a)*
centrípeto	centripetal	centripète
cepa	strain	entorse
cerebelo	cerebellum	cervelet
cerebral	cerebral	cérébral
cerebro	brain, cerebrum	cerveau
cerebroespinal	cerebrospinal	cérébrospinal
cerebrovascular	cerebrovascular	cérébrovasculaire
cerumen	ear wax	cérumen
cervical	cervical	cervical
cesárea	caesarean section (Eng), cesarean section (Am)	césarienne
cetoacidosis	ketoacidosis	céto-acidose
cetogénesis	ketogenesis	cétogenèse
cetonuria	ketonuria	cétonurie
cetosis	ketosis	cétose
chalacio	chalazion	chalazion
chancro	chancre	chancre
cianosis	cyanosis	cyanose
ciática	sciatica	sciatique
ciático	sciatic	sciatique
cicatriz	scar	cicatrice
ciclo	cycle	cycle
ciego	caecum (Eng), cecum (Am)	caecum
ciesis	cyesis	grossesse

ITALIAN	GERMAN	SPANISH
caustico (n)	Ätzmittel (n), Kaustikum (n)	cáustico (n)
caustico (a)	ätzend (a), brennend (a)	cáustico (a)
cauterizzare	kauterisieren, ätzen, brennen	cauterizar
cavernoso	kavernös	cavernoso
cavità	Höhle	cavidad
cavità amniotica	Amnionhöhle	cavidad amniótica
depressioni puntiformi, fovea	Dellenbildung	cavitación
ciecostomia	Zökostomie	cecostomía
mal di testa	Kopfschmerzen	cefalea
cefalea muscolotensiva	Spannungskopfschmerz	cefalea por tensión
cefalico	Kopf-, Schädel-	cefálico
cefalometria	Kephalometrie, Schädelmessung	cefalometría
amaurosi, cecità	Amaurose, Blindheit	ceguera
cecità ai colori, acromatopsia	Farbenblindheit	ceguera de colores
emeralopia	Nachtblindheit	ceguera nocturna
arcata sopracciliare, sopracciglio	Augenbraue	ceja
celiaco	abdominal	celíaco
cellula	Zelle	célula
cellulite	Zellulitis	celulitis
centigrado	Celsiusgrad	centígrado
centrifugare	zentrifugieren	centrifugar
centrifuga (n)	Zentrifuge (n)	centrífugo (n)
centrifugo (a)	zentrifugal (a)	centrífugo (a)
centripeto	zentripetal	centrípeto
tensione	Anstrengung, Belastung	cepa
cervelletto	Cerebellum, Kleinhirn	cerebelo
cerebrale	zerebral, Gehirn-	cerebral
cervello	Gehirn, Verstand, Großhirn	cerebro
cerebrospinale	zerebrospinal	cerebroespinal
cerebrovascolare	zerebrovaskulär	cerebrovascular
cerume	Zerumen, Ohrenschmalz	cerumen
cervicale	zervikal	cervical
taglio cesareo	Kaiserschnitt, Sectio	cesárea
chetoacidosi	Ketoazidose	cetoacidosis
chetogenesi	Ketogenese	cetogénesis
chetonuria	Ketonurie	cetonuria
chetosi	Ketose	cetosis
calazion	Chalazion, Hagelkorn	chalacio
cancroide, ulcera venerea	Schanker	chancro
cianosi	Zyanose	cianosis
sciatica	Ischias	ciática
sciatico	ischiadicus	ciático
cicatrice	Narbe	cicatriz
ciclo	Zyklus	ciclo
intestino cieco	Zökum	ciego
gravidanza	Schwangerschaft	ciesis

SPANISH	ENGLISH	FRENCH
cifolordosis	kypholordosis	cypholordose
cifoscoliosis	kyphoscoliosis	cyphoscoliose
cifosis	kyphosis	cyphose
cigoma	zygoma	zygoma
cigoto	zygote	zygote
ciliar	ciliary	ciliaire
cilios	cilia	cils
cinasa	kinase	kinase
cintura	girdle	ceinture
cintura escapular	shoulder girdle	ceinture scapulaire
cintura pélvica	pelvic girdle	ceinture pelvienne
circinado	circinate	circinal
circulación	circulation	circulation
circulación colateral	collateral circulation	circulation collatérale
circulación fetal	fetal circulation	circulation foetale
circulación portal	portal circulation	hypertension porte
circulación sistémica	systemic circulation	circulation systémique
circumoral	circumoral	péribuccal
circuncisión	circumcision	circoncision
cirrosis	cirrhosis	cirrhose
cirugía	surgery	chirurgie
cirujano	surgeon	chirurgien
cistitis	cystitis	cystite
cistocele	cystocele	cystocèle
cistometría	cystometry	cystométrie
cistopexia	cystopexy	cystopexie
citología	cytology	cytologie
citomegalovirus	cytomegalovirus (CMV)	cytomégalovirus
citoscopía	cystoscopy	cystoscopie
citoscopio	cystoscope	cystoscope
citotóxico	cytotoxic	cytotoxique
claudicación	claudication	claudication
claustrofobia	claustrophobia	claustrophobie
clavícula	clavicle	clavicule
clavo de Steinmann	Steinmann's pin	broche de Steinmann
climatérico	climacteric	climatérique
clínico	clinical	clinique
clítoris	clitoris	clitoris
cloasma	chloasma, liver spot	chloasma, tache hépatique
clono	clone, clonus	clone, clonus
clonus	clonus	clonus
coadyuvante	adjuvant	adjuvant
coagulación de la sangre	blood clotting, blood coagulation	coagulation du sang, coagulation sanguine
coagulación intravascular diseminada (CID)	disseminated intravascular coagulation (DIC)	coagulation intravasculaire disséminée (CID)
coagular	clot	coaguler

ITALIAN	GERMAN	SPANISH
cifolordosi	Kypholordose	cifolordosis
cifoscoliosi	Kyphoskoliose	cifoscoliosis
cifosi	Kyphose	cifosis
zigomo, osso zigomatico	Zygoma, Jochbein	cigoma
zigote	Zygote	cigoto
ciliare	ziliar, Wimpern-	ciliar
ciglia	Zilien, Wimpern	cilios
chinasi	Kinase	cinasa
cintura	Gürtel	cintura
cingolo scapolare	Schultergürtel	cintura escapular
cingolo pelvico	Beckengürtel	cintura pélvica
circinato	kreisförmig	circinado
circolazione	Kreislauf, Zirkulation, Durchblutung	circulación
circolazione collaterale	Kollateralkreislauf	circulación colateral
circolazione fetale	fetaler Kreislauf	circulación fetal
circolazione portale	Portalkreislauf, Pfortaderkreislauf	circulación portal
circolazione sistemica	Großer Kreislauf	circulación sistémica
circumorale	zirkumoral	circumoral
circoncisione	Zirkumzision, Beschneidung	circuncisión
cirrosi	Zirrhose	cirrosis
chirurgia	Chirurgie	cirugía
chirurgo	Chirurg	cirujano
cistite	Zystitis, Blasenentzündung	cistitis
cistocele	Zystozele	cistocele
cistometria	Zystometrie, Blasendruckmessung	cistometría
cistopessia	Zystopexie	cistopexia
citologia	Zytologie	citología
citomegalovirus	Zytomegalie-Virus (CMV)	citomegalovirus
cistoscopia	Zystoskopie, Blasenspiegelung	citoscopía
cistoscopio	Zystoskop, Blasenspiegel	citoscopio
citotossico	zytotoxisch, zellschädigend	citotóxico
claudicazione	Hinken, Claudicatio	claudicación
claustrofobia	Klaustrophobie	claustrofobia
clavicola	Schlüsselbein	clavícula
chiodo per estensione di Steinmann	Steinmann Knochennagel	clavo de Steinmann
climaterio	Klimakterium, Wechseljahre	climatérico
clinico	klinisch	clínico
clitoride	Klitoris	clítoris
cloasma	Chloasma, Hyperpigmentierung, Leberfleck	cloasma
clone, clono	Klonus	clono
clono	Klonus	clonus
adiuvante	Adjuvans	coadyuvante
coagulazione ematica, coagulazione del sangue	Blutgerinnung	coagulación de la sangre
coagulazione intravascolare disseminata (CID)	disseminierte intravasale Gerinnung (DIC)	coagulación intravascular diseminada (CID)
coagulare	gerinnen, koagulieren	coagular

SPANISH	ENGLISH	FRENCH
coágulo	clot	caillot
coalescer	coalesce	se combiner
coartación	coarctation	coarctation
cóccix	coccyx	coccyx
cóclea	cochlea	limaçon osseux
codo del tenista	tennis elbow	'tennis elbow'
cognición	cognition	cognition
coiloniquia	koilonychia	koïlonychie
coito	coitus, intercourse, sexual intercourse	coït, rapports, rapports sexuels
colágeno	collagen	collagène
colangiografía	cholangiography	cholangiographie
colangiopancreatografía endoscópica retrógrada	endoscopic retrograde cholangiopancreatography (ERCP)	cholangio-pancréatographie rétrograde endoscopique (CPRE)
colangitis	cholangitis	cholangite
colapsar	collapse	s'affaisser
colapso	collapse	affaissement
colecistectomía	cholecystectomy	cholécystectomie
colecistitis	cholecystitis	cholécystite
colecistografía	cholecystography	cholécystographie
colectomía	colectomy	colectomie
coledocografía	choledochography	cholédochographie
coledocolitiasis	choledocholithiasis	cholédocholithiase
colelitiasis	cholelithiasis	cholélithiase
cólera	cholera	choléra
colestasis	cholestasis	cholestase
colesteatoma	cholesteatoma	cholestéatome
colesterol	cholesterol (chol)	cholestérol
colesterol unido a las lipoproteínas de alta densidad (HDLC)	high density lipoprotein cholesterol (HDLC)	cholestérol composé de lipoprotéines de haute densité
colgajo	flap	lambeau
cólico	colic	colique
cólico intestinal	gripe	colique
coliforme	coliform	coliforme
colinérgico	cholinergic	cholinergique
colitis	colitis	colite
coloboma	coloboma	colobome, coloboma
coloide	colloid	colloïde
colon	colon	côlon
colon ascendente	ascending colon	côlon ascendant
colon descendente	descending colon	côlon descendant
colonizar	colonize	coloniser
colonoscopia	colonoscopy	coloscopie
colon transverso	transverse colon	côlon transversal
colorrectal	colorectal	colorectal
colostomía	colostomy	colostomie
colporrafia	colporrhaphy	colporraphie

coagulo	Blutgerinnsel, Koagel	coágulo
aggregarsi	zusammenwachsen	coalescer
coartazione	Coarctatio	coartación
coccige	Steißbein	cóccix
coclea	Cochlea, Schnecke	cóclea
epicondilite radio-omerale, gomito del tennista	Tennisellenbogen	codo del tenista
cognizione	Erkennungsvermögen, Wahrnehmung	cognición
coilonichia	Koilonychie, Löffelnagel	coiloniquia
coito	Koitus, Geschlechtsverkehr	coito
collageno	Kollagen	colágeno
colangiografia	Cholangiographie	colangiografía
colangio-pancreatografia retrograda endoscopica (ERCP)	endoskopische retrograde Cholangiopankre	colangiopancreatografía endoscópica retrógrada
colangite	Cholangitis	colangitis
collassarsi, crollare	kollabieren	colapsar
collasso	Kollaps	colapso
colecistectomia	Cholezystektomie	colecistectomía
colecistite	Cholezystitis	colecistitis
colecistografia	Cholezystographie	colecistografía
colectomia	Kolektomie, Kolonresektion	colectomía
coledocografia	Choledochographie	coledocografía
coledocolitiasi	Choledocholithiasis	coledocolitiasis
colelitiasi	Cholelithiasis, Gallensteinleiden	colelitiasis
colera	Cholera	cólera
colestasi	Cholestase, Gallenstauung	colestasis
colesteatoma	Cholesteatom	colesteatoma
colesterolo	Cholesterin	colesterol
colesterolo legato a lipoproteina ad alta densità	high density lipoprotein-cholesterol (HDL-Cholesterol)	colesterol unido a las lipoproteínas de alta densidad (HDLC)
lembo, innesto	Lappen, Hautlappen	colgajo
colica	Kolik	cólico
colica addominale	Kolik, Bauchschmerzen	cólico intestinal
coliforme	coliform	coliforme
colinergico	cholinergisch	colinérgico
colite	Kolitis	colitis
coloboma	Kolobom	coloboma
colloide	Kolloid	coloide
colon	Kolon	colon
colon ascendente	Colon ascendens	colon ascendente
colon discendente	Colon descendens	colon descendente
colonizzare	kolonisieren	colonizar
colonscopia	Koloskopie	colonoscopia
colon trasverso	Colon transversum	colon transverso
colorettale	kolorektal	colorrectal
colostomia	Kolostomie	colostomía
colporrafia	Kolporrhaphie	colporrafia

SPANISH	ENGLISH	FRENCH
colposcopio	colposcope	colposcope
columna vertebral	vertebral column	colonne vertébrale
colutorio	gargle	gargarisme
coma	coma	coma
comadrona	midwife	sage-femme
comatoso	comatose	comateux
comidas preparadas poco nutritivas	junk food	aliments non nutritifs
comisura	commissure	commissure
compás	caliper	armature orthopédique
compatibilidad	compatibility	compatibilité
compensación	compensation	compensation
complejo primario	primary complex	complexe primaire
complejo relacionado con SIDA	AIDS-related complex	para-SIDA
complemento	complement	complément
comportamiento	behavior (Am), behaviour (Eng)	comportement
compos mentis	compos mentis	compos mentis
compresión	compression	compression
compresión digital	digital compression	compression digitale
comprimido	tablet	comprimé
comprimido entérico	enteric-coated tablet (ECT)	dragée entérosoluble, comprimé à délitement entérique
compuesto	compound	composé
compulsión	compulsion	compulsion
concepción	conception	conception
concusión	concussion	commotion
condón	condom	préservatif
condritis	chondritis	chondrite
condroma	chondroma	chondrome
condromalacia	chondromalacia	chondromalacie
conducto	duct	conduit
conducto ileal	ileal conduit	conduit iléal
conducto semicircular	semicircular canal	canal semi-circulaire
confusión	confusion	confusion
congelación	frostbite	gelure
congénito	congenital	congénital
congestión	congestion	congestion
conjugado (n)	conjugate (n)	diamètre conjugué (n)
conjugado (a)	conjugate (a)	conjugué (a)
conjuntiva	conjunctiva	conjonctive
conjuntivitis	conjunctivitis, pinkeye	conjonctivite, conjonctivite aiguë contagieuse
conjuntivitis de inclusion por tracomas	trachoma inclusion conjunctivitis (TRIC)	conjonctivite à inclusions trachomateuses
consciente	conscious	conscient
consejo	counselling	consultation
consolidación	consolidation	consolidation

ITALIAN	GERMAN	SPANISH
colposcopio	Kolposkop	colposcopio
colonna vertebrale	Wirbelsäule, Rückgrat	columna vertebral
gargarismi	Gurgelmittel	colutorio
coma	Koma	coma
levatrice	Hebamme	comadrona
comatoso	komatös	comatoso
cibo contenente additivi chimici	ungesunde Nahrung	comidas preparadas poco nutritivas
commessura	Kommissur	comisura
compasso per pelvi-craniometria	Schiene	compás
compatibilità	Kompatibilität, Verträglichkeit	compatibilidad
compenso	Kompensation, Entschädigung	compensación
complesso primario, complesso di Ghon	Primärkomplex	complejo primario
complesso AIDS-correlato	AIDS-related complex	complejo relacionado con SIDA
complemento	Komplement	complemento
comportamento	Verhalten	comportamiento
mentalmente sano	zurechnungsfähig	compos mentis
compressione	Kompression	compresión
compressione digitale	Fingerdruck	compresión digital
pasticca, compressa	Tablette	comprimido
compressa enterica rivestita (passano lo stomaco senza sciogliersi)	magensaftresistente Tablette	comprimido entérico
composto	Verbindung, Zusammensetzung	compuesto
compulsione	Zwang	compulsión
concepimento	Empfängnis	concepción
commozione	Erschütterung, Commotio	concusión
profilattico maschile	Kondom, Präservativ	condón
condrite	Chondritis	condritis
condroma	Chondrom	condroma
condromalacia	Chondromalazie	condromalacia
dotto	Ductus, Gang	conducto
vescica ileale (protesi mediante segmento ileale)	Ileumconduit	conducto ileal
canale semicircolare	Bogengang	conducto semicircular
confusione	Verwirrung	confusión
congelamento	Erfrierung	congelación
congenito	angeboren	congénito
congestione	Stauung	congestión
coniugata (n)	Beckendurchmesser (n)	conjugado (n)
coniugato (a)	konjugiert (a)	conjugado (a)
congiuntiva	Konjunktiva, Bindehaut	conjuntiva
congiuntivite, congiuntivite batterica acuta contagiosa, congiuntivite catarrale	Konjunktivitis, Bindehautentzündung, epidemische Konjunktivitis	conjuntivitis
congiuntivite tracomatosa	Trachom, Einschluß(körperchen)-konjunktivitis	conjuntivitis de inclusion por tracomas
conscio	bewußt, bei Bewußtsein	consciente
consulenza eugenetica	Beratung	consejo
solidificazione, addensamento	Konsolidierung, Festigung	consolidación

SPANISH	ENGLISH	FRENCH
constricción	constriction	constriction
consulta psicológica	counselling	consultation
consunción	consumption, wasting away	consommation, dépérissement
contacto	contact	contact
contagioso	contagious	contagieux
contracción	contraction	contraction
contractura	contracture	contracture
contractura isquémica de Volkmann	Volkmann's ischaemic contracture (Eng), Volkmann's ischemic contracture (Am)	contracture ischémique de Volkmann
contragolpe	contrecoup	contrecoup
contraindicación	contraindication	contre-indication
contralateral	contralateral	controlatéral
contundir	bruise	contusionner
contusión	bruise	contusion
contusión violenta	concussion	commotion
convulsión	convulsion	convulsion
corazón	heart	coeur
cordón	cord	cordon
cordón umbilical	umbilical cord	cordon ombilical
cordotomía	cordotomy	cordotomie
cordura	sanity	santé mentale
corea	chorea	chorée
corea de Huntington	Huntington's chorea	chorée de Huntington
corion	chorion	chorion
coriza	coryza	coryza
córnea	cornea	cornée
coroides	choroid	choroïde
coroiditis	choroiditis	choroïdite
coronario (n)	coronary (n)	coronaire (n)
coronario (a)	coronary (a)	coronaire (a), coronarien (a)
cor pulmonale	cor pulmonale	coeur pulmonaire
corpúsculo	corpuscle	corpuscule
corteza	cortex	cortex
corticosteroide	corticosteroid	corticostéroïde
costal	costal	costal
costilla	rib	côte
costocondral	costochondral	costochondral
costocondritis	costochondritis	costochondrite
costra	scab, eschar	croûte, escarre
costra láctea	cradle cap	casque séborrhéique
cráneo	cranium, skull	boîte crânienne, crâne
craneosinostosis	cranio-synostosis	craniosynostose
craurosis vulvar	kraurosis vulvae	kraurosis de la vulve
creatina	creatine	créatine
creatinina	creatinine	créatinine

ITALIAN	GERMAN	SPANISH
costrizione	Konstriktion, Einengung	constricción
consulenza eugenetica	Beratung	consulta psicológica
consunzione, cachessia	Konsum, Verbrauch, Schwinden	consunción
contatto	Kontakt, Berührung	contacto
contagioso	kontagiös, ansteckend	contagioso
contrazione	Kontraktion	contracción
contrattura	Kontraktur	contractura
paralisi ischemica di Volkmann	Volkmann-Kontraktur	contractura isquémica de Volkmann
contraccolpo	contre coup	contragolpe
controindicazione	Kontraindikation, Gegenanzeige	contraindicación
controlaterale	kontralateral	contralateral
ammaccare	stoßen, quetschen	contundir
contusione	Quetschung, Prellung	contusión
commozione	Erschütterung, Commotio	contusión violenta
convulsione	Krampf, Zuckung, Konvulsion	convulsión
cuore	Herz	corazón
corda, cordone, notocorda	Strang, Schnur, Ligament	cordón
cordone ombelicale	Nabelschnur	cordón umbilical
cordotomia	Stimmbandresektion	cordotomía
sanità	geistige Gesundheit	cordura
corea	Chorea, Veitstanz	corea
corea di Huntington	Chorea Huntington	corea de Huntington
corion	Chorion	corion
coriza	Koryza, Schnupfen	coriza
cornea	Kornea, Hornhaut (des Auges)	córnea
coroide	Choroidea, Aderhaut	coroides
coroidite	Choroiditis	coroiditis
coronaria (n)	Koronararterie (n)	coronario (n)
coronarico (a)	koronar (a)	coronario (a)
cuore polmonare	Cor pulmonale	cor pulmonale
corpuscolo	Corpusculum	corpúsculo
corteccia	Cortex, Rinde	corteza
corticosteroide	Kortikosteroide	corticosteroide
costale	kostal, Rippen-	costal
costa	Rippe	costilla
costocondrale	Rippenknorpel-	costocondral
costocondrite	Tietze Syndrom	costocondritis
crosta, escara	Schorf, Kruste, Brandschorf	costra
stecca, rima di frattura	Milchschorf	costra láctea
cranio	Schädel, Kranium	cráneo
craniosinostosi	Kraniosynostose	craneosinostosis
craurosi vulvare	Craurosis vulvae	craurosis vulvar
creatina	Kreatin	creatina
creatinina	Kreatinin	creatinina

crecimiento	growth	croissance
crepitación	crepitation	crépitation
cretinismo	cretinism	crétinisme
criba	screening	dépistage
cricoideo	cricoid	cricoïde
criocirugía	cryosurgery	cryochirurgie
crioterapia	cryotherapy	cryothérapie
cripta	crypt	crypte
criptogénico	cryptogenic	cryptogène
criptomenorrea	cryptomenorrhea (Am), cryptomenorrhoea (Eng)	cryptoménorrhée
crisis	crisis	crise
crisis miasténica	myasthenic crisis	crise myasthénique
crisis tirotóxica	thyrotoxic crisis	crise thyrotoxique
cristalino	lens	lentille
cromatografía	chromatography	chromatographie
cromosoma	chromosome	chromosome
crónico	chronic	chronique
crup	croup	croup
cuádriceps	quadriceps	quadriceps
cuadriplejía	quadriplegia	quadriplégie
cualitativo	qualitative	qualitatif
cuantitativo	quantitative	quantitatif
cuarentena	quarantine	quarantaine
cuartana	quartan	quarte
cúbito	ulna	cubitus
cucharilla de legrado	curette (Eng), curet (Am)	curette
cuello	neck	cou
cuello uterino	cervix	cou
cuerda	cord	cordon
cuerda vocal	vocal cord	corde vocale
cuero cabelludo	scalp	épicrâne
cuerpo	corpus	corps
cuerpo de Leishman-Donovan	Leishman-Donovan body	Leishmania donovani
cuerpo pineal	pineal body	glande pinéale
cuidados postoperatorios	aftercare	postcure
cuidados terminales	terminal care	soins pour malades en phase terminale
cuidar	nurse	soigner
cultivo	culture	culture
cumplimiento del paciente	patient compliance	observance du patient
cura	dressing	pansement
curación	healing	curatif
curas para heridas	wound dressing	pansements
cureta	curette (Eng), curet (Am)	curette
curetaje	curettage	curetage
cutáneo	cutaneous	cutané
cutícula	cuticle	cuticule

ITALIAN	GERMAN	SPANISH
crescita	Wachstum, Zunahme, Geschwulst, Tumor	crecimiento
crepitazione	Krepitation, Rasseln	crepitación
cretinismo	Kretinismus	cretinismo
selezione	Screening, Reihenuntersuchung	criba
cricoide	krikoid	cricoideo
criochirurgia	Kryochirurgie	criocirugía
crioterapia	Kryotherapie	crioterapia
cripta	Krypte	cripta
criptogenico	kryptogenetisch, unbekannten Ursprungs	criptogénico
criptomenorrea	Kryptomenorrhoe	criptomenorrea
crisi	Krise	crisis
crisi miastenica	myasthenische Krise	crisis miasténica
crisi tireotossica	thyreotoxische Krise	crisis tirotóxica
lente	Linse	cristalino
cromatografia	Chromatographie	cromatografía
cromosoma	Chromosom	cromosoma
cronico	chronisch	crónico
ostruzione laringea	Krupp	crup
quadricipite	Quadrizeps	cuádriceps
tetraplegia	Tetraplegie	cuadriplejía
qualitativo	qualitativ	cualitativo
quantitativo	quantitativ	cuantitativo
quarantena	Quarantäne	cuarentena
quartana	quartana (Malaria)	cuartana
ulna	Ulna, Elle	cúbito
curette, cucchiaio chirurgico	Kürette	cucharilla de legrado
collo	Nacken, Hals	cuello
cervice	Zervix, Gebärmutterhals	cuello uterino
corda, cordone, notocorda	Strang, Schnur, Ligament	cuerda
corda vocale	Stimmband	cuerda vocal
cuoio capelluto	Kopfhaut	cuero cabelludo
corpo	Corpus	cuerpo
corpi di Leishman-Donovan	Leishman-Donovan-Körper	cuerpo de Leishman-Donovan
ghiandola pineale	Epiphyse	cuerpo pineal
assistenza post-operatoria	Nachbehandlung, Nachsorge	cuidados postoperatorios
cura terminale	Pflege Sterbender	cuidados terminales
assistere	stillen, pflegen	cuidar
coltura	Bakterienkultur, Kultur	cultivo
acquiescenza alle prescrizioni	Compliance	cumplimiento del paciente
medicazione	Verband, Umschlag	cura
cicatrizzazione, guarigione	Heilung	curación
medicazione di ferita	Verbandmaterial	curas para heridas
curette, cucchiaio chirurgico	Kürette	cureta
curettage, raschiamento	Kürettage, Ausschabung	curetaje
cutaneo	kutan, Haut-	cutáneo
cuticola	Cuticula, Häutchen	cutícula

D

SPANISH	ENGLISH	FRENCH
dacriocistitis	dacryocystitis	dacryocystite
daltonismo	color blindness (Am), colour blindness (Eng)	daltonisme
debilidad	debility, weakness	débilité, faiblesse
decidua	decidua	caduque
dedo de la mano	finger	doigt
dedo del pie	toe	orteil
dedo en gatillo	trigger finger	index
dedo gordo del pie	hallux	hallux
dedos en palillo de tambor	clubbing	hippocratisme digital
dedos hipocráticos	clubbing	hippocratisme digital
de espíritu sano	compos mentis	compos mentis
defecación	defaecation (Eng), defecation (Am)	défécation
defecto	defect	anomalie, défaut
defecto del septum auricular	atrial septal defect (ASD)	communication auriculaire
degeneración	degeneration	dégénération
degeneración grasa	fatty degeneration	dégénérescence graisseuse
dehiscencia	dehiscence	déhiscence
delirio	delirium, delusion	délire, hallucination
deltoides	deltoid	deltoïde
demarcación	demarcation	démarcation
demencia	dementia, insanity	démence, aliénation
demencia presenil	presenile dementia	démence présénile
demografia	demography	démographie
denervación	denervation	énervation
dengue	dengue	dengue
dentadura	denture	dentier
dentario	odontic	dentaire
dentición	dentition	dentition
dentista	dentist	dentiste
de pie	recumbent	couché
deposición	stool	selle
depresión	depression	dépression
depresión agitada	agitated depression	dépression anxieuse
derivación	shunt	dérivation
dermatitis	dermatitis	dermatite
dermatitis del cuero cabelludo	cradle cap	casque séborrhéique
dermatitis seborréica	seborrheic dermatitis (Am), seborrhoeic dermatitis (Eng)	eczéma
dermatología	dermatology	dermatologie
dermatólogo	dermatologist	dermatologue
dermatomiositis	dermatomyositis	dermatomyosite
dermátomo	dermatome	dermatome
dermatosis	dermatosis	dermatose

ITALIAN	GERMAN	SPANISH
dacriocistite	Dakryozystitis	dacriocistitis
cecità ai colori, acromatopsia	Farbenblindheit	daltonismo
debilità, debolezza	Schwäche	debilidad
decidua	Dezidua	decidua
dito	Finger	dedo de la mano
dito del piede	Zehe	dedo del pie
dito a scatto	schnellender Finger	dedo en gatillo
alluce	Hallux, Großzeh	dedo gordo del pie
dita a clava, ippocratismo	Trommelschlegelfinger	dedos en palillo de tambor
dita a clava, ippocratismo	Trommelschlegelfinger	dedos hipocráticos
mentalmente sano	zurechnungsfähig	de espíritu sano
defecazione	Defäkation, Darmentleerung	defecación
difetto	Defekt, Mangel, Störung	defecto
difetto atriosettale	Vorhofseptumdefekt	defecto del septum auricular
degenerazione	Degeneration, Verfall	degeneración
degenerazione grassa	fettige Degeneration, Verfettung	degeneración grasa
deiscenza	Dehiszenz, Schlitz	dehiscencia
delirio, allucinazione, fissazione	Delirium, Fieberwahn, Wahn, Wahnvorstellung	delirio
deltoide	Deltoides, Deltamuskel	deltoides
demarcazione	Demarkation	demarcación
demenza, pazzia	Demenz, Geisteskrankheit	demencia
demenza presenile	präsenile Demenz	demencia presenil
demografia	Demographie	demografía
denervazione	Denervierung	denervación
dengue, infezione da Flavivirus ('febbre rompiossa')	Denguefieber	dengue
dentiera	Gebiß	dentadura
dentario	Odonto-, Zahn-	dentario
dentizione	Dentition, Zahnung	dentición
dentista	Zahnarzt	dentista
supino, sdraiato	liegend, ruhend	de pie
feci	Stuhl, Stuhlgang, Kot	deposición
depressione	Depression	depresión
depressione agitata	agitierte Depression	depresión agitada
derivazione	Shunt	derivación
dermatite	Dermatitis	dermatitis
stecca, rima di frattura	Milchschorf	dermatitis del cuero cabelludo
dermatite seborroica	seborrhoisches Ekzem	dermatitis seborréica
dermatologia	Dermatologie	dermatología
dermatologo	Dermatologe	dermatólogo
dermatomiosite	Dermatomyositis	dermatomiositis
dermatomo	Dermatom, Hautmesser	dermátomo
dermatosi	Dermatose, Hauterkrankung	dermatosis

SPANISH	ENGLISH	FRENCH
dermis	dermis	derme
dermoide	dermoid	dermoïde
derrame	effusion	effusion
desarticulación	disarticulation	désarticulation
desbridamiento	debridement	débridement
descerebrado	decerebrate	décérébré
descompensación	decompensation	décompensation
descompresión	decompression	décompression
descongestivo	decongestant	décongestionnant
desdentado	edentulous	édenté
desensibilización	desensitization	désensibilisation
desequilibrio	imbalance	déséquilibre
desescamación	desquamation	desquamation
desesfacelación	desloughing	curetage
desfibrilación	defibrillation	défibrillation
desfibrilador	defibrillator	défibrillateur
deshidratación	dehydration	déshydratation
desimpactación	disimpaction	désimpaction
desinfección	disinfection	désinfection
desinfectante	disinfectant	désinfectant
desinfectar	disinfect	désinfecter
desinfestación	disinfestation	désinfestation
desmayar	faint	s'évanouir
desmedro	failure to thrive (FTT)	absence de développement pondéro-statural normal
desmielinización	demyelination	démyélinisation
desnutrición	malnutrition	malnutrition
desobliteración	rebore	désobstruction
desodorante (n)	deodorant (n)	déodorant (n)
desodorante (a)	deodorant (a)	déodorant (a)
desorientación	disorientation	désorientation
desoxigenación	deoxygenation	désoxygénation
despistaje	screening	dépistage
desprendimiento de retina	detached retina	rétine décollée
desprendimiento prematuro de la placenta	placental abruption	rupture placentaire
desrealización	derealization	déréalisation
destemplanza	malaise	malaise
desvanecimiento	dizziness	étourdissement
desviado	aberrant	aberrant
detergente	detergent	détergent
deterioro	deterioration	détérioration
dextrocardia	dextrocardia	dextrocardie
diabetes	diabetes	diabète
diabetes insípida	diabetes insipidus	diabète insipide
diabetes mellitus	diabetes mellitus (DM)	diabète sucré
diabetes mellitus insulinodependiente	insulin dependent diabetes mellitus (IDDM)	diabète sucré insulinodépendant

derma	Haut	dermis
dermoide	Dermoid, Dermoidzyste	dermoide
effusione	Erguß	derrame
disarticolazione	Exartikulation	desarticulación
sbrigliamento	Debridement, Wundtoilette	desbridamiento
decerebrato	dezerebriert	descerebrado
decompensazione	Dekompensation, Insuffizienz	descompensación
decompressione	Dekompression, Drucksenkung	descompresión
decongestionante	Dekongestionsmittel	descongestivo
edentulo	zahnlos	desdentado
desensibilizzazione	Desensibilisierung	desensibilización
squilibrio	Gleichgewichtsstörung	desequilibrio
desquamazione	Desquamation, Schuppung	desescamación
rimozione di escara da una ferita	Schorfabtragung	desesfacelación
defibrillazione	Defibrillierung	desfibrilación
defibrillatore	Defibrillator	desfibrilador
deidratazione	Dehydration, Flüssigkeitsmangel	deshidratación
riduzione	Fragmentlösung	desimpactación
disinfezione	Desinfektion	desinfección
disinfettante	Desinfektionsmittel	desinfectante
disinfettare	desinfizieren	desinfectar
disinfestazione	Entwesung, Entlausung	desinfestación
svenire	ohnmächtig werden	desmayar
marasma infantile	Gedeihstörung	desmedro
demielinizzazione	Demyelinisierung, Entmarkung	desmielinización
malnutrizione	Unterernährung, Fehlernährung	desnutrición
disobliterazione	Desobliteration	desobliteración
deodorante (n)	Deodorant (n)	desodorante (n)
deodorante (a)	desodorierend (a)	desodorante (a)
disorientamento	Desorientiertheit	desorientación
deossigenazione	Desoxydation, Sauerstoffentzug	desoxigenación
selezione	Screening, Reihenuntersuchung	despistaje
distacco di retina	abgelöste Netzhaut	desprendimiento de retina
distacco prematuro della placenta	Plazentaablösung	desprendimiento prematuro de la placenta
derealizzazione	Derealisation	desrealización
indisposizione, malessere	Unwohlsein	destemplanza
stordimento, capogiro, vertigini	Schwindel	desvanecimiento
aberrante	aberrans, abartig	desviado
detergente	Reinigungsmittel	detergente
deterioramento	Verschlechterung	deterioro
destrocardia	Dextrokardie	dextrocardia
diabete	Diabetes	diabetes
diabete insipido	Diabetes insipidus	diabetes insípida
diabete mellito	Diabetes mellitus, Zuckerkrankheit	diabetes mellitus
diabete mellito insulinodipendente	insulinabhängiger Diabetes mellitus	diabetes mellitus insulinodependiente

SPANISH	ENGLISH	FRENCH
diabetes mellitus no insulinodependiente	non-insulin dependent diabetes mellitus (NIDDM)	diabète sucré non insulinodépendant
diáfisis	diaphysis	diaphyse
diaforesis	diaphoresis	diaphorèse
diafragma	diaphragm, midriff	diaphragme
diagnóstico (n)	diagnosis (n)	diagnostic (n)
diagnóstico (a)	diagnostic (a)	diagnostique (a)
diagnóstico diferencial	differential diagnosis	diagnostic différentiel
diálisis	dialysis	dialyse
diálisis peritoneal	peritoneal dialysis	dialyse péritonéale
dializado	dialysate	dialysat
dializador	dialyser (Eng), dialyzer (Am)	dialyseur
diarrea	diarrhea (Am), diarrhoea (Eng)	diarrhée
diarrea y vómitos	diarrhea and vomiting (D & V) (Am), diarrhoea and vomiting (D & V) (Eng)	diarrhées et vomissements
diastasis	diastasis	diastasis
diástole	diastole	diastole
diatermia	diathermy	diathermie
diente	tooth	dent
dientes	teeth	dents
dieta cetógena	ketogenic diet	régime cétogène
dietética	dietetics	diététique
dietista	dietitian	diététicien
difteria	diphtheria	diphtérie
difteria laríngea	croup	croup
digestión	digestion	digestion
digital	digitalis	digitale
digitalización	digitalization	digitalisation
dilatación	dilatation (Eng), dilation (Am)	dilatation
dilatación y raspado/legrado	dilatation and curettage (D & C) (Eng), dilation and curettage (D & C) (Am)	dilatation et curetage
diplejía	diplegia	diplégie
diplopia	diplopia	diplopie
disartria	dysarthria	dysarthrie
discariosis	dyskaryosis	dyskaryose
discinesia	dyskinesia	dyskinésie
disco de Petri	Petri dish	boîte de Pétri
discrasia	dyscrasia	dyscrasie
discreto	discrete	discret
disección	dissection	dissection
diseminado	disseminated	disséminé
disentería	dysentery	dysenterie
disfagia	dysphagia	dysphagie
disfasia	dysphasia	dysphasie
disfunción	dysfunction	dysfonctionnement
dislexia	dyslexia	dyslexie

ITALIAN	GERMAN	SPANISH
diabete mellito non insulinodipendente	Diabetes mellitus Typ II, non-insulin dependent diabetes mellitus (NIDDM)	diabetes mellitus no insulinodependiente
diafisi	Diaphyse, Knochenschaft	diáfisis
diaforesi	Diaphorese, Schweißabsonderung	diaforesis
diaframma, parte bassa del torace	Diaphragma, Zwerchfell	diafragma
diagnosi (n)	Diagnose (n)	diagnóstico (n)
diagnostico (a)	diagnostisch (a)	diagnóstico (a)
diagnosi differenziale	Differentialdiagnose	diagnóstico diferencial
dialisi	Dialyse	diálisis
dialisi peritoneale	Peritonealdialyse	diálisis peritoneal
dialisato	Dialysat	dializado
dializzatore	Dialysator	dializador
diarrea	Diarrhoe, Durchfall	diarrea
diarrea e vomito	Brechdurchfall	diarrea y vómitos
diastasi, amilasi	Diastase	diastasis
diastole	Diastole	diástole
diatermia	Diathermie	diatermia
dente	Zahn	diente
denti	Zähne, Gebiß	dientes
dieta chetogenica	ketogene Ernährung	dieta cetógena
dietetica	Diätlehre, Ernährungskunde	dietética
dietista, dietologo	Diätspezialist	dietista
difterite	Diphtherie	difteria
ostruzione laringea	Krupp	difteria laríngea
digestione	Verdauung	digestión
digitale	Digitalis, Fingerhut	digital
digitalizzazione	Digitalisierung	digitalización
dilatazione	Dilatation, Erweiterung	dilatación
dilatazione e raschiamento	Dilatation und Kürettage	dilatación y raspado/legrado
diplegia	Diplegie, doppelseitige Lähmung	diplejía
diplopia	Diplopie, Doppelsehen	diplopia
disartria	Dysarthrie	disartria
discariosi	Kernanomalie, Dysplasie	discariosis
discinesia	Dyskinesie	discinesia
capsula di Petri	Petrischale	disco de Petri
discrasia	Dyskrasie	discrasia
discreto	diskret	discreto
dissezione	Sektion, Obduktion	disección
disseminato	disseminiert, verstreut	diseminado
dissenteria	Dysenterie, Ruhr	disentería
disfagia	Dysphagie, Schluckbeschwerden	disfagia
disfasia	Dysphasie	disfasia
disfunzione	Dysfunktion, Funktionsstörung	disfunción
dislessia	Dyslexie	dislexia

SPANISH	ENGLISH	FRENCH
dislocación	dislocation	dislocation
dismenorrea	dysmenorrhea (Am), dysmenorrhoea (Eng)	dysménorrhée
dismenorrea espasmódica	spasmodic dysmenorrhoea	dysménorrhée spasmodique
disminución	handicap	handicapé
disnea	dyspnea (Am), dyspnoea (Eng), shortness of breath	dyspnée, essoufflement
disociación	dissociation	dissociation
disolvente	solvent	solvant
dispareunia	dyspareunia	dyspareunie
dispepsia	dyspepsia	dyspepsie
displasia	dysplasia	dysplasie
dispositivo intrauterino anticonceptivo (DIU)	intrauterine contraceptive device (IUD, IUCD)	dispositif intra-utérin (DIU), stérilet
dispraxia	dyspraxia	dyspraxie
disquectomía	discectomy (Eng), diskectomy (Am)	discectomie
disritmia	dysrhythmia	dysrythmie
distal	distal	distal
distrofia	dystrophy	dystrophie
distrofia muscular	muscular dystrophy	dystrophie musculaire
disuria	dysuria	dysurie
diuresis	diuresis	diurèse
diurético (n)	diuretic (n)	diurétique (n)
diurético (a)	diuretic (a)	diurétique (a)
diverticulitis	diverticulitis	diverticulite
divertículo	diverticulum	diverticulum
divertículo de Meckel	Meckel's diverticulum	diverticule de Meckel
diverticulosis	diverticulosis	diverticulose
dolor	dolor, pain	douleur
doloroso	sore	douloureux
dolor referido	referred pain	douleur irradiée
dominante	dominant	dominant
donante	donor	donneur
dopamina	dopamine	dopamine
dorsal	dorsal	dorsal
dorsiflexión	dorsiflexion	dorsiflexion
dosis diaria recomendada	recommended daily allowance (RDA)	taux quotidien recommandé
drenaje	drain	drain
drenar	drain	drainer
ducha	douche	douche
ductus arteriosus	ductus arteriosus	canal artériel
duodenitis	duodenitis	duodénite
duodeno	duodenum	duodénum

ITALIAN	GERMAN	SPANISH
dislocazione	Dislokation, Verrenkung	dislocación
dismenorrea	Dysmenorrhoe	dismenorrea
dismenorrea spastica	spastische Dysmenorrhoe	dismenorrea espasmódica
handicappato, minorato	Behinderung	disminución
dispnea, respiro affannoso	Dyspnoe, Atemnot, Kurzatmigkeit	disnea
dissociazione	Dissoziation, Trennung	disociación
solvente	Lösungsmittel	disolvente
dispareunia	Dyspareunie	dispareunia
dispepsia	Dyspepsie, Verdauungsstörung	dispepsia
displasia	Dysplasie, Fehlbildung	displasia
dispositivo anticoncezionale intrauterino (IUD)	Intrauterinpessar (IUP)	dispositivo intrauterino anticonceptivo (DIU)
disprassia	Dyspraxie	dispraxia
discectomia, asportazione di disco intervertebrale	Diskektomie	disquectomía
disritmia	Dysrhythmie, Rhythmusstörung	disritmia
distale	distal	distal
distrofia	Dystrophie	distrofia
distrofia muscolare	Muskeldystrophie	distrofia muscular
disuria	Dysurie	disuria
diuresi	Diurese	diuresis
diuretico (n)	Diuretikum (n)	diurético (n)
diuretico (a)	diuretisch (a)	diurético (a)
diverticolite	Divertikulitis	diverticulitis
diverticolo	Divertikel	divertículo
diverticolo di Meckel	Meckel-Divertikel	divertículo de Meckel
diverticolosi	Divertikulose	diverticulosis
dolore	Schmerz	dolor
dolente	wund, schmerzhaft	doloroso
dolore riferito	ausstrahlender Schmerz, fortgeleiteter Schmerz	dolor referido
dominante	dominant, vorherrschend	dominante
donatore	Spender	donante
dopammina	Dopamin	dopamina
dorsale	dorsal, Rücken-	dorsal
dorsiflessione	Dorsalflexion	dorsiflexión
dose giornaliera raccomandata	empfohlene Tagesdosis	dosis diaria recomendada
drenaggio	Drain	drenaje
drenare	drainieren	drenar
lavanda vaginale	Dusche, Spülung	ducha
dotto arterioso	Ductus arteriosus	ductus arteriosus
duodenite	Duodenitis, Zwölffingerdarmentzündung	duodenitis
duodeno	Duodenum, Zwölffingerdarm	duodeno

E

eccema	eczema	eczéma
eclampsia	eclampsia	éclampsie
ecocardiografía	echocardiography	échocardiographie
ecoencefalografía	echoencephalography	écho-encéphalographie
ecografía	ultrasonography	échographie
ecolalia	echolalia	écholalie
ectodermo	ectoderm	ectoderme
ectoparásito	ectoparasite	ectoparasite
ectópico	ectopic	ectopique
ectropión	ectropion	ectropion
edema	edema (Am), oedema (Eng)	oedème
edema angioneurótico (sólido)	angioneurotic edema (solidus) (Am), angioneurotic oedema (solidus) (Eng)	oedème angioneurotique
efecto secundario	side effect	effet latéral
efectos secundarios extrapiramidales	extrapyramidal side effects	effets latéraux extrapyramidaux
efedrina	ephedrine	éphédrine
eferente	efferent	efférent
eje	axis	axe
elastina	elastin	élastine
electrocardiograma (ECG)	electrocardiogram (ECG)	électrocardiogramme (ECG)
electrochoqueterapia (ECT)	electroconvulsive therapy (ECT)	électrochoc
electrodo	electrode	électrode
electroencefalograma (EEG)	electroencephalogram (EEG)	électroencéphalogramme (EEG)
electrólisis	electrolysis	électrolyse
electrólito	electrolyte	électrolyte
electromiografía	electromyography	électromyographie
elefantiasis	elephantiasis	éléphantiasis
elevador	levator	releveur
eliminación	elimination	élimination
eliptocitosis	elliptocytosis	elliptocytose
elixir	elixir	élixir
emaciación	emaciation	émaciation
embarazo	cyesis, pregnancy	grossesse
embarazo a término	full-term	à terme
embarazo ectópico	ectopic pregnancy	grossesse ectopique
embarazo fantasma	phantom pregnancy	fausse grossesse
embolia	embolism	embolisme
embólico	embolic	embolique
embolismo pulmonar	pulmonary embolism (PE)	embolie pulmonaire (EP)
émbolo	embolus	embole
embriología	embryology	embryologie
embrión	embryo	embryon
embriopatía	embryopathy	embryopathie

eczema	Ekzem	eccema
eclampsia	Eklampsie	eclampsia
ecocardiografia	Echokardiographie	ecocardiografía
ecoencefalografia	Echoenzephalographie	ecoencefalografía
ultrasonografia, ecografia	Sonographie, Ultraschallmethode	ecografía
ecolalia	Echolalie	ecolalia
ectoderma	Ektoderm	ectodermo
ectoparassita	Ektoparasit	ectoparásito
ectopico	ektop	ectópico
ectropion	Ektropion	ectropión
edema	Ödem, Flüssigkeitsansammlung	edema
edema angioneurotico	Quincke-Ödem	edema angioneurótico (sólido)
effetto collaterale	Nebenwirkung	efecto secundario
reazioni collaterali extrapiramidali da farmaci	extrapyramidale Nebenwirkungen	efectos secundarios extrapiramidales
efedrina	Ephedrin	efedrina
efferente	efferent	eferente
asse, colonna vertebrale	Achse	eje
elastina	Elastin	elastina
elettrocardiogramma (ECG)	Elektrokardiogramm (EKG)	electrocardiograma (ECG)
terapia elettroconvulsiva, elettroshock	Elektroschocktherapie	electrochoqueterapia (ECT)
elettrodo	Elektrode	electrodo
elettroencefalogramma (EEG)	Elektroenzephalogramm (EEG)	electroencefalograma (EEG)
elettrolisi	Elektrolyse	electrólisis
elettrolito	Elektrolyt	electrólito
elettromiografia	Elektromyographie	electromiografía
elefantiasi	Elephantiasis	elefantiasis
muscolo elevatore	Levator	elevador
eliminazione	Elimination, Ausscheidung	eliminación
ellissocitosi	Elliptozytose	eliptocitosis
elisir	Elixier	elixir
emaciazione	Auszehrung	emaciación
gravidanza	Schwangerschaft, Gravidität	embarazo
gravidanza a termine	ausgetragen	embarazo a término
gravidanza ectopica	ektope Schwangerschaft	embarazo ectópico
pseudociesi	Scheinschwangerschaft, hysterische Schwangerschaft	embarazo fantasma
embolia	Embolie	embolia
embolico	embolisch	embólico
embolia polmonare (EP)	Lungenembolie	embolismo pulmonar
embolo	Embolus	émbolo
embriologia	Embryologie	embriología
embrione	Embryo	embrión
embriopatia	Embryopathie	embriopatía

SPANISH	ENGLISH	FRENCH
emesis	emesis	vomissement
emético (n)	emetic (n)	émétique (n)
emético (a)	emetic (a)	émétique (a)
eminencia hipotenar	hypothenar eminence	éminence hypothénar
emoción	emotion	émotion
emocional	emotional	émotionnel
emoliente (n)	emollient (n)	émollient (n)
emoliente (a)	emollient (a)	émollient (a)
empatía	empathy	empathie
empeine	instep	tarse
empiema	empyema	empyème
empírico	empirical	empirique
emulsión	emulsion	émulsion
enanismo	dwarfism	nanisme
encapsulación	encapsulation	capsulage
encefalina	encephalin (Eng), enkephalin (Am)	encéphaline
encefalitis	encephalitis	encéphalite
encefalitis espongiforme bovina	bovine spongiform encephalitis (BSE)	encéphalite spongiforme bovine
encefalomielitis	encephalomyelitis	encéphalomyélite
encefalomielitis miálgica	myalgic encephalomyelitis (ME)	encéphalomyélite myalgique
encefalopatía	encephalopathy	encéphalopathie
encía	gingiva	gencive
encopresis	encopresis	encoprésie
endarterectomía	endarterectomy	endartériectomie
endarteritis	endarteritis	endartérite
endémico (n)	endemic (n)	endémie (n)
endémico (a)	endemic (a)	endémique (a)
endocarditis	endocarditis	endocardite
endocarditis bacteriana subaguda	subacute bacterial endocarditis (SBE)	endocardite lente
endocervical	endocervical	endocervical
endocrino	endocrine	endocrine
endocrinología	endocrinology	endocrinologie
endógeno	endogenous	endogène
endometrio	endometrium	endomètre
endometriosis	endometriosis	endométriose
endometritis	endometritis	endométrite
endoneuro	endoneurium	endonèvre
endoparásito	endoparasite	endoparasite
endorfina	endorphin	endorphine
endoscopia	endoscopy	endoscopie
endoscopio	endoscope	endoscope
endotelio	endothelium	endothélium
endotoxina	endotoxin	endotoxine
endotraqueal	endotracheal	endotrachéique
enema	enema	lavement
enema de bario	barium enema	lavement au baryte

vomito, emesi	Erbrechen	emesis
emetico (n)	Emetikum (n), Brechmittel (n)	emético (n)
emetico (a)	emetisch (a)	emético (a)
eminenza ipotenar	Antithenar	eminencia hipotenar
emozione	Emotion, Gefühl	emoción
emotivo	emotional	emocional
emoliente (n)	Emollientium (n)	emoliente (n)
emoliente (a)	erweichend (a)	emoliente (a)
immedesimazione, identificazione	Empathie, Einfühlungsvermögen	empatía
dorso del piede	Fußrücken, Spann	empeine
empiema	Empyem	empiema
empirico	empirisch	empírico
emulsione	Emulsion	emulsión
nanismo	Zwergwuchs	enanismo
incapsulamento	Verkapselung	encapsulación
encefalina	Enzephalin	encefalina
encefalite	Enzephalitis	encefalitis
encefalite spongiforme bovina	Rinderwahnsinn, Bovine Spongiforme Enzephalitis (BSE)	encefalitis espongiforme bovina
encefalomielite	Enzephalomyelitis	encefalomielitis
encefalomielite mialgica	myalgische Enzephalomyelitis	encefalomielitis miálgica
encefalopatia	Enzephalopathie	encefalopatía
gengiva	Gingiva, Zahnfleisch	encía
encopresi	Enkopresis, Einkoten	encopresis
endoarterectomia	Endarteriektomie	endarterectomía
endoarterite	Endarteriitis	endarteritis
endemia (n)	Endemie (n)	endémico (n)
endemico (a)	endemisch (a)	endémico (a)
endocardite	Endokarditis	endocarditis
endocardite batterica subacuta	Endocarditis lenta	endocarditis bacteriana subaguda
endocervicale	endozervikal	endocervical
endocrino	endokrin	endocrino
endocrinologia	Endokrinologie	endocrinología
endogeno	endogen	endógeno
endometrio	Endometrium	endometrio
endometriosi	Endometriose	endometriosis
endometrite	Endometritis	endometritis
endonevrio	Endoneurium	endoneuro
endoparassita	Endoparasit	endoparásito
endorfina	Endorphin	endorfina
endoscopia	Endoskopie	endoscopia
endoscopio	Endoskop	endoscopio
endotelio	Endothel	endotelio
endotossina	Endotoxin	endotoxina
endotracheale	endotracheal	endotraqueal
clistere	Klistier, Einlauf	enema
clisma opaco	Bariumeinlauf	enema de bario

SPANISH	ENGLISH	FRENCH
enfermedad	disease, illness	maladie
enfermadad arterial coronaria	coronary artery disease (CAD)	coronaropathie, cardiopathie ischémique, insuffisance coronarienne globale
enfermedad autoinmune	autoimmune disease	maladie auto-immune
enfermedad coronaria	coronary heart disease (CHD)	insuffisance coronarienne cardiaque
enfermedad de Addison	Addison's disease	maladie d'Addison
enfermedad de Alzheimer	Alzheimer's disease	maladie d'Alzheimer
enfermedad de Bornholm	Bornholm disease	maladie de Bornholm
enfermedad declarable	notifiable disease	maladie à déclaration obligatoire
enfermedad de Crohn	Crohn's disease	mal de Crohn
enfermedad de Graves	Graves' disease	goitre exophtalmique
enfermedad de Hashimoto	Hashimoto's disease	maladie d'Hashimoto
enfermedad de Hirschsprung	Hirschsprung's disease	maladie de Hirschsprung
enfermedad de Hodgkin	Hodgkin's disease	maladie de Hodgkin
enfermedad de la membrana hialina	hyaline membrane disease	maladie des membranes hyalines
enfermedad del legionario	legionnaires' disease	maladie des légionnaires
enfermedad de Lyme	Lyme disease	arthrite de Lyme, maladie de Lyme
enfermedad de Ménière	Ménière's disease	syndrome de Ménière
enfermedad de Osgood-Schlatter	Osgood-Schlatter disease	maladie d'Osgood-Schlatter
enfermedad de Paget	Paget's disease	maladie de Paget
enfermedad de Perthes	Perthes' disease	coxa plana
enfermedad de Peyronie	Peyronie's disease	maladie de La Peyronie
enfermedad de Pott	Pott's disease	mal de Pott
enfermedad de Raynaud	Raynaud's disease	maladie de Raynaud
enfermedad de Schlatter	Schlatter's disease	maladie d'Osgood-Schlatter
enfermedad de Still	Still's disease	maladie de Still
enfermedad de Tay-Sachs	Tay-Sachs disease	maladie de Tay-Sachs
enfermedad de transmisión sexual (ETS)	sexually transmitted disease (STD)	maladie sexuellement transmissible (MST)
enfermedad de von Recklinghausen	von Recklinghausen's disease	maladie de von Recklinghausen
enfermedad de von Willebrand	von Willebrand's disease	maladie de von Willebrand
enfermedad de Weil	Weil's disease	maladie de Weil
enfermedad de Wilson	Wilson's disease	maladie de Wilson
enfermedad hemolítica del recién nacido	haemolytic disease of the newborn (HDN) (Eng), hemolytic disease of the newborn (HDN) (Am)	hémolyse des nouveau-nés
enfermedad hemorrágica neonatal	haemorrhagic disease of the newborn (Eng), hemorrhagic disease of the newborn (Am)	hémorragies des nouveau-nés
enfermedad industrial	industrial disease	maladie professionnelle
enfermedad infecciosa	infectious disease	maladie infectieuse
enfermedad inflamatoria de la pelvis	pelvic inflammatory disease (PID)	pelvipéritonite
enfermedad obstructiva crónica de las vias respiratorias	chronic obstructive airway disease (COAD)	bronchopneumopathie chronique obstructive, syndrome respiratoire obstructif chronique
enfermedad periodontal	periodontal disease	paradontolyse

ITALIAN	GERMAN	SPANISH
malattia, affezione, infermità	Krankheit, Leiden	enfermedad
malattia delle arterie coronarica (MAC)	Koronaropathie	enfermadad arterial coronaria
malattia autoimmune	Autoimmunerkrankung	enfermedad autoinmune
malattia cardiaca coronarica (MCC)	koronare Herzkrankheit (KHK)	enfermedad coronaria
morbo di Addison	Addison Krankheit	enfermedad de Addison
morbo di Alzheimer	Alzheimer Krankheit	enfermedad de Alzheimer
malattia di Bornholm, mialgia epidemica	Bornholm-Krankheit	enfermedad de Bornholm
malattia da denunciare alle autorità sanitarie	meldepflichtige Erkrankung	enfermedad declarable
malattia di Crohn	Morbus Crohn	enfermedad de Crohn
morbo di Graves	Basedow-Krankheit	enfermedad de Graves
tiroidite di Hashimoto	Hashimoto-Struma	enfermedad de Hashimoto
malattia di Hirschsprung	Hirschsprung-Krankheit	enfermedad de Hirschsprung
malattia di Hodgkin	Morbus Hodgkin	enfermedad de Hodgkin
malattia delle membrane ialine	Hyalinmembrankrankheit	enfermedad de la membrana hialina
malattia dei legionari	Legionärskrankheit	enfermedad del legionario
malattia di Lyme	Lyme-Arthritis, Lyme-Borreliose	enfermedad de Lyme
sindrome di Ménière	Morbus Ménière	enfermedad de Ménière
malattia di Osgood-Schlatter	Osgood-Schlatter Krankheit	enfermedad de Osgood-Schlatter
malattia di Paget	Morbus Paget	enfermedad de Paget
malattia di Perthes	Perthes-Krankheit	enfermedad de Perthes
malattia di Peyronie	Induratio penis plastica	enfermedad de Peyronie
malattia di Pott	Malum Potti	enfermedad de Pott
malattia di Raynaud	Raynaud-Krankheit	enfermedad de Raynaud
malattia di Schlatter	Schlatter-Krankheit	enfermedad de Schlatter
malattia di Still	Still-Krankheit	enfermedad de Still
malattia di Tay-Sachs	Tay-Sachs-Krankheit	enfermedad de Tay-Sachs
malattia a trasmissione sessuale (STD)	Geschlechtskrankheit	enfermedad de transmisión sexual (ETS)
malattia di von Recklinghausen, neurofibromatosi	Morbus von Recklinghausen	enfermedad de von Recklinghausen
malattia di von Willebrand	Willebrand-Krankheit	enfermedad de von Willebrand
malattia di Weil	Weil Krankheit	enfermedad de Weil
malattia di Wilson	Wilson-Krankheit	enfermedad de Wilson
ittero dei neonati, eritroblastosi fetale (da incompatibilità Rh)	Morbus haemolyticus neonatorum	enfermedad hemolítica del recién nacido
malattia emorragica del neonato	Morbus haemorrhagicus neonatorum	enfermedad hemorrágica neonatal
malattia industriale	Berufskrankheit	enfermedad industrial
malattia infettiva	Infektionskrankheit	enfermedad infecciosa
malattia infiammatoria della pelvi (PID)	Salpingitis	enfermedad inflamatoria de la pelvis
malattia ostruttiva cronica delle vie respiratorie	chronische obstruktive Lungenerkrankung	enfermedad obstructiva crónica de las vias respiratorias
periodontopatia	Periodontitis, Wurzelhautentzündung	enfermedad periodontal

857

enfermedad profesional	occupational disease	maladie professionnelle
enfermedad respiratoria febril aguda	acute febrile respiratory disease/illness (AFRD/I)	affection/maladie respiratoire fébrile aiguë
enfermedad sin pulso	pulseless disease	syndrome de Takayashu
enfermedad tropical	tropical disease	maladie tropicale
enfermedad venérea	venereal disease (VD)	maladie vénérienne (MV)
enfermera	nurse	infirmière
enfermería por aislamiento	barrier nursing	nursage de protection
enfisema	emphysema	emphysème
enoftalmos	enophthalmos	énophtalmie
enteral	enteral	entéral
entérico	enteric	entérique
enteritis	enteritis	entérite
enteroanastómosis	enteroanastomosis	entéro-anastomose
enterobius vermincularis	threadworm	ascaride
enterocele	enterocele	entérocèle, hernie intestinale
enterocolitis	enterocolitis	entérocolite
enterocolitis necrotizante	necrotizing enterocolitis (NEC)	entérocolite nécrosante
enteropatía provocada por glúten	gluten-induced enteropathy	maladie coeliaque
enterostomía	enterostomy	entérostomie
enterovirus	enterovirus	entérovirus
entropión	entropion	entropion
entuertos	afterpains	tranchées utérines
enucleación	enucleation	énucléation
enuresis	enuresis	énurèse
enuresis nocturna	bedwetting	incontinence nocturne
envejecimiento	ageing	vieillissement
envenenar	poison	empoisonner
enyesado	cast	plâtre
enzima	enzyme	enzyme
enzima proteolítico	proteolytic enzyme	enzyme protéolytique
enzimología	enzymology	enzymologie
eosinofilia	eosinophilia	éosinophilie
eosinófilo (n)	eosinophil (n)	éosinophile (n)
eosinófilo (a)	eosinophil (a)	éosinophile (a)
ependimoma	ependymoma	épendymome
epicanto	epicanthus	épicanthus
epicardio	epicardium	épicarde
epidemia	epidemic	épidémie
epidémico	epidemic	épidémique
epidemiología	epidemiology	épidémiologie
epidermis	epidermis	épiderme
epididimitis	epididymitis	épididymite
epidídimo	epididymis	épididyme
epididimoorquitis	epididymo-orchitis	orchi-épididymite
epidural	epidural	épidural
epífisis	epiphysis	épiphyse

ITALIAN	GERMAN	SPANISH
malattia professionale	Berufskrankheit	enfermedad profesional
malattia respiratoria acuta febbrile	Atemwegsinfekt (akut fieberhaft)	enfermedad respiratoria febril aguda
sindrome dell'arco aortico	Pulsloskrankheit	enfermedad sin pulso
malattia tropicale	Tropenkrankheit	enfermedad tropical
malattia venerea (MV)	Geschlechtskrankheit	enfermedad venérea
infermiere	Krankenschwester, Schwester, Pflegerin	enfermera
isolamento	Isolierung (auf Isolierstation)	enfermería por aislamiento
enfisema	Emphysem	enfisema
enoftalmo	Enophtalmus	enoftalmos
enterale, intestinale	enteral	enteral
enterico	enterisch	entérico
enterite	Enteritis	enteritis
enteroanastomosi	Enteroanastomose	enteroanastómosis
ossiuro	Fadenwurm	enterobius vermincularis
enterocele	Enterozele	enterocele
enterocolite	Enterokolitis	enterocolitis
enterocolite necrotizzante	nekrotisierende Enterokolitis	enterocolitis necrotizante
enteropatia da glutine	Zöliakie	enteropatía provocada por glúten
enterostomia	Enterostomie	enterostomía
enterovirus	Enterovirus	enterovirus
entropion	Entropion	entropión
contrazioni uterine post partum	Nachwehen	entuertos
enucleazione	Enukleation, Ausschälung	enucleación
enuresi	Enuresis, Bettnässen	enuresis
enuresi notturna	Bettnässen	enuresis nocturna
senescenza, invecchiamento	Altern	envejecimiento
avvelenare	vergiften	envenenar
ingessatura, steccatura	Abdruck, Gipsverband	enyesado
enzima	Enzym	enzima
enzima proteolitico, proteasi	proteolytisches Enzym	enzima proteolítico
enzimologia	Enzymologie	enzimología
eosinofilia	Eosinophilie	eosinofilia
eosinofilo (n)	Eosinophiler (n)	eosinófilo (n)
eosinofilo (a)	eosinophil (a)	eosinófilo (a)
ependimoma	Ependymom	ependimoma
epicanto	Epikanthus	epicanto
epicardio	Epikard	epicardio
epidemia	Epidemie	epidemia
epidemico	epidemisch	epidémico
epidemiologia	Epidemiologie	epidemiología
epidermide	Epidermis	epidermis
epididimite	Epididymitis, Nebenhodenentzündung	epididimitis
epididimo	Epididymis, Nebenhoden	epidídimo
epididimo-orchite	Epididymoorchitis	epididimoorquitis
epidurale	epidural	epidural
epifisi	Epiphyse, Zirbeldrüse	epífisis

SPANISH	ENGLISH	FRENCH
epífisis desplazada	slipped epiphysis	épiphysiolyse
epigastrio	epigastrium	épigastre
epiglotis	epiglottis	épiglotte
epiglotitis	epiglottitis	épiglottite
epilepsia	epilepsy	épilepsie
epiléptico	epileptic	épileptique
epileptiforme	epileptiform	épileptiforme
epileptógeno	epileptogenic	épileptogène
epinefrina	epinephrine	adrénaline, épinéphrine
epiplón	omentum	épiploon
episclera	episclera	épisclérotique
escleritis	episcleritis	épisclérite
episiotomía	episiotomy	épisiotomie
epistaxis	epistaxis, nosebleed	épistaxis, saignement de nez
epitelio	epithelium	épithélium
epitelioma	epithelioma	épithélioma
equímosis	bruise, ecchymosis	contusion, ecchymose
erección	erection	érection
eréctil	erectile	érectile
erisipela	erysipelas	érysipèle
eritema	erythema	érythème
eritroblasto	erythroblast	érythroblaste
eritrocito	erythrocyte, red blood cell (RBC)	érythrocyte, globule rouge
eritrodermia	erythroderma	érythroderme
eritropoyesis	erythropoiesis	érythropoïèse
eritropoyetina	erythropoietin	érythropoïétine
eructo	belching	éructation
erupción	eruption	éruption
escafoides	scaphoid	scaphoïde
escaldadura	scald	échaudure
escalpelo	scalpel	scalpel
escamoso	squamous	squameux
escara	eschar	escarre
escarlatina	scarlet fever	scarlatine
escayola	plaster of Paris	sulfate de calcium hydraté, plâtre
escleredema	scleredema (Am), scleredoema (Eng)	scléroderme
escleritis	scleritis	sclérite
escleroderma	scleroderma	scléroderme
esclerosis	sclerosis	sclérose
esclerosis múltiple	multiple sclerosis (MS)	sclérose en plaques
esclerosis tuberosa	tuberous sclerosis	sclérose tubéreuse du cerveau
escleroterapia	sclerotherapy	sclérothérapie
esclerótica	sclera	sclérotique
esclerótico	sclerotic	sclérotique
escoliosis	scoliosis	scoliose
escorbuto	scurvy	scorbut

ITALIAN	GERMAN	SPANISH
distacco epifisario	Epiphyseolyse	epífisis desplazada
epigastrio	Epigastrium, Oberbauch	epigastrio
epiglottide	Epiglottis	epiglotis
epiglottite	Epiglottitis	epiglotitis
epilessia	Epilepsie	epilepsia
epilettico	epileptisch	epiléptico
epilettiforme	epileptiform	epileptiforme
epilettogeno	epileptogen	epileptógeno
adrenalina	Adrenalin	epinefrina
omento	Omentum, Netz	epiplón
episclera	Episklera	episclera
episclerite	Episkleritis	episcleritis
episiotomia	Episiotomie, Dammschnitt	episiotomía
epistassi	Epistaxis, Nasenbluten	epistaxis
epitelio	Epithel	epitelio
epitelioma	Epitheliom	epitelioma
contusione, ecchimosi	Quetschung, Prellung, Ekchymose	equímosis
erezione	Erektion	erección
erettile	erektil	eréctil
erisipela	Erysipel, Wundrose	erisipela
eritema	Erythem	critema
eritroblasto	Erythroblast	eritroblasto
eritrocito, globulo rosso (RBC)	Erythrozyt, rotes Blutkörperchen	eritrocito
eritrodermia	Erythrodermie	eritrodermia
eritropoiesi	Erythropoese	eritropoyesis
eritropoietina	Erythropoetin, erythropoetischer Faktor	eritropoyetina
eruttazione	Aufstoßen	eructo
eruzione	Ausbruch, Ausschlag	erupción
scafoide	Scaphoid	escafoides
scottatura	Verbrühung, Brandwunde	escaldadura
bisturi	Skalpell	escalpelo
squamoso	squamös, schuppig	escamoso
escara	Brandschorf	escara
scarlattina	Scharlach	escarlatina
gesso di Parigi (calcio solfato diidrato)	Gips	escayola
scleredema	Sklerödem	escleredema
sclerite	Skleritis	escleritis
sclerodermia	Sklerodermie	escleroderma
sclerosi	Sklerose	esclerosis
sclerosi multipla	multiple Sklerose (MS)	esclerosis múltiple
sclerosi tuberosa	tuberöse Sklerose	esclerosis tuberosa
scleroterapia	Sklerotherapie	escleroterapia
sclera, sclerotica	Sklera	esclerótica
sclerotico	sklerotisch, Sklera-	esclerótico
scoliosi	Skoliose	escoliosis
scorbuto	Skorbut	escorbuto

SPANISH	ENGLISH	FRENCH
escotoma	scotoma	scotome
escrófula	scrofula	scrofule
escroto	scrotum	scrotum
esencia	essence	essence
esfacelo	slough	escarre
esfenoides	sphenoid	sphénoïde
esferocitosis	spherocytosis	sphérocytose
esfigmomanómetro	sphygmomanometer	sphygmomanomètre
esfínter	sphincter	sphincter
esguince	sprain	foulure
esmalte	enamel	émail
esofágico	esophageal (Am), oesophageal (Eng)	oesophagien
esofagitis	esophagitis (Am), oesophagitis (Eng)	oesophagite
esófago	esophagus (Am), oesophagus (Eng)	oesophage
espacio subaracnoideo	subarachnoid space	espace sous-arachnoïdien
espasmo	cramp, spasm	crampe, spasme
espástico	spastic	spastique
espátula	spatula	spatule
especie	species	espèce
específico	specific	spécifique
espéculo	speculum	spéculum
espéculo de Sim	Sims' speculum	spéculum de Sim
esperma	sperm	sperme
espermático	spermatic	spermatique
espermatocele	spermatocele	spermatocèle
espermicida	spermicide	spermicide
espesado	inspissated	épaissir
espica	spica	spica
espícula	spicule	spicule
espina bífida	spina bifida	spina bifida
espinal	spinal	spinal
espiración	expiration	expiration
espirografía	spirograph	spirographe
espirómetro	spirometer	spiromètre
espiroqueta	spirochaete (Eng), spirochete (Am)	spirochète
esplácnico	splanchnic	splanchnique
esplenectomía	splenectomy	splénectomie
esplenomegalia	splenomegaly	splénomégalie
espondilitis	spondylitis	spondylite
espondilolistesis	spondylolisthesis	spondylolisthésis
esponjoso	cancellous	spongieux
esporádico	sporadic	sporadique
esprue	sprue	sprue
esputo	sputum	salive

ITALIAN	GERMAN	SPANISH
scotoma	Skotom, Gesichtsfeldausfall	escotoma
scrofola, linfadenite tubercolare	Skrofula, Lymphknotentuberkulose	escrófula
scroto	Skrotum, Hodensack	escroto
essenza	Essenz	esencia
crosta, escara	Schorf	esfacelo
sfenoide	Sphenoid, Keilbein	esfenoides
sferocitosi	Sphärozytose, Kugelzellanämie	esferocitosis
sfigmomanometro	Blutdruckmeßgerät	esfigmomanómetro
sfintere	Sphinkter, Schließmuskel	esfínter
distorsione	Verstauchung	esguince
smalto	Emaille	esmalte
esofageo	ösophageal	esofágico
esofagite	Ösophagitis	esofagitis
esofago	Ösophagus, Speiseröhre	esófago
spazio subaracnoideo	Subarachnoidalraum	espacio subaracnoideo
crampo, spasmo	Krampf, Spasmus	espasmo
spastico	spastisch, krampfhaft	espástico
spatola	Spatel	espátula
specie	Spezies, Art	especie
specifico	spezifisch, speziell	específico
speculum	Spekulum, Spiegel	espéculo
speculum di Sim	Sims-Spekulum	espéculo de Sim
sperma	Sperma, Samen	esperma
spermatico	Sperma-, Samen-	espermático
spermatocele	Spermatozele	espermatocele
spermicida	Spermizid	espermicida
inspessito	kondensiert, eingedickt	espesado
spiga	Kornährenverband, Sporn	espica
spicola, picco	Spikulum	espícula
spina bifida	Spina bifida	espina bífida
spinale	spinal, Rückenmarks-, Wirbelsäulen-	espinal
espirazione, termine	Exspiration, Ausatmen	espiración
spirografo	Spirograph	espirografía
spirometro	Spirometer	espirómetro
spirocheta	Spirochäte	espiroqueta
splancnico	viszeral, Eingeweide-	esplácnico
splenectomia	Splenektomie	esplenectomía
splenomegalia	Splenomegalie	esplenomegalia
spondilite	Spondylitis	espondilitis
spondilolistesi	Spondylolisthesis	espondilolistesis
spugnoso, trabecolare	spongiös, schwammartig	esponjoso
sporadico	sporadisch	esporádico
sprue	Sprue	esprue
sputo, escreato	Sputum, Auswurf	esputo

SPANISH	ENGLISH	FRENCH
esqueleto	skeleton	squelette
esquistosomiasis	schistosomiasis	schistosomiase
esquizofrenia	schizophrenia	schizophrénie
esquizofrenia paranoica	paranoid schizophrenia	schizophrénie paranoïaque
estancamiento	engorgement	engorgement
estapedectomía	stapedectomy	stapédectomie
estasis	stasis	stase
esteatorrea	steatorrhea (Am), steatorrhoea (Eng)	stéatorrhée
estenosis	stenosis	sténose
estéril	sterile	stérile
esterilización	sterilization	stérilisation
esternocostal	sternocostal	sternocostal
esternón	sternum	sternum
esteroide	steroid	stéroïde
estetoscopio	stethoscope	stéthoscope
estigmas	stigmata	stigmate
estilbestrol	stilbestrol (Am), stilboestrol (Eng)	stilboestrol
estiloides	styloid	styloïde
estimulante (n)	analeptic (n), stimulant (n)	analeptique (n), stimulant (n)
estimulante (a)	analeptic (a), stimulant (a)	analeptique (a), stimulant (a)
estoma	stoma	stoma
estómago	stomach	estomac
estomatitis	stomatitis	stomatite
estornudar	sneeze	éternuer
estornudo	sneeze	éternuement
estrabismo	squint, strabismus	strabisme
estradiol	estradiol (Am), oestradiol (Eng)	oestradiol
estrangulación	strangulation	strangulation
estranguria	strangury	strangurie
estrato	stratum	couche
estreñimiento	constipation	constipation
estrés	stress	stress
estrias	striae	stries
estribo	stapes	étrier
estrictura	stricture	rétrécissement
estridor	stridor	stridor
estriol	estriol (Am), oestriol (Eng)	oestriol
estrógeno	estrogen (Am), oestrogen (Eng)	oestrogène
estupor	stupor	stupeur
etiología	aetiology	étiologie
etmoides	ethmoid	ethmoïde
étnico	ethnic	ethnique
euforia	euphoria	euphorie
eutanasia	euthanasia	euthanasie
evacuación	evacuation	évacuation
evaporar	evaporate	évaporer

864

ITALIAN	GERMAN	SPANISH
scheletro	Skelett	esqueleto
schistosomiasi	Schistosomiasis, Bilharziose	esquistosomiasis
schizofrenia	Schizophrenie	esquizofrenia
schizofrenia paranoide	paranoide Schizophrenie	esquizofrenia paranoica
congestione	Stauung, Anschoppung	estancamiento
stapedectomia	Stapedektomie	estapedectomía
stasi, ristagno	Stase	estasis
steatorrea, seborrea	Steatorrhoe, Fettstuhl	esteatorrea
stenosi	Stenose	estenosis
sterile	steril, keimfrei, unfruchtbar	estéril
sterilizzazione	Sterilisation, Sterilisierung	esterilización
sternocostale	sternokostal	esternocostal
sterno	Sternum, Brustbein	esternón
steroide	Steroid	esteroide
stetoscopio	Stethoskop	estetoscopio
stigmate	Stigmata, Kennzeichen	estigmas
stilbestrolo	Diäthylstilboestrol	estilbestrol
stiloide, stiloideo	Styloid-	estiloides
analettico (n), stimolante (n)	Analeptikum (n), Stimulans (n)	estimulante (n)
analettico (a), stimolante (a)	analeptisch (a), stimulierend (a)	estimulante (a)
stoma, orifizio	Stoma, Mund	estoma
stomaco	Magen	estómago
stomatite	Stomatitis, Mundhöhlenentzündung	estomatitis
starnutire	niesen	estornudar
starnuto	Niesen	estornudo
strabismo	Schielen, Strabismus	estrabismo
estradiolo	Östradiol	estradiol
strangolamento	Strangulation, Einklemmung	estrangulación
stranguria	Harnzwang	estranguria
strato	Stratum, Schicht	estrato
stipsi	Verstopfung	estreñimiento
stress	Belastung, Streß	estrés
stria	Striae, Streifen	estrias
staffa	Stapes, Steigbügel	estribo
stenosi, restringimento	Striktur	estrictura
stridore	Stridor	estridor
estriolo	Östriol	estriol
estrogeno	Östrogen	estrógeno
stupore	Stupor, Benommenheit	estupor
eziologia	Ätiologie	etiología
etmoide	Ethmoid, Siebbein	etmoides
etnico	ethnisch, rassisch	étnico
euforia	Euphorie	euforia
eutanasia	Euthanasie, Sterbehilfe	eutanasia
evacuazione	Ausleerung, Stuhlgang	evacuación
evaporare	verdampfen, verdunsten	evaporar

SPANISH	ENGLISH	FRENCH
eversión	eversion	éversion
exacerbación	exacerbation	exacerbation
exantema	rash	rash
exantema del pañal	diaper rash (Am), napkin rash (Eng)	érythème fessier du nourrisson, érythème papulo-érosif
excisión	ablation, excision	ablation, excision
excitabilidad	excitability	excitabilité
excitación	excitation	excitation
excoriación	excoriation	excoriation
excreción	excretion	excrétion
exéresis de tumores benignos de la mama	lumpectomy	exérèse locale d'une tumeur du sein
exfoliación	exfoliation, peeling	exfoliation, desquamation
exhibicionismo	exhibitionism	exhibitionnisme
exocrino	exocrine	exocrine
exoftalmía	exophthalmos	exophthalmie
exógeno	exogenous	exogène
exónfalo	exomphalos	exomphale
exostosis	exostosis	exostose
exotoxina	exotoxin	exotoxine
expectorante (n)	expectorant (n)	expectorant (n)
expectorante (a)	expectorant (a)	expectorant (a)
exploración	exploration, scan	exploration, échogramme
expresión	expression	expression
expulsión de la placenta y membranas	afterbirth	arrière-faix
extensión	extension	extension
extensor	extensor	extenseur
extraarticular	extra-articular	extra-articulaire
extracción	extraction	extraction
extracción con ventosa	ventouse extraction	extraction par ventouse
extracelular	extracellular	extracellulaire
extractor al vacío	vacuum extractor	ventouse obstétricale
extradural	extradural	extradural
extramural	extramural	extramural
extrasístole	extrasystole	extrasystole
extrauterino	extrauterine	extra-utérin
extravasación	extravasation	extravasation
extremidad	limb	membre
extrínseco	extrinsic	extrinsèque
exudado	exudate	exsudat
eyaculación	ejaculation	éjaculation

eversione, estrofia	Auswärtskehrung, Umstülpung	eversión
esacerbazione	Verschlimmerung	exacerbación
eruzione cutanea	Ausschlag, Hautausschlag	exantema
eruzione cutanea da pannolino	Windeldermatitis	exantema del pañal
ablazione, escissione	Ablatio, Absetzung, Exzision	excisión
eccitabilità	Reizbarkeit, Erregbarkeit	excitabilidad
eccitazione	Reizung, Erregung	excitación
escoriazione	Exkoriation, Abschürfung	excoriación
escrezione	Exkretion, Ausscheidung	excreción
mastectomia parziale	Lumpektomie	exéresis de tumores benignos de la mama
esfoliazione, desquamazione	Exfoliation, Schälen (Haut), Schuppung	exfoliación
esibizionismo	Exhibitionismus	exhibicionismo
esocrino	exokrin	exocrino
esoftalmo	Exophthalmus	exoftalmía
csogeno	exogen	exógeno
crnia ombelicale, protrusione dell'ombelico	Exomphalos, Nabelbruch	exónfalo
esostosi	Exostose	exostosis
esotossina	Exotoxin	exotoxina
espettorante (n)	Expektorans (n), Sekretolytikum (n)	expectorante (n)
espettorante (a)	schleimlösend (a)	expectorante (a)
esplorazione, ecografia, scintigrafia	Exploration, Scan	exploración
espressione	Expressio	expresión
secondine, membrane fetali e placenta	Plazenta, Nachgeburt	expulsión de la placenta y membranas
estensione	Extension, Streck-	extensión
estensore	Extensor, Streckmuskel	extensor
extraarticolare	extraartikulär	extraarticular
estrazione	Extraktion	extracción
estrazione con ventosa ostetrica	Schröpfkopf	extracción con ventosa
extracellulare	extrazellulär	extracelular
ventosa ostetrica, ventosa cefalica	Vakuumextraktor, Saugglocke	extractor al vacío
cxtradurale	extradural	extradural
extramurale	extramural	extramural
extrasistole	Extrasystole	extrasístole
extrauterino	extrauterin	extrauterino
stravaso	Extravasat	extravasación
braccio	Glied, Extremität	extremidad
estrinseco	exogen	extrínseco
essudato	Exsudat	exudado
eiaculazione	Ejakulation, Samenerguß	eyaculación

F

Spanish	English	French
faceta	facet	facette
facial	facial	facial
facies	facies	faciès
factor liberador de la hormona luteinizante	LH-releasing factor (LHRF)	substance libératrice de l'hormone lutéotrope
factor Rhesus	Rhesus factor	facteur Rhésus
facultativo	facultative, physician	facultatif, médecin
fagocito	phagocyte	phagocyte
fagocitosis	phagocytosis	phagocytose
faja	drawsheet	alèse
falanges	phalanges	phalanges
falciforme	falciform	falciforme
falo	phallus	phallus
familiar	familial	familial
faringe	pharynx	pharynx
faringitis	pharyngitis	pharyngite
faringotomía	pharyngotomy	pharyngotomie
farmacéutico (n)	pharmacist (n)	pharmacien (n)
farmacéutico (a)	pharmaceutical (a)	pharmaceutique (a)
fármaco	drug	médicament
fármaco antiinflamatorio no esteroide (AINE)	non-steroidal anti-inflammatory drug (NSAID)	anti-inflammatoire non stéroïdien
farmacocinética	pharmacokinetics	pharmacocinétique
fármaco controlado	controlled drug	médicament contrôlé
farmacogenético	pharmacogenetics	pharmacogénétique
farmacología	pharmacology	pharmacologie
farmacos antiparkinsonianos	antiparkinson(ism) drugs	médicaments contre la maladie de Parkinson
fascia	fascia	fascia
fasciculación	fasciculation	fasciculation
fatiga	fatigue	fatigue
fauces	fauces	fosse gutturale
febril	febrile	fébrile
fecal	faecal (Eng), fecal (Am)	fécal
fecalito	faecalith (Eng), fecalith (Am)	concrétion fécale
fecha de concepción	date of conception (DOC)	date du rapport fécondant
fecha de nacimiento	date of birth (DOB)	date de naissance
fecha esperada del parto	expected date of confinement (EDC)	date présumée de l'accouchement
fecha probable del parto (FPP)	expected date of delivery (EDD)	date présumée de l'accouchement
fecha última regla (FUR)	last menstrual period (LMP)	dernières règles
fémur	femur	fémur
fenestración	fenestration	fenestration
fenilcetonuria	phenylketonuria (PKU)	phénylcétonurie
fenotipo	phenotype	phénotype
feocromocitoma	phaeochromocytoma (Eng), pheochromocytoma (Am)	phéochromocytome
ferroso	ferrous (Eng), ferrus (Am)	ferreux

ITALIAN	GERMAN	SPANISH
faccetta	Facette	faceta
facciale	Gesichts-	facial
facies	Facies, Gesicht	facies
releasing factor dell'ormone LH	LH-luteinizing hormone releasing factor (LHRF)	factor liberador de la hormona luteinizante
fattore Rh	Rhesusfaktor	factor Rhesus
facoltativo, medico	fakultativ, Arzt	facultativo
fagocito	Phagozyt	fagocito
fagocitosi	Phagozytose	fagocitosis
traversa	Unterziehtuch	faja
falangi	Fingerglieder, Zehenglieder	falanges
falciforme	falciformis	falciforme
fallo	Phallus, Penis	falo
familiare	familiär	familiar
faringe	Pharynx, Rachen	faringe
faringite	Pharyngitis	faringitis
faringotomia	Pharyngotomie	faringotomía
farmacista (n)	Apotheker (n), Pharmazeut (n)	farmacéutico (n)
farmaceutico (a)	pharmazeutisch (a), Apotheker- (a)	farmacéutico (u)
farmaco, medicinale, droga	Arzneimittel, Rauschgift	fármaco
farmaco antinfiammatorio non steroideo (FANS)	nichtsteroidales Antiphlogistikum	fármaco antiinflamatorio no esteroide (AINE)
farmacocinetica	Pharmakokinetik	farmacocinética
farmaco sottoposto a controllo	Betäubungsmittel (gemäß BTM)	fármaco controlado
farmacogenetica	Pharmakogenetik	farmacogenético
farmacologia	Pharmakologie	farmacología
farmaci antiparkinsoniani	Antiparkinsonmittel	farmacos antiparkinsonianos
fascia	Faszie	fascia
fascicolazione	Faszikulation	fasciculación
stanchezza, astenia	Ermüdung	fatiga
fauci	Rachen, Schlund	fauces
febbrile	Fieber-, fieberhaft	febril
fecale	fäkal, kotig	fecal
fecalito	Kotstein	fecalito
data del concepimento	Empfängnisdatum	fecha de concepción
data di nascita	Geburtsdatum	fecha de nacimiento
data presunta delle doglie	errechneter Geburtstermin	fecha esperada del parto
data prevista per il parto	errechneter Geburtstermin	fecha probable del parto (FPP)
ultimo periodo mestruale	letzte Menstruationsperiode	fecha última regla (FUR)
femore	Femur	fémur
fenestrazione	Fensterung	fenestración
fenilchetonuria	Phenylketonurie (PKU)	fenilcetonuria
fenotipo	Phänotyp	fenotipo
feocromocitoma	Phäochromozytom	feocromocitoma
ferroso	Eisen-	ferroso

SPANISH	ENGLISH	FRENCH
fertilización	fertilization	fertilisation
fertilización in vitro (FIV)	in vitro fertilization (IVF)	fertilisation in vitro
feto	fetus	foetus
fetoscopia	fetoscopy	fétoscopie
fibra	fiber (Am), fibre (Eng)	fibre
fibra alimentaria	roughage	ballant intestinal
fibra dietética	dietary fiber (Am), dietary fibre (Eng)	fibre alimentaire
fibrilación	fibrillation	fibrillation
fibrilación auricular	atrial fibrillation	fibrillation auriculaire
fibrilla	fibril	fibrille
fibrina	fibrin	fibrine
fibrinógeno	fibrinogen	fibrinogène
fibroadenoma	fibroadenoma	fibroadénome
fibroblasto	fibroblast	fibroblaste
fibrocístico	fibrocystic	fibrokystique
fibroma	fibroma	fibrome
fibromioma	fibromyoma	fibromyome
fibroplasia retrolental	retrolental fibroplasia	fibroplasie rétrolentale
fibrosarcoma	fibrosarcoma	fibrosarcome
fibrosis	fibrosis	fibrose
fibrosis quística	cystic fibrosis (CF)	fibrose cystique
fibrositis	fibrositis	fibrosite
fiebre	fever, pyrexia	fièvre, pyrexie
fiebre amarilla	yellow fever	fièvre jaune
fiebre de Lassa	Lassa fever	fièvre de Lassa
fiebre del heno	hay fever	rhume des foins
fiebre de origen desconocido	pyrexia of unknown origin (PUO, FUO)	fièvre d'origine inconnue
fiebre glandular	glandular fever	fièvre glandulaire
fiebre hemoglobinúrica	blackwater fever	hématurie
fiebre manchada de las Montañas Rocosas	Rocky Mountain spotted fever	fièvre pourprée des montagnes Rocheuses
fiebre paratifoidea	paratyphoid fever	fièvre paratyphoïde
fiebre Q	Q fever	fièvre Q
fiebre reumática	rheumatic fever	rhumatisme articulaire aigu
fiebre tifoidea	typhoid fever	fièvre typhoïde
fijación	fixation	fixation
filariasis	filariasis	filariose
filtración	filtration	filtration
filtrado	filtrate	filtrat
fimbria	fimbria	fimbria
fimosis	phimosis	phimosis
fisiológico	physiological	physiologique
fisión	fission	fission

fertilizzazione	Befruchtung	**fertilización**
fertilizzazione in vitro	In-vitro-Fertilisation	**fertilización in vitro (FIV)**
feto	Fetus	**feto**
fetoscopia	Fetoskopie	**fetoscopia**
fibra	Faser	**fibra**
alimento ricco di fibre	Ballaststoff	**fibra alimentaria**
fibra dietetica	Ballaststoff	**fibra dietética**
fibrillazione	Fibrillieren	**fibrilación**
fibrillazione atriale	Vorhofflimmern	**fibrilación auricular**
fibrilla	Fibrille, Fäserchen	**fibrilla**
fibrina	Fibrin	**fibrina**
fibrinogeno	Fibrinogen	**fibrinógeno**
fibroadenoma	Fibroadenom	**fibroadenoma**
fibroblasto	Fibroblast	**fibroblasto**
fibrocistico	fibrozystisch	**fibrocístico**
fibroma	Fibrom	**fibroma**
fibromioma	Fibromyom	**fibromioma**
fibroplasia retrolenticolare	retrolentale Fibroplasie	**fibroplasia retrolental**
fibrosarcoma	Fibrosarkom	**fibrosarcoma**
fibrosi	Fibrose	**fibrosis**
mucoviscidosi, malattia fibrocistica del pancreas	Mukoviszidose	**fibrosis quística**
fibrosite	Fibrositis, Bindegewebsentzündung	**fibrositis**
febbre, piressia	Fieber	**fiebre**
febbre gialla	Gelbfieber	**fiebre amarilla**
febbre di Lassa	Lassafieber	**fiebre de Lassa**
febbre da fieno, raffreddore da fieno	Heuschnupfen	**fiebre del heno**
piressia di origine sconosciuta (POS)	Fieber unklarer Genese	**fiebre de origen desconocido**
mononucleosi infettiva	Mononukleose, Pfeiffersches Drüsenfieber	**fiebre glandular**
febbre emoglobinurica da Plasmodium falciparum	Schwarzwasserfieber	**fiebre hemoglobinúrica**
febbre purpurica delle Montagne Rocciose	Rocky Mountain spotted fever	**fiebre manchada de las Montañas Rocosas**
febbre paratifoide	Paratyphus	**fiebre paratifoidea**
febbre Q	Q-Fieber	**fiebre Q**
febbre reumatica	rheumatisches Fieber	**fiebre reumática**
febbre tifoide, tifo addominale, ileotifo	Typhus	**fiebre tifoidea**
fissazione	Fixation, Fixierung	**fijación**
filariasi	Filariasis, Fadenwurmbefall	**filariasis**
filtrazione	Filtrieren, Filtration	**filtración**
filtrato	Filtrat	**filtrado**
fimbria	Fimbrie	**fimbria**
fimosi	Phimose	**fimosis**
fisiologico	physiologisch	**fisiológico**
fissione	Spaltung	**fisión**

SPANISH	ENGLISH	FRENCH
fístula	fistula	fistule
fláccido	flaccid	mou
flato	flatus	flatuosité
flatulencia	flatulence, wind	flatulence, gaz
flebectomía	phlebectomy	phlébectomie
flebitis	phlebitis	phlébite
flebolito	phlebolith	phlébolithe
flebotomía	phlebotomy	phlébotomie
flema	phlegm	phlegme
flexión	flexion	flexion
flexionar	flex	fléchir
flexor	flexor	fléchisseur
flexura	flexure	angle
flictena	blister	ampoule
flora	flora	flore
florido	florid	coloré
flotadores	floaters	flottants
fluctuación	fluctuation	variation
flujo sanguíneo renal (FSR)	renal blood flow (RBF)	débit sanguin rénal
flúor	fluoride	fluorure
fluoresceína	fluorescein	fluorescéine
fobia	phobia	phobie
focomelia	phocomelia	phocomélie
foliculitis	folliculitis	folliculite
folículo	follicle	follicule
folículo de De Graaf	Graafian follicle	follicule de De Graaf
folículos de Naboth	nabothian follicles	oeufs de Naboth
fontanela	fontanelle	fontanelle
foramen	foramen	orifice
fórceps	forceps	forceps
formación de imágenes por resonancia magnética	magnetic resonance imaging (MRI)	imagerie par résonance magnétique
formar una costra	scab	former une croûte
fórmula	formula	formule
fórmula leucocitaria	differential blood count	formule leucocytaire
formulario	formulary	formulaire
fórnix	fornix	fornix
forúnculo	boil, furuncle	furoncle
fosa nasale	nostril	narine
fotofobia	photophobia	photophobie
fotosensible	photosensitive	photosensible
fototerapia	phototherapy	photothérapie
fóvea	fovea	fovea
fractura	fracture	fracture
fractura con hundimiento	depressed fracture	enfoncement localisé
fractura conminuta	comminuted fracture	fracture esquilleuse

fistola	Fistel	fístula
flaccido	schlaff	fláccido
flatulenza, gas intestinale	Flatus, Wind	flato
flatulenza, ventosità	Flatulenz, Blähung, Wind	flatulencia
flebectomia	Phlebektomie	flebectomía
flebite	Phlebitis, Venenentzündung	flebitis
flebolito	Phlebolith	flebolito
flebotomia	Venae sectio	flebotomía
flemma	Phlegma	flema
flessione	Flexion, Beugung	flexión
flettere	beugen, flektieren	flexionar
flessore	Flexor, Beugemuskel	flexor
flessura	Flexur	flexura
vescicola, bolla	Blase, Hautblase, Brandblase	flictena
flora	Flora	flora
florido	floride	florido
corpuscoli vitreali sospesi visibili	Mouches volantes	flotadores
fluttuazione	Fluktuation	fluctuación
perfusione renale	Nierendurchblutung, renaler Blutfluß (RBF)	flujo sanguíneo renal (FSR)
fluoruro	Fluorid	flúor
fluoresceina	Fluorescin	fluoresceína
fobia	Phobie	fobia
focomelia	Phokomelie	focomelia
follicolite	Follikulitis	foliculitis
follicolo	Follikel	folículo
follicolo di Graaf	Graaf-Follikel	folículo de De Graaf
follicoli di Naboth	Naboth-Eier	folículos de Naboth
fontanella	Fontanelle	fontanela
foramen	Foramen	foramen
forcipe	Zange, Pinzette, Klemme	fórceps
indagine morfologica con risonanza magnetica	Kernspintomographie (NMR)	formación de imágenes por resonancia magnética
ricoprirsi di croste	verkrusten	formar una costra
formula	Formel, Milchzusammensetzung	fórmula
formula leucocitaria	Differentialblutbild	fórmula leucocitaria
formulario	Formelnbuch	formulario
fornice	Fornix	fórnix
foruncolo	Furunkel, Eiterbeule	forúnculo
narice	Nasenloch	fosa nasale
fotofobia	Photophobie, Lichtscheue	fotofobia
fotosensibile	lichtempfindlich	fotosensible
fototerapia	Phototherapie	fototerapia
fovea	Fovea	fóvea
frattura	Fraktur, Knochenbruch	fractura
frattura con infossamento dei frammenti	Impressionsfraktur	fractura con hundimiento
frattura comminuta	Splitterbruch	fractura conminuta

SPANISH	ENGLISH	FRENCH
fractura de Colles	Colles' fracture	fracture de Pouteau-Colles
fractura de Pott	Pott's fracture	fracture de Pott
fractura en tallo verde	greenstick fracture	fracture incomplète
fractura patológica	pathological fracture	fracture spontanée
fracturar	fracture	fracturer
franja	fimbria	fimbria
frecuencia cardíaca fetal (FCF)	fetal heart rate (FHR)	fréquence cardiaque foetale
frémito	thrill	murmure respiratoire
frénico	phrenic	psychique
frenillo	frenum	frein
frenillo pudendo	fourchette	fourchette
frenotomía	frenotomy	frénotomie
frente	forehead	front
friable	friable	friable
fricción	friction	friction
frigidez	frigidity	frigidité
frío	cold	froid
frontal	frontal	frontal
frotis	smear	frottis
fuga	fugue	fugue
fuga de ideas	flight of ideas	fuite des idées
fulguración	fulguration	fulguration
fulminante	fulminant	fulminant
función	function	fonction
funcionar	function	fonctionner
fundoplicatura	fundoplication	fundoplication
fundus	fundus	fond

ITALIAN	GERMAN	SPANISH
frattura di Colles	distale Radiusfraktur	fractura de Colles
frattura di Pott	Pott-Fraktur	fractura de Pott
frattura a legno verde	Grünholzfraktur	fractura en tallo verde
frattura patologica	pathologische Fraktur	fractura patológica
fratturare	frakturieren, brechen	fracturar
fimbria	Fimbrie	franja
battito cardiaco fetale	fetale Herzfrequenz	frecuencia cardíaca fetal (FCF)
fremito	Vibrieren, Schwirren	frémito
frenico (diaframmatico mentale)	diaphragmatisch, Zwerchfell-	frénico
freno	Frenulum	frenillo
forchetta	hintere Schamlippenkommissur	frenillo pudendo
frenulotomia	Frenotomie, Zungenbändchendurchtrennung	frenotomía
fronte	Stirn	frente
friabile	bröckelig, brüchig	friable
attrito, frizione	Friktion, Reibung	fricción
frigidità	Frigidität, Kälte	frigidez
freddo	kalt	frío
frontale	Stirn-, frontal	frontal
striscio	Belag, Abstrich	frotis
fuga	Fugue	fuga
fuga delle idee	Ideenflucht	fuga de ideas
folgorazione	Fulguration	fulguración
fulminante	fulminant	fulminante
funzione	Funktion	función
funzionare	funktionieren	funcionar
fundoplicazione	Fundoplikatio(n)	fundoplicatura
fondo	Fundus, Augenhintergrund	fundus

G

galactogogo	galactagogue	galactagogue
galactorrea	galactorrhea (Am), galactorrhoea (Eng)	galactorrhée
galactosa	galactose	galactose
galactosemia	galactosaemia (Eng), galactosemia (Am)	galactosémie
gameto	gamete	gamète
gammaglobulina	gammaglobulin	gamma-globuline
gammaglobulina humana	human gamma globulin (HGG)	gamma-globuline humaine (GGH), globuline humaine
gamma glutamil transferasa (GGT)	gamma glutamyl transferase (GGT)	gamma-glutamyl-transférase (GGT)
ganglio	ganglion	ganglion
ganglio linfático	lymph node	ganglion lymphatique
ganglios basales	basal ganglia	noyau lenticulaire, noyau caudé, avant-mur et noyau amygdalien
gangrena	gangrene	gangrène
gargajear	gargle	se gargariser
gárgara	gargle	gargarisme
garrapata	tick	tique
garrotillo	croup	croup
gas	gas	gaz
gasa	gauze	gaze
gastrectomía	gastrectomy	gastrectomie
gástrico	gastric	gastrique
gastrina	gastrin	gastrine
gastritis	gastritis	gastrite
gastrocnemio	gastrocnemius	gastrocnémien
gastrocólico	gastrocolic	gastrocolique
gastrodinia	gastrodynia	gastrodynie
gastroenteritis	gastroenteritis	gastro-entérite
gastroenterología	gastroenterology	gastro-entérologie
gastroenteropatía	gastroenteropathy	gastro-entéropathie
gastroenterostomía	gastroenterostomy	gastro-entérostomie
gastroesofágico	gastroesophageal (Am), gastro-oesophageal (Eng)	gastro-oesophagien
gastrointestinal	gastrointestinal	gastro-intestinal
gastroscopio	gastroscope	gastroscope
gastrosquisis	gastroschisis	gastroschisis
gastrotomía	gastrostomy	gastrostomie
gastroyeyunostomía	gastrojejunostomy	gastrojéjunostomie
gaznate	gullet	oesophage
gelatina	gelatine (Eng), gelatin (Am)	gélatine
gemelos	gastrocnemius	gastrocnémien
gemelos idénticos	identical twins	jumeaux univitellins
gen	gene	gène
generador	generative	génératif

Italian	German	Spanish
galattagogo	Galaktagogum	galactogogo
galattorrea	Galaktorrhoe	galactorrea
galattosio	Galaktose	galactosa
galattosemia	Galaktosämie	galactosemia
gamete	Gamete	gameto
gammaglobulina	Gammaglobulin	gammaglobulina
gammaglobulina umana	Human-Gammaglobulin	gammaglobulina humana
transaminasi, transferasi glutammica	Gammaglutamyltransferase (gGT)	gamma glutamil transferasa (GGT)
ganglio	Ganglion, Überbein	ganglio
linfonodo	Lymphknoten	ganglio linfático
gangli basali	Basalganglien	ganglios basales
gangrena	Gangrän	gangrena
gargarizzare	gurgeln	gargajear
gargarismi	Gurgelmittel	gárgara
zecca	Zecke	garrapata
ostruzione laringea	Krupp	garrotillo
gas	Gas, Wind	gas
garza	Gaze, Mull	gasa
gastrectomia	Magenresektion	gastrectomía
gastrico	gastrisch, Magen-	gástrico
gastrina	Gastrin	gastrina
gastrite	Gastritis, Magenschleimhautentzündung	gastritis
gastrocnemio	gastrocnemius	gastrocnemio
gastrocolico	gastrokolisch	gastrocólico
gastrodinia	Magenschmerz	gastrodinia
gastroenterite	Gastroenteritis	gastroentcritis
gastroenterologia	Gastroenterologie	gastroenterología
gastroenteropatia	Gastroenteropathie	gastroenteropatía
gastroenterostomia	Gastroenterostomie	gastroenterostomía
gastroesofageo	gastroösophageal	gastroesofágico
gastrointestinale	gastrointestinal, Magendarm-	gastrointestinal
gastroscopio	Gastroskop, Magenspiegel	gastroscopio
gastroschisi	Gastroschisis	gastrosquisis
gastrostomia	Gastrostomie	gastrotomía
gastrodigiunostomia	Gastrojejunostomie	gastroyeyunostomía
esofago (gola)	Speiseröhre	gaznate
gelatina	Gelatine, Gallerte	gelatina
gastrocnemio	gastrocnemius	gemelos
gemelli omozigoti	eineiige Zwillinge	gemelos idénticos
gene	Gen	gen
riproduttivo	fertil, Fortpflanzungs-	generador

SPANISH	ENGLISH	FRENCH
genérico *(n)*	generic *(n)*	dénomination commune d'un médicament *(n)*
genérico *(a)*	generic *(a)*	générique *(a)*
género	genus	genre
genética	genetics	génétique
genético	genetic	génétique
genital	genital	génital
genitales	genitalia	organes génitaux
genitourinario	genitourinary (GU)	génito-urinaire (GT)
genoma	genome	génome
genotipo	genotype	génotype
genu valgum	genu valgum, knock-knee	genu valgum, genou cagneux
genu varum	genu varum	genu varum
gérmen	germ	germe
geriatra	geriatrician	gériatre
geriatría	geriatrics	gériatrie
geriátrico	geriatric	gériatrique
gestación	gestation	gestation
gestacional	gravitational	gravitationnel
giardiasis	giardiasis	giardiase
ginecología	gynaecology (Eng), gynecology (Am)	gynécologie
ginecomastia	gynaecomastia (Eng), gynecomastia (Am)	gynécomastie
gingivitis	gingivitis	gingivite
glándula	gland	glande
glándula apocrina	apocrine gland	glande apocrine
glándula parótida	parotid gland	glande parotide
glándula paratiroidea	parathyroid gland	glande parathyroïde
glándula salivar	salivary gland	glande salivaire
glándulas de Bartolino	Bartholin's glands	glandes de Bartholin
glaucoma	glaucoma	glaucome
glenohumeral	glenohumeral	gléno-huméral
glenoide	glenoid	glénoïde
glioma	glioma	gliome
globo histérico	globus hystericus	boule hystérique
glóbulo rojo	red blood cell (RBC)	globule rouge
glomerulitis	glomerulitis	glomérulite
glomérulo	glomerulus	glomérule
glomerulonefritis	glomerulonephritis	glomérulonéphrite
glomerulosclerosis	glomerulosclerosis	glomérulosclérose
glositis	glossitis	glossite
glosodinia	glossodynia	glossodynie
glosofaríngeo	glossopharyngeal	glossopharyngien
glotis	glottis	glotte
glucagón	glucagon	glucagon
glucemia	blood sugar	glycémie
glucemia en ayunas	fasting blood sugar (FBS)	glycémie à jeun

ITALIAN	GERMAN	SPANISH
medico generico (n)	Substanznahme (n), Generic (n)	genérico (n)
generico (a)	generisch (a)	genérico (a)
genere	Genus, Gattung	género
genetica	Genetik	genética
genetico	genetisch	genético
genitale	genital, Geschlechts-	genital
organi genitali	Genitalien	genitales
genito-urinario	urogenital	genitourinario
genoma	Genom	genoma
genotipo	Genotyp	genotipo
ginocchio valgo	Genu valgum, X-Bein	genu valgum
ginocchio varo	Genu varum, O-Bein	genu varum
germe	Erreger, Keim, Bazillus	gérmen
geriatra	Geriater	geriatra
geriatria	Geriatrie	geriatría
geriatrico	geriatrisch	geriátrico
gestazione	Gestation, Schwangerschaft	gestación
gravitazionale	Gravitations-	gestacional
giardiasi	Lambliasis	giardiasis
ginecologia	Gynäkologie, Frauenheilkunde	ginecología
ginecomastia	Gynäkomastie	ginecomastia
gengivite	Gingivitis, Zahnfleischentzündung	gingivitis
ghiandola	Glandula, Drüse	glándula
ghiandola apocrina	apokrine Drüse	glándula apocrina
ghiandola parotide	Parotis, Ohrspeicheldrüse	glándula parótida
ghiandola paratiroide	Nebenschilddrüse, Parathyreoidea	glándula paratiroidea
ghiandola salivare	Speicheldrüse	glándula salivar
ghiandole di Bartolini	Bartolini-Drüsen	glándulas de Bartolino
glaucoma	Glaukom, grüner Star	glaucoma
gleno-omerale	glenohumeral	glenohumeral
glenoide	Schultergelenk-	glenoide
glioma	Gliom	glioma
bolo isterico	Globus hystericus, Globusgefühl	globo histérico
eritrocito, globulo rosso (RBC)	Erythrozyt	glóbulo rojo
glomerulite	Glomerulitis	glomerulitis
glomerulo	Glomerulus	glomérulo
glomerulonefrite	Glomerulonephritis	glomerulonefritis
glomerulosclerosi	Glomerulosklerose	glomerulosclerosis
glossite	Glossitis	glositis
glossodinia	Glossodynie, Zungenschmerz	glosodinia
glossofaringeo	glossopharyngeal	glosofaríngeo
glottide	Glottis, Stimmritze	glotis
glucagone	Glukagon	glucagón
glicemia	Blutzucker	glucemia
glicemia a digiuno	Nüchternblutzucker (NBZ)	glucemia en ayunas

glucocorticoide	glucocorticoid	glucocorticoïde
glucogénesis	glucogenesis, glycogenesis	glucogenèse, glycogenèse
glucolisis	glycolysis	glycolyse
gluconeogénesis	gluconeogenesis	gluconéogenèse
glucosa	glucose	glucose
glucosuria	glycosuria	glycosurie
gluten	gluten	gluten
glúteo	gluteal	fessier
goma	gumma	gomme
gónada	gonad	gonade
gonadotropina	gonadotrophin (Eng), gonadotropin (Am)	gonadotrophine
gonadotropina coriónica humana (GCH)	human chorionic gonadotrophin (HCG) (Eng), human chorionic gonadotropin (HCG) (Am)	gonadotrophine chorionique humaine (GCH)
gonorrea	gonorrhea (Am), gonorrhoea (Eng)	gonorrhée
gota	gout	goutte
gota a gota intravenoso	drip	perfusion
gran mal	grand mal	grand mal
grano	pimple	bouton
granulación	granulation	granulation
granulocito	granulocyte	granulocyte
granuloma	granuloma	granulome
grasa	fat	graisse
graso	fat, adipose	gras, obèse, adipeux
gravedad	gravity	gravité
grupo sanguíneo	blood group	groupe sanguin
grupos de Lancefield	Lancefield's groups	groupes de streptocoques suivant la classification de Lancefield

ITALIAN	GERMAN	SPANISH
glicocorticoide	Glukokortikoid	glucocorticoide
glucogenesi, glicogenesi	Glukogenese, Glykogenese	glucogénesis
glicolisi	Glykolyse, Glukoseabbau	glucolisis
gluconeogenesi	Glukoneogenese	gluconeogénesis
glucosio	Glukose, Traubenzucker	glucosa
glicosuria	Glykosurie, Glukoseausscheidung im Urin	glucosuria
glutine	Gluten	gluten
gluteo	gluteal	glúteo
gomma	Gumma	goma
gonade	Gonade	gónada
gonadotropina	Gonadotropin	gonadotropina
gonadotropina corionica umana (GCU)	Choriongonadotropin (HCG)	gonadotropina coriónica humana (GCH)
gonorrea	Gonorrhoe, Tripper	gonorrea
gotta	Gicht	gota
fleboclisi	Tropfinfusion	gota a gota intravenoso
grande male	Grand mal	gran mal
pustola, piccolo foruncolo	Pickel, Mitesser	grano
granulazione	Granulation	granulación
granulocita	Granulozyt	granulocito
granuloma	Granulom, Granulationsgeschwulst	granuloma
adipe	Fett	grasa
grasso, adiposo	fett, fetthaltig, adipös, fettleibig	graso
gravità	Schwere (der Erkrankung)	gravedad
gruppo sanguigno	Blutgruppe	grupo sanguíneo
gruppi di Lancefield	Lancefield-Gruppen	grupos de Lancefield

H

habilidad	ability	capacité, aptitude, compétence
hábito	habit	habitude
habituación	habituation	accoutumance
halitosis	halitosis	halitose
hambre	hunger	faim
hebefrenia	hebephrenia	hébéphrénie
heces	faeces (Eng), feces (Am)	fèces
hemangioma	haemangioma (Eng), hemangioma (Am)	hémangiome
hemartrosis	haemarthrosis (Eng), hemarthrosis (Am)	hémarthrose
hematemesis	haematemesis (Eng), hematemesis (Am)	hématémèse
hematocolpos	haematocolpos (Eng), hematocolpos (Am)	hématocolpos
hematócrito	haematocrit (Eng), hematocrit (Am)	hématocrite
hematología	haematology (Eng), hematology (Am)	hématologie
hematoma	haematoma (Eng), hematoma (Am)	hématome
hematoma cefálico	cephalhaematoma (Eng), cephalhematoma (Am)	céphalhématome
hematuria	haematuria (Eng), hematuria (Am)	hématurie
hembra	female	femelle
hemiparesia	hemiparesis	hémiparésie
hemiplejía	hemiplegia	hémiplégie
hemocolectomía	hemicolectomy	hémicolectomie
hemocromatosis	haemochromatosis (Eng), hemochromatosis (Am)	hémochromatose
hemocultivo	blood culture	hémoculture
hemodiálisis	haemodialysis (Eng), hemodialysis (Am)	hémodialyse
hemofilia	haemophilia (Eng), hemophilia (Am)	hémophilie
hemoglobina (Hb)	haemoglobin (Hb) (Hg) (Eng), hemoglobin (Hb) (Hg) (Am)	hémoglobine (Hb) (Hg)
hemoglobinopatía	haemoglobinopathy (Eng), hemoglobinopathy (Am)	hémoglobinopathie
hemoglobinuria	haemoglobinuria (Eng), hemoglobinuria (Am)	hémoglobinurie
hemograma completo	complete blood count (CBC)	numération globulaire
hemólisis	haemolysis (Eng), hemolysis (Am)	hémolyse
hemoneumotórax	haemopneumothorax (Eng), hemopneumothorax (Am)	hémopneumothorax
hemopericardio	haemopericardium (Eng), hemopericardium (Am)	hémopéricarde
hemoperitoneo	haemoperitoneum (Eng), hemoperitoneum (Am)	hémopéritoine

abilità, capacità	Fähigkeit	habilidad
abitudine	Gewohnheit	hábito
assuefazione	Habituation, Gewöhnung	habituación
alitosi	Foetor ex ore, Mundgeruch	halitosis
fame	Hunger	hambre
ebefrenia	Hebephrenie	hebefrenia
feci	Fäzes, Kot	heces
emangioma	Hämangiom	hemangioma
emartrosi	Hämarthros	hemartrosis
ematemesi	Hämatemesis, Bluterbrechen	hematemesis
ematocolpo	Hämatokolpos	hematocolpos
ematrocrito	Hämatokrit (HKT)	hematócrito
ematologia	Hämatologie	hematología
ematoma	Hämatom, Bluterguß	hematoma
cefaloematoma	Kephalhämatom	hematoma cefálico
ematuria	Hämaturie, Blut im Urin	hematuria
femmina	weiblich	hembra
emiparesi	Hemiparese, unvollständige Halbseitenlähmung	hemiparesia
emiplegia	Hemiplegie, Halbseitenlähmung	hemiplejía
emicolectomia	Hemikolektomie	hemocolectomía
emocromatosi	Hämochromatose, Bronzediabetes	hemocromatosis
emocoltura	Blutkultur	hemocultivo
emodialisi	Hämodialyse	hemodiálisis
emofilia	Hämophilie, Bluterkrankheit	hemofilia
emoglobina (E)	Hämoglobin	hemoglobina (Hb)
emoglobinopatia	Hämoglobinopathie	hemoglobinopatía
emoglobinuria	Hämoglobinurie	hemoglobinuria
esame emocromocitometrico	großes Blutbild	hemograma completo
emolisi	Hämolyse	hemólisis
emopneumotorace	Hämatopneumothorax	hemoneumotórax
emopericardio	Hämatoperikard	hemopericardio
emoperitoneo	Hämatoperitoneum	hemoperitoneo

SPANISH	ENGLISH	FRENCH
hemopoyesis	haemopoiesis (Eng), hemopoiesis (Am)	hémopoïèse
hemoptisis	haemoptysis (Eng), hemoptysis (Am)	hémoptysie
hemorragia	haemorrhage (Eng), hemorrhage (Am)	hémorragie
hemorragia subaracnoidea	subarachnoid haemorrhage (Eng), subarachnoid hemorrhage (Am)	hémorragie sous-arachnoïdienne
hemorragia uterina funcional	dysfunctional uterine bleeding (DUB)	ménométrorragies fonctionnelles
hemorroide	haemorrhoid (Eng), hemorrhoid (Am)	hémorroïde
hemorroidectomía	haemorrhoidectomy (Eng), hemorrhoidectomy (Am)	hémorroïdectomie
hemorroides	piles	hémorroïdes
hemostasis	haemostasis (Eng), hemostasis (Am)	hémostase
hemotórax	haemothorax (Eng), hemothorax (Am)	hémothorax
hepático	hepatic	hépatique
hepatitis	hepatitis	hépatite
hepatitis vírica	viral hepatitis	hépatite virale
hepatocelular	hepatocellular	hépatocellulaire
hepatoma	hepatoma	hépatome
hepatomegalia	hepatomegaly	hépatomégalie
hepatosplenomegalia	hepatosplenomegaly	hépatosplénomégalie
hepatotóxico	hepatotoxic	hépatotoxique
hereditario	hereditary	héréditaire
herencia	heredity	hérédité
herida	wound	plaie
herida penetrante	penetrating wound	plaie par pénétration
hermafrodita	hermaphrodite	hermaphrodite
hermano no gemelo	sibling	frère ou soeur
hernia	hernia	hernie
hernia de disco	slipped disc	hernie discale
hernia estrangulada	strangulated hernia	hernie étranglée
hernia umbilical	exomphalos, umbilical hernia	exomphale, hernie ombilicale
herniorrafia	herniorraphy	herniorrhaphie
herniotomía	herniotomy	herniotomie
herpes	herpes	herpès
herpes labial	cold sore	herpès
herpes zóster	shingles	zona
heterogéneo	heterogenous	hétérogène
heterosexual	heterosexual	hétérosexuel
hialitis	hyalitis	hyalite
hialoide	hyaloid	hyaloïde
hidramnios	hydramnios	hydramnios
hidratar	hydrate	hydrater
hidrato	hydrate	hydrate
hidrato de carbono	carbohydrate (CHO)	glucide
hidrocéfalo	hydrocephalus	hydrocéphale
hidrocele	hydrocele	hydrocèle
hidrólisis	hydrolysis	hydrolyse
hidronefrosis	hydronephrosis	hydronéphrose

ITALIAN	GERMAN	SPANISH
ematopoiesi	Hämatopoese	hemopoyesis
cartilagine costale	Hämoptoe, Bluthusten	hemoptisis
emorragia	Hämorrhagie, Blutung	hemorragia
emorragia subaracnoidea	Subarachnoidalblutung	hemorragia subaracnoidea
sanguinamento uterino funzionale	dysfunktionale Uterusblutung	hemorragia uterina funcional
emorroide	Hämorrhoide	hemorroide
emorroidectomia	Hämorrhoidektomie, Hämorrhoidenoperation	hemorroidectomía
emorroidi	Hämorrhoiden	hemorroides
emostasi	Hämostase, Blutgerinnung	hemostasis
emotorace	Hämatothorax	hemotórax
epatico	hepatisch, Leber-	hepático
epatite	Hepatitis	hepatitis
epatite virale	Virushepatitis	hepatitis vírica
epatocellulare	hepatozellulär	hepatocelular
epatoma	Hepatom	hepatoma
epatomegalia	Hepatomegalie	hepatomegalia
epatosplenomegalia	Hepatosplenomegalie	hepatosplenomegalia
epatotossico	leberschädigend	hepatotóxico
ereditario	hereditär, erblich	hereditario
eredità	Erblichkeit, Vererbung	herencia
ferita	Wunde, Verletzung	herida
ferita penetrante	penetrierende Verletzung	herida penetrante
ermafrodito	Hermaphrodit, Zwitter	hermafrodita
fratello germano	Geschwister	hermano no gemelo
ernia	Hernie, Bruch	hernia
ernia discale	Bandscheibenvorfall	hernia de disco
ernia strozzata	inkarzerierte Hernie	hernia estrangulada
ernia ombelicale, protrusione dell'ombelico	Exomphalos, Nabelbruch	hernia umbilical
erniorrafia	Bruchoperation	herniorrafia
erniotomia	Herniotomie	herniotomía
herpes	Herpes, Bläschenausschlag	herpes
herpes, labialis	Herpes	herpes labial
herpes zoster	Herpes zoster, Gürtelrose	herpes zóster
eterogenico	heterogen	heterogéneo
eterosessuale	heterosexuell	heterosexual
ialinite	Hyalitis	hialitis
ialoideo	Glaskörper-	hialoide
idramnios	Hydramnion	hidramnios
idratare	hydrieren, hydratisieren	hidratar
idrato	Hydrat	hidrato
carboidrato	Kohlenhydrat, Kohlenwasserstoff	hidrato de carbono
idrocefalo	Hydrozephalus	hidrocéfalo
idrocele	Hydrozele, Wasserbruch	hidrocele
idrolisi	Hydrolyse	hidrólisis
idronefrosi	Hydronephrose	hidronefrosis

SPANISH	ENGLISH	FRENCH
hidrosálpinx	hydrosalpinx	hydrosalpinx
hidrosis	hidrosis	transpiration
hígado	liver	foie
higiene	hygiene	hygiène
higiene profesional	occupational health	hygiène du travail
higroma	hygroma	hygroma
hilio	hilum	hile
himen	hymen	hymen
himenectomía	hymenectomy	hymenectomie
hinchado	swollen	enflé
hioides	hyoid	hyoïde
hipema	hyphaema (Eng), hyphema (Am)	hyphéma
hiperacidez	hyperacidity	hyperacidité
hiperactividad	hyperactivity	hyperactivité
hiperalgesia	hyperalgesia	hyperalgie, hyperalgésie
hiperbilirrubinemia	hyperbilirubinaemia (Eng), hyperbilirubinemia (Am)	hyperbilirubinémie
hipercalcemia	hypercalcaemia (Eng), hypercalcemia (Am)	hypercalcémie
hipercalciuria	hypercalciuria	hypercalciurie
hipercaliemia	hyperkalaemia (Eng), hyperkalemia (Am)	hyperkaliémie
hipercapnia	hypercapnia	hypercapnie
hipercolesterolemia	hypercholesterolaemia (Eng), hypercholesterolemia (Am)	hypercholestérolémie
hiperemesis	hyperemesis	hyperémèse
hiperemia	hyperaemia (Eng), hyperemia (Am)	hyperémie
hiperestesia	hyperaesthesia (Eng), hyperesthesia (Am)	hyperesthésie
hiperextensión	hyperextension	hyperextension
hiperflexión	hyperflexion	hyperflexion
hiperglucemia	hyperglycaemia (Eng), hyperglycemia (Am)	hyperglycémie
hiperhidrosis	hyperidrosis	hyperhidrose
hiperlipemia	hyperlipaemia (Eng), hyperlipemia (Am)	hyperlipémie
hiperlipoproteinemia	hyperlipoproteinaemia (Eng), hyperlipoproteinemia (Am)	hyperlipoprotéinémie
hipermetropía	hypermetropia	hypermétropie
hipernefroma	hypernephroma	hypernéphrome
hiperparatiroidismo	hyperparathyroidism	hyperparathyroïdisme
hiperpirexia	hyperpyrexia	hyperpyrexie
hiperplasia	hyperplasia	hyperplasie
hiperpnea	hyperpnea (Am), hyperpnoea (Eng)	hyperpnoïa
hipersensibilidad	hypersensitive	hypersensibilité
hipertelorismo	hypertelorism	hypertélorisme
hipertensión	hypertension	hypertension
hipertensión portal	portal hypertension	circulation porte
hipertermia	hyperthermia	hyperthermie

ITALIAN	GERMAN	SPANISH
idrosalpinge	Hydrosalpinx	hidrosálpinx
idrosi, sudorazione	Hidrosis, Schweißabsonderung	hidrosis
fegato	Leber	hígado
igiene	Hygiene	higiene
medicina del lavoro	Gewerbehygiene	higiene profesional
igroma	Hygrom	higroma
ilo	Hilus	hilio
imene	Hymen	himen
imenectomia	Hymenektomie	himenectomía
gonfio, tumefatto	geschwollen, vergrößert	hinchado
ioide	Os hyeoideum	hioides
ifema	Hyphaema	hipema
iperacidità	Hyperazidität	hiperacidez
iperattività	Überaktivität	hiperactividad
iperalgesia	Hyperalgesie	hiperalgesia
iperbilirubinemia	Hyperbilirubinämie	hiperbilirrubinemia
ipercalcemia	Hyperkalzämie	hipercalcemia
ipercalciuria	Hyperkalziurie	hipercalciuria
iperkaliemia, iperpotassiemia	Hyperkaliämie	hipercaliemia
ipercapnia	Hyperkapnie	hipercapnia
ipercolesterolemia	Hypercholesterinämie	hipercolesterolemia
iperemesi	Hyperemesis	hiperemesis
iperemia	Hyperämie	hiperemia
iperestesia	Hyperästhesie	hiperestesia
iperestensione	Überdehnung, Überstreckung	hiperextensión
iperflessione	Hyperflexion	hiperflexión
iperglicemia	Hyperglykämie	hiperglucemia
iperidrosi	Hyperhidrosis	hiperhidrosis
iperlipemia	Hyperlipämie	hiperlipemia
iperlipoproteinemia	Hyperlipoproteinämie	hiperlipoproteinemia
ipermetropia	Hypermetropie, Weitsichtigkeit	hipermetropía
ipernefroma	Hypernephrom	hipernefroma
iperparatiroidismo	Hyperparathyreoidismus	hiperparatiroidismo
iperpiressia	Hyperpyrexie	hiperpirexia
iperplasia	Hyperplasie	hiperplasia
iperpnea	Hyperpnoe	hiperpnea
ipersensitività, ipersensibilità	Hypersensibilität, Überempfindlichkeit	hipersensibilidad
ipertelorismo	Hypertelorismus	hipertelorismo
ipertensione	Hypertonie	hipertensión
ipertensione portale	Pfortaderhochdruck	hipertensión portal
ipertermia	Hyperthermie	hipertermia

SPANISH	ENGLISH	FRENCH
hipertiroidismo	hyperthyroidism	hyperthyroïdisme
hipertonía	hypertonia	hypertonie
hipertónico	hypertonic	hypertonique
hipertrofia	hypertrophy	hypertrophie
hiperventilación	hyperventilation	hyperventilation
hipervolemia	hypervolaemia (Eng), hypervolemia (Am)	hypervolémie
hipnosis	hypnosis	hypnose
hipnoterapia	hypnotherapy	hypnothérapie
hipnótico (n)	hypnotic (n)	hypnotique (n)
hipnótico (a)	hypnotic (a)	hypnotique (a)
hipo	hiccup	hoquet
hipocalcemia	hypocalcaemia (Eng), hypocalcemia (Am)	hypocalcémie
hipocaliemia	hypokalaemia (Eng), hypokalemia (Am)	hypokalémie
hipocapnia	hypocapnia	hypocapnie
hipocondría	hypochondria	hypocondrie
hipocondrio	hypochondrium	hypocondre
hipocrómico	hypochromic	hypochromique
hipodérmico	hypodermic	hypodermique
hipoestesia	hypoaesthesia (Eng), hypoesthesia (Am)	hypoesthésie, hypesthésie
hipofaringe	hypopharynx	hypopharynx
hipófisis	pituitary gland	hypophyse
hipofunción	hypofunction	hypofonction
hipogastrio	hypogastrium	hypogastre
hipogloso	hypoglossal nerve	hypoglosse
hipoglucemia	hypoglycaemia (Eng), hypoglycemia (Am)	hypoglycémie
hipohidrosis	hypoidrosis	hypohidrose
hipomanía	hypomania	hypomanie
hipoparatiroidismo	hypoparathyroidism	hypoparathyroïdisme
hipopión	hypopyon	hypopyon
hipopituitarismo	hypopituitarism	hypopituitarisme
hipoplasia	hypoplasia	hypoplasie
hipopnea	hypopnea (Am), hypopnoea (Eng)	hypopnée
hipoproteinemia	hypoproteinaemia (Eng), hypoproteinemia (Am)	hypoprotéinémie
hiposecreción	hyposecretion	hyposécrétion
hiposensibilidad	hyposensitive	hyposensibilité
hipospadias	hypospadias	hypospadias
hipostasis	hypostasis	hypostase
hipotálamo	hypothalamus	hypothalamus
hipotensión	hypotension	hypotension
hipotensor (n)	antihypertensive (n)	antihypertenseur (n)

ipertiroidismo	Hyperthyreoidismus, Schilddrüsenüberfunktion	hipertiroidismo
ipertonia	Hypertension, Hypertonus	hipertonía
ipertonico	hyperton	hipertónico
ipertrofia	Hypertrophie	hipertrofia
iperventilazione	Hyperventilation	hiperventilación
ipervolemia	Hypervolämie	hipervolemia
ipnosi	Hypnose	hipnosis
ipnoterapia	Hypnotherapie	hipnoterapia
ipnotico (n)	Schlafmittel (n), Hypnotikum (n)	hipnótico (n)
ipnotico (a)	hypnotisch (a)	hipnótico (a)
singhiozzo	Schluckauf	hipo
ipocalcemia	Hypokalzämie	hipocalcemia
ipokalemia	Hypokaliämie	hipocaliemia
ipocapnia	Hypokapnie	hipocapnia
ipocondria	Hypochondrie	hipocondría
ipocondrio	Hypochondrium	hipocondrio
ipocromico	hypochrom, farbarm	hipocrómico
ipodermico	subkutan	hipodérmico
ipoestesia	Hypästhesie	hipoestesia
ipofaringe	Hypopharynx	hipofaringe
ghiandola pituitaria, ipofisi	Hypophyse	hipófisis
ipofunzione	Unterfunktion	hipofunción
ipogastrio	Hypogastrium	hipogastrio
ipoglosso	Nervus hypoglossus	hipogloso
ipoglicemia	Hypoglykämie	hipoglucemia
ipoidrosi	Hypohidrosis, Schweißmangel	hipohidrosis
ipomania	Hypomanie	hipomanía
ipoparatiroidismo	Hypoparathyreoidismus	hipoparatiroidismo
ipopion	Hypopyon	hipopión
ipopituitarismo	Hypopituitarismus	hipopituitarismo
ipoplasia	Hypoplasie	hipoplasia
ipopnea	flache Atmung	hipopnea
ipoproteinemia	Hypoproteinämie	hipoproteinemia
iposecrezione	Sekretionsmangel, Sekretionsschwäche	hiposecreción
iposensitività, iposensibilità	hyposensibel, unterempfindlich	hiposensibilidad
ipospadia	Hypospadie	hipospadias
ipostasi	Hypostase	hipostasis
ipotalamo	Hypothalamus	hipotálamo
ipotensione	Hypotonie	hipotensión
anti-ipertensivo (n)	Antihypertonikum (n), Antihypertensivum (n)	hipotensor (n)

SPANISH	ENGLISH	FRENCH
hipotensor *(a)*	antihypertensive *(a)*	antihypertensif *(a)*
hipotermia	hypothermia	hypothermie
hipotiroidismo	hypothyroidism	hypothyroïdisme
hipotonía	hypotonia	hypotonie
hipotónico	hypotonic	hypotonique
hipoventilación	hypoventilation	hypoventilation
hipovolemia	hypovolaemia *(Eng)*, hypovolemia *(Am)*	hypovolémie
hipoxemia	hypoxaemia *(Eng)*, hypoxemia *(Am)*	hypoxémie
hipoxia	hypoxia	hypoxie
hirsutismo	hirsuties, hirsutism	hirsutisme
histerectomía	hysterectomy	hystérectomie
histeria	hysteria	hystérie
histerosalpingectomía	hysterosalpingectomy	hystérosalpingectomie
histerosalpingografía	hysterosalpingography	hystérosalpingographie
histerotomía	hysterotomy	hystérotomie
histiocito	histiocyte	histiocyte
histiocitoma	histiocytoma	histiocytome
histólisis	histolysis	histolyse
histología	histology	histologie
hombro	shoulder	épaule
hombro congelado/rígido	frozen shoulder	épaule ankylosée
homeopatía	homeopathy *(Am)*, homoeopathy *(Eng)*	homéopathie
homeostasis	homeostasis	homéostasie
homicidio	homicide	homicide
homocigoto	homozygous	homozygote
homogéneo	homogeneous *(Eng)*, homogenous *(Am)*	homogène
homólogo	homologous	homologue
homónimo	homonymous	homonyme
homosexual *(n)*	homosexual *(n)*	homosexuel *(n)*
homosexual *(a)*	homosexual *(a)*	homosexuel *(a)*
hongo	fungus	mycète
hormona	hormone	hormone
hormona adrenocorticotropa (ACTH)	adrenocorticotrophic hormone (ACTH)	hormone adrénocorticotrope (ACTH)
hormona corticosuprarrenal (HCS)	adrenal cortical hormone (ACH)	hormone cortico-surrénale
hormona del crecimiento (HC)	growth hormone (GH)	hormone de croissance (HGH), somatotrophine (STH)
hormona estimulante del folículo (FSH)	follicle stimulating hormone (FSH)	hormone folliculo-stimulante, gonadotrophine A
hormona estimulante del tiroides (TSH)	thyroid stimulating hormone (TSH)	thyrotrophine, thyréostimuline
hormona luteinizante (LH)	luteinizing hormone (LH)	hormone lutéinisante (HL)
horquilla	fourchette	fourchette
hospicio	hospice	hospice, asile

ITALIAN	GERMAN	SPANISH
anti-ipertensivo *(a)*	blutdrucksenkend *(a)*, antihypertensiv *(a)*	hipotensor *(a)*
ipotermia	Hypothermie	hipotermia
ipotiroidismo	Hypothyreose	hipotiroidismo
ipotonia	Hypotonie	hipotonía
ipotonico	hypoton	hipotónico
ipoventilazione	Hypoventilation	hipoventilación
ipovolemia	Hypovolämie	hipovolemia
ipossiemia	Hypoxämie	hipoxemia
ipossia	Hypoxie	hipoxia
irsutismo	Hirsutismus	hirsutismo
isterectomia	Hysterektomie	histerectomía
isteria	Hysterie	histeria
isterosalpingectomia	Hysterosalpingektomie	histerosalpingectomía
isterosalpingografia	Hysterosalpingographie	histerosalpingografía
isterotomia	Hysterotomie	histerotomía
istiocito	Histiozyt	histiocito
istiocitoma	Histiozytom	histiocitoma
istolisi	Histolyse	histólisis
istologia	Histologie	histología
spalla	Schulter	hombro
'spalla congelata', periartrite scapoloomerale	Frozen shoulder, Periarthritis humeroscapularis	hombro congelado/rígido
omeopatia	Homöopathie	homeopatía
omeostasi	Homöostase	homeostasis
omicidio	Totschlag, Mord	homicidio
omozigote	homozygot	homocigoto
omogeneo	homogen	homogéneo
omologo	homolog	homólogo
omonimo	homonym	homónimo
omosessuale *(n)*	Homosexueller *(n)*	homosexual *(n)*
omosessuale *(a)*	homosexuell *(a)*	homosexual *(a)*
fungo	Pilz	hongo
ormone	Hormon	hormona
ormone corticotropo (ACTH)	adrenokortikotropes Hormon (ACTH)	hormona adrenocorticotropa (ACTH)
ormone corticosurrenale	Nebennierenrindenhormon (ACH)	hormona corticosuprarrenal (HCS)
ormone della crescita (GH)	Wachstumshormon	hormona del crecimiento (HC)
ormone follicolostimolante (FSH)	follikelstimulierendes Hormon (FSH)	hormona estimulante del folículo (FSH)
ormone tireotropo (TSH)	Thyreotropin	hormona estimulante del tiroides (TSH)
ormone luteinizzante (LH)	luteinisierendes Hormon	hormona luteinizante (LH)
forchetta	hintere Schamlippenkommissur	horquilla
ricovero	Hospiz	hospicio

SPANISH	ENGLISH	FRENCH
hospital	hospital	hôpital
hospital de día	day hospital	hôpital de jour
huesecillos	ossicle	osselet
hueso	bone	os
hueso coxal o ilíaco	hip bone	os coxal
huésped	host	hôte
huevo	egg	oeuf
huez de Adán	Adam's apple	pomme d'Adam
húmero	humerus	humérus
hydrops fetal	hydrops fetalis	anasarque foeto-placentaire

ITALIAN	GERMAN	SPANISH
ospedale	Krankenhaus, Hospital	hospital
ospedale diurno	Tagesklinik	hospital de día
ossicino	Gehörknöchelchen, Ossikel	huesecillos
osso	Knochen, Gräte	hueso
osso iliaco	Hüftknochen	hueso coxal o ilíaco
ospite	Wirt	huésped
uovo	Ei, Ovum	huevo
pomo di Adamo	Adamsapfel	huez de Adán
omero	Humerus, Oberarmknochen	húmero
idrope fetale	Hydrops fetalis	hydrops fetal

I

ictericia	icterus, jaundice	ictère, jaunisse
ictericia nuclear	kernicterus	ictère cérébral
ictiosis	ichthyosis	ichthyose
ictus	stroke	apoplexie
id	id	ça
idea	idea	idée
idea delusiva	delusion	hallucination
identificación	identification	identification
idiopático	idiopathic	idiopathique
idiosincrasia	idiosyncrasy	idiosyncrasie
ileítis	ileitis	iléite
ileítis regional	regional ileitis	iléite régionale
íleo	ileus	iléus
ileocecal	ileocaecal (Eng), ileocecal (Am)	iléocaecal
ileoctomía	ileectomy	iléoctomie
ileón	ileum	iléon
ileostomía	ileostomy	iléostomie
ilíaco	iliac	iliaque
ilion	ilium	ilion
ilusión	illusion	illusion
impactado	impacted	enclavé
imperforado	imperforate	imperforé
impétigo	impetigo	impétigo
implantación	implantation	implantation
implantar	implant	implanter
implante	implant	implant
impotencia	impotence	impotence
impulso	impulse	impulsion
inadaptación	maladjustment	inadaptation
incarcerado	incarcerated	incarcéré
incesto	incest	inceste
incidencia	incidence	fréquence
incipiente	incipient	débutant
incisión	incision	incision
incisivo	incisor	incisive
inclinado	prone	en pronation
incompatibilidad	incompatibility	incompatibilité
incompatibilidad Rhesus	Rhesus incompatibility	incompatibilité Rhésus
incompetencia	incompetence	incompétence
inconsciente	unconscious	sans connaissance
incontinencia	incontinence	incontinence
incoordinación	incoordination	incoordination
incubación	incubation	incubation
incubadora	incubator	incubateur

ITALIAN	GERMAN	SPANISH
ittero	Ikterus, Gelbsucht	ictericia
ittero nucleare	Kernikterus	ictericia nuclear
ittiosi	Ichthyosis	ictiosis
ictus, colpo apoplettico, accidente cerebrovascolare	Schlag, Schlaganfall	ictus
incoscio	Es	id
idea	Gedanke, Vorstellung	idea
allucinazione, fissazione	Wahn, Wahnvorstellung	idea delusiva
indentificazione	Identifizierung	identificación
idiopatico	idiopathisch, essentiell	idiopático
idiosincrasia	Idiosynkrasie	idiosincrasia
ileite	Ileitis	ileítis
ileite regionale	Ileitis regionalis	ileítis regional
ileo, occlusione intestinale acuta	Ileus, Darmverschluß	íleo
ileocecale	ileozäkal	ileocecal
ileectomia	Ileumresecktion	ileoctomía
ileo	Ileum	íleón
ileostomia	Ileostomie	ileostomía
iliaco	ileo-	ilíaco
ilio, osso dell'anca	Os ilium	ilion
illusione	Illusion	ilusión
impatto, compresso, incuneato	impaktiert	impactado
imperforato	nicht perforiert	imperforado
impetigine	Impetigo	impétigo
impianto	Implantation	implantación
impiantare	implantieren	implantar
impianto chirurgico sottocutaneo di farmaci	Implantat	implante
impotenza	Impotenz	impotencia
impulso	Impuls, Reiz	impulso
assestamento difettoso	Fehlanpassung	inadaptación
incarcerato	inkarzeriert, eingeklemmt	incarcerado
incesto	Inzest	incesto
incidenza	Inzidenz	incidencia
incipiente	beginnend	incipiente
incisione	Inzision, Einschnitt	incisión
incisore	Schneidezahn	incisivo
prono	veranlagt, empfänglich	inclinado
incompatibilità	Inkompatibilität, Unverträglichkeit	incompatibilidad
incompatibilità Rh	Rh-Unverträglichkeit	incompatibilidad Rhesus
incompetenza	Insuffizienz	incompetencia
inconscio	bewußtlos	inconsciente
incontinenza	Inkontinenz	incontinencia
incoordinazione	Inkoordination	incoordinación
incubazione	Inkubation	incubación
incubatore	Inkubator, Brutkasten	incubadora

SPANISH	ENGLISH	FRENCH
incumplimiento	noncompliance	non observance
incus	incus	enclume
indicador	indicator	indicateur
índice de Apgar	Apgar score	indice d'Apgar
índice de masa corporal (IMC)	body mass index (BMI)	indice de masse corporelle (IMC)
indice de tiroxina libre	free thyroxine index (FTI)	index de thyroxine libre
indígena	indigenous	indigène
indigestión	indigestion	indigestion
inducción	induction	induction
induración	induration	induration
inercia	inertia	inertie
inervación	innervation	innervation
infantil	infantile	infantile
infarto	infarction	infarcissement
infarto de miocardio (IM)	myocardial infarction (MI)	infarctus du myocarde
infección	infection	infection
infección de las vías respiratorias altas	upper respiratory tract infection (URTI)	infection des voies respiratoires supérieures
infección de las vías respiratorias bajas	lower respiratory tract infection (LRTI)	infection du poumon profond
infección de las vías urinarias (IVU)	urinary tract infection (UTI)	infection des voies urinaires
infección oportunista	opportunistic infection	infection opportuniste
infeccioso	infective	infectieux
inferior	inferior	inférieur
infertilidad	infertility	infertilité
infestación	infestation	infestation
infiltración	infiltration	infiltration
inflamación	inflammation	inflammation
influenza	influenza	grippe
infundir	drip	perfuser
infusión	infusion	infusion
ingestión	ingestion	ingestion
ingle	groin	aine
inguinal	inguinal	inguinal
inhalación	inhalation	inhalation
inhalación de pegamento	glue sniffing	intoxication par inhalation de solvant
inhalador spinhaler	spinhaler	turbo-inhalateur
inhalar	inhale	inhaler
inherente	inherent	inhérent
inhibición	inhibition	inhibition
inhibidor de la monoaminooxidasa (IMAO)	monoamine oxidase inhibitor (MAOI)	inhibiteur de la monoamine-oxydase (IMAO)
injertar	graft	greffer
injerto	flap, graft	lambeau, greffe
injerto corneal	corneal graft	greffe de la cornée
injerto óseo	bone graft	greffe osseuse

ITALIAN	GERMAN	SPANISH
inadempienza a prescrizioni	Noncompliance	incumplimiento
incudine	Incus, Amboß	incus
indicatore	Indikator	indicador
indice di Apgar	Apgar-Index	índice de Apgar
indice di massa corporea (IMC)	Körpermassenindex	índice de masa corporal (IMC)
indice di tiroxina libera	freier Thyroxinindex (FTi)	indice de tiroxina libre
indigeno	eingeboren, einheimisch	indígena
indigestione	Verdauungsstörung, Magenverstimmung	indigestión
induzione	Induktion, Einleitung	inducción
indurimento	Induration, Verhärtung	induración
inerzia	Trägheitsmoment, Untätigkeit	inercia
innervazione	Innervation	inervación
infantile	infantil, kindlich	infantil
infarto	Infarzierung	infarto
infarto miocardico	Myokardinfarkt, Herzinfarkt	infarto de miocardio (IM)
infezione	Infektion	infección
infezione del tratto respiratorio superiore (URTI)	Atemwegsinfekt	infección de las vías respiratorias altas
infezione del tratto respiratorio inferiore (LRTI)	Atemwegsinfekt (untere)	infección de las vías respiratorias bajas
infezione delle vie urinarie (IVU)	Harnwegsinfekt	infección de las vías urinarias (IVU)
infezione opportunista	opportunistische Infektion	infección oportunista
infettivo	infektiös, ansteckend	infeccioso
inferiore	tiefer gelegen, minderwertig	inferior
infertilità	Infertilität	infertilidad
infestazione	Befall	infestación
infiltrazione	Infiltration	infiltración
infiammazione	Entzündung	inflamación
influenza	Influenza, Grippe	influenza
gocciolare, far gocciolare	tröpfeln, tropfen	infundir
infusione	Infusion	infusión
ingestione	Einnahme, Aufnahme	ingestión
inguine	Leiste	ingle
inguinale	inguinal, Leisten-	inguinal
inalazione	Inhalation, Einatmen	inhalación
inalazione di toluene o collanti	Schnüffeln, Leimschnüffeln	inhalación de pegamento
nebulizzatore per farmaci	Drehinhaliergerät	inhalador spinhaler
inalare	inhalieren, einatmen	inhalar
inerente	eigen, angeboren	inherente
inibizione	Inhibierung, Hemmung	inhibición
inibitore monoaminoossidasi (IMAO)	Monoaminoxydase-Hemmer	inhibidor de la monoaminooxidasa (IMAO)
trapiantare	transplantieren, übertragen	injertar
lembo, innesto, trapianto	Lappen, Hautlappen, Transplantat, Transplantation, Plastik	injerto
trapianto corneale	Korneaplastik	injerto corneal
trapianto osseo	Osteoplastik, Knochentransplantation	injerto óseo

SPANISH	ENGLISH	FRENCH
inmediatamente después del comienzo	immediately after onset (IAO)	immédiatement après le début
inmune	immune	immun
inmunidad	immunity	immunité
inmunización	immunization	immunisation
inmunodeficiencia	immunodeficiency	immunodéficience
inmunoensayo	immunoassay	dosage immunologique, immunodosage
inmunofluorescencia	immunofluorescence	immunofluorescence
inmunoglobulina (Ig)	immunoglobulin (Ig)	immunoglobuline (lg)
inmunología	immunology	immunologie
inmunosupresión	immunosuppression	immunosuppression
innato	innate	endogène
inocente	innocent	innocent
inoculación	inoculation	inoculation
inocuo	innocuous	inoffensif
inorgánico	inorganic	inorganique
inotrópico	inotropic	inotrope
inseminación	insemination	insémination
inseminación artificial	artificial insemination (AI)	insémination artificielle (IA)
inseminación artificial por donante (AID)	artificial insemination by donor (AID)	insémination hétérologue
insensible	insensible	insensible
inserción	insertion	insertion
insidioso	insidious	insidieux
in situ	in situ	in situ
insolación	heatstroke, sunstroke	coup de chaleur, insolation
insomnio	insomnia	insomnie
inspiración	inspiration	inspiration
instilación	instillation	instillation
instinto	instinct	instinct
institucionalización	institutionalization	institutionalisation
insuficiencia cardíaca	heart failure	cardiopathie, maladie du coeur
insuficiencia cardíaca congestiva (ICC)	congestive cardiac failure (CCF), congestive heart failure (CHF)	insuffisance cardiaque globale
insuficiencia coronaria	coronary heart failure (CHF)	insuffisance coronarienne cardiaque
insuficiencia coronaria crónico	chronic coronary insufficiency (CCI)	insuffisance coronarienne chronique
insuficiencia placentaria	placental insufficiency	insuffisance placentaire
insuficiencia respiratoria	respiratory failure	insuffisance respiratoire
insuficiencia vertebrobasilar	vertebrobasilar insufficiency (VBI), basilar-vertebral insufficiency	insuffisance vertébro-basilaire, insuffisance basilaire vertébrale
insuflación	insufflation	insufflation
insulina	insulin	insuline
intelecto	intellect	intellect
inteligencia	intelligence	intelligence
interacción	interaction	interaction
interarticular	interarticular	interarticulaire
intercostal	intercostal	intercostal
intercurrente	intercurrent	intercurrent

ITALIAN	GERMAN	SPANISH
immediatamente dopo l'attacco	unmittelbar nach Krankheitsausbruch	inmediatamente después del comienzo
immune	immun	inmune
immunità	Immunität	inmunidad
immunizzazione	Immunisierung, Schutzimpfung	inmunización
immunodeficienza	Immundefekt	inmunodeficiencia
dosaggio immunologico	Immunoassay	inmunoensayo
immunofluorescenza	Immunfluoreszenz	inmunofluorescencia
immunoglobulina (Ig)	Immunglobulin	inmunoglobulina (Ig)
immunologia	Immunologie	inmunología
immunosoppressione	Immunsuppression	inmunosupresión
innato	kongenital, angeboren	innato
innocente	unschuldig, unschädlich	inocente
inoculazione	Impfung	inoculación
innocuo	unschädlich, harmlos	inocuo
inorganico	anorganisch	inorgánico
inotropo	inotrop	inotrópico
inseminazione	Befruchtung	inseminación
inseminazione artificiale	künstliche Befruchtung	inseminación artificial
fecondazione artificiale tramite donatore	heterologe Insemination	inseminación artificial por donante (AID)
insensibile	bewußtlos, unempfindlich	insensible
inserzione	Insertion	inserción
insidioso	heimtückisch, schleichend	insidioso
in situ	in situ	in situ
colpo di calore, colpo di sole	Hitzschlag, Sonnenstich	insolación
insonnia	Schlaflosigkeit	insomnio
inspirazione	Inspiration, Einatmung	inspiración
istillazione	Einträufelung, Einflößung	instilación
istinto	Instinkt	instinto
istituzionalizzazione	Institutionalisierung	institucionalización
scompenso cardiaco	Herzinsuffizienz, Herzversagen	insuficiencia cardíaca
insufficienza cardiaca congestizia, scompenso cardiaco congestizio	Stauungsherz, Herzinsuffizienz mit Stauungszeichen	insuficiencia cardíaca congestiva (ICC)
insufficienza cardiaca coronarica	Herzinfarkt	insuficiencia coronaria
insufficienza coronarica cronica	chronische Koronarinsuffizienz	insuficiencia coronaria crónico
insufficienza placentare	Plazentainsuffizienz	insuficiencia placentaria
insufficienza respiratoria	respiratorische Insuffizienz	insuficiencia respiratoria
insufficienza vertebrobasilare	vertebrobasiläre Insuffizienz, Basilarvertebralinsuffizienz	insuficiencia vertebrobasilar
insufflazione	Insufflation	insuflación
insulina	Insulin	insulina
intelletto	Intellekt	intelecto
intelligenza	Intelligenz	inteligencia
interazione	Wechselwirkung	interacción
interarticolare	interartikulär	interarticular
intercostale	interkostal	intercostal
intercorrente	interkurrent	intercurrente

SPANISH	ENGLISH	FRENCH
interespinoso	interspinous	interépineux
interleucina	interleukin	interleukine
intermenstrual	intermenstrual	intermenstruel
intermitente	intermittent	intermittent
interno	internal	interne
interóseo	interosseous	interosseux
interrupción del embarazo	termination of pregnancy (TOP)	interruption de grossesse (IG)
intersticial	interstitial	interstitiel
intertrigo	intertrigo	intertrigo
intertrocantéreo	intertrochanteric	intertrochantérien
intervención quirúrgica	operation	opération
intervertebral	intervertebral	intervertébral
intestino	bowel, gut, intestine	intestin
íntima	intima	intima
intolerancia	intolerance	intolérance
intoxicación alimentaria	food poisoning	intoxication alimentaire
intraabdominal	intra-abdominal	intra-abdominal
intraarterial	intra-arterial	intra-artériel
intracapsular	intracapsular	intracapsulaire
intracelular	intracellular	intracellulaire
intradérmico	intradermal	intradermique
intramural	intramural	intramural
intramuscular (im)	intramuscular (IM)	intramusculaire (IM)
intranasal	intranasal	intranasal
intraocular	intraocular	intra-oculaire
intraoral	intraoral	intra-oral
intra partum	intrapartum	intrapartum
intraperitoneal	intraperitoneal	intrapéritonéal
intratecal	intrathecal	intrathécal
intrauterino	intrauterine	intra-utérin
intravaginal	intravaginal	intravaginal
intravenoso (IV)	intravenous (IV)	intraveineux (IV)
intrínseco	intrinsic	intrinsèque
introito	introitus	orifice
introspección	introspection	introspection
introversión	introversion	introversion
introvertido	introvert	introverti
intubación	intubation	intubation
intususcepción	intussusception	intussusception
invaginación	invagination	invagination
invasión	invasion	invasion
inversión	inversion	inversion
in vitro	in vitro	in vitro
in vivo	in vivo	in vivo
involución	involution	involution
involuntario	involuntary	involontaire
inyección	injection	injection

ITALIAN	GERMAN	SPANISH
interspinoso	interspinal	interespinoso
interleuchina	Interleukin	interleucina
intermestruale	intermenstruel	intermenstrual
intermittente	intermittierend	intermitente
interno	intern, innerlich	interno
interosseo	interossär	interóseo
interruzione di gravidanza (IG)	Schwangerschaftsabbruch	interrupción del embarazo
interstiziale	interstitiell	intersticial
intertrigine	Intertrigo	intertrigo
intertrocanterico	intertrochantär	intertrocantéreo
operazione	Operation, Einwirkung, Eingriff	intervención quirúrgica
intervertebrale	intervertebral, Zwischenwirbel-	intervertebral
intestino	Darm	intestino
intima	Intima	íntima
intolleranza	Intoleranz, Unverträglichkeit	intolerancia
avvelenamento alimentare	Nahrungsmittelvergiftung	intoxicación alimentaria
intra-addominale	intraabdominal	intraabdominal
intra-arterioso	intraarteriell	intraarterial
intracapsulare	intrakapsulär	intracapsular
intracellulare	intrazellulär	intracelular
intradermico	intradermal, intrakutan	intradérmico
intramurale	intramural	intramural
intramuscolare (IM)	intramuskulär	intramuscular (im)
intranasale	intranasal	intranasal
intraoculare	intraokulär	intraocular
intraorale	intraoral	intraoral
intraparto	intra partum	intra partum
intraperitoneale	intraperitoneal	intraperitoneal
intratecale	intrathekal	intratecal
intrauterino	intrauterin	intrauterino
intravaginale	intravaginal	intravaginal
endovenoso (EV)	intravenös, endovenös	intravenoso (IV)
intrinseco	intrinsisch, endogen	intrínseco
introito	Introitus	introito
introspezione	Introspektion	introspección
introversione	Introversion	introversión
introverso	Introvertierter	introvertido
intubazione	Intubation	intubación
intussuscezione	Intussuszeption	intususcepción
invaginazione	Invagination	invaginación
invasione	Invasion	invasión
inversione	Inversion, Umkehrung	inversión
in vitro	in vitro	in vitro
in vivo	in vivo	in vivo
involuzione	Involution, Rückbildung	involución
involontario	unabsichtlich, unwillkürlich	involuntario
iniezione	Injektion, Spritze	inyección

SPANISH	ENGLISH	FRENCH
inyectar	inject	injecter
ión	ion	ion
ipsilateral	ipsilateral	ipsilatéral
iris	iris	iris
iritis	iritis	iritis
irradiación	irradiation	irradiation
irreductible	irreducible	irréductible
irrigación	irrigation	irrigation
irritable	irritable	irritable
irritante	irritant	irritant
islotes de Langerhans	islets of Langerhans	îlots de Langerhans, îlots pancréatiques
islotes pancreáticos	pancreatic islets	îlots pancréatiques, îlots de Langerhans
isoinmunización	isoimmunization	iso-immunisation
isométrico	isometric	isométrique
isotónico	isotonic	isotonique
isquemia	ischaemia (Eng), ischemia (Am)	ischémie
isquión	ischium	ischion
isquiorrectal	ischiorectal	ischio-rectal
istmo	isthmus	isthme

J

jadeo	wheeze	wheezing
jeringuilla	syringe	seringue
juanete	bunion	hallux valgus
jubilado	old age pensioner (OAP)	retraité(e)

K

kala-azar	kala-azar	kala-azar
kwashiorkor	kwashiorkor	kwashiorkor

ITALIAN	GERMAN	SPANISH
iniettare	injizieren, spritzen	**inyectar**
ione	Ion	**ión**
ipsilaterale, omolaterale	ipsilateral	**ipsilateral**
iride	Iris	**iris**
irite	Iritis	**iritis**
irradiazione	Bestrahlung	**irradiación**
irriducibile	unreduzierbar	**irreductible**
irrigazione	Spülung	**irrigación**
irritabile	reizbar, erregbar	**irritable**
irritante	reizend	**irritante**
isole di Langerhans	Langerhans-Inseln	**islotes de Langerhans**
isolotti pancreatici	Langerhans-Inseln	**islotes pancreáticos**
isoimmunizzazione	Isoimmunisierung	**isoinmunización**
isometrico	isometrisch	**isométrico**
isotonico	isotonisch	**isotónico**
ischemia	Ischämie	**isquemia**
ischio	Ischium, Sitzbein	**isquión**
ischiorettale	ischiorektal	**isquiorrectal**
istmo	Isthmus, Verengung	**istmo**
sibilo	Giemen	**jadeo**
siringa	Spritze	**jeringuilla**
borsite dell'alluce	entzündeter Fußballen	**juanete**
anziano pensionato	Rentner	**jubilado**
kala-azar	Kala-Azar	**kala-azar**
kwashiorkor	Kwashiorkor	**kwashiorkor**

L

SPANISH	ENGLISH	FRENCH
la belle indifférence	'belle indifference'	indifférence
laberintitis	labyrinthitis	labyrinthite
laberinto	labyrinth	labyrinthe
lábil	labile	labile
labilidad	lability	labilité
labio	lip	lèvre
labio leporino	harelip	bec-de-lièvre
labios	labia	lèvres
lacerado	lacerated	lacéré
lactación	lactation	lactation
lactante	infant	enfant, nourrisson
lactasa	lactase	lactase
lactato	lactate	lactate
lactosa	lactose	lactose
lactulosa	lactulose	lactulose
lagrimal	lacrimal	lacrymal
lágrimas	tears	larmes
lámina	lamina	lame
laminectomía	laminectomy	laminectomie
lanugo	lanugo	lanugo
laparoscopia	laparoscopy	coelioscopie
laparotomía	laparotomy	laparotomie
laringe	larynx	larynx
laríngeo	laryngeal	laryngien
laringitis	laryngitis	laryngite
laringología	laryngology	laryngologie
laringoscopio	laryngoscope	laryngoscope
laringospasmo	laryngospasm	laryngospasme
laringotraqueobronquitis	laryngotracheobronchitis	laryngotrachéobronchite
láser	laser	laser
lateral	lateral	latéral
latigazo	whiplash	coup de fouet
lavado	lavage	lavage
laxante *(n)*	aperient *(n)*, laxative *(n)*	laxatif *(n)*
laxante *(a)*	aperient *(a)*	laxatif *(a)*
laxativo	laxative	laxatif
leche	milk	lait
lecitina	lecithin	lécithine
legrado	curettage	curetage
legrar	curette (Eng), curet (Am)	cureter
leishmaniasis	leishmaniasis	leishmaniose
lengua	glossa, tongue	langue
lente de contacto	contact lens	verre de contact
lentigo	lentigo	lentigo

ITALIAN	GERMAN	SPANISH
'belle indifference'	belle indifference	la belle indifférence
labirintite	Labyrinthitis	laberintitis
labirinto	Labyrinth	laberinto
labile	labil	lábil
labilità	Labilität	labilidad
labbro	Lippe	labio
labbro leporino	Hasenscharte	labio leporino
labbra	Labia	labios
lacerato	eingerissen, zerrissen	lacerado
lattazione	Laktation, Milchbildung, Stillen	lactación
infante	Kleinkind, Säugling	lactante
lattasi	Laktase	lactasa
lattato	Laktat	lactato
lattosio	Laktose, Milchzucker	lactosa
lattulosio	Laktulose	lactulosa
lacrimale	Tränen-, Tränengangs-	lagrimal
lacrime	Tränen	lágrimas
lamina	Lamina	lámina
laminectomia	Laminektomie, Wirbelbogenresektion	laminectomía
lanugine	Lanugo	lanugo
laparoscopia	Laparoskopie, Bauchspiegelung	laparoscopia
laparotomia	Laparotomie	laparotomía
laringe	Larynx, Kehlkopf	laringe
laringeo	laryngeal, Kehlkopf-	laríngeo
laringite	Laryngitis	laringitis
laringologia	Laryngologie	laringología
laringoscopio	Laryngoskop, Kehlkopfspiegel	laringoscopio
laringospasmo	Laryngospasmus	laringospasmo
laringotracheobronchite	Laryngo-Tracheobronchitis	laringotraqueobronquitis
laser	Laser	láser
laterale	lateral, seitlich	lateral
colpo di frusta	Peitschenhiebsyndrom, Mediansyndrom	latigazo
lavaggio	Spülung	lavado
lassativo (n)	Abführmittel (n), Laxans (n)	laxante (n)
lassativo (a)	abführend (a), laxierend (a)	laxante (a)
lassativo	laxierend, abführend	laxativo
latte	Milch	leche
lecitina	Lezithin	lecitina
curettage, raschiamento	Kürettage, Ausschabung	legrado
raschiare, scarificare	kürettieren	legrar
leishmaniosi	Leishmaniose	leishmaniasis
lingua	Zunge	lengua
lente a contatto	Kontaktlinse	lente de contacto
lentiggine	Lentigo	lentigo

SPANISH	ENGLISH	FRENCH
lepra	leprosy	lèpre
leptospirosis	leptospirosis	leptospirose
lesbiana	lesbian	lesbien
lesión	injury, lesion	blessure, lésion
lesión no accidental	non-accidental injury (NAI)	traumatisme non accidentel
letal	lethal	létal, léthal
letargo	lethargy	léthargie
leucemia	leukaemia (Eng), leukemia (Am)	leucémie
leucemia por virus humano de las células T	human T-cell leukaemia virus (HTLV) (Eng), human T-cell leukemia virus (HTLV) (Am)	leucémie humaine à lymphocytes T
leucocito	leucocyte (Eng), leukocyte (Am)	leucocyte
leucocitosis	leucocytosis (Eng), leukocytosis (Am)	leucocytose
leucopenia	leucopenia (Eng), leukopenia (Am)	leucopénie
leucoplasia	leucoplakia (Eng), leukoplakia (Am)	leucoplasie
leucorrea	leucorrhea (Eng), leukorrhea (Am)	leucorrhée
leucotomía	leucotomy (Eng), leukotomy (Am)	leucotomie
levadura	yeast	levure
líbido	libido	libido
libras por pulgada cuadrada (psi)	pounds per square inch (psi)	livres par pouce carré (psi)
licor	liquor	liquide
liendre	nit	lente
ligadura	ligature	ligature
ligamento	ligament	ligament
ligamento ancho	broad ligament	ligaments larges
ligar	ligate	ligaturer
linctus	linctus	linctus
línea	linea	ligne
linfa	lymph	lymphe
linfadenectomía	lymphadenectomy	lymphadénectomie
linfadenitis	lymphadenitis	lymphadénite
linfadenopatía	lymphadenopathy	lymphadénopathie
linfangitis	lymphangitis	lymphangite
linfático	lymphatic	lymphatique
linfedema	lymphedema (Am), lymphoedema (Eng)	lymphoedème
linfoblasto	lymphoblast	lymphoblaste
linfocinesis	lymphokine	lymphokine
linfocito	lymphocyte	lymphocyte
linfocitosis	lymphocytosis	lymphocytose
linfogranuloma inguinal	lymphogranuloma inguinale	lymphogranulome vénérien
linfoma	lymphoma	lymphome
linfosarcoma	lymphosarcoma	lymphosarcome
linimento	liniment	liniment
lipasa	lipase	lipase
lipemia	lipaemia (Eng), lipemia (Am)	lipémie
lípido	lipid	lipide
lipidosis	lipidosis	lipidose, dyslipoïdose

ITALIAN	GERMAN	SPANISH
lebbra	Lepra, Aussatz	lepra
leptospirosi	Leptospirose	leptospirosis
lesbismo	lesbisch	lesbiana
lesione	Verletzung, Läsion	lesión
lesione non accidentale	nicht unfallbedingte Verletzung	lesión no accidental
letale	letal, tödlich	letal
letargia	Lethargie	letargo
leucemia	Leukämie	leucemia
virus della leucemia a cellule T	human T-cell leukemia virus (HTLV)	leucemia por virus humano de las células T
leucocito	Leukozyt	leucocito
leucocitosi	Leukozytose	leucocitosis
leucopenia	Leukopenie	leucopenia
leucoplachia	Leukoplakie	leucoplasia
leucorrea	Leukorrhoe	leucorrea
leucotomia	Leukotomie	leucotomía
lievito	Hefe, Hefepilz	levadura
desiderio sessuale	Libido	líbido
libbre per pollici quadrati	pounds per square inch (psi)	libras por pulgada cuadrada (psi)
liquido	Liquor, Flüssigkeit	licor
lendine	Nisse	liendre
legatura	Ligatur, Gefäßunterbindung	ligadura
ligamento	Ligament, Band	ligamento
legamento largo	ligamentum latum uteri	ligamento ancho
legare	abbinden	ligar
sciroppo	Linctus	linctus
linea	Linea, Linie	línea
linfa	Lymphe	linfa
linfoadenectomia	Lymphadenektomie	linfadenectomía
linfadenite	Lymphadenitis	linfadenitis
linfadenopatia	Lymphadenopathie	linfadenopatía
linfangite	Lymphangitis	linfangitis
linfatico	lymphatisch, Lymph-	linfático
linfedema	Lymphödem	linfedema
linfoblasto	Lymphoblast	linfoblasto
linfochina	Lymphokine	linfocinesis
linfocito	Lymphozyt	linfocito
linfocitosi	Lymphozytose	linfocitosis
linfogranuloma inguinale	Lymphogranuloma inguinale	linfogranuloma inguinal
linfoma	Lymphom	linfoma
linfosarcoma	Lymphosarkom	linfosarcoma
linimento	Liniment, Einreibemittel	linimento
lipasi	Lipase	lipasa
lipemia	Lipämie	lipemia
lipide	Lipid	lípido
lipoidosi	Lipidose	lipidosis

SPANISH	ENGLISH	FRENCH
lipocondrodistrofia	lipochondrodystrophy	maladie de Hurler, lipochondrodystrophie
lipodistrofia	lipodystrophy	lipodystrophie
lipolisis	lipolysis	lipolyse
lipoma	lipoma	lipome
lipoproteína	lipoprotein	lipoprotéine
lipoproteína de alta densidad (HDL)	high density lipoprotein (HDL)	lipoprotéine de haute densité (LHD)
lipoproteína de baja densidad (LDL)	low density lipoprotein (LDL)	lipoprotéine de basse densité (LBD)
lipoproteína de muy baja densidad (VLDL)	very low density lipoprotein (VLDL)	lipoprotéine de très faible densité
lipotrófico	lipotrophic	hormone lipotrope hypophysaire
líquen	lichen	lichen
liquenificación	lichenification	lichénification
líquido amniótico	amniotic fluid	liquide amniotique
líquido cefalorraquídeo (LCR)	cerebrospinal fluid (CSF)	liquide céphalo-rachidien
líquido sinovial	synovial fluid	fluide synovial
lisis	lysis	lyse
lisosoma	lysosome	lysosome
lisozima	lysozyme	lysozyme
lista de espera	waiting list	liste d'attente
litonefrotomía	lithonephrotomy	lithonéphrotomie
litotomía	lithotomy	lithotomie
litotripsia	lithotripsy	lithotripsie, lithotritie
litotriptor	lithotriptor	lithotriteur
litotritor	lithotrite	lithotriteur
lívido	livid	livide
lobectomía	lobectomy	lobectomie
lobotomía	lobotomy	lobotomie
lóbulo	lobe, lobule	lobe, lobule
localizar	localize	localiser
locomotor	locomotor	locomoteur
loculado	loculated	loculé
locura	insanity	aliénation
logopedia	speech therapy	orthophonie
lombriz	worm	ver
lomo	loin	région lombaire
loquios	lochia	lochies
lordosis	lordosis	lordose
lúcido	lucid	lucide
lumbago	lumbago	lumbago
lumbalgia	low back pain	douleurs lombaires basses
lumbar	lumbar	lombaire
lumbosacro	lumbosacral	lombo-sacré
lupus	lupus	lupus
lupus eritematoso	lupus erythematosus	lupus érythémateux

ITALIAN	GERMAN	SPANISH
lipocondrodistrofia	Lipochondrodystrophie	lipocondrodistrofia
lipodistrofia	Lipodystrophie	lipodistrofia
lipolisi	Lipolyse	lipolisis
lipoma	Lipom	lipoma
lipoproteina	Lipoprotein	lipoproteína
lipoproteina ad alta densità (LAD)	high density lipoprotein (HDL)	lipoproteína de alta densidad (HDL)
lipoproteina a bassa densità (LBD)	low density lipoprotein (LDL)	lipoproteína de baja densidad (LDL)
lipoproteina a bassissima densità	Lipoprotein sehr geringer Dichte	lipoproteína de muy baja densidad (VLDL)
lipotrofico	lipotroph	lipotrófico
lichene	Lichen	líquen
lichenificazione	Lichenifikation	liquenificación
fluido amniotico	Amnionflüssigkeit, Fruchtwasser	líquido amniótico
liquido cerebrospinale (LCS)	Liquor	líquido cefalorraquídeo (LCR)
liquido sinoviale	Synovialflüssigkeit	líquido sinovial
lisi	Lysis	lisis
lisosoma	Lysosom	lisosoma
lisozima	Lysozym	lisozima
lista d'attesa	Warteliste	lista de espera
litonefrotomia	Nephrolithotomie	litonefrotomía
litotomia	Lithotomie	litotomía
litotripsia	Lithotripsie	litotripsia
litotritore	Lithotriptor	litotriptor
litotritore	Lithotriptor	litotritor
livido	livide, bleich	lívido
lobectomia	Lobektomie, Lungenlappenresektion	lobectomía
lobotomia	Lobotomie, Leukotomie	lobotomía
lobo, lobulo	Lappen (Organ-), Lobulus, Läppchen	lóbulo
localizzare	lokalisieren	localizar
locomotore	fortbewegend, Bewegungs-	locomotor
loculato	gekammert	loculado
pazzia	Geisteskrankheit	locura
terapia del linguaggio	Sprachtherapie	logopedia
verme	Wurm	lombriz
regione lombare	Lende	lomo
lochi puerperali	Lochien, Wochenfluß	loquios
lordosi	Lordose	lordosis
lucido	glänzend, bei Bewußtsein	lúcido
lombaggine	Lumbago, Hexenschuß	lumbago
rachialgia lombosacrale	Kreuzschmerzen	lumbalgia
lombare	Lumbal-, Lenden-	lumbar
lombosacrale	lumbosakral	lumbosacro
lupus	Lupus	lupus
lupus eritematoso	Lupus erythematodes	lupus eritematoso

SPANISH	ENGLISH	FRENCH
lupus eritematoso sistémico (LES)	systemic lupus erythematosus (SLE)	lupus érythémateux systémique
lúteo	luteum	corps jaune
luz	lumen	lumière

ITALIAN	GERMAN	SPANISH
lupus eritematoso sistemico (LES)	systemischer Lupus erythematodes, Lupus erythematodes visceralis (SLE)	**lupus eritematoso sistémico (LES)**
luteo	Luteom, Luteinom	**lúteo**
lume	Lumen, Durchmesser	**luz**

M

maceración	maceration	macération
macrocefalia	macrocephaly	macrocéphalie
macrocito	macrocyte	macrocyte
macrófago	macrophage	macrophage
macroscópico	macroscopic	macroscopique
mácula	macula, macule	macule
maculopapular	maculopapular	maculopapuleux
magullar	bruise	contusionner
mal	mal	mal
malabsorción	malabsorption	malabsorption
malacia	malacia	malacie
malar	malar	malaire
malathion	malathion	malathion
mal de altura	altitude sickness	mal d'altitude, mal des montagnes
mal de pinto	pinta	pinta
maléolo	malleolus	malléole
malestar	malaise	malaise
malformación	malformation	malformation
malformación de Arnold-Chiari	Arnold-Chiari malformation	malformation d'Arnold Chiari
malignidad	malignancy	malignité
maligno	malignant	malin
maloclusión	malocclusion	malocclusion
malposición	malposition	malposition
malpraxis	malpractice	faute professionnelle
malpresentación	malpresentation	présentation vicieuse
maltosa	maltose	maltose
mama	breast	sein
mamografía	mammography	mammographie
mamoplastia	mammoplasty	mammoplastie
mancha	spot	bouton
mancha ciega	blind spot	tache aveugle
mancha de nacimiento	birthmark	naevus, envie
manchas de Koplik	Koplik's spots	points de Koplik
mandíbula	jaw-bone, mandible	mâchoire, mandibule
manía	mania	manie
manipulación	manipulation	manipulation
mano	hand	main
manubrio	manubrium	manubrium
máquina de circulación extracorpórea	heart-lung machine	poumon d'acier
marasmo	failure to thrive (FTT), marasmus	absence de développement pondéro-statural normal, athrepsie
marcapasos	pacemaker	stimulateur cardiaque
marcha	gait	démarche

Italian	German	Spanish
macerazione	Mazeration	maceración
macrocefalia	Makrozephalie	macrocefalia
macrocito	Makrozyt	macrocito
macrofago	Phagozyt	macrófago
macroscopico	makroskopisch	macroscópico
macula	Makula, Fleck	mácula
maculopapulare	makulopapulär	maculopapular
ammaccare	stoßen, quetschen	magullar
male, malattia	Übel, Leiden	mal
malassorbimento	Malabsorption	malabsorción
malacia	Malazie, Erweichung	malacia
malare	Backe betr, Backen-	malar
malathion	Malathion	malathion
mal di montagna	Höhenkrankheit	mal de altura
pinta, spirochetosi discromica	Pinta	mal de pinto
malleolo	Malleolus, Knöchel	maléolo
indisposizione, malessere	Unwohlsein	malestar
malformazione	Mißbildung	malformación
sindrome di Arnold Chiari	Arnold-Chiari-Mißbildung	malformación de Arnold Chiari
neoplasia maligna	Malignität, Bosartigkeit	malignidad
maligno	maligne, bösartig	maligno
malocclusione	Malokklusion	maloclusión
malposizione	Lageanomalie	malposición
pratica errata o disonesta	Kunstfehler	malpraxis
presentazione fetale anomala	anomale Kindslage	malpresentación
maltosio	Maltose	maltosa
mammella	Brust	mama
mammografia	Mammographie	mamografía
mammoplastica	Mammaplastik	mamoplastia
foruncolo	Flecken, Pickel	mancha
punto cieco	blinder Fleck, Papille	mancha ciega
nevo congenito	Muttermal, Storchenbiß	mancha de nacimiento
segni di Koplik	Koplik-Flecken	manchas de Koplik
osso mandibolare, mandibola	Kieferknochen, Mandibula, Unterkiefer	mandíbula
mania	Manie	manía
manipolazione	Manipulation, Handhabung	manipulación
mano	Hand	mano
manubrio	Manubrium	manubrio
macchina cuore-polmone	Herzlungenmaschine	máquina de circulación extracorpórea
marasma infantile, marasma	Gedeihstörung, Marasmus	marasmo
pacemaker	Schrittmacher	marcapasos
andatura	Gang	marcha

SPANISH	ENGLISH	FRENCH
mareado	giddy	pris de vertige
mareo	dizziness	étourdissement
marsupialización	marsupialization	marsupialisation
martillo	malleus	marteau
masaje	massage	massage
mastalgia	mastalgia	mastalgie, mammalgie
mastectomía	mastectomy	mastectomie
masticación	mastication	mastication
mastitis	mastitis	mastite
mastoidectomía	mastoidectomy	mastoïdectomie
mastoideo	mastoid	mastoïde
mastoiditis	mastoiditis	mastoïdite
masturbación	masturbation	masturbation
material de legrado	curetting	curetages
matriz	matrix, womb	matrice, utérus
maxilar	maxilla	maxillaire
maxilofacial	maxillofacial	maxillofacial
meconio	meconium	méconium
medial	medial	interne
mediana	median	médian
mediastinitis	mediastinitis	médiastinite
mediastino	mediastinum	médiastin
medicado	medicated	médicamenté
medicamento	medicament	médicament
medicamento de liberación lenta	slow release drug	médicament retard
medicina	medicine	médecine
medicina alternativa	alternative medicine	médecine complémentaire
medicina complementaria	complementary medicine	traitement complémentaire
medicina forense	forensic medicine	médecine légale
médico	doctor, physician	médecin
médico forense	coroner	médecin légiste
médicolegal	medicolegal	médico-légal
médicosocial	medicosocial	médico-social
médico-social	sociomedical	sociomédical
medida de la velocidad máxima del flujo espiratorio	peak expiratory flow meter (PEFM)	appareil de mesure du débit expiratoire de pointe
medio	medium	milieu
médula	medulla	moelle
médula espinal	cord	cordon
médula ósea	bone marrow	moelle osseuse
meduloblastoma	medulloblastoma	médulloblastome
megacolon	megacolon	mégacôlon
megaloblasto	megaloblast	mégaloblaste
meiossis	meiosis	méiose
mejilla	cheek	joue
mejoría	amelioration	amélioration

ITALIAN	GERMAN	SPANISH
stordito, affetto da vertigini o capogiro	schwindlig	mareado
stordimento, capogiro, vertigini	Schwindel	mareo
marsupializzazione	Marsupialisation	marsupialización
martello	Malleus, Hammer	martillo
massaggio	Massage	masaje
mastalgia	Mastodynie	mastalgia
mastectomia	Mastektomie, Brustamputation	mastectomía
masticazione	Kauen, Kauvermögen	masticación
mastite	Mastitis, Brustdrüsenentzündung	mastitis
mastoidectomia	Mastoidektomie	mastoidectomía
mastoide, mastoideo	mastoideus	mastoideo
mastoidite	Mastoiditis	mastoiditis
masturbazione	Masturbation, Selbstbefriedigung	masturbación
curettage, raschiamento	Kürettage, Ausschabung	material de legrado
matrice, utero	Matrix, Uterus, Gebärmutter	matriz
mascella superiore	Maxilla, Oberkieferknochen	maxilar
maxillofacciale	maxillofazial	maxilofacial
meconio	Mekonium	meconio
mediale	medial	medial
mediano	Median-	mediana
mediastinite	Mediastinitis	mediastinitis
mediastino	Mediastinum	mediastino
medicato, medicamentoso	medizinisch	medicado
medicamento	Medikament, Arzneimittel	medicamento
farmaco a lenta dismissione	Retardmittel	medicamento de liberación lenta
medicina	Medizin, Arznei	medicina
medicina alternativa	Alternativmedizin	medicina alternativa
medicina complementare	komplementäre Medizin	medicina complementaria
medicina forense	Gerichtsmedizin, Rechtsmedizin	medicina forense
dottore, medico	Arzt	médico
medico legale	Leichenbeschauer	médico forense
medicolegale	rechtsmedizinisch	médicolegal
medicosociale	sozialmedizinisch	médicosocial
sociosanitario	sozialmedizinisch	médico-social
misuratore del flusso espiratorio massimo	Peak-Flowmeter	medida de la velocidad máxima del flujo espiratorio
mezzo	Medium	medio
midollo	Medulla, Mark	médula
corda, cordone, notocorda	Strang, Schnur, Ligament	médula espinal
midollo osseo	Knochenmark	médula ósea
medulloblastoma	Medulloblastom	meduloblastoma
megacolon	Megacoloncongenitum, Hirschsprung-Krankheit	megacolon
megaloblasto	Megaloblast	megaloblasto
meiosi	Meiose	meiossis
guancia	Wange, Backe	mejilla
miglioramento	Besserung	mejoría

melancolía	melancholia	mélancolie
melanina	melanin	mélanine
melanoma	melanoma	mélanome
melena	melaena (Eng), melena (Am)	méléna
mellizo	twin	jumeau
membrana	membrane	membrane
membrana celular	cell membrane	membrane cellulaire
membrana sinovial	synovial membrane	membrane synoviale
memoria	memory	mémoire
menarquía	menarche	établissement de la menstruation
meninges	meninges	méninges
meningioma	meningioma	méningiome
meningismo	meningism	méningisme
meningitis	meningitis	méningite
meningocele	meningocele	méningocèle
meningoencefalitis	meningoencephalitis	méningo-encéphalite
meniscectomía	meniscectomy	méniscectomie
menisco	meniscus	ménisque
menopausia	menopause	ménopause
menorragia	menorrhagia	ménorrhagie
menorrea	menorrhea (Am), menorrhoea (Eng)	ménorrhée
menstruación	menstruation	menstruation
menstrual	menstrual	menstruel
mental	mental	mental
mentoanterior	mentoanterior	posture antéromentonnière
mentón	mentum	menton
mentoposterior	mentoposterior	posture postmentonnière
mercurio	mercury	mercure
mesencéfalo	midbrain	mésencéphale
mesenterio	mesentery	mésentère
mesotelioma	mesothelioma	mésothéliome
metabólico	metabolic	métabolique
metabolismo	metabolism	métabolisme
metabolito	metabolite	métabolite
metacarpo	metacarpus	métacarpe
metacarpofalángico	metacarpophalangeal	métacarpophalangien
metahemoglobina	methaemoglobin (Eng), methemoglobin (Am)	méthémoglobine
metahemoglobinemia	methaemoglobinaemia (Eng), methemoglobinemia (Am)	méthémoglobinémie
metástasis	metastasis	métastase
metatarsalgia	metatarsalgia	métatarsalgie
metatarso	metatarsus	métatarse
metatarsofalángico	metatarsophalangeal	métatarsophalangien
metilcelulosa	methylcellulose	méthylcellulose
metropatía hemorrágica	metropathia haemorrhagica (Eng), metropathia hemorrhagica (Am)	métropathie hémorragique
metrorragia	metrorrhagia	métrorragie

ITALIAN	GERMAN	SPANISH
melanconia	Melancholie	melancolía
melanina	Melanin	melanina
melanoma	Melanom	melanoma
melena	Meläna, Blutstuhl	melena
gemello	Zwilling	mellizo
membrana	Membran	membrana
membrana cellulare	Zellmembran	membrana celular
membrana sinoviale	Synovia	membrana sinovial
memoria	Gedächtnis, Erinnerungsvermögen	memoria
menarca	Menarche	menarquía
meningi	Meningen, Hirnhäute	meninges
meningioma	Meningiom	meningioma
meningismo	Meningismus	meningismo
meningite	Meningitis, Gehirnhautentzündung	meningitis
meningocele	Meningozele	meningocele
meningoencefalite	Meningoenzephalitis	meningoencefalitis
meniscectomia	Meniskusentfernung	meniscectomía
menisco	Meniskus	menisco
menopausa	Menopause, Wechseljahre	menopausia
menorragia	Menorrhagie	menorragia
menorrea	Monatsblutung, Menstruation	menorrea
mestruazione	Menstruation, Monatsblutung	menstruación
mestruale	menstruell	menstrual
mentale	geistig, seelisch	mental
mentoanteriore	mentoanterior	mentoanterior
mento	Kinn	mentón
mentoposteriore	mentoposterior	mentoposterior
mercurio	Quecksilber	mercurio
mesencefalo	Mittelhirn	mesencéfalo
mesentere	Mesenterium	mesenterio
mesotelioma	Mesotheliom	mesotelioma
metabolico	metabolisch, Stoffwechsel-	metabólico
metabolismo	Metabolismus, Stoffwechsel	metabolismo
metabolita	Metabolit, Stoffwechselprodukt	metabolito
metacarpo	Metakarpus, Mittelhand	metacarpo
metacarpofalangeo	metakarpophalangeal	metacarpofalángico
metemoglobina	Methämoglobin	metahemoglobina
metemoglobinemia	Methämoglobinämie	metahemoglobinemia
metastasi	Metastase	metástasis
metatarsalgia	Metatarsalgie	metatarsalgia
metatarso	Metatarsus, Mittelfuß	metatarso
metatarsofalangeo	metatarsophalangeal	metatarsofalángico
metilcellulosa	Methylzellulose	metilcelulosa
metropatia emorragica	Metropathia haemorrhagica	metropatía hemorrágica
metrorragia	Metrorrhagie, Zwischenblutung	metrorragia

SPANISH	ENGLISH	FRENCH
mezcla de Brompton	Brompton's mixture	liquide de Brompton
mialgia	myalgia	myalgie
miastenia	myasthenia	myasthénie
micción	micturition	micturition
micosis	mycosis	mycose
microbiología	microbiology	microbiologie
microcefalia	microcephaly	microcéphalie
microcirculación	microcirculation	microcirculation
microcirugía	microsurgery	microchirurgie
microcito	microcyte	microcyte
microfilaria	microfilaria	microfilaire
microorganismo	microorganism	micro-organisme
microscópico	microscopic	microscopique
microscopio	microscope	microscope
microscopio quirúrgico	operating microscope	microscope opératoire
microvellosidad	microvilli	micropoils
midriasis	mydriasis	mydriase
midriático *(n)*	mydriatic *(n)*	mydriatique *(n)*
midriático *(a)*	mydriatic *(a)*	mydriatique *(a)*
mielina	myelin	myéline
mielitis	myelitis	myélite
mielofibrosis	myelofibrosis	myélofibrose
mielografía	myelography	myélographie
mieloide	myeloid	myéloïde
mieloma	myeloma	myélome
mielomatosis	myelomatosis	myélomatose
mielomeningocele	meningomyelocele	méningomyélocèle
mielopatía	myelopathy	myélopathie
migraña	migraine	migraine
miliar	miliary	miliaire
miliaria	miliaria	miliaire
miliequivalente (mEq)	milliequivalent (mEq)	milliéquivalent (mEq)
mineralocorticoide	mineralocorticoid	minéralocorticoïde
minusvalía	handicap	handicapé
miocardio	myocardium	myocarde
miocardiopatía	cardiomyopathy	cardiomyopathie
miocarditis	myocarditis	myocardite
miofibrosis	myofibrosis	myofibrose
mioma	myoma	myome
miomectomía	myomectomy	myomectomie
miometrio	myometrium	myomètre
miopatía	myopathy	myopathie
miope	myope	myope
miopía	myopia	myopie
miosis	miosis	myosis
miositis	myositis	myosite

ITALIAN	GERMAN	SPANISH
soluzione di Brompton	Brompton-Lösung (Alkohol, Morphin, Kokain)	mezcla de Brompton
mialgia	Myalgie, Muskelschmerz	mialgia
miastenia	Myasthenie, Muskelschwäche	miastenia
minzione	Wasserlassen, Blasenentleerung	micción
micosi	Mykose, Pilzinfektion	micosis
microbiologia	Mikrobiologie	microbiología
microcefalia	Mikrozephalie	microcefalia
microcircolazione	Mikrozirkulation	microcirculación
microchirurgia	Mikrochirurgie	microcirugía
microcita	Mikrozyt	microcito
microfilaria	Mikrofilarie	microfilaria
microoganismo	Mikroorganismus	microorganismo
microscopico	mikroskopisch	microscópico
microscopio	Mikroskop	microscopio
microscopio chirurgico	Operationsmikroskop	microscopio quirúrgico
microvilli	Mikrovilli	microvellosidad
midriasi	Mydriasis, Pupillenerweiterung	midriasis
midriatico (n)	Mydriatikum (n)	midriático (n)
midriatico (a)	mydriatisch (a), pupillenerweiternd (a)	midriático (a)
mielina	Myelin	mielina
mielite	Myelitis	mielitis
mielofibrosi	Myelofibrose	mielofibrosis
mielografia	Myelographie	mielografía
mieloide	myeloisch	mieloide
mieloma, plasmacitoma maligno	Myelom	mieloma
mielomatosi	Myelomatose	mielomatosis
meningomielocele	Meningomyelozele	mielomeningocele
mielopatia	Myelopathie	mielopatía
emicrania	Migräne	migraña
miliare	miliar	miliar
miliaria, esantema miliare	Miliaria	miliaria
milliequivalente (mEq)	Milli-Aquivalent	miliequivalente (mEq)
mineralcorticoide	Mineralokortikoid	mineralocorticoide
handicappato, minorato	Behinderung	minusvalía
miocardio	Myokard, Herzmuskel	miocardio
cardiomiopatia	Kardiomyopathie	miocardiopatía
miocardite	Myokarditis, Herzmuskelentzündung	miocarditis
miosite	Myofibrose	miofibrosis
leiomioma dell'utero, mioma	Myom	mioma
miomectomia	Myomektomie	miomectomía
miometrio	Myometrium	miometrio
miopatia	Myopathie, Muskelerkrankung	miopatía
miope	Myoper, Kurzsichtiger	miope
miopia	Myopie, Kurzsichtigkeit	miopía
miosi	Miosis, Pupillenverengung	miosis
miosite	Myositis	miositis

SPANISH	ENGLISH	FRENCH
miringotomía	myringotomy	myringotomie
mitocondria	mitochondrion	mitochondrie
mitosis	mitosis	mitose
mitral	mitral	mitral
mittelschmerz	mittelschmerz	crise intermenstruelle
mixedema	myxedema (Am), myxoedema (Eng)	myxoedème
mixoma	myxoma	myxome
mixovirus	myxovirus	myxovirus
moco	mucous (Eng), mucus (Am)	muqueux
mola hidatidiforme	hydatidiform mole	hydatidiforme
molar	molar	molaire
molécula	molecule	molécule
molusco	molluscum	molluscum
monocromato	monochromat	monochromat
mononuclear	mononuclear	mononucléaire
mononucleosis	mononucleosis	mononucléose
mononucleosis infecciosa	infectious mononucleosis	mononucléose infectieuse
monoplegia	monoplegia	monoplégie
morbilidad	morbidity	morbidité
morbiliforme	morbilliform	morbilliforme
morfología	morphology	morphologie
moribundo	moribund	moribond
mortalidad	mortality	mortalité
mortinato	stillborn	mort-né
mosca tsetsé	tsetse	mouche tsé-tsé
motor	motor	moteur
móvil	motile	mobile
movimiento	motion	mouvement
movimiento rápido de los ojos (REM)	rapid eye movement (REM)	période des mouvements oculaires
mucina	mucin	mucine
mucocele	mucocele (Am), mucocoele (Eng)	mucocèle
mucocutáneo	mucocutaneous	mucocutané
mucoide	mucoid	mucoïde
mucolítico	mucolytic	mucolytique
mucopolisacaridosis	mucopolysaccharidosis	mucopolysaccharidose
mucopurulento	mucopurulent	mucopurulent
mucosa	mucosa	muqueuse
muela del juicio	wisdom tooth	dent de sagesse
muerte	death	mort
muerte en la cuna	cot death	mort subite de nourrisson
muerte súbita infantil	cot death	mort subite de nourrisson
muerto	dead	mort
muerto al llegar	dead on arrival (DOA)	mort à l'arrivée

ITALIAN	GERMAN	SPANISH
miringotomia	Parazentese	miringotomía
mitocondrio	Mitochondrium	mitocondria
mitosi	Mitose	mitosis
mitrale, mitralico	mitral	mitral
dolore intermestruale	Mittelschmerz	mittelschmerz
mixedema	Myxödem	mixedema
mixoma	Myxom	mixoma
myxovirus	Myxovirus	mixovirus
mucoso	mukös, schleimig	moco
idatiforme	Blasenmole	mola hidatidiforme
molare	molar	molar
molecula	Molekül	molécula
mollusco	Molluscum	molusco
monocromatico	Monochromat, monochrom Farbenblinder	monocromato
mononucleare	mononukleär	mononuclear
mononucleosi	Mononukleose, Pfeiffersches Drüsenfieber	mononucleosis
mononucleosi infettiva	Pfeiffersches Drüsenfieber, infektiöse Mononukleose	mononucleosis infecciosa
monoplegia	Monoplegie	monoplegia
morbilità	Morbidität, Krankhaftigkeit	morbilidad
morbilliforme	morbilliform, masernähnlich	morbiliforme
morfologia	Morphologie	morfología
moribondo	moribund, sterbend	moribundo
mortalità	Mortalität, Sterblichkeit	mortalidad
nato morto	totgeboren	mortinato
tse-tse	Tsetsefliege	mosca tsetsé
motore	motorisch	motor
mobile	bewegungsfähig, beweglich	móvil
movimento	Bewegung, Stuhlgang	movimiento
fase REM del sonno, movimento oculare rapido	rapid eye movement (REM)	movimiento rápido de los ojos (REM)
mucina	Muzin	mucina
mucocele	Mukozele	mucocele
mucocutaneo	mukokutan	mucocutáneo
mucoide	mukoid	mucoide
mucolitico	schleimlösendes Mittel	mucolítico
mucopolisaccaridosi	Mukopolysaccharidose	mucopolisacaridosis
mucopurulento	mukopurulent, schleimig-eitrig	mucopurulento
mucosa	Mukosa, Schleimhaut	mucosa
dente del giudizio	Weisheitszahn	muela del juicio
morte	Tod, Todesfall	muerte
sindrome da morte improvvisa del lattante	plötzlicher Säuglingstod	muerte en la cuna
sindrome da morte improvvisa del lattante	plötzlicher Säuglingstod	muerte súbita infantil
morto	tot	muerto
deceduto all'arrivo in ospedale	tot bei Einlieferung	muerto al llegar

SPANISH	ENGLISH	FRENCH
muestra de orina de la parte media de la micción	midstream urine specimen (MUS)	urine du milieu du jet
muguet	thrush	aphte
multilocular	multilocular	multiloculaire
multípara	multigravida	multigeste
muñeca	wrist	poignet
mural	mural	pariétal
músculo	muscle	muscle
musculocutáneo	musculocutaneous	musculo-cutané
musculoesquelético	musculoskeletal	musculo-squelettique
músculo esternocleidomastoideo	sternocleidomastoid muscle	muscle sternocléidomastoïdien
músculos glúteos	gluteus muscles	muscles fessiers
músculos peroneos	peroneus muscles	muscles péroniers
músculos trapecios	trapezius muscles	muscles trapèzes
mutación	mutation	mutation
mutágeno	mutagen	mutagène
mutante	mutant	mutant
mutilación	mutilation	mutilation
mutismo	mutism	mutisme

ITALIAN	GERMAN	SPANISH
campione urinario del mitto intermedio (CUM)	Mittelstrahlurin	muestra de orina de la parte media de la micción
stomatite de Candida albicans, mughetto	Soor, Sprue	muguet
multiloculare	multilokulär	multilocular
plurigravida	Multigravida	multípara
polso	Handgelenk, Karpus	muñeca
murale, parietale	mural	mural
muscolo	Muskel	músculo
muscolocutaneo	muskulokutan	musculocutáneo
muscoloscheletrico	Skelettmuskulatur betr	musculoesquelético
muscolo sternocleidomastoideo	Musculus sternocleidomastoideus	músculo esternocleidomastoideo
muscoli glutei	Glutealmuskulatur, Gesäßmuskulatur	músculos glúteos
muscoli peronei	Musculi peronei	músculos peroneos
muscoli trapezi	Musculi trapezii	músculos trapecios
mutazione	Mutation	mutación
mutageno	Mutagen	mutágeno
mutante	Mutante	mutante
mutilazione	Verstümmelung	mutilación
mutismo	Mutismus, Stummheit	mutismo

N

SPANISH	ENGLISH	FRENCH
nacido muerto	stillborn	mort-né
nacimiento	birth	naissance
nalga	buttock	fesse
nalgas	breech	siège
narcolepsia	narcolepsy	narcolepsie
narcosis	narcosis	narcose
narcótico (n)	narcotic (n)	narcotique (n)
narcótico (a)	narcotic (a)	narcotique (a)
nariz	nose	nez
nasal	nasal	nasal
nasofaringe	nasopharynx	rhinopharynx
nasogástrico	nasogastric	nasogastrique
nasolacrimal	nasolacrimal	nasolacrymal
náusea	nausea	nausée
nauseabundo	queasy	indigeste, délicat
náuseas matinales	morning sickness	nausées matinales
nebulizador	nebulizer	nébuliseur
necrosis	necrosis	nécrose
necrosis tubular	tubular necrosis	nécrose tubulaire
nefralgia	nephralgia	néphralgie
nefrectomía	nephrectomy	néphrectomie
nefritis	nephritis	néphrite
nefrógeno	nephrogenic	d'origine rénale
nefrología	nephrology	néphrologie
nefrona	nephron	néphron
nefrosis	nephrosis	néphrose
nefrostomía	nephrostomy	néphrostomie
nefrotóxico	nephrotoxic	néphrotoxique
negligencia	negligence	négligence
nematodo	nematode	nématode
neonato (n)	neonate (n), newborn (n)	nouveau-né (n)
neonato (a)	neonate (a), newborn (a)	nouveau-né (a)
neoplasia	neoplasia	néoplasie
neoplasia intraepitelial cervical	cervical intraepithelial neoplasia (CIN)	néoplasie intra-épithéliale cervicale
neoplasma	neoplasm	néoplasme
nervio	nerve	nerf
nervio ciático	sciatic nerve	nerf grand sciatique
nervio craneal	cranial nerve	nerf crânien
nervio motor	motor nerve	nerf moteur
nervio peroneo	peroneal nerve	nerf péronier
nervioso	neural	neural
nervios vasomotores	vasomotor nerves	nerfs vasomoteurs

ITALIAN	GERMAN	SPANISH
nato morto	totgeboren	nacido muerto
nascita	Geburt	nacimiento
natica	Gesäßbacke	nalga
natica	Steiß, Gesäß	nalgas
narcolessia	Narkolepsie	narcolepsia
narcosi	Narkose, Anästhesie	narcosis
narcotico (n)	Narkosemittel (n), Betäubungsmittel (n), Rauschgift (n)	narcótico (n)
narcotico (a)	narkotisch (a)	narcótico (a)
naso	Nase	nariz
nasale	nasal	nasal
nasofaringe	Nasopharynx, Nasenrachenraum	nasofaringe
nasogastrico	nasogastrisch	nasogástrico
nasolacrimale	nasolakrimal	nasolacrimal
nausea	Nausea, Übelkeit, Brechreiz	náusea
nauseabondo, nauseato, a disagio	unwohl, übel	nauseabundo
malessere mattutino	morgendliche Übelkeit der Schwangeren	náuseas matinales
nebulizzatore, atomizzatore	Zerstäuber, Vernebler	nebulizador
necrosi	Nekrose	necrosis
necrosi tubulare	Tubulusnekrose	necrosis tubular
nevralgia	Nephralgie	nefralgia
nefrectomia	Nephrektomie	nefrectomía
nefrite	Nephritis, Nierenentzündung	nefritis
nefrogenico	nephrogen	nefrógeno
nefrologia	Nephrologie	nefrología
nefrone	Nephron	nefrona
nefrosi, nefropatia	Nephrose	nefrosis
nefrostomia	Nephrostomie	nefrostomía
nefrotossico	nephrotoxisch, nierenschädigend	nefrotóxico
negligenza	Nachlässigkeit	negligencia
nematode	Nematode, Fadenwurm	nematodo
neonato (n)	Neugeborenes (n)	neonato (n)
neonato (a)	neugeboren (a)	neonato (a)
neoplasia	Neoplasie	neoplasia
neoplasia intraepiteliale della cervice uterina (CIN)	zervikale intraepitheliale Neoplasie (CIN)	neoplasia intraepitelial cervical
neoplasma	Neoplasma, Tumor	neoplasma
nervo	Nerv	nervio
nervo sciatico	Ischiasnerv, Nervus ischiadicus	nervio ciático
nervo craniale	Hirnnerv	nervio craneal
nervo motore	motorischer Nerv	nervio motor
nervo peroneo	Nervus peroneus	nervio peroneo
neurale	neural	nervioso
nervi vasomotori	vasomotorische Nerven	nervios vasomotores

SPANISH	ENGLISH	FRENCH
neumaturia	pneumaturia	pneumaturie
neumocéfalo	pneumocephalus	pneumo-encéphale, pneumocéphale
neumocito	pneumocyte	cellule alvéolaire
neumoconiosis	pneumoconiosis	pneumoconiose
neumonectomía	pneumonectomy	pneumonectomie
neumonía	pneumonia	pneumonie
neumonitis	pneumonitis	pneumonite
neumoperitoneo	pneumoperitoneum	pneumopéritoine
neumotórax	pneumothorax	pneumothorax
neuralgia	neuralgia	névralgie
neurastenia	burnout syndrome, neurasthenia	syndrome de 'surmenage', neurasthénie
neuritis	neuritis	névrite
neuroblastoma	neuroblastoma	neuroblastome
neurocirugía	neurosurgery	neurochirurgie
neurofarmacología	neuropharmacology	neuropharmacologie
neurofibromatosis	neurofibromatosis	neurofibromatose
neurógeno	neurogenic	neurogène
neurolema	neurolemma	neurilemme
neuroléptico (n)	neuroleptic (n)	neuroleptique (n)
neuroléptico (a)	neuroleptic (a)	neuroleptique (a)
neurología	neurology	neurologie
neuromuscular	neuromuscular	neuromusculaire
neurona	neuron	neurone
neurona motora	motor neurone	neurone moteur
neuropatia	neuropathy	neuropathie
neuropraxia	neurapraxia	neurapraxie
neuropsiquiatría	neuropsychiatry	neuropsychiatrie
neurosífilis	neurosyphilis	neurosyphilis
neurosis	neurosis	névrose
neurosis obsesiva	obsessional neurosis	névrose obsessionnelle
neurotrópico	neurotropic	neurotrope
neutrófilo (n)	neutrophil (n)	polynucléaire neutrophile (n)
neutrófilo (a)	neutrophil (a)	neutrophile (a)
neutropenia	neutropenia	neutropénie
nevo	mole, naevus (Eng), nevus (Am)	naevus
nicotina	nicotine	nicotine
nictalgia	nyctalgia	nyctalgie
nicturia	nocturia, nycturia	nycturie
nido	nidus	foyer morbide
niño azul	blue baby	enfant bleu, enfant atteint de la maladie bleue
nistagmo	nystagmus	nystagmus
nocturno	nocturnal	nocturne
nodo	node	noeud
nodo sinoauricular	sinoatrial node	noeud sinusal de Keith et Flack
nódulo	nodule	nodule

ITALIAN	GERMAN	SPANISH
pneumaturia	Pneumaturie	neumaturia
pneumocefalo	Pneumozephalus	neumocéfalo
pneumocito	Pneumozyt	neumocito
pneumoconiosi	Pneumokoniose, Staublunge	neumoconiosis
pneumonectomia	Pneumonektomie, Lungenresektion	neumonectomía
polmonite	Pneumonie, Lungenentzündung	neumonía
polmonite	Pneumonitis	neumonitis
pneumoperitoneo	Pneumoperitoneum	neumoperitoneo
pneumotorace	Pneumothorax	neumotórax
nevralgia	Neuralgie	neuralgia
incapacità ad agire, sindrome di esaurimento professionale, neuroastenia	Helfer-Syndrom, Neurasthenie	neurastenia
neurite	Neuritis, Nervenentzündung	neuritis
neuroblastoma	Neuroblastom	neuroblastoma
neurochirurgia	Neurochirurgie	neurocirugía
neurofarmacologia	Neuropharmakologie	neurofarmacología
neurofibromatosi	Neurofibromatose	neurofibromatosis
neurogenico	neurogen	neurógeno
neurilemma	Neurolemm	neurolema
neurolettico (n)	Neuroleptikum (n)	neuroléptico (n)
neurolettico (a)	neuroleptisch (a)	neuroléptico (a)
neurologia	Neurologie	neurología
neuromuscolare	neuromuskulär	neuromuscular
neurone	Neuron	neurona
neurone motore	Motoneuron	neurona motora
neuropatia	Neuropathie	neuropatia
neuroaprassia	Neurapraxie	neuropraxia
neuropsichiatria	Neuropsychiatrie	neuropsiquiatría
neurosifilide	Neurosyphilis	neurosífilis
nevrosi	Neurose	neurosis
nevrosi ossessiva	Zwangsneurose	neurosis obsesiva
neurotropo	neurotrop	neurotrópico
granulocito neutrofilo (n)	Neutrophiler (n)	neutrófilo (n)
neutrofilo (a)	neutrophil (a)	neutrófilo (a)
neutropenia	Neutropenie	neutropenia
neo, nevo	Mole, Muttermal, Nävus	nevo
nicotina	Nikotin	nicotina
nictalgia	Nyktalgie	nictalgia
nicturia	Nykturie	nicturia
nido	Nidus	nido
'blue baby' (cianosi da cardiopatia congenita)	zyanotisches Neugeborenes	niño azul
nistagmo	Nystagmus	nistagmo
notturno	nächtlich, Nacht-	nocturno
nodo	Knoten	nodo
nodo sinoatriale	Sinusknoten	nodo sinoauricular
nodulo	Nodulus, Knötchen	nódulo

SPANISH	ENGLISH	FRENCH
nódulos de Osler	Osler's nodes	nodules d'Osler
no invasivo	non-invasive	non invasif
nombre de patente	proprietary name	nom de marque
noradrenalina	noradrenaline	noradrénaline
norepinefrina	norepinephrine	norépinéphrine, noradrénaline
normoblasto	normoblast	normoblaste
normocito	normocyte	normocyte
normoglucémico	normoglycaemic (Eng), normoglycemic (Am)	normoglycémique
normotónico	normotonic	normotonique
nuca	nape	nuque
núcleo	nucleus	noyau
nudillo	knuckle	jointure
nulípara	nullipara	nullipare
nutrición	nutrition	nutrition
nutrición parenteral total	total parenteral nutrition (TPN)	alimentation parentérale totale
nutriente (n)	nutrient (n)	nutriment (n)
nutriente (a)	nutrient (a)	nourricier (a)

ITALIAN	GERMAN	SPANISH
noduli di Osler	Osler-Knötchen	nódulos de Osler
non invasivo	nichtinvasiv	no invasivo
marchio depositato	Markenname	nombre de patente
noradrenalina	Noradrenalin	noradrenalina
norepinefrina	Norepinephrin, Noradrenalin	norepinefrina
normoblasto	Normoblast	normoblasto
normocito	Normozyt	normocito
normoglicemico	Normoglykämie	normoglucémico
normotonico	normoton	normotónico
nuca	Nacken	nuca
nucleo	Nukleus, Kern	núcleo
articolazione interfalangea	Knöchel	nudillo
nullipara	Nullipara	nulípara
nutrizione	Ernährung	nutrición
nutrizione parenterale totale	parenterale Ernährung	nutrición parenteral total
sostanza nutritiva (n)	Nahrungsmittel (n)	nutriente (n)
nutriente (a)	nahrhaft (a)	nutriente (a)

O

obesidad	obesity	obésité
obstetricia	obstetrics	obstétrique
obstructivo	obstructive	obstructif
obturador	obturator	obturateur
occipital	occipital	occipital
occipitoanterior	occipitoanterior	occipito-antérieur
occipito anterior izquierdo	left occipito-anterior (LOA)	occipito-antérieur gauche
occipitofrontal	occipitofrontal	occipito-frontal
occipitoposterior	occipitoposterior	occipito-postérieur
occipucio	occiput	occiput
oclusión	occlusion	occlusion
ocular	ocular	oculaire
oculógiro	oculogyric	oculogyre
oculomotor	oculomotor	oculomoteur
oculta	occult	occulte
odontoides	odontoid	odontoïde
odontologia	dentistry	médecine dentaire, dentisterie
oftalmía	ophthalmia	ophtalmie
oftálmico	ophthalmic	ophtalmique
oftalmología	ophthalmology	ophtalmologie
oftalmoplejía	ophthalmoplegia	ophtalmoplégie
oftalmoscopio	ophthalmoscope	ophtalmoscope
oído	ear, hearing	oreille, audition
ojo	eye	oeil
olécranon	olecranon (process)	olécrane
olfatorio	olfactory	olfactif
oligohemia	oligaemia (Eng), oligemia (Am)	hypovolémie
oligomenorrea	oligomenorrhea (Am), oligomenorrhoea (Eng)	spanioménorrhée
oliguria	oliguria	oligurie
ombligo	navel, umbilicus	nombril
omoplato	scapula	omoplate
oncocerciasis	onchocerciasis	onchocercose
oncocerciasis ocular	river blindness	cécité des rivières
oncogén	oncogene	oncogène
oncología	oncology	oncologie
onicogriposis	onychogryphosis	onychogryphose
onicólisis	onycholysis	onycholyse
ooforectomía	oophorectomy	ovariectomie
opacidad	opacity	opacité
opaco	opaque	opaque
operación de Billroth	Billroth's operation	opération de Billroth
operación de Caldwell-Luc	Caldwell-Luc operation	opération de Caldwell-Luc
operación de Ramstedt	Ramstedt's operation	opération de Ramstedt

ITALIAN	GERMAN	SPANISH
obesità	Adipositas, Obesitas	obesidad
ostetricia	Geburtshilfe	obstetricia
ostruttivo	obstruktiv	obstructivo
otturatorio	Obturator, Gaumenverschlußplatte	obturador
occipitale	okzipital	occipital
occipitoanteriore	vordere Hinterhauptslage	occipitoanterior
occipitoanteriore sinistro (OAS)	linke vordere Hinterhauptslage	occipito anterior izquierdo
occipitofrontale	okzipitofrontal	occipitofrontal
occipitoposteriore	hintere Hinterhauptslage	occipitoposterior
occipite	Okziput, Hinterkopf	occipucio
occlusione	Okklusion, Verschluß	oclusión
oculare	okular	ocular
oculogiro	Bewegung der Augen betr	oculógiro
oculomotore	Oculomotorius-	oculomotor
occulto	okkult	oculta
odontoide	odontoid	odontoides
odontoiatria	Zahnheilkunde, Zahntechnik	odontologia
oftalmia	Ophthalmie	oftalmía
oftalmico	Augen-	oftálmico
oftalmologia	Ophthalmologie, Augenheilkunde	oftalmología
oftalmoplegia	Ophthalmoplegie, Augenmuskellähmung	oftalmoplejía
oftalmoscopio	Ophthalmoskop, Augenspiegel	oftalmoscopio
orecchio, udito	Ohr, Gehör, Hören	oído
occhio	Auge	ojo
olecrano	Olekranon, Ellenbozen	olécranon
olfattorio	olfaktorisch	olfatorio
oligoemia	Oligämie, Blutmangel	oligohemia
oligomenorrea	Oligomenorrhoe	oligomenorrea
oliguria	Oligurie	oliguria
ombelico	Nabel	ombligo
scapola	Skapula, Schulterblatt	omoplato
oncocerchiasi	Onchozerkose	oncocerciasis
oncocerchiasi, cecità fluviale	Flußblindheit	oncocerciasis ocular
oncogene	Onkogen	oncogén
oncologia	Onkologie	oncología
onicogrifosi	Onychogryposis	onicogriposis
onicolisi	Onycholyse, Nagelablösung	onicólisis
ovariectomia, ooforectomia	Oophorektomie	ooforectomía
opacità	Opazität	opacidad
opaco	undurchsichtig, verschattet (radiolog)	opaco
operazione di Billroth	Billroth-Magenresektion	operación de Billroth
operazione di Caldwell-Luc	Caldwell-Luc-Operation	operación de Caldwell-Luc
intervento di Ramstedt, piloromiotomia	Weber-Ramstedt-Operation, Ramstedt-(Weber)-Operation	operación de Ramstedt

SPANISH	ENGLISH	FRENCH
operación de Shirodkar	Shirodkar's operation	opération de Shirodkar
óptico *(n)*	optician *(n)*	opticien *(n)*
óptico *(a)*	optic *(a)*	optique *(a)*
óptimo	optimum	optimum
oral	oral	oral
órbita	orbit	orbite
orgánico	organic	organique
organismo	organism	organisme
orgasmo	orgasm	orgasme
orientación	orientation	orientation
orificio	orifice	orifice
origen	origin	origine
orina	urine	urine
orofaringe	oropharynx	oropharynx
orquidectomía	orchidectomy	orchidectomie
orquidopexia	orchidopexy	orchidopexie
orquidotomía	orchidotomy	orchodotomie
orquiopexia	orchiopexy	orchidopexie
orquitis	orchitis	orchite
ortodoncia	orthodontics	orthodontie
ortopedia	orthopaedic (Eng), orthopedic (Am)	orthopédique
ortopnea	orthopnea (Am), orthopnoea (Eng)	orthopnée
ortóptica	orthoptics	orthoptique
ortosis	orthosis	orthèse
ortostático	orthostatic	orthostatique
orzuelo	chalazion, stye	chalazion, orgelet
oscilación	oscillation	oscillation
óseo	osseous	osseux
osmolalidad	osmolality	osmolalité
osmolaridad	osmolarity	osmolarité
osmosis	osmosis	osmose
osteítis	osteitis	ostéite
osteoartritis	osteoarthritis (OA)	ostéo-arthrite
osteoartropatía	osteoarthropathy	ostéo-arthropathie
osteoblasto	osteoblast	ostéoblaste
osteocito	osteocyte	ostéocyte
osteoclasto	osteoclast	ostéoclaste
osteocondritis	osteochondritis	ostéochondrite
osteocondroma	osteochondroma	ostéochondrome
osteocondrosis	osteochondrosis	ostéochondrose
osteodistrofia	osteodystrophy	ostéodystrophie
osteofito	osteophyte	ostéophyte
osteogénico	osteogenic	ostéogène
osteolítico	osteolytic	ostéolytique
osteoma	osteoma	ostéome
osteomalacia	osteomalacia	ostéomalacie

intervento di Shirodkar	Shirodkar-Operation	operación de Shirodkar
ottico (n)	Optiker (n)	óptico (n)
ottico (a)	optisch (a), Seh- (a)	óptico (a)
optimum	optimal	óptimo
orale	oral	oral
orbita	Orbita, Augenhöhle	órbita
organico	organisch	orgánico
organismo	Organismus, Keim	organismo
orgasmo	Orgasmus	orgasmo
orientamento	Orientierung	orientación
orifizio	Öffnung	orificio
origine	Ursprung	origen
urina	Urin, Harn	orina
orofaringe	Mundrachenhöhle	orofaringe
orchidectomia	Orchidektomie	orquidectomía
orchidopessia	Orchidopexie	orquidopexia
orchidectomia	Orchidotomie	orquidotomía
orchidopessia	Orchipexie	orquiopexia
orchite	Orchitis	orquitis
ortodonzia	Kieferorthopädie	ortodoncia
ortopedia	orthopädisch	ortopedia
ortopnea	Orthopnoe	ortopnea
ortottica	Orthoptik	ortóptica
raddrizzamento, correzione di una deformità	Orthose	ortosis
ortostatico	orthostatisch	ortostático
calazion, orzaiolo	Chalazion, Hagelkorn, Hordeolum, Gerstenkorn	orzuelo
oscillazione	Oszillation, Schwankung	oscilación
osseo	knöchern, Knochen-	óseo
osmolalità	Osmolalität	osmolalidad
osmolarità	Osmolarität	osmolaridad
osmosi	Osmose	osmosis
osteite	Ostitis, Knochenentzündung	osteítis
osteoartrosi (OA)	Osteoarthritis	osteoartritis
osteoartropatia	Osteoarthrose	osteoartropatía
osteoblasto	Osteoblast	osteoblasto
osteocito	Osteozyt	osteocito
osteoclasto	Osteoklast	osteoclasto
osteocondrite	Osteochondritis	osteocondritis
osteocondroma	Osteochondrom	osteocondroma
osteocondrosi	Osteochondrose	osteocondrosis
osteodistrofia	Osteodystrophie	osteodistrofia
osteofito	Osteophyt	osteofito
osteogenico	osteogen	osteogénico
osteolitico	osteolytisch	osteolítico
osteoma	Osteom	osteoma
osteomalacia	Osteomalazie	osteomalacia

SPANISH	ENGLISH	FRENCH
osteomielitis	osteomyelitis	ostéomyélite
osteopatía	osteopathy	ostéopathie
osteopetrosis	osteopetrosis	ostéopétrose
osteoplastia	bone graft	greffe osseuse
osteoporosis	osteoporosis	ostéoporose
osteosarcoma	osteosarcoma	ostéosarcome
osteosclerosis	osteosclerosis	ostéosclérose
osteotomía	osteotomy	ostéotomie
ostomía	ostomy	ostéotomie
otalgia	otalgia	otalgie
otitis	otitis	otite
otitis media exudativa crónica	glue ear	otite moyenne adhésive
otolaringología	otolaryngology	otolaryngologie
otología	otology	otologie
otorrea	otorrhea (Am), otorrhoea (Eng)	otorrhée
otorrinolaringología (ORL)	ear nose and throat (ENT)	oto-rhino-laryngologie (ORL)
otosclerosis	otosclerosis	otospongiose
otoscopio	otoscope	otoscope
ototóxico	ototoxic	ototoxique
ovárico	ovarian	ovarien
ovario	ovary	ovaire
ovulación	ovulation	ovulation
óvulo	ovum	ovule, ovocyte de premier ordre, oeuf
oxidación	oxidation	oxydation
oxigenación	oxygenation	oxygénation
oxitocina	oxytocin	oxytocine
oxiuros	threadworm	ascaride

ITALIAN	GERMAN	SPANISH
osteomielite	Osteomyelitis, Knochenmarksentzündung	osteomielitis
osteopatia	Osteopathie	osteopatía
osteoporosi	Osteopetrose	osteopetrosis
trapianto osseo	Osteoplastik, Knochentransplantation	osteoplastia
osteoporosi	Osteoporose	osteoporosis
sarcoma osteogenico	Osteosarkom, Knochensarkom	osteosarcoma
osteosclerosi	Osteosklerose, Eburnifikation	osteosclerosis
osteotomia	Osteotomie	osteotomía
otalgia	Osteotomie	ostomía
otite	Otalgie, Ohrenschmerz	otalgia
otite	Otitis, Mittelohrentzündung	otitis
cerume nell orecchio	glue ear	otitis media exudativa crónica
otolaringologia	Otolaryngologie	otolaringología
otologia	Otologie, Ohrenheilkunde	otología
otorrea	Otorrhoe, Ohrenfluß	otorrea
orecchio naso e gola, otorinolaringoiatria	Hals- Nasen- Ohren-	otorrinolaringología (ORL)
otosclerosi	Otosklerose	otosclerosis
otoscopio	Otoskop, Ohrenspiegel	otoscopio
ototossico	ototoxisch	ototóxico
ovarico	ovarial, Eierstock	ovárico
ovaio	Ovarium, Eierstock	ovario
ovulazione	Ovulation, Eisprung	ovulación
uovo, gamete femminile	Ovum, Ei	óvulo
ossidazione	Oxydation	oxidación
ossigenazione	Sauerstoffsättigung, Oxygenierung	oxigenación
ossitocina	Oxytozin	oxitocina
ossiuro	Fadenwurm	oxiuros

P

SPANISH	ENGLISH	FRENCH
pabellón de la oreja	pinna	pavillon de l'oreille
paciente inmunocomprometido	immunocompromised patient	malade à déficit immunitaire
paciente inmunosuprimido	immunosuppressed patient	malade à suppression immunitaire
paladar	palate	palais
paladar blando	soft palate	voile du palais
paladar hendido	cleft palate	fente palatine
palatino	palatine	palatin
paliativo (n)	palliative (n)	palliatif (n)
paliativo (a)	palliative (a)	palliatif (a)
palidez	pallor	pâleur
palma	palm	paume
palmar	palmar	palmaire
palpable	palpable	palpable
palpación	palpation	palpation
palpitación	palpitation	palpitation
paludismo	malaria	paludisme
panadizo	whitlow	panaris
pancitopenia	pancytopenia	pancytopénie
páncreas	pancreas	pancréas
pancreatitis	pancreatitis	pancréatite
pandémico (n)	pandemic (n)	pandémie (n)
pandémico (a)	pandemic (a)	pandémique (a)
pantorrilla	calf	mollet
paperas	mumps	oreillons
papilar	papillary	papillaire
papiledema	papilledema (Am), papilloedema (Eng)	oedème papillaire
papiloma	corn, papilloma	cor, papillome
pápula	papule	papule
paracentesis	tapping	ponction
parafimosis	paraphimosis	paraphimosis
parafrenia	paraphrenia	paraphrénie
parálisis	palsy, paralysis	paralysie
parálisis bilateral	diplegia	diplégie
parálisis cerebral	cerebral palsy, general paralysis of the insane	infirmité motrice cérébrale, paralysie générale des aliénés
parálisis de Bell	Bell's palsy	paralysie de Bell
paralítico	paralytic	paralytique
paramédico	paramedical	paramédical
paranoia	paranoia	paranoïa
paraplejía	paraplegia	paraplégie
parasimpático	parasympathetic	parasympathique
parásito	parasite	parasite
parasuicidio	parasuicide	parasuicide
parathormona	parathormone	parathormone
paratiroidectomía	parathyroidectomy	parathyroïdectomie

padiglione auricolare	Ohrmuschel	pabellón de la oreja
paziente immunocompromesso	immungestörter Patient	paciente inmunocomprometido
paziente immunosoppresso	immunsupprimierter Patient	paciente inmunosuprimido
palato	Gaumen	paladar
palato molle	weicher Gaumen	paladar blando
palatoschisi	Gaumenspalte	paladar hendido
palatale, palatino	palatal	palatino
palliativo (n)	Palliativum (n)	paliativo (n)
palliativo (a)	palliativ (a)	paliativo (a)
pallore	Blässe	palidez
palmo	Handinnenfläche	palma
palmare	palmar	palmar
palpabile	palpabel, tastbar	palpable
palpazione	Palpation	palpación
palpitazione	Palpitation, Herzklopfen	palpitación
malaria	Malaria	paludismo
patereccio	Panaritium	panadizo
pancitopenia	Panzytopenie	pancitopenia
pancreas	Pankreas, Bauchspeicheldrüse	páncreas
pancreatite	Pankreatitis, Bauchspeicheldrüsenentzündung	pancreatitis
pandemia (n)	Pandemie (n)	pandémico (n)
pandemico (a)	pandemisch (a)	pandémico (a)
polpaccio	Wade	pantorrilla
parotite epidemica	Mumps, Ziegenpeter	paperas
papillare	papillär	papilar
papilledema	Papillenödem	papiledema
callo, papilloma	Klavus, Hühnerauge, Papillom	papiloma
papula	Papel, Knötchen	pápula
aspirazione di fluido	Abzapfen, Punktieren, Perkutieren	paracentesis
parafimosi	Paraphimose	parafimosis
parafrenia	Paraphrenie	parafrenia
paralisi	Paralyse, Lähmung	parálisis
diplegia	Diplegie, doppelseitige Lähmung	parálisis bilateral
paralisi cerebrale, paralisi progressiva luetica	Zerebralparese, progressive Paralyse	parálisis cerebral
paralisi di Bell	Bell-Fazialisparese	parálisis de Bell
paralitico	paralytisch, gelähmt	paralítico
paramedico	paramedizinisch	paramédico
paranoia	Paranoia	paranoia
paraplegia	Paraplegie, Querschnittslähmung	paraplejía
parasimpatico	parasympathisch	parasimpático
parassita	Parasit, Schmarotzer	parásito
suicidio figurato	parasuizidale Handlung	parasuicidio
paratormone	Parathormon	parathormona
paratiroidectomia	Parathyreoidektomie	paratiroidectomía

SPANISH	ENGLISH	FRENCH
paravertebral	paravertebral	paravertébral
parénquima	parenchyma	parenchyme
parenteral	parenteral	parentéral
paresia	paresis	parésie
parestesia	paraesthesia (Eng), paresthesia (Am)	paresthésie
pareunia	pareunia	coït
paridad	parity	parité
parietal	parietal	pariétal
parir	parous	poreux
parkinsonismo	parkinsonism	parkinsonisme
paroniquia	paronychia	panaris superficiel
parotiditis	parotitis	parotite
paroxístico	paroxysmal	paroxysmal
párpado	palpebra	paupière
partes por millón (ppm)	parts per million (ppm)	parties par million (ppm)
parto	birth, delivery, labor (Am), labour (Eng), parturition	naissance, livraison, accouchement, travail, parturition
parturición	parturition	parturition
parturienta	parturient	parturient
pasivo	passive	passif
pasta	paste	pâte
pasteurización	pasteurization	pasteurisation
pastilla	lozenge	pastille
patido cardíaco	heartbeat	pulsation (de coeur)
patogenia	pathogenesis	pathogenèse
patogenicidad	pathogenicity	pouvoir pathogène
patógeno	pathogen	pathogène
patognomónico	pathognomonic	pathognomonique
patología	pathology	pathologie
pecho	breast	sein
pectoral	pectoral	pectoral
pedal	pedal	pédieux
pediatría	paediatrics (Eng), pediatrics (Am)	pédiatrie
pediculosis	pediculosis	pédiculose
pedúnculo	peduncle	pédoncule
pelagra	pellagra	pellagre
pelo	hair	poil
peloteo	ballottement	ballottement
pelvimetría	pelvimetry	pelvimétrie
pelvis	pelvis	pelvis
péndulo	pendulous	pendant
pene	penis	pénis
pénfigo	pemphigus	pemphigus
penfigoide	pemphigoid	pemphigoïde
pepsina	pepsin	pepsine
péptico	peptic	peptique
péptido	peptide	peptide

938

paravertebrale	paravertebral	**paravertebral**
parenchima	Parenchym	**parénquima**
parenterale	parenteral	**parenteral**
paresi	Parese, Lähmung	**paresia**
parestesia	Parästhesie	**parestesia**
coito	Koitus, Geschlechtsverkehr	**pareunia**
parità, numero di gravidanze pregresse	Gebärfähigkeit, Ähnlichkeit	**paridad**
parietale	parietal, wandständig	**parietal**
che ha avuto figli	geboren habend	**parir**
parkinsonismo	Parkinsonismus	**parkinsonismo**
paronichia	Paronychie	**paroniquia**
parotite	Parotitis	**parotiditis**
parossistico	paroxysmal, krampfartig	**paroxístico**
palpebra	Palpebra, Lid	**párpado**
parti per milione (ppm)	ppm, mg/l	**partes por millón (ppm)**
nascita, parto, travaglio di parto	Geburt, Entbindung, Wehen, Gebären	**parto**
parto	Gebären, Geburt	**parturición**
partoriente	gebärend	**parturienta**
passivo	passiv, teilnahmslos	**pasivo**
pasta, pasta gelificante	Paste, Salbe	**pasta**
pastorizzazione	Pasteurisierung	**pasteurización**
pastiglia	Pastille	**pastilla**
battito cardiaco	Herzschlag	**patido cardíaco**
patogenesi	Pathogenese	**patogenia**
patogeneticità	Pathogenität	**patogenicidad**
patogeno	Krankheitserreger, Erreger	**patógeno**
patognomonico	pathognomonisch	**patognomónico**
patologia	Pathologie	**patología**
mammella	Brust	**pecho**
pettorale	pektoral, Brust-	**pectoral**
del piede	Fuß-	**pedal**
pediatria	Pädiatrie, Kinderheilkunde	**pediatría**
pediculosi	Pedikulose, Läusebefall	**pediculosis**
peduncolo	Stiel	**pedúnculo**
pellagra	Pellagra	**pelagra**
pelo, capello	Haar	**pelo**
ballottamento	Ballottement	**peloteo**
pelvimetria	Pelvimetrie	**pelvimetría**
pelvi	Pelvis, Becken	**pelvis**
pendulo	hängend, gestielt	**péndulo**
pene	Penis	**pene**
pemfigo	Pemphigus	**pénfigo**
pemfigoide	pemphigoid	**penfigoide**
pepsina	Pepsin	**pepsina**
peptico	peptisch	**péptico**
peptide	Peptide	**péptido**

percepción	perception	perception
percusión	percussion	percussion
percutáneo	percutaneous	percutané
pérdida de peso	weight loss	perte de poids
perforación	perforation	perforation
perfusión	perfusion	perfusion
perianal	perianal	périanal
pericardio	pericardium	péricarde
pericarditis	pericarditis	péricardite
pericondrio	perichondrium	périchondre
periférico	peripheral	périphérique
perinatal	perinatal	périnatal
perineo	perineum	périnée
periódico	recurrence	répétition, réapparition
período neonatal	neonatal period	période néonatale
perioperatorio	perioperative	périopératoire
perioral	perioral	périoral
periostio	periosteum	périoste
peristalsis	peristalsis	péristaltisme
peritoneo	peritoneum	péritoine
peritonitis	peritonitis	péritonite
periumbilical	periumbilical ´	périombilical
permeable	patent, permeable	libre, perméable
peroné	fibula	fibula
peroral	circumoral, peroral	péribuccal, peroral
perseverancia	perseveration	persévération
persona autística	autistic	autiste
personalidad	personality	personnalité
personalidad antisocial	antisocial personality	personnalité psychopathique
personalidad esquizoide	schizoid personality	personnalité schizoïde
personalidad psicopática	psychopathic personality	personnalité psychopathique
pesario	pessary	pessaire
peso atómico	atomic weight (at wt)	poids atomique
peso corporal total	total body weight (TBW)	poids corporel total
pestaña	lash	mèche, lanière
peste	plague	peste
petequia	petechia	pétéchie
petit mal	petit mal	petit mal
pezón	nipple	mamelon
pian	yaws	pian
piartrosis	pyarthrosis	pyarthrose
pica	pica	pica
picadura	sting	piqûre
picor	itch	démangeaison
pie	foot	pied
pie de atleta	athlete's foot	pied d'athlète

ITALIAN	GERMAN	SPANISH
percezione	Perzeption, Wahrnehmung	percepción
percussione	Perkussion	percusión
percutaneo	perkutan	percutáneo
perdita di peso	Gewichtsverlust	pérdida de peso
perforazione	Perforation	perforación
perfusione	Durchblutung	perfusión
perianale	perianal	perianal
pericardio	Perikard, Herzbeutel	pericardio
pericardite	Perikarditis	pericarditis
pericondrio	Perichondrium, Knorpelhaut	pericondrio
periferico	peripher	periférico
perinatale	perinatal	perinatal
perineo	Perineum, Damm	perineo
recidiva	Rezidiv	periódico
periodo neonatale	Neonatalperiode, Neugeborenenperiode	período neonatal
perioperatorio	perioperativ	perioperatorio
periorale	perioral	perioral
periostio	Periost, Knochenhaut	periostio
peristalsi	Peristaltik	peristalsis
peritoneo	Peritoneum, Bauchfell	peritoneo
peritonite	Peritonitis	peritonitis
periombelicale	periumbilikal	periumbilical
aperto, esposto, permeabile	offen, durchgängig, permeabel, durchlässig	permeable
fibula	Fibula, Wadenbein	peroné
circumorale, perorale	zirkumoral, peroral	peroral
perseverazione	Perseveration	perseverancia
autistico	autistisch	persona autística
personalità	Persönlichkeit	personalidad
personalità antisociale	asoziale Persönlichkeit	personalidad antisocial
personalità schizoide	schizoide Persönlichkeit	personalidad esquizoide
personalità psicopatica	psychopathische Persönlichkeit	personalidad psicopática
pessario	Pessar	pesario
peso atomico	Atomgewicht	peso atómico
peso corporeo totale	Körpergewicht	peso corporal total
ciglio	Wimper	pestaña
peste	Pest, Seuche	peste
petecchia	Petechie	petequia
piccolo male	Petit mal	petit mal
capezzolo	Brustwarze, Mamille	pezón
framboesia, pian	Frambösie	pian
pioartrosi, piartro	Pyarthrose, eitrige Gelenkentzündung	piartrosis
picacismo	Pica	pica
dolore acuto, puntura	Stachel, Stich	picadura
prurito	Jucken	picor
piede	Fuß	pie
piede di atleta	Fußpilz	pie de atleta

SPANISH	ENGLISH	FRENCH
pie de trinchera	trench foot	pied gelé
piel	skin	peau
piel de naranja	peau d'orange	peau d'orange
pielitis	pyelitis	pyélite
pielografía	pyelography	pyélographie
pielograma intravenoso	intravenous pyelogram (IVP)	urographie intraveineuse (UIV)
pielonefritis	pyelonephritis	pyélonéphrite
piemia	pyaemia (Eng), pyemia (Am)	septicopyohémie
pierna	leg	jambe
pie plano	flat-foot	pied plat
pie zambo	club-foot	pied bot
pigmentación	pigmentation	pigmentation
pigmento	pigment	pigment
píldora	pill	pilule
pilonidal	pilonidal	pilonidal
píloro	pylorus	pylore
piloromiotomía	pyloromyotomy	pylorotomie
piloroplastia	pyloroplasty	pyloroplastie
pilorospasmo	pylorospasm	pylorospasme
pinchar	puncture	ponctionner
pinguécula	pinguecula	pinguécula
pioderma	pyoderma	pyodermie
piógeno	pyogenic	pyogène
piojo	louse	pou
piómetra	pyometra	pyométrie
pionefrosis	pyonephrosis	pyonéphrose
piosalpinx	pyosalpinx	pyosalpinx
piramidal	pyramidal	pyramidal
pirexia	pyrexia	pyrexie
pirosis	heartburn, pyrosis	aigreurs, pyrosis
pitiriasis	pityriasis	pityriasis
piuria	pyuria	pyurie
placa	plaque	plaque
placas de Peyer	Peyer's patches	plaques de Peyer
placebo	placebo	placebo
placenta	placenta	placenta
plaga	plague	peste
planificación familiar	family planning	contrôle des naissances
plantar	plantar	plantaire
plaqueta	platelet	plaquette
plasma	plasma	plasma
plasmaféresis	plasmapheresis	plasmaphérèse
plétora	plethora	pléthore
pleura	pleura	plèvre
pleuresia	pleurisy (pleuritis)	pleurésie
pleuritis	pleurisy (pleuritis)	pleurésie

ITALIAN	GERMAN	SPANISH
piede da trincea	Schützengrabenfuß	pie de trinchera
pelle	Haut	piel
buccia d'arancia	Orangenhaut	piel de naranja
pielite	Pyelitis, Nierenbeckenentzündung	pielitis
pielografia	Pyelographie	pielografía
pielografia endovenosa (PE)	i.v. − Pyelogramm	pielograma intravenoso
pielonefrite	Pyelonephritis	pielonefritis
piemia	Pyämie	piemia
arto, gamba, membro	Bein	pierna
piede piatto	Plattfuß	pie plano
piede torto	Klumpfuß	pie zambo
pigmentazione	Pigmentierung, Färbung	pigmentación
pigmento	Pigment, Farbstoff	pigmento
pillola	Pille	píldora
pilonidale	pilonidal	pilonidal
piloro	Pylorus	píloro
piloromiotomia, intervento di Ramstedt	Pyloromyotomie	piloromiotomía
piloroplastica	Pyloroplastik	piloroplastia
pilorospasmo	Pylorospasmus	pilorospasmo
pungere	stechen, injizieren	pinchar
pinguecula	Pinguekula	pinguécula
piodermite, pioderma	Pyodermie	pioderma
piogenico	pyogen	piógeno
pidocchio	Laus	piojo
piometra	Pyometra	piómetra
pionefrosi	Pyonephrose	pionefrosis
piosalpinge	Pyosalpinx	piosalpinx
piramidale	pyramidal	piramidal
piressia	Fieber	pirexia
pirosi	Sodbrennen	pirosis
pitiriasi	Pityriasis	pitiriasis
piuria	Pyurie	piuria
placca	Plaque, Zahnbelag	placa
placche di Peyer	Peyer Plaques	placas de Peyer
placebo	Plazebo	placebo
placenta	Plazenta, Nachgeburt	placenta
peste	Pest, Seuche	plaga
controllo delle nascite	Familienplanung	planificación familiar
plantare	plantar	plantar
piastrina	Thrombozyt, Blutplättchen	plaqueta
plasma	Plasma	plasma
plasmaferesi	Plasmapherese	plasmaféresis
pletora	Plethora	plétora
pleura	Pleura	pleura
pleurite	Pleuritis, Rippenfellentzündung	pleuresia
pleurite	Pleuritis, Rippenfellentzündung	pleuritis

pleurodesis	pleurodesis	pleurodèse
pleurodinia	pleurodynia	pleurodynie
plexo	plexus	plexus
plexo solar	solar plexus	plexus solaire
plicatura	plication	plicature
plomo	lead	plomb
plumbismo	plumbism	saturnisme
podología	chiropody	chiropodie
podólogo	chiropodist	pédicure
poliarteritis	polyarteritis	polyartérite
poliartralgia	polyarthralgia	polyarthralgie
poliartritis	polyarthritis	polyarthrite
policitemia	polycythaemia (Eng), polycythemia (Am)	polycythémie
polidipsia	polydipsia	polydipsie
polifarmacia	polypharmacy	polypharmacie
polimialgia reumática	polymyalgia rheumatica	polymyalgie rhumatismale
polimiositis	polymyositis	polymyosite
polineuritis	polyneuritis	polynévrite
poliomielitis	poliomyelitis	poliomyélite
poliovirus	poliovirus	poliovirus
polipectomía	polypectomy	polypectomie
pólipo	polyp	polype
poliposis	polyposis	polypose
poliquístico	polycystic	polykystique
polisacárido	polysaccharide	polysaccharide
poliuria	polyuria	polyurie
ponfólix	pompholyx	pompholyx
poplíteo	popliteal, popliteus	poplité
porfiria	porphyria	porphyrie
porfirinas	porphyrin	porphyrine
poro	pore	pore
porta	porta	porte
portador	carrier	porteur
portocava	portacaval	porto-cave
portohepatitis	portahepatitis	porto-hépatite
posición de Sim	Sims' position	position de Sim
postcoital	postcoital	après rapport
postencefalítico	postencephalitic	postencéphalitique
posterior	posterior	postérieur
posthepático	posthepatic	posthépatique
postherpético	postherpetic	postherpétique
postmaduro	postmaturity	postmature
postmenopáusico	postmenopausal	postménopausique
postmortem	post-mortem	post mortem
postnasal	postnasal	rétronasal
postnatal	postnatal	postnatal

ITALIAN	GERMAN	SPANISH
pleurodesi	Pleurodese	pleurodesis
pleurodinia	Pleuralgie	pleurodinia
plesso	Plexus	plexo
plesso solare, plesso celiaco	Solarplexus	plexo solar
plicazione, piegatura	Faltenbildung	plicatura
piombo derivazione	Ableitung	plomo
intossicazione da piombo	Bleivergiftung	plumbismo
chiropodia	Pediküre, Fußpflege	podología
callista	Fußpfleger	podólogo
poliarterite	Polyarteritis	poliarteritis
poliartralgia	Polyarthralgie	poliartralgia
poliartrite	Polyarthritis	poliartritis
policitemia	Polyzythämie	policitemia
polidipsia	Polydipsie	polidipsia
prescrizione multipla di farmaci, abuso di farmaci	Polypragmasie	polifarmacia
polimialgia reumatica	Polymyalgia rheumatica	polimialgia reumática
polimiosite	Polymyositis	polimiositis
polineurite	Polyneuritis	polineuritis
poliomielite	Poliomyelitis, Kinderlähmung	poliomielitis
virus della poliomielite	Poliovirus	poliovirus
polipectomia	Polypektomie	polipectomía
polipo	Polyp	pólipo
poliposi	Polyposis	poliposis
policistico	polyzystisch	poliquístico
polisaccaride	Polysaccharid	polisacárido
poliuria	Polyurie	poliuria
ponfolice (disidrosi vescicolare)	Pompholyx	ponfólix
popliteo	popliteal, popliteus	poplíteo
porfiria	Porphyrie	porfiria
porfirina	Porphyrin	porfirinas
poro	Pore	poro
porta	Eingang	porta
portatore	Ausscheider, Trägerstoff	portador
portocavale	portokaval	portocava
portaepatite	Porta hepatis, Leberpforte	portohepatitis
posizione di Sim	Sims-Lage	posición de Sim
postcoitale	Postkoital-	postcoital
postencefalitico	postenzephalitisch	postencefalítico
posteriore	posteriore, hintere, Gesäß-	posterior
postepatico	posthepatisch	posthepático
posterpetico	postherpetisch	postherpético
postmaturo, ipermaturo	Überreife	postmaduro
postmenopausale	postmenopausal	postmenopáusico
post mortem	postmortal	postmortem
retronasale	postnasal	postnasal
postnatale	postnatal	postnatal

SPANISH	ENGLISH	FRENCH
postoperatorio	postoperative	postopératoire
postpartum	postpartum	postpartum
postprandial	postprandial	postprandial
postración	bearing down	efforts expulsifs
postural	postural	postural
precanceroso	precancerous	précancéreux
preconceptual	preconceptual	préconceptuel
precordial	precordial	précordial
precursor	precursor	précurseur
predisposición	predisposition	prédisposition
preeclampsia	pre-eclampsia	éclampsisme
prematuro	premature	prématuré
premedicación	premedication	prémédication
premenstrual	premenstrual	prémenstruel
prenatal	prenatal	prénatal
preoperatorio	preoperative	préopératoire
preparto	ante-partum	ante partum
prepubertal	prepubertal	prépubertaire
prepucio	foreskin, prepuce	prépuce
prerrenal	prerenal	prérénal
presentación	presentation	présentation
presentación de nalgas	breech-birth presentation	présentation, naissance par le siège
presión arterial (PA)	blood pressure (BP)	tension artérielle (TA)
presión capilar pulmonar (PCP)	pulmonary capillary pressure (PCP)	pression capillaire pulmonaire (PCP), pression artérielle bloquée moyenne
presión continua positiva de las vías respiratorias	continuous positive airway pressure (CPAP)	ventilation spontanée en pression positive continue
presión intracraneal (PIC)	intracranial pressure (ICP)	pression intracrânienne
presión osmótica	osmotic pressure	pression osmotique
presión parcial	partial pressure	pression partielle
presión venosa central (PVC)	central venous pressure (CVP)	tension veineuse centrale
presor	pressor	pressif
primeros auxilios	first aid	secourisme, premiers soins
primigrávida	primigravida	primigeste
primípara	primipara	primipare
probar	test	tester
procidencia	procidentia	procidence
proctalgia	proctalgia	proctalgie
proctitis	proctitis	rectite
proctocolectomia	proctocolectomy	proctocolectomie
proctocolitis	proctocolitis	rectocolite
proctoscopio	proctoscope	rectoscope
prodrómico	prodromal	prodromique
profármaco	pro-drug	précurseur de médicament
profilaxis	prophylaxis	prophylaxie
prolapso	prolapse	prolapsus
proliferar	proliferate	proliférer

946

ITALIAN	GERMAN	SPANISH
postoperatorio	postoperativ	postoperatorio
post partum	post partum	postpartum
postprandiale	postprandial	postprandial
fase espulsiva del parto	Pressen	postración
posturale	Lage-	postural
precanceroso	präkanzerös	precanceroso
precedente il concepimento	vor Empfängnis	preconceptual
precordiale, epigastrico	präkordial	precordial
precursore	Vorzeichen, Vorstufe, Präkursor	precursor
predisposizione	Prädisposition, Anfälligkeit	predisposición
preeclampsia	Präeklampsie, Eklampsiebereitschaft	preeclampsia
preamaturo	frühreif, vorzeitig	prematuro
premedicazione, preanestesia	Prämedikation	premedicación
premestruale	prämenstruell	premenstrual
prenatale	pränatal, vorgeburtlich	prenatal
preoperatorio	präoperativ	preoperatorio
preparto	ante partum, vor der Entbindung	preparto
prepubertale	Präpubertäts-	prepubertal
prepuzio	Präputium, Vorhaut	prepucio
prerenale	prärenal	prerrenal
presentazione	Lage, Kindslage	presentación
presentazione podalica	Steißlage	presentación de nalgas
pressione arteriosa	Blutdruck	presión arterial (PA)
pressione polmonare di incuneamento	Lungenkapillardruck	presión capilar pulmonar (PCP)
pressione continua positiva delle vie aeree	kontinuierlich positiver Atemwegsdruck	presión continua positiva de las vías respiratorias
pressione intracranica	Hirndruck, intrakranieller Druck	presión intracraneal (PIC)
pressione osmotica	osmotischer Druck	presión osmótica
pressione parziale	Partialdruck	presión parcial
pressione venosa centrale	zentraler Venendruck (ZVD)	presión venosa central (PVC)
pressorio	blutdruckerhöhend, vasopressorisch	presor
pronto soccorso	Erste Hilfe	primeros auxilios
primigravida	Primigravida	primigrávida
primipara	Primipara, Erstgebärende	primípara
valutare	testen, untersuchen	probar
procidenza	Prolaps, Vorfall	procidencia
proctalgia	Proktalgie	proctalgia
proctite	Proktitis	proctitis
proctocolectomia, rettocolectomia	Proktokolektomie	proctocolectomia
proctocolite	Proktokolitis	proctocolitis
proctoscopio	Rektoskop	proctoscopio
prodromico	prodromal	prodrómico
profarmaco (precursore inattivo)	pro-drug (Pharmakon-Vorform)	profármaco
profilassi	Prophylaxe, Vorbeugung	profilaxis
prolasso	Prolaps, Vorfall	prolapso
proliferare	proliferieren	proliferar

SPANISH	ENGLISH	FRENCH
pronador	pronator	pronateur
pronar	pronate	mettre en pronation
prono	prone	en pronation
pronóstico	prognosis	pronostic
proptosis	proptosis	proptose
prostaglandina	prostaglandin	prostaglandine
próstata	prostate	prostate
prostatectomía	prostatectomy	prostatectomie
prostatismo	prostatism	prostatisme
proteína	protein	protéine
proteína C-reactiva	C-reactive protein (CRP)	test de protéine C-réactive
proteína de Bence-Jones	Bence-Jones protein (BJ)	protéine de Bence Jones (BJ)
proteína de unión con el hierro	iron binding protein (IBP)	sidérophyline
proteinuria	proteinuria	protéinurie
prótesis	prosthesis	prothèse
protozoos	protozoa	protozoaires
proximal	proximal	proximal
prueba	test	test
prueba auditiva	hearing test	test auditif
prueba calórica	caloric test	essai calorique
prueba de función hepática	liver function test (LFT)	test de la fonction hépatique (TFH)
prueba de función respiratoria	respiratory function test	test de la fonction respiratoire
prueba de Guthrie	Guthrie test	test de Guthrie
prueba de Heaf	Heaf test	cuti-réaction de Heaf
prueba de Kveim	Kveim test	test de Kveim
prueba de la agregación plaquetaria	platelet aggregation test (PAT)	test d'agrégation plaquettaire (PAT)
prueba de la tolerancia a la insulina	insulin tolerance test (ITT)	épreuve de tolérance à l'insuline
prueba del parche	patch test	tache, plaque, pièce
prueba del sudor	sweat test	test de sueur
prueba de Paul-Bunnell	Paul-Bunnell test	réaction de Paul et Bunnell
prueba de resistencia a la insulina	glucose insulin tolerance test (GITT)	épreuve de tolérance au glucose et à l'insuline
prueba de Schick	Schick test	réaction de Schick
prueba de tinción de Papanicolaou	Papanicolaou's stain test (Pap test)	test de Papanicolaou
prueba de tolerancia a la glucosa	glucose tolerance test (GTT)	épreuve d'hyperglycémie provoquée
prueba radioalergosorbente (RAST)	radioallergosorbent test (RAST)	technique du RAST
prurito	pruritus	prurit
pseudopoliposis	pseudopolyposis	pseudopolypose
psicoanálisis	psychoanalysis	psychanalyse
psicodinámica	psychodynamics	psychodynamique
psicógeno	psychogenic	psychogène
psicogeriátrico	psychogeriatric	psychogériatrique
psicología	psychology	psychologie
psicomotor	psychomotor	psychomoteur
psicópata	psychopath	psychopathe

ITALIAN	GERMAN	SPANISH
pronatore	Pronator	pronador
pronare	pronieren	pronar
prono	veranlagt, empfänglich	prono
prognosi	Prognose	pronóstico
proptosi	Vorfall, Exophthalmus	proptosis
prostaglandina	Prostaglandine	prostaglandina
prostata	Prostata	próstata
prostatectomia	Prostatektomie	prostatectomía
prostatismo	chronisches Prostataleiden	prostatismo
proteina	Protein	proteína
proteina C reattiva	C-reaktives Protein (CRP)	proteína C-reactiva
proteina di Bence-Jones	Bence-Jones-Proteine	proteína de Bence-Jones
proteina che lega il ferro	eisenbindendes Protein	proteína de unión con el hierro
proteinuria	Proteinurie	proteinuria
protesi	Prothese	prótesis
protozoi	Protozoe	protozoos
prossimale	proximal	proximal
test, prova	Test, Untersuchung	prueba
test audiometrici	Hörtest	prueba auditiva
test calorico	kalorische Prüfung	prueba calórica
test di funzionalità epatica (TFE)	Leberfunktionstest	prueba de función hepática
test di funzionalità respiratoria	Atemfunktionstest	prueba de función respiratoria
test di Guthrie per la fenilchetonuria	Guthrie-Test	prueba de Guthrie
test alla tubercolina	Heaf-Test	prueba de Heaf
test di Kveim	Kveim-Test	prueba de Kveim
test di aggregazione piastrinico	Plättchen-Aggregations-Test (PAT)	prueba de la agregación plaquetaria
test di tolleranza all' insulina	Insulintoleranztest	prueba de la tolerancia a la insulina
test epicutaneo	Läppchenprobe, Einreibeprobe	prueba del parche
test del sudore, prova del sudore	Schweißtest	prueba del sudor
test di Paul-Bunnell	Paul-Bunnell-Reaktion	prueba de Paul-Bunnell
test insulinico di tolleranza al glucosio	Glukose-Insulin-Toleranztest	prueba de resistencia a la insulina
test di Schick	Schick-Test	prueba de Schick
test di Papanicolaou (Pap test)	Papanicolaou-Färbung (Pap)	prueba de tinción de Papanicolaou
test di tolleranza al glucosio (TTG)	Glukose-Toleranztest	prueba de tolerancia a la glucosa
test di radioallergoassorbimento (RAST)	Radio-Allergo-Sorbent-Test (RAST)	prueba radioalergosorbente (RAST)
prurito	Pruritus, Jucken	prurito
pseudopoliposi	Pseudopolypse	pseudopoliposis
psicoanalisi	Psychoanalyse	psicoanálisis
psicodinamica	Psychodynamik	psicodinámica
psicogenico	psychogen	psicógeno
psicogeriatrico	gerontopsychiatrisch	psicogeriátrico
psicologia	Psychologie	psicología
psicomotorio	psychomotorisch	psicomotor
psicopatico	Psychopath	psicópata

SPANISH	ENGLISH	FRENCH
psicopatía	psychopathy	psychopathie
psicopatología	psychopathology	psychopathologie
psicosis	psychosis	psychose
psicosis de Korsakoff	Korsakoff's psychosis	psychose de Korsakoff
psicosis maniacodepresiva	manic-depressive psychosis	psychose maniacodépressive
psicosomático	psychosomatic	psychosomatique
psicoterapia	psychotherapy	psychothérapie
psicotrópico	psychotropic	psychotrope
psiquiatría	psychiatry	psychiatrie
psiquiátrico	psychiatric	psychiatrique
psíquico	psychic	psychique
psitacosis	psittacosis	psittacose
psoas	psoas	psoas
psoralen	psoralen	psoralène
psoriasis	psoriasis	psoriasis
pterigión	pterygium	ptérygion
ptosis	ptosis	ptose
pubertad	puberty	puberté
pubis	pubis	pubis
puerperal	puerperal	puerpéral
puerperio	puerperium	puerpérium
pulga	flea	puce
pulgar	thumb	pouce
pulmón	lung	poumon
pulmonar	pulmonary	pulmonaire
pulsación	pulsation	pulsation
pulsátil	pulsatile	pulsatile
pulso	pulse	pouls
pulso alternante	pulsus alternans	pouls alternant
pulso paradójico	pulsus paradoxus	pouls paradoxal
punción	puncture	ponction
punción esternal	sternal puncture	ponction sternale
punción lumbar (PL)	lumbar puncture (LP)	ponction lombaire
punto de McBurney	McBurney's point	point de McBurney
punto de presión	pressure point	point particulièrement sensible
punto de sutura	stitch	point de suture
pupila	pupil	pupille
pupilar	pupillary	pupillaire
purga	purgative	purgatif
purgante	purgative	purgatif
púrpura	purpura	purpura
púrpura de Schönlein-Henoch	Henoch-Schönlein purpura	purpura rhumatoïde
purulento	purulent	purulent
pus	pus	pus
pústula	pustule	pustule
putrefacción	putrefaction	putréfaction

ITALIAN	GERMAN	SPANISH
psicopatia	Psychopathie	psicopatía
psicopatologia	Psychopathologie	psicopatología
psicosi	Psychose	psicosis
psicosi di Korsakoff	Korsakow-Psychose	psicosis de Korsakoff
psicosi maniaco-depressiva	manisch-depressive Psychose	psicosis maniacodepresiva
psicosomatico	psychosomatisch, Leib-Seele-	psicosomático
psicoterapia	Psychotherapie	psicoterapia
psicotropo	psychotrop	psicotrópico
psichiatria	Psychiatrie	psiquiatría
psichiatrico	psychiatrisch	psiquiátrico
psichico	psychisch, seelisch	psíquico
psittacosi	Psittakose, Ornithose	psitacosis
psoas	Psoas	psoas
psoralene	Psoralen	psoralen
psoriasi	Psoriasis, Schuppenflechte	psoriasis
pterigio, eponichio	Pterygium	pterigión
ptosi	Ptose	ptosis
pubertà	Pubertät	pubertad
pube	Os pubis, Schambein	pubis
puerperale	puerperal, Kindbett-	puerperal
puerperio	Wochenbett, Puerperium	puerperio
pulce	Floh	pulga
pollice	Daumen	pulgar
polmoni	Lunge	pulmón
polmonare	Lungen-	pulmonar
pulsazione	Pulsieren, Pulsschlag	pulsación
pulsatile	pulsierend	pulsátil
polso	Puls	pulso
polso alternante	Pulsus alternans	pulso alternante
polso paradosso	Pulsus paradoxus	pulso paradójico
puntura	Stich, Injektion	punción
puntura sternale	Sternalpunktion	punción esternal
puntura lombare, rachicentesi	Lumbalpunktion	punción lumbar (PL)
punto di McBurney	McBurney-Punkt	punto de McBurney
punto cutaneo sensibile alla pressione	Druckpunkt, Dekubitus	punto de presión
punto	Stechen	punto de sutura
pupilla	Pupille	pupila
pupillare	pupillar, Pupillen-	pupilar
lassativo	Purgativum, Abführmittel	purga
purgante	purgierend, abführend	purgante
porpora	Purpura	púrpura
porpora di Schönlein-Henoch	Purpura Schönlein-Henoch	púrpura de Schönlein-Henoch
purulento	purulent, eitrig	purulento
pus	Eiter	pus
pustola	Pustel, Pickel	pústula
putrefazione	Verwesung, Fäulnis	putrefacción

Q

queilosis	cheilosis	chéilose
quelantes	chelating agent	agent chélateur
queloide	keloid	chéloïde
quemadura	burn	brûlure
quemar	burn	brûler
quemosis	chemosis	chémosis
queratina	keratin	kératine
queratinización	keratinization	kératinisation
queratitis	keratitis	kératite
queratocele	keratocele	kératocèle
queratoconjuntivitis	keratoconjunctivitis	kératoconjonctivite
queratoma	keratome	kératome
queratomalacia	keratomalacia	kératomalacie
queratosis	keratosis	kératose
quiasma	chiasma	chiasma
quilo	chyle	chyle
quimioprofilaxis	chemoprophylaxis	chimioprophylaxie
quimiorreceptor	chemoreceptor	chimiorécepteur
quimiotaxis	chemotaxis	chimiotaxie
quimioterapia	chemotherapy	chimiothérapie
quiropráctica	chiropractic	chiropractique
quiropractor	chiropractor	chiropracteur
quiste	cyst	kyste
quistectomía	cystectomy	cystectomie
quiste de chocolate	chocolate cyst	kyste chocolat
quiste hidatídico	hydatid	kyste hydatique

ITALIAN	GERMAN	SPANISH
cheilosi	Mundeckenschrunden	**queilosis**
agente chelante	Chelatbildner	**quelantes**
cheloide	Keloid	**queloide**
ustione, scottatura	Verbrennung, Brandwunde	**quemadura**
bruciare	brennen, verbrennen	**quemar**
chemosi	Chemosis	**quemosis**
cheratina	Keratin	**queratina**
cheratinizzazione	Keratinisation, Verhornung	**queratinización**
cheratite	Keratitis, Hornhautentzündung	**queratitis**
cheratocele	Keratozele	**queratocele**
cheratocongiuntivite	Keratokonjunktivitis	**queratoconjuntivitis**
cheratomo	Keratotom	**queratoma**
cheratomalacia	Keratomalazie	**queratomalacia**
cheratosi	Keratose	**queratosis**
chiasma	Chiasma	**quiasma**
chilo	Chylus	**quilo**
chemioprofilassi	Chemoprophylaxe	**quimioprofilaxis**
chemorecettore	Chemorezeptor	**quimiorreceptor**
chemiotassi	Chemotaxis	**quimiotaxis**
chemioterapia	Chemotherapie	**quimioterapia**
chiropratica	Chiropraktik	**quiropráctica**
chiropratico	Chiropraktiker	**quiropractor**
cisti	Zyste	**quiste**
cistectomia	Zystektomie, Zystenentfernung	**quistectomía**
cisti cioccolato (c. emosiderinica dell'endometriosi)	Schokoladenzyste, Teerzyste	**quiste de chocolate**
cisti idatidea	Hydatide	**quiste hidatídico**

R

rabia	rabies	rage
radiactivo	radioactive	radioactif
radical	radical	radical
radio	radius	radius
radiografía	radiograph, radiography	radiographe, radiographie
radioisótopo	radioisotope	radio-isotope
radiología	radiology	radiologie
radiopaco	radio-opaque	radio-opaque
radiosensible	radiosensitive	radiosensible
radioterapia	radiotherapy	radiothérapie
raquis	spine	colonne vertébrale
raquitismo	rickets	rachitisme
rasgo	trait	trait
raspado	curettage	curetage
raspados	curetting	curetages
rayos X	X-rays	rayons X
reacción	reaction	réaction
reacción adversa a un medicamento	adverse drug reaction (ADR)	réaction médicamenteuse indésirable
reacción anafiláctica	anaphylactic reaction	réaction anaphylactique
reacción de Wassermann	Wassermann reaction	réaction de Wassermann
reacción de Widal	Widal reaction	réaction de Widal
reacción inmunológica	immune reaction	réaction immunitaire
reactivo	reagent	réactif
recaer	relapse	rechuter
receptor	receptor	récepteur
recesivo	recessive	récessif
receta	formula, prescription	formule, ordonnance
rechazo	rejection	rejet
recidiva	relapse	rechute
recipiente	recipient	receveur
recordar	recall	évoquer
recto	rectum	rectum
rectocele	rectocele	rectocèle
recuento de glóbulos rojos	red blood cell count (RBC)	numération érythrocytaire
recuento de leucocitos	white blood cell count (WBC)	nombre de globules blancs (NGB)
recuento sanguíneo	blood count	dénombrement des hématies
recuerdo	recall	évocation
recumbente	recumbent	couché
reflejo	reflex	réflexe
reflejo condicionado	conditioned reflex	réflexe conditionné
reflejo de Babinski	Babinski's reflex	réflexe de Babinski
reflejo de Moro	Moro reflex	réflexe de Moro

ITALIAN	GERMAN	SPANISH
rabbia	Tollwut	rabia
radioattivo	radioaktiv	radiactivo
radicale	radikal, Wurzel-	radical
radio	Radius, Halbmesser	radio
immagine radiologica, radiografia	Röntgenaufnahme, Röntgen	radiografía
radioisotopo	Radioisotop	radioisótopo
radiologia	Radiologie, Röntgenologie	radiología
radioopaco	röntgendicht	radiopaco
radiosensibile	strahlenempfindlich	radiosensible
radioterapia	Strahlentherapie, Radiotherapie	radioterapia
spina	Wirbelsäule, Rückgrat	raquis
rachitismo	Rachitis	raquitismo
tratto, carattere ereditario	Zug, Charakterzug, Eigenschaft	rasgo
curettage, raschiamento	Kürettage, Ausschabung	raspado
curettage, raschiamento	Kürettage, Ausschabung	raspados
raggi X	Röntgenstrahlen, Röntgenaufnahmen	rayos X
reazione	Reaktion	reacción
reazione dannosa (indesiderata) da farmaci	unerwünschte Arzneimittelreaktion	reacción adversa a un medicamento
reazione anafilattica	anaphylaktische Reaktion	reacción anafiláctica
reazione di Wassermann	Wassermann-Reaktion	reacción de Wassermann
reazione di Widal	Widal-Reaktion	reacción de Widal
immunoreazione, reazione immune	Immunreaktion	reacción inmunológica
reagente	Reagens	reactivo
recidivare	rezidivieren, Rückfall erleiden	recaer
recettore	Rezeptor	receptor
recessivo	rezessiv	recesivo
formula, prescrizione, ricetta	Formel, Milchzusammensetzung, Rezept, Verschreibung	receta
rigetto	Abstoßung	rechazo
ricaduta, recidiva	Rückfall, Rezidiv	recidiva
ricevente	Empfänger	recipiente
ricordare	(sich) erinnern	recordar
retto	Rektum	recto
rettocele	Rektozele	rectocele
conteggio dei globuli rossi (CGR)	rotes Blutbild	recuento de glóbulos rojos
conteggio dei globuli bianchi (CGB, WBC)	weißes Blutbild	recuento de leucocitos
emocitometria	Blutbild	recuento sanguíneo
memoria	Errinerung, Errinerungsvermögen	recuerdo
supino, sdraiato	liegend, ruhend	recumbente
riflesso	Reflex	reflejo
riflesso condizionato	bedingter Reflex, konditionierter Reflex	reflejo condicionado
riflesso di Babinski	Babinski-Reflex	reflejo de Babinski
riflesso di Moro	Moro-Reflex	reflejo de Moro

reflujo	reflux	reflux
refracción	refraction	réfraction
refractario	refractory	réfractaire
regeneración	regeneration	régénération
régimen	diet, regimen	régime
regresión	regression	régression
regurgitación	regurgitation	régurgitation
regurgitación láctea del neonato	posseting	régurgitation
rehabilitación	rehabilitation	réadaptation
relajante (n)	relaxant (n)	relaxant (n)
relajante (a)	relaxant (a)	relaxant (a)
remisión	remission	rémission
remitente	remittent	rémittent
renal	renal	rénal
renina	renin	rénine
repermeabilización	rebore	désobstruction
represión	repression	répression
resección	resection	résection
resectoscopio	resectoscope	résectoscope
resfriado	cold	rhume
residual	residual	résiduel
resistente al alcohol	alcohol-fast	résistant à l'alcool
resolución	resolution	résolution
resonancia	resonance	résonance
resorción	resorption	résorption
respiración	respiration	respiration
respiración anaerobia	anaerobic respiration (Eng), anerobic respiration (Am)	respiration anaérobie
respiración boca a boca	mouth to mouth resuscitation	réanimation au bouche-à-bouche
respiración de Cheyne-Stokes	Cheyne-Stokes respiration	dyspnée de Cheyne-Stokes
respirador	respirator	respirateur
resucitación	resuscitation	ressuscitation
resucitación cardiopulmonar	cardiopulmonary resuscitation (CPR)	réanimation cardiorespiratoire
retención	retention	rétention
reticulado	cancellous	spongieux
reticular	reticular	réticulaire
reticulocito	reticulocyte	réticulocyte
reticulocitosis	reticulocytosis	réticulocytose
retina	retina	rétine
retinitis	retinitis	rétinite
retinoblastoma	retinoblastoma	rétinoblastome
retinopatía	retinopathy	rétinopathie
retráctil	retractile	rétractile
retractor	retractor	rétracteur
retraso	retardation	retard
retrobulbar	retrobulbar	rétrobulbaire
retrocecal	retrocaecal (Eng), retrocecal (Am)	rétrocaecal

ITALIAN	GERMAN	SPANISH
reflusso	Reflux	reflujo
rifrazione	Refraktion, Brechung	refracción
refrattario	refraktär	refractario
rigenerazione	Regeneration	regeneración
regime, dieta, prescrizione dietetica	Ernährung, Diät	régimen
regressione	Regression, Rückbildung	regresión
regurgito	Regurgitieren	regurgitación
rigurgito	Regurgitation bei Säuglingen	regurgitación láctea del neonato
riabilitazione	Rehabilitation	rehabilitación
rilassante (n)	Relaxans (n)	relajante (n)
rilassante (a)	entspannend (a), relaxierend (a)	relajante (a)
remissione	Remission	remisión
remittente	remittierend, abfallend	remitente
renale	renal, Nieren-	renal
renina	Renin	renina
disobliterazione	Desobliteration	repermeabilización
repressione	Unterdrückung, Verdrängung	represión
resezione	Resektion	resección
resettore endoscopico	Resektoskop, Resektionszystoskop	resectoscopio
raffreddore	Kälte, Erkältung	resfriado
residuo	Residual	residual
alcool-resistente	alkoholresistent	resistente al alcohol
risoluzione	Auflösung, Rückgang	resolución
risonanza	Resonanz, Schall	resonancia
riassorbimento	Resorption	resorción
respirazione	Respiration, Atmung	respiración
respirazione anaerobica	anaerobe Respiration	respiración anaerobia
rianimazione bocca a bocca	Mund-zu-Mund-Wiederbelebung	respiración boca a boca
respiro di Cheyne-Stokes	Cheyne-Stokes-Atmung	respiración de Cheyne-Stokes
respiratore	Respirator, Beatmungsgerät	respirador
rianimazione	Reanimation, Wiederbelebung	resucitación
rianimazione cardiorespiratoria	Herz-Lungen-Wiederbelebung, Reanimation	resucitación cardiopulmonar
ritenzione	Retention	retención
spugnoso, trabecolare	spongiös, schwammartig	reticulado
reticolare	retikulär	reticular
reticolocito	Retikulozyt	reticulocito
reticolocitosi	Retikulozytose	reticulocitosis
retina	Retina, Netzhaut	retina
retinite	Retinitis, Netzhautentzündung	retinitis
retinoblastoma	Retinoblastom	retinoblastoma
retinopatia	Retinopathie	retinopatía
retrattile	retraktionsfähig	retráctil
divaricatore	Wundhaken, Spreizer, Retraktor	retractor
ritardo mentale, psicomotorio	Verzögerung, Hemmung	retraso
retrobulbare	retrobulbär	retrobulbar
retrociecale	retrozökal	retrocecal

retrofaríngeo	retropharyngeal	rétropharyngien
retrógrado	retrograde	rétrograde
retroperitoneal	retroperitoneal	rétropéritonéal
retroplacentario	retroplacental	rétroplacentaire
retrosternal	retrosternal	rétrosternal
retroversión	retroversion	rétroversion
reumatismo	rheumatism	rhumatisme
reumatoide	rheumatoid	rhumatoïde
reumatología	rheumatology	rhumatologie
revascularización	revascularization	revascularisation
rhesus negativo (Rh−)	rhesus negative (Rh−)	rhésus négatif (Rh−)
rhesus positivo (Rh+)	rhesus positive (Rh+)	rhésus positif (Rh+)
rigor	rigor	rigor
rinitis	rhinitis	rhinite
rinofima	rhinophyma	rhinophyma
riñón	kidney	rein
rinoplastia	rhinoplasty	rhinoplastie
rinorrea	rhinorrhea (Am), rhinorrhoea (Eng)	rhinorrhée
rinovirus	rhinovirus	rhinovirus
rodilla	knee	genou
rollos	rouleaux	rouleaux
roncar	snore	ronfler
roncus	rhonchus	ronchus
ronquido	snore	ronflement
rosácea	rosacea	acné rosacée
rosario raquítico	rickety rosary	chapelet costal
roséola	roseola	roséole
rotatorio	rotator	rotateur
rotavirus	rotavirus	rotavirus
rótula	patella	rotule
rubéola	German measles, rubella	rubéole
rubor	flush, rubor	rougeur
ruptura	rupture	hernie

retrofaringeo	retropharyngeal	retrofaríngeo
retrogrado	retrograd, rückläufig	retrógrado
retroperitoneale	retroperitoneal	retroperitoneal
retroplacentare	retroplazentar	retroplacentario
retrosternale	retrosternal	retrosternal
retroversione	Retroversion	retroversión
reumatismo	Rheumatismus	reumatismo
reumatoide	rheumatisch	reumatoide
reumatologia	Rheumatologie	reumatología
rivascolarizzazione	Revaskularisation	revascularización
Rh negativo (Rh−)	Rh-negativ	rhesus negativo (Rh−)
Rh positivo (Rh+)	Rh-positiv	rhesus positivo (Rh+)
rigor, ipertonia extrapiramidale	Rigor, Starre	rigor
rinite	Rhinitis	rinitis
rinofima	Rhinophym	rinofima
rene	Niere	riñón
rinoplastica	Rhinoplastik	rinoplastia
rinorrea	Rhinorrhoe	rinorrea
rhinovirus	Rhinovirus	rinovirus
ginocchio	Knie	rodilla
colonne di eritrociti	Geldrollenagglutination	rollos
russare	schnarchen	roncar
ronco	Rhonchus, Rasselgeräusch	roncus
russo	Schnarchen	ronquido
rosacea, acne rosacea	Rosacea	rosácea
rosario rachitico	rachitischer Rosenkranz	rosario raquítico
roseola	Roseole	roséola
muscolo rotatore	Rotator	rotatorio
rotavirus	Rotavirus	rotavirus
patella, rotula	Patella, Kniescheibe	rótula
rosolia	Rubella, Röteln	rubéola
eritema vasomotorio, arrossamento infiammatorio	Flush, Rubor, Rötung	rubor
rottura	Riß, Bruch	ruptura

S

SPANISH	ENGLISH	FRENCH
sabañón	chilblain, frostbite	engelure, gelure
saco	sac	sac
sacral	sacral	sacré
sacro	sacrum	sacrum
sacrococcígeo	sacrococcygeal	sacrococcygien
sacroileítis	sacroiliitis	sacro-ilite
sacrofliaco	sacroiliac	sacro-iliaque
safeno	saphenous	saphène
sagital	sagittal	sagittal
salino	saline	salin
saliva	saliva	salive
salivazo	spittle	crachat
salpingectomía	salpingectomy	salpingectomie
salpingitis	salpingitis	salpingite
salud	health	santé
salvado	bran	son
sangrar	bleed	saigner
sangre	blood	sang
sangre oculta	occult blood	sang occulte
sangre oculta fecal	faecal occult blood (FOB) (Eng), fecal occult blood (FOB) (Am)	sang occulte fécal
sarampión	measles	rougeole
sarampión parotiditis y rubéola	measles mumps and rubella (MMR)	oreillons rougeole et rubéole
sarcoideo	sarcoid	sarcoïde
sarcoidosis	sarcoidosis	sarcoïdose
sarcoma	sarcoma	sarcome
sarcoma de Ewing	Ewing's tumour	tumeur d'Ewing
sarcoma de Kaposi	Kaposi's sarcoma	sarcome de Kaposi
sarna	scabies	gale
saturnismo	plumbism	saturnisme
sebáceo	sebaceous	sébacé
sebo	sebum	sébum
seborrea	seborrhea (Am), seborrhoea (Eng)	séborrhée
secreción	secretion	sécrétion
secretorio	secretory	sécréteur
secuela	sequela	séquelle
secuestro	sequestrum	séquestre
secundinas	afterbirth	arrière-faix
sed	thirst	soif
sedación	sedation	sédation
sedante (n)	sedative (n)	sédatif (n)
sedante (a)	sedative (a)	sédatif (a)
sedentario	sedentary	sédentaire
segmento	segment	segment
semen	semen	sperme

ITALIAN	GERMAN	SPANISH
gelone, congelamento	Frostbeule, Pernio, Erfrierung	sabañón
sacco, sacca	Sack, Beutel	saco
sacrale	sakral, Kreuzbein-	sacral
sacro	Sakrum, Kreuzbein	sacro
sacrococcigeo	sakrokokkygeal	sacrococcígeo
sacroiliite	Sakroiliitis	sacroileítis
sacroiliaco	Iliosakral-	sacroíliaco
safeno	saphenus	safeno
sagittale	sagittal	sagital
salino	salinisch	salino
saliva	Speichel	saliva
saliva	Speichel	salivazo
salpingectomia	Salpingektomie	salpingectomía
salpingite	Salpingitis, Eileiterentzündung	salpingitis
salute	Gesundheit	salud
crusca	Kleie	salvado
sanguinare	bluten	sangrar
sangue	Blut	sangre
sangue occulto	okkultes Blut	sangre oculta
sangue occulto fecale	okkultes Blut (im Stuhl)	sangre oculta fecal
morbillo	Masern	sarampión
parotide epidemica morbillo e rosolia	Masern Mumps und Röteln	sarampión parotiditis y rubéola
sarcoideo	fleischähnlich	sarcoideo
sarcoidosi	Sarkoidose, Morbus Boeck	sarcoidosis
sarcoma	Sarkom	sarcoma
tumore di Ewing	Ewing-Sarkom	sarcoma de Ewing
sarcoma di Kaposi	Kaposi-Sarkom	sarcoma de Kaposi
scabbia	Skabies, Krätze	sarna
intossicazione da piombo	Bleivergiftung	saturnismo
sebaceo	Talg-, talgig	sebáceo
sebo	Talg	sebo
seborrea	Seborrhoe	seborrea
secrezione	Sekretion	secreción
secretorio	sekretorisch	secretorio
sequela	Folgeerscheinung, Folgezustand	secuela
sequestro	Sequester	secuestro
secondine, membrane fetali e placenta	Plazenta, Nachgeburt	secundinas
sete	Durst	sed
sedazione	Sedierung	sedación
sedativo (n)	Sedativum (n), Beruhigungsmittel (n)	sedante (n)
sedativo (a)	sedierend (a), beruhigend (a)	sedante (a)
sedentario	sitzend, seßhaft	sedentario
segmento	Segment	segmento
seme	Samen	semen

semilunar	semilunar	semi-lunaire
seminal	seminal	séminal, spermatique
seminoma	seminoma	séminome
semiótica	semeiotic	sémiologique
semipermeable	semipermeable	semi-perméable
semisoluble	partly soluble (p.sol)	partiellement soluble
'señal sanguinolenta menstrual'	'show'	eaux de l'amnios
senescencia	senescence	sénescence
senil	senile	sénile
seno	sinus	sinus
sensación	sensation	sensation
sensibilidad	sensitivity	sensibilité
sensibilización	sensitization	sensibilisation
sensible	sensitive	sensible
sensorineural	sensorineural	de perception
sensorio	sensory	sensitif
sentido	sense	sens
separar con aguja	tease	défilocher
sepsis	sepsis	septicémie
septicemia	septicaemia (Eng), septicemia (Am)	septicémie
septo	septum	septum
serología	serology	sérologie
seropositivo	seropositive	séropositif
serosa	serosa	séreuse
seroso	serous	séreux
servicio de urgencias/traumatologia	emergency treatment/trauma unit (ETU)	service des urgences/des traumatismes
shock	shock	choc
sien	temple	tempe
sífilis	syphilis	syphilis
sigmoideo	sigmoid	sigmoïde
sigmoidoscopio	sigmoidoscope	sigmoïdoscope
sigmoidostomía	sigmoidostomy	sigmoïdostomie
signo	sign	signe
signo de Chvostek	Chvostek's sign	signe de Chvostek
signo de Kernig	Kernig's sign	signe de Kernig
signo de Trendelenburg	Trendelenburg sign	signe de Trendelenburg
silicosis	silicosis	silicose
simbiosis	symbiosis	symbiose
simpatectomía	sympathectomy	sympathectomie
simpaticomimético (n)	sympathomimetic (n)	sympathomimétique (n)
simpaticomimético (a)	sympathomimetic (a)	sympathomimétique (a)
simulación de síntomas	malingering	simulation
sinapsis	synapse	synapse
síncope	syncope, faint	syncope
síndrome	syndrome	syndrome
síndrome alcohólico	alcohol syndrome	syndrome d'alcoolisme

ITALIAN	GERMAN	SPANISH
semilunare	semilunar, halbmondförmig	semilunar
seminale	Samen-, Spermien-	seminal
seminoma	Seminom	seminoma
semiotico	semiotisch	semiótica
semipermeabile	semipermeabel	semipermeable
parzialmente solubile	teilweise löslich	semisoluble
perdita ematica che precede il parto o la mestruazione	Geburtsbeginn (Anzeichen)	'señal sanguinolenta menstrual'
senescenza	Seneszenz, Altern	senescencia
senile	senil, Alters-	senil
seno, fistula suppurante	Sinus, Nebenhöhle	seno
sensazione, sensibilità	Sinneswahrnehmung, Gefühl	sensación
sensibilità	Empfindlichkeit, Feingefühl	sensibilidad
sensibilizzazione	Sensitivierung, Allergisierung	sensibilización
sensibile	sensitiv, empfindlich	sensible
neurosensoriale	Sinne u Nerven betr	sensorineural
sensoriale	sensorisch, Sinnes-	sensorio
sensi	Sinn	sentido
dissociare i tessuti	zupfen	separar con aguja
sepsi	Sepsis	sepsis
setticemia	Septikämie	septicemia
setto	Septum, Scheidewand	septo
sierologia	Serologie	serología
siero-positivo	seropositiv	seropositivo
sierosa, membrana sierosa	Serosa	serosa
sieroso	serös, Serum-	seroso
pronto soccorso	Notfallstation	servicio de urgencias/traumatologia
shock	Schock	shock
tempia	Schläfe	sien
sifilide	Syphilis, Lues	sífilis
sigmoide	sigmoid	sigmoideo
sigmoidoscopio	Sigmoidoskop	sigmoidoscopio
sigmoidostomia	Sigmoidostomie	sigmoidostomía
segno	Zeichen, Symptom	signo
segno di Chvostek	Chvostek-Zeichen	signo de Chvostek
segno di Kernig	Kernig Zeichen	signo de Kernig
segno di Trendelenburg	Trendelenburg-Zeichen	signo de Trendelenburg
silicosi	Silikose	silicosis
simbiosi	Symbiose	simbiosis
simpatectomia, simpaticectomia	Sympathektomie	simpatectomía
simpaticomimetico (n)	Sympathomimetikum (n)	simpaticomimético (n)
simpaticomimetico (a)	sympathomimetisch (a)	simpaticomimético (a)
simulazione di malattia	scheinkrank	simulación de síntomas
sinapsi, giunzione	Synapse	sinapsis
sincope, svenimento	Synkope, Ohnmacht	síncope
sindrome	Syndrom	síndrome
sindrome da alcool	Alkoholsyndrom	síndrome alcohólico

síndrome alcohólico fetal	fetal alcohol syndrome	syndrome d'alcoolisme foetal
síndrome carcinoide	carcinoid syndrome	syndrome carcinoïde
síndrome cerebral crónico	chronic brain syndrome (CBS)	syndrome chronique du cerveau
síndrome de Behçet	Behçet syndrome	syndrome de Behçet
síndrome de Cushing	Cushing's syndrome	syndrome de Cushing
síndrome de distress respiratorio	respiratory distress syndrome (RDS)	syndrome de membrane hyaline et de souffrance respiratoire
síndrome de Down	Down's syndrome	trisomie 21
síndrome de dumping	dumping syndrome	syndrome de chasse
síndrome de Horner	Horner's syndrome	syndrome de Bernard-Horner, syndrome oculaire sympathique
síndrome de inmunodeficiencia adquirida (SIDA)	acquired immune deficiency syndrome (AIDS)	syndrome d'immuno-déficience acquise (SIDA)
síndrome de Klinefelter	Klinefelter's syndrome	syndrome de Klinefelter
síndrome de la articulación temporomandibular	temporomandibular joint syndrome	syndrome de Costen
síndrome del asa ciega	blind loop syndrome	syndrome de l'anse borgne
síndrome del intestino irritable	irritable bowel syndrome	syndrome de l'intestin irritable
síndrome del niño apaleado	battered baby syndrome	syndrome des enfants maltraités
síndrome del túnel carpiano	carpal tunnel syndrome	syndrome du canal carpien
síndrome del vaciamiento en gastrectomizados	dumping syndrome	syndrome de chasse
síndrome de Mendelson	Mendelson's syndrome	syndrome de Mendelson
síndrome de muerte súbita infantil	sudden infant death syndrome (SIDS)	syndrome de mort subite de nourrisson
síndrome de Münchhausen	Münchhausen's syndrome	syndrome de Münchhausen
síndrome de piernas inquietas	restless legs syndrome	syndrome d'impatience musculaire
síndrome de Ramsay-Hunt	Ramsay Hunt syndrome	maladie de Ramsay Hunt
síndrome de Reiter	Reiter's syndrome	syndrome de Fiessinger-Leroy-Reiter
síndrome de Reye	Reye's syndrome	syndrome de Reye
síndrome de shock tóxico	toxic shock syndrome	syndrome de choc toxique staphylococcique
síndrome de Sjögren	Sjögren-Larsson syndrome	syndrome de Sjögren
síndrome de Stein-Leventhal	Stein-Leventhal syndrome	syndrome de Stein-Leventhal
síndrome de Stevens-Johnson	Stevens-Johnson syndrome	syndrome de Stevens-Johnson
síndrome de Stokes-Adams	Stokes-Adams syndrome	syndrome de Stokes-Adams
síndrome de Turner	Turner's syndrome	syndrome de Turner
síndrome de vibración	vibration syndrome	syndrome de vibrations
síndrome hemolítico urémico	haemolytic uraemic syndrome (HUS) (Eng), hemolytic uremic syndrome (HUS) (Am)	hémolyse urémique des nouveau-nés
síndrome hipercinético	hyperkinetic syndrome	syndrome hyperkinétique
síndrome nefrótico	nephrotic syndrome	syndrome néphrotique
síndrome uretral	urethral syndrome	syndrome urétral
sinequia	synechia	synéchie
sinergia	synergy	synergie
sínfisis	symphysis	symphyse

ITALIAN	GERMAN	SPANISH
sindrome da alcolismo materno	fetales Alkoholsyndrom	síndrome alcohólico fetal
sindrome da carcinoide	Karzinoid-Syndrom	síndrome carcinoide
sindrome cerebrale cronica	chronisches Gehirnsyndrom	síndrome cerebral crónico
sindrome di Behçet	Behçet-Syndrom	síndrome de Behçet
sindrome di Cushing	Cushing-Syndrom	síndrome de Cushing
sindrome di sofferenza respiratoria	Respiratory-distress-Syndrom, Atemnotsyndrom	síndrome de distress respiratorio
mongoloidismo, sindrome di Down	Down-Syndrom, Mongolismus	síndrome de Down
sindrome del gastroresecato	Dumping-Syndrom	síndrome de dumping
sindrome di Horner	Horner-Syndrom	síndrome de Horner
sindrome da immunodeficienza acquisita (AIDS)	erworbenes Immundefektsyndrom (AIDS)	síndrome de inmunodeficiencia adquirida (SIDA)
sindrome di Klinefelter	Klinefelter-Syndrom	síndrome de Klinefelter
sindrome dell'articolazione temporomandibolare	Costen-Syndrom	síndrome de la articulación temporomandibular
sindrome dell'ansa cieca	Syndrom der blinden Schlinge	síndrome del asa ciega
sindrome dell'intestino irritabile	Reizdarm	síndrome del intestino irritable
sindrome del bambino maltrattato	Kindesmißhandlung (Folgen)	síndrome del niño apaleado
sindrome del tunnel carpale	Karpaltunnelsyndrom	síndrome del túnel carpiano
sindrome del gastroresecato	Dumping-Syndrom	síndrome del vaciamiento en gastrectomizados
sindrome di Mendelson	Mendelson-Syndrom	síndrome de Mendelson
sindrome della morte neonatale improvvisa (SIDS)	plötzlicher Säuglingstod, Sudden-infant-death-Syndrom (SIDS)	síndrome de muerte súbita infantil
sindrome di Münchhausen	Münchhausen-Syndrom	síndrome de Münchhausen
sindrome delle gambe irrequiete, sindrome di Ekbom	Wittmaack-Ekbom-Syndrom	síndrome de piernas inquietas
sindrome di Ramsay Hunt	Ramsay-Hunt-Syndrom	síndrome de Ramsay-Hunt
sindrome di Reiter	Reiter-Syndrom	síndrome de Reiter
sindrome di Reye	Reye-Syndrom	síndrome de Reye
sindrome da shock tossico	toxisches Schocksyndrom (TSS)	síndrome de shock tóxico
sindrome di Sjögren-Larsson (eritrodermia ittiosiforme con oligofrenia spastica)	Sjögren-Syndrom	síndrome de Sjögren
sindrome di Stein-Leventhal	Stein-Leventhal-Syndrom	síndrome de Stein-Leventhal
sindrome di Stevens-Johnson	Stevens-Johnson-Syndrom	síndrome de Stevens-Johnson
sindrome di Stokes-Adams	Morgagni-Stokes-Adams-Syndrom	síndrome de Stokes-Adams
sindrome di Turner, disgenesia gonadica	Turner-Syndrom	síndrome de Turner
sindrome vibratoria	Vibrationssyndrom	síndrome de vibración
sindrome emolitico-uremica	hämolytisch-urämisches Syndrom	síndrome hemolítico urémico
sindrome ipercinetica	hyperkinetisches Syndrom	síndrome hipercinético
sindrome nefrosica	nephrotisches Syndrom	síndrome nefrótico
sindrome uretrale	Urethralsyndrom	síndrome uretral
sinechia, aderenza	Synechie, Verwachsung	sinequia
sinergia	Synergie	sinergia
sinfisi	Symphyse	sínfisis

SPANISH	ENGLISH	FRENCH
sin receta médica	over the counter (OTC)	spécialités pharmaceutiques grand public
sin sentido	unconscious	sans connaissance
síntoma	symptom	symptôme
sinusitis	sinusitis	sinusite
siringomielia	syringomyelia	syringomyélie
sistema nervioso central (SNC)	central nervous system (CNS)	système nerveux central (CNS)
sistema nervioso simpático	sympathetic nervous system	système nerveux sympathique
sistema reticuloendotelial (SRE)	reticuloendothelial system (RES)	système réticulo-endothélial
sístole	systole	systole
solución	solution	solution
solución de Hartmann	Hartmann's solution	liquide de Hartmann
solución salina	saline	solution physiologique
somático	somatic	somatique
somatomamotropina corionica humana	human chorionic somatomammotrophin (HCS) (Eng), human chorionic somatomammotropin (HCS, HPL) (Am)	somatomammotropine chorionique humaine (HCS), somatoprolactine chorionique humain
sonambulismo	somnambulism	somnambulisme
sonido	sound	son
soplo	murmur	murmure
soplo sistólico	systolic murmur	murmure systolique
soporífero (n)	soporific (n)	soporifique (n)
soporífero (a)	soporific (a)	soporifique (a)
soporte de vida básico	basic life support	équipement de survie
sordera	deafness	surdité
sordo	deaf	sourd
status	status	statut
stress	stress	stress
subagudo	subacute	subaigu
subclavia	subclavian	sous-clavier
subclínico	subclinical	sous-clinique
subconjuntival	subconjunctival	sous-conjonctival
subconsciente	subconscious	subconscient
subcostal	subcostal	sous-costal
subcutáneo (SC)	subcutaneous (SC, SQ)	sous-cutané (SC)
subdural	subdural	sous-dural
subfertilidad	subfertility	sous-fertilité
subfrénico	subphrenic	sous-phrénique
subjetivo	subjective	subjectif
sublimado	sublimate	sublimé
subliminal	subliminal	subliminal
sublingual	sublingual	sublingual
subluxación	subluxation	subluxation
submandibular	submandibular	submandibulaire
submucosa	submucosa	tissu sous-muqueux
subnormalidad	subnormality	subnormalité
suboccipital	suboccipital	sous-occipital

ITALIAN	GERMAN	SPANISH
(farmaco) ottenibile senza prescrizione medica	rezeptfrei	sin receta médica
inconscio	bewußtlos	sin sentido
sintomo	Symptom	síntoma
sinusite	Sinusitis	sinusitis
siringomielia	Syringomyelie	siringomielia
sistema nervoso centrale	Zentralnervensystem (ZNS)	sistema nervioso central (SNC)
sistema nervoso simpatico	sympathisches Nervensystem	sistema nervioso simpático
sistema reticoloendoteliale (RES)	retikuloendotheliales System	sistema reticuloendotelial (SRE)
sistole	Systole	sístole
soluzione	Lösung, Auflösung	solución
soluzione di Hartmann	Hartmann-Lösung	solución de Hartmann
soluzione fisiologica	Kochsalzlösung	solución salina
somatico	somatisch, körperlich	somático
somatomammotropina corionica umana	human chorionic somatomammotropin (HCS)	somatomamotropina corionica humana
sonnambulismo	Somnambulismus, Schlafwandeln	sonambulismo
suono	Ton, Klang	sonido
soffio, rullio	Herzgeräusch, Geräusch	soplo
soffio sistolico	systolisches Geräusch, Systolikum	soplo sistólico
ipnotico (n)	Schlafmittel (n)	soporífero (n)
ipnotico (a)	einschläfernd (a)	soporífero (a)
mantenimento delle funzioni vitali	Vitalfunktionserhaltung	soporte de vida básico
sordità	Taubheit, Schwerhörigkeit	sordera
sordo	taub, schwerhörig	sordo
stato	Status, Zustand	status
stress	Belastung, Streß	stress
subacuto	subakut	subagudo
succlavio, sottoclavicolare	Subklavia-	subclavia
subclinico	subklinisch	subclínico
sottocongiuntivale	subkonjunktival	subconjuntival
subconscio	unterbewußt	subconsciente
sottocostale	subkostal	subcostal
sottocutaneo	subkutan	subcutáneo (SC)
subdurale, sottodurale	subdural	subdural
subfertilità	Subfertilität	subfertilidad
subfrenico, sottodiaframmatico	subdiaphragmatisch	subfrénico
soggettivo	subjektiv	subjetivo
sublimato	Sublimat, Quicksilberchlorid	sublimado
subliminale	unterschwellig	subliminal
sublinguale	sublingual	sublingual
sublussazione	Subluxation	subluxación
sottomandibolare	submandibulär	submandibular
sottomucosa	Submukosa	submucosa
subnormalità	Subnormalität	subnormalidad
suboccipitale	subokzipital	suboccipital

SPANISH	ENGLISH	FRENCH
sucusión	succussion	succussion
sudar	sweat	suer
sudor	perspiration, sweat	perspiration, sueur
sudoración nocturna	night sweat	sueurs nocturnes
suelo de la pelvis	pelvic floor	plancher pelvien
sueño	sleep	sommeil
sueño REM	REM sleep	sommeil paradoxal
suero	serum	sérum
sugestión	suggestion	suggestion
suicidio	suicide	suicide
sulfonamida	sulfonamide (Am), sulphonamide (Eng)	sulfamide
sulfonilurea	sulfonylurea (Am), sulphonylurea (Eng)	sulfonylurée
superior	superior	supérieur
supinador	supinator	supinateur
supinar	supination	supination
supino	supine	en supination
supositorio	suppository	suppositoire
supraclavicular	supraclavicular	supraclaviculaire
supracondilar	supracondylar	supracondylaire
supraesternal	suprasternal	suprasternal
suprapúbico	suprapubic	suprapubien
supresión	suppression, withdrawal	suppression, retrait, sevrage
supuración	suppuration	suppuration
surco	sulcus	sillon, gouttière, scissure
surmenage	burnout syndrome	syndrome de 'surmenage'
susceptibilidad	susceptibility	susceptibilité
sutura	suture	suture
suturar	suture	suturer

ITALIAN	GERMAN	SPANISH
succussione, scuotimento	Erschütterung, Schütteln	sucusión
sudare	schwitzen	sudar
perspirazione, sudore	Schweiß	sudor
sudorazione notturna	Nachtschweiß	sudoración nocturna
pavimento pelvico	Beckenboden	suelo de la pelvis
sonno	Schlaf	sueño
sonno REM, fase dei movimenti oculari rapidi	REM-Schlaf	sueño REM
siero	Serum, Blutserum	suero
suggestione	Vorschlag, Suggestion	sugestión
suicidio	Suizid, Selbstmord	suicidio
sulfonammide	Sulfonamid	sulfonamida
sulfonilurea	Sulfonylharnstoff	sulfonilurea
superiore	oben, überlegen	superior
supinatore	Supinator	supinador
supinazione	Supination	supinar
supino	supiniert	supino
supposta	Suppositorium, Zäpfchen	supositorio
sopraclavicolare	supraklavikulär	supraclavicular
sopracondiloideo, epicondiloideo	suprakondylär	supracondilar
soprasternale	suprasternal	supraesternal
soprapubico	suprapubisch	suprapúbico
soppressione, ritiro, astinenza, sospensione	Unterdrückung, Verdrängung, Entzug	supresión
suppurazione	Suppuration, Eiterung	supuración
solco	Sulcus, Furche	surco
incapacità ad agire, sindrome di esaurimento professionale	Helfer-Syndrom	surmenage
suscettibilità	Anfälligkeit, Empfindlichkeit	susceptibilidad
sutura	Naht	sutura
suturare, cucire	nähen	suturar

T

tabes	tabes	tabès
tabique	septum	septum
táctil	tactile	tactile
tálamo	thalamus	thalamus
talasemia	thalassaemia (Eng), thalassemia (Am)	thalassémie
talco	talc	talc
talipes	talipes	pied bot
talón	heel	talon
taponamiento	tamponade	tamponnement
tapon de oído	glue ear	otite moyenne adhésive
taquicardia	tachycardia	tachycardie
taquipnea	tachypnea (Am), tachypnoea (Eng)	tachypnée
tarsalgia	tarsalgia	tarsalgie
tarso	tarsus	tarse
tarsorrafia	tarsorrhaphy	tarsorraphie
tartamudeo	stammer	bégaiement
tasa de filtración glomerular (FG)	glomerular filtration rate (GFR)	taux de filtration glomérulaire
tasa de metabolismo basal (MB)	basal metabolic rate (BMR)	taux du métabolisme basal
técnica aséptica	aseptic technique	technique aseptique
técnica de ultrasonidos Doppler	Doppler ultrasound technique	échographie de Doppler
tejido	tissue	tissu
telangiectasia	telangiectasis	télangiectasie
temblor	tremor	tremblement
temblor fino	fine tremor	tremblement fin
temperamento	temperament	tempérament
temporal	temporal	temporal
tenar	thenar	thénar
tendinitis	tendinitis (Am), tendonitis (Eng)	tendinite
tendón	tendon	tendon
tendón de Aquiles	Achilles tendon	tendon d'Achille
tendón del hueso poplíteo	hamstring	tendon du jarret
tenesmo	tenesmus	ténesme
tenia	Taenia	ténia
tenia solitaria	tapeworm	ténia
tenosinovitis	tenosynovitis	ténosynovite
tenotomía	tenotomy	ténotomie
tensión premenstrual	premenstrual tension (PMT)	syndrome de tension prémenstruelle
tensoactivo	surfactant	surfactant
terapéutica	therapeutics, therapy	thérapeutique, thérapie
terapéutica de reposición de hormonas	hormone replacement therapy (HRT)	traitement hormonal substitutif, hormonothérapie supplétive
terapéutica ocupacional	occupational therapy	ergothérapie
teratógeno	teratogen	tératogène

tabe dorsale	Auszehrung, Schwindsucht	**tabes**
setto	Septum, Scheidewand	**tabique**
tattile	taktil, tastbar	**táctil**
talamo	Thalamus	**tálamo**
talassemia	Thalassämie, Mittelmeeranämie	**talasemia**
talco	Talkum	**talco**
piede talo	Klumpfuß, pes equinovarus	**talipes**
tallone	Ferse	**talón**
tamponamento	Tamponade	**taponamiento**
cerume nell orecchio	glue ear	**tapon de oído**
tachicardia	Tachykardie	**taquicardia**
tachipnea	Tachypnoe	**taquipnea**
tarsalgia	Tarsalgie	**tarsalgia**
tarso	Fußwurzel, Lidknorpel	**tarso**
tarsorrafia	Tarsorrhaphie	**tarsorrafia**
balbuzie	Stottern	**tartamudeo**
volume di filtrazione glomerulare (VFG)	glomeruläre Filtrationsrate (GFR)	**tasa de filtración glomerular (FG)**
indice del metabolismo basale (MB)	Grundumsatz	**tasa de metabolismo basal (MB)**
tecnica asettica	aseptische Technik	**técnica aséptica**
tecnica ultrasonografica Doppler	Doppler-Sonographie	**técnica de ultrasonidos Doppler**
tessuto	Gewebe	**tejido**
telangectasia	Teleangiektasie	**telangiectasia**
tremore	Tremor	**temblor**
tremore fino	feinschlägiger Tremor	**temblor fino**
temperamento	Temperament, Gemütsart	**temperamento**
temporale	temporal, Schläfen-	**temporal**
pertinente al palmo della mano	Thenar-	**tenar**
tendinite	Tendinitis, Sehnenentzündung	**tendinitis**
tendine	Sehne	**tendón**
tendine di Achille	Achillessehne	**tendón de Aquiles**
tendine del ginocchio	Kniesehne	**tendón del hueso poplíteo**
tenesmo	Tenesmus	**tenesmo**
Tenia	Bandwurm, Tänia	**tenia**
cestode	Bandwurm, Tänia	**tenia solitaria**
tenosinovite	Tendovaginitis, Tendosynovitis, Sehnenscheidenentzündung	**tenosinovitis**
tenotomia	Tenotomie	**tenotomía**
tensione premenstruale	prämenstruelles Syndrom	**tensión premenstrual**
tensioattivo, surfattante	Surfactant-Faktor	**tensoactivo**
terapia	Therapeutik, -therapie, Therapie, Behandlung	**terapéutica**
terapia sostitutiva ormonale	Hormonsubstitutionstherapie	**terapéutica de reposición de hormonas**
ergoterapia	Beschäftigungstherapie	**terapéutica ocupacional**
teratogeno	Teratogen	**teratógeno**

SPANISH	ENGLISH	FRENCH
teratoma	teratoma	tératome
terciario	tertiary	tertiaire
termal	thermal	thermique
terminación nerviosa	nerve ending	terminaison nerveuse
termómetro	thermometer	thermomètre
testículo	orchis, testis	testicule
testículos no descendidos	undescended testes	ectopie testiculaire
tetania	tetany	tétanie
tétanos	tetanus	tétanos
tetralogía de Fallot	Fallot's tetralogy, tetralogy of Fallot	trilogie de Fallot, tétralogie de Fallot
tetraplejía	tetraplegia	tétraplégie
tibia	shin bone, tibia	tibia
tibioperoneo	tibiofibular	tibiofibulaire
tic	tic	tic
tic doloroso	tic douloureux	tic douloureux
tiempo de sangría	'bleeding time'	temps de saignement
tifus	typhus	typhus
timo	thymus	thymus
timpánico	tympanic	tympanique
tímpano	eardrum, tympanum	tympan
timpanoplastia	tympanoplasty	tympanoplastie
tiña	ringworm, tinea	dermatophytose, teigne
tinción de Gram	Gram stain	coloration de Gram
tinnitus	tinnitus	tintement
tipo	type	type
tirogloso	thyroglossal	thyroglossien
tiroidectomía	thyroidectomy	thyroïdectomie
tiroides	thyroid	thyroïde
tiroiditis	thyroiditis	thyroïdite
tirotoxicosis	thyrotoxicosis	thyrotoxicose
tiroxina libre	free thyroxine (FT)	thyroxine libre (TL)
tisis	consumption	consommation
titulación	titration	titrage
titulo	titer (Am), titre (Eng)	titre
tobillo	ankle	cheville
tococardiógrafo	cardiotocograph	cardiotocographe
todavía no diagnosticado	not yet diagnosed (NYD)	non encore diagnostiqué
tofo	tophus	tophus
tolerancia	tolerance	tolérance
tomografía axial computerizada (TAC)	computerized axial tomography (CAT)	tacographie
tomografía computerizada	computerized tomography	tomographie avec ordinateur, scanographie
tónico	tonic	tonique
tono	tone	tonus
tonómetro	tonometer	tonomètre
tonsilectomía	tonsillectomy	amygdalectomie

ITALIAN	GERMAN	SPANISH
teratoma	Teratom	teratoma
terziario	tertiär, dritten Grades	terciario
termale	thermal, Wärme-	termal
terminazione nervosa	Nervenendigung	terminación nerviosa
termometro	Thermometer	termómetro
testicolo	Hoden	testículo
testicoli ritenuti	Kryptorchismus	testículos no descendidos
tetania	Tetanie	tetania
tetano	Tetanus, Wundstarrkrampf	tétanos
tetralogia di Fallot	Fallot-Tetralogie	tetralogía de Fallot
tetraplegia	Tetraplegie	tetraplejía
tibia	Schienbein, Tibia	tibia
tibiofibulare	tibiofibular	tibioperoneo
tic	Tic	tic
tic doloroso, nevralgia del trigemino	Tic douloureux	tic doloroso
tempo di sanguinamento	Blutungszeit	tiempo de sangría
tifo	Typhus, Fleckfieber	tifus
timo	Thymus	timo
timpanico, risonante	Trommelfell-	timpánico
timpano	Trommelfell, Tympanon	tímpano
timpanoplastica	Tympanoplastik	timpanoplastia
tricofizia, tinea, tigna	Tinea, Fadenpilzerkrankung, Onchozerkose	tiña
colorazione di Gram	Gramfärbung	tinción de Gram
tinnito	Tinnitus	tinnitus
tipo	Typ, Art	tipo
tireoglosso	thyreoglossus	tirogloso
tiroidectomia	Thyreoidektomie	tiroidectomía
tiroide	Thyreoidea, Schilddrüse	tiroides
tiroidite	Thyreoiditis	tiroiditis
tireotossicosi, ipertiroidismo	Thyreotoxikose	tirotoxicosis
tiroxina libera (FT)	freies Thyroxin (FT)	tiroxina libre
consunzione	Konsum, Verbrauch	tisis
titolazione	Titration	titulación
titolo	Titer	titulo
caviglia	Knöchel, Talus	tobillo
cardiotocografia	Kardiotokograph	tococardiógrafo
non ancora diagnosticato	noch nicht diagnostiziert	todavía no diagnosticado
tofo, concrezione tofacea	Tophus, Gichtknoten	tofo
tolleranza	Toleranz	tolerancia
tomografia assiale computerizzata (TAC)	axiale Computertomographie	tomografía axial computerizada (TAC)
tomografia computerizzata	Computertomographie (CT)	tomografía computerizada
tonico	Tonikum, Stärkungsmittel	tónico
tono	Ton, Laut	tono
tonometro	Tonometer	tonómetro
tonsillectomia	Tonsillektomie, Mandelentfernung	tonsilectomía

SPANISH	ENGLISH	FRENCH
tópico	topical	topique
torácico	thoracic	thoracique
toracoplastia	thoracoplasty	thoracoplastie
toracotomía	thoracotomy	thoracotomie
tórax	thorax	thorax
tórax de pichón	pigeon chest	thorax en carène
torcer	sprain	se fouler
tornasol	litmus	tournesol
torniquete	tourniquet	tourniquet
torsión	torsion	torsion
tortícolis	wry-neck	torticolis
torunda	swab	tampon
tos	cough	toux
toser	cough	tousser
tos ferina	pertussis, whooping cough	pertussis, coqueluche
toxemia	toxaemia (Eng), toxemia (Am)	toxémie
toxicidad	toxicity	toxicité
tóxico	toxic	toxique
toxicomanía	addiction	accoutumance
toxina	toxin	toxine
toxoide	toxoid	toxoïde
toxoplasmosis	toxoplasmosis	toxoplasmose
tracción	traction	traction
tracoma	trachoma	trachome
tragar	swallow	avaler
tranquilizante	tranquilizer	tranquillisant
transabdominal	transabdominal	transabdominal
transamniótico	transamniotic	transamniotique
transcutáneo	transcutaneous	transcutané
transección	transection	transsection
transfusión	transfusion	transfusion
translocación	translocation	translocation
translúcido	translucent	translucide
transmural	transmural	transmural
transtorácico	transthoracic	transthoracique
transuretral	transurethral	transurétral
tráquea	trachea, windpipe	trachée
traqueitis	tracheitis	trachéite
traqueoesofágico	tracheoesophageal (Am), tracheo-oesophageal (Eng)	trachéo-oesophagien
traqueostomía	tracheostomy	trachéostomie
traqueotomía	tracheotomy	trachéotomie
trasmisible	contagious	contagieux
trasplantar	transplant	transplanter
trasplante	transplant	transplantation
trastorno funcional	functional disorder	fonctionnel

ITALIAN	GERMAN	SPANISH
topico, locale	topisch, örtlich	tópico
toracico	thorakal, Brust-	torácico
toracoplastica	Thorakoplastik	toracoplastia
toracotomia	Thorakotomie	toracotomía
torace	Thorax, Brustkorb	tórax
torace carenato	Hühnerbrust	tórax de pichón
distorcere	verstauchen	torcer
tornasole	Lackmus	tornasol
laccio emostatico	Tourniquet	torniquete
torsione	Torsion	torsión
torcicollo	Tortikollis, (angeborener) Schiefhals	tortícolis
tampone	Tupfer, Abstrichtupfer	torunda
tosse	Husten	tos
tossire	husten	toser
pertosse	Pertussis, Keuchhusten	tos ferina
tossiemia	Toxämie, Toxikämie, Blutvergiftung	toxemia
tossicità	Toxizität	toxicidad
tossico	toxisch, giftig	tóxico
tossicomania	Sucht, Gewöhnung	toxicomanía
tossina	Toxin	toxina
tossoide	Toxoid	toxoide
toxoplasmosi	Toxoplasmose	toxoplasmosis
trazione, attrazione	Traktion, Zug	tracción
tracoma	Trachom, ägyptische Augenkrankheit	tracoma
inghiottire	schlucken	tragar
tranquillante	Tranquilizer, Beruhigungsmittel	tranquilizante
transaddominale	transabdominal	transabdominal
transamniotico	transamniotisch	transamniótico
percutaneo	transkutan	transcutáneo
sezione trasversale	Querschnitt	transección
trasfusione	Transfusion, Bluttransfusion	transfusión
traslocazione	Translokation	translocación
translucido	durchscheinend, durchsichtig	translúcido
transmurale	transmural	transmural
transtoracico	transthorakal	transtorácico
transuretrale	transurethral	transuretral
trachea	Trachea, Luftröhre	tráquea
tracheite	Tracheitis	traqueitis
tracheoesofageo	Tracheoösophageal-	traqueoesofágico
tracheostomia	Tracheostomie	traqueostomía
tracheotomia	Tracheotomie, Luftröhrenschnitt	traqueotomía
contagioso	kontagiös, ansteckend	trasmisible
trapiantare	transplantieren	trasplantar
trapianto	Transplantat, Transplantation	trasplante
disturbo funzionale	funktionelle Störung	trastorno funcional

trasudado	transudate	transsudat
tratamiento con oxígeno hiperbárico	hyperbaric oxygen treatment	oxygénothérapie hyperbase
tratamiento por aversión	aversion therapy	cure de dégoût
trauma	trauma	traumatisme
trazador	tracer	traceur
trematodo	fluke	douve
trepanar	trephine	trépaner
trépano	trephine	tréphine
triage	triage	triage
tríceps	triceps	triceps
trichuris trichiura	whipworm	flagellé
tricotilomanía	trichotillomania	trichotillomanie
tricúspide	tricuspid	tricuspide
trigémino	trigeminal	trigéminal
trimestre	trimester	trimestre
tripanosomiasis	trypanosomiasis	trypanosomiase
trismo	lock jaw	tétanos
trisomía	trisomy	trisomie
trocánter	trochanter	trochanter
trombectomía	thrombectomy	thrombectomie
trombo	thrombus	thrombus
trombocitemia	thrombocythaemia (Eng), thrombocythemia (Am)	thrombocytémie
trombocito	thrombocyte	thrombocyte
trombocitopenia	thrombocytopenia	thrombopénie
trombocitosis	thrombocytosis	thrombocytose
tromboembólico	thromboembolic	thrombo-embolique
tromboflebitis	thrombophlebitis	thrombophlébite
trombolítico	thrombolytic	thrombolytique
trombosis	thrombosis	thrombose
trombosis venosa profunda	deep vein thrombosis (DVT)	thrombose veineuse profonde (TVP)
trompa de Eustaquio	Eustachian tube	trompe d'Eustache
trompa de Falopio	Fallopian tube	trompe de Fallope
tubárico	tubal	tubaire
tubérculo	tubercle	tubercule
tuberculoide	tuberculoid	tuberculoïde
tuberculosis (TB)	tuberculosis (TB)	tuberculose (TB)
tuberosidad	tuberosity	tubérosité
tubo de ensayo	test tube	tube à essai, éprouvette
túbulo	tubule	tube
tumescencia	tumescence	tumescence
tumor	tumor (Am), tumour (Eng)	tumeur
tumor de Wilms	Wilms' tumor (Am), Wilms' tumour (Eng)	tumeur de Wilms
turbinado	turbinate	cornet
túrgido	turgid	enflé

ITALIAN	GERMAN	SPANISH
trasudato	Transsudat	trasudado
ossigenoterapia iperbarica	hyperbare Sauerstoffbehandlung	tratamiento con oxígeno hiperbárico
decondizionamento	Aversionstherapie	tratamiento por aversión
trauma	Trauma	trauma
tracciante	Tracer	trazador
trematode, Digeneum	Trematode	trematodo
trapanare	trepanieren	trepanar
trapano	Trepan	trépano
selezione e distribuzione dei malati	Triage	triage
tricipite	Trizeps	tríceps
verme a frusta, tricocefalo	Oxyuris, Peitschenwurm	trichuris trichiura
tricotíllomania	Trichotillomanie	tricotilomanía
tricuspide	Trikuspidal	tricúspide
trigemino	Trigeminus-	trigémino
trimestre	Trimester	trimestre
tripanosomiasi	Trypanosomiasis	tripanosomiasis
tetano, trisma	Kiefersperre	trismo
trisomia	Trisomie	trisomía
trocantere	Trochanter	trocánter
trombectomia	Thrombektomie	trombectomía
trombo	Thrombus	trombo
trombocitemia	Thrombozythämie	trombocitemia
trombocito	Thrombozyt, Blutplättchen	trombocito
trombocitopenia	Thrombopenie	trombocitopenia
trombocitosi	Thrombozytose	trombocitosis
tromboembolico	thromboembolisch	tromboembólico
tromboflebite	Thrombophlebitis	tromboflebitis
trombolitico	thrombolytisch	trombolítico
trombosi	Thrombose	trombosis
trombosi venosa profonda (TVP)	tiefe Venenthrombose	trombosis venosa profunda
tuba d'Eustachio	Eustachische Röhre	trompa de Eustaquio
tuba di Falloppio	Tube, Eileiter	trompa de Falopio
tubarico	Tuben-, Eileiter-	tubárico
tubercolo	Tuberkel	tubérculo
tubercoloide	tuberkuloid	tuberculoide
tubercolosi (TBC)	Tuberkulöse	tuberculosis (TB)
tuberosità	Tuberositas	tuberosidad
provetta	Reagenzglas	tubo de ensayo
tubulo	Tubulus, Röhrchen	túbulo
tumefazione	Tumeszenz, diffuse Anschwellung	tumescencia
tumore, tumefazione	Tumor	tumor
tumore di Wilms	Wilms-Tumor	tumor de Wilms
turbinato	Nasenmuschel	turbinado
turgido	geschwollen	túrgido

U

SPANISH	ENGLISH	FRENCH
úlcera	ulcer	ulcère
úlcera corrosiva	rodent ulcer	ulcus rodens
úlcera de decúbito	pressure sore	plaie de décubitus
úlcera dendrítica	dendritic ulcer	ulcère dendritique
úlcera duodenal	duodenal ulcer	ulcère duodénal
úlcera por decúbito	bedsore	escarre de décubitus
ulcerativo	ulcerative	ulcératif
úlcera trófica	trophic ulcer	ulcère trophique
ultrasonografía	ultrasonography	échographie
ultravioleta (UV)	ultraviolet (UV)	ultraviolet (UV)
uña	nail	ongle
ungüento	ointment, salve	pommade
unidad de cuidados coronarios (UCC)	coronary care unit (CCU)	unité de soins intensifs coronaires
unidad de cuidados especiales	special care unit (SCU)	unité de soins spéciaux
unidad de cuidados intensivos (UCI)	intensive care unit (ICU), intensive therapy unit (ITU)	unité de soins intensifs, service de réanimation
unidad de cuidados intensivos para recién nacidos	neonatal intensive care unit (NICU) (Am)	service de soins intensifs néonatals
unidad para cuidados especiales neonatales	special care baby unit (SCBU)	pavillon de soins spéciaux aux nouveau-nés
unilateral	unilateral	unilatéral
uniocular	uniocular	unioculé
unión defectuosa	malunion	cal vicieux
urato	urate	urate
urea	urea	urée
urea sérica	blood urea	urée du sang
uremia	uraemia (Eng), uremia (Am)	urémie
uréter	ureter	uretère
ureterocólico	ureterocolic	urétérocolique
uretra	urethra	urètre
uretritis	urethritis	urétrite
uretritis inespecífica	non-specific urethritis (NSU)	urétrite aspécifique
uretritis no gonocócica	non-gonococcal urethritis (NGU)	urétrite non gonococcique
uretrocele	urethrocele	urétrocèle
uricemia	uricaemia (Eng), uricemia (Am)	uricémie
uricosúrico	uricosuria	uricosurique
urinálisis	urinalysis	analyse d'urine
urografía	urography	urographie
urología	urology	urologie
urticaria	hives, nettle rash, urticaria	éruption, urticaire
útero	uterus	utérus
útero pequeño para la edad gestacional	small-for-dates (SFD)	présentant un retard de croissance
uterosacro	uterosacral	utéro-sacré

ITALIAN	GERMAN	SPANISH
ulcera	Ulkus, Geschwür	úlcera
ulcus rodens, basalioma	Ulcus rodens	úlcera corrosiva
ulcera da decubito	Druckgeschwür, Dekubitus	úlcera de decúbito
ulcera dendritica	verzweigtes Geschwür	úlcera dendrítica
ulcera duodenale	Duodenalulkus, Zwölffingerdarmgeschwür	úlcera duodenal
piaga da decubito	Dekubitus, Durchliegen	úlcera por decúbito
ulcerativo, ulceroso	ulzerierend, geschwürig	ulcerativo
ulcera trofica	trophisches Ulkus	úlcera trófica
ultrasonografia, ecografia	Sonographie, Ultraschallmethode	ultrasonografía
ultravioletto (UV)	ultraviolett	ultravioleta (UV)
unghia	Nagel	uña
unguento	Salbe	ungüento
reparto coronarico	Infarktpflegestation	unidad de cuidados coronarios (UCC)
unità pediatrica di cure speciali	Intensivstation	unidad de cuidados especiales
unità di cura intensiva, unità di terapia intensiva	Intensivstation	unidad de cuidados intensivos (UCI)
reparto di terapia intensiva neonatale	Frühgeborenen-Intensivstation	unidad de cuidados intensivos para recién nacidos
unità di cure speciali pediatriche	Säuglings-Intensivstation	unidad para cuidados especiales neonatales
unilaterale	einseitig	unilateral
monoculare	einäugig	uniocular
unione difettosa	Fehlstellung (Frakturenden)	unión defectuosa
urato	Urat	urato
urea, carbammide	Urea, Harnstoff	urea
azotemia	Blutharnstoff	urea sérica
uremia	Urämie, Harnvergiftung	uremia
uretere	Ureter, Harnleiter	uréter
ureterocolico	Ureterkolik	ureterocólico
uretra	Urethra, Harnröhre	uretra
uretrite	Urethritis	uretritis
uretrite aspecifica	unspezifische Urethritis	uretritis inespecífica
uretrite non gonococcica	nicht durch Gonokokken bedingte Urethritis	urethritis no gonocócica
uretrocele	Urethrozele	uretrocele
uricemia	Urikämie	uricemia
uricuria	Urikosurie	uricosúrico
esame dell'urina	Urinanalyse, Urinuntersuchung	urinálisis
urografia	Urographie	urografía
urologia	Urologie	urología
orticaria	Ausschlag, Nesselfieber, Urtikaria, Nesselsucht	urticaria
utero	Uterus, Gebärmutter	útero
basso peso alla nascita	termingemäß klein	útero pequeño para la edad gestacional
uterosacrale	uterosakral	uterosacro

SPANISH	ENGLISH	FRENCH
uterovesical	uterovesical	utéro-vésical
uveitis	uveitis	uréite
úvula	uvula	uvule
uvulitis	uvulitis	uvulite

ITALIAN	GERMAN	ENGLISH	SPANISH
uterovescicale	uterovesikal		uterovesical
uveite	Uveitis		uveitis
ugola	Uvula, Zäpfchen		úvula
stafilite	Uvulitis		uvulitis

V

vacuna	vaccine	vaccin
vacunación	vaccination	vaccination
vacuna triple	triple vaccine	triple vaccin
vagal	vagal	vague
vagina	vagina	vagin
vaginismo	vaginismus	vaginisme
vaginitis	vaginitis	vaginite
vagotomía	vagotomy	vagotomie
vahído	faint	syncope
valgus	valgus	valgus
valvotomía	valvotomy	valvulotomie
válvula	valve	valve
varicela	chickenpox, varicella	varicelle
varices	varicose veins	varices
varilla de Harrington	Harrington rod	tige de Harrington
varus	varus	varus
vascular	vascular	vasculaire
vasculitis	vasculitis	vasculite
vasculopatia pulmonar	pulmonary vascular disease (PVD)	pneumopathie vasculaire
vasectomía	vasectomy	vasectomie
vaso	vessel	vaisseau
vasoconstrictor *(n)*	vasoconstrictor *(n)*	vasoconstricteur *(n)*
vasoconstrictor *(a)*	vasoconstrictor *(a)*	vasoconstricteur *(a)*
vasodilatador *(n)*	vasodilator *(n)*	vasodilatateur *(n)*
vasodilatador *(a)*	vasodilator *(a)*	vasodilatateur *(a)*
vasopresor *(n)*	vasopressor *(n)*	vasopresseur *(n)*
vasopresor *(a)*	vasopressor *(a)*	vasopresseur *(a)*
vasospasmo	vasospasm	spasme d'un vaisseau
vector	vector	vecteur
vejiga	bladder	vessie
vellosidad	villus	villosité
vellosidades coriónicas	chorionic villi	villosités du chorion
velocidad de sedimentación globular (VSG)	blood sedimentation rate (BSR), erythrocyte sedimentation rate (ESR), sedimentation rate (SR)	vitesse de sédimentation sanguine, vitesse de sédimentation globulaire, vitesse de sédimentation (VS)
velocidad espiratoria máxima (VEM)	peak expiratory velocity (PEV)	volume expiratoire maximum (VEM)
velocidad máxima del flujo espiratorio (VMFE)	peak expiratory flow rate (PEFR)	débit expiratoire de pointe
vena	vein	veine
vena cava	vena cava	veine cave
vena cubital	cubital vein	veine de l'avant-bras
vena femoral	femoral vein	veine fémorale
vena porta	portal vein	veine porte
vena radial	radial vein	veine radiale

ITALIAN	GERMAN	SPANISH
vaccino	Vakzine, Impfstoff	vacuna
vaccinazione	Impfung, Vakzination	vacunación
triplo vaccino	Dreifachimpfstoff	vacuna triple
vagale	vagal, Vagus-	vagal
vagina	Vagina, Scheide	vagina
vaginismo	Vaginismus	vaginismo
vaginite	Vaginitis	vaginitis
vagotomia	Vagotomie	vagotomía
svenimento	Ohnmacht	vahído
valgo	valgus	valgus
valvulotomia	Valvotomie	valvotomía
valvola	Klappe, Ventil	válvula
varicella	Varizellen, Windpocken	varicela
vene varicose	Varizen, Krampfadern	varices
bastoncello retiníco (per anestetizzare la dentina)	Harrington Stab	varilla de Harrington
varo	varus	varus
vascolare	vaskulär, Gefäß-	vascular
vasculite	Vaskulitis	vasculitis
vasculopatia polmonare	Lungengefäßerkrankung	vasculopatia pulmonar
vasectomia	Vasektomie, Vasoresektion	vasectomía
vaso	Gefäß, Ader	vaso
vasocostrittore (n)	Vasokonstriktor (n)	vasoconstrictor (n)
vasocostrittore (a)	vasokonstriktorisch (a)	vasoconstrictor (a)
vasodilatatore (n)	Vasodilatator (n)	vasodilatador (n)
vasodilatatore (a)	vasodilatatorisch (a)	vasodilatador (a)
vasopressore (n)	Vasopressor (n)	vasopresor (n)
vasopressore (a)	vasopressorisch (a)	vasopresor (a)
vasospasmo, angiospasmo	Vasospasmus	vasospasmo
vettore	Überträger, Vektor	vector
vescica	Blase, Harnblase	vejiga
villo	Zotte	vellosidad
villi coriali	Chorionzotten	vellosidades coriónicas
velocità di eritrosedimentazione (VES)	Blutkörperchen-Senkungsgeschwindigkeit (BSG, BKS)	velocidad de sedimentación globular (VSG)
velocità espiratoria massima (VEM)	maximale exspiratorische Atemgeschwindigkeit	velocidad espiratoria máxima (VEM)
tasso di picco del flusso espiratorio	maximale exspiratorische Atemstromstärke	velocidad máxima del flujo espiratorio (VMFE)
vena	Vene	vena
vena cava	Vena cava	vena cava
vena cubitale	Unterarmvene	vena cubital
vena femorale	Vena femoralis	vena femoral
vena porta	Pfortader	vena porta
vena radiale	Vena radialis	vena radial

vena yugular	jugular vein	veine jugulaire
vendaje	bandage, dressing	bandage, pansement
vendaje de yeso	cast	plâtre
veneno	poison	poison
venéreo	venereal	vénérien
venereología	venereology	vénéréologie
venipuntura	venipuncture	ponction d'une veine
venisección	venesection	phlébotomie
venografía	venography	phlébographie
venopuntura	venepuncture	ponction d'une veine
ventilación con presión positiva	positive pressure ventilation	ventilation à pression positive
ventilador	ventilator	appareil de ventilation artificielle
ventosidad	wind	gaz
ventral	ventral	ventral
ventrículo	ventricle	ventricule
ventrofijación	ventrofixation	hystéropexie abdominale
ventrosuspensión	ventrosuspension	ventro-suspension
vénula	venule	veinule
verdugón	weal	marque
verruga	verruca, wart	verrue
versión	version	version
versión cefálica externa	external cephalic version (ECV)	version céphalique externe
vértebra	vertebra	vertèbre
vértice	vertex	vertex
vértigo	vertigo	vertige
vesicoureteral	vesicoureteric	vésico-urétérique
vesicovaginal	vesicovaginal	vésico-vaginal
vesícula	bleb, blister, vesicle	phlyctène, ampoule, vésicule
vesícula biliar	gall bladder	vésicule biliaire
vestíbulo	vestibule	vestibule
viable	viable	viable
víal	ampoule (Eng), ampule (Am)	ampoule
vías respiratorias y circulación	airway breathing and circulation (ABC)	intubation ventilation et circulation
vientre	belly	ventre
vinculación	bonding	attachement
vinculado al sexo	sex-linked	lié au sexe
viremia	viraemia (Eng), viremia (Am)	virémie
virilismo	virilism	virilisme
virología	virology	virologie
viruela	smallpox	variole
virulencia	virulence	virulence
virus	virus	virus
virus Coxsackie	Coxsackie virus	virus Coxsackie
virus de Epstein-Barr	Epstein-Barr virus (EBV)	virus d'Epstein-Barr
virus de la inmunodeficiencia humana (VIH)	human immunodeficiency virus (HIV)	virus de l'immunodéficience humaine

ITALIAN	GERMAN	SPANISH
vena giugulare	Vena jugularis	vena yugular
benda, medicazione	Verband, Umschlag	vendaje
ingessatura, steccatura	Abdruck, Gipsverband	vendaje de yeso
veleno	Gift	veneno
venereo	venerisch	venéreo
venereologia	Venerologie	venereología
puntura di vena	Venenpunktion	venipuntura
flebotomia	Venae sectio	venisección
flebografia	Phlebographie	venografía
puntura di vena	Venenpunktion	venopuntura
ventilazione a pressione positiva	Überdruckbeatmung	ventilación con presión positiva
ventilatore	Ventilator	ventilador
flatulenza, ventosità	Blähung, Wind	ventosidad
ventrale	ventral, Bauch-	ventral
ventricolo	Ventrikel, Kammer	ventrículo
ventro-fissazione	Hysteropexie	ventrofijación
ventrosospensione, ventrofissazione	Ventrofixation, Ligamentopexie	ventrosuspensión
venula	Venula	vénula
pomfo	Schwiele, Striemen	verdugón
verruca, verruca volgare	Warze, Verruca	verruga
versione	Versio, Wendung	versión
versione cefalica esterna	äußere Wendung auf den Kopf	versión cefálica externa
vertebra	Wirbel	vértebra
vertice	Vertex, Scheitel	vértice
vertigine	Schwindel, Vertigo	vértigo
vescicoureterale	vesikoureteral	vesicoureteral
vescicovaginale	vesikovaginal	vesicovaginal
vescichetta, flittena, vescicola, bolla	Blase, Hautblase, Brandblase, Vesikula, Bläschen	vesícula
cistifellea	Gallenblase	vesícula biliar
vestibolo	Vestibulum, Vorhof	vestíbulo
vitale, in grado di vivere	lebensfähig	viable
ampolla, fiala	Ampulle	vial
ventilazione e respirazione nelle vie respiratorie	Luftwege Atmung und Kreislauf (ABC-Regel)	vías respiratorias y circulación
addome, ventre	Bauch	vientre
legame	Bindung	vinculación
legato al sesso	geschlechtsgebunden	vinculado al sexo
viremia	Virämie	viremia
virilismo	Virilismus	virilismo
virologia	Virologie	virología
vaiolo	Variola, Pocken	viruela
virulenza	Virulenz	virulencia
virus	Virus	virus
virus Coxsackie	Coxsackie-Virus	virus Coxsackie
virus di Epstein Barr	Epstein-Barr-Virus (EBV)	virus de Epstein-Barr
virus dell'immunodeficienza umana (HIV)	human immunodeficiency virus (HIV), AIDS-Virus	virus de la inmunodeficiencia humana (VIH)

SPANISH	ENGLISH	FRENCH
virus del herpes simple (VHS)	herpes simplex virus (HSV)	virus de l'herpès simplex (HSV)
virus ECHO	echovirus	échovirus
virus semejante al del herpes (HLV)	herpes-like virus (HLV)	virus de type herpétique (HLV)
virus sincitial respiratorio (VSR)	respiratory syncytial virus (RSV)	virus respiratoire syncytial
visceras	viscera	viscères
viscoso	viscid	visqueux
visión binocular	binocular vision	vision binoculaire
visión doble	double vision	double vision
visual	visual	visuel
vitamina	vitamin	vitamine
vitíligo	vitiligo	vitiligo
vítreo	vitreous body	vitré
volet torácico	flail chest	volet thoracique
volumen corpuscular medio (VCM)	mean corpuscular volume (MCV)	volume globulaire moyen (VGM)
volumen de células agregadas	packed cell volume (PCV)	hématocrite
volumen espiratorio forzado (VEF)	forced expiratory volume (FEV)	volume expiratoire maximum (VEM)
volumen hemático	blood volume (BV)	masse sanguine
vólvulo	volvulus	volvulus
vomitar	vomit	vomir
vómito cíclico	cyclical vomiting	vomissement cyclique
vulva	vulva	vulve
vulvitis	vulvitis	vulvite
vulvovaginal	vulvovaginal	vulvo-vaginal

ITALIAN	GERMAN	SPANISH
virus herpes simplex	Herpes simplex-Virus (HSV)	virus del herpes simple (VHS)
echovirus	ECHO-Virus	virus ECHO
virus della famiglia dell'herpes	Herpes-ähnlicher Virus	virus semejante al del herpes (HLV)
virus respiratorio sinciziale (RSV)	RS-Virus	virus sincitial respiratorio (VSR)
visceri	Eingeweide, Viszera	visceras
viscido	zäh, klebrig	viscoso
visione binoculare	binokulares Sehen, beidäugiges Sehen	visión binocular
diplopia	Doppelsehen, Diplopie	visión doble
visivo	visuell, Seh-	visual
vitamina	Vitamin	vitamina
vitiligine	Vitiligo	vitíligo
corpo vitreo	Glaskörper	vítreo
anomala motilità respiratoria della cassa toracica in conseguenza di fratture	Flatterbrust	volet torácico
volume corpuscolare medio (VCM)	mittleres Erythrozytenvolumen (MCV)	volumen corpuscular medio (VCM)
volume cellulare (VC)	Hämatokrit (HKT)	volumen de células agregadas
volume espiratorio forzato	forciertes Exspirationsvolumen, Atemstoßwert	volumen espiratorio forzado (VEF)
volume sanguigno	Blutvolumen	volumen hemático
volvolo	Volvulus	vólvulo
vomitare	sich übergeben, erbrechen	vomitar
vomito ciclico	zyklisches Erbrechen	vómito cíclico
vulva	Vulva	vulva
vulvite	Vulvitis	vulvitis
vulvovaginale	vulvovaginal	vulvovaginal

X

xantelasma	xanthelasma	xanthélasma
xantemia	xanthaemia (Eng), xanthemia (Am)	xanthémie, caroténémie
xantoma	xanthoma	xanthome
xeroderma	xeroderma	xérodermie
xeroftalmia	xerophthalmia	xérophtalmie

Y

yatrógeno	iatrogenic	iatrogène
yaws	yaws	pian
yeso	gypsum, plaster	gypse, plâtre
yeyuno	jejunum	jéjunum
yodo	iodine	iode
yunque	incus	enclume

Z

zona de decúbito	pressure area	zone particulièrement sensible
zoonosis	zoonosis	zoonose
zóster	zoster	zona
zurdo	left-handed	gaucher

ITALIAN	GERMAN	SPANISH
xantelasma	Xanthelasma	**xantelasma**
xantemia	Xanthämie	**xantemia**
xantoma, malattia di Rayer	Xanthom	**xantoma**
xerodermia	Xerodermie	**xeroderma**
xeroftalmia	Xerophthalmie	**xeroftalmia**
iatrogeno	iatrogen	**yatrógeno**
framboesia, pian	Frambösie	**yaws**
gesso, solfato di calcio	Gips, Pflaster	**yeso**
digiuno	Jejunum	**yeyuno**
iodio	Jod	**yodo**
incudine	Incus, Amboß	**yunque**
area di pressione	Druckfläche	**zona de decúbito**
zoonosi	Zoonose, Tierkrankheit	**zoonosis**
herpes zoster	Herpes zoster, Gürtelrose	**zóster**
mancino	linkshändig	**zurdo**

ABRÉVIATIONS ESPAGNOLES
SPANISCHE ABKÜRZUNGEN
ABBREVIAZIONI SPAGNOLE
ABREVIATURAS ESPAÑOLAS

ACTH	hormona adrenocorticotropa
ACV	accidente vascular cerebral
ADN	ácido desoxirribonucléico
AFP	alfafetoproteína
AID	inseminación artificial por donante
AINE	fármaco antiinflamatorio no esteroide
AIT	ataque isquémico transitorio
AR	artritis reumatoide
ARN	ácido ribonucléico
AV	aurículo-ventricular
AVM	ácido vanilmandélico
BCG	bacilo de Calmette-Guérin
BHE	barrera hematoencefálica
CID	coagulación intravascular diseminada
CPT	capacidad pulmonar total
DIU	dispositivo intrauterino anticonceptivo
ECG	electrocardiograma
ECT	electrochoqueterapia
EEG	electroencefalograma
ETS	enfermedad de transmisión sexual
FCF	frecuencia cardíaca fetal
FG	tasa de filtración glomerular
FIV	fertilización in vitro
FPP	fecha probable del parto
FSH	hormona estimulante del folículo
FSR	flujo sanguíneo renal
FUR	fecha última regla
GCH	gonadotropina coriónica humana
GGT	gamma glutamil transferasa
Hb	hemoglobina
HC	hormona del crecimiento
HCS	hormona corticosuprarrenal
HDL	lipoproteína de alta densidad
HDLC	colesterol unido a las lipoproteínas de alta densidad
HLA	antígeno linfocitario humano
HLV	virus semejante al del herpes
ICC	insuficiencia cardíaca congestiva
Ig	inmunoglobulina
IM	infarto de miocardio
im	intramuscular
IMAO	inhibidor de la monoaminooxidasa
IMC	índice de masa corporal
IV	intravenoso
IVU	infección de las vías urinarias
LCR	líquido cefalorraquídeo
LDL	lipoproteína de baja densidad
LES	lupus eritematoso sistémico
LH	hormona luteinizante
MB	tasa de metabolismo basal

mEq	miliequivalente
ORL	otorrinolaringología
PA	presión arterial
PCP	presión capilar pulmonar
PIC	presión intracraneal
PL	punción lumbar
ppm	partes por millón
psi	libras por pulgada cuadrada
PVC	presión venosa central
RAST	prueba radioalergosorbente
REM	movimiento rápido de los ojos
Rh−	rhesus negativo
Rh+	rhesus positivo
SC	subcutáneo
SIDA	síndrome de inmunodeficiencia adquirida
SNC	sistema nervioso central
SRE	sistema reticuloendotelial
TAC	tomografía axial computerizada
TB	tuberculosis
TSH	hormona estimulante del tiroides
UCC	unidad de cuidados coronarios
UCI	unidad de cuidados intensivos
UV	ultravioleta
VCM	volumen corpuscular medio
VEF	volumen espiratorio forzado
VEM	velocidad espiratoria máxima
VHS	virus del herpes simple
VIH	virus de la inmunodeficiencia humana
VLDL	lipoproteína de muy baja densidad
VMFE	velocidad máxima del flujo espiratorio
VSG	velocidad de sedimentación globular
VSR	virus sincitial respiratorio

Anatomical drawings
Dessins anatomiques
Anatomische Zeichnungen
Disegni anatomici
Dibujos anatómicos

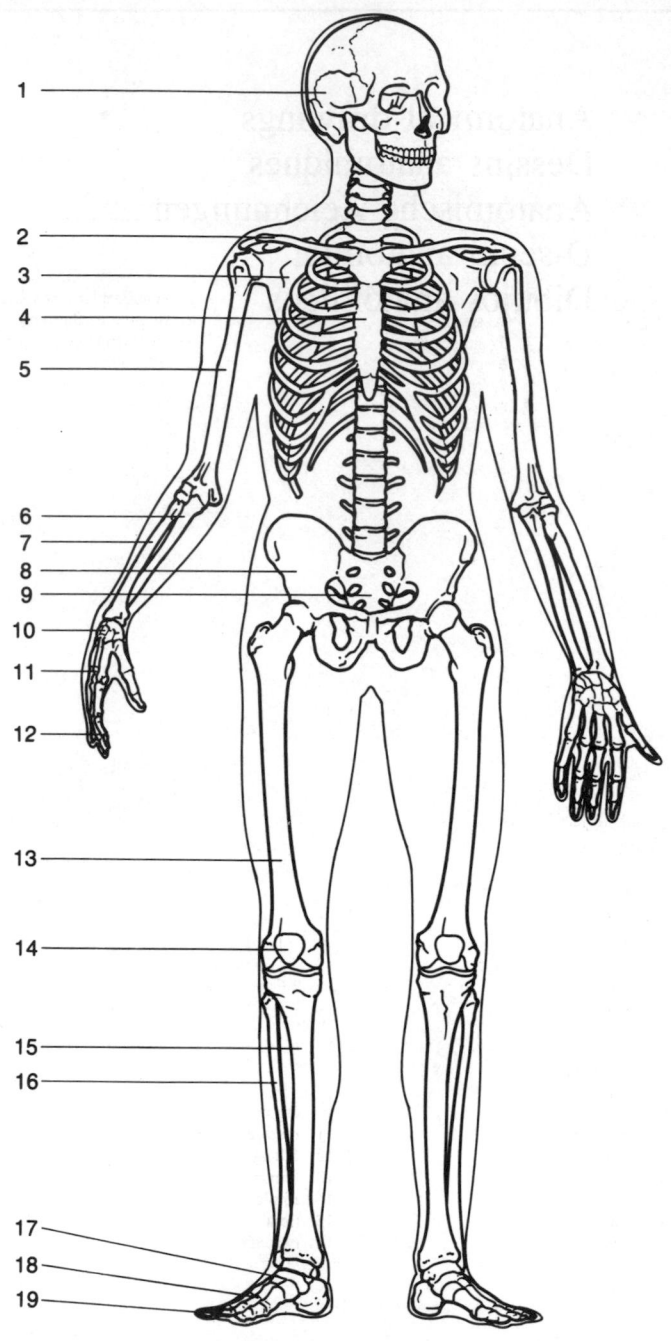

Skeleton — front view
Skelette — vue avant
Skelett — Vorderansicht
Scheletro — visione anteriore
Esqueleto — vista frontal

English	French	German
Anglais	*Français*	*Allemand*
Englisch	*Französisch*	*Deutsch*
Inglese	*Francese*	*Tedesco*
Inglés	*Francés*	*Alemán*

English	French	German
1. skull	1. crâne	1. Schädel, Cranium
2. clavicle	2. clavicule	2. Schlüsselbein, Clavicula
3. scapula	3. scapule	3. Schulterblatt, Scapula
4. sternum	4. sternum	4. Brustbein, Sternum
5. humerus	5. humérus	5. Oberarmknochen, Humerus
6. ulna	6. cubitus	6. Elle, Ulna
7. radius	7. radius	7. Speiche, Radius
8. hip bone	8. os iliaque	8. Os coxae
9. sacrum	9. sacrum	9. Kreuzbein, Os sacrum
10. carpus	10. carpe	10. Handwurzelknochen, Ossa carpalia
11. metacarpals	11. métacarpes	11. Mittelhandknochen, Ossa metacarpalia
12. phalanges	12. phalanges	12. Phalangen
13. femur	13. fémur	13. Oberschenkelknochen, Femur
14. patella	14. rotule	14. Kniescheibe, Patella
15. tibia	15. tibia	15. Schienbein, Tibia
16. fibula	16. péroné	16. Wadenbein, Fibula
17. tarsus	17. tarse	17. Fußwurzel, Tarsus
18. metatarsals	18. métatarses	18. Mittelfußknochen, Ossa metatarsalia
19. phalanges	19. phalanges	19. Phalangen

Italian	Spanish
Italien	*Espagnol*
Italienisch	*Spanisch*
Italiano	*Spagnolo*
Italiano	*Español*

Italian	Spanish
1. cranio	1. cráneo
2. clavicola	2. clavícula
3. scapola	3. omoplato
4. sterno	4. esternón
5. omero	5. húmero
6. ulna	6. cúbito
7. radio	7. radio
8. osso iliaco	8. hueso coxal
9. osso sacro	9. sacro
10. carpo	10. carpo
11. metacarpo	11. metacarpianos
12. falangi	12. falanges
13. femore	13. fémur
14. rotula	14. rótula
15. tibia	15. tibia
16. fibula	16. peroné
17. tarso	17. tarso
18. metatarso	18. metatarsianos
19. falangi	19. falanges

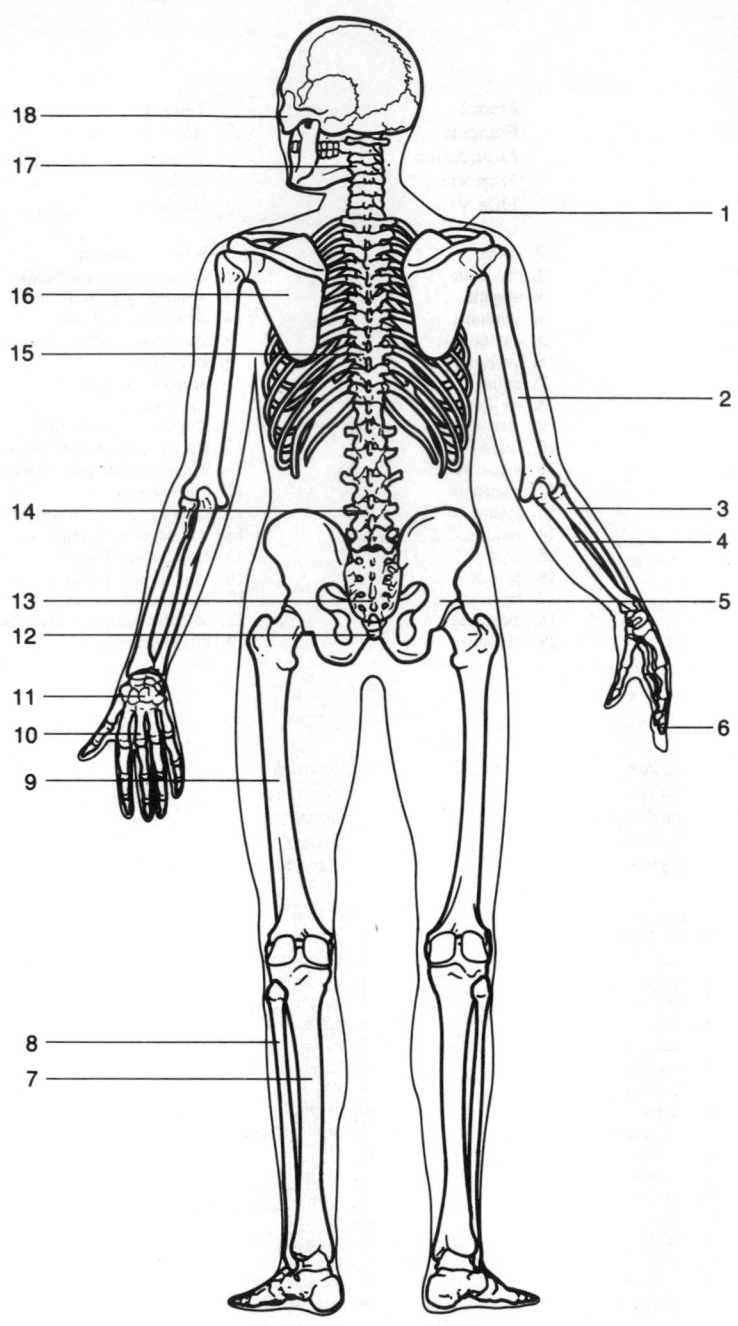

Skeleton — back view
Skelette — vue arrière
Skelett — Rückansicht
Scheletro — visione posteriore
Esqueleto — vista posterior

English	French	German
Anglais	*Français*	*Allemand*
Englisch	*Französisch*	*Deutsch*
Inglese	*Francese*	*Tedesco*
Inglés	*Francés*	*Alemán*

1. clavicle	1. clavicule	1. Schlüsselbein, Clavicula
2. humerus	2. humérus	2. Oberarmknochen, Humerus
3. radius	3. radius	3. Speiche, Radius
4. ulna	4. cubitus	4. Elle, Ulna
5. hip bone	5. os iliaque	5. Os coxae
6. phalanges	6. phalanges	6. Phalangen
7. tibia	7. tibia	7. Schienbein, Tibia
8. fibula	8. péroné	8. Wadenbein, Fibula
9. femur	9. fémur	9. Oberschenkelknochen, Femur
10. metacarpals	10. métacarpes	10. Mittelhandknochen, Ossa metacarpalia
11. carpus	11. carpe	11. Handwurzelknochen, Ossa carpalia
12. coccyx	12. coccyx	12. Steißbein, Os coccygis
13. sacrum	13. sacrum	13. Kreuzbein, Os sacrum
14. lumbar vertebrae	14. vertèbres lombaires	14. Lendenwirbel, Vertebrae lumbales
15. thoracic vertebrae	15. vertèbres dorsales	15. Brustwirbel, Vertebrae thoracicae
16. scapula	16. scapule	16. Schulterblatt, Scapula
17. cervical vertebrae	17. vertèbres cervicales	17. Halswirbel, Vertebrae cervicales
18. skull	18. crâne	18. Schädel, Cranium

Italian	Spanish
Italien	*Espagnol*
Italienisch	*Spanisch*
Italiano	*Spagnolo*
Italiano	*Español*

1. clavicola	1. clavícula
2. omero	2. húmero
3. radio	3. radio
4. ulna	4. cúbito
5. osso iliaco	5. hueso coxal
6. falangi	6. falanges
7. tibia	7. tibia
8. fibula	8. peroné
9. femore	9. fémur
10. metacarpo	10. metacarpianos
11. carpo	11. carpo
12. coccige	12. cóccix
13. osso sacro	13. sacro
14. vertebre lombari	14. vértebras lumbares
15. vertebre toraciche	15. vértebras toracicas
16. scapola	16. omoplato
17. vertebre cervicali	17. vértebras cervicales
18. cranio	18. cráneo

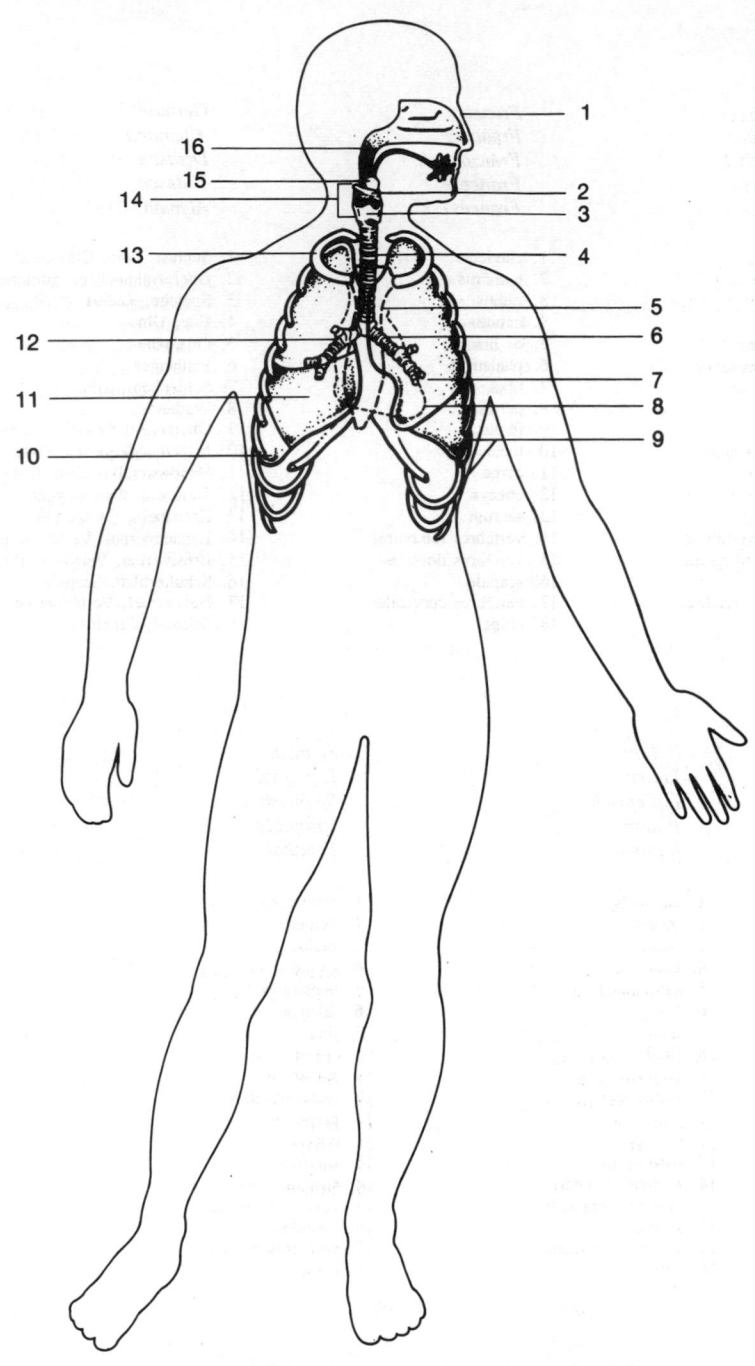

Respiratory system and related structures
Appareil respiratoire
Atemwege
Sistema respiratorio
Sistema respiratorio

English	French	German
English	*French*	*German*
Anglais	*Français*	*Allemand*
Englisch	*Französisch*	*Deutsch*
Inglese	*Francese*	*Tedesco*
Inglés	*Francés*	*Alemán*

1. nose	1. nez	1. Nase
2. hyoid bone	2. os hyoïde	2. Zungenbein, Os hyoideum
3. thyroid cartilage	3. cartilage thyroïde	3. Schildknorpel, Cartilago thyroidea
4. trachea	4. trachée	4. Luftröhre, Trachea
5. sternum	5. sternum	5. Brustbein, Sternum
6. left bronchus	6. bronche gauche	6. linker Hauptbronchus
7. left lung	7. pumon gauche	7. linke Lunge
8. heart	8. coeur	8. Herz
9. ribs	9. côtes	9. Rippen
10. base of lung	10. base du poumon	10. Lungenbasis
11. right lung	11. poumon droit	11. rechte Lunge
12. right bronchus	12. bronche droit	12. rechter Hauptbronchus
13. first rib	13. 1ère côte	13. 1. Rippe
14. larynx	14. larynx	14. Kchlkopf, Larynx
15. epiglottis	15. épiglotte	15. Kehldeckel, Epiglottis
16. pharynx	16. pharynx	16. Schlund, Pharynx

Italian	Spanish
Italian	*Spanish*
Italien	*Espagnol*
Italienisch	*Spanisch*
Italiano	*Spagnolo*
Italiano	*Español*

1. naso	1. nariz
2. osso ioide	2. hueso hioides
3. cartilagine tiroide	3. cartílago tiroides
4. trachea	4. tráquea
5. sterno	5. esternón
6. bronco sinistro	6. bronquio izquierdo
7. polmone sinistro	7. pulmón izquierdo
8. cuore	8. corazón
9. coste	9. costillas
10. base polmonare	10. base del pulmón
11. polmone destro	11. pulmón derecho
12. bronco destro	12. bronquio derecho
13. prima costa	13. 1a costilla
14. laringe	14. laringe
15. epiglottide	15. epiglotis
16. faringo	16. faringe

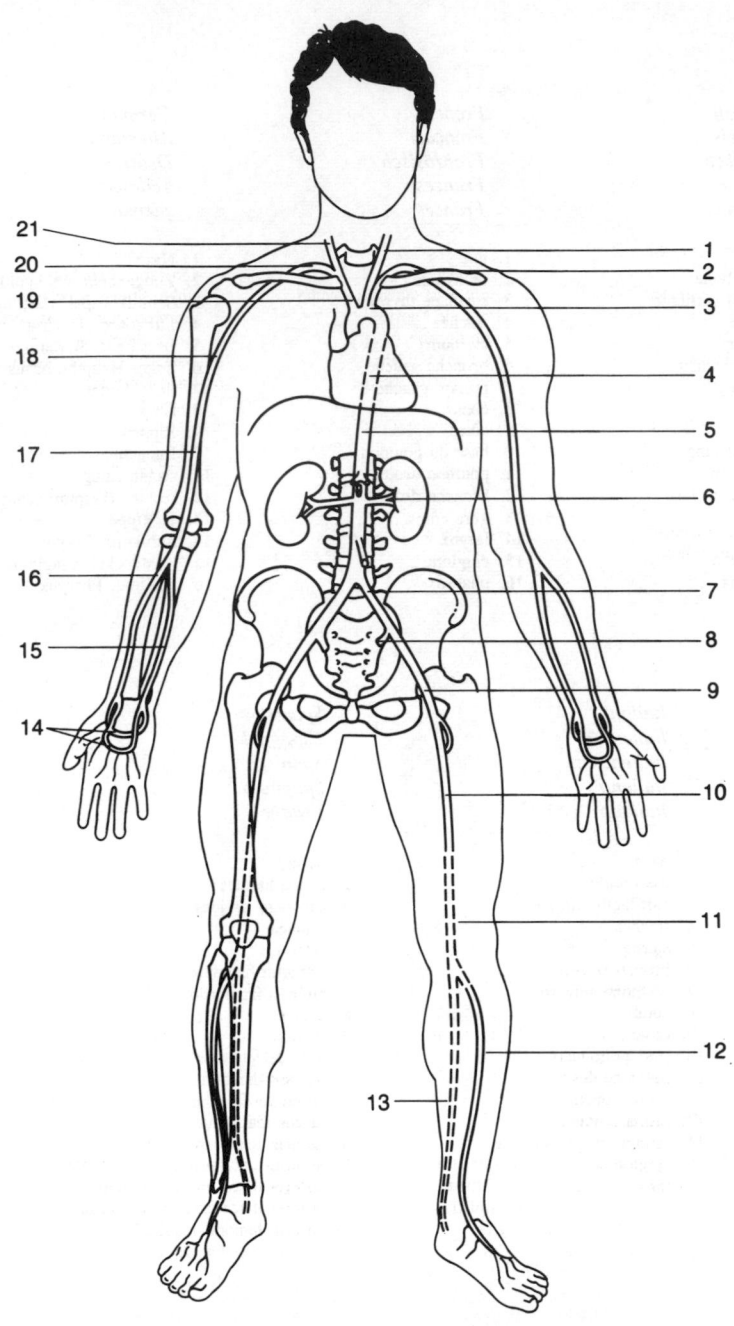

Circulatory system – arteries
Appareil circulatoire – artères
Gefäßsystem – Arterien
Sistema circolatorio – arterie
Sistema circulatorio – arterias

English	French	German
Anglais	*Français*	*Allemand*
Englisch	*Französisch*	*Deutsch*
Inglese	*Francese*	*Tedesco*
Inglés	*Francés*	*Alemán*

1. left common carotid artery
2. left subclavian artery
3. arch of aorta
4. thoracic aorta
5. abdominal aorta
6. left renal artery
7. left common iliac artery
8. left internal iliac artery
9. left external iliac artery
10. left femoral artery
11. left popliteal artery
12. left anterior tibial artery
13. left posterior tibial artery
14. right palmar arches
15. right ulnar artery
16. right radial artery
17. right brachial artery
18. right axillary artery
19. brachiocephalic artery
20. right subclavian artery
21. right common carotid artery

1. artère carotide commune gauche
2. artère sous-clavière gauche
3. crosse de l'aorte
4. aorte dorsale
5. aorte abdominale
6. artère rénale gauche
7. artère iliaque commune gauche
8. artère iliaque interne gauche
9. artère iliaque externe gauche
10. artère fémorale gauche
11. artère poplitée gauche
12. artère tibiale antérieure gauche
13. artère tibiale postérieure gauche
14. voûtes palmaires droites
15. artère cubitale droite
16. artère radiale droite
17. artère brachiale droite
18. artère axillaire droite
19. artère brachio-céphalique
20. artère sous-clavière droite
21. artère carotide commune droite

1. linke Halsschlagader, linke Arteria carotis communis
2. linke Arteria subclavia
3. Aortenbogen, Arcus aortae
4. Aorta thoracica
5. Bauchschlagader, Aorta abdominalis
6. linke Nierenarterie, linke Arteria renalis
7. linke Arteria iliaca communis
8. linke Arteria iliaca interna
9. linke Arteria iliaca externa
10. linke Oberschenkelarterie, linke Arteria femoralis
11. linke Arteria poplitea
12. linke Arteria tibialis anterior
13. linke Arteria tibialis posterior
14. rechte Palmarbögen
15. rechte Arteria ulnaris
16. rechte Arteria radialis
17. rechte Arteria brachialis
18. rechte Arteria axillaris
19. Arteria brachiocephalica
20. rechte Arteria subclavia
21. rechte Halsschlagader, rechte Arteria carotis communis

Italian	Spanish
Italien	*Espagnol*
Italienisch	*Spanisch*
Italiano	*Spagnolo*
Italiano	*Español*

1. arteria carotide comune sinistra
2. arteria succlavia sinistra
3. arco dell'aorta
4. aorta toracica
5. aorta addominale
6. arteria renale sinistra
7. arteria iliaca comune sinistra
8. arteria iliaca interna sinistra
9. arteria iliaca esterna sinistra
10. arteria femorale sinistra
11. arteria poplitea sinistra
12. arteria tibiale anteriore sinistra
13. arteria tibiale posteriore sinistra
14. arcate palmari destre
15. arteria ulnare destra
16. arteria radiale destra
17. arteria brachiale destra
18. arteria ascellare destra
19. arteria brachiocefalica destra
20. arteria succlavia destra
21. arteria carotide comune destra

1. arteria carótida primitiva izquierda
2. arteria subclavia izquierda
3. cayado aórtico
4. aorta torácica
5. aorta abdominal
6. arteria renal izquierda
7. arteria ilíaca primitiva izquierda
8. arteria ilíaca interna izquierda
9. arteria ilíaca externa izquierda
10. arteria femoral izquierda
11. arteria poplítea izquierda
12. arteria tibial anterior izquierda
13. arteria tibial posterior izquierda
14. arcos palmares derechos
15. arteria cubital derecha
16. arteria radial derecha
17. arteria humeral derecha
18. arteria axilar derecha
19. tronco braquiocefálico
20. arteria subclavia derecha
21. arteria carótida primitiva derecha

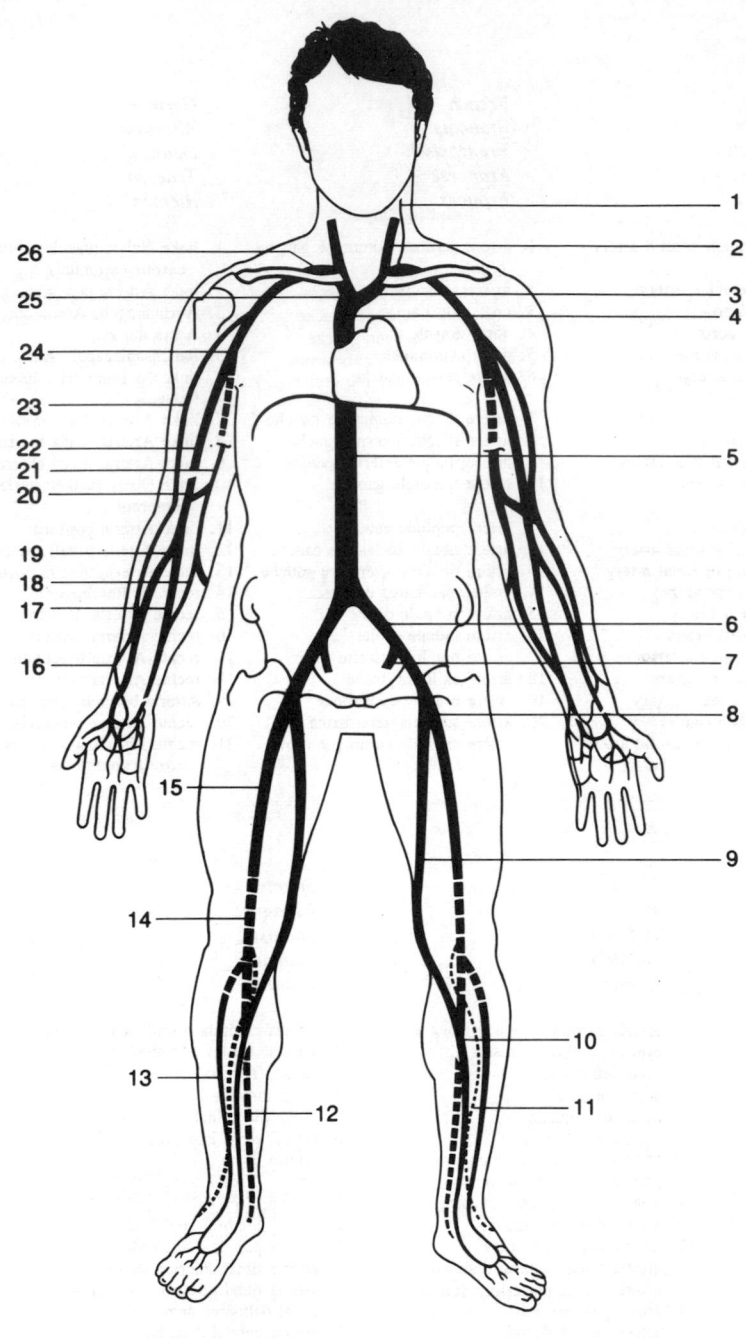

Circulatory system − veins
Appareil circulatoire − veines
Gefäßsystem − Venen
Sistema circolatorio − vene
Sistema circulatorio − venas

English / Anglais / Englisch / Inglese / Inglés	French / Français / Französisch / Francese / Francés	German / Allemand / Französisch / Deutsch / Tedesco / Alemán
1. left external jugular vein	1. veine jugulaire externe gauche	1. linke Vena jugularis externa
2. left internal jugular vein	2. veine jugulaire interne gauche	2. linke Vena jugularis interna
3. left braciocephalic vein	3. tronc brachio-céphalique gauche	3. linke Vena brachiocephalica
4. superior vena cava	4. veine cave supérieure	4. obere Hohlvene, Vena cava superior
5. inferior vena cava	5. veine cave inférieure	5. untere Hohlvene, Vena cava inferior
6. left common iliac vein	6. veine iliaque commune gauche	6. linke Vena iliaca communis
7. left internal iliac vein	7. veine iliaque interne gauche	7. linke Vena iliaca interna
8. left external iliac vein	8. veine iliaque externe gauche	8. linke Vena iliaca externa
9. left long saphenous vein	9. veine grande saphène gauche	9. linke magna Vena saphena
10. left long saphenous vein	10. veine grande saphène gauche	10. linke magna Vena saphena
11. left short saphenous vein	11. veine petite saphène gauche	11. linke parva Vena saphena
12. right posterior tibial vein	12. veine tibiale postérieure droite	12. rechte Vena tibialis posterior
13. right anterior tibial vein	13. veine tibiale antérieure droite	13. rechte Vena tibialis anterior
14. right popliteal vein	14. veine poplitée droite	14. rechte Vena poplitea
15. right femoral vein	15. veine fémorale droite	15. rechte Oberschenkelvene, rechte Vena femoralis
16. right cephalic vein	16. veine céphalique droite	16. rechte Vena cephalica
17. right ulnar vein	17. veine cubitale droite	17. rechte Vena ulnaris
18. right median vein	18. veine médiane droite	18. rechte Vena mediana
19. right radial vein	19. veine radiale droite	19. rechte Vena radialis
20. right median cubital vein	20. veine médiane cubitale droite	20. rechte Vena mediana cubiti
21. right basilic vein	21. veine basilique droite	21. rechte Vena basilica
22. right brachial vein	22. veine brachiale droite	22. rechte Vena brachialis
23. right cephalic vein	23. veine céphalique droite	23. rechte Vena cephalica
24. right axillary vein	24. veine axillaire droite	24. rechte Vena axillaris
25. right brachiocephalic vein	25. tronc brachio-céphalique droit	25. rechte Vena brachiocephalica
26. right subclavian vein	26. veine sous-clavière	26. rechte Vena subclavia

Italian / Italien / Italienisch / Italiano / Italiano	Spanish / Espagnol / Spanisch / Spagnolo / Español
1. vena giugulare esterna sinistra	1. vena yugular externa izquierda
2. vena giugulare interna sinistra	2. vena yugular interna izquierda
3. vena brachiocefalica sinistra	3. tronco venoso braquiocefálico izquierdo
4. vena cava superiore	4. vena cava superior
5. vena cava inferiore	5. vena cava inferior
6. vena iliaca comune sinistra	6. vena ilíaca primitiva izquierda
7. vena iliaca interna sinistra	7. vena ilíaca interna izquierda
8. vena iliaca esterna sinistra	8. vena ilíaca externa izquierda
9. vena safena sinistra	9. vena safena interna izquierda
10. vena safena sinistra	10. vena safena interna izquierda
11. vena safena accessoria sinistra	11. vena safena externa izquierda
12. vena tibiale posteriore destra	12. vena tibial posterior derecha
13. vena tibiale anteriore destra	13. vena tibial anterior derecha
14. vena poplitea destra	14. vena poplítea derecha
15. vena formorale destra	15. vena femoral derecha
16. vena cefalica destra	16. vena cefálica derecha
17. vena ulnare destra	17. vena cubital derecha
18. vena mediana destra	18. vena mediana derecha
19. vena radiale destra	19. vena radial izquierda
20. vena mediana cubitale destra	20. vena mediana cubital derecha
21. vena basilica destra	21. vena basílica derecha
22. vena brachiale destra	22. vena humeral derecha
23. vena cefalica destra	23. vena cefálica derecha
24. vena ascellare destra	24. vena axilar derecha
25. vena brachiocefalica destra	25. tronco venoso braquiocefálico derecho
26. vena succlavia destra	26. vena subclavia derecha

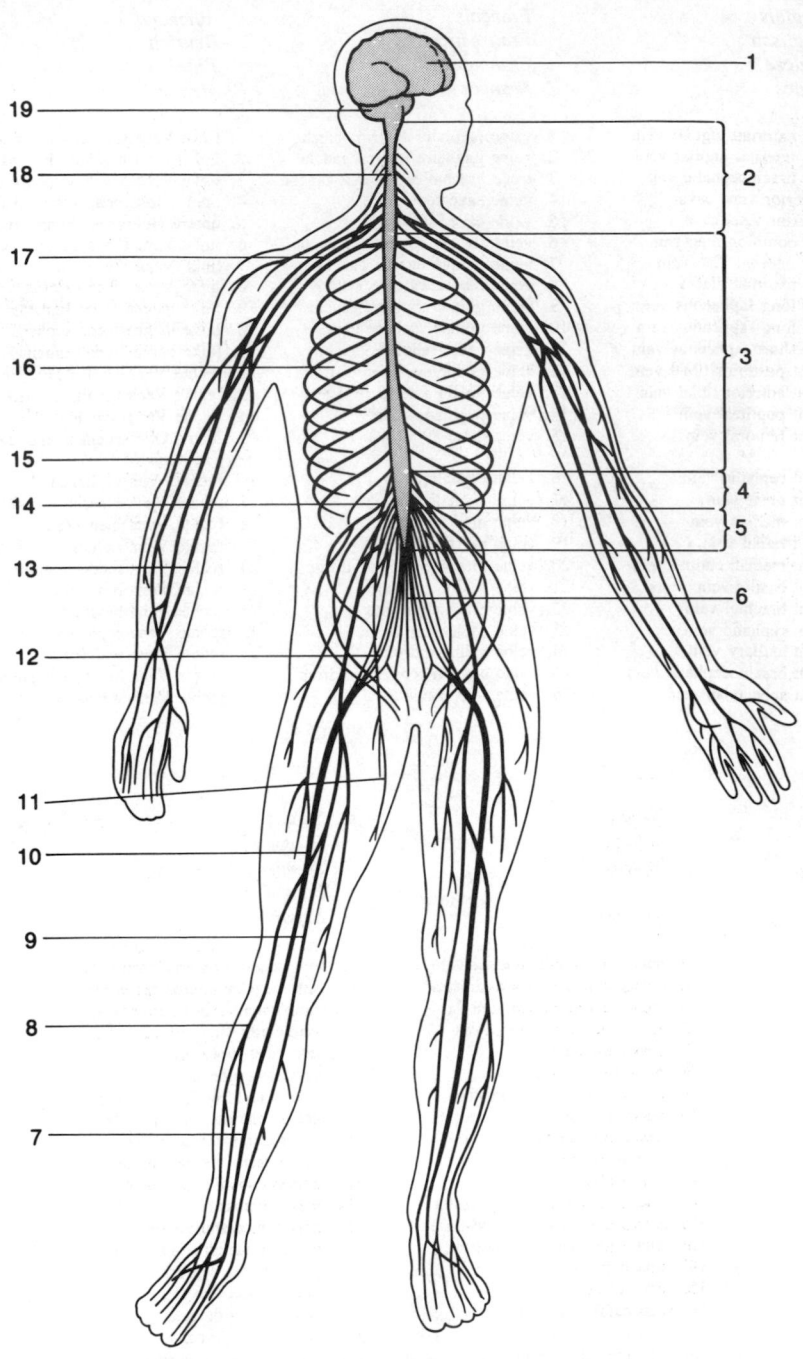

Nervous system
Système nerveux
Nervensystem
Sistema nervoso
Sistema nervioso

English	French	German
Anglais	Français	Allemand
Englisch	Französisch	Deutsch
Inglese	Francese	Tedesco
Inglés	Francés	Alemán

1. cerebrum
2. cervical nerve roots
3. thoracic nerve roots
4. lumbar nerve roots
5. sacral nerve roots
6. coccygeal nerve root
7. tibial nerve
8. common peroneal nerve
9. saphenous nerve
10. sciatic nerve
11. obturator nerve
12. sacral plexus
13. ulnar nerve
14. lumbar plexus
15. median nerve
16. thoracic nerve
17. brachial plexus
18. spinal cord
19. cerebellum

1. hemisphères cérébraux
2. racines des nerfs cervicaux
3. racines des nerfs dorsaux
4. racines des nerfs lombaires
5. racines des nerfs sacrés
6. racine du nerf coccygien
7. nerf sciatique poplité interne
8. nerf sciatique poplité externe
9. nerf saphène interne
10. nerf sciatique
11. nerf obturateur
12. nerf du plexus sacré
13. nerf cubital
14. nerf du plexus lombaire
15. nerf médian
16. nerf thoracique
17. nerf du plexus brachial
18. moelle épinière
19. cervelet

1. Gehirn, Cerebrum
2. Nervenwurzeln der Halswirbelsäule
3. Nervenwurzeln der Brustwirbelsäule
4. Nervenwurzeln der Lendenwirbelsäule
5. Nervenwurzeln des Kreuzbeins
6. Nervenwurzel des Steißbeins
7. Nervus tibialis
8. Nervus peronaeus communis
9. Nervus saphenus
10. Nervus ischiadicus
11. Nervus obturatorius
12. Plexus sacralis
13. Nervus ulnaris
14. Plexus lumbaris
15. Nervus medianus
16. Nervus thoracicus
17. Plexus brachialis
18. Rückenmark, Medulla spinalis
19. Kleinhirn, Cerebellum

Italian	Spanish
Italien	Espagnol
Italienisch	Spanisch
Italiano	Spagnolo
Italiano	Español

1. cervello
2. radici dei nervi cervicali
3. radici dei nervi toracici
4. radici dei nervi lombari
5. radici dei nervi sacrali
6. radice del nervo coccigeo
7. nervo tibiale
8. nervo peroneo comune
9. nervo safeno
10. nervo sciatico
11. nervo otturatorio
12. plesso sacrale
13. nervo ulnare
14. plesso lombare
15. nervo mediano
16. nervo toracico
17. plesso brachiale
18. midollo spinale
19. cervelletto

1. cerebro
2. raices nerviosas cervicales
3. raices nerviosas torácicas
4. raices nerviosas lumbares
5. raices nerviosas sacras
6. raice nerviosa coccígca
7. nervio tibial
8. ciatico poplíteo externo
9. nervio safeno
10. nervio ciático
11. obturador
12. plexo sacro
13. nervio cubital
14. plexo lumbar
15. nervio mediano
16. nervio torácico
17. plexo braquial
18. médula espinal
19. cerebelo

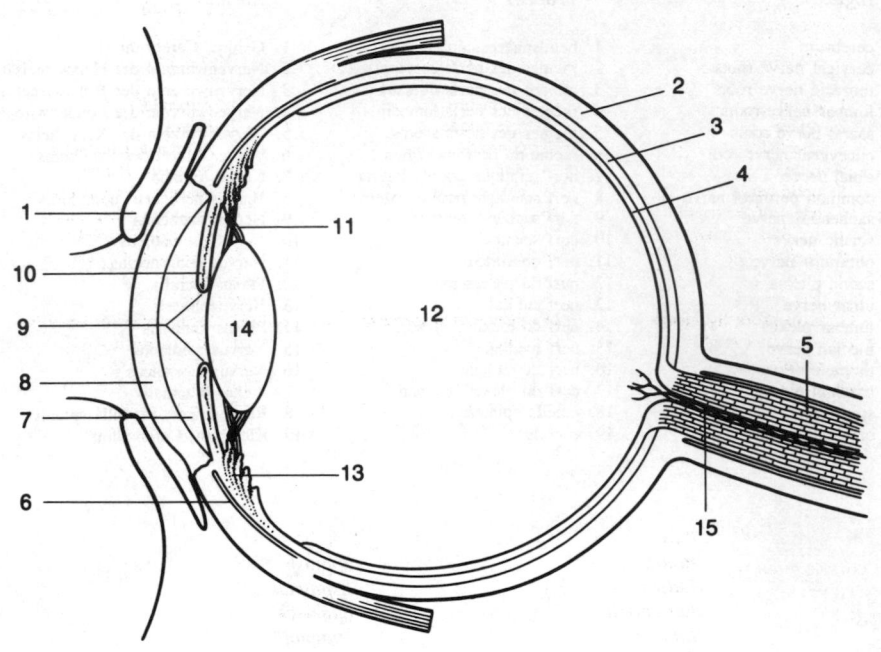

Eye
Oeil
Auge
Occhio
Ojo

English	French	German
Anglais	Français	Allemand
Englisch	Französisch	Deutsch
Inglese	Francese	Tedesco
Inglés	Francés	Alemán

1. eyelid	1. paupière	1. Augenlid
2. sclera	2. sclérotique	2. Sklera
3. choroid	3. choroïde	3. Aderhaut, Choroidea
4. retina	4. rétine	4. Netzhaut, Retina
5. optic nerve	5. nerf optique	5. Sehnerv, Nervus opticus
6. canal of Schlemm	6. canal scléral	6. Schlemm'scher Kanal
7. aqueous humour	7. humeur aqueuse	7. wässrige Flüssigkeit
8. cornea	8. cornée	8. Hornhaut, Cornea
9. pupil	9. pupille	9. Pupille
10. iris	10. iris	10. Iris
11. suspensory ligaments	11. ligaments suspenseurs	11. Ligamentae suspensoriae
12. vitreous humour	12. humeur vitreuse	12. Glaskörperflüssigkeit
13. ciliary body	13. corps ciliaire	13. Ziliarkörper
14. lens	14. cristallin	14. Linse
15. blood vessels in retina	15. vaisseaux sanguins allant vers la rétine	15. Netzhautgefäße

Italian	Spanish
Italien	Espagnol
Italienisch	Spanisch
Italiano	Spagnolo
Italiano	Español

1. palpebra	1. párpado
2. sclera	2. esclerótica
3. coroide	3. coroides
4. retina	4. retina
5. nervo ottico	5. nervio optico
6. canale di Schlemm	6. conducto de Schlemm
7. umore acqueo	7. humor acuoso
8. cornea	8. córnea
9. pupilla	9. pupila
10. iride	10. iris
11. legamenti sospensori del cristallino	11. ligamentos suspensores
12. corpo vitreo	12. humor vítreo
13. corpo ciliare	13. cuerpo ciliar
14. cristallino	14. cristalino
15. vasi della retina	15. vasos sanguíneos de la retina

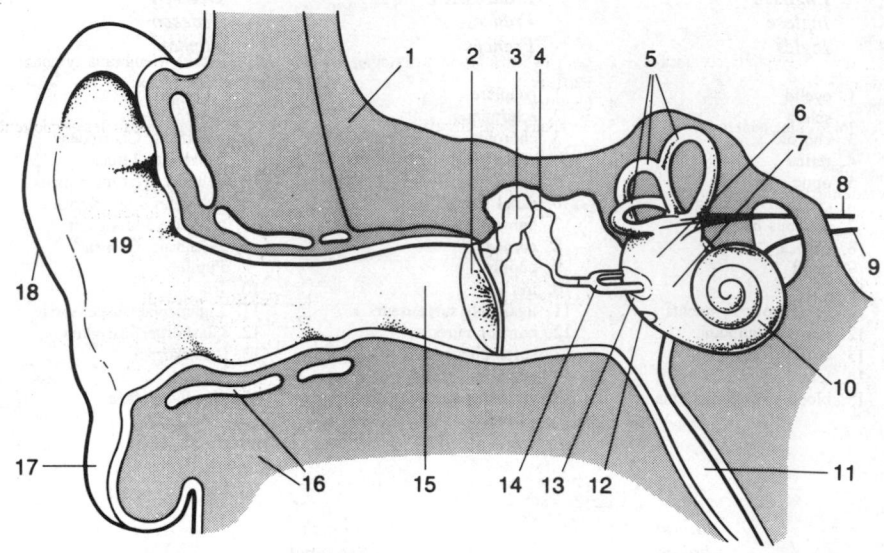

Ear
Oreille
Ohr
Orecchio
Oido

English	French	German
Anglais	*Français*	*Allemand*
Englisch	*Französisch*	*Deutsch*
Inglese	*Francese*	*Tedesco*
Inglés	*Francés*	*Alemán*

1. bony wall	1. paroi osseuse	1. knöcherne Wand
2. ear drum (tympanic membrane)	2. tympan (membrane du tympan)	2. Trommelfell, Membrana tympani
3. malleus	3. marteau	3. Hammer, Malleus
4. incus	4. enclume	4. Amboß, Incus
5. 3 semicircular canals	5. 3 canaux semi-circulaires	5. 3 Bogengänge, 3 canales semicirculares
6. utricle	6. utricule	6. Utriculus
7. saccule	7. petit sac	7. Sacculus
8. vestibular nerve	8. nerf vestibulaire	8. Nervus vestibularis
9. acoustic nerve	9. nerf auditif	9. Hörnerv, Nervus acusticus
10. cochlea	10. limaçon	10. Schnecke, Cochlea
11. eustachian tube	11. trompe d'Eustache	11. Eustachische Röhre
12. round window	12. fenêtre ronde	12. Fenestra cochleae
13. oval window	13. fenêtre ovale	13. Fenestra vestibuli
14. stapes	14. étrier	14. Steigbügel, Stapes
15. auditory canal	15. conduit auditif	15. Gehörgang, Meatus acusticus
16. cartilage and bone	16. cartilage et os	16. Knorpel und Knochen
17. lobe	17. lobe	17. Ohrläppchen
18. helix	18. hélix	18. Helix
19. pinna	19. pavillon	19. Ohrmuschel

Italian	Spanish
Italien	*Espagnol*
Italienisch	*Spanisch*
Italiano	*Spagnolo*
Italiano	*Español*

1. parete ossea	1. pared ósea
2. membrana timpanica	2. timpano (membrana timpánica)
3. martello	3. martillo
4. incudine	4. yunque
5. 3 canali semicircolari	5. 3 canales semicirculares
6. utricolo	6. utrículo
7. sacculo	7. sáculo
8. nervo vestibolare	8. nervio vestibular
9. nervo acustico	9. nervio acústico
10. coclea	10. cóclea
11. tromba d'Eustachio	11. trompa de Eustaquio
12. finestra rotonda della coclea	12. ventana redonda
13. finestra ovale/finestra del vestibolo	13. ventana oval
14. staffa	14. estribo
15. meato acustico	15. conducto auditivo
16. cartilagine ed osso	16. cartílago y hueso
17. lobo	17. lóbulo
18. elice	18. hélix
19. padiglione auricolare	19. pabellón

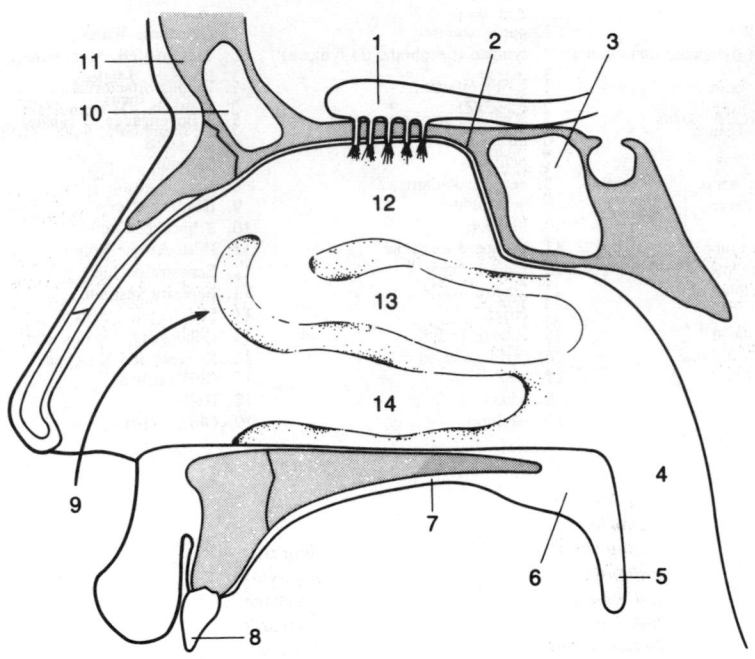

Nose
Nez
Nase
Naso
Nariz

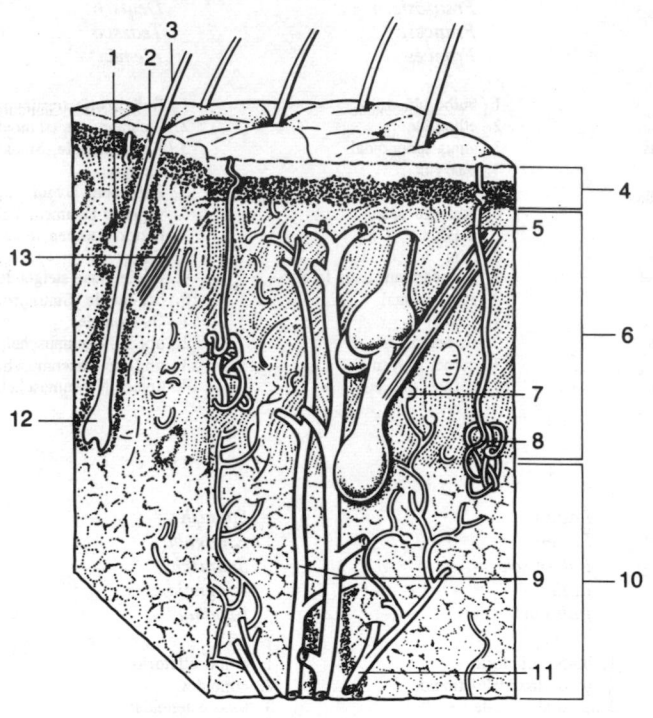

Skin
Peau
Haut
Cute
Piel

English	French	German
English	*French*	*German*
Anglais	*Français*	*Allemand*
Englisch	*Französisch*	*Deutsch*
Inglese	*Francese*	*Tedesco*
Inglés	*Francés*	*Alemán*

1. sebaceous gland	1. glande sébacée	1. Talgdrüse, Glandula sebacea
2. hair root	2. racine d'un poil	2. Haarwurzel
3. hair shaft	3. tige de poil	3. Haarschaft
4. epidermis	4. épiderme	4. Epidermis
5. sweat gland duct	5. canal de la glande sudoripare	5. Ausführungsgang einer Schweißdrüse
6. dermis	6. derme	6. Dermis, Corium
7. nerve endings	7. terminaisons nerveuses	7. Nervenendigung
8. sweat gland	8. glande sudoripare	8. Schweißdrüse, Glandula sudorifera
9. blood vessels	9. vaisseaux sanguins	9. Blutgefäße
10. sub-cutaneous tissue	10. tissu sous-cutané	10. Subkutangewebe
11. cutaneous nerve	11. nerf cutané	11. Hautnerv
12. hair bulb	12. bulbe pileux	12. Haarfollikel
13. arrector pilorum muscle	13. muscle arrecteur des poils	13. Musculus arrector pili

Italian	Spanish
Italian	*Spanish*
Italien	*Espagnol*
Italienisch	*Spanisch*
Italiano	*Spagnolo*
Italiano	*Español*

1. ghiandola sebacea	1. glándula sebácea
2. radice del pelo	2. raíz pilosa
3. fusto del pelo	3. tallo piloso
4. epidermide	4. epidermis
5. dotto sudorifero	5. conducto de la glándula sudorípara
6. derma	6. dermis
7. terminazioni nervose	7. terminaciones nerviosas
8. ghiandola sudorifera	8. glándula sudorípara
9. vasi sanguigni	9. vasos sanguíneos
10. tessuto sottocutaneo	10. tejido subcutáneo
11. nervo cutaneo	11. nervio cutáneo
12. bulbo pilifero	12. bulbo piloso
13. muscolo erettore del pelo	13. músculo erector del pelo

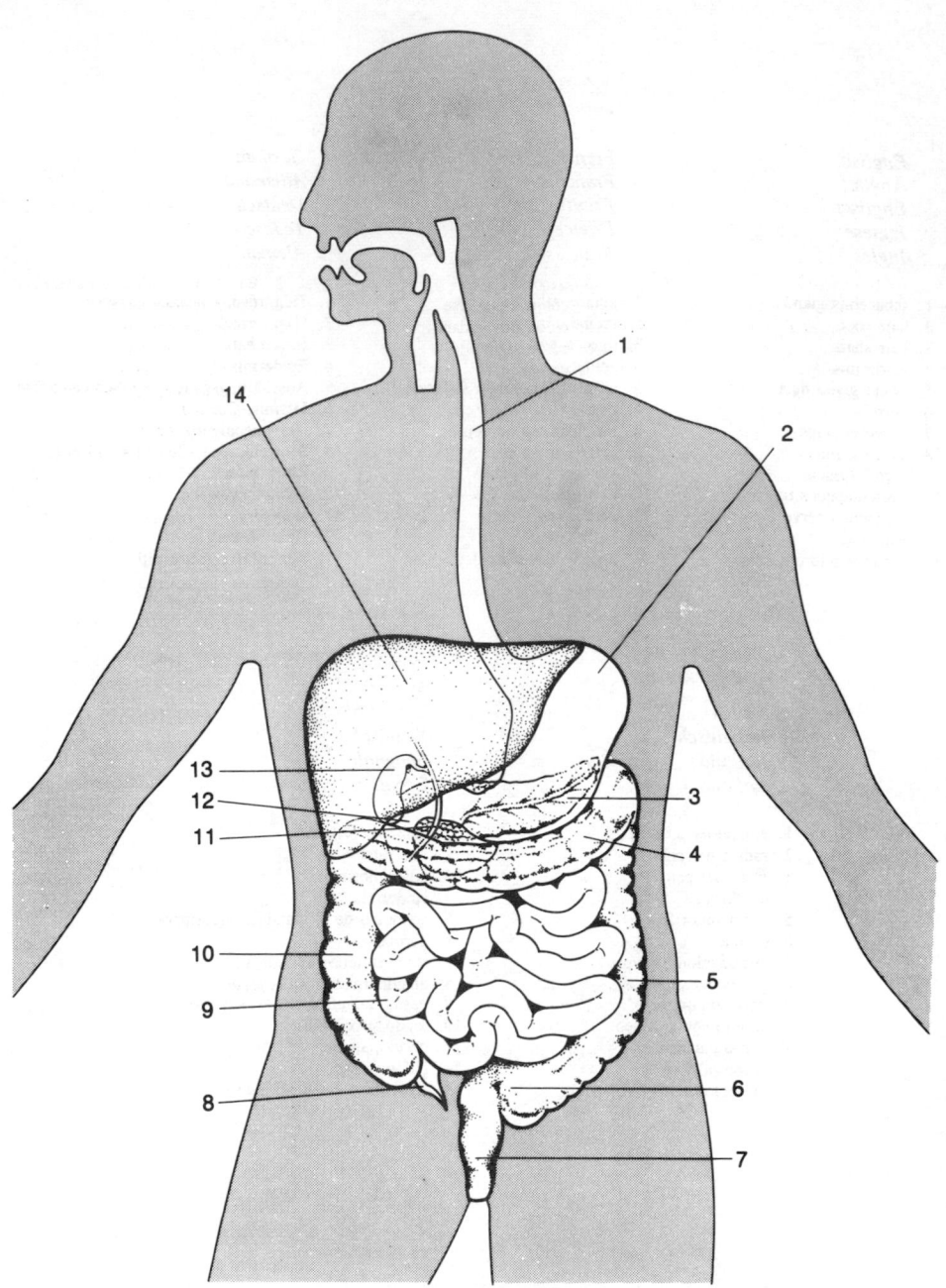

Digestive system
Appareil digestif
Verdauungstrakt
Apparato digerente
Sistema digestivo

English	French	German
Anglais	Français	Allemand
Englisch	Französisch	Deutsch
Inglese	Francese	Tedesco
Inglés	Francés	Alemán

1. oesophagus	1. oesophage	1. Speiseröhre, Ösophagus
2. stomach	2. estomac	2. Magen
3. pancreas	3. pancréas	3. Bauchspeicheldrüse, Pankreas
4. transverse colon	4. côlon transverse	4. Colon transversum
5. descending colon	5. côlon descendant	5. Colon descendens
6. sigmoid colon	6. côlon sigmoïde	6. Colon sigmoideum
7. rectum	7. rectum	7. Mastdarm, Rectum
8. appendix	8. appendice	8. Wurmfortsatz, Appendix
9. small intestine	9. intestin grêle	9. Dünndarm
10. ascending colon	10. côlon ascendant	10. Colon ascendens
11. common bile duct	11. canal cholédoque	11. Choledochus
12. duodenum	12. duodénum	12. Zwölffingerdarm, Duodenum
13. gallbladder	13. vésicule biliaire	13. Gallenblase
14. liver	14. foie	14. Leber

Italian	Spanish
Italien	Espagnol
Italienisch	Spanisch
Italiano	Spagnolo
Italiano	Español

1. esofago	1. esófago
2. stomaco	2. estómago
3. pancreas	3. pancreas
4. colon trasverso	4. colon transverso
5. colon discendente	5. colon descendente
6. colon sigmoideo	6. colon sigmoide
7. retto	7. recto
8. appendice	8. apéndice
9. intestino tenue	9. intestino delgado
10. colon ascendente	10. colon ascendente
11. coledoco	11. conducto biliar común
12. duodeno	12. duodeno
13. cistifellea/colecisti	13. vesícula biliar
14. fegato	14. hígado

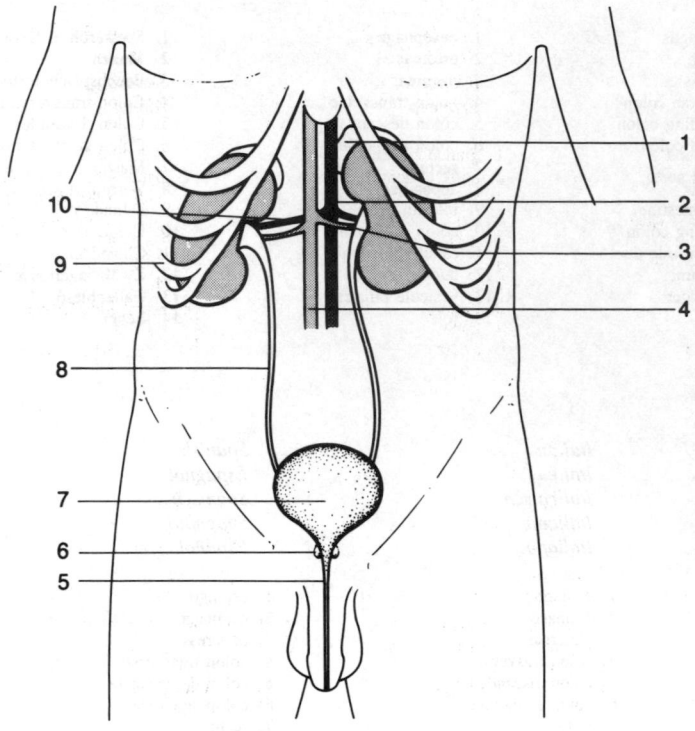

Urinary system
Appareil urinaire
Niere und ableitende Harnwege
Apparato urinario
Aparato urinario

English	French	German
Anglais	*Français*	*Allemand*
Englisch	*Französisch*	*Deutsch*
Inglese	*Francese*	*Tedesco*
Inglés	*Francés*	*Alemán*

1. adrenal gland	1. glande surrénale	1. Nebenniere
2. abdominal aorta	2. aorte abdominale	2. Bauchaorta, Aorta abdominalis
3. renal vein	3. veine rénale	3. Nierenvene, Vena renalis
4. inferior vena cava	4. veine cave inférieure	4. untere Hohlvene, Vena cava inferior
5. urethra	5. urètre	5. Harnröhre, Urethra
6. sphincter muscle	6. sphincter	6. Schließmuskel, Musculus sphincter
7. bladder	7. vessie	7. Blase
8. ureter	8. uretère	8. Harnleiter, Ureter
9. ribs	9. côtes	9. Rippen
10. renal artery	10. artère rénale	10. Nierenarterie, Arteria renalis

Italian	Spanish
Italien	*Espagnol*
Italienisch	*Spanisch*
Italiano	*Spagnolo*
Italiano	*Español*

1. ghiandola surrenale	1. glándula suprarrenal
2. aorta addominale	2. aorta abdominal
3. vena renale	3. vena renal
4. vena cava inferiore	4. vena cava inferior
5. uretra	5. uretra
6. sfintere	6. esfínter
7. vescica urinaria	7. vejiga
8. uretere	8. uréter
9. coste	9. costillas
10. arteria renale	10. arteria renal

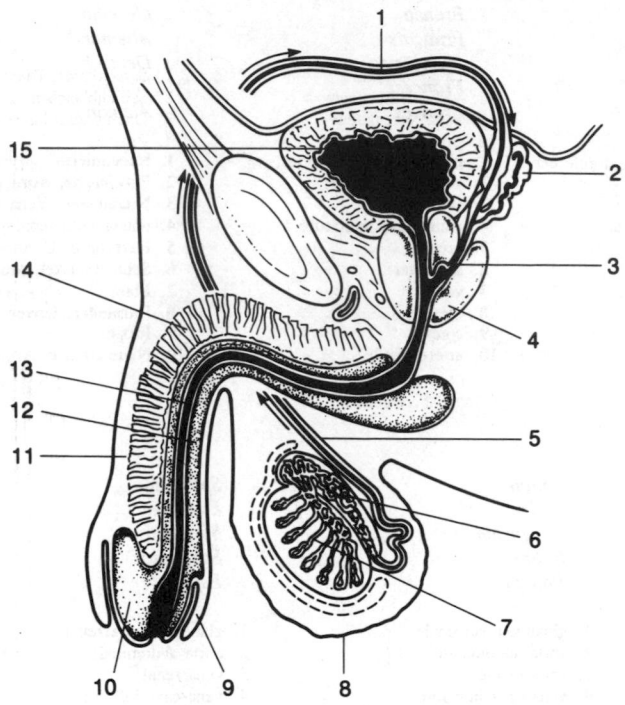

Male reproductive system
Appareil reproducteur de l'homme
Männliches Genitale
Apparato riproduttivo maschile
Aparato reproductor masculino

English	French	German
Anglais	*Français*	*Allemand*
Englisch	*Französisch*	*Deutsch*
Inglese	*Francese*	*Tedesco*
Inglés	*Francés*	*Alemán*

1. deferent duct	1. canal déférent	1. Samenleiter, Ductus deferens
2. seminal vesicle	2. vésicule séminale	2. Samenbläschen
3. ejaculatory duct	3. canal éjaculateur	3. Ductus ejaculatorius
4. prostate gland	4. prostate	4. Prostata
5. spermatic cord and deferent duct	5. cordon spermatique et canal déférent	5. Samenstrang und Samenleiter, Funiculus spermaticus und Ductus deferens
6. epididymis	6. épididyme	6. Nebenhoden, Epididymis
7. testis	7. testicules	7. Hoden, Testis
8. scrotum	8. scrotum	8. Hodensack, Skrotum
9. prepuce	9. prépuce	9. Vorhaut, Präputium
10. glans penis	10. gland du pénis	10. Eichel, Glans penis
11. penis	11. pénis	11. Penis
12. corpus spongiosum	12. corps spongieux	12. Corpus spongiosum
13. urethra	13. urètre	13. Harnröhre, Urethra
14. corpus cavernosa	14. corps caverneux	14. Corpus cavernosum
15. urinary bladder	15. vessie	15. Harnblase

Italian	Spanish
Italien	*Espagnol*
Italienisch	*Spanisch*
Italiano	*Spagnolo*
Italiano	*Español*

1. dotto deferente	1. conducto deferente
2. vesscicola seminale	2. vesícula seminal
3. dotto ejaculatore	3. conducto eyaculador
4. prostata	4. prostata
5. cordone spermatico e dotto deferente	5. cordon espermatico y conducto deferente
6. epididimo	6. epidídimo
7. testicolo	7. testículo
8. scroto	8. escroto
9. prepuzio	9. prepucio
10. glande	10. glande
11. pene	11. pene
12. corpo spugnoso	12. cuerpo esponjoso
13. uretra	13. uretra
14. corpo cavernoso	14. cuerpo cavernoso
15. vescica urinaria	15. vejiga

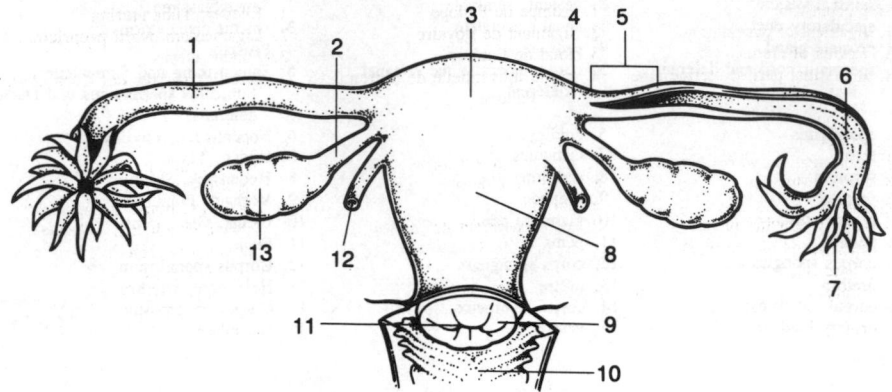

Female reproductive system
Appareil reproducteur de la femme
Weibliches Genitale
Apparato riproduttivo femminile
Aparato reproductor femenino

English	French	German
Anglais	*Français*	*Allemand*
Englisch	*Französisch*	*Deutsch*
Inglese	*Francese*	*Tedesco*
Inglés	*Francés*	*Alemán*

1. uterine tube	1. trompe de Fallope	1. Eileiter, Tuba uterina
2. ligament of ovary	2. ligament de l'ovaire	2. Ligamentum ovarii proprium
3. fundus of uterus	3. fond de l'utérus	3. Fundus uteri
4. interstitial part of uterine tube	4. partie interstitielle de la trompe de Fallope	4. pars interstitialis der Tuba uterina
5. isthmus	5. isthme	5. Isthmus
6. ampulla	6. ampoule	6. Ampulla
7. infundibulum with fimbrae	7. pavillon avec franges	7. Infundibulum mit Fimbriae
8. body of uterus	8. corps de l'utérus	8. Corpus uteri
9. cervix	9. col	9. Gebärmutterhals, Zervix
10. vagina showing rugae	10. vagin montrant des crêtes	10. Scheide (Vagina) mit Rugae
11. external os of cervix	11. os externe de col	11. äußerer Muttermund
12. round ligament	12. ligament rond	12. Ligamentum rotundum uteri
13. ovary	13. ovaire	13. Eierstock, Ovar

Italian	Spanish
Italien	*Espagnol*
Italienisch	*Spanisch*
Italiano	*Spagnolo*
Italiano	*Español*

1. tuba uterina	1. trompa de Falopio
2. legamento ovarico	2. ligamento del ovario
3. fondo uterino	3. fondo del utero
4. parte interstiziale della tuba uterina	4. parte intersticial de la trompa de Falopio
5. istmo	5. istmo
6. ampolla	6. ampolla
7. infundibolo con frangie	7. infundibulo con fimbrias
8. corpo dell'utero	8. cuerpo del utero
9. cervice	9. cuello uterino
10. vagina con pliche	10. vagina mostrando los pliegues
11. orifizio esterno della cervice	11. orificio externo del cuello uterino
12. legamento rotondo	12. ligamento redondo
13. ovaio	13. ovario

Figs 1, 2, 6, 7, 8, 9, 11 and 12 are reproduced with permission from the Royal Society of Medicine *Family Medical Guide* (Longman).

Figs. 3, 4, 5, 10, 13 and 14 are reproduced with permission from Ross & Wilson's *Foundations of Anatomy and Physiology* (Churchill Livingstone, Edinburgh).

Les figures 1, 2, 6, 7, 8, 9, 11 et 12 sont extraites de Royal Society of Medicine, *Family Medical Guide*, avec l'autorisation des éditions Longman.

Les figures 3, 4, 5, 10, 13 et 14 sont extraites de Ross and Wilson's *Foundations of Anatomy and Physiology*, avec l'autorisation des éditions Churchill Livingstone, Edinburgh.

Die Abbildungen Nr. 1, 2, 6, 7, 8, 9, 11 und 12 wurden entnommen aus: The Royal Society of Medicine, *Family Medical Guide*. Harlow: Longman. Abdruck mit freundlicher Genehmigung.

Die Abbildungen Nr. 3, 4, 5, 10, 13 und 14 wurden entnommen aus: Ross, J. und Wilson, K. *Foundations of Anatomy and Physiology*, 5. Auflage. Edinburgh: Churchill Livingstone. Abdruck mit freundlicher Genehmigung.

Le figure 1, 2, 6, 7, 8, 9, 11 e 12 sono riproduzioni autorizzate dalla *Family Medical Guide* della Royal Society of Medicine (ed. Longman).

Le figure 3, 4, 5, 10, 13 e 14 sono riproduzioni autorizzate da Ross e Wilson, *Foundations of Anatomy and Physiology* (ed. Churchill Livingstone).

Las Figs 1, 2, 6, 7, 8, 9, 11 y 12 están reproducidas, con el permiso de la Real Sociedad de Medicina, de *Family Medical Guide* (Longman).

Las Figs 3, 4, 5, 10, 13 y 14 están reproducidas, con el permiso de Ross & Wilson, de *Foundations of Anatomy and Physiology* (Churchill Livingstone, Edinburgh).